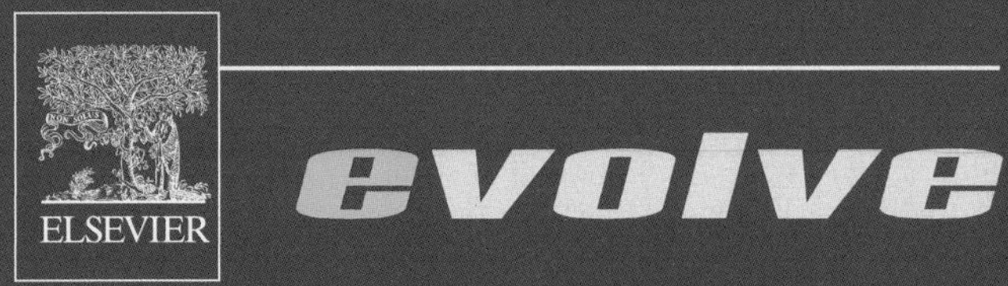

To access your Student Resources, visit the Web address below:

http://evolve.elsevier.com/Fritz/essential

- **3-Dimensional Anatomical Art**
  Review anatomical structures by viewing this additional art!
- **Content Updates**
  Read about the latest related news and research findings from the author.
- **Range of Motion Image Collection**
  View images not included in the book to further study range of motion!
- **Crossword Puzzles and Labeling Exercises**
  Reinforce medical terminology definitions and body system structures through these fun, interactive activities!
- **Critical Thinking Questions**
  Review concepts from the body by thinking through and answering these additional critical thinking questions.
- **Case Studies**
  Read the case studies and then apply knowledge from the chapters in order to answer the questions.

Evolve activities are indicated in the book with this icon: 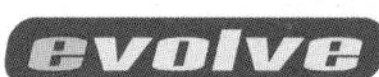

MOSBY'S

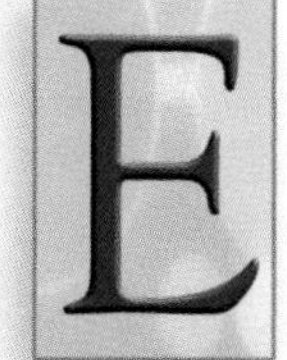

ESSENTIAL SCIENCES *for* THERAPEUTIC MASSAGE

Anatomy, Physiology, Biomechanics, and Pathology

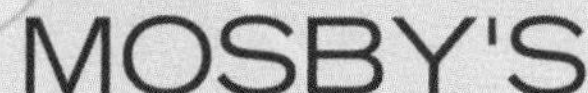
MOSBY'S

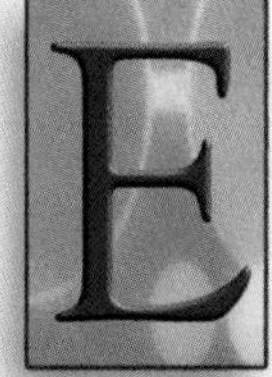

ESSENTIAL SCIENCES *for* THERAPEUTIC MASSAGE

Anatomy, Physiology, Biomechanics, and Pathology

Second Edition

SANDY FRITZ, MS, NCTMB
Founder, Owner, Director, and Head Instructor
Health Enrichment Center
School of Therapeutic Massage and Bodywork
Lapeer, Michigan

M. JAMES GROSENBACH, EDD
Clinical Psychologist
Director of Education
Health Enrichment Center
School of Therapeutic Massage and Bodywork
Lapeer, Michigan

With 690 illustrations

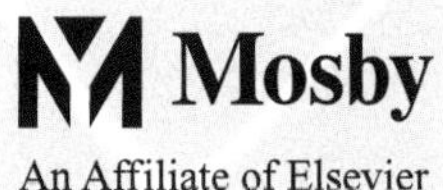

An Affiliate of Elsevier

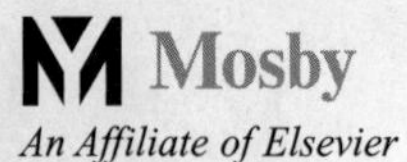

An *Affiliate of Elsevier*

11830 Westline Industrial Drive
St. Louis, Missouri 63146

MOSBY'S ESSENTIAL SCIENCES FOR THERAPEUTIC MASSAGE, SECOND EDITION

NOTICE

Massage Therapy is an ever-changing field. Standard safety precautions must be followed, but as new research and clinical experience broaden our knowledge, changes in treatment and drug therapy may become necessary or appropriate. Readers are advised to check the most current product information provided by the manufacturer of each drug to be administered to verify the recommended dose, the method and duration of administration, and contraindications. It is the responsibility of the licensed prescriber, relying on experience and knowledge of the patient, to determine dosages and the best treatment for each individual patient. Neither the publisher nor the author assumes any liability for any injury and/or damage to persons or property arising from this publication.

Second Edition

Publishing Director: Linda Duncan
Editor: Kellie Fitzpatrick
Developmental Editor: Jennifer Watrous
Editorial Assistant: Kendra Bailey
Publishing Services Manager: Linda McKinley
Project Manager: Rich Barber
Senior Designer: Julia Dummitt
Original Illustrations: Don O'Connor, Graphic World
Inside Back Cover Art: From LaFleur Brooks M: *Exploring medical language: a student-directed approach*, ed 5, St Louis, 2002 Mosby

ISBN-13: 978-0-323-02027-5
ISBN-10: 0-323-02027-5

Printed in Canada

Last digit is the print number: 9 8 7 6 5 4

Second Edition Dedication

To Dedo and the Instructing Staff, Roxanne, Pat, Dianne, and Dennis for keeping it all happening, and to Amy, for her persistence and being able to read my writing.

First Edition Dedication

To all of those who read and read and read.

And to the Health Enrichment Center School of Therapeutic Massage and Bodywork's graduating class of 1998—for being guinea pigs.

FOREWORD

In order to become a competent therapeutic massage professional, it is an essential prerequisite that therapists have a sound understanding of the territory on, and with which, they are working. There is an absolute requirement for an intimate familiarity with structural patterns, attachments and functions of the muscles, ligaments, tendons, fascia and joints being treated, as well as with the body systems they support and which service them.

It is obvious that it is not necessary to understand the intimate workings of an automobile in order to drive one; however, there would be little confidence in an auto mechanic who did not fully understand the construction and functioning of the motor he or she was attempting to repair. Where human health and well-being are concerned it is clear that many individuals understand their own body workings as imperfectly as do many drivers and their cars. The massage therapist, however, must have a sufficient degree of knowledge in order to ensure safety and efficacy in what is being offered therapeutically.

What the authors have achieved in the second edition of this landmark text is to set out all the ingredients required for the entry level and advanced level student to experience the wonderful adventure and exploration of the interrelated systems and subsystems of the body. They have managed to make this material come alive, to lift it out of the mere presentation of facts, without compromising on the scientific and academic requirements of such a text. They have also done something quite remarkable in producing the information in an easily accessible manner while at the same time encouraging a personal growth experience as the reader is challenged to relate what is being discussed to themselves and their own experience.

It is one thing to present information and quite another to do so and to ask the reader to explore both the topic and its relationship to health and disease as well as to their own belief systems, health status, and understanding of how the body works. From such challenges, which are peppered throughout the book, only one result can be anticipated of anyone who diligently works their way through the systematic unfolding of this anatomy and physiology exploration—a sound understanding of how the body works, where the constituent parts are to be found and how they interact in health and disease. With this knowledge and the tools that are available to the skilled modern soft tissue or movement therapist, the future of these emerging professions will become far more assured.

This is a most important time for these professions, as realization of their value becomes established through research and as national standards are evaluated and improved. As the soft tissue and movement professions encroach on territory that other professions hold to be their own, it is vital for training standards to be enhanced, reinforced, and constantly upgraded so that critics and potentially hostile professional organizations are denied the ammunition that weak standards offer.

The existence of this text, following on from the superb *Mosby's Fundamentals of Therapeutic Massage,* is precisely the ammunition needed to counter any attempt at denigration of these modalities as such. There remain major tasks in the arena of educational, personal, and professional growth; however, this book makes such effort far less arduous. Mosby and the authors are to be congratulated on the effort that has gone into the writing and production of this important text.

Leon Chaitow ND, DO
Senior Lecturer
University of Westminster, London

PREFACE

Mosby's Essential Sciences for Therapeutic Massage, second edition, presents the science basics—anatomy, physiology, biomechanics, and pathology, with clinical application—to a specific population—future massage professionals. This population views the body in a holistic manner. Because philosophy and practices from ancient healing wisdom often form the basis for massage modalities, an introduction to the common thread of ancient healing wisdom is carried through the text. This wisdom is related directly to body structure and function and does not represent any particular spiritual discipline.

Two themes are woven through this text:

1. Dynamic balance or homeostasis
2. Analysis and reasoning that honors both the scientific model of cause and effect and the larger picture of intuition, possibilities, and the feelings of the people involved

This textbook presents the objective facts and information about human beings as they currently exist. Information is not static, but dynamic and like life, ever-changing. Teachers and students are encouraged to question and explore the information to make it their own. The information was selected to best serve the beginning and intermediate student of therapeutic massage and to reflect current competencies of the profession. Decisions were made as to what to include based on the authors' experiences of many years of training entry- and intermediate-level therapeutic massage students, and several expert reviewers who analyzed the original manuscript content.

This book has been developed to serve two roles. It can be used as follows:

1. As a complete essential science textbook/workbook combination—this book can stand alone without the use of additional support materials for the muscles/skeletal system and other key topics.

or

2. As a companion text to a more general anatomy and physiology book—as a companion, this text will guide the learning and application of the material specifically for the therapeutic massage student.

ABOUT THIS BOOK

New to this edition are several key additions that will aid in student learning. These additions include, but are not limited to, the following: All chapters have been revised and updated to reflect changes in curriculum standards and to include new research. The student learning from this book can feel confident in using it as a reference to study for the National Certification Exam. Content within the book is applicable to the test questions, and it keeps pace with changes in therapeutic massage education, as mandated by the Commission on Massage Therapy Accreditation (COMTA).

The entire book is presented in full color for this edition, and it corresponds directly with the design of *Mosby's Fundamentals of Therapeutic Massage,* ed. 3, allowing students using both textbooks to feel comfortable moving from one text to the next with ease.

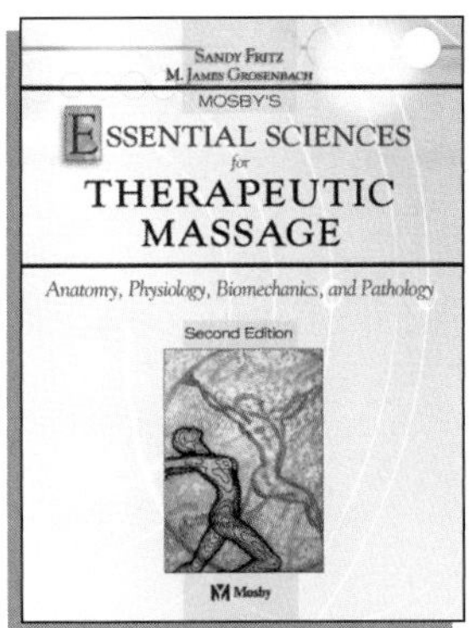

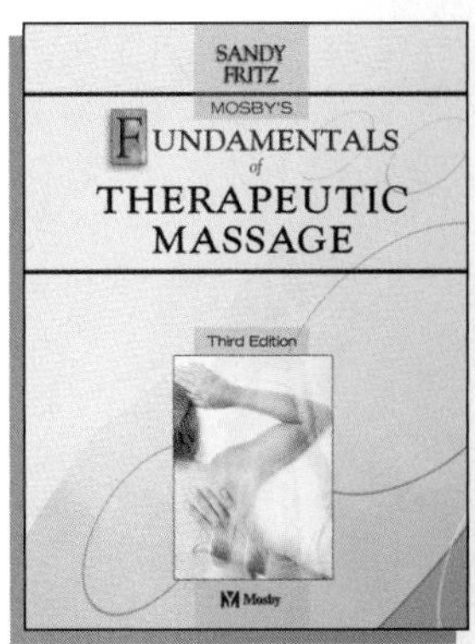

Content has been significantly expanded in Section IV, specifically in the areas of digestive, circulatory, and lymphatic systems.

Clinical reasoning activities (labeled Activity within the text) have been re-worked and improved in response to student feedback.

ACTIVITY 3-2

Using the abbreviations in Table 3-4, decipher the message below. (The answers can be found on p. 94.)

Your Turn

In the am ______________ evaluate Hx ______________
and ADL ______________ . Use this information ad lib
______________ to CC ______________
of GI ______________ and ABD ______________
meds ______________ . Use ROM ______________
as tol ______________ on the h ______________
as PT ______________ on the ft ______________
to assist R ______________ . Monitor T ______________
and P ______________ in the pm ______________
and provide H_2O ______________ and TLC ______________
as requested for OB ______________ clients.

This second edition, now in full color, is highly illustrated, with approximately 100 new figures, all geared specifically toward the massage therapy student.

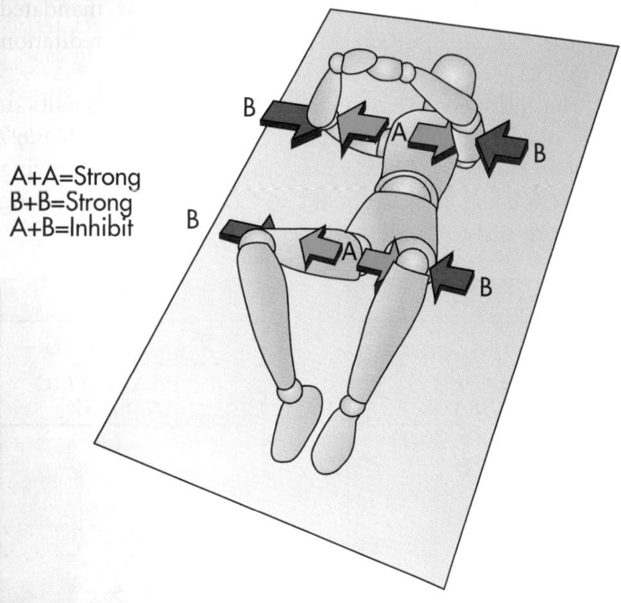

The art in the muscle chapter, Chapter 9, besides being converted to full color, has been enlarged for a more in-depth view of the muscles.

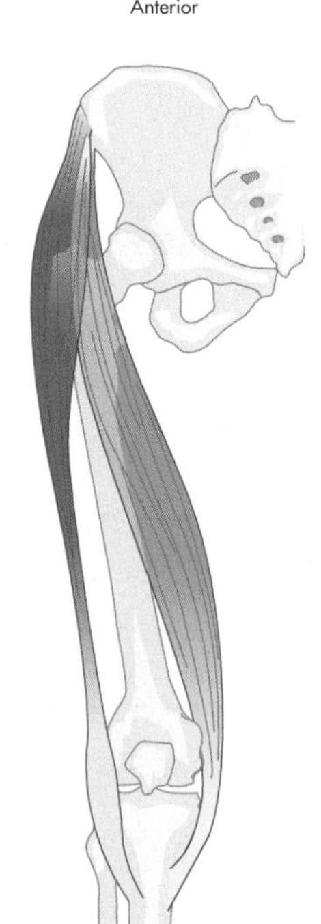

Finally, new to this edition is the accompanying EVOLVE website. Within each chapter, placed directly before the Workbook section, is an EVOLVE exercise for the student to complete online in order to enhance the learning of one or more of the chapter topics. For example, Chapter 9's EVOLVE exercise directs the student to three-dimensional art on the website that will aid in the understanding of the muscles. Other EVOLVE activities include crossword puzzles, mini-quizzes, Internet articles, and weblinks for additional reading and research.

evolve

Several activities on the Fritz EVOLVE site reinforce the anatomy lessons taught in Chapter 9. Log on to your student account, and explore the dissection atlas as well as the anatomy weblinks that are located under the Chapter 9 Course Material section.

The format of this text has been designed to address various learning styles. Throughout the text are the activities that assist the student in transferring new information from short-term to long-term memory and developing clinical reasoning skills. These activities do not have only one correct answer. Instead they are designed for the student to use what is familiar from past experiences as a vehicle to transport the new or unfamiliar information to a level of understanding through a gentle and effective learning process. This enhances the student's ability to utilize creative problem-solving skills. Because there is seldom only one correct way to do anything, developing a process to determine the most effective decision at the time is important. This more gray approach, while more like the body, professional practice, and life, is not the familiar black/white textbook format. This may seem uncomfortable for some at first. An example of the various activities is often provided to give the student direction.

Understanding is the learning goal of this text. Memorization is not the goal. Instead, the activities identify the fundamental material and ask the student to manipulate it in a personal way to enhance the learning process. The bulk of the text is designed as reference material.

The workbook section at the end of each chapter can act as a self-evaluation if desired, or as a reinforcement of the information presented. The answers to these sections are provided at the end of each chapter.

170 SECTION II: SYSTEMS OF CONTROL

WORKBOOK SECTION

SHORT ANSWER

1. Define the peripheral nervous system.
2. List the components of the peripheral nervous system.
3. List the cranial nerves and describe the general function of each.
6. Compare and contrast a dermatome and a myotome.
7. Explain reflex mechanisms and sensory receptor reflex arcs and their relationship to therapeutic massage and movement therapies.
8. Identify the two divisions of the autonomic nervous system.

A conversational tone has been used whenever possible, and supported by metaphors and practical applications. Indications and contraindications for clinical massage practice have also been included. The word indications in the context of this book is defined as when treatment is appropriate and beneficial. The word contraindications encompasses both avoidance and cautions for the application of treatment. This practical feature allows the student to take the knowledge from the classroom straight into actual therapy. The result is a user-friendly text that relates to daily professional life for the massage therapist.

INDICATIONS CONTRAINDICATIONS

For Therapeutic Massage

After these conditions are diagnosed, stress management can be an important part of ongoing therapeutic management. ■

Another way in which this text can be used as a direct reference when practicing massage therapy is its inclusion of Practical Applications, which are scattered throughout each chapter.

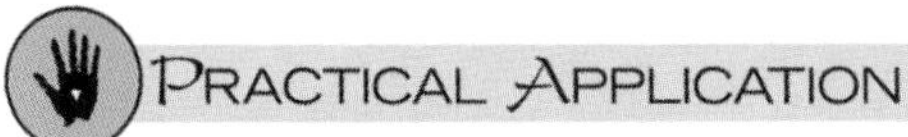

PRACTICAL APPLICATION

Stimulation of the peripheral nervous system (PNS) and the responses elicited by this stimulation constitute one of the main physiologic modes by which massage and bodywork benefit the client. Those who practice these therapies must understand thoroughly the anatomy and physiology of the PNS and comprehend the way soft tissue and movement methods interact with the PNS. ■

The workbook exercises and activities presented do not represent any specific curriculum design or learning mode other than to address various learning styles. Instead, an attempt has been made to be as generic and as inclusive as possible to allow the instructor and student to individualize the application of the material.

The linear flow of the text begins with a section that includes the fundamentals and a big picture look at the body, health, disease, terminology, and a clinical reasoning model.

The second section presents the mechanisms of physiologic function and control by the nervous system and endocrine system. This is a major deviation from traditional presentations and is presented based on over 20 years of teaching experience indicating that if the systems of control are understood first, then it is much easier to understand the rest of the body's anatomy and physiology.

Section III represents the core portion of the text from a movement science perspective, and the learning includes the musculoskeletal system, kinesiology, and biomechanics. Should this information flow seem out of order, the instructor may decide to simply switch the presentation of Sections II and III.

The last section covers the remainder of the body systems, including the integumentary, cardiovascular, lymphatic, and immune systems, as well as the digestive, respiratory, urinary, and reproductive systems. Only the information most applicable to the therapeutic massage student is presented in these chapters.

Each chapter in the book contains an outline, key terms with definitions, and chapter objectives.

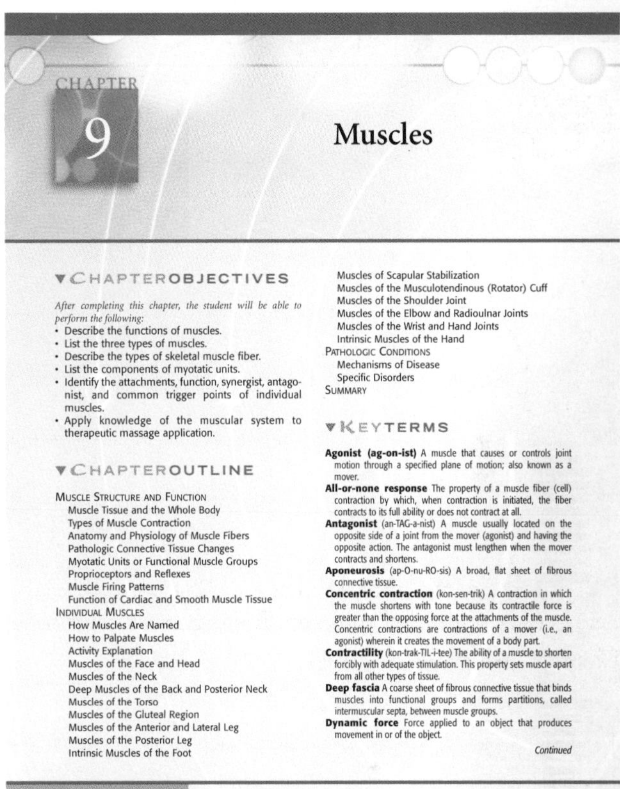

CHAPTER 9

Muscles

CHAPTER OBJECTIVES

After completing this chapter, the student will be able to perform the following:

- Describe the functions of muscles.
- List the three types of muscles.
- Describe the types of skeletal muscle fiber.
- List the components of myotatic units.
- Identify the attachments, function, synergist, antagonist, and common trigger points of individual muscles.
- Apply knowledge of the muscular system to therapeutic massage application.

CHAPTER OUTLINE

MUSCLE STRUCTURE AND FUNCTION
- Muscle Tissue and the Whole Body
- Types of Muscle Contraction
- Anatomy and Physiology of Muscle Fibers
- Pathologic Connective Tissue Changes
- Myotatic Units or Functional Muscle Groups
- Proprioceptors and Reflexes
- Muscle Firing Patterns
- Function of Cardiac and Smooth Muscle Tissue

INDIVIDUAL MUSCLES
- How Muscles Are Named
- How to Palpate Muscles
- Activity Explanation
- Muscles of the Face and Head
- Muscles of the Neck
- Deep Muscles of the Back and Posterior Neck
- Muscles of the Torso
- Muscles of the Gluteal Region
- Muscles of the Anterior and Lateral Leg
- Muscles of the Posterior Leg
- Intrinsic Muscles of the Foot
- Muscles of Scapular Stabilization
- Muscles of the Musculotendinous (Rotator) Cuff
- Muscles of the Shoulder Joint
- Muscles of the Elbow and Radioulnar Joints
- Muscles of the Wrist and Hand Joints
- Intrinsic Muscles of the Hand

PATHOLOGIC CONDITIONS
- Mechanisms of Disease
- Specific Disorders

SUMMARY

KEY TERMS

Agonist (ag-on-ist) A muscle that causes or controls joint motion through a specified plane of motion; also known as a mover.

All-or-none response The property of a muscle fiber (cell) contraction by which, when contraction is initiated, the fiber contracts to its full ability or does not contract at all.

Antagonist (an-TAG-a-nist) A muscle usually located on the opposite side of a joint from the mover (agonist) and having the opposite action. The antagonist must lengthen when the mover contracts and shortens.

Aponeurosis (ap-O-nu-RO-sis) A broad, flat sheet of fibrous connective tissue.

Concentric contraction (kon-sen-trik) A contraction in which the muscle shortens with tone because its contractile force is greater than the opposing force at the attachments of the muscle. Concentric contractions are contractions of a mover (i.e., an agonist) wherein it creates the movement of a body part.

Contractility (kon-trak-TIL-i-tee) The ability of a muscle to shorten forcibly with adequate stimulation. This property sets muscle apart from all other types of tissue.

Deep fascia A coarse sheet of fibrous connective tissue that binds muscles into functional groups and forms partitions, called intermuscular septa, between muscle groups.

Dynamic force Force applied to an object that produces movement in or of the object.

Continued

308

A glossary appears at the end of the book for quick reference.

GLOSSARY

Abduction Lateral movement away from the midline of the trunk.

Absorption The movement of food molecules from the digestive tract to the circulatory or lymphatic systems.

Acetylcholine A neurotransmitter that stimulates the parasympathetic nervous system and the skeletal muscles and is involved in memory.

Acne A chronic inflammation of the sebaceous glands and hair follicles caused by interactions between bacteria, sebum, and sex hormones.

Active transport The transport of substances into or out of a cell using energy.

Acupuncture The practice of inserting needles at specific points on meridians, or channels, to stimulate or sedate energy flow to regulate or alter body function. A branch of Chinese medicine, acupuncture is the art and science of manipulating the flow of Qi, the basic life force, and xue, the blood, body fluids, and nourishing essences. Western medicine uses acupuncture primarily to reduce pain. Acupressure, which uses digital pressure, follows the same Asian principles.

Acute disease Disease that has a specific beginning, signs, and symptoms that develop quickly, last a short time, and then disappear.

Acute pain Pain that is usually temporary, of sudden onset, and easily localized. Acute pain can be a symptom of a disease process or a temporary aspect of medical treatment. Acting as a warning signal, acute pain activates the sympathetic nervous system.

Adduction A medial movement toward the midline of the body.

lipids, proteins, and nucleic acids. The processes require energy supplied from adenosine triphosphate.

Anaplasia Meaning without shape, the term describes abnormal or undifferentiated cells that fail to mature into specialized cell types. Anaplasia is a characteristic of malignant cells.

Anatomic position A standard position in which the person stands upright with the feet slightly apart, arms hanging at the sides, and palms facing forward with thumbs outward.

Anatomic range of motion (ROM) The amount of motion available to a joint based on the structure of the joint and determined by the shape of the joint surfaces, joint capsule, ligaments, muscle bulk, and surrounding musculotendinous and bony structures.

Anatomy The study of the structures of the body and the relationship of its parts.

Androgens Male sex hormones.

Anemia A decrease in the normal number of red blood cells or in the amount of hemoglobin or iron in the blood.

Aneurysm A permanent dilation of part of a blood vessel caused by weakness or damage to its structure. The most common sites of aneurysms are the aorta and the arteries of the brain.

Antagonist A muscle usually located on the opposite side of a joint from the agonist and having the opposite action.

Anterior pelvic rotation Anterior movement of the upper pelvis; the iliac crest tilts forward in a sagittal plane.

Antibody A specific protein produced to destroy or suppress antigens.

Of course, there is no single correct way to use this book. The sections do not need to be presented in any specific order; however, Chapter 1 does set the stage for learning. The activities, exercises, and workbook sections can all be used at your discretion.

This text is designed for a 500 to 1500 hour curriculum (approximately 15 to 30 credits). A more generalized approach will need to be taken with the shorter curriculums, while additional class time will allow for a more in-depth integration process. Since the text is student-friendly and self-directed, much of the work can be assigned in a self-study format.

It is our greatest hope that the material in this book will come alive with the careful guidance of a skilled teacher and with the patient commitment of a dedicated student.

Have fun with the book.

Sandy Fritz
M. James Grosenbach

ACKNOWLEDGMENTS

This text is written by teachers seeking a more efficient and gentle way to help students understand and use this information. Credit and appreciation is given to the authors of the reference texts consulted in the development of this textbook. Without their efforts, this book never could have been written. Thanks also goes to those who reviewed the manuscript. Their dedicated attention added to the quality of this text.

Special thanks goes to the following people/groups:

To Joe Muscolino for his review of the muscle chapter (Chapter 9), also to the advanced practitioner students, and the Class of 2003 for reviewing the entire text.

To Jessica Smith for all of her proofreading and to Michael McPharlin, BSN, NCBTMB, for his review of the muscle firing patterns.

To the athletes I work with for constantly challenging me to dig into the anatomy and physiology to figure out what to do with all of their assorted bumps, bruises, sprains, strains, breaks, performance stresses, and personalities.

To the Detroit Lions organization and IMG/IPI for supporting the educational partnership with Health Enrichment Center. To the Detroit Marathon organizers, the University of Michigan Athletic Department, the VA Hospital in Detroit, Michigan, and all of the veterans there, and all of the residents and staff at Suncrest Regional Care Facility, and hospice.

And to the staff at Mosby, especially Rich Barber, for all of their wonderful support.

CONTENTS

DETAILED CONTENTS

MOSBY'S

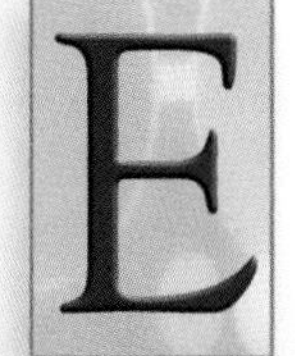

ESSENTIAL SCIENCES for THERAPEUTIC MASSAGE

Anatomy, Physiology, Biomechanics, and Pathology

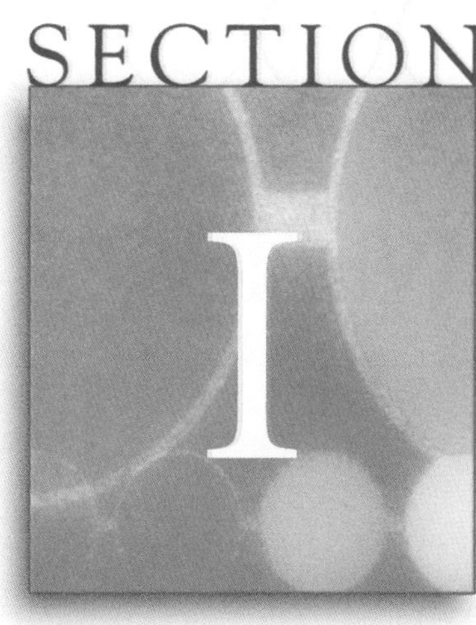

Fundamentals

Section I lays the foundation for the study of functional anatomy and physiology that the massage professional must have. The study begins in Chapter 1 with the big picture—a look at the body as a whole. This chapter explores functional balance and the ability of the body to maintain a relatively constant internal environment, regardless of external influences. Chapter 2 discusses mechanisms of health and disease. Stress, a primary factor in imbalances in the body, is highlighted, because stress management is a major benefit of massage therapy.

The ability to speak the language of another is essential for effective communication. In Chapter 3, the student will study Western-based scientific language and will be introduced to the language of systems based on ancient healing wisdom.

The first major theme of this text is understanding self-regulating mechanisms, which allow the body to maintain homeostasis, or dynamic balance.

The second major theme is using clinical reasoning, which enables the student to apply the information learned to the therapeutic setting. Without the ability to reason clinically and to solve problems, information becomes little more than a collection of facts. What is a fact? Decision making begins with gathering facts. This book is full of facts (information) currently seen as true; however, things change and change brings a revelation of the reliability of the facts. Are the facts truth, absolute concrete pieces of information, or are the facts changeable as knowledge expands? Sometimes we see decisions as answers, and although we all seek answers, few answers exist. Therefore, formulating reliable and accurate decision-making skills and practicing to develop an inquiring mind is necessary.

The journey begins.

Identify three personal goals that will motivate you during the study of anatomy and physiology. An example is provided to get you started.

Example: I will learn about my body so that I can age well and remain vital into my elder years.

Your Turn

1. ______________________________

2. ______________________________

3. ______________________________

CHAPTER 1

The Body as a Whole

▼ CHAPTER OBJECTIVES

After completing this chapter, the student will be able to perform the following:

- Define the terms *anatomy* and *physiology*.
- Explain the importance of understanding the relationship of the structure and function of the body as a whole.
- Compare the yin/yang theory to anatomy and physiology.
- Define the characteristics of life.
- List and discuss the levels of organization of the body.

▼ CHAPTER OUTLINE

▼ KEY TERMS

Active transport The transport of substances into or out of a cell using energy.

Adenosine triphosphate (ATP) (ah-DEN-o-seen tri-FOS-fate) A compound that stores energy in the muscles. When ATP is broken down during catabolic reactions, it releases energy.

Anabolism (ah-NAB-o-lizm) Chemical processes in the body that join simple compounds to form more complex compounds of carbohydrates, lipids, proteins, and nucleic acids. The processes require energy supplied from adenosine triphosphate.

Anatomy (ah-NAT-o-mee) The study of the structures of the body and the relationship of its parts.

Apical surface The surface of epithelial cells that is exposed to the external environment.

Atom The smallest particle of an element that retains and exhibits the properties of that element. Atoms are made up of protons, neutrons, and electrons.

Atrophy (AT-ro-fee) A decrease in the size of a body part or organ caused by a decrease in the size of the cells.

Basal surface (BA-sal) The tissue surface that faces the inside of the body.

Basement membrane A permeable membrane that attaches epithelial tissues to the underlying connective tissues.

Carbohydrates (kar-bo-HY-drates) Sugars, starches, and cellulose composed of carbon, hydrogen, and oxygen.

Cardiac muscle fibers (kar-DE-ak) Smaller, striated, involuntary muscle fibers (cells) in the heart that contract to pump blood.

Catabolism (kah-TAB-o-lizm) Chemical processes in the body that release energy as complex compounds are broken down into simpler ones.

Cell The basic structural unit of a living organism. A cell contains a nucleus and cytoplasm and is surrounded by a membrane.

Collagen (KOL-ah-jen) A protein substance composed of small fibrils that combine to create the connective tissue of fasciae, tendons, and ligaments. When combined with water, it forms gelatin. Collagen constitutes approximately one fourth of the protein in the body.

Collagenous fibers Strong fibers with little capacity for stretch. They have a high degree of tensile strength, which allows them to withstand longitudinal stress.

Connective tissue The most abundant type of tissue in the body, connective tissue supports and holds together the body and its parts, protects the body from foreign matter, and is organized to transport substances throughout the body.

Cytosol (SI-to-sol) The fluid that surrounds the nucleus or organelles inside the cell membrane.

Cytoplasm (SI-to-plasm) Material enclosed by the cell membrane.

Cytoskeleton (SI-TO-skel-e-ton) A framework of proteins inside the cell providing flexibility and strength.

Continued

Diffusion (di-FU-zhun) Movement of ions and molecules from an area of higher concentration to that of a lower concentration.

Deoxyribonucleic acid (DNA) (dee-ok-see-rye-bo-noo-KLEE-ik) Genetic material of the cell that carries the chemical "blueprint" of the body.

Elastic fibers Connective tissue fibers that are extensible and elastic. They are made of a protein called elastin, which returns to its original length after being stretched.

Element (el-E-ment) Substance containing only a single kind of atom.

Endocytosis (en-DO-SI-TO-sis) The cellular process of engulfing particles located outside the cell membrane into a cell by forming vesicles.

Endoplasmic reticulum (en-DO-plas-mic re-TIC-u-lum) A network of intracellular membranes in the form of tubes that is connected to the nuclear membrane.

Energy The capacity to work, and work is movement or a change in the physical structure of matter.

Epithelial tissues (ep-i-THEE-lee-al) A specialized group of tissues that cover and protect the surface of the body and its parts, line body cavities, and form glands. Epithelial tissue usually is found in areas that move substances into and out of the body during secretion, absorption, and excretion.

Exocytosis (ex-O-SY-TO-sis) The movement of substances out of a cell.

Gross anatomy The study of body structures visible to the naked eye.

Homeostasis (ho-me-o-STA-sis) The relatively constant state of the internal environment of the body that is maintained by adaptive responses.

High-energy bonds Covalent bonds created in specific organic substrates in the presence of enzymes.

Hypertrophy (hye-PER-tro-fee) An increase in the size of a cell, which results in an increase in the size of a body part or organ.

Impermeable The quality of not permitting entry of a substance.

Inorganic compounds Chemical structures that do not have carbon and hydrogen atoms as the primary structure.

Interphase (IN-ter-faze) The period during which a cell grows and carries on its activities.

Ion pumps Carriers that transport substances into or out of a cell using energy.

Lipids (LIP-idz) Organic compounds that have carbon, hydrogen, and oxygen atoms but in a different proportion than that of carbohydrates.

Lysosome (LY-SO-som) Cell organelle that is part of the intracellular digestive system.

Matrix (MAY-triks) The basic substance between the cells of a tissue. Matrix is composed of amorphous ground substance consisting of molecules that expand when water molecules and electrolytes bind to them. As much as 90% of connective tissue is ground substance. Fibers make up the other component of matrix.

Meiosis (my-O-sis) A type of cell division in which each daughter cell receives half the normal number of chromosomes, forming two reproductive cells.

Membrane A thin, sheetlike layer of tissue that covers a cell, an organ, or some other structure; that lines a tube or a cavity; or that divides or separates one part from another.

Metabolism (me-TAB-o-lizm) Chemical processes in the body that convert food and air into energy to support growth, distribution of nutrients, and elimination of waste.

Metabolites (me-TAB-o-lyts) Molecules synthesized or broken down inside the body by chemical reactions.

Microvilli (MI-KRO-vil-li) Small projections of the cell membrane that increase the surface area of the cell.

Mitochondria (MIT-O-kon-DRE-a) Cell organelles of rod or oval shape that provide energy for cellular activity.

Mitosis (my-TOE-sis) Cell division in which the cell duplicates its DNA and divides into two identical daughter cells.

Molecule (MOL-e-kyool) A combination of two or more atoms. A molecule is the smallest portion of a substance that can exist separately without losing the physical and chemical properties of that substance.

Muscle tissue A specialized form of tissue that contracts and shortens to provide movement, maintain posture, and produce heat.

Nervous tissue A specialized tissue that coordinates and regulates body activity. It can develop more excitability and conductivity than other types of tissue.

Nutrients Essential elements and molecules obtained from the diet that are required by the body for normal body function.

Organelles (or-gan-NELLZ) The basic components of a cell that perform specific functions within the cell.

Organic compounds Substances that have carbon and hydrogen as part of their basic structure.

Osmosis Diffusion of water from a region of lower concentration of solution to a region of higher concentration of solution across the semipermeable membrane of a cell.

Passive transport Transportation of substance across the cell membrane without the use of energy.

Phagocytosis (fag-O-SY-TO-sis) The process of endocytosis followed by digestion of the vescicle contents by enzymes present in the cytoplasm.

Phospholipid bilayer (fos-FO-li-pid) Cell membrane made up of lipids, carbohydrates, and proteins.

Physiology (fiz-ee-OL-o-jee) The study of the processes and functions of the body involved in supporting life.

Proteins (PRO-teens) Substances formed from amino acids.

Regional anatomy The study of the structures of a particular area of the body.

Reticular fibers Delicate, connective tissue fibers that occur in networks and support small structures such as capillaries, nerve fibers, and the basement membrane. Reticular fibers are made of a specialized type of collagen called reticulin.

Ribonucleic acid (RNA) A type of nucleic acid.

Skeletal muscle fibers Large, cross-striated cells that are connected to the skeleton and under voluntary control of the nervous system.

Smooth muscle fibers Muscle fibers that are neither striated nor voluntary. These muscle cells help regulate blood flow through the cardiovascular system, propel food through the gut, and squeeze secretions from glands.

Surface anatomy The study of internal organs and structures as they can be recognized and related to external features.

Systemic anatomy The study of the structure of a particular body system.

Tissue (TISH-yoo) A group of similar cells combined to perform a common function.

The study of the human body in its structure and function is fascinating. For students of massage the body is the territory of our work. This text provides a map of our territory. A map is a representation of an object, but the map is not the object, any more than this textbook is your body. Our goal is to offer information on which to make decisions as you work with each person you touch. As practitioners, the more familiar we are with the body and its functions, the better able we are to provide the methods used to relax, encourage, and nurture clients with the approaches of therapeutic massage. This first chapter provides information about the body as a whole. Because massage professionals deal with the wholeness of each client they serve, this seems to be the best place to begin.

ANATOMY AND PHYSIOLOGY

Anatomy and physiology are two distinct yet interrelated biologic studies that combine to present the operation of the body as a whole organism. **Anatomy** is the scientific study of the structures of the body and the relationship of its parts. **Physiology** is the scientific study of the processes and functions of the body that support life.

The word *anatomy* means to cut apart. Anatomy is a broad field with many subdivisions, each of which is a comprehensive study in itself. The following categories are some of these divisions and subdivisions:

Developmental anatomy: How anatomy changes over the life cycle

Gross anatomy: The study of body structures large enough to be visible to the naked eye

Regional anatomy: The study of all the structures of a particular area

Systemic anatomy: The study of the body divided into its systems that contribute to the same function

Surface anatomy: The study of the internal organs and structures as they are recognized from and related to the overlying skin surface

The term *physiology* is a combination of two Greek words: *physis,* which means nature, and *logos,* which means science. Physiology, the study of the way the body works, can be divided into three fields:

Organizational physiology: The study of the body organization (e.g., cellular physiology)

Pathophysiology: The study of disease

Systemic physiology: The study of body systems (e.g., cardiophysiology)

Structure (anatomy) and function (physiology) cannot be separated any more than a person can be separated into body, mind, or spirit. Structure and function form a continuum; structure guides function, and function can modify structure.

The concepts of anatomy and physiology are examples of the duality of wholeness, a duality also represented in the yin and yang concept expressed in Asian terminology. Yin corresponds to structure and yang to function, opposite but complementary qualities.

Yang (Sympathetic—using intermittent function, protective and supportive function)
Yin (Parasympathetic—restoring constant function, vital function)

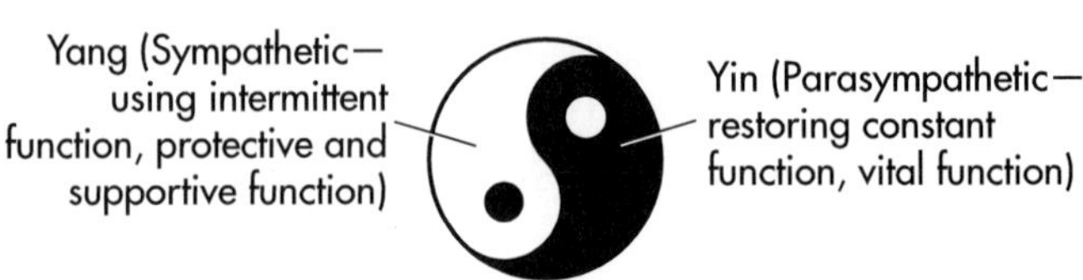

Figure 1-1
Yin and yang. (From Fritz S: *Mosby's fundamentals of therapeutic massage,* ed 3, St Louis, 2004, Mosby.)

The idea of wholeness is presented in many cultures and religions as well as in science. We use terminology such as yin and yang to represent physiological function, not a spiritual approach (Figure 1-1).

The dual aspects of yin and yang combine to form a dynamic unit; they are complementary. Yang is said to contain the seed of yin, and yin the seed of yang. These seeds are represented by the small black and white spots in the yin/yang symbol (Figure 1-1). Nothing can be totally yin or totally yang (Table 1-1).

The human body and all its functions can be understood through this concept of the relationship of opposites that creates wholeness. We will use this concept as one of the main themes throughout this text (Activity 1-1).

PRACTICAL APPLICATION

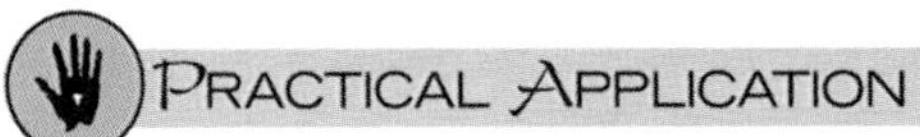

Students of therapeutic massage must be well versed in gross anatomy. The most effective application of massage methods depends on the practitioner's ability to locate,

TABLE 1-1
Yang Qualities Versus Yin Qualities

YANG QUALITIES	YIN QUALITIES
Day	Night
Immaterial	Material
Produces energy	Produces form
Hot	Cold
Sun	Moon
Expansion	Contraction
Energy	Matter
Above	Below
Fire	Water
Hollow	Solid
Hard	Soft
Superior	Inferior

ACTIVITY 1-1

Taking no more than 60 seconds, list as many examples as you can of sets of opposites that together reflect wholeness. Two examples are given to get you started.

Example: Black/white
Flexion/extension

Your Turn

recognize, and understand the structure the hands are manipulating. We also must have a working understanding of organizational and systemic physiology to understand how and why methods of bodywork are beneficial. Although we touch the anatomy, the physiology produces the benefits of the massage. Knowing the location of a muscle is not enough; we also must know how it functions, and what effects massage or other soft tissue approaches have on the function of that muscle, as well as the effect of the muscle on the whole body. We need to understand how stimulating physiologic changes can influence structure as part of the dynamic process of change that unfolds constantly in our bodies and in our lives as a whole (Activity 1-2). ■

Characteristics of Life

What constitutes life? No single criterion defines it. Instead, characteristics of life consist of the following:

Maintenance of boundaries: Keeping the internal environment distinct from the external environment
Movement: The ability to transport the entire being, as well as internal components, throughout the body

ACTIVITY 1-2

Consider this statement: As the tree is bent, so it grows. How does the statement reflect the influence of the function on structure?

Your Turn

Responsiveness: The ability to sense, monitor, and respond to changes in the external environment
Conductivity: The movement of energy from one point to another
Growth: A normal increase in size and/or number of cells
Respiration: The absorption, transport, and use or exchange of respiratory gases (oxygen and carbon dioxide)
Digestion: The process by which food products are broken down into simple substances to be used by individual cells
Absorption: The transport and use of nutrients
Secretion: The production and delivery of specialized substances for diverse functions
Excretion: The removal of waste products
Circulation: The movement of fluids, nutrients, secretions, and waste products from one area of the body to another
Reproduction: The formation of a new being; also, the formation of new cells in the body to permit growth, repair, and replacement
Metabolism: A chemical reaction that occurs in cells to effect transformation, production, or consumption of energy

Each characteristic of life is related to the sum of all the physical and chemical reactions that occur in the body. Physiology, or function, characterizes life.

We can study form (structure) without life, such as in cadaver dissection, but we can study physiology only in terms of living dynamics. This text represents the study of life and the dynamic process of living. Therefore anatomy and physiology are presented together (Activity 1-3).

Organization of Body Structure

From the simplest to the most complex, the structures of the body are able to perform their functions in a logical and well-coordinated manner. This organization is one of the vital characteristics of body structure and function.

Patterns of dysfunction also present a logical order of progression in a well-coordinated manner. Disease processes usually begin at the most basic level and, if left uninterrupted, progress to complex, multisystem involvement. On careful assessment the logic of the progression can be identified. With this information an intervention process can interrupt the dysfunctional process effectively and move the body toward logical, well-coordinated patterns of health. Our bodies work toward balance, which reflects a logical progression of cause and effect. When we understand the patterns of effective function and dysfunction, we can create a map to follow for a return to balance and health.

All living and nonliving things are made of the same components. For this reason, a study of anatomy and physiology must begin with an investigation of the basic chemical and physical components.

ACTIVITY 1-3

Reflect on the characteristics of life as a metaphor of characteristics of your personal life. Then answer the following:

Your Turn

1. Maintenance of boundaries. What are your professional (external) and personal (internal) boundaries?

____

2. Movement. How efficient is your movement along the path of life?

____

3. Responsiveness. How do you recognize, monitor, and respond to changes in your life?

____

4. Conductivity. What is your explanation for how you make something happen? How do you energize?

____

5. Growth. How would you measure personal and professional growth?

____

6. Respiration. How effectively do you breathe?

____

7. Digestion. Describe how you take large, complex concepts and break them into smaller, more understandable pieces.

____

8. Absorption. How do you learn? How do you use your learning?

____

9. Secretion. How do you teach? How do you reach a diverse population?

____

10. Excretion. How do you dispose of those aspects of life that no longer serve you?

____

11. Circulation. How do you move physically and mentally in professional relationships?

____

12. Reproduction. How do you maintain, restore, and permit new growth in yourself?

____

13. Metabolism. How do you create your energy and adjust your use of energy in your life?

____

Chemical Level

Every substance has chemical and physical properties that give it a unique identity. Chemical properties are those that demonstrate the way the substance reacts with other substances or the way it responds to a change in the environment. Physical properties are characteristics such as color, taste, texture, and odor.

Atoms and Molecules

An **atom** is a small particle of an **element**, which is a substance composed of a single kind of atom. Atoms are made up of smaller particles called protons, neutrons, and electrons. Protons, which carry a positive charge (yang), and neutrons, which have a neutral charge, form the nucleus of an atom. They attract electrons, which are negatively charged particles (yin) that travel around the nucleus in specific orbital patterns. The atoms most commonly found in living things are hydrogen, carbon, nitrogen, and oxygen.

Electrons are involved in all chemical reactions that bond atoms to make a **molecule,** a combination of two or more atoms. Molecules can form elements (substances composed of a single type of atom) or compounds (substances made up of different types of atoms). In elements the number of protons in the nucleus of an atom remains the same. This consistency of protons gives the element its identity and its atomic number. The number of protons and neutrons in the nucleus combine to create the atomic weight (Table 1-2). (Because electrons are extremely light, their weight is not a factor.)

Chemical Bonds

The most important structural feature in a chemical reaction is the stability of the outer shell of the atom, where the electrons are located. Shells, or electron shells, are envelopes or layers of electron orbit patterns. If the outer shell is full and does not react chemically, the atom is inert. If the outer shell is not full, the atom is chemically reactive. An atom can achieve a state of maximal stability by forming one of the following three types of bonds to fill the outer electron shell (Activity 1-4):

Ionic bond: An atom can gain or lose electrons to fill or empty its outer shell. When this happens, the atom is no longer electrically neutral, because the ratio of protons to electrons is no longer equal. The atom becomes an electrically charged ion with a negative charge (anion) or a positive charge (cation). Negatively and positively charged ions attract each other to form a stable union. Soluble negatively charged molecules with ions that

TABLE 1-2
Elements Found in the Body: Their Symbols and Percentage of Body Weight

Element (Atomic Number)	Symbol	Percentage of Body Weight
Oxygen (8)	O	65
Carbon (6)	C	18.6
Hydrogen (1)	H	9.7
Nitrogen (7)	N	3.2
Calcium (20)	Ca	1.8
Phosphorus (15)	P	1.0
Potassium (19)	K	0.4
Sodium (11)	Na	0.2
Chlorine (17)	Cl	0.2
Magnesium (12)	Mg	0.06
Sulfur (16)	S	0.04
Iron (26)	Fe	0.007
Iodine (53)	I	0.0002

ACTIVITY 1-4

Describe a professional, social, or personal relationship that represents the properties of each of the three types of bonds.

Example
Polar covalent bond: A stray cat lives in my barn. The cat feeds with my other barn cats, but I don't think of the cat as part of my family. The weak bond that we have could be broken easily if the cat were drawn to the neighbor's barn and chose to leave.

Your Turn
1. Ionic bond

2. Covalent bond

3. Polar covalent bond

conduct electrical currents are called electrolytes. This type of bond is important in nerve and brain function.

Covalent bond: When two or more atoms share electrons, a covalent bond is created, the most stable kind of association that atoms can form with one another. This sharing completes the outer shell. CO_2, carbon dioxide, is an example.

Polar covalent bond: Molecules with polar covalent bonds, called polar molecules, are electrically neutral because they have the same number of protons and electrons. However, the electrons can be arranged in the shells so that one side of the molecule is more negative and the other side more positive. Water is an example of a polar molecule. Polar molecules attract each other, with the positive side of one attracting the negative side of a different molecule. These weak polar covalent bonds, sometimes referred to as hydrogen bonds, are abundant in nature. They help create larger molecules such as **proteins** and **deoxyribonucleic acid (DNA).**

Two or more atoms joined by chemical bonds create a molecule. A molecule is the smallest part of a substance that can exist independently without losing the physical and chemical properties of that substance. If the atoms are of the same type, the result is an element. Atoms of two or more different elements combine to make a compound. **Inorganic compounds** are chemical structures that do not have carbon and hydrogen atoms. **Organic compounds** are chemical structures that have carbon and hydrogen atoms. The function of a molecule is related to its structures. The structure of a molecule depends on the patterns of the chemical bonds.

Chemical reactions take place when chemical bonds are broken and new ones are formed. In a chemical reaction the number of atoms remains the same, but the atoms become linked in a different way, forming a new substance (Figure 1-2). Matter exists as a solid, liquid, or gas depending on attraction of the molecules. When the molecules exist close together, the substance is solid; conversely, when molecules are farthest apart, they form a gas.

Metabolism

Metabolism is the word we use to describe all the physiologic processes that take place in our bodies to convert the

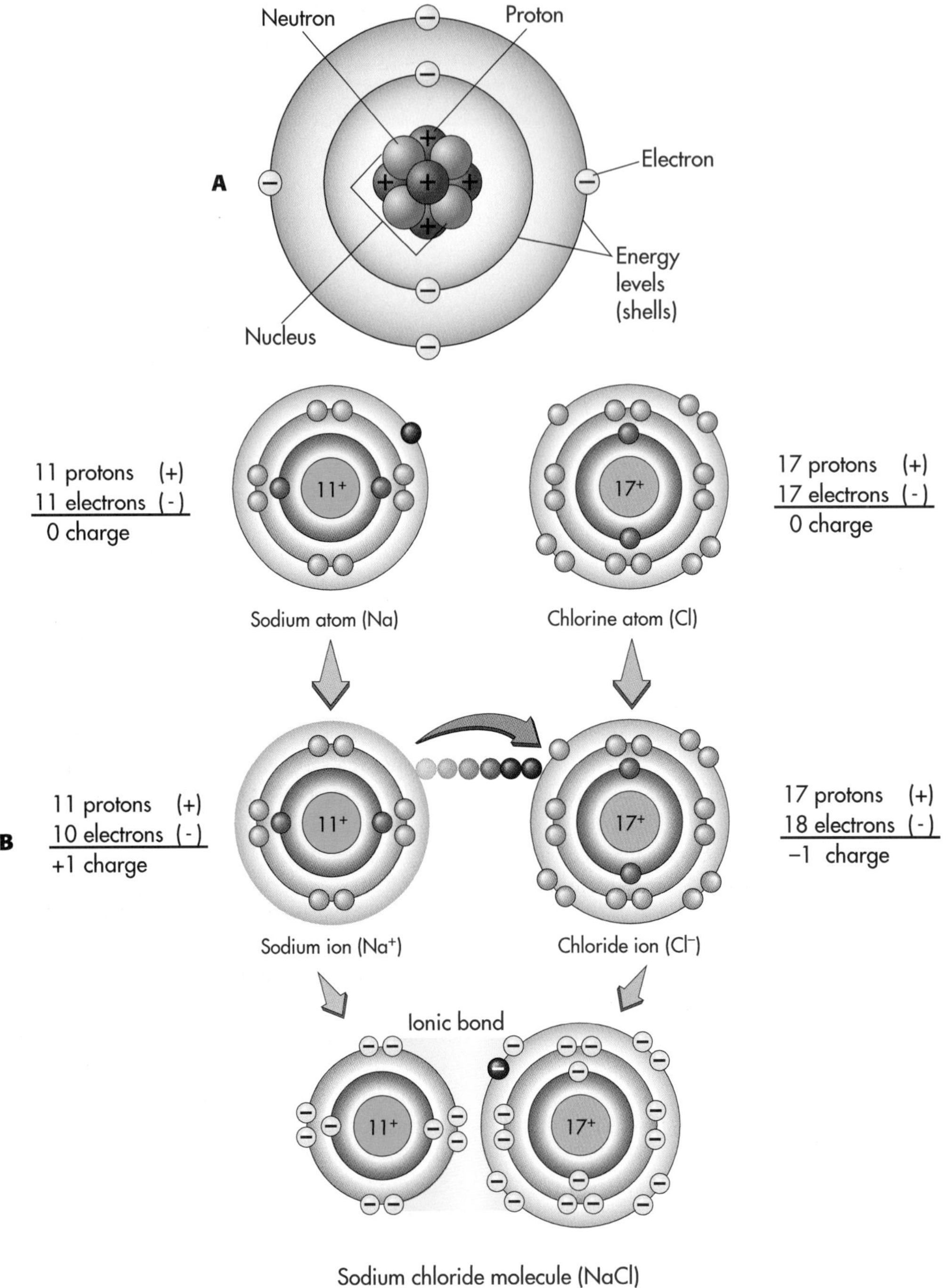

Figure 1-2
A, Model of the atom. The nucleus, made up of protons (+) and neutrons, is at the core. Electrons (–) inhabit outer regions called energy levels. **B,** Ionic bonding. The sodium atom donates the single electron in its outer energy level to a chlorine atom that has seven electrons in its outer level; now each atom has eight electrons in its outer shell. Because the electron-to-proton ratio changes, the sodium atom becomes a positive sodium ion and the chlorine atom becomes a negative chloride ion. The positive-negative attraction between these oppositely charged ions is called an ionic bond.

food we eat and the air we breathe into the energy we need to function.

Energy is the capacity to work. Work is defined as a movement or a change in the physical structure of matter. Energy exists in two forms: potential and kinetic. If an elastic band is held in a stretched position, it has the potential energy to return to its original shape. Kinetic energy occurs when the elastic band actually moves. Energy is constant and not lost and is converted from one form to another.

In the body, during chemical reactions, most of the energy is converted to heat and maintains the core body temperature. If the body is cold, the muscles contract and relax quickly, increasing the metabolism (chemical reactions) and producing more heat.

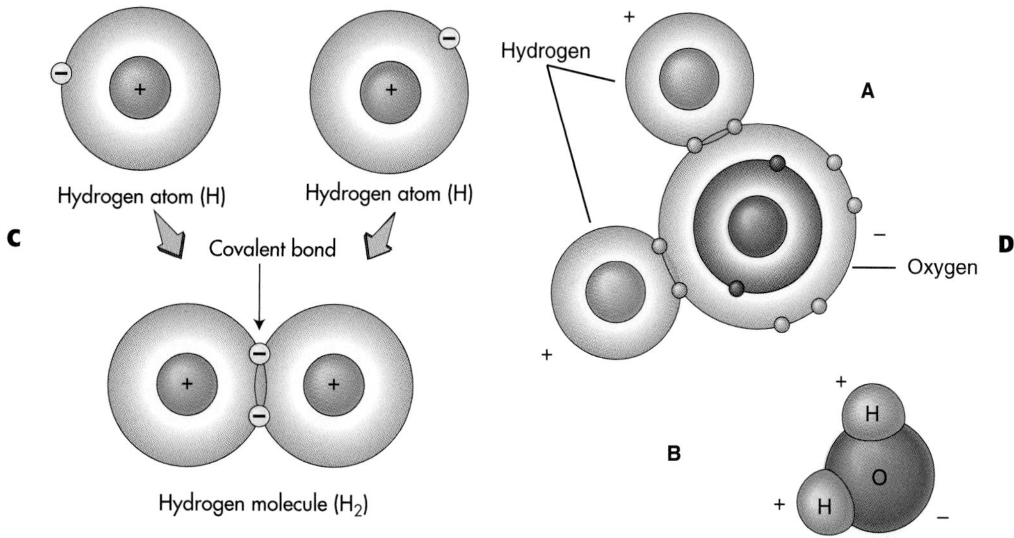

Figure 1-2, cont'd.
C, Covalent bonding. Two hydrogen atoms move together, resulting in overlapping of their energy levels. Neither atom gains or loses an electron; rather, the two atoms share the electrons, forming a covalent bond. **D,** Water is a polar molecule, as shown in the diagram. The two hydrogen atoms are nearer one end of the molecule, giving that end a partial positive charge. The opposite end of the molecule has a partial negative charge. (**A** to **C** from Thibodeau GA, Patton KT: *Structure and function of the body,* ed 11, St Louis, 2000, Mosby. **D** from Thibodeau GA, Patton KT: *Anatomy and physiology,* ed 5, St Louis, 2003, Mosby.)

The body stores potential energy as high-energy compounds. Chemical reactions form these compounds or break them down. The two forms of chemical reactions are as follows:

Anabolism: Chemical reactions that use energy as they join simple molecules to form more complex molecules of **carbohydrates, lipids,** proteins, and **nucleic acids;** the energy for this process comes from **adenosine triphosphate (ATP).**

Catabolism: Chemical reactions that release energy as they break down complex compounds. ATP contains many **high-energy bonds** that, when broken during catabolism, supply energy for the work of the body. Hydrolysis is a catabolic reaction that uses water to break down larger molecules. Dehydration is an anabolic reaction involving the removal of water while small molecules combine to create larger ones.

Enzymes are proteins that speed up chemical reactions but are not consumed or altered in the process. Enzyme activity is altered by factors such as temperature, acidity, or alkalinity. Enzyme activity often is reduced in acidic conditions. Cold and acid environments are used in food preservation such as freezing and pickling. When muscle activity increases and oxygen is inadequate, lactic acid forms and the muscle environment becomes acidic. Enzyme activity slows down and muscle fatigue results. **Metabolites** are molecules synthesized or broken down inside the body by chemical reactions. **Nutrients** are the essential elements and molecules obtained from the diet that are required by the body for normal function.

Acidity and alkalinity. The body has to maintain a balance of acidity/alkalinity to support normal function. The acidity/alkalinity of a solution is measured in terms of pH. The pH is actually a measure of hydrogen ion concentration in the body fluid. Water is considered to be a pH of 7, which is neutral. If the pH is lower than 7, the fluid has more hydrogen ions and is acidic. If a solution has a pH higher than 7, it has fewer hydrogen ions and is alkaline.

The pH of the body is 7.4, which is slightly alkaline. For the enzymes of the body to be active and for the chemical reactions to proceed normally, the pH needs to be maintained at this level.

Buffers are compounds that help maintain the hydrogen ion concentration. Proteins, hemoglobin, and a combination of bicarbonate and carbonic acid compounds are examples of buffers present in body fluids.

Organic compounds have the elements carbon, hydrogen, and oxygen. Four organic compounds are important in the body: carbohydrates, proteins, fats or lipids, and nucleic acids.

Carbohydrates. Carbohydrates make up 2% to 3% of our body weight. Sugars and starches are examples. Carbohydrates supply most of the energy for cells and may be simple or complex.

Simple sugars, such as glucose and fructose, dissolve easily in water and are transported easily in blood. Complex sugars are formed by the combination of two or more simple sugars and need to be broken down by the digestive tract before being absorbed into the body.

Lipids. Lipids make up 10% to 12% of our body weight. Lipids are insoluble in water and have to be transported in the blood by special mechanisms. Lipids are used to form important structures such as cell membranes and certain hormones and are an important source of energy. When lipid supply exceeds demand, lipids are stored as fat reserves for future use or as important body insulators. (Fatty acids, glycerides, steroids and phospholipids are examples of lipids found in the body.)

Proteins. Proteins make up about 20% of the body weight. Proteins consist of chains of organic molecules known as amino acids with chains of amino acids called peptides. In our bodies about 20 amino acids are significant. Each amino acid has a different chemical structure that alters its properties. Proteins form the structural framework for the body. All proteins contain carbon, hydrogen, oxygen, and nitrogen.

Enzymes that facilitate chemical reactions are proteins, as are buffers. The blood contains proteins in the plasma, and they are used to transport gases (hemoglobin) and hormones (plasma proteins). The antibodies are proteins, too. Many hormones are proteins.

Nucleic acids. Nucleic acid is the major component of ova and sperm and conveys information about the genetic cycle. Two types of nucleic acid exist: DNA and **ribonucleic acid (RNA).**

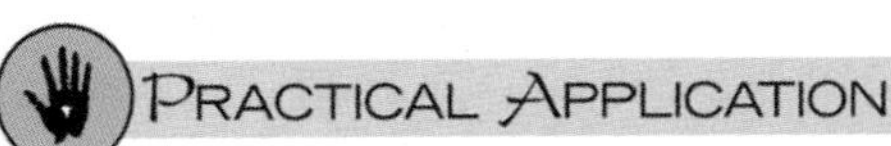

In the study of therapeutic massage the student must remain mindful of the basic chemical foundations of life and the dynamic processes of change. Change is balanced by the stability of constancy represented in the metaphor of yin and yang, as reflected in the electron and proton relationship. We function in a continual process of old bonds being broken and new ones being formed every millisecond of our lives, whether in cellular functions or social relationships. Each time we apply massage to a client's body, we become part of the stimulus pattern that is the activation process for chemical reactions within the body. ■

Subtle or energetic forms of bodywork may be reflected by the electrical bonding of negatives and positives during chemical reactions that seem to generate the energy of life. The yin and yang concept of a balance of positives and negatives and the duality of wholeness that provides stability during change also is related to the balance of chemical relationships. A more detailed study of the electrical and chemical levels of life, beyond this basic overview, would be valuable not only for an appreciation of the elegance of the simple physical basis of life but also for an understanding of the metaphor of the way we relate to our clients, our families and friends, and the peoples of this world.

Organelle Level

Molecules combine in specific ways to form **organelles,** the basic structures found in cells (Figure 1-3). Each type of

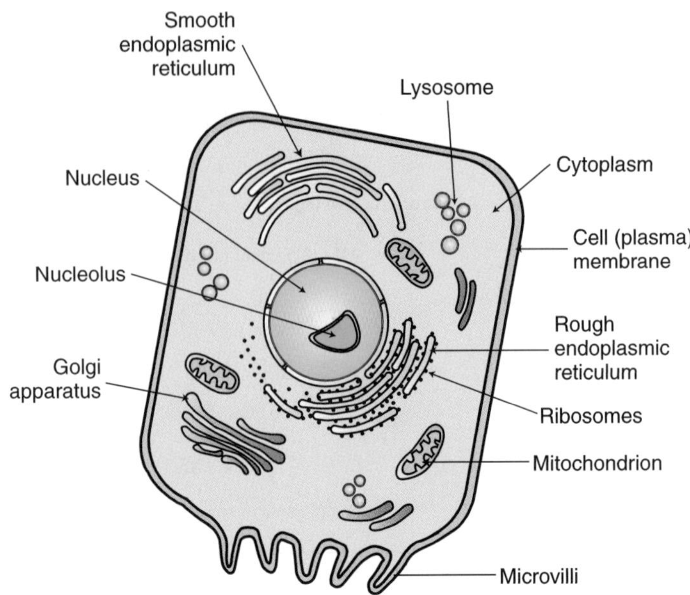

Figure 1-3
Generalized cell.

organelle performs a specific function within the **cell.** More than two dozen organelles have been identified, but the following list includes only the most common ones (Activity 1-5):

Cell membrane: Also known as the plasma membrane, the cell **membrane** is the outer boundary of the cell. The membrane is composed of lipids, carbohydrates, and proteins and is called the **phospholipid bilayer,** with molecules arranged in such a way that they resemble a sandwich. The function of the cell membrane is to contain the inside of the cell and allow transport of certain substances into and out of the cell through various proteins embedded in the cell membrane. Proteins on the surface of the cell act as markers that identify the cell or work as receptors for chemical signals.

The cell membrane is **impermeable** if it does not allow substances to pass through and is selectively permeable if it stops one substance from entering the cell and freely allows another to pass through. Electrical charge, chemical composition, and the size and shape of a substance determine whether the cell membrane will allow it to pass through.

Transport of substances across the cell membrane without use of energy is called **passive transport.** Types of passive transport are diffusion, osmosis, filtration, carrier-mediated transport, and vesicular transport. **Diffusion** is the movement of ions and molecules from an area of higher concentration to that of a lower concentration. **Osmosis** is the diffusion of water from a region of lower solution concentration to a region of higher solution concentration across a semipermeable membrane.

During **filtration,** hydrostatic pressure forces water across a semipermeable membrane. This occurs in the body

ACTIVITY 1-5

Develop a metaphor for each organelle (think of its function).

Example: The nucleus is the mom of the cell, or the nucleus holds the building plans for a house.

Your Turn

1. Nucleus
2. Ribosomes
3. Endoplasmic reticulum
4. Mitochondria
5. Lysosomes
6. Golgi apparatus
7. Cytoplasm
8. Cytosol
9. Cytoskeleton

when filtration moves fluid out of capillaries and into the renal tubules of the kidney to form urine. **Carrier-mediated transport** occurs when integral proteins bind to specific ions or other substances such as glucose and amino acids and carry them across the cell membrane into the cell. During **vesicular transport,** small membrane-lined sacs form as the cell membrane folds to form vescicles that surround substances and move it into or out of the cell. Bringing substances into the cell by forming vesicles is **endocytosis,** and transporting of substances out of the cell is **exocytosis.**

Active transport of substances across the cell membrane requires energy in the form of ATP. Active transport uses energy to create **ion pumps.** The most common ion pump is the sodium-potassium pump. Under normal circumstances the extracellular fluid contains more sodium than the intracellular fluid and vice versa for potassium. The sodium-potassium pump, by using energy, pumps sodium out and potassium in to maintain **homeostasis.** Cells are negatively charged inside and positively charged outside. This difference in charges, known as the transmembrane potential, is maintained by ionic pumps that move substances by active transport . The maintenance of transmembrane potential is important and necessary for many functions, such as transmission of nerve impulses, muscle contraction, and secretion from glands.

Cytoplasm: The material enclosed by the cell membrane is called **cytoplasm,** which contains the nucleus and organelles. The fluid portion of the cytoplasm is called intracellular fluid or **cytosol.** Cytoplasm, which is not classified as an organelle, is the medium that surrounds all the organelles. The fluid portion, or cytosol, contains many protein enzymes, which function as catalysts in the cell processes. The **cytoskeleton** is an internal scaffolding that anchors the organelles and allows the cells to move and to maintain or change their shape.

Endoplasmic reticulum: **Endoplasmic reticulum** is a network of interconnected tubes, flattened sacs, and channels distributed throughout the cytoplasm. Rough endoplasmic reticulum is found in cells in which large amounts of proteins are made. Smooth endoplasmic reticulum usually is involved in the metabolism of lipids (fats); it also assists in the detoxification of drugs and the deactivation of steroids. Smooth endoplasmic reticulum of muscle cells (sarcoplasmic reticulum) uses large amounts of calcium to trigger muscle contractions.

Golgi apparatus (or complex): The Golgi **apparatus** process and package protein and some carbohydrates for distribution to other parts of the cell or for secretion from the cell.

Lysosomes: **Lysosomes** contain enzymes that function as the digestive system of the cell. These enzymes are enclosed in membranes to keep them from breaking down the cell itself.

Microvilli: **Microvilli** are small fingerlike projections of the cell membrane that serve to increase the surface area. They are found in cells that are involved in absorbing substances from the extracellular fluid.

Mitochondria: The **mitochondria** may be the largest and one of the most numerous of the organelles. They produce ATP, which provides energy for cell activity.

Nucleus: Usually the largest of the organelles, the **nucleus** contains the chromosomes (threads of DNA). DNA is a double-helix strand held together by hydrogen bonds. Inside the nucleus is the nucleolus, which contains RNA structures that form ribosomes. The nucleus controls the daily activities of the cell and all cellular reproduction. The nucleus has the information needed for the manufacture of more than 100,000 proteins and controls which proteins are synthesized and in what amounts in a given time.

The nitrogenous bases adenine, thymine, cytosine, and guanine are arranged in different ways to form the genetic code of DNA. The lineup of bases that code for a specific protein is known as a gene, and a gene exists for every type of protein manufactured in the body.

Peroxisomes: **Peroxisomes** are similar to lysosomes, except that they help to detoxify substances such as alcohol and hydrogen peroxide in the cell.

Ribosomes: Often the most numerous of the organelles, **ribosomes** are the sites where amino acids are combined to create various proteins.

Cellular Level

A cell is the basic structural unit of an organism and is also the primary functional unit with properties that reflect the characteristics of life. Cells reproduce by cell division. They are surrounded by a dilute saltwater solution called interstitial fluid. Cells are self-regulating, which allows them to adjust to constant changes and to interact with their surroundings. The specific activities of any organism depend on the individual and collective activities of the cells.

Chemically, a cell is composed of carbon, hydrogen, nitrogen, oxygen, and trace amounts of several other elements. Cells are made of approximately 15% protein, 3% lipids, 1% carbohydrates, 1% nucleic acids, and 80% water. Although cells are diverse in size and shape, they almost all have the same parts and general form. Cells are surrounded by a cell membrane, and all contain cytoplasm and organelles.

Cell metabolism involving catabolism (breaking down) and anabolism (building up) can be identified and measured in terms of our recurring theme, the duality of wholeness.

The life cycle of a cell follows a series of changes from the time the cell is formed until it reproduces. The cycle can be divided into two major periods:

1. Growth, or **interphase,** in which the cell carries on most of its activities.
2. Reproduction (**mitosis**), or cell division, in which the cell reproduces itself. **Meiosis** is a form of mitosis that halves the number of chromosomes (threads of DNA) in reproductive cells before they combine and multiply.

The cell division is regulated by growth factors in the extracellular fluid that bind to receptors in the cell membrane to trigger cell division. The main growth factors are growth hormone, nerve growth factor, epidermal growth factor, and erythropoietin.

Cell division is suppressed by repressor genes. If the rate of growth exceeds that of repression, tissue enlarges. If cell growth is uncontrolled, a tumor or neoplasm results.

Cells change size in response to hormones, nutrient availability, and changes in their function. **Atrophy** is a decrease in the size of a cell; **hypertrophy** is an increase in the size of a cell. Muscle cells in particular can adapt their size to their function. Hypertrophy most often occurs when a person is continually using muscle cells, such as in weight training; atrophy occurs in underused muscle cells, such as when a muscle is immobilized so that a broken bone can heal.

No matter what a cell does or where it is located in the body, its basic maintenance functions are the same. These are nutrition, metabolism, respiration, excretion, organization, and irritability. When a cell needs to adapt to perform specialized duties, the structure of the cell and in turn some of the specialized functions are modified; this form of specialization is referred to as cell differentiation. For example, fat cells are modified to store energy, but they have lost the functions of contraction and secretion. Muscle cells have well-developed functions of contractility but diminished functions of secretion and reproduction. Cells that specialize in certain functions form tissues. As mentioned before, disease most likely appears when cellular homeostasis (internal balance) has been lost.

Tissue Level

A **tissue** is a group of similar cells that are specialized for a specific function. The cells of a tissue are embedded in or surrounded by nonliving material called the **matrix**. The amount and configuration of matrices differ with the type of tissue and the amount of containment or support needed for the tissue.

In most cases, cells directly connect with one another, which allows for better, more stable intercellular communication. Blood plasma, which is a matrix, maintains tissue structure but does not hold it in a solid mass. Desmosomes are small contact points of filaments between cells that act like welds. Gap junctions are formed when channels of the cell membranes adhere to each other. Tight junctions are the type of configuration their name suggests: whole membranes fused together around the cells to create nonpermeable structures.

The four principal types of tissue—epithelial, connective, muscle, and nervous—can be identified by their structures and functions.

Epithelial Tissue

Epithelial tissues cover and protect the surface of the body and its parts (Figure 1-4). They line cavities, form glands, and specialize in moving substances into and out of the blood during secretion, absorption, and excretion. Because they endure a considerable amount of wear and tear, epithelial cells reproduce actively. If a person is suffering from stress overload or any homeostatic imbalance, the condition often is first seen in the epithelial tissues because of the fast turnover of cells.

Typically, little matrix material is found in epithelial tissues. The matrix present tends to form continuous sheets of cells, with the cells held closely together. The surface of most epithelial tissue is not in contact with other tissues but rather is exposed to the external or internal environment. This surface is the **apical surface.** The other surface faces the inside of the body and is known as the **basal surface.** A permeable, thin **basement membrane** attaches epithelial tissues to the underlying **connective tissues.** Because epithelial tissues contain no blood vessels, they must obtain oxygen and other nutrients by diffusion from capillaries in the connective tissue.

The epithelial tissues make up three types of membranes, each formed with epithelial tissue on the surface and a specialized connective tissue layer underneath. A membrane is a thin, sheetlike layer of tissue that covers a cell, an organ,

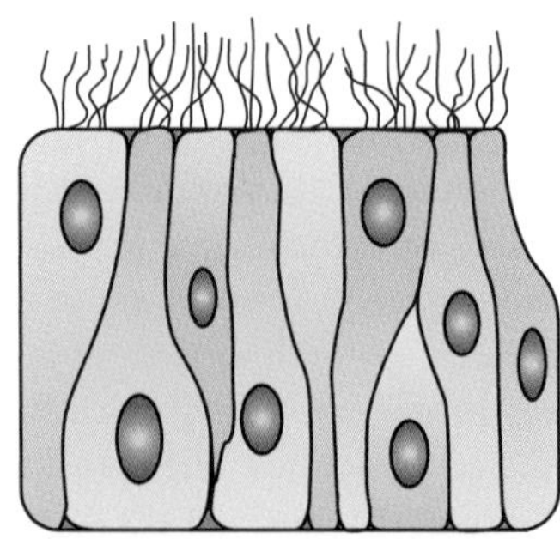

Figure 1-4
Epithelial tissue.

or a structure; that lines tubes or cavities; or that divides and separates one part from another. The three types of membranes are as follows:

Cutaneous membranes cover the surface of the body, which is exposed to the external environment. The largest cutaneous membrane, more commonly known as our skin, accounts for about 16% of our body weight.

Serous membranes line body cavities not open to the external environment and cover many of the organs. These membranes secrete a thin, watery fluid that lubricates organs to reduce friction as they rub against one another and against the walls of the cavities. Serous membranes line the peritoneal, pleural, and pericardial cavities.

Mucous membranes are found on the surface of tubes that open directly to the exterior, such as those lining the respiratory, digestive, urinary, and reproductive tracts. The film of mucus secreted by these membranes coats and protects the underlying cells.

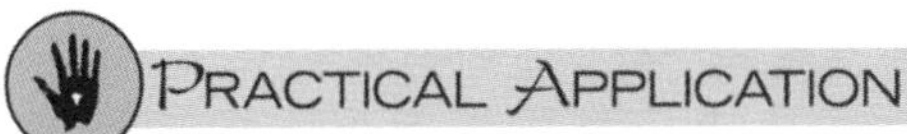

Therapeutic massage focuses on the skin as the primary point of touch. Of particular importance is the sensory function of the touch receptors in the skin. Touch is discussed more extensively in Chapter 11. Passive and active joint movement methods support normal function of the synovial membranes, which are connective tissue membranes. The synovial membranes, which secrete the synovial fluid, line all synovial joints. ■

Connective Tissue

Connective tissue is the most abundant tissue in the body and is the most widely distributed of the four primary types of tissue. Connective tissue is specialized to support and hold together the body and its parts, transport substances through the body, and protect the body from foreign substances. All forms of connective tissue are made of matrix, fibers, and cells. The properties of the connective tissue cells and the composition and arrangement of the matrix elements account for the amazing diversity of connective tissues.

Connective tissue cells often are spaced far apart, and the space between cells is filled with large amounts of nonliving matrix. Within the matrix of connective tissue is a shapeless ground substance containing molecules that expand when combined with electrolytes and water molecules. The matrix of connective tissue may be 90% ground substance. The remainder is made up mainly of one or more of the following fibers:

Collagenous fibers: Collagenous fibers are tough and strong and have minimal stretch capability. They have a high degree of tensile strength, which allows them to withstand longitudinal stress. These fibers occur in bundles. Because of their color, they are referred to as white fibers. **Collagen** makes up more than one quarter of the protein in the body. As we age, the molecular structure of collagen changes, which accounts for the appearance of changes in our tissues.

Reticular fibers: Reticular fibers are delicate fibers found in networks that support small structures such as capillaries, nerve fibers, and the basement membrane. These fibers are made of a form of collagen called reticulin.

Elastic fibers: Elastic fibers are extensible and elastic. Found in the stretchy tissues, they are made from a protein called elastin, which has the ability to return to its original length, much like an elastic band does after being stretched. Because of their color, these fibers are called yellow fibers.

Each major type of connective tissue has a fundamental cell type that secretes the matrix and fibers (Table 1-3).

A watery ground substance creates a fluid connective tissue such as blood. By changing the proportion of collagen and elastic and reticular fibers, the tissue can be made as tough as tendons or as flexible as the tissue that covers muscles. Calcium salts added to the ground substance make the tissue become rigid, such as bone.

Connective tissue can be manipulated by application of heat, cold, stretch, and activity. Connective tissue is thixotropic, which makes substances solidify when cold or left undisturbed and become more fluid when warmed or stirred. Gelatin is an example. If not stretched and warmed by muscular activity, connective tissue tends to stiffen and become less flexible.

Therapeutic massage stretches, strokes, and moves tissue and generates heat to make connective tissue more fluid, allowing greater mobility and encouraging blood flow.

The collagen fibers of connective tissue tend to bind together by hydrogen bonding with disuse and chronic pressure. Inflammation is a factor in the bonding process called adhesions. Nerves and blood vessels may get caught in adhesions, and range of motion often is reduced or pain results. Massage manipulation helps slow down formation of adhesions and also aids the alignment of the collagen fibers, reducing friction and allowing more optimal movement.

Although connective tissue is found in all areas of the body, some areas contain more than others. The brain has little connective tissue, whereas ligaments, tendons, and skin

TABLE 1-3
Connective Tissue Cell Types

Cell Type	Matrix and Fibers
Fibroblast	Connective tissue
Chondroblast	Cartilage
Osteoblast	Bone
Hemocytoblast (hematopoietic stem cell)	Blood

have high concentrations. The number of blood vessels in connective tissue varies. Cartilage has none, but other types of connective tissue have a large number of blood vessels. Connective tissue contains cells that help with repair, healing, and storage as well as other cells that help with defense. Fibroblasts and mesenchymal cells repair injured tissue. Connective tissue disease is discussed more in Chapter 8.

Three other types of cells also are found commonly in connective tissue:

Macrophages are large, irregularly shaped cells. They develop in the bone marrow and move throughout the connective tissue, searching for microorganisms, damaged cells, and foreign particles. When these targets are found, the macrophages dispose of them by ingesting and digesting them, a process known as **phagocytosis.**

Mast cells also develop in bone marrow. Their functions focus on releasing chemicals (heparin and histamine) as part of the inflammatory response, allergic response, and pain.

Adipose cells are large cells stored in white or brown fat in the dermis, in the deep layer of the skin, in the gut, and in the colon. When clustered together, they are known as adipose tissue.

Types of connective tissue. Descriptions of the structure and function of four types of connective tissue follow.

Dense regular connective tissue (Figure 1-5)

Structure: The matrix consists mainly of collagen fibers produced by fibroblasts, with fibers oriented in parallel. The ligaments and tendons formed by this type of tissue have a small number of cells, and blood flow to the area is limited.

Function: Dense regular connective tissue provides strength and resistance while allowing some degree of stretch.

Dense irregular connective tissue (Figure 1-6)

Structure: Collagen and elastin fibers are interwoven and oriented in an irregular pattern to create the matrix. The tissue has little blood flow and is concentrated in the dermis, joint capsules and surrounding muscles, and in some organs.

Function: Dense irregular connective tissue can withstand intense pulling forces and resist impact.

Loose (areolar) tissue (Figure 1-7)

Structure: A loose, irregular configuration of fibroblastic cells, macrophages, and lymphocytes is contained within a fine network of mostly collagen and elastin. Fluid-filled spaces separate the cells and fibers from one another.

Function: Areolar tissue is distributed throughout the body and is the substance on which most epithelium rests. Areolar tissue is the packing material between glands, muscles, and nerves; attaches the skin to the underlying tissues; and supplies nourishment because of its high vascularity.

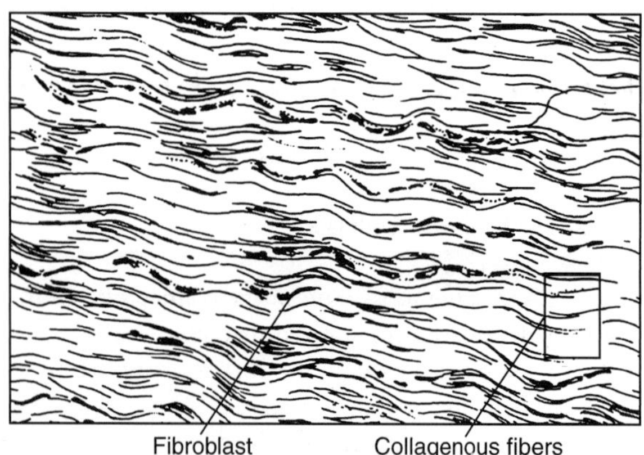

Figure 1-5
Dense regular connective tissue. (From Thibodeau GA, Patton KT: *Anatomy and physiology,* ed 5, St Louis, 2003, Mosby.)

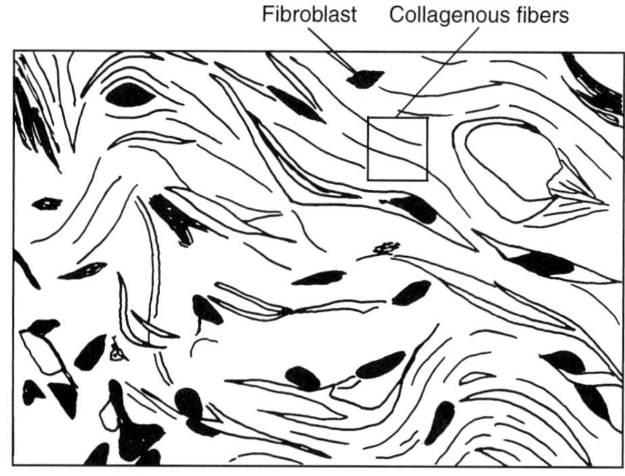

Figure 1-6
Dense irregular connective tissue. (From Thibodeau GA, Patton KT: *Anatomy and physiology,* ed 5, St Louis, 2003, Mosby.)

Bundle of collagenous fibers

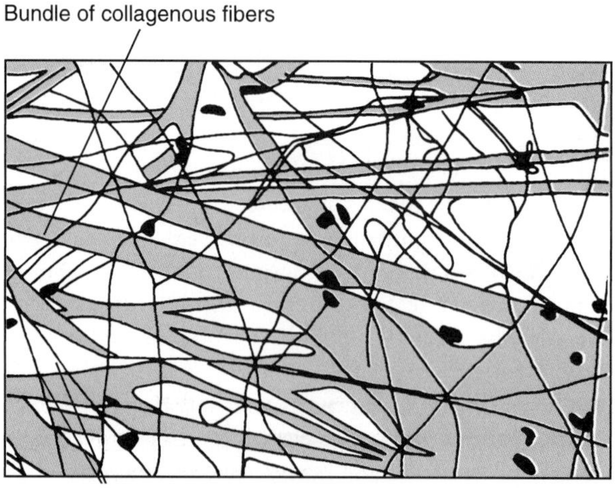

Figure 1-7
Loose (areolar) tissue. (From Thibodeau GA, Patton KT: *Anatomy and physiology,* ed 5, St Louis, 2003, Mosby.)

Adipose tissue (Figure 1-8)

Structure: Adipose tissue is composed of fat cells with little matrix between the cells. Support is provided by reticular and collagenous fibers. Adipose tissue is associated closely with the capillaries of the blood and lymph. Most adipose tissue is found in the buttocks, anterior abdominal wall, breasts, arms, and thighs.

Function: The storage and release of fat are regulated by stimulation from hormones and the nervous system. Adipose tissue is a source of fuel, helps to insulate and pad organs and tissues, and stores fat-soluble vitamins.

Types of cartilage. Cartilage is composed of chondrocytes surrounded by an extensive matrix. Collagen gives cartilage its flexibility, and the strength and water-binding capacity of the ground substance make cartilage rigid yet able to spring back when compressed. Because cartilage has little blood flow, it heals slowly. The three types of cartilage are hyaline cartilage, fibrocartilage, and elastic cartilage.

Hyaline cartilage (Figure 1-9)

Structure: Hyaline cartilage is semitransparent and has a milky bluish color; has a strong and solid matrix; and is flexible and insensitive.

Function: Hyaline cartilage is found at the end of bones in most synovial joints, where it provides additional weight-bearing support or attaches to other bones such as with costal cartilage. Hyaline cartilage provides the support and flexibility found in the trachea, lungs, and nose.

Fibrocartilage (Figure 1-10)

Structure: Fibrocartilage is composed of large amounts of dense fibrous tissue and small amounts of matrix, an arrangement that creates a more rigid structure than hyaline cartilage. Fibrocartilage is found mainly in the symphysis pubis, intervertebral disks, and tendon attachments.

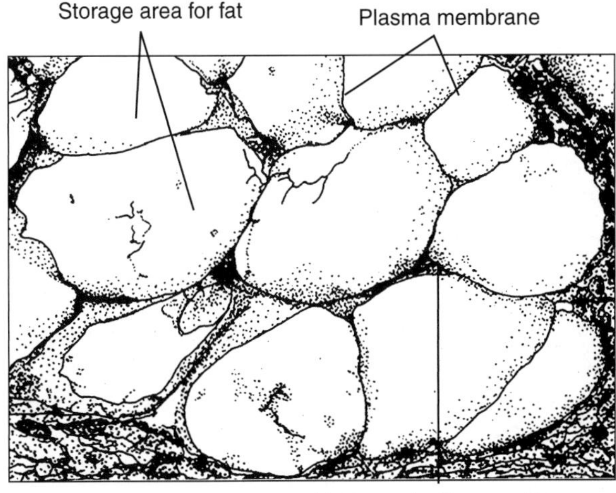

Figure 1-8
Adipose tissue. (From Thibodeau GA, Patton KT: *Anatomy and physiology,* ed 5, St Louis, 2003, Mosby.)

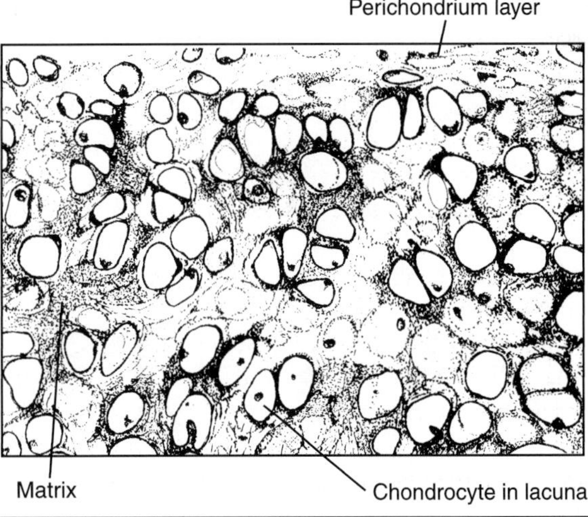

Figure 1-9
Hyaline cartilage. (From Thibodeau GA, Patton KT: *Anatomy and physiology,* ed 5, St Louis, 2003, Mosby.)

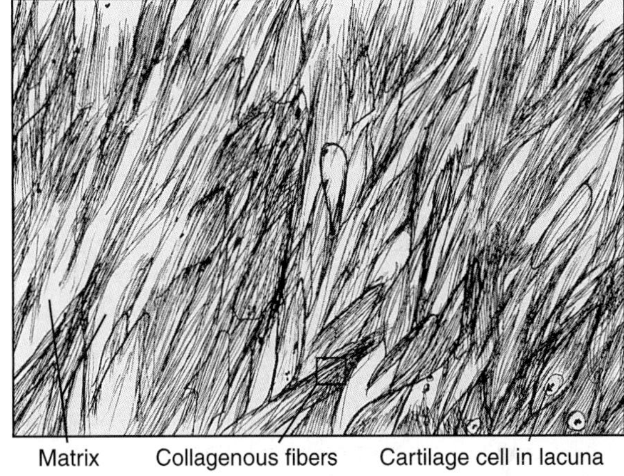

Figure 1-10
Fibrocartilage. (From Thibodeau GA, Patton KT: *Anatomy and physiology,* ed 5, St Louis, 2003, Mosby.)

Function: Fibrocartilage can withstand compression and impact forces, diffusing the force so that it is not focused on specific areas of the bone.

Elastic cartilage (Figure 1-11)

Structure: As its name implies, elastic cartilage is a flexible form of hyaline cartilage with a large concentration of elastic fibers.

Function: Elastic cartilage provides flexibility and support to the external ear and the larynx.

Other forms of connective tissue

Bone (Figure 1-12)

Structure: Bone is the most rigid of the connective tissues because of its hard, mineralized matrix.

Function: Bone provides the framework for supporting the body, protects the internal organs, serves as storage for minerals, and produces blood cells.

Blood (Figure 1-13)

Structure: Blood cells float within an extremely loose matrix, a fluid known as plasma, which contains no fibers.

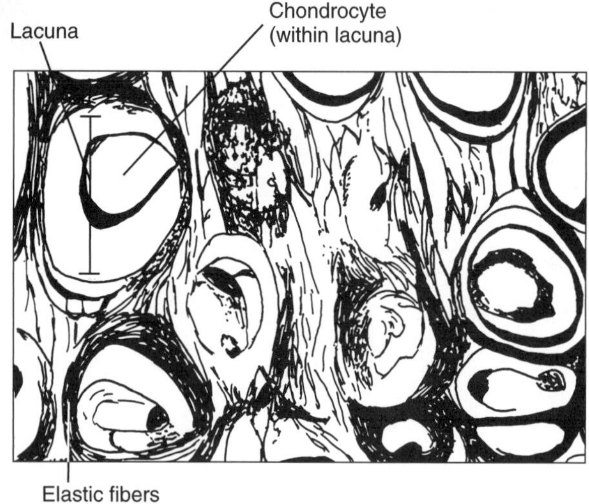

Figure 1-11
Elastic cartilage. (From Thibodeau GA, Patton KT: *Anatomy and physiology,* ed 5, St Louis, 2003, Mosby.)

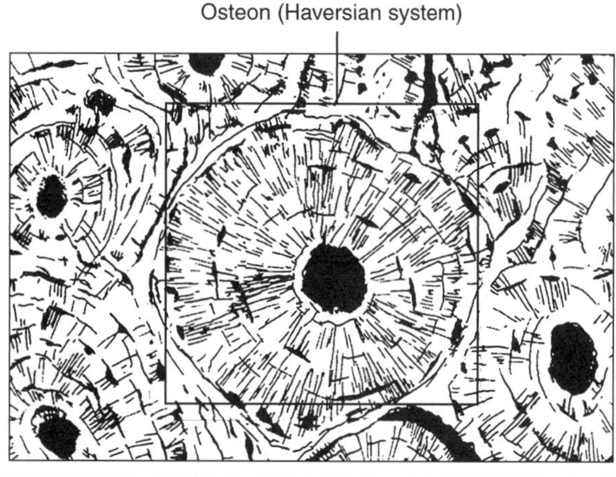

Figure 1-12
Bone tissue. (From Thibodeau GA, Patton KT: *Anatomy and physiology,* ed 5, St Louis, 2003, Mosby.)

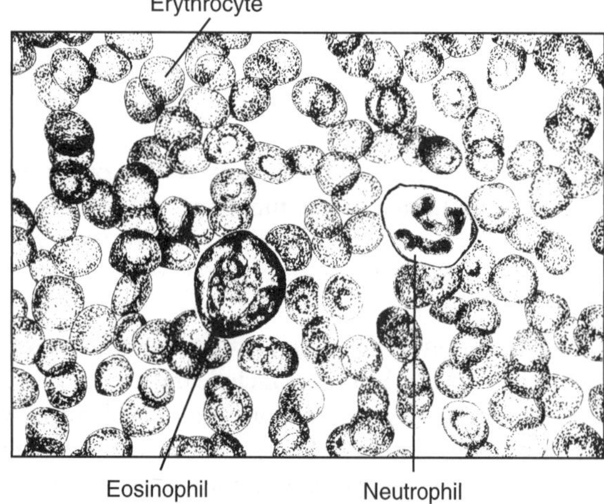

Figure 1-13
Blood. (From Thibodeau GA, Patton KT: *Anatomy and physiology,* ed 5, St Louis, 2003, Mosby.)

Function: Blood helps maintain homeostasis by transporting substances, resisting infection, and maintaining heat.

Connective tissue membranes. Connective tissue membranes are composed exclusively of various types of connective tissue. They are classified as synovial membranes.

Synovial membranes line the joint spaces in the mobile synovial joints. This type of membrane also is found in bursae, which are protective sacs found near joints; between layers of muscle and connective tissue; and wherever the body needs extra protection. Synovial fluid is a thick lubricant secreted by these membranes to keep themselves slippery.

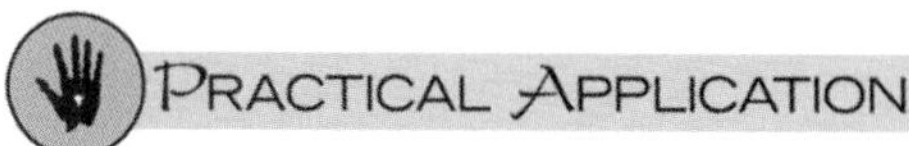

Many of the benefits of massage and bodywork therapies derive from the effects of these treatments on the connective tissue. Most methods affect the consistency of the ground substance and the directional pattern of the fiber configuration and networks. The gel of the ground substance is considered thixotropic, which means that it liquefies when agitated and returns to a gel state as it stands. Manipulating connective tissue seems to soften the ground substance and increase the water-binding capacity, which makes the tissue more pliable (i.e., induces a more liquid state).

When an electrical current is passed through collagen, a slight deforming of the structure results because of the piezoelectric property of the collagen. When collagen itself is compressed, stretched, or twisted, it produces minute electrical currents. Researchers recognize that some forms of electrical stimulation enhance bone growth, but the exact reason why bodywork methods could cause this effect on collagen is under investigation. The innate ability of the body to generate electrical current may provide some insight into the inherent energy flow of the body, what can be called Qi, or Prana, among other names and may be considered life force, or enlivening energy. ■

Muscle Tissue

The main characteristic of **muscle tissue** is its ability to provide movement by shortening through contraction. Contraction assists in maintaining posture and produces heat. Contraction results from the action of contractile proteins found inside muscle cells. Muscle cells are longer than they are wide, creating a distinctive pattern that resembles fibers; for this reason the cells often are referred to as muscle fibers.

Muscle tissues (Figure 1-14) may be categorized by their appearance, function, and location as follows:

- ***Skeletal muscle fibers*** are large, cross-striated cells connected to the skeleton. They are controlled by the nervous system, and their actions are voluntary.

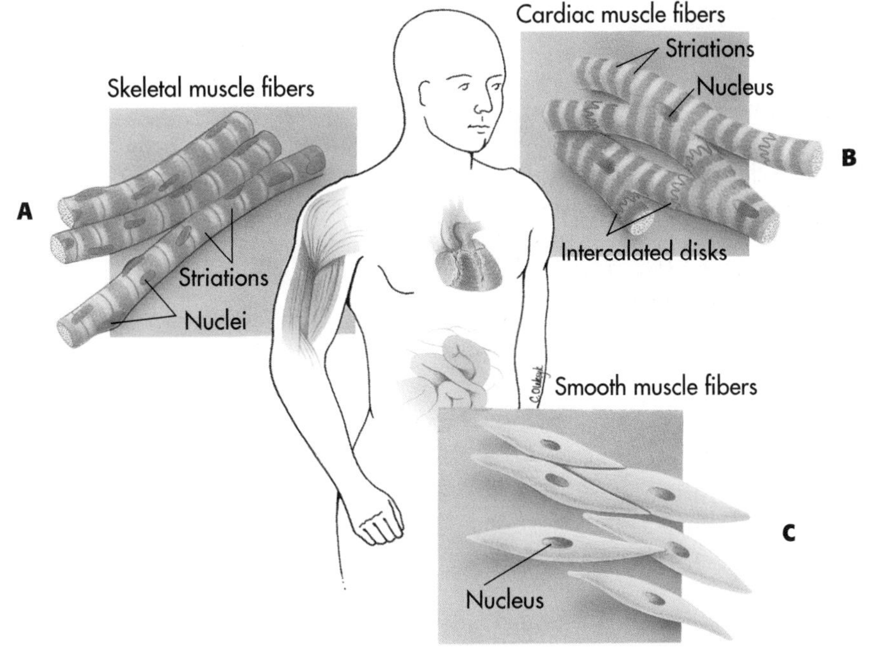

Figure 1-14
Muscle tissue. **A,** Skeletal muscle. **B,** Cardiac muscle. **C,** Smooth muscle. (From Thibodeau GA, Patton KT: *Anatomy and physiology,* ed 5, St Louis, 2003, Mosby.)

- ***Cardiac muscle fibers,*** which are found in the heart, are smaller, striated fibers. Their structure is not as organized as that of skeletal muscles.
- ***Smooth muscle fibers*** are neither striated nor voluntary. Found in the organs and viscera, they help regulate blood flow through the cardiovascular system, move substances such as food and waste through the intestines, and squeeze secretions from glands.

Muscle tissue is discussed in greater detail in Chapter 9.

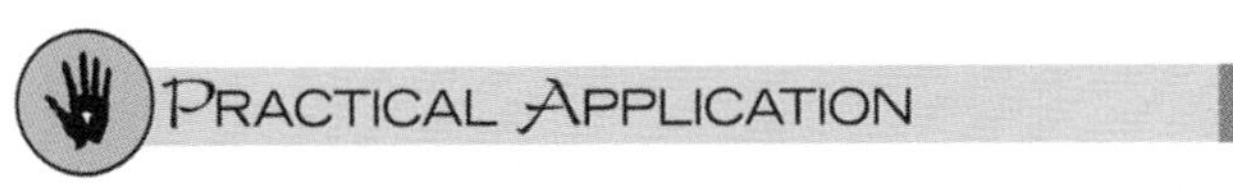

The major element of soft tissue is the muscle and its associated connective tissue. Muscle tissue provides the active aspect of movement. Soft tissue and movement approaches seek to maintain or restore effective movement patterns. ■

Nervous (Neural) Tissue

The functions of **nervous tissue** (Figure 1-15) are to coordinate and regulate body activity. Nervous tissue does this well because it has specialized to develop more excitability and conductivity than other types of tissue. Nerve cells are divided into two types: neurons, which are the actual functional units, and neuroglia, which connect and support the neurons. Nervous tissue is discussed in depth in Chapters 4 and 5.

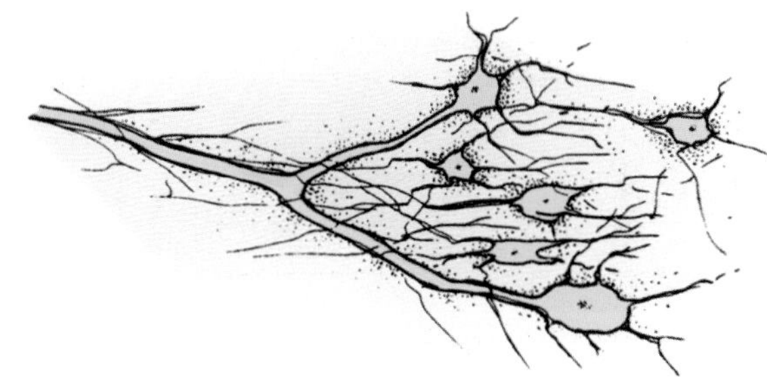

Figure 1-15
Nervous tissue. (From LaFleur Brooks M: *Exploring medical language: a student-directed approach,* ed 5, St Louis, 2002, Mosby.)

Organ Level

Organs are groups of two or more kinds of tissue that combine to perform a special function.

According to Asian healing theories, the function of the organs can be associated with energy patterns. Organs that are hollow and work intermittently are thought of as yang organs. Extensions of the yang organs make contact with the exterior of the body. Examples include the stomach, with the mouth opening to the exterior, and the bladder, which empties through the urethra. Organs that are solid and must work all the time to maintain homeostasis are yin organs. Instead of filling and emptying, they store the various essences of life extracted from the food and air. Examples include the heart and lungs. The relationships of the organs are presented in the five-element (phases) meridian theory, which is explained in Chapter 3.

System Level

Organs that combine to perform more complex body functions are referred to as systems. The number and types of organs found in a system depend on its functions. The 11 systems of the human body are the integumentary, skeletal, muscular, nervous, endocrine, cardiovascular, lymphatic and immune, respiratory, digestive, urinary, and reproductive systems.

Organism Level: The Body as a Whole

We are more than the sum of our parts. Each part of the body works with the other parts to support the whole. The mutually dependent nature of cells and the organization of complex systems allow us the endless possibilities of diversity that we experience. The cooperation, interdependence, and respect the body displays for itself could be a wise metaphor for the larger organism of the world in which we are the cells—a fundamental unit of life.

After the overview information has been developed in Chapters 1, 2, and 3, this text discusses each of the systems individually. Organizing the book in this manner allows the student to use other anatomy and physiology references developed on a systems approach to expand on the knowledge presented in this text.

SUMMARY

This chapter has laid the foundation for the study of anatomy and physiology. The relationship of structure, function, and homeostasis, in terms of Western and Asian thought, was presented. The biologic organization of life, from the parts of the atom to the systems of the body, was laid out sequentially, and each level comprising the components that build the next level of body organization. If a massage therapist is going to plan and organize competently an effective session to meet outcome goals for clients' massages, then the therapist must have knowledge of the structure and function of the human body. On this foundation we will continue to build levels of knowledge as our study of the human body progresses.

evolve

Log on to the Mosby's Essential Sciences for Therapeutic Massage, ed. 2, EVOLVE website at http://evolve.elsevier.com, and set up a password for your account, to be used whenever you log on to the site.

WORKBOOK SECTION

SHORT ANSWER

1. Explain the importance of understanding the relationship of anatomy (structure) and physiology (function) of the body as a whole.

____
____
____
____
____

2. Explain the relationship of yin and yang to anatomy and physiology.

____
____
____
____
____

3. List and define the 13 characteristics of life.

____
____
____
____
____
____
____
____
____
____
____
____
____

4. List and explain the seven levels of organization of the body.

____
____
____
____
____
____
____

FILL IN THE BLANK

(1) ______________ is the scientific study of the (2) ______________ of the body and the relationship of its parts. (3) ______________ is the scientific study of the processes and (4) ______________ of the body that support life.

(5) ______________ is the study of body structures large enough to be visible to the naked eye. (6) ______________ is the study of all of the structures of a particular area. (7) ______________ is the study of the body divided into its systems. (8) ______________ is the study of internal body structures as they can be recognized and related to the overlying skin surface.

An (9) ______________ is the smallest particle of an element that retains the properties of that element. (10) ______________ are the smallest parts of a substance that can exist independently without losing the physical and chemical properties of that substance.

(11) ______________ refers to the chemical reactions in the body. A chemical reaction that releases energy as it breaks down complex compounds into simpler ones is (12) ______________. (13) ______________ is a chemical reaction that uses energy as it joins simple molecules together to form more complex molecules. Anabolism requires energy supplied from the molecule adenosine triphosphate, or (14) ______________.

(15) ______________ are proteins that speed up chemical reactions but are not consumed or altered in the process. (16) The ______________ / ______________ of a solution is measured in terms of pH. (17) ______________ are the basic structures of the cells, and they perform specific functions within the cell. (18) ______________ is the movement of ions and molecules from an area of higher concentration to that of a lower concentration. Bringing substances into the cell by forming vesicles is (19) ______________, and

WORKBOOK SECTION

transporting of substances out of the cell is (20) _______________.

A (21) _______________ is the basic structural and functional unit of a living organism. (22) _______________ is the period when the cell grows and carries on most of its activities. (23) _______________ occurs when the cell divides, the process by which the cell (24) _______________ itself.

(25) _______________ is a special form of mitosis that halves the number of chromosomes in (26) _______________ cells. (27) _______________ is an increase in the size of a cell; (28) _______________ is a decrease in cell size.

A (29) _______________ is a group of similar cells that usually have a similar embryologic origin and that are specialized for a particular function. The tissue surface that faces the inside of the body is known as the (30) _______________ surface. (31) _______________ tissue covers and protects the surfaces of the body; lines body cavities; specializes in moving substances into and out of the blood during secretion, excretion, and absorption; and forms many glands. A (32) _______________ is a thin, sheetlike layer of tissue that covers a cell, an organ, or a structure; that lines tubes or cavities; or that divides and separates one part from another.

(33) _______________ tissue is specialized to support and hold together the body and its parts, to transport substances through the body, and to protect it from foreign substances. Within the (34) _______________ of connective tissue is a shapeless or amorphous ground substance containing molecules that expand when bound with electrolytes and water molecules. Of all the hundreds of different protein compounds in the body, (35) _______________ is the most abundant, accounting for more than one fourth of the protein in the body.

(36) _______________ fibers are strong fibers with minimal stretch capacity. They have a high degree of tensile strength, which allows them to withstand longitudinal stress. (37) _______________ fibers are delicate connective tissue fibers that occur in networks, which support small structures such as capillaries, nerve fibers, and the basement membrane.

(38) _______________ fibers are extensible and elastic. They are made from a protein called elastin, which returns to its original length after being stretched.

(39) _______________ tissue provides movement, maintains posture, and produces heat. (40) _______________ muscle fibers are made up of large, cross-striated cells connected to the skeleton and under voluntary control of the nervous system. (41) _______________ muscle fibers are small, striated, involuntary fibers that enable the heart to pump blood.

(42) _______________ muscle fibers are neither striated nor voluntary. They help regulate blood flow through the cardiovascular system, propel food through the gut, and squeeze secretions from glands.

WORKBOOK SECTION

PROBLEM SOLVING

Read the problem presented. There is no correct answer; rather, the exercise assists the student in developing the analytical and decision-making skills necessary in professional practice.

After reading the problem through, follow the six steps given below:

1. Identify the facts presented in the information.
2. Identify the possibilities presented ("what if" statements), or develop your own possibilities that relate to the facts.
3. Evaluate each possibility in terms of the logical cause and effect and pros and cons.
4. Consider the effect on the persons involved.
5. Write each answer in the space provided.
6. Develop your solution by answering the question posed.

PROBLEM

The study of anatomy, physiology, and the mechanisms of health and disease can be fascinating and frustrating. The student must absorb and understand a tremendous amount of information and remember many details. Textbooks do not always agree, and new research results change the information constantly. Students may find themselves lost in the magnitude of all the information and the implications of what can happen when they delve into this study. If this happens, a student may give up and study merely to pass a test instead of to learn and understand.

Frequently, the information does not seem relevant to the career choice or the broader topic the student is studying. As a result, the wonder, fascination, and importance of the information about the body often is replaced with the dread of learning new terms and understanding complex concepts. Unless a direct correlation is established between the acquisition and application of the information they are to learn, students may store data in their minds as interesting but irrelevant facts. When the time comes actually to use the information, it may not be available because it was never integrated as part of a whole process.

QUESTION

What can you do to avoid becoming overwhelmed and to remain excited as you learn about the body?

The first response is provided as a guide to get you started. Fill in at least two more statements.

FACTS

1. The student must learn a tremendous amount of information.
2. ______
3. ______

POSSIBILITIES

1. The student may not know what should be committed to memory.
2. ______
3. ______

LOGICAL CAUSE AND EFFECT

1. The student studies only to pass the test.
2. ______
3. ______

EFFECT

1. The student feels overwhelmed.
2. ______
3. ______

What can you do to avoid becoming overwhelmed and to remain excited as you learn about the body? ______

______

FURTHER STUDY

Using additional resource material (see Works Consulted list at the back of this book), identify the chapters that pertain to the information presented in this chapter. Locate the information presented in this text and then elaborate on it by writing a paragraph of additional information on each of the following:

Atom

______

______

______

______

______

Molecules

______

______

______

______

______

______

WORKBOOK SECTION

Chemical bonds

Metabolism

Adenosine triphosphate (ATP)

Organelles

Cell

Tissue types

Membrane types

WORKBOOK SECTION

Answer Key

SHORT ANSWER

1. Anatomy and physiology are two distinct yet interrelated biologic studies that combine to present the operation of the body as a whole organism. Structure (anatomy) and function (physiology) cannot be separated. Structure and function form a continuum; structure guides function, and function can modify structure. The concept of anatomy and physiology is an example of the duality of wholeness.
2. Yin and Yang represent opposite but complementary qualities; they form a whole unit. Yin corresponds to structure, or anatomy, and yang to function, or physiology. Yang contains the seed of yin and vice versa. Nothing is totally yin or totally yang; yang transforms into yin and yin into yang. The human body and its functions can be understood by following this concept of the relationship of opposites that creates wholeness.
3. (1) Maintenance of boundaries: Keeping the internal environment distinct from the external environment
   (2) Movement: The ability to transport the entire being, as well as internal components
   (3) Responsiveness: The ability to sense, monitor, and respond to changes in the external environment
   (4) Conductivity: The movement of energy from one point to another
   (5) Growth: A normal increase in the size or number (or both) of cells
   (6) Respiration: The absorption, transport, and use or exchange of respiratory gases (oxygen and carbon dioxide)
   (7) Digestion: The process by which food products are broken down into simple substances to be used by individual cells
   (8) Absorption: The transport and use of nutrients
   (9) Secretion: The production and delivery of specialized substances for diverse functions
   (10) Excretion: The removal of waste products
   (11) Circulation: The movement of fluids, nutrients, secretions, and waste products from one area of the body to another
   (12) Reproduction: The formation of a new being; also, the formation of new cells in the body to permit growth, repair, and replacement
   (13) Metabolism: A chemical reaction that occurs in cells to effect transformation, production, or consumption of energy
4. (1) Chemical level (atoms and molecules): The chemical properties of a substance have to do with the way it reacts with other substances or responds to a change in the environment. Molecules are the smallest part of a substance that can exist independently without losing the physical and chemical properties of the substance. Atoms combine to form molecules. The atoms most commonly found in living things are hydrogen, carbon, nitrogen, and oxygen. An atom can achieve a state of maximal stability by gaining or losing electrons to fill or empty its outer shell. Chemical reactions or chemical change results in the breakdown of substances and the formation of new ones.
   (2) Organelle level: Molecules combine in specific ways to form organelles, the basic structures found in cells. Organelles perform specific functions within the cell; the sum property of these structures allows each cell to live. More than two dozen organelles have been identified.
   (3) Cellular level: A cell is the basic structural and functional unit of a living organism. Cells are self-regulating, which allows them to adjust to change by attempting to remain constant and maintain homeostasis.
   (4) Tissue level: A tissue is a group of similar cells that usually have a similar embryologic origin and are specialized for a particular function.
   Epithelial tissue covers and protects the surfaces of the body; lines cavities; specializes in moving substances into and out of the blood during secretion, excretion, and absorption; and forms many glands.
   Connective tissue is specialized to support and hold together the body and its parts, to transport substances through the body, and to protect the body from foreign substances.
   Muscle tissue has the ability to effect movement by shortening through contraction. Muscle tissue enables the body to move, maintain posture, and produce heat.
   Nervous tissue is able to regulate and coordinate body activity quickly. Nervous tissue has developed more excitability and conductivity than other types of tissue.
   (5) Organ level: Organs are more complex than tissue. An organ is a group of two or more kinds of tissues arranged so that they can perform a special function.
   (6) System level: Organs that work together to perform more complex bodily functions are called systems. The 11 systems of the human body are the integumentary, skeletal, muscular, nervous, endocrine, cardiovascular, lymphatic and immune, respiratory, digestive, urinary, and reproductive systems.
   (7) Organism level: The body as a whole is an organism. Each part of the body works with the other parts to support the whole. The mutually dependent nature of the cells and the organization of complex systems allow us the endless possibilities of diversity that we experience.

WORKBOOK SECTION

FILL IN THE BLANK

1. Anatomy
2. structures
3. Physiology
4. functions
5. Gross anatomy
6. Regional anatomy
7. Systemic anatomy
8. Surface anatomy
9. atom
10. Molecules
11. Metabolism
12. catabolism
13. Anabolism
14. ATP
15. Enzymes
16. acidity/alkalinity
17. Organelles
18. Diffusion
19. endocytosis
20. exocytosis
21. cell
22. Interphase
23. Mitosis
24. reproduces
25. Meiosis
26. reproductive
27. Hypertrophy
28. atrophy
29. tissue
30. basal
31. Epithelial
32. membrane
33. Connective
34. matrix
35. collagen
36. Collagenous
37. Reticular
38. Elastic
39. Muscle
40. Skeletal
41. Cardiac
42. Smooth

CHAPTER 2

Mechanisms of Health and Disease

CHAPTER OBJECTIVES

After completing this chapter, the student will be able to perform the following:

- Define homeostasis, self-regulatory mechanisms, and body rhythms in relationship to bodywork modalities and Asian and Ayurvedic theories of health.
- Discuss and contrast the mechanisms of disease and health.
- Define disease terminology.
- List disturbances in homeostasis.
- Discuss risk factors in disease development.
- List the four primary signs of the inflammatory response.
- Define pain and list the types of pain.
- Discuss the pain-spasm-pain cycle in relationship to bodywork methods.
- Identify viscerally referred pain patterns.
- Define phantom pain.
- List the factors influencing health.
- Identify factors contributing to the stress response.
- List the stages in the cycle of life.

CHAPTER OUTLINE

KEY TERMS

Acute pain Pain that is usually temporary, of sudden onset, and easily localized. Acute pain can be a symptom of a disease process or a temporary aspect of medical treatment. Acting as a warning signal, acute pain activates the sympathetic nervous system.

Afferent (AF-er-ent) Toward a center or point of reference.

Anaplasia (an-ah-PLAY-zee-a) Meaning without shape, the term describes abnormal or undifferentiated cells that fail to mature into specialized cell types. Anaplasia is a characteristic of malignant cells.

Benign (be-NINE) Usually describing a noncancerous tumor that is contained and does not spread.

Biologic rhythms The internal, periodic timing component of an organism, also known as a biorhythm. Circadian rhythms work on a 24-hour period to coordinate internal functions such as sleep. Ultradian rhythms repeat themselves from every 90 minutes to every few hours, whereas seasonal rhythms are annual functions.

Cancer Malignant, nonencapsulated cells that invade surrounding tissue. They often break away, or metastasize, from the primary tumor and form secondary cancer masses.

Chronic pain Pain that continues or recurs over a prolonged time, usually for more than 6 months. The onset may be obscure, and the character and quality of the pain change over time. Chronic pain usually is poorly localized and not as intense as acute pain, although for some the pain is exhausting and depressing.

Dosha Physiologic function.

Efferent (EF-er-ent) Away from a center or point of reference.

Entrainment (en-TRAIN-ment) A coordination or synchronization to an internal or external rhythm, especially when a person responds to certain patterns by moving in a coordinated manner to those patterns.

Continued

Etiology (e-tee-OL-o-jee) The study of the factors involved in the development of disease, including the nature of the disease and the susceptibility of the person.

Fistula (fis-tu-la) A track that is open at both ends through which abnormal connections occur between two surfaces.

Health A condition of homeostasis resulting in a state of physical, emotional, social, and spiritual well-being.

Homeostasis (ho-me-o-STA-sis) The relatively constant state of the internal environment of the body that is maintained by adaptive responses. Specific control and feedback mechanisms are responsible for adjusting body systems to maintain this state.

Hyperplasia (hye-per-PLAY-zee-a) An uncontrolled increase in the number of cells of a body part.

Inflammation (in-flah-MAY-shun) A protective response of the tissues to irritation or injury that may be chronic or acute. The four primary signs are redness, heat, swelling, and pain.

Kapha dosha Physiologic function that blends the water and earth elements.

Neoplasm (NEE-o-plazm) The abnormal growth of new tissue. Also called a tumor, a neoplasm may be benign or malignant.

Opportunistic pathogens Organisms that cause disease only when the immunity is low in a host

Pain An unpleasant sensation. Pain is a complex, private experience with physiologic, psychologic, and social aspects. Because pain is subjective, it is often difficult to explain or describe.

Pathogenicity (path-O-jen-i-ci-TE) The ability of the infectious agent to cause disease.

Pathology (pah-THOL-o-jee) The study of disease as observed in the structure and function of the body.

Phantom pain A form of pain or other sensation experienced in the missing extremity after a limb amputation.

Pitta dosha Physiologic function that combines fire and water.

Sinus A tract leading from a cavity to the surface.

Somatic pain (so-MA-tik) Pain that arises from the body as opposed to the viscera. Superficial somatic pain comes from the stimulation of receptors in the skin, whereas deep somatic pain arises from stimulation of receptors in skeletal muscles, joints, tendons, and fasciae.

Stress Any external or internal stimulus that requires a change or response to prevent an imbalance in the internal environment of the body, mind, or emotions. Stress may be any activity that makes demands on mental and emotional resources. Some responses to stress may stimulate neurons of the hypothalamus to release corticotropin-releasing hormone.

Vata dosha Physiologic function formed from ether and air.

Virulent (vir-U-lent) A quality of organisms that readily cause disease.

Visceral pain (VIS-er-al) Pain that results from the stimulation of receptors or an abnormal condition in the viscera (internal organs).

Chapter 1 sets the stage as an overview and introduction to the study of the body in structure and function. This chapter provides a big picture view of how anatomy and physiology affect each of us in daily life. Once we show the importance of anatomy and physiology in relationship to how we function, the relevance of the more detailed study in future chapters becomes clear.

HOMEOSTASIS

Our body cells survive and thrive in a healthy condition only when the temperature, pressure, and chemical composition of their fluid environment remains relatively constant. The overall structure of our body does not change noticeably from moment to moment. When you go to bed at night, unless major trauma has occurred, your body looks pretty much the same as it did when you woke up. This consistency is due to the constant balancing activities of our physiology.

Homeostasis is the relatively constant state maintained by the physiology of the body. We have our own regulatory mechanisms that constantly adjust and adapt to keep the temperature and chemical composition in balance in the fluid environment contained inside our skin. When this balance is interrupted, homeostasis is altered, and the body is more susceptible to a disease process. Homeostasis is the delicate maintenance of the balance of yin and yang we saw in Chapter 1. No matter how complicated, the signs and symptoms in disease can be explained in terms of yin and yang (Box 2-1).

Most healing arts describe the balanced state of homeostasis in their own terminology. Besides the organ relationship of yin and yang, the Asian five-element theory is a metaphor of the life elements of fire, earth, metal, water, and wood. They are found in nature, and their characteristics are reflected in our bodies.

The ancient healing model of Ayurveda says that an individual is made up of five primary elements. The elements differ from the Asian model, but the whole picture of balance is similar. The Ayurvedic elements are ether (space), air, fire, water, and earth.

Certain elements can combine to create various physiologic *functions,* called **doshas.** The ***Vata dosha*** is formed from ether and air. Vata governs the *principles of movement*

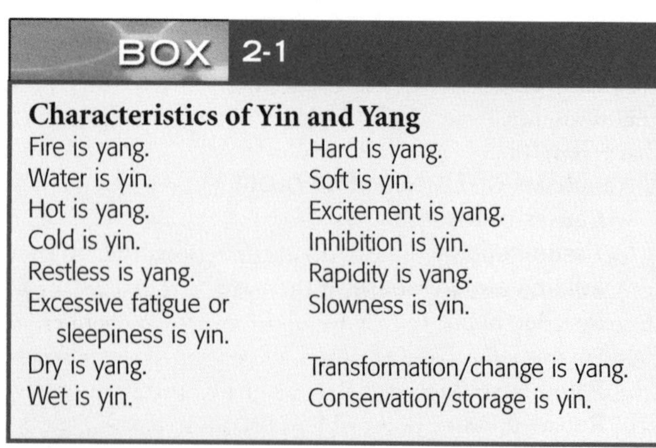

BOX 2-1

Characteristics of Yin and Yang

Fire is yang.	Hard is yang.
Water is yin.	Soft is yin.
Hot is yang.	Excitement is yang.
Cold is yin.	Inhibition is yin.
Restless is yang.	Rapidity is yang.
Excessive fatigue or sleepiness is yin.	Slowness is yin.
Dry is yang.	Transformation/change is yang.
Wet is yin.	Conservation/storage is yin.

Modified from Maciocia G: *The foundations of Chinese medicine,* New York, 1994, Churchill Livingstone.

and is seen in nerve impulses, circulation, respiration, and elimination.

The ***Pitta dosha*** is a combination of fire and water and represents the *process of transformation.* Metabolic transformation begins at a cellular level and moves up through all body functions. One example of Pitta is the transformation of food into usable nutrients.

The ***Kapha dosha*** blends the water and earth elements. These elements *hold our cells together* and build our muscles, fat, and bones. They also form some of the protective lining and fluids, such as the mucosal stomach lining and cerebrospinal fluid.

We are created with our own unique proportions of Vata, Pitta, and Kapha, which allows for the great diversity of human beings. The three doshas and the five elements must be balanced for us to maintain healthy bodies. Our character is an expression of the harmonious and smooth interaction between them. The same concept is the foundation of the body/mind relationship of **health** and disease that has developed in recent years in Western science.

Feedback Loop

Every system in our body contributes to maintaining homeostasis, but the nervous and endocrine systems are the most important. For the interaction and communication necessary for the self-regulation to succeed, a well-developed control system is necessary. This system is called a *feedback loop.* Nerve impulses or chemical messengers transmit the information needed to maintain homeostasis through these feedback loops.

One definition of **stress** states that stress is any stimulus, internal or external, that creates an imbalance in our internal environment. If we are exposed to such a stress, certain mechanisms attempt to counteract the responses to the stress and bring the conditions back into balance. Thus the body of a person exposed to stress could respond before any awareness of the stress occurs and bring itself back to a balanced state—homeostasis.

Each feedback loop is made up of the following:

1. A *sensor mechanism* that generates an impulse in response to an **afferent** electrical or chemical signal
2. An *integration/control center* that analyzes and integrates all signals received and, if needed, initiates a response (**efferent**)
3. An *effector mechanism* that actualizes the efferent response from the control center

The terms *afferent* and *efferent* are directional terms. They are used to describe movement of a signal from a sensor to an integrating or control center or, in reverse, movement of a signal from the control center to some type of effector mechanism. *Afferent* means that a signal is traveling toward a particular center or point of reference, and *efferent* means that a signal is traveling away from a particular center or point of reference.

Imagine that we put a person in a controlled situation in which we measured the activities that took place during a stress response. When a stress, the stimulus, disturbs homeostasis, receptors immediately send input to an integration center. These signals are interpreted, and corrective responses are sent to effectors.

Negative feedback refers to the feedback that reverses the original stimulus, stabilizes physiologic function, and helps us maintain our constant internal environment. Most systems are this type. For example, increasing and maintaining the tension in a muscle helps us later to relax the muscle. During massage, when applying muscle energy approaches, this is the feedback mechanism used by postisometric relaxation (a muscle energy technique that first contracts a muscle and then lengthens it) to help with lengthening and stretching the tissue.

Positive feedback enhances the original stimulus and thus maintains or accelerates a disturbed state of homeostasis. In doing so, positive feedback does not maintain a stable internal environment. The few forms of positive feedback that our bodies use serve a specific purpose, such as maintaining contractions during labor and delivery or more commonly continuing a cycle that may become harmful if it does not cease when the cycle no longer serves a purpose. An example of this is a muscle spasm causing **pain,** which results in increased spasm. The pain-spasm-pain cycle (pain creates protective spasm, which in turn increases pain) is a positive feedback loop (Figure 2-1).

One premise of Ayurveda is that our body is a projection of our consciousness. Other healing practices have similar underlying principles, including behavioral medicine and mind/body approaches. Self-correcting systems use feedback loops to influence their own expression. Our bodies can use this to coordinate our activities (negative feedback), allowing us to remain in a relatively constant state while being immersed in the waves of change (Activity 2-1).

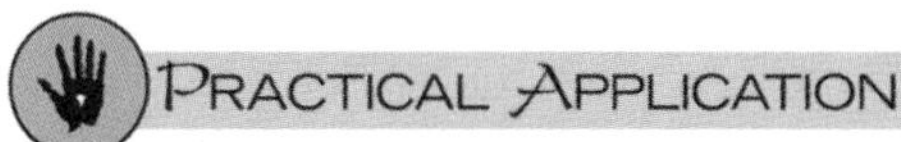

Therapeutic massage approaches can support or stimulate homeostatic processes. The stimuli from these methods are received by the receptors of the nervous or endocrine systems that send signals through afferent pathways for interpretation in the control centers of the central nervous system. Messages are returned by way of efferent pathways to the effector targets, where the response is to reestablish balanced function, such as relaxing or

ACTIVITY 2-1

Many mechanical systems in our homes, automobiles, and work environment have feedback mechanisms. Identify one and on a separate piece of paper, diagram the flow pattern, labeling the sensor mechanism, control center, and effector mechanism. Show afferent and efferent message pathways.

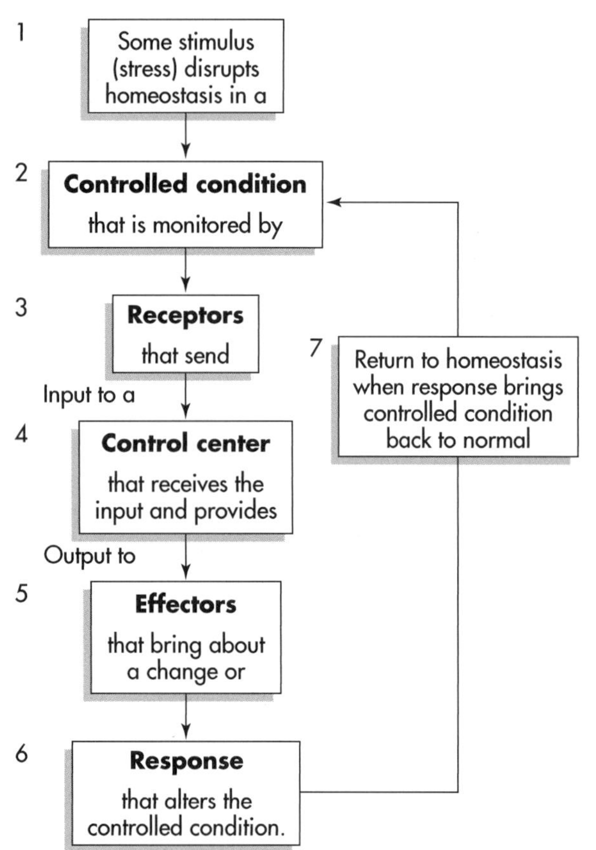

Figure 2-1
Components of a negative feedback system (loop).

tightening a muscle, softening or firming connective tissue, or reducing or increasing arousal responses of the autonomic nervous system, whichever restores homeostasis. Massage approaches are often nonspecific; the stimuli used usually disrupt the general existing homeostatic pattern, which requires a response through the feedback mechanism. The objective is to reestablish homeostasis the same way we push a reset button on a machine. ■

BODY RHYTHMS

Biologic rhythms are the internal, periodic timing components of an organism generated within the body. *Circadian rhythms* work on a 24-hour period to coordinate internal functions such as sleep. *Ultradian rhythms* repeat themselves every 90 minutes to every few hours, whereas *seasonal rhythms* are annual functions. Some forms of depressive disorders—as well as many sleep, neurologic, cardiovascular, and endocrine disorders—recently have been associated with biologic rhythm dysfunction. Many of the conveniences we use have put us out of sync with the natural rhythms of light, dark, the seasons, and the cycles of the moon (Activity 2-2).

ACTIVITY 2-2

Map your own body rhythms for a 24-hour period.
Write in any other rhythms you recognize.

Rhythm	Time
Waking	________
Elimination (bladder and bowel)	________
Food	________
Alert phase (mental and physical peak)	________
Fatigue phase (mental and physical low)	________
Elimination	________
Food	________
Alert phase	________
Fatigue phase	________
Elimination	________
Food	________
Alert phase	________
Fatigue phase	________
Elimination	________
Food	________
Alert phase	________
Fatigue phase	________
Elimination	________
Sleep	________

Our biologic rhythms are interconnected. The synchronization of the rhythms of our heart, respiration, and digestion promotes this balance, or homeostasis, to support a healthy body. A balance between sympathetic and parasympathetic portions of the autonomic nervous system influences the sinus nodes of the heart and vascular systems, which in turn modulate heart rate and blood pressure. Our nasal reflexes, stimulated by the movement of air through the nose, rhythmically interact with the heart, lung, and diaphragm (Timmons, 1994).

Our body rhythms are kept balanced through negative feedback loops. When a change occurs in our heart rate, blood pressure, and respiratory rate, efferent nerve receptors called baroreceptors respond to changes in pressure in these systems. The various mental or emotional stressors we encounter daily stimulate the sympathetic system (the part of the nervous system that responds by fight-or-flight reactions). The central nervous system integrates the

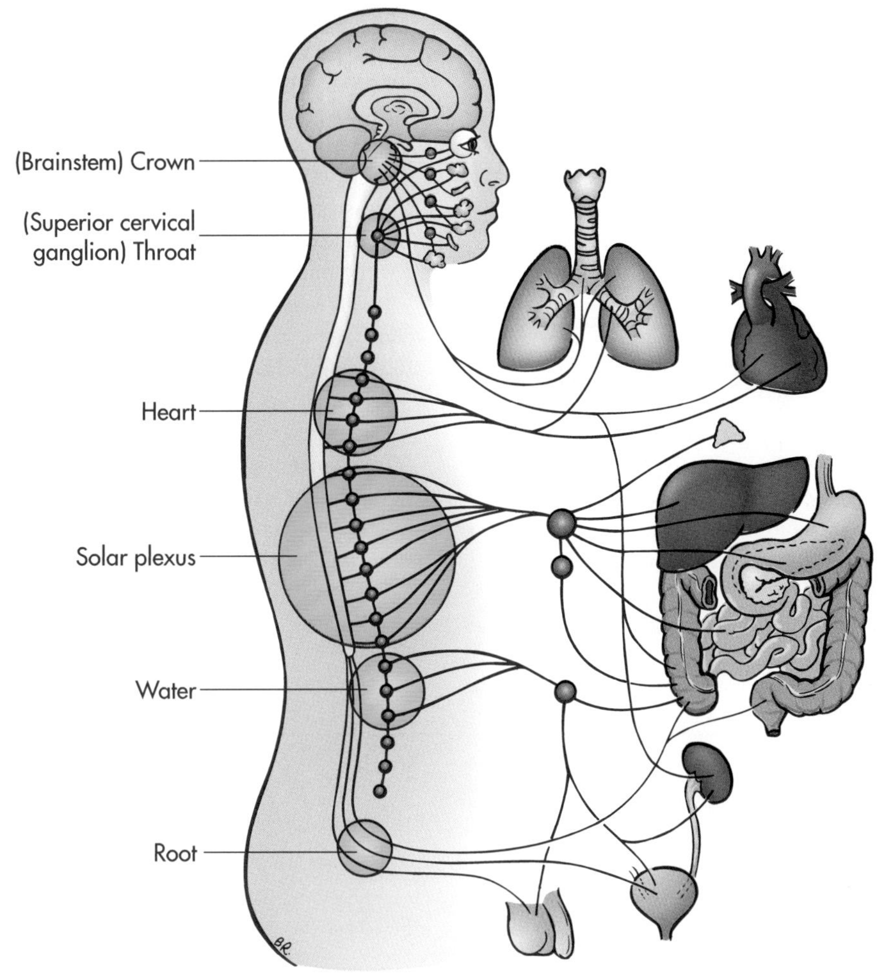

Figure 2-2
Comparison of the autonomic nervous system, traditional energy chakra centers, and biologic oscillators. (From Fritz S: *Mosby's fundamentals of therapeutic massage,* ed 3, St Louis, 2004, Mosby.)

information, slows down our brain waves, and decreases the release of cortisol (a steroid hormone of the sympathetic system), thus increasing parasympathetic (relaxation and restoration) activity. Balance is maintained in this manner.

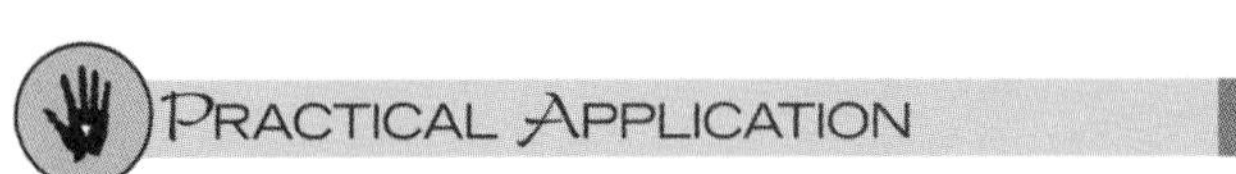

Practical Application

When a person experiences positive emotional states, the tendency is for the biologic rhythms naturally to begin to oscillate together, which is called entrainment. Research on entrainment dates back to 1665 when Dutch scientist Christian Huygens noticed that clock pendulums were synchronized. **Entrainment** is the physical phenomenon of resonance tendency for oscillating bodies to move in a synchronized, harmonic manner. We also can enhance entrainment processes with techniques that shift our consciousness to our breathing patterns and heart rate. Many disciplines quiet the mind and body during meditation. Examples include yoga focusing attention on the breath, whereas Qigong focuses on the point below the navel. These systems center attention on body areas that have known biologic oscillators. The location of the chakra system correlates with biologic oscillators (Figure 2-2). ■

Biologic rhythms can be affected by the rhythm of music or other repetitive sound action or visual movement pattern. Chaotic or abrupt noise can be a disruptive factor, whereas surf or other similar nature sounds usually have a calming effect. Studies have shown that the rhythmic physiologic patterns of a dog's or cat's breathing or heart rate can benefit elderly persons. The rhythmic patterns of drumming, clapping, singing, chanting, and movement in our religious and social rituals interact with biologic patterns, resulting in a calming or exciting organization or disruption of body rhythms.

The rhythmic and ordered approach used in massage and bodywork methods would seem to have effects similar to those just mentioned, especially when provided by a calm and focused practitioner (the same effect as found in dog and cat studies). The length of application seems to be important as well. A session that lasts between 45 and 90 minutes falls within the ultradian rhythm pattern, thus working within the natural balance of the body.

We may not understand the magnitude of influences that affect our body rhythms for many years. Current research is being done regarding the possibility of disease processes resulting from disruption in body rhythms, as well as the effects of work environments that directly disturb or alter natural body rhythms (Activity 2-3).

MECHANISMS OF DISEASE: PATHOLOGY

Massage, other forms of soft tissue bodywork, exercise, and movement therapies focus on maintaining health or a balanced state of physical, emotional, social, and spiritual well-being—homeostasis. Health results from the effective adaptation of the organism to change. Disease occurs when the demand to adapt exceeds the ability of the body and imbalance results. Massage therapies support the body in maintaining or returning it to a healthy state—homeostasis. To accomplish both, massage and bodywork professionals require a knowledge base and understanding of the normal function of the body and the abnormal body functions of disease states:

Disease can be described as an abnormality in functions of the body, especially when the abnormality threatens well-being.

Pathology is the study of disease.

Congenital disease is something present at birth, not something accrued in life, whereas *inherited* disease is acquired naturally, not as a result of circumstance.

Epidemiology is the field of science that studies the frequency, transmission, occurrence, and distribution of disease in human beings.

Pharmacology deals with the preparation and action of medications and their use to treat or prevent a disease.

ACTIVITY 2-3

The following exercise demonstrates the entrainment process as part of your understanding of your own body rhythm.

First, take your pulse to measure heart rate.

Next, measure your respiration rate by counting the number of breaths taken in a 60-second period.

Now play some music and listen to it for about 5 minutes.

Retake your pulse and recount your respiration rate.

Notice if any change occurs.

Repeat the exercise two more times with different types and tempos of music.

Preassessment

Pulse rate ________________

Respiration rate ________________

Music

Type ________________

Beats per minute ________________

Postassessment

Pulse rate ________________

Respiration rate ________________

Describe the change ________________

____

____

____

____

Music

Type ________________

Beats per minute ________________

Postassessment

Pulse rate ________________

Respiration rate ________________

Describe the change ________________

____

____

____

Music

Type ________________

Beats per minute ________________

Postassessment

Pulse rate ________________

Respiration rate ________________

Describe the change ________________

____

____

____

Signs are objective changes that can be seen or measured by someone other than the client.

Symptoms are the subjective changes noticed or felt only by the client.

A *syndrome* is a group of signs and symptoms that identify a pathologic condition, especially when they have a common cause.

Acute disease has a specific beginning, signs, and symptoms that develop quickly, last a short time, and then disappear.

Chronic disease has a vague onset, develops slowly, and lasts for a long time, sometimes for life.

Subacute refers to diseases with characteristics between acute and chronic.

Communicable diseases can be transmitted from one person to another.

Etiology is the study of all the factors involved in causing a disease.

Idiopathic describes diseases with undetermined causes.

Prognosis is the expected outcome of a disease.

Pathogenesis follows the development of a disease. For example, flu begins with a latent or nonactive stage, during which the virus becomes established. When a disease is infectious, this stage is called the *incubation* stage. After the disease develops and has run its course, body functions return to normal during the *convalescence* stage.

Structural lesion is an altered organic structure such as macules, vesicles, blebs or bullae, chancres, pustules, papules, tubercles, wheals, and tumors.

Biochemical lesion is a lesion caused by any biochemical compound such as an antigen, antibody, abnormal enzyme, or hormone that is altered sufficiently in a disease to serve as an aid in diagnosing or in predicting susceptibility to the disease.

Remission is a reversal of signs and symptoms that occurs in chronic diseases. This can be a temporary or permanent condition.

Diagnosis occurs when a licensed medical professional categorizes disease by identifying its signs and symptoms.

As stated previously, homeostasis is the relatively constant state of the internal environment of the body. If a disease process disturbs homeostasis, a variety of feedback mechanisms usually attempt to return the body to health. A disease condition exists when homeostasis cannot be easily restored. In acute conditions the body recovers its homeostatic balance quickly. In chronic diseases a normal state of balance may never be restored (Thibodeau, 2002).

Causes of Disease

Disease results from the action of various injurious agents on cells and tissues, causing biochemical or structural damage (lesion). Disease may be caused by impaired energy production, that is, reduced nutrition or reduced availability of oxygen to tissues.

According to Thibodeau and Patton (2002), disturbances in homeostasis may occur from many different sources:

1. *Genetic mechanisms:* Altered or mutated genes can cause abnormality. Predisposition is the tendency toward disease development. Genetic disease is caused directly by genetic abnormality.
2. *Physical and chemical agents:* Toxic or destructive chemicals, extreme heat or cold, mechanical injury, radiation, and metabolic agents such as alcohol, cigarettes, and drugs can affect the normal homeostasis of the body.
3. *Malnutrition:* Insufficient or imbalanced intake of nutrients can cause a variety of diseases.
4. *Degeneration:* Tissues sometimes break apart or degenerate. The cause is unknown. Degeneration is a normal consequence of aging. Degeneration of tissues also can result from disease.
5. *Hypersensitivity of the immune system:* Some diseases result from the immune system attacking the body (autoimmunity) and from mistakes or overreactions of the immune response. Allergy is the hypersensitivity of the immune system to relatively harmless environmental antigens. Steroids often are used to treat autoimmune disease.
6. *Immune suppression or immune deficiency:* Some diseases are caused by the failure of the immune system to defend against pathogens. The chief characteristic of immune deficiency is the development of unusual or recurring severe infections or **cancer.**
7. *Pathogenic organisms and infectious agents:* An organism that lives in or on another organism to obtain nutrients from it is called a parasite. The ability of infectious agents to cause disease is called **pathogenicity.** Organisms that easily cause disease are **virulent,** and organisms that cause disease only when the immunity is low are **opportunistic pathogens.** The presence of microscopic or larger parasites may interfere with normal body functions of the host and cause disease. Pathogenic organisms include the following:

   Viruses: Microscopic, intracellular parasites that consist of a nucleic acid core with a protein coat. Viruses invade a host cell and take over the cell function to produce more viruses.

   Bacteria, rickettsiae, and chlamydiae: Tiny cells without nuclei that secrete toxins, eat body cells, or form colonies.

   Fungi: Simple, plantlike organisms that lack chlorophyll. Fungi are generally molds or yeast.

   Protozoa: Large, one-celled organisms having organized nuclei such as amebae.

   Pathogenic animals: Large multicellular organisms such as roundworms, flatworms, flukes, mites, and lice.

   Medications and herbs used to treat pathogenic organisms are classified by type:

   Bacteria: Antibiotics
   Viruses: Antivirals and vaccines
   Fungi: Antifungals

Worms: Anthelmintics
Lice: Pediculicides
Scabies: Scabicides

8. *Tumors and cancer:* Abnormal tissue growths from uncontrolled cell division called **hyperplasia** results in a **neoplasm** or tumor. Tumors can cause a variety of physiologic disruptions. The tumor is named from the tissue type—lipoma, for example—which is a **benign** tumor of adipose (fat) tissue. Osteosarcoma is cancer of the bone.

   The benign tumor is contained and encapsulated. Benign tumors are relatively harmless, remain localized within the tissue from which they arose, and usually grow slowly. Interference with function is caused by crowding or blocking of functional tissue or pressing on pain-sensitive structures.

   A malignant tumor (cancer) is a nonencapsulated mass that invades surrounding tissue rather than pushing it aside. In addition, malignant cells have the devastating ability to break away from the primary tumor and form secondary cancer masses. This ability of cells to break away is called metastasis. Malignant or cancerous tumors tend to spread to other regions of the body. The cells most commonly migrate by way of the lymphatic system or blood vessels. Cancer cells that do not metastasize can spread another way by growing rapidly and extending the tumor into nearby tissues. Malignant tumors can replace part of a vital organ with abnormal tissues, a life-threatening situation (Figure 2-3).

   Generally speaking, cells that divide many times display increased mutation rates. Cells in the lymphatic system, epidermis, bone marrow, and gastrointestinal tract are more prone to develop cancer than cells of organs that do not divide rapidly, such as nerve and muscle tissue.

   The mechanism of all cancers is a mistake or problem in cell division called **anaplasia,** which is the reproduction of abnormal and undifferentiated cells that fail to mature into specialized cell types. The result is tissue not related to the needs of the body nor contributing to the body. Mature specialized cell types display boundary recognition, and therefore they do not invade surrounding tissue. Abnormal undifferentiated cancer cells lack the ability to recognize boundaries and therefore invade and destroy surrounding tissue.

   Certainly a life metaphor is reflected in mature versus undifferentiated cell behavior. Even at the cellular level, growing up and following a life purpose is important, living in a way that respects the boundaries of others. When we do not know who we are, we have no purpose in life and act in an immature manner that invades others' boundaries; we function like a cancer in their lives.

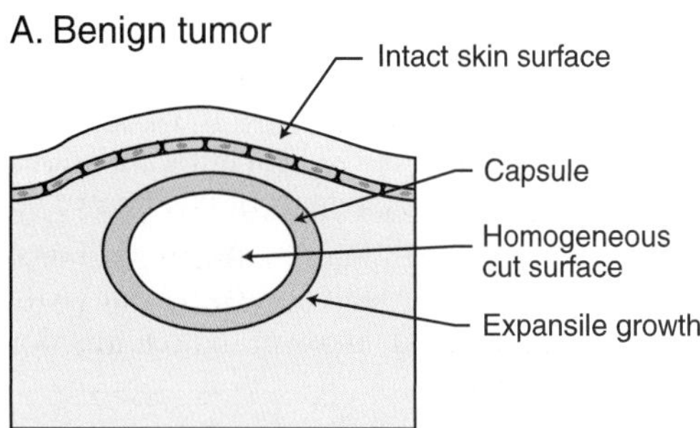

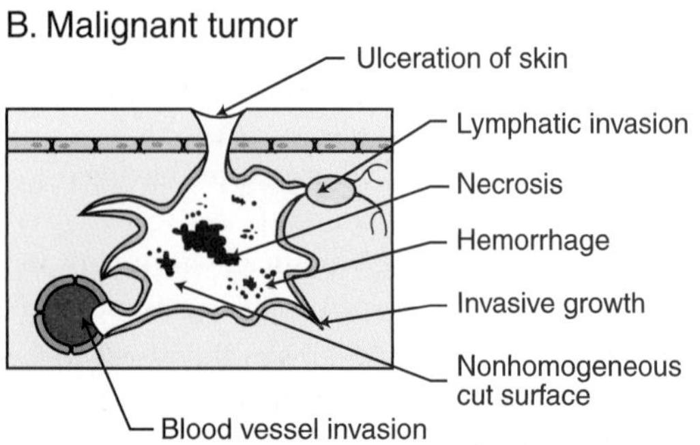

Figure 2-3
Gross appearance of benign (**A**) and malignant (**B**) tumors.

At present, the following factors are known to play a role in the development of cancer:

1. *Genetic factors:* More than a dozen forms of cancer are known to be inherited. Cancers with known genetic risk factors include basal cell carcinoma (a type of skin cancer), breast cancer, and neuroblastoma (a cancer of nerve tissue).
2. *Carcinogens:* Carcinogens are chemicals that affect genetic activity in some way, causing abnormal cell reproduction. Many industrial products are carcinogens. A variety of natural vegetable and animal materials are also carcinogenic.
3. *Age:* Certain cancers are found primarily in young people (e.g., leukemia) and others primarily in older adults (e.g., colon cancer). The age factor may result from changes in the genetic activity of cells over time or from accumulated effects of cell damage.
4. *Environment:* Exposure to damaging types of radiation, chronic mechanical injury, or virus and chronic irritants can cause cancer. For example, sunlight can cause skin cancer, and breathing asbestos fibers can cause lung cancer (Thibodeau, 2002).

Cancer specialists, or oncologists, have summarized some major signs of early stages of cancer. Early detection of cancer is important because the stages of development of primary tumors, before metastasis and the development of secondary tumors have begun, are when cancer is most treatable. Several warning signs of cancer are listed in Box 2-2.

Chemotherapy medications used to treat cancer are called antineoplastics. Most of the drugs in this category prevent the growth of rapidly dividing cells. One of the side effects is that they affect epithelial cells, which also rapidly divide, and as a result, antineoplastic drugs interfere with the function of the epithelial tissues and

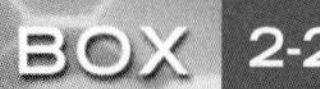 2-2

Warning Signs of Cancer
Sores that do not heal
Unusual bleeding
A change in a wart or mole
A lump or thickening in any tissue
Persistent hoarseness or cough
Chronic indigestion
A change in bowel or bladder function

From Thibodeau GA, Patton KT: *The human body in health and disease,* ed 3, St Louis, 2002, Mosby.

tissue repair. Surgery, radiation, and medication usually are used in a cancer treatment program.

9. *Inflammatory response:* The body often responds to homeostatic disturbances with the inflammatory response. **Inflammation** may occur as a response to any tissue injury. The inflammatory response is a normal mechanism that usually speeds recovery from an infection or injury. Disease symptoms can occur when the inflammatory response activates at inappropriate times or is abnormally prolonged or severe, resulting in damage to normal tissues.

   The inflammatory response is a combination of processes that attempt to minimize injury to tissues, thus maintaining homeostasis. Inflammation also may accompany specific immune system reactions. Inflammation occurs only in living tissues. Necrotic or dead tissue cannot mount an inflammatory response. For example, a gangrenous foot cannot become inflamed. Because the body cannot combat infection in necrotic tissue, a foot that is affected by gangrene must be amputated.

   The inflammatory response has four primary signs (Figure 2-4):

   Heat and redness: As tissue cells are damaged, they release inflammation chemicals such as histamine, prostaglandins, and compounds called kinins. Some inflammation mediators (histamine and bradykinin) cause blood vessels to dilate, increasing blood volume in the tissue. Increased blood volume produces the heat and redness of inflammation. This response is important because it allows immune system cells (white blood cells: neutrophils, monocytes, and macrophages) in the blood to travel quickly and easily to the site of injury. These cells attach themselves to the pathogens to be destroyed, especially if tagged with antibodies (proteins that mark pathogens).

   Swelling and pain: Some inflammation mediators increase the permeability of blood vessel walls. As water leaks out of the vessel, tissue swelling or edema results. The pressure caused by edema triggers pain receptors. The fluid that accumulates in inflamed tissue is called inflammatory exudate and has the beneficial effect of diluting the irritant. Inflammatory exudate is removed slowly by lymphatic vessels. Bacteria and damaged cells are held in the lymph nodes and destroyed by white blood cells. This causes the lymph nodes to enlarge when they process a large amount of infectious material.

Exudates vary in their composition of proteins, fluid, and cell contents, and types of cells. If the skin is slightly burned, a blister forms that is filled with clear exudate, indicating a low-protein content. These are known as serous exudates. Sometimes, inflammation results in fibrous exudates that are thick and sticky because of a meshwork of proteins present in the exudates. This type of inflammation can increase adhesion and scar tissue in the area. Yellow-white fluid in an infected inflamed area is called pus or purulent exudate. Purulent exudates may collect in different ways, such as a capsule surrounding the injury to form an abscess. If the immunity is low, the purulent exudates may spread over a large surface of tissue. If the fluid that collects is blood-tinged, the blood vessels are injured or the tissue is crushed, resulting in hemorrhagic exudates.

Inflammatory Process

Inflammation is a complex process that involves (1) changes in blood circulation, (2) changes in vessel wall permeability, (3) a white blood cell response, and (4) the release of inflammatory mediators.

Circulatory Change

Changes in blood flow represent the first response of the body to injury.

The relaxation of smooth muscle cells allows arterial blood to move into capillaries, creating redness, swelling, and warmth of the tissue. The first response of arterioles to an injurious stimulus is vasoconstriction, which lasts only a few seconds and is followed by vasodilation, which results in flooding of the capillary network with arterial blood. The influx of blood dilates the capillaries, which cannot regulate blood flow actively. From the capillaries the pressure is transmitted to venules, small veins. Increased pressure in the capillaries and venules forces plasma filtration through the vessel wall, leading to edema.

The blood flow in dilated capillaries and venules is slow, which leads to congestion. The white blood cells become sticky, adhering to the lining of the capillaries and venules. This adhesion is accomplished by surface adhesion molecules, which are normally present on leukocytes and vascular cells and which are activated by soluble mediators of inflammation, the best known of which are interleukins. Small amounts of interleukin are normally present in the blood. The concentration of interleukins is increased, however, at the site of inflammation. These mediators are derived in part from platelets and from leukocytes. The adhesion of white blood cells is one of the most common triggers for the release of mediators of inflammation.

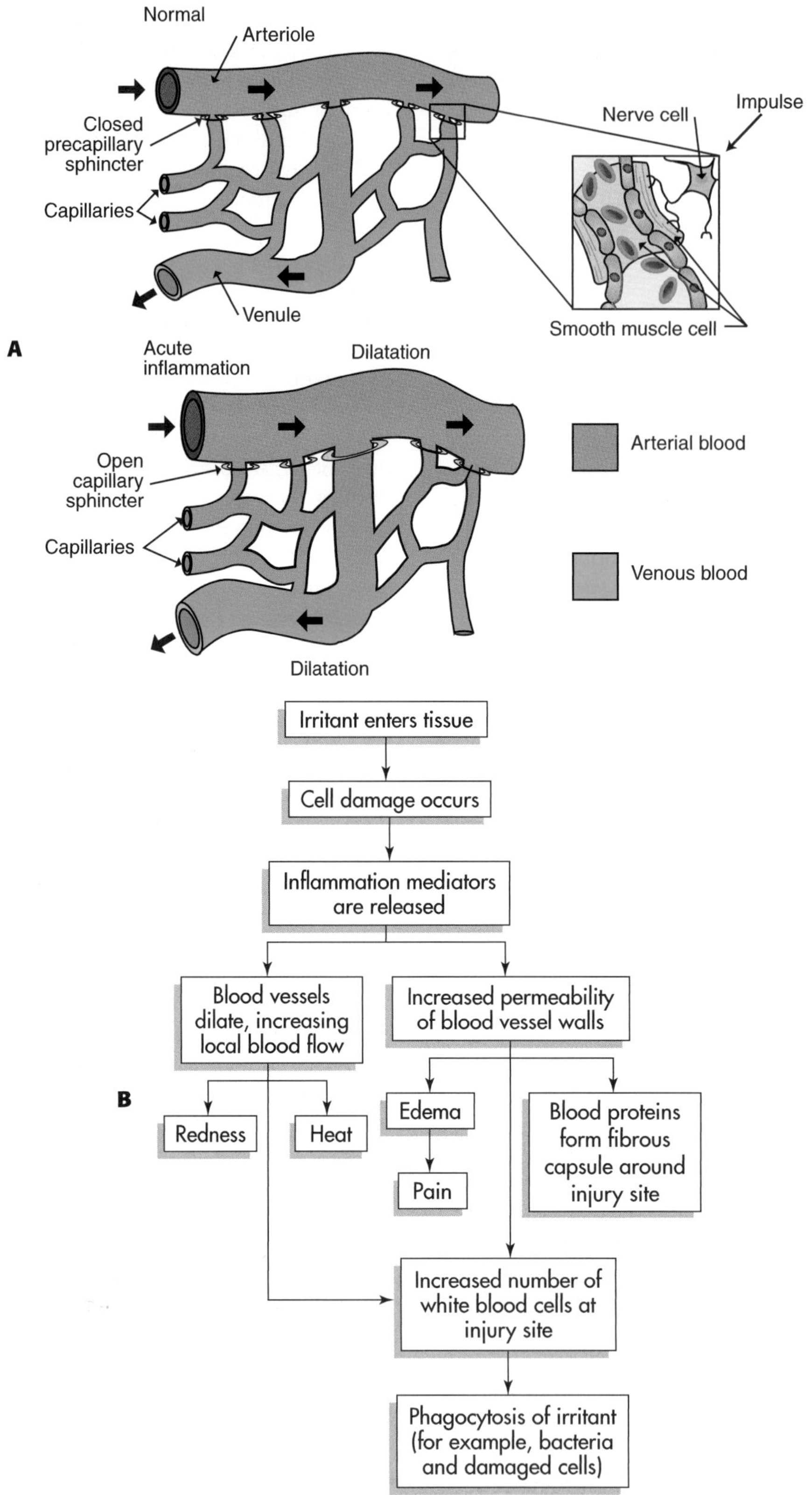

Figure 2-4
A, Circulatory changes in inflammation. Relaxation of the precapillary sphincter in the arterioles results in flooding of the capillary network and dilation of capillaries and postcapillary venules. **B,** Inflammatory response. (**A** modified from Damjanov I: *Pathology for the health-related professions*, ed 2, Philadelphia, 2000, Saunders.)

Vessel Wall Changes

The permeability of the capillaries and postcapillary venules of the vessel wall changes in response to inflammation because of (1) increased pressure inside the congested blood vessels; (2) slowing of the circulation, which reduces the supply of oxygen and nutrients to cells; (3) adhesion of white blood cells and platelets to vessel walls; and (4) the release of inflammatory mediators.

Inflammatory Mediators

The most important and common inflammatory mediators are histamines (increasing blood vessel permeability), bradykinin (which among other functions elicits pain), and arachidonic acid derivatives such as prostaglandins. They have numerous effects on blood vessels, inflammatory cells, and other cells in the body. The most important effects are vasodilation or vasoconstriction, altered vascular permeability, activation of inflammatory cells, chemotaxis, cytotoxicity, degradation of tissue, pain, and fever.

Arachidonic acid derivatives are involved in all stages of inflammation and are generated in large amounts from various sources. The process of prostaglandin synthesis can be blocked by aspirin, which is a potent inhibitor of cyclooxygenase. The antiinflammatory effects of corticosteroid hormones are particularly caused by the inhibition of arachidonic acid formation. (More information on the inflammatory response is present in Chapter 11.)

Tissue Repair

The processes of inflammation eventually eliminate the irritant, and tissue repair can begin. Tissues have two cell types: *parenchymal cells* perform the tissue functions and *stromal cells* provide the tissue structure. Tissue repair is the replacement of dead cells with living cells. In a type of tissue repair called regeneration (parenchymal cells), the new cells are similar to those that they replace. Another type of tissue repair is replacement (stromal cells). The new cells are formed from connective tissue. These stromal cells are different from those they replace, resulting in a scar. Collagen is the chief constituent of scar tissue. Factors that promote collagen formation and health are vitamin C and adequate nutrition, in particular protein intake. Often, fibrous connective tissue replaces the damaged tissue, resulting in a condition called fibrosis. Most tissue repairs are a combination of regeneration and replacement.

Cells regenerate to different degrees and at different rates. *Labile cells* regenerate easily and quickly, such as cells of the lymphatic system, epidermis, bone marrow, and gastrointestinal tract. *Stable cells,* the most common cell type, regenerate at slower rates, such as cells of the parenchymal or epithelial portion of an organ or gland and the connective tissue or stroma. For example, intestinal cells regenerate in 1 to 2 days, liver cells in 3 to 5 days, and kidney cells in 7 to 14 days.

Total tissue repair can take 4 weeks or longer. *Permanent cells,* such as nerve and muscle cells, do not regenerate well if at all, and when they do, the process is slow, taking months. Bone regenerates extremely well. Massage practitioners should wait at least 30 to 45 days before working deeply on an area of tissue repair so as not to disturb the repair formation.

A goal in the healing process is to promote regeneration and keep replacement to a minimum (Figure 2-5).

Inflammatory Disease

Local inflammation occurs in a small area. If the irritant spreads throughout the body or causes changes in other areas, the inflammation is called systemic. When inflammation becomes chronic and stays active for a longer period than benefits the body or is more intense than seems necessary, it may be called an inflammatory disease. Such systemic inflammations that may become diseases include arthritis, asthma, eczema, and bronchitis.

Chronic Inflammation

Chronic inflammation persists from 6 weeks to years. Medically, inflammation is considered chronic if the area is infiltrated by lymphocytes and macrophages, if growth of new capillaries occurs, and if fibroblasts are in the area. Chronic inflammation is implicated in many disease processes from arthritis to autoimmune disease. Chronic inflammation may develop fibrosis, or an ulcer, **sinus,** or **fistula.**

The fibroblasts produce collagen and fibrous tissue, causing fibrosis resulting in scar tissue and adhesion formation.

Chronic inflammation may lead to ulcer formation when the surface covering of an organ or tissue is lost because of cell deaths and is replaced by inflammatory tissue. The most common locations of ulcers are the gut and skin.

Chronic inflammation may produce a sinus or fistula. A *sinus* is a tract leading from a cavity to the surface. A *fistula* is a tract that is open at both ends through which abnormal connection occurs between two surfaces. For example, fistulae may form between the bladder and the vagina.

Treatments

Antiinflammatory and steroid medications are used to treat inflammation. Antihistamines and aspirin can be used to suppress inflammatory responses.

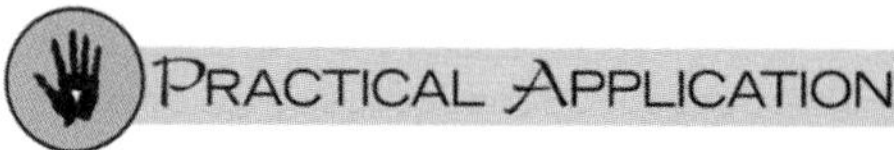

Some soft tissue methods can be used deliberately to create mild and controlled inflammation. Methods such as transverse friction create a localized inflammatory response to stimulate tissue reorganization in areas of adhesion and scarring. Acupuncture and moxibustion cause mild inflammation. Certain connective tissue methods and stretching methods can pull apart microadhesions in the soft tissue, resulting in inflammation that signals the tissue repair process. ■

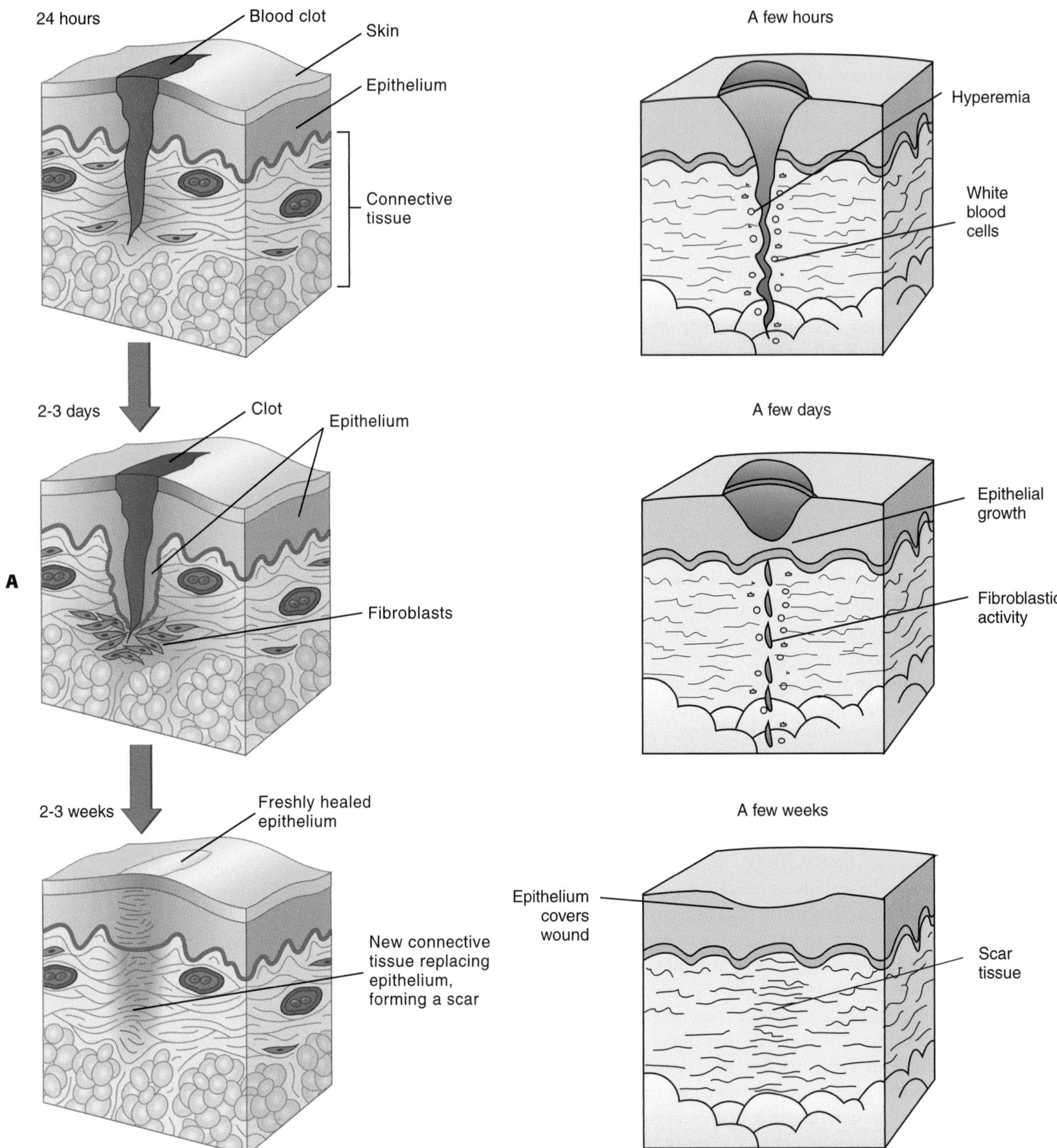

Figure 2-5
Wound healing. Healing of skin wounds reflects mechanisms of healing in general. **A** & **B** illustrate healing of superficial wounds by primary intention and deeper wounds by second intention. Wound healing is accelerated by bringing the edges of the wound together, through the use of bandaging and sutures. If this were a muscle injury (strain), muscle spasming around the site of the injury brings the ends closer together to encourage healing. (**A** modified from Thibodeau GA, Patton KT: *Anatomy and physiology,* ed 5, St Louis, 2003, Mosby.)

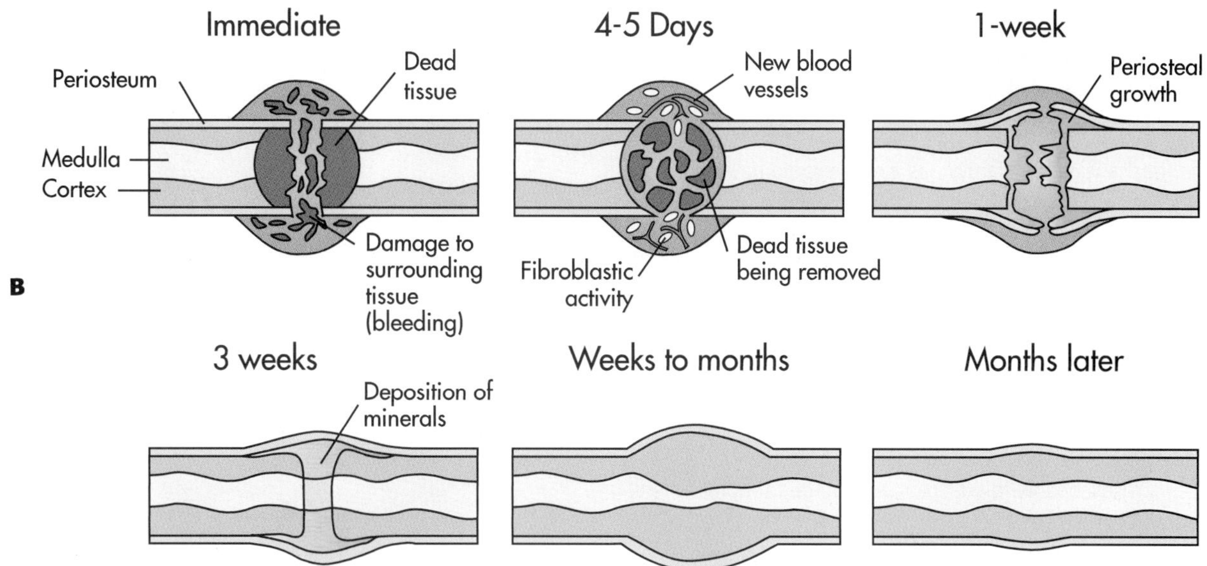

Figure 2-5, cont'd.
Wound healing. Healing of skin wounds reflects mechanisms of healing in general. The basic mechanisms involved in healing of bone fractures (**B**) are similar to skin or other tissue healing. Adequate blood supply, nutrition, and rest are necessary for appropriate healing. Deficiency of protein, essential fatty acids, vitamin C, and zinc delay healing. The acute inflammatory process also supports healing; therefore, the use of antinflammatory medicine in the first week after the injury can slow down the healing process.

The controlled use of therapeutic inflammation also is used to stabilize lax ligaments caused by overstretching, degeneration, or injury. Injection with a solution that creates inflammation signals the tissue repair process to lay down additional connective tissue fibers, reinforcing the ligament. Transverse friction massage can be used as well in areas that are accessed easily from the surface of the body. Sometimes creating controlled inflammation over an area of chronic soft tissue inflammation can jump-start the body into a resolution process and support healing. The controlled use of inflammation can stimulate healing and, coupled with appropriate rehabilitation, is an effective approach in dealing with these situations.

The key in these methods is to use just enough therapeutic inflammation to encourage the body to restore homeostasis and avoid overstressing the system. These methods should not be used on someone with systemic inflammation, such as systemic lupus erythematosus, or when tissue repair mechanisms are compromised, such as in fibromyalgia. Proper training in these methods must include a clear understanding of anatomy to provide specificity, exact application of technique to obtain the desired results, and an understanding of the physiology of the inflammation and healing processes.

Risk Factors

Certain predisposing conditions may make a disease more likely to develop. Usually called risk factors, these conditions may put one at risk for a disease but often do not actually cause a disease.

Some major types of risk factors follow (Thibodeau, 2002) (Activity 2-4):

1. *Genetic factors:* Several types of genetic risk factors exist. An inherited trait can put a person at a greater than normal risk, or predisposition, for a specific disease. Family history of a disease process and causes of death usually can reveal possible familial genetic traits. Steps can be taken to support the body against the genetic tendency toward a disease process (e.g., changes in diet and lifestyle).
2. *Age:* Biologic and behavioral factors increase the risk for certain diseases to develop at certain times in life. For example, musculoskeletal problems are common between ages 30 and 50.
3. *Lifestyle:* The way we live and work can put us at risk for some diseases. Some researchers believe that the high-fat, low-fiber diet common among persons in the developed nations increases their risk of certain types of cancer. Smoking, excessive use of alcohol, lack of exercise, and poor sleep habits are examples of negative lifestyles.
4. *Stress:* Stress may be defined as any substantial change in your routine or any activity that causes the body to adapt. Stress makes demands on mental and emotional resources. Research has shown that as stresses accumulate, an individual becomes increasingly susceptible to physical, mental, and emotional problems and accidental injuries.
5. *Environment:* Some environmental situations put us at greater risk for getting certain diseases. For example, living in high concentrations of air pollution may

ACTIVITY 2-4

Using the aforementioned factors disrupting homeostasis and risk factors, do a personal health assessment.

Example

Genetic mechanisms: My family has a tendency to have strokes, heart attacks, and joint problems.
Physical and chemical agents: I grew up in an environment with heavy secondary cigarette smoke.
Nutrition: I do not eat enough fresh vegetables, and I eat on the run all the time.
Degeneration: I have degenerative disk problems.
Immune hypersensitivity: I have some allergies to pollens.
Immune deficiency: I get upper respiratory problems when my immune system is depressed.
Viruses: I am susceptible to flu, colds, and herpes simplex when stressed and tired.
Fungi: I used to get yeast infections in my teens and 20s.
Protozoa: N/A.
Pathogenic animals: N/A.
Tumors and cancer: N/A.
Inflammatory response: I have chronic inflammation in my back.
Environment: I work in a clean environment with natural light. I live in an area I like, but my sleep is sometimes interrupted from highway noise.
Age: I am in my 40s and am experiencing age-related hormone changes and weight gain.
Lifestyle: My lifestyle is extremely busy with demands from many persons. I work 60 to 70 hours per week, but I am able to maintain a regular sleep schedule. I exercise moderately, eat too much fat, have never smoked, and do not drink alcohol or use drugs.
Stress: I am a single parent of three. I have many persons in my life with many different needs. I have many agencies to answer to and feel stressed by the bureaucratic expectations.
Preexisting conditions: I have disk dysfunction, an endocrine problem, and inner ear balance syndrome, breathing pattern disorder, and dyslexia.
Considering this information, how would you rate your personal health history on a scale of 1 to 10, with 10 being excellent health? To what types of disease processes do you feel you are most susceptible? What could you do to support your personal homeostasis?

Example

In general my health is good, an 8 on the scale. The inner ear problem creates physiologic confusion and nausea that adds to my stress levels. The back and endocrine problems have stabilized but have to be managed. The breathing pattern disorder is under control. I take fairly good care of myself and use some nutritional supplements to balance my diet. If I get enough sleep and exercise, I do better. I feel that I am most susceptible to cardiovascular disease, joint problems, and osteoporosis. Continued attention to diet and exercise, coupled with therapeutic massage to manage my back and stress level, seems to be working.

Your Turn

Genetic mechanisms:

Physical and chemical agents:

Nutrition:

Degeneration:

Immune hypersensitivity:

Immune deficiency:

Viruses:

Fungi:

Protozoa:

Pathogenic animals:

Tumors and cancer:

Inflammatory response:

Environment:

Age:

Lifestyle:

Stress:

Preexisting conditions:

Considering this information, how would you rate your personal health history on a scale of 1 to 10, with 10 being excellent health? To what types of disease processes do you feel you are most susceptible? What could you do to support your personal homeostasis?

increase the risk for respiratory problems.

6. *Preexisting conditions:* A primary (preexisting) condition can put a person at risk of a secondary condition. For example, a viral infection can compromise the immune system and make the person more susceptible to bacterial infection.

Pain

Pain is a complex, private, abstract experience that is difficult to explain or describe. Pain is the number one symptom or complaint that causes persons to seek health care, and its effective management is a major challenge. Defining pain in descriptive and measurable terms is not easy because pain has physiologic, psychologic, and social aspects.

Pain Sensations

We need the sensations we get from pain to live a normal life. These sensations provide us enough information about potential tissue damage to help us protect ourselves from greater damage. Pain often initiates one's search for medical assistance. The subjective description and indication of the location of the pain helps to pinpoint the underlying cause of disease.

The receptors for pain, called nociceptors, are simply the branching ends of the dendrites (projections from the nerve cell body) of certain sensory neurons. Pain receptors are found in practically every tissue of the body, and they may respond to any type of stimulus. When stimuli for other sensations, such as touch, pressure, heat, and cold, reach a certain intensity, they may cause the sensation of pain as well. Injured tissue releases bradykinin, which causes the release of inflammatory chemicals such as histamine and prostaglandins, making peripheral nociceptors more sensitive to the normal pain response. This increased sensitivity to pain is called hyperalgesia.

As stated previously, excessive stimulation of a sensory organ causes pain. Additional or excessive stimuli for pain receptors includes distention or dilation of a structure, prolonged muscular contractions, muscle spasms, inadequate blood flow to an organ, or the presence of certain chemical substances. Pain receptors, because of their sensitivity to all stimuli, perform a protective function by identifying changes that may endanger the body. Pain receptors adapt only slightly or not at all. Adaptation is the decrease or disappearance of the perception of a sensation even though the stimulus is still present. An example is getting used to our clothes soon after dressing. If adaptation to pain occurred, the stimuli would cease to be sensed and irreparable damage could result.

Sensory impulses for pain are controlled by the central nervous system along spinal and cranial nerves to the reticular activating system and hypothalamus to change awareness and arousal and to the thalamus for transmission to the cerebral cortex for interpretation. From there the impulses may be relayed to the parietal lobe. Recognition of the kind and intensity of most pain ultimately is localized in the cerebral cortex. Some awareness of pain also occurs at subcortical (under the cortex) levels.

Acute pain is a symptom of a disease condition or a temporary aspect of medical treatment. Acute pain acts as a warning signal because it can activate the sympathetic (fight or flight) nervous system. Acute pain is usually temporary, of sudden onset, and easily localized. The person frequently can describe the pain, which often subsides with or without treatment.

Chronic pain is also a symptom of a disease condition but is identified as a major health problem, with about 25% of the population being affected. Chronic pain is a symptom that persists or recurs for indefinite periods, usually for more than 6 months. Chronic pain frequently has an obscure onset, and the character and quality of the pain change over time. The pain usually is diffused, poorly localized, and often requires the efforts of a multidisciplinary health care team for its effective management.

Intractable pain occurs when chronic pain persists even if treatment is provided or when chronic pain exists without active disease. This represents the greatest challenge to all health care providers. Temporary symptomatic relief from this type of pain may be provided by soft tissue approaches.

Specific types of pain include the following:

1. *Pricking or bright pain:* This type of pain exists when the skin is cut or jabbed with a sharp object. The pain is short-lived but intense and easily localized and sometimes is termed *superficial* ***somatic pain.***
2. *Burning pain:* This type of pain is slower to develop, lasts longer, and is localized less accurately (e.g., when the skin is burned). This type of pain often stimulates cardiac and respiratory activity.
3. *Aching pain:* Aching pain occurs when the visceral organs are stimulated. The pain is constant, not well localized, and often is referred to areas of the body distant from where the damage may be occurring. Aching pain is important because it may be a sign of a life-threatening disorder of a vital organ.
4. *Deep pain:* The main difference between superficial and deep pain is the nature of the pain evoked by noxious stimuli. Unlike superficial pain, deep pain is poorly localized, nauseating, and frequently associated with sweating and changes in blood pressure. Deep pain initiates reflex contraction of nearby skeletal muscles. This reflex contraction is similar to the muscle spasm associated with injuries to bones, tendons, and joints. The steadily contracting muscles become ischemic (lacking in oxygen), and ischemia stimulates the pain receptors in the muscles. The pain in turn initiates more spasms, setting up a vicious circle (Figure 2-6).
5. *Muscle pain:* If a muscle contracts rhythmically in the presence of an adequate blood supply, pain usually does not result. However, if the blood supply to a muscle is occluded (closed off), the same rhythmic contraction

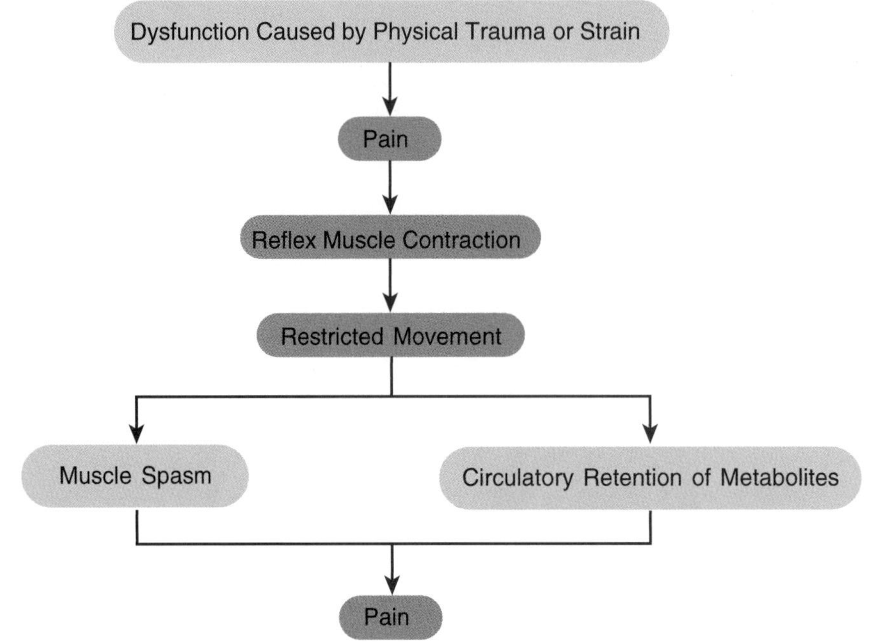

Figure 2-6
Muscle pain spasm cycle.

soon causes pain. The pain persists even after the contraction until blood flow is reestablished. If a muscle with a normal blood supply is made to contract continuously without periods of relaxation, it also begins to ache because the maintained contraction compresses the blood vessels supplying the muscle, reducing the blood supply.

Let us look at pain in two other ways: somatic and visceral. Somatic pain arises from stimulation of receptors in the skin (superficial somatic pain) or from stimulation of receptors in skeletal muscles, joints, tendons, and fasciae (deep somatic pain). **Visceral pain** results from stimulation of receptors in the viscera (any of our internal organs).

Superficial somatic pain is transmitted along finely myelinated A delta nerve fibers at a fast rate. Deep somatic pain and most visceral pain are transmitted slowly by unmyelinated C nerve fibers. This difference in transmission of pain signals is why superficial somatic stimulation transmitted on A delta fibers can block or mask deep somatic or visceral pain. Stimulation of more A fibers than C fibers blocks the C fiber transmission from entering the spinal cord. If the signal does not enter the spinal cord, it cannot be felt as pain. Methods of touch and pressure and most methods of movement are transmitted on A fibers; any stimuli of this type increases A-fiber transmission. Treating pain in this way is called counterirritation (Figure 2-7).

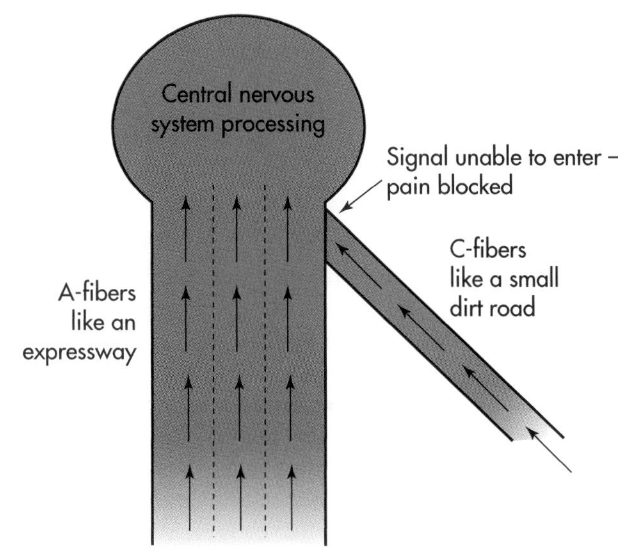

Figure 2-7
Gate-control theory of pain (based on Melzack and Wall's gate-control theory of pain).

Referred Pain

The ability of the cerebral cortex to locate the origin of pain is related to past experience. In most instances of somatic pain and in some instances of visceral pain, the cortex accurately projects the pain back to the stimulated area.

The pain also may be felt in a surface area far from the stimulated organ. This phenomenon is called referred pain. In general, the area to which the pain is referred and the visceral organ that is stimulated receive their innervation from the same segment of the spinal cord. Because of this association the cortex may misinterpret the source. The following are examples. The pain of a heart attack is typically felt in the skin over the heart and along the left arm. The same factor is at work with the referred pain in the shoulder

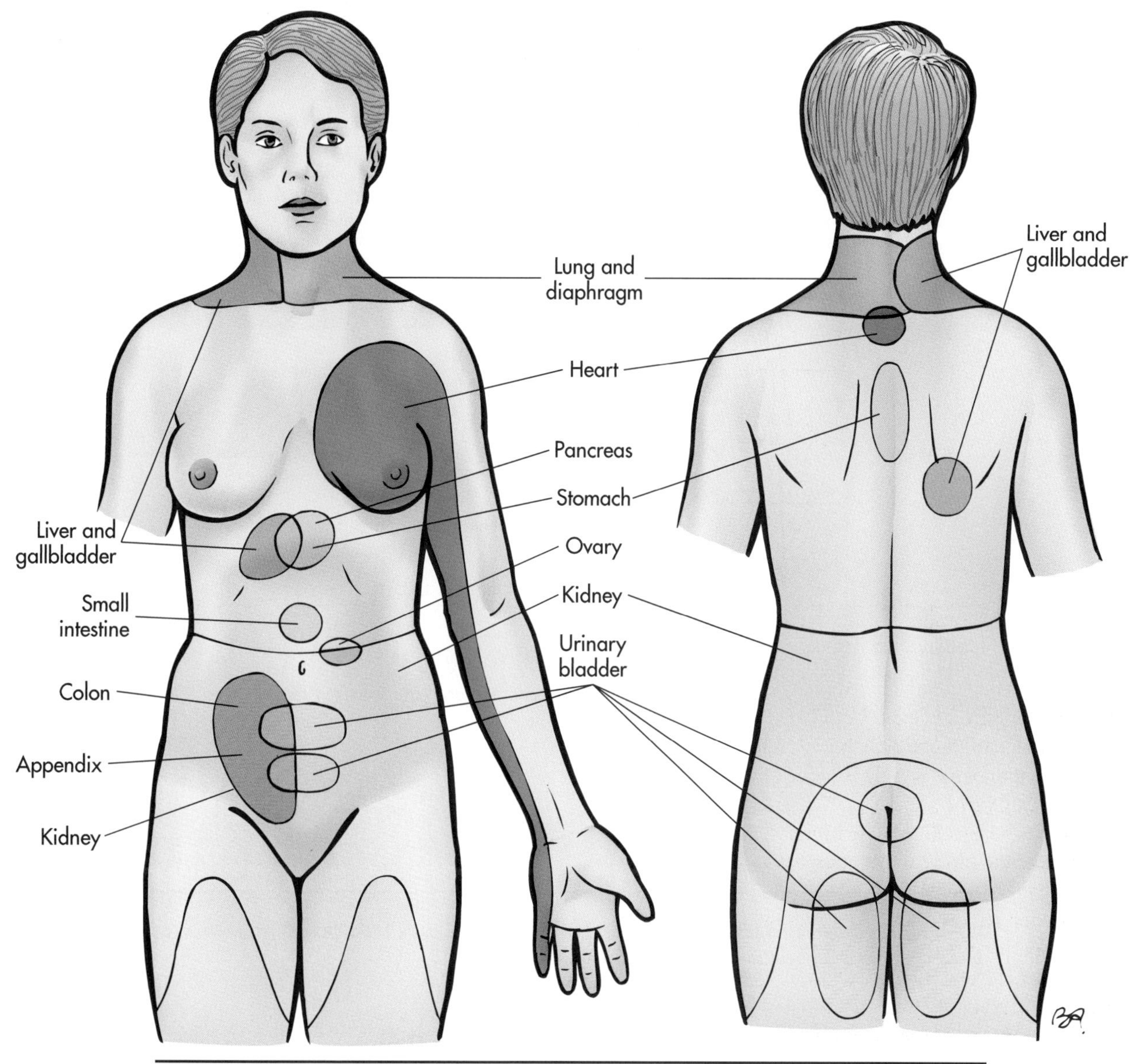

Figure 2-8
Referred pain. The diagram indicates cutaneous areas to which visceral pains may be referred. The professional encountering pain in these areas needs to refer the client for diagnosis to rule out visceral dysfunction. (From Fritz S: *Mosby's fundamentals of therapeutic massage,* ed 3, St Louis, 2004, Mosby.)

caused by gallstone pain. Figure 2-8 illustrates cutaneous (skin) regions to which visceral pain may be referred. If the client has a recurring pain pattern that resembles patterns on the chart, the client should be referred to a physician for an accurate diagnosis.

As already stated, irritation of the viscera frequently produces pain that is felt not in the viscera but in some somatic structure that may be a considerable distance from the viscera. Such pain is said to be referred to the somatic structure. Deep somatic pain also may be referred, but superficial pain is not. When visceral pain is local and referred, it sometimes seems to spread (radiate) from the local to the distant site.

Visceral pain, like deep somatic pain, initiates reflex contraction of nearby skeletal muscle. Because somatic pain is much more common than visceral pain, the brain has learned to project the pain to the somatic area and initiate the reflex contraction there.

Obviously, knowledge of referred pain and the common sites of pain referral from each of the viscera are important to massage practitioners and other health care professionals. The most common example of referred pain is that of a heart attack, which often appears as chest pain. Another example is pain in the tip of the shoulder, which may be due to irritation in the central portion of the diaphragm. However, one must remember that sites of reference are not stereotyped, and unusual reference sites occur with considerable frequency. Heart pain, for instance, may be experienced as purely abdominal, may be referred to the right arm, and even may be referred to the neck.

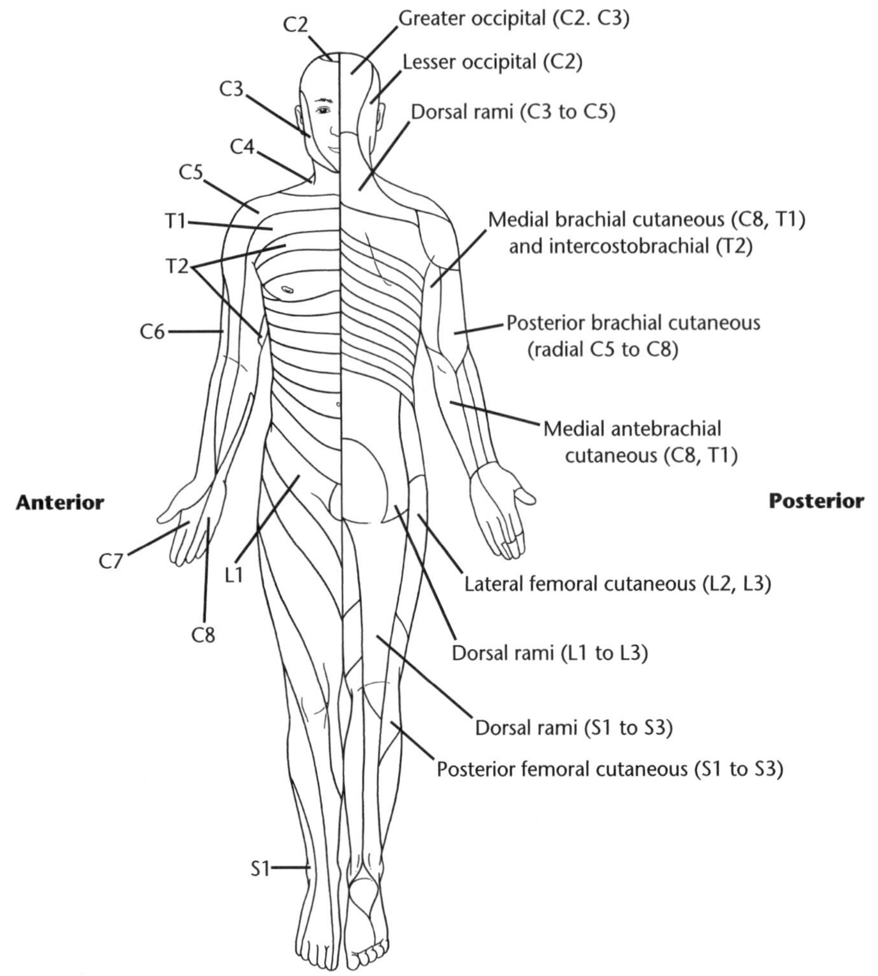

Figure 2-9
Dermatomal map (anterior view) and cutaneous nerve distribution (posterior view) of the human body. (From Greenstein GM: *Clinical assessment of neuromusculoskeletal disorders,* St Louis, 1997, Mosby.)

As previously noted, past experience plays an important role in referred pain. Although pain originating in an inflamed abdominal organ usually is referred to the midline, in clients who have had previous abdominal surgery, the pain of an inflamed abdominal organ frequently is referred to their surgical scars. Pain originating in the maxillary sinus usually is referred to nearby teeth, but in clients with a history of traumatic dental work, such pain regularly is referred to the previously traumatized teeth. This is true even if the teeth are distant from the sinus.

When pain is referred, the reference is usually to a structure that developed from the same embryonic segment or is located in the same dermatome as the structure in which the pain originates. For example, during embryonic development, the diaphragm moves from the neck to its adult location in the abdomen and takes its nerve supply, the phrenic nerve, with it. One third of the fibers in the phrenic nerve are afferent, and they enter the spinal cord at the level of the second to fourth cervical segments, the same location at which afferent nerves from the tip of the shoulder enter. Similarly, the heart and the arm have the same embryonic segmental origin (Fritz, 2004) (Figure 2-9).

Phantom Pain

A kind of pain frequently experienced by persons who have had a limb amputated is called **phantom pain.** They experience pain or other sensations in the extremity as if the limb were still there. Phantom pain is suspected to occur because the remaining proximal portions of the sensory nerves that previously received impulses from the limb are being stimulated by the trauma of the amputation. Stimuli from these nerves are interpreted by the brain as coming from the nonexistent (phantom) limb.

Pain Threshold and Tolerance

Pain may be brought on by mechanical, electrical, thermal, or chemical stimuli. We do not appear to adapt to pain or to accommodate it. We all have about the same threshold for pain. A **pain threshold** is when stimulation becomes intense enough to initiate the firing of pain receptors. Pain tolerance is how we respond to pain (Activity 2-5). **Pain tolerance** varies considerably and is influenced greatly by cultural and psychologic factors. Pain tolerance is modified by age and

ACTIVITY 2-5

List three personal factors that could change your pain tolerance.

Examples
Things that could increase pain tolerance
1. Reading a good book
2. Going for a walk
3. Practicing relaxation techniques

Things that could decrease pain tolerance
1. Being tired and upset with the kids
2. Driving in heavy traffic
3. Loud music

Your Turn
Things that could increase my pain tolerance

Things that could decrease my pain tolerance

emotional and mental state. Subjective measurements of pain intensity are more reliable than the observable ones. Only the person in pain can determine the amount of severity experienced. Pain is rarely the same at all times. Pain is felt (perceived) differently over time and differs with various precipitating and aggravating factors. Pain can range from excruciating to mild and may be difficult for the person to verbalize.

The cause of severity and type of pain has to be identified to treat it best. Assessing the severity and degree of pain is difficult because pain cannot be measured objectively, so a thorough history has to be obtained and a systematic physical assessment carried out. Some questions to ask are these:
Is the pain acute or chronic?
What is the location of the pain?
What is the quality of pain (sharp, burning, pricking, etc.)?
How intense is the pain?
When does the pain occur; that is, the timing?
What factors affect the intensity of the pain?

Pain Management

Acute pain usually is caused by tissue injury. Inflammation is often present, and rest (speeds up healing), ice (numbs pain receptors, constricts blood vessels, and reduces edema), compression (reduces bleeding, if any, and edema), and elevation (allows gravity to help with lymphatic drainage and reduces edema) play important parts in management. Short-term use of an analgesic is effective.

Chronic pain management is more difficult. Some options work for certain individuals and not for others. These strategies can be used alone or in combination.

Transcutaneous Electric Nerve Stimulation

Electrodes attached to a small portable unit are used to stimulate the skin surface over the area of pain. Transcutaneous electric nerve stimulation stimulates large A delta fibers of the skin, and according to the gate-control theory, the fibers inhibit pain-conducting fibers in the spinal cord. Research has shown that low-voltage doses of electricity increase the levels of endogenous opioids such as endorphins, enkephalins, and denorphins in the body.

Acupuncture

Acupuncture is done by inserting a thin needle into the skin along acupuncture meridians. One of the ways acupuncture works is by releasing endogenous opioids.

Acupressure

Acupressure stimulates acupuncture points without using needles. Pressure is applied to the points with the thumb, finger, or any blunt instrument. The physiologic explanations are the same as for acupuncture.

Placebo Response

Placebo response is the use of any treatment process that produces a positive response. Because of the person's belief that the treatment will be effective, rather than painkilling properties of the method, 20% to 40% of persons on whom pain has been induced by stimuli have reported pain relief with the use of placebos.

Distraction and Imagery

Distraction is focusing the attention on stimuli other than that of pain. Imagery consists of using the imagination to create or remember a mental picture that is relaxing and pain relieving.

Biofeedback

Biofeedback is a technique in which the person is made aware of body function by external measuring equipment such as a computer-generated image of blood pressure to control the function at the conscious level. Nerve fibers from the cerebral cortex that can inhibit the impulses ascending in the pain pathways produce pain relief. This kind of treatment is especially useful in treating migraines, tension headaches or other forms of pain in which muscle tension is involved.

Aromatherapy

Essential oils stimulate the olfactory nerve, which has many important connections that link into the limbic system (emotions) and hypothalamus (endocrine function). Therefore aromas can have profound effects on the mind and emotions. The oils are lipid extracts from different parts of plants and can penetrate the skin quickly. Essential oils can be used as compresses, for inhalation, in baths, and with massage oils.

Music Therapy

Music has been used to reduce pain. The pain relief may be because of a reduction in anxiety, inhibition of pain pathways, distraction, or increase in endorphins produced by music. Music therapy can aggravate pain; therefore preferences need to be considered before using music during massage.

Hypnosis

Hypnotic techniques alter the focus of attention and enhance imagery by using suggestions. Individuals vary widely in their ability to be hypnotized.

Heat

Heat can be used to reduce pain. Heat dilates local blood vessels and increases the blood flow. The increase in blood flow can reduce pain by washing away pain-producing chemicals. Temperature receptors are stimulated by heat, and the impulses are carried by large myelinated nerve fibers that may inhibit the pain fibers. Heat softens collagen fibers, making them more pliable, allowing joints, tendons, and ligaments to be stretched further before stimulating the pain receptors.

Cold

Cold application relieves pain by decreasing swelling by vasoconstriction, decreasing stimulation of pain nerve endings, and stimulating release of endogenous opioids.

Massage

Massage has an analgesic effect. The various methods used help speed up the drainage of pain-producing substances from the area. Release of histamine and direct stimulation cause local blood vessels to dilate and wash away toxins, remove edema, and bring oxygen to the area. Massage can reduce muscle spasm, improve blood flow, and remove pressure on pain receptors. The touch and pressure sensations carried by large myelinated fibers can inhibit pain fibers. Massage also is used for distraction. The relaxation music that is often used also helps. Special techniques that help reduce adhesions can free nerves that may be producing the pain.

Other Forms of Therapy

Art, prayer, meditation, and laughter are other forms of therapy that are being used effectively for pain management.

Medication

Painkilling medications are called analgesics. Oral analgesics such as aspirin reduce inflammation and inhibit transmission of pain impulses. They are nonaddictive. Narcotic analgesics have an effect like morphine and can be addictive, and tolerance may develop. Narcotics (opioids) are used in individuals in whom relief cannot be obtained by other means, especially those suffering from cancer pain or those whose life expectancy is limited.

Surgical Techniques

Surgical techniques are used to remove the cause or block the transmission of pain. Because damage to nerve cell bodies produces irreversible changes, surgery is used as a last resort.

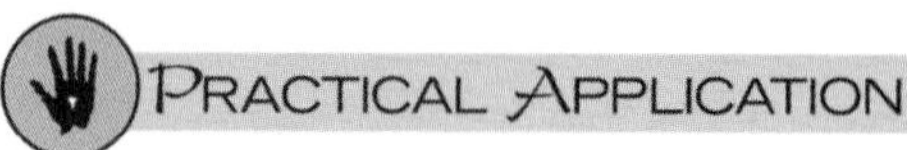

Pain is a complex problem with physical, psychologic, social, and financial components. The vast difference in the experience of pain in human beings suggests that natural neural mechanisms must exist to modulate pain transmission and perception. Beta-endorphins, enkephalins, and denorphins are natural opiates, are released in the body when we are in pain, and reduce our perception of pain. Stimulus-induced forms of analgesia such as acupuncture, massage, and other forms of bodywork, hydrotherapy, and exercise are believed to tap into these natural opiate pathways. Counterirritations from touch and movement therapies are viable explanations for why these approaches are effective in pain management, because they release endorphins and enkephalins. ■

Alleviation of pain can be accomplished in many ways. The massage professional, as part of a health care team, can contribute valuable manual therapy for various painful conditions with direct tissue manipulation and reflex stimulation of the nervous system and the circulation. Touch and movement, when used as a therapeutic intervention, may help reduce the need for pain medication, thus reducing its side effects. Clients in intense pain must have their therapy monitored by a physician or other appropriate health care professional. Most persons experience less extreme pain occasionally throughout life. Massage approaches may provide temporary symptomatic relief for moderate pain brought on by daily stress, reducing or eliminating use of over-the-counter pain medications, but if any pain persists, the client should be referred to a physician.

Note: For sufficient information to deal with pain situations presented by clients, a pathology text and a reference text of pharmaceuticals would be helpful. Texts written for nurses often provide the most useful information on pathology and pharmaceuticals. Suggestions are included in the Works Consulted list at the back of this book.

MECHANISMS OF HEALTH

A state of health is supported by a balanced lifestyle. Disease reflects states of the "too much" or "not enough" ends of the continuum of imbalance; health is that state of "just right," or homeostasis.

Health is influenced by many factors, including inherited and constitutional conditions. Lifestyle, activity level, rest, loving relationships, exercise, diet, empowering beliefs and attitudes, self-esteem, authentic personality, and freedom from self-hindering patterns all support health.

Individuals need to understand their own bodies, minds, and spiritual selves as they seek balance to allow the body to maintain a dynamic state of homeostasis (Activity 2-6).

ACTIVITY 2-6

This activity affords you an extensive look at your health profile. Complete the following statements by providing three different responses to each statement.

Example

My lifestyle supports health in the following ways:

1. I am involved in work that I love.
2. I am surrounded by information.
3. I am financially stable.

My lifestyle does not support health in the following ways:

1. I work too many hours.
2. I am overwhelmed with too much to know and understand.
3. I have a lot of debt.

Your Turn

My lifestyle supports health in the following ways:

1. ______
2. ______
3. ______

My lifestyle does not support health in the following ways:

1. ______
2. ______
3. ______

My activity level supports health in the following ways:

1. ______
2. ______
3. ______

My activity level does not support health in the following ways:

1. ______
2. ______
3. ______

My rest pattern supports health in the following ways:

1. ______
2. ______
3. ______

My rest pattern does not support health in the following ways:

1. ______
2. ______
3. ______

My relationships support health in the following ways:

1. ______
2. ______
3. ______

My relationships do not support health in the following ways:

1. ______
2. ______
3. ______

My aerobic exercise supports health in the following ways:

1. ______
2. ______
3. ______

My aerobic exercise does not support health in the following ways:

1. ______
2. ______
3. ______

My diet supports health in the following ways:

1. ______
2. ______
3. ______

My diet does not support health in the following ways:

1. ______
2. ______
3. ______

My beliefs and attitudes support health in the following ways:

1. ______
2. ______
3. ______

My beliefs and attitudes do not support health in the following ways:

1. ______
2. ______
3. ______

My self-esteem supports health in the following ways:

1. ______
2. ______
3. ______

ACTIVITY 2-6—cont'd

My self-esteem does not support health in the following ways:

1. ______

2. ______

3. ______

My personality supports health in the following ways:

1. ______

2. ______

3. ______

My personality does not support health in the following ways:

1. ______

2. ______

3. ______

STRESS MANAGEMENT

Maintaining and supporting health requires us to manage stress and stressors effectively. A stressor is not always a negative event. A wedding and a funeral may be equally stressful.

Exposures to intense or extreme stressors (too much) and deprivation of necessary stimuli (too little) can cause imbalance and thus many problems. Too much heat, cold, noise, activity, exercise, food, or social demands, or not enough food, touch, social interaction, or sleep can be detrimental to health. Our continued need to respond or change to maintain homeostasis increases the effects of stress (Figure 2-10, *A* to *D*).

Stress

Hans Selye called the response of the body to stress the **general adaptation syndrome,** which he suggested be divided into three stages. The first stage is the alarm reaction, also called the fight-or-flight response, which is the initial reaction of the body to the perceived stressor. The second stage is known as the resistance reaction, which through the secretion of regulating hormones allows the body to continue fighting a stressor long after the effects of the alarm reaction have dissipated (cortisol). The third stage is the exhaustion reaction, which takes place if the stress response continues without relief. General adaptation is a uniform, consistent general response to the perceived stimuli.

The autonomic nervous system is responsible for the monitoring, regulating, and coordinating of almost all systems of the body such as temperature of the body, pH, oxygen levels, volume of blood, blood pressure, intake of food, digestion and absorption of food and water, and excretion of waste products. The response of the autonomic nervous system can be summed up as the fight-or-flight response and is brought about by an increase in the activity of the sympathetic nervous system. Some of the manifestations of sympathetic arousal are dilation of the pupil, increased heart rate and blood pressure, increased respiratory rate, dry mouth, and sweating hands. Gastrointestinal tract activity is diminished. One of the manifestations of stress is the tensing of muscles, particularly in the neck, shoulders, and torso. Prolonged tension causes responses such as stiffness of the neck, backache, headaches, and clenching of the teeth. Therapeutic massage is particularly helpful in managing this aspect of stress.

Stress situations inhibit the thyroid, reproductive, and growth hormones to conserve energy.

Our perception of a stressor is important. Anything we perceive as a threat, whether real or imagined, arouses fear or anxiety. How we respond is influenced by other conditions, some of which are under our conscious control and some of which are not. Our physical and mental health; hereditary predisposition and genetics; past experiences; current coping habits, learned and inborn; diet; environment; and social support determine which stimuli are interpreted as stressors.

Hans Selye's groundbreaking research on stress began in 1935 and was formalized in his book *The Stress of Life,* published in 1956. Selye's research laid the foundation for current concepts about stress.

The word *stress* currently is used to refer to any stimulus that directly or indirectly stimulates neurons of the hypothalamus to release corticotropin-releasing hormone. Many hormones regulated by the hypothalamus come into play during stress. The hypothalamus has connections with the cortex and limbic system, and situations perceived as stressful have an effect on the hypothalamus. The hypothalamus controls the pituitary, and the pituitary gland regulates secretions of hormones from the thyroid gland, adrenal cortex, ovaries, and testes. Stress easily becomes an event affecting the whole body. One of the hormones secreted by the adrenal cortex is cortisol. Cortisol maintains blood glucose levels, facilitates fat metabolism, and affects protein and collagen synthesis. Increased cortisol secretion in stressful situations reduces the immune reaction, and the antiinflammatory effect of cortisol can slow down healing as well. In generalized stress conditions the hypothalamus acts on the anterior pituitary gland to cause the release of adrenocorticotropic hormone, which in turn stimulates the adrenal cortex to secrete glucocorticoid. Glucocorticoids are a class of adrenal cortical hormones that work to protect our bodies against stress and aid in protein and carbohydrate metabolism. Cortisol is an example. Glucocorticoids also

A
ME
B
ME
Homeostasis—ability to adapt—but at limit
High stress load
C
ME
ME
SOCIAL SUPPORT
D
TRASH
Falling apart—too much to carry and manage
Stress coping. Reduce the load—eliminate some stressors and add social support

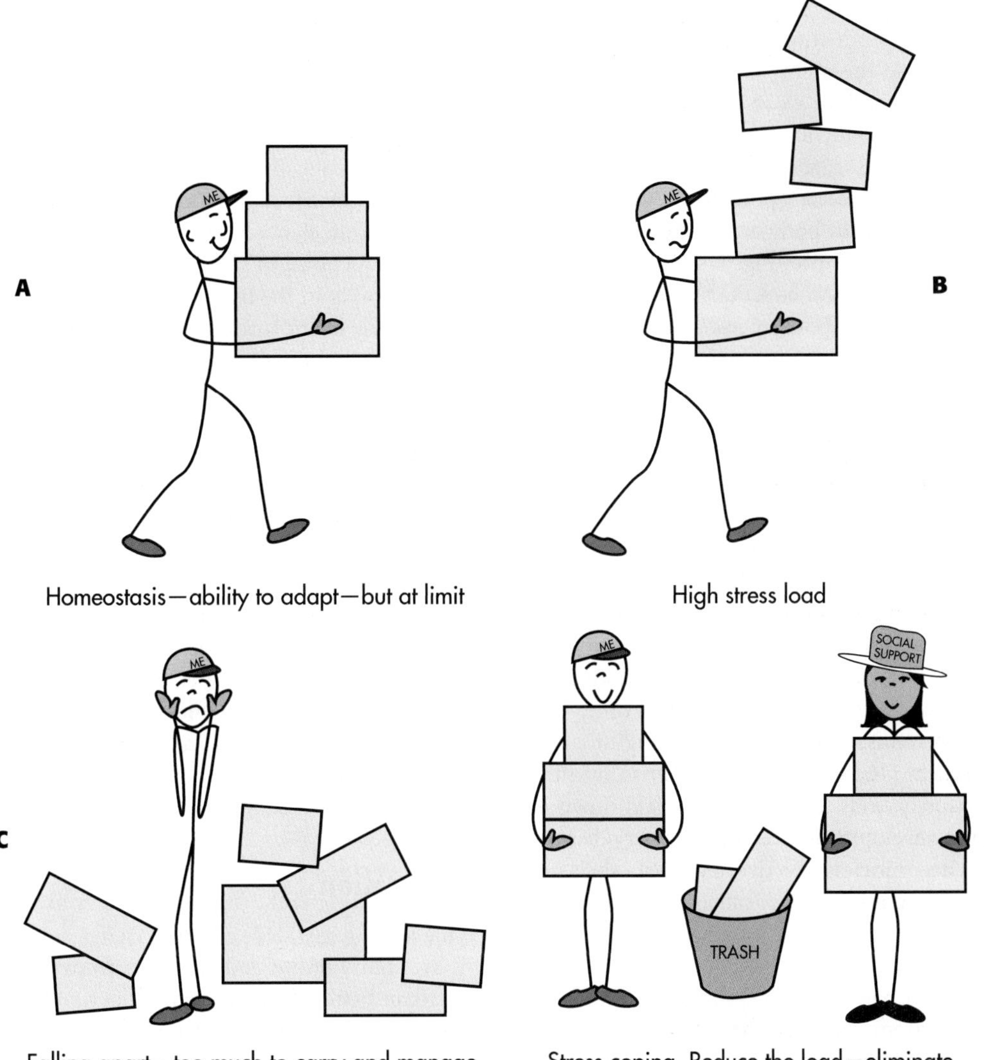

It is not always the type of stress that causes problems, although some types of stress are more demanding than others. It is more the amount of the stress load and the need to balance many different things that cause breakdown. Many stressors cannot be easily altered, but the stress load can be managed through physical mechanisms such as exercise, diet, and relaxation methods that allow the body to better cope with those things that cannot be changed. The stress load can be lightened by eliminating those stressors possible and asking for help from social support such as family, friends and co-workers.

Activity:

In *A*, fill in the boxes with those stressors that you can manage. In *B*, again fill in the stressors from *A*, and add some additional stressors. In *C*, fill in the stressors you listed in *B* and add two more that would make the load too heavy. In *D*, identify the stressors that you can manage yourself. Write those in the boxes carried by the figure representing you. Identify two stressors that can be eliminated by putting them in the trash basket. Then identify two stressors that you can have someone help you with and write them in the boxes carried by the figure representing social support.

Figure 2-10
A to **D,** Stress load.

work to provide an antiinflammatory effect, assist in the release of amino acids from muscle, mobilize fatty acids from fat stores, increase the ability of skeletal muscles to maintain contraction and thus avoid fatigue, and increase adenosine triphosphate production.

In addition to causing glucocorticoid release, the adrenal medulla stimulates the release of epinephrine (adrenaline) and norepinephrine to help the body in its response to stress. However, during periods of prolonged stress, continued release of these hormones may have harmful side effects, such as decreased immune response, lowered blood glucose levels, and altered protein and fat metabolism, which in turn decreases our resistance to stress. Therefore the continued release of epinephrine and norepinephrine increase the possibility of high blood pressure, decreased digestion, reduced tissue repair, and more (Figure 2-11).

Persons who experience excessive or ongoing stress often express being overwhelmed by tension, anger, fear, and frustration, resulting in feelings of anxiety. This causes adrenaline levels to rise, blood pressure and heart rate to increase, and breathing to change. Overbreathing often results in overoxygenation of the blood, reducing carbon dioxide levels, which then leads to hyperventilation syndrome. (See Chapter 12.) This response can be the beginning of panic attacks. Blood levels of glucose and fatty acids rise, and the combination eventually leads to plaque being laid down in the arteries and the development of coronary artery disease. Immune function becomes less effective, and the body is not as able to deal with pathogens or cancer cells. Often a decrease in memory and the ability to concentrate or solve problems occurs; susceptibility to infection increases; and complaints of stomach pain, heart palpitation, fatigue, and muscle aches are common. Sleep disorders and depression frequently accompany long-term stress. All these changes in our bodies are the result of prolonged stress.

Mood and behavior are affected by stress as well, and an ongoing interplay between physiologic and psychologic stress occurs that is best described by the chicken and the egg question of "Which came first?" Certainly, psychologic stress can result in physiologic response, and the physiologic stress response alters perception, mood, thought processes, and behavior, thus creating psychologic stress.

When we see how many of our organs and glands are innervated by the autonomic nervous system, such vast consequences to autonomic system disturbances are not surprising. This is especially true of stress-induced diseases. A prolonged or excessive physiologic response to stress, the fight-or-flight response, can disrupt normal functioning—homeostasis—throughout the body. This reaction increases the strength and rate of the heartbeat, causes a rise in blood pressure, and results in hyperglycemia, pallor, coolness of skin, sweaty palms, and dry mouth. Water retention and increases in blood volume are caused by the increase in antidiuretic hormone and aldosterone secretion, which result from stress.

Stress is considered a contributing or risk factor in many conditions. The following is a list of various areas susceptible to stress-related diseases, although the exact cause-and-effect relationship is often unclear:

Digestive tract: Diseases that may be caused or aggravated by stress include gastritis, stomach and duodenal ulcers, ulcerative colitis, and irritable colon.

Reproductive organs: Stress-related problems include difficult conception or infertility, menstrual disorders or lack of menstrual periods in women, and impotence and premature ejaculation in men.

Bladder: A common stress response is sensitivity or irritability in the bladder, causing bladder urgency, bed-wetting, or incontinence.

Brain: Many mental and emotional problems—among them anxiety, psychosis, and depression—may be triggered by stress.

Hair: Some forms of hair loss and baldness have been linked to high levels of stress.

Mouth: Sores, ulcers, and oral lichen planus (thrush) often seem to develop under stress.

Lungs: Asthma symptoms often worsen under high levels of mental or emotional stress.

Heart: Heart rate disturbances and angina attacks often occur during or after periods of stress.

Muscles: Muscle tension and its associated pain are often the result of stress, as are an increase in muscle twitches and nervous tics. The muscular tremor of Parkinson's disease is also more marked at such times.

Adaptation

One of the remarkable effects of change, internal and external, is the ability of the body to adapt to stress. The body is able to adapt better if changes are brought on gradually. Sudden changes, along with a diminished physiologic reserve, can have dramatic negative effects on the body.

The effect of stress on the body also is determined by the genetic makeup. The genetic makeup of a person is responsible for how well the different organs adapt and respond to stressful situations.

With age, the ability to adapt is diminished. Individuals who are fit mentally and physically are able to adapt to stress placed on them much more easily than others. Those who are motivated to live are well known to survive the worst onslaughts made on their minds and bodies.

Studies have shown that sleep and proper nutrition are important for restoring energy, regenerating tissue, and coping with stress. Poor nutrition is a stress-causing agent, and irregular cycles of sleep and wakefulness can reduce immunity and physical and psychological function.

The psychological stresses can be combated by a supportive social network. More and more persons seek medical assistance to help sort out and identify stress-related symptoms. Because each of us responds to stress in different ways, the possibility of an accurate diagnosis becomes difficult. This lack of specificity has led to frustration in clients and health care providers. As more research is done in the area of stress coping, this situation is continuing to improve. Contemporary health care now recognizes exces-

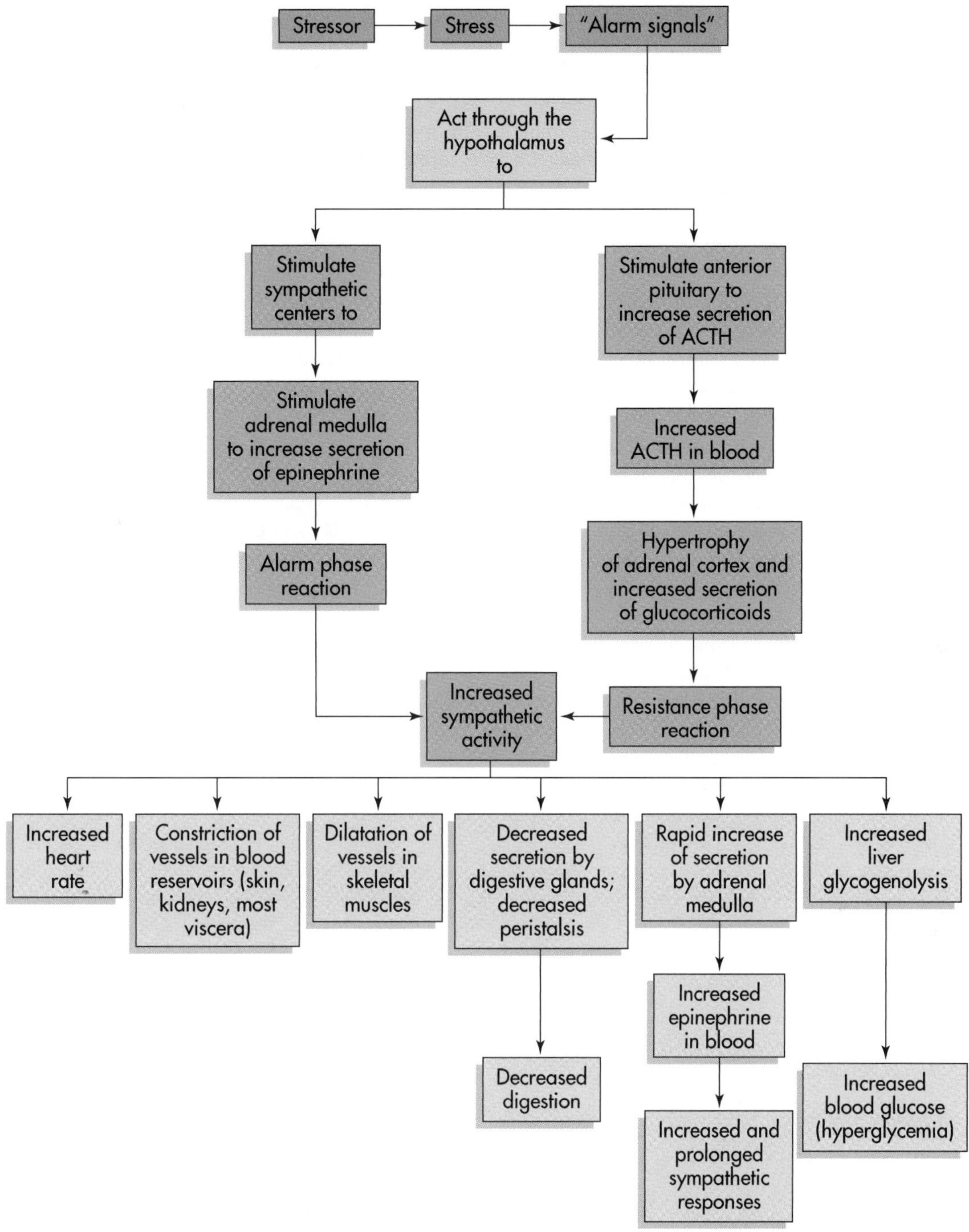

Figure 2-11
Stress response. The word *stress* currently is used to refer to any stimulus that directly or indirectly stimulates neurons of the hypothalamus to release corticotropin-releasing hormone. Many hormones regulated by the hypothalamus come into play during stress. The main stress response of the autonomic nervous system can be summed up as the fight-or-flight response and is brought about by an increase in the activity of the sympathetic nervous system. Some of the manifestations of sympathetic arousal are dilation of the pupils, increased heart rate and blood pressure, increased respiratory rate, dry mouth, and sweating hands. One of the manifestations of stress is the tensing of muscles, particularly in the neck, shoulders, and torso. Prolonged tension causes effects such as stiffness of the neck, backache, headaches, and clenching of the teeth.

sive and long-term stress as an important and widespread cause of disease because stress disrupts homeostasis in numerous psychologic and physiologic control systems. Psychophysiology is the study of the interplay between psychologic and physiologic stressors and neuroimmunology, sometimes referred to as psychoneuroimmunology, or the study of the mind-immunity link in uncovering the interaction of the mind/body connection.

Modern stress must be managed to support health. An increased openness, respect, and understanding of approaches—such as massage and other forms of bodywork, along with acupuncture, meditation, and relaxation methods using breathing, biofeedback, music therapy, hypnosis, exercise, and other forms of movement therapy—provide mechanisms for managing stress response. Many of these approaches are described on pages 43-44 as pain management strategies. The ancient health wisdom of indigenous peoples is now being understood through investigation by Western scientific methods (Fritz, 2004).

Therapeutic massage has been shown to reduce cortisol levels and decrease arousal of the sympathetic nervous system, resulting in reestablishment of homeostatic balance.

Massage therapy is postulated to introduce a different sort of stress (stimuli) into the system to which the body can respond and resolve through physiologic coping mechanisms. Because unresolved stress increases the intensity of the stress syndrome, the signals introduced by massage help reset the system, allowing for a more effective state of balance. Massage methods often have a pleasurable and comforting quality to them. They also can provide a soothing rhythmic pattern to which the recipient's body can entrain (organize and synchronize biologic rhythms). Massage is based on the premise of safe touch providing balanced sensory stimulation, which in turn supports health for its recipients.

Therefore massage can be an effective stress management tool. Remembering that the primary reason for the stress may require a multidisciplinary approach for resolution or effective long-term management is important, but massage modalities can play a part. Considering the amount of stress, not the type of stress, coupled with a person's perception of the events, anything that can change the perception of threat to one of safety or reduce the intensity of the physical stress response is going to promote mechanisms of health. These supportive changes include effective sleep, reduction in pain perception, and a sense of affiliation that supports effective social contact and support, and enhancement of the restorative and self-regulating processes of the body.

The stress response and stress syndrome are discussed throughout the text as they relate to each system studied. Because therapeutic massage effectively deals with stress management, a thorough understanding of stress, stressors, and the stress response or syndrome is important (Activity 2-7).

THE LIFE CYCLE

A human being is conceived by the joining of two cells, reinforcing the underlying concept of two opposites blending to make a whole. Cells multiply, divide, and differentiate, forming the organism. Birth brings forth an independent organism, which remains in a dependent functioning state while accelerated growth and development occur. The homeostatic mechanisms of infants and young children are less regular because they are in the process

ACTIVITY 2-7

List three major stressors in your life:

Example: Losing car keys

Your Turn

1. ______________________________

2. ______________________________

3. ______________________________

Now complete the following for each of the listed stressors: When (the stressor) happens, I feel (What are the physical and emotional sensations you experience?). The result is (What do you do about the feelings?). What I could do to alleviate the stress response is (Identify an activity that would restore homeostasis.).

Example

When I lose my car keys, I feel anxious and frustrated. My neck tenses up and I start to hyperventilate, which makes me feel light-headed, confused, and panicky. The result is that I begin to look frantically for my keys and start to holler at anyone around. What I could do to alleviate the stress response is use a breathing method to reestablish the oxygen/carbon dioxide balance and reverse the overbreathing.

Your Turn

Choose three different stressful situations and fill in the information.

When ________________ happens:

I feel ________________.

The result is ________________.

What I could do to alleviate the stress response is ________.

When ________________ happens:

I feel ________________.

The result is ________________.

What I could do to alleviate the stress response is ________.

When ________________ happens:

I feel ________________.

The result is ________________.

What I could do to alleviate the stress response is ________.

of creating their bodies. From adolescence through middle adulthood we have the most efficient bodily functions. Normal aging affects repair and replacement of the structural components of the body. During the extremes of life, infancy and old age, the body is presented with its greatest challenges for homeostasis. Advancing age creates changes in cell number and ability to function effectively. Changes occur in the production of hormones and the receptors in target tissue that bind these hormones. Some hormonal levels increase, whereas others remain unchanged or decrease. Many theories on aging exist, but the actual mechanics remain elusive to research. Three areas of research look to the physiologic mechanics of aging, which seem to be associated with cellular changes produced by genetic and environmental factors, changes in cellular regularity and central process, and degenerative extracellular and vascular changes. Examples of decreased functional ability include muscle atrophy; loss of elasticity of the skin; and changes in the cardiovascular, respiratory, and skeletal systems. The term *atrophy* describes the wasting effect of advancing age. In addition to structural atrophy the function of many physiologic control mechanisms also decreases and becomes less precise with advancing age. The aging process is cumulative, progressive, and natural.

Any behavior that supports cellular function enhances longevity. Many who live to advanced years have lived simple lives with a sense of purpose, physical work, and social support. Currently, the maximal life span of human beings is between 80 and 100 years, with many more in a society with stable sanitation, proper nutrition, and health care living beyond 100 years.

Life expectancy, or one's average life span, has increased with women reaching between the ages of 80 and 100, the fastest growing segment of many populations. Women in general live longer than men because of genetic, hormonal, immune, and social role influences.

Death can be thought of as the separation of structure (yin) and function (yang). In its purest form, yang is totally immaterial and corresponds to pure energy. Yin in its coarsest and most dense form is totally material and corresponds to matter. Yin and yang are essentially an expression of duality in time. Dying and gestation, death and birth are similar processes. Metaphorically speaking, birth is anabolic and death is catabolic. The cycle of life is a balance of yin and yang: conception, gestation, birth, living, dying, and death.

SUMMARY

In this chapter, we looked at homeostasis and factors influencing health and disease. Homeostasis consists of balancing mechanisms in constant communication with each other in a feedback loop system. Many factors can disrupt homeostasis, and yet in most situations the body is able to respond effectively and restore efficient functioning. We are equipped with the ability to deal with many different types of stressors. However, stress-coping mechanisms can be overloaded with an accumulated heavy load of unresolved stress, which contributes to the development of disease and pain patterns. We can be educators in wellness and coaches in the ongoing dynamic of homeostasis by being competent and able to recognize and support health mechanisms in ourselves and the clients we serve. We must assess for and identify disease, must be able to refer clients effectively as necessary, and must develop appropriate treatment plans for clients with disease processes. Proficiently integrating our skills with the health care community when supervised by medical professionals is also important. Massage can be a valuable tool to the treatment and management of many health concerns, especially those related to stress.

The information in this chapter is essential for the massage professional to be able to plan and organize an effective therapeutic massage session.

Many reasons, types, and ways to manage pain exist. Acute pain can be a friend by alerting us to emergency situations. Even chronic pain can be a gauge by which to monitor the effectiveness of therapy and the return to health or as near health as possible. As stated, the perception of a threat often makes the difference in the response of the body to life events. Perception is something that can be altered with diligent work and awareness coupled with professional assistance when necessary. We are conceived, born, live, and die. As we travel through life, each event is equally important in the total experience of being. Physical, emotional, and spiritual health are our objectives.

evolve

Two links to web articles dealing with the effect of stress on the body's health status are posted on the EVOLVE site to accompany this book. Read over these articles and apply them to the concepts presented in this chapter.

WORKBOOK SECTION

SHORT ANSWER

1. Define homeostasis, self-regulatory mechanisms, and body rhythms in relationship to bodywork modalities and Asian and Ayurvedic theories of health.

2. Discuss and contrast the mechanisms of disease and health.

Define these terms:

1. Disease
2. Pathology
3. Etiology
4. Health
5. Pharmacology
6. Signs
7. Symptoms
8. Syndrome
9. Acute
10. Chronic
11. Subacute
12. Communicable diseases
13. Pathogenesis
14. Incubation
15. Convalescence
16. Remission
17. Carcinogens
18. Oncologist

19. Tissue repair

____

20. Regeneration

____

21. Replacement

____

EXERCISE

1. List sources that may disturb homeostasis.

____

2. List the major risk factors in disease development.

____

3. List the four primary signs of the inflammatory response.

____

4. Define pain and list the general and specific types of pain.

____

5. Identify viscerally referred pain patterns.

____

6. Explain phantom pain.

____

7. List the factors influencing health.

____

8. Identify factors contributing to the stress response and the response of the body to stress.

____

9. List the stages in the cycle of life.

____

FILL IN THE BLANK

(1) _______________ is the relatively constant state maintained by the physiology of the body. (2) _______________ signals move toward a particular center or point of reference, whereas (3) _______________ signals move away from a particular center or point of reference.

(4) _______________ are the internal, periodic timing of an organism generated within the body. (5) _______________ is the synchronization of rhythms.

(6) _______________ is the study of disease. (7) _______________ disease is something present at birth not something accrued during life, whereas (8) _______________ disease is acquired naturally, not as a result of

circumstance. (9) ________________ is the study of all the factors involved in causing a disease. (10) ________________ lesion is an altered organic structure such as macules, vesicles, blebs or bullae, chancres, pustules, papules, tubercles, wheals, and tumors.

Uncontrolled cell division is (11) ________________ and can result in a (12) ________________ or abnormal growth of new tissue called a tumor. A (13) ________________ tumor is a contained and encapsulated neoplasm. (14) ________________ is the reproduction of abnormal and undifferentiated cells that fail to mature into specialized cell types. (15) ________________ is a nonencapsulated malignant cell mass that invades surrounding tissue. The cells have the devastating ability to break away from the primary tumor and form secondary cancer masses, called (16) ________________.

(17) ________________ is a protective response of the tissues to irritation or injury. The inflammatory response has four primary signs: heat, redness, swelling, and pain.

Chronic inflammation may produce a sinus or (18) ________________. A (19) ________________ is a tract leading from a cavity to the surface. (20) ________________ is an unpleasant complex, private, abstract experience. (21) ________________ pain can be a symptom of a disease condition or a temporary aspect of medical treatment. The pain acts as a warning signal, activating the sympathetic nervous system, and is usually temporary, of sudden onset, and easily localized. (22) ________________ pain persists or recurs for indefinite periods, usually for more than 6 months. The pain frequently has an obscure onset, and the character and quality of the pain change over time. The pain is usually diffuse and poorly localized.

(23) ________________ pain arises from stimulation of receptors in the skin, in which case it is called (24) ________________ somatic pain, or from stimulation of receptors in skeletal muscles, joints, tendons, and fasciae, in which case it is (25) ________________ somatic pain. (26) ________________ pain results from stimulation of receptors in the (27) ________________ or internal organs. (28) ________________ pain frequently is experienced by persons who have had a limb amputated and experience pain or other sensations in the extremity as if the limb were still there. Pain may be brought on by mechanical, electrical, thermal, or chemical stimuli.

WORKBOOK SECTION

PROBLEM SOLVING

Read the problem presented. There is no correct answer; rather the exercise assists the student in developing analytical and decision-making skills necessary in professional practice.

1. Identify the facts presented in the information.
2. Identify the possibilities presented ("what if" statements), or develop your own possibilities that relate to the facts.
3. Evaluate each possibility in terms of the logical cause and effect and pros and cons.
4. Consider the effect on the persons involved.
5. Write each answer in the space provided.
6. Develop your solution by answering the question posed.

Problem

Supporting health is a lifetime commitment. Many factors encountered in day-to-day life threaten the homeostatic mechanism of the body. Not only do inherent genetic strengths and weaknesses predispose us to disease, but also our learned behaviors influence our perception of events and can determine whether we respond with survival fight-or-flight actions. Behavior often is determined by attempting to manage stress. Sometimes the behavior is resourceful, bringing resolution to the situation or understanding that no answer to the problem exists and developing effective coping strategies. When this happens, persons feel effective, empowered, and resourceful. However, if stress is managed with unresourceful behavior, such as the use of alcohol or temper tantrums, not only does the person feel out of control but also those they interact with may feel uncomfortable, helpless, or afraid. In general, persons seem to respond to stress management better if they understand the physical, mental, and spiritual components that contribute to health and a disruption in health. If more education were provided on these topics, maybe we could learn to cope better with what seems to be the increasing stress load in our societies. If the body were better understood, maybe we would take better care of it. Regardless, the inability to cope effectively with stress is becoming a major health concern, the result of which is renewed interest in drugless approaches to dealing with stress and pain management. Such interest will likely create an environment in which bodywork methods are seen as important components in stress management programs.

Questions

What information would you need to become an effective educator about stress management methods?

The first response is provided as a guide to get you started. Fill in at least two more statements.

Facts:

1. Supporting health is a lifelong commitment.
2. ______________________
3. ______________________

Possibilities:

1. We could compromise our health by responding in ways that activate the fight-or-flight response.
2. ______________________
3. ______________________

Logical cause and effect:

1. The person may develop behaviors such as alcohol abuse.
2. ______________________
3. ______________________

Impact on persons:

1. The person may feel out of control.
2. ______________________
3. ______________________

FURTHER STUDY

Using additional resource material (see Works Consulted list at the back of this book), identify the chapters that pertain to the information presented in this chapter. As a study guide, locate the information presented in this text and elaborate by writing a paragraph of additional information on each of the following:

1. Feedback mechanism

____

____

____

____

____

____

____

____

WORKBOOK SECTION

2. Tumor development and types

3. Inflammatory response

4. Gate-control theory of pain and Melzack and Wall

5. Pain-spasm-pain cycle

6. General adaptation syndrome and Hans Selye

7. Breathing pattern disorder

8. Life cycle

Answer Key

SHORT ANSWER

1. Homeostasis is the relatively constant state maintained by the physiology of the body. Specific regulatory mechanisms constantly adjust and adapt our body systems to maintain homeostasis. The concept of balance—homeostasis—reflects the opposition of the yin/yang balance.

   In the ancient healing art of Ayurveda, an individual is made up of five primary elements. This model is similar to the five-element theory of the Asian model. When any of these elements are present in the environment, they in turn have an influence on us. Biologic systems have the ability to influence their own expression from moment to moment.

   When we genuinely experience positive emotional states, a tendency exists for the biologic rhythm to oscillate naturally together or to entrain. In addition, the entrainment process can be facilitated with specific techniques that shift conscious attention to the breath, heart, and abdomen.

   Massage and other soft tissue approaches support or stimulate homeostatic processes. Bodywork is generally nonspecific in that the stimulus disrupts the general existing homeostatic balance, requiring a response through the feedback mechanism. The objective is to reestablish homeostasis.
2. Disease is an abnormality in the functioning of the body that disrupts a person's physical, mental, or social well-being. Health is not a static condition but rather a condition of constant changes and adaptations to stress and stressors to maintain homeostasis. Health is the success of the organism to adapt continuously and effectively to change.

   Stress is any external or internal stimulus or substantial change in routine that causes the body to adapt. If a stressor acts on the body, mechanisms attempt to counteract the effects of the stress and bring the condition back to normal.

1. An abnormality in the functioning of the body, any part or system, especially when the abnormality threatens well-being
2. The study of disease
3. The study of the factors involved in causing a disease
4. The success of the organism to adapt continuously and effectively to change
5. The preparation, use, and action of prescription medications
6. Objective changes that can be seen or measured by someone other than the person
7. Subjective changes noticed or felt only by the person.
8. A group of signs and symptoms that identify a pathologic condition
9. A disease or process the signs and symptoms of which develop quickly, last a short time, and then disappear
10. Diseases or processes that develop slowly and last for a long time, sometimes for life
11. Diseases with characteristics between acute and chronic
12. Can be transmitted from one person to another
13. The pattern of the development of a disease
14. The latent stage in infectious diseases
15. The time when body functions return to normal and recovery occurs
16. A temporary or permanent reversal in chronic diseases
17. Chemicals that affect genetic activity in some way, causing abnormal cell reproduction
18. Doctor specializing in the treatment of cancer
19. The replacement of dead cells with living cells
20. New cells used for tissue repair are similar to those that they replace
21. The new cells in tissue repair are formed from connective tissue, resulting in a scar

EXERCISE

1. Genetic mechanisms, pathogenic organisms, tumors and cancer, physical and chemical agents, malnutrition, hypersensitivity, immunity, immune deficiency, inflammatory response, degeneration
2. Genetic factors, age, lifestyle, stress, environment, preexisting conditions
3. Heat, redness, pain, edema, or swelling
4. Pain is a complex, private, abstract experience, difficult to explain or describe. Pain has physiologic, psychologic, and social aspects. Types of pain are acute pain, chronic pain, intractable pain, pricking or bright pain, burning pain, aching pain, deep pain, muscle pain, somatic pain, visceral pain, and referred pain.
5. When pain is referred, it is usually to a structure that developed from the same embryonic segment or dermatome as the structure in which the pain originates.
6. A kind of pain frequently experienced by persons who have had a limb amputated. Phantom pain is suspected to occur because the remaining proximal portions of the sensory nerves that previously received impulses from the limb are being stimulated by the trauma of the amputation. Stimuli from these nerves are interpreted by the brain as coming from the nonexistent (phantom) limb.
7. Inherited and constitutional conditions, lifestyle, activity, rest, loving relationships, exercise, diet, empowering beliefs and attitudes, self-esteem, authentic personality, and freedom from self-hindering patterns
8. Stressors are extreme stimuli: too much or too little of almost anything. The three stages of the general adaptation syndrome are the first stage of alarm, the fight-or-flight response, which is the initial reaction of the body to the perceived stressor; the second stage, known as the resistance reaction, that through the secretion of regulating hormone allows the body to continue fighting a stressor long after the effects of the alarm reaction have dissipated; the third stage, the stage of exhaustion, in which the stress response continues without relief. Unfortunately, during periods of prolonged stress, glucocorticosteroids may have harmful side effects that include decreased immune response, decreased blood glucose levels, altered protein and fat metabolism, and decreased resistance to stress. Prolonged or frequent activation of the sympathetic division of the autonomic nervous system also results in increased likelihood of high blood pressure, decreased digestion, reduced tissue repair, and more.

   Persons experiencing excessive or ongoing accumulating stress often are overwhelmed by tension, anger, fear, and frustration. This results in feelings of anxiety. Adrenaline levels

WORKBOOK SECTION

rise, blood pressure and heart rate increase, and breathing changes. Overbreathing often results in overoxygenation of the blood and the reduction of carbon dioxide levels, leading to hyperventilation syndrome. Panic attacks can result. Blood levels of glucose and fatty acids rise. This combination over time leads to plaque being laid down in arteries and coronary artery disease developing. Immune function becomes less effective, and the body is not as able to deal with pathogens or cancer cells. Often a decrease in memory and the ability to concentrate or solve problems exists; susceptibility to infection increases; and complaints of stomach pain, heart palpitations, fatigue, and muscle aches are common. Sleep disorders and depression frequently accompany long-term stress. Mood and behavior are affected.

9. Conception, gestation, birth, living, dying, and death

FILL IN THE BLANK

1. Homeostasis
2. Afferent
3. efferent
4. Biologic rhythms
5. Entrainment
6. Pathology
7. Congenital
8. Inherited
9. Etiology
10. Structural
11. hyperplasia
12. neoplasm
13. benign
14. Anaplasia
15. Cancer
16. metastases
17. Inflammation
18. fistula
19. sinus
20. Pain
21. Acute
22. Chronic
23. Somatic
24. superficial
25. deep
26. Visceral
27. viscera
28. Phantom

CHAPTER 3

Medical Terminology

▼ CHAPTER OBJECTIVES

After completing this chapter, the student will be able to perform the following:

- Identify three word elements used in medical terms.
- Combine word elements into medical terms.
- Identify abbreviations used in health care and their meanings.
- Use a charting method that incorporates a clinical reasoning/problem-solving model.
- Define terms used to describe the positions of the body in relation to other body parts.
- Identify terminology from an ancient Chinese healing model.

▼ CHAPTER OUTLINE

▼ KEY TERMS

Acupuncture The practice of inserting needles at specific points on meridians, or channels, to stimulate or sedate energy flow to regulate or alter body function. A branch of Chinese medicine, acupuncture is the art and science of manipulating the flow of Qi, the basic life force, and xue, the blood, body fluids, and nourishing essences. Western medicine uses acupuncture primarily to reduce pain. Acupressure, which uses digital pressure, follows the same Asian principles.

Biomechanics The principles and methods of mechanics applied to the structure and function of the human body.

Charting The process of keeping a written record of a client or patient. The most effective charting methods follow clinical reasoning, which emphasizes a problem-solving approach. Many systems of charting are used, but these models all have similar components: POMR (problem-oriented medical record) and SOAP (subjective, objective, analysis, and plan–the four parts of the written record).

Combining vowel A vowel added between two roots or a root and a suffix to make pronunciation of the word easier.

Disharmony Distortions in health that result when the functions or systems are neither balanced nor working at their optimum. In Chinese medicine, disharmony can be created by the imbalance of the Six Pernicious Influences or the Seven Emotions.

Kinematics (kin-i-ma-tics) A branch of mechanics that involves the time, space, and mass aspects of a moving system.

Kinesiology (ki-NE-SE-ol-O-JE) The study of movement.

Kinetics (ki-ne-tics) Those forces causing movement in a system.

Mechanics The branch of physics dealing with the study of forces and the motion produced by their actions.

Prefix A word element added to the beginning of a root to change the meaning of the word.

Qi Also known as Chi, Qi refers to the life force.

Root A word element that contains the basic meaning of the word.

Suffix A word element added to the end of a root to change the meaning of the word.

Word elements The parts of a word; the prefix, root, and suffix.

Yin/yang *Yin* and *yang* are terms used to describe polar relationships. Yin/yang refers to the dynamic balance between opposing forces and the continual process of creation and destruction. Yin/yang reflects the natural order and duality of the whole universe and everything in it, including the individual.

Professionals who use anatomy and physiology must have a standard terminology. Without a common language, health care practitioners cannot communicate. Professionals have an ethical responsibility to learn to communicate with their clients in a common language, to understand and communicate across disciplines with other health professionals, and to identify with language cross-culturally to appreciate a different perspective of the anatomic map of the body. This chapter introduces the student to the basic concepts necessary to enable fluent communication in generalized medical terms, to use a clinical reasoning approach in client care, and to consider a model of cross-cultural terminology.

LANGUAGE OF SCIENCE AND MEDICINE

Most scientific and medical terms are derived from Latin and Greek fundamental **word elements,** the commonly accepted language base. These elements are combined to form medical terms. A term can be interpreted easily by separating the word into its elements: **prefix, root,** and **suffix.**

Each of the following sections includes a list of some of the more common word elements. These lists are not meant to be all-encompassing, but they provide enough examples for you to gain a general understanding of most of the terms encountered by therapeutic professionals.

Prefixes

A prefix is an element placed at the beginning of a word to change the meaning of the word. A prefix cannot stand alone; it must be combined with another word element. A vowel, called a **combining vowel,** often is used to join word elements. The combining vowel most often used is *o,* but occasionally *i* or some other vowel is used. Table 3-1 presents a list of the more common prefixes and some examples of accompanying combining vowels. These prefixes will help you recognize and understand scientific and medical terminology.

Roots

The root (or stem) word element provides the fundamental meaning of the word. Roots are combined with prefixes and suffixes to form medical and scientific terms. In medicine the root word often refers to a part of the body. As with prefixes, a combining vowel often is added when two roots are combined or when a suffix is added to a root. The combining vowel usually is *o,* but occasionally it is *i.* Table 3-2 on p. 63 presents a list of some of the more common root words and their accompanying combining vowels.

Suffixes

A suffix is a word element that is added to the end of a root to change the meaning of the word. Suffixes cannot stand alone. In interpreting scientific terms, the suffix is the starting point. Roots that end in a consonant require a combining vowel when a suffix is added. If the root ends with a vowel and the suffix begins with a vowel, the vowel at the end of the root is deleted. Table 3-3 on p. 64 presents a list of some of the more common suffixes.

The ability to use a medical dictionary is a necessary skill; the amount of information that can be found in a quality medical dictionary is amazing. The dictionary is the place to begin research or to clarify the meaning of a word or topic. With the condensed information gathered from the dictionary, the investigation can proceed. When selecting a medical dictionary, the student should look for one that is encyclopedic and illustrated. The table of contents indicates how expansive the dictionary is. The dictionary often contains a special section for medical terminology.

Activity 3-1 on p. 65 gives you a chance to create some medical terms of your own.

Abbreviations

Abbreviations are shortened forms of words or phrases. They are used primarily in written communication to save time and space. Table 3-4 on p. 65 presents a list of some abbreviations. Most medical dictionaries have a more extensive list of accepted abbreviations. In **charting** and keeping records, if you are unsure whether an abbreviation is acceptable, write the term out in full to ensure accuracy.

Activity 3-2 on p. 66 gives you a chance to put your knowledge of medical abbreviations into practice.

Using too many abbreviations creates confusion. If you use abbreviations in charting, you should provide an abbreviation key with the clinical notes. Abbreviations are not understood universally, and a key ensures accurate interpretation of your notes by the client or a fellow health care professional (Activity 3-3 on p. 67).

CLINICAL REASONING AND CHARTING

Effective assessment, analysis, and decision making are essential to meeting the needs of each client. In attempting to individualize treatment, the practitioner often finds routines or recipe-type applications of massage and bodywork treatments of limited value or even ineffective, because clients' circumstances vary so widely. The mark of an experienced professional is skill in effective reasoning.

As the volume of knowledge grows and as massage and bodywork treatments become part of the health care system,

TABLE 3-1
Common Prefixes and Their Meanings

Prefix	Meaning	Prefix	Meaning	Prefix	Meaning
A-, an-	Without or not	Febr(i, o)-	Fever, boil	Onc(o)-	Tumor, mass
Ab-	Away from	Fract-	Break, broken	Ortho(o)-	Straight, erect, correct
Acr(o)-	Extremity, tip	Fund-	Base, bottom	Osm(io, o)-	Smell, odor
Ad-	Toward	Gen-	Beginning, origin, produce	Oxy-	Sharp, acute, acid
Alba-	White	Gluc-	Sweet, sugar, glucose	Palp-	Touch, feel
Ambi-	Both, on sides	Gyn(a, e, eco, o)-	Female	Pan-	All
Ana-	Upward, backward, excessive, through	Hemi-	Half	Para-	Abnormal, near
Andr(o)	Male	Heter-	Other, different	Path(o)-	Disease, suffering
Ankyl(o)-	Crooked, fused, stiff	Hol-	Whole, all	Pept(o)-	Digestion
Ante-	Before, forward	Hom(eo, o)-	Unchanged, alike, same	Per-	By, through
Anti-	Against, opposed	Hyg(ei, ie)-	Health	Peri-	Around
Audi-	Hear	Hyper-	Excessive, too much, high	Phag(o)-	Eat, consume
Auto-	Self	Hypo-	Under, decreased, less than normal	Pharmaco-	Drugs, poison, medication
Bi-	Double, two	Iatr(o)-	Physician	Physio-	Natural, physical agents
Bio-	Life, living matter	Idio-	Distinct, peculiar to the individual	Poly-	Many, much
Brach-	Short	Immuno-	Protection	Post-	After, behind
Brady(o)-	Slow, short, dull	In-	In, into, within, not	Pre-	Before, in front of, prior to
Carcin(o)-	Cancer, malignant	Infra-	Beneath	Pro-	Before, in front of
Cata-	Down, negative, under, against, lower	Inter-	Between	Pseudo-	False
Caud-	Tail, inferior	Intra-	Within	Quadr(a, i)-	Four
Cent(i)-	Hundred	Intro-	Into, within	Re-	Again
Chron(i, o, us)-	Time, long time	Iso-	Equal, like, identical	Retro-	Backward
Circum-	Around	Juxta-	Adjoining, near to	Schist(o)-	Split, divided
Contra-	Against, opposite	Kyph(o)-	Bend, hump	Scler(o)-	Hard
Counter-	Against, opposite	Lact(o)-	Milk	Semi-	Half
Cry(mo, o)	Cold	Later(al, o)-	Side	Sepsi-	Putrid, rotten
De-	Down, from, away from, not	Leuk-	White	Son(o)-	Sound
Dext-	Right	Levo-	Left	Steno-	Contracted, narrow
Di-	Two, double, twice	Macro-	Large	Strat(i)-	Layer
Dia-	Across, through, apart	Mal-	Bad, illness, disease	Sub-	Under
Dis-	Separation, away from	Mega-	Large	Super-	Above, over, excess

TABLE 3-1—cont'd

PREFIX	MEANING	PREFIX	MEANING	PREFIX	MEANING
Dys-	Bad, difficult, abnormal	Micro-	Small	Supra-	Above, over
Ecto-	Outer, outside	Mono-	One, single	Therm-	Warm
En-	In, into, within	Morph(o)-	Form, shape	Tort(i, o)-	Twisted
Endo-	Inner, inside	Multi-	Many	Tract-	Pull down
Epi-	Over, on, upon	Necr(o)-	Death, destruction, corpse	Trans-	Across
Eryth-	Red	Neo-	New	Ultr(a, o)-	Excessive, extreme, beyond
Esthesi-	Sensation	Noct(i, o)-	Night	Uni-	One
Etio-	Cause	Non-	Not	Zyg(o, us)-	Yoke, join, together
Ex-	Out, out of, from, away from	Olig-	Small, scanty		

Modified from Fritz S: *Mosby's fundamentals of therapeutic massage,* ed 3, St Louis, 2004, Mosby.

the practitioner will find it increasingly important to be able to think through an intervention process and to justify the effectiveness of a massage intervention. Clinical reasoning skills enable massage practitioners to be able to gather information effectively, analyze the information and determine the type or appropriateness of a therapeutic intervention, and evaluate and justify the benefits derived from the intervention. This skill has to be learned.

Charting is the process of keeping a written record of professional interactions. Effective charting is more than writing down what happened. Charting represents a clinical reasoning methodology that emphasizes a problem-solving approach to client care. Clinical problems are varied and not necessarily related to dysfunction; rather the problem involves how to achieve therapeutic outcomes for the massage.

To reason clinically and chart effectively, a practitioner must have a comprehensive knowledge of medical terms, abbreviations, and anatomy and physiology in balanced and altered states of functioning. Assessment procedures identify deviations from the effective and normal functioning. Information obtained during the assessment serves as the basis for developing a care plan, identifying any contraindications to therapy, and evaluating the need for referral.

A commonly used method of charting is the problem-oriented medical record (POMR) as reflected in the process of (SOAP) *subjective* data from the client, *objective* data from observation, palpation or other form of *assessment* and *analysis* of the data, and *planning* guidelines for the next session. In this method, the written account of the health assessment is divided into four parts for clarity and completeness.

Because the method is based on an analytic process, after one has learned it, the method can be adapted easily to any other charting method. The key point is the ability to reason through a massage session rationally and comprehensively. A charting method can provide a structure for and a record of the process.

Any problem-solving charting method must begin with a database, which is collected before the process of identifying the client's problems and goals actually has begun. The **database** consists of all the information available that contributes to therapeutic interaction and can be divided into two parts, which are created with information obtained from a history-taking interview with the client and other pertinent persons, prior records, health care treatment orders (subjective), and the physical assessment (objective).

The first part of the database, the history-taking interview, provides information about the client's health history and the reason for the visit, a descriptive profile of the client, a history of the client's current condition, a history of past illness and health, and a history of family illness. The history also contains an account of the client's current health practices.

The physical assessment makes up the second part of the database. The extent and depth of this assessment vary from setting to setting, practitioner to practitioner, and according to the client's situation. Practitioners of therapeutic massage generally use some sort of visual assessment to look for bilateral symmetry and deviations. Functional assessment reveals restricted, exaggerated, painful, or otherwise altered movement patterns. Palpation is used to identify changes in tissue texture and temperature, to locate energy changes, and to identify areas of tenderness. Various manual tests may be used to distinguish soft tissue problems from other conditions, such as joint dysfunction.

After collecting the information, the practitioner analyzes it. The practitioner identifies goals to be achieved, problems to be addressed, and outcomes of the massage based on a conclusion or decision that results from examination, inves-

TABLE 3-2
Common Root Words and Their Meanings

Root (Combining Vowel)	Meaning	Root (Combining Vowel)	Meaning	Root (Combining Vowel)	Meaning
Abdomin(o)-	Abdomen	Hemat(o)-	Blood	Psych(o)-	Mind
Aden(o)-	Gland	Hepat(o)-	Liver	Pulm(o)-	Lung
Adren(o)-	Adrenal gland	Hydr(o)-	Water	Py(o)-	Pus
Angi(o)-	Vessel	Hyster(o)-	Uterus	Rect(o)-	Rectum
Arteri(o)-	Artery	Ile(o)-, ili(o)-	Ileum	Rhin(o)-	Nose
Arthr(o)-	Joint	Laryng(o)-	Larynx	Salping(o)-	Eustachian tube, uterine tube
Bronch(o)-	Bronchus, bronchi	Mamm(o)-	Breast, mammary gland	Splen(o)-	Spleen
Card-, cardi(o)-	Heart	Mast(o)-	Mammary gland, breast	Sten(o)-	Narrow, constriction
Cephal(o)-	Head	Men(o)-	Menstruation	Stern(o)-	Sternum
Chondr(o)-	Cartilage	My(o)-	Muscle	Stomat(o)-	Mouth
Col(o)-	Colon	Myel(o)-	Spinal cord, bone marrow	Therm(o)-	Heat
Cost(o)-	Rib	Nephr(o)-	Kidney	Thorac(o)-	Chest
Crani(o)-	Skull	Neur(o)-	Nerve	Thromb(o)-	Clot, thrombus
Cyan(o)-	Blue	Ocul(o)-	Eye	Thyr(o)-	Thyroid
Cyst(o)-	Bladder, cyst	Ophthalm(o)-	Eye	Tox(o)-	Poison
Cyt(o)-	Cell	Orth(o)-	Straight, normal, correct	Toxic(o)-	Poison, poisonous
Derma-	Skin	Oste(o)-	Bone	Trache(o)-	Trachea
Duoden(o)-	Duodenum	Ot(o)-	Ear	Ur(o)-	Urine, urinary tract, urination
Encephal(o)-	Brain	Ped(o)-	Child, foot	Urethr(o)-	Urethra
Enter(o)-	Intestines	Pharyng(o)-	Pharynx	Urin(o)-	Urine
Fibr(o)	Fiber, fibrous	Phleb(o)-	Vein	Uter(o)-	Uterus
Gastr(o)-	Stomach	Pnea-	Breathing, respiration	Vas(o)-	Blood vessel, vas deferens
Gloss(o)-	Tongue	Pneum(o)-	Lung, air, gas	Ven(o)-	Vein
Gyn-, gyne-, gynec(o)-	Woman	Proct(o)-	Rectum	Vertebr(o)-	Spine, vertebrae
Hem-, hema-, hem(o)-	Blood				

Modified from Fritz S: *Mosby's fundamentals of therapeutic massage,* ed 3, St Louis, 2004, Mosby.

tigation, and analysis of the data collected. The practitioner then makes a decision on a care or treatment plan, recording at each session any action taken, its effectiveness, and the outcome.

You should remember that not all therapeutic goals relate to dysfunction. Clients commonly use therapeutic massage to maintain health, manage stress, and fulfill pleasure needs. The same analytic process is used to determine the methods that best meet the client's goals.

With the SOAP charting method, the following pattern is used:

S Subjective information from the client
O Objective data from inspection, palpation, and testing and a record of interventions performed

TABLE 3-3
Common Suffixes and Their Meanings

SUFFIX	MEANING	SUFFIX	MEANING	SUFFIX	MEANING
-able	Capable of, suitable for	-graph	Diagram, recording instrument	-phylaxis	Protection
-ago	Disease	-graphy	Making a recording	-plasty	Surgical repair or reshaping
-algesia	Pain	-hood	State, quality of, condition	-plegia	Paralysis
-algia	Pain	-iasis	Condition of	-pnea	To breathe
-ase	Enzyme	-ician	One skilled in, one who practices	-porosis	Passage
-asis	State or condition of, usually abnormal	-ism	Condition	-ptosis	Falling, sagging, dropping, down
-cele	Hernia, herniation, pouching	-itis	Inflammation	-rrhage, -rrhagia	Excessive flow
-cide	Kill, causing death	-ity	Quality of, state of	-rrhea	Profuse flow, discharge
-cule	Very small	-ive	Having power to, that which performs	-sclerosis	Dryness, hardness
-cyte	Cell	-ize	To treat by a special method	-scoliosis	Curvature, crooked
-dom	State of being	-kinesis	Motion	-scope	Examination instrument
-duct	Tube, channel	-lemma	Sheath, covering	-scopy	Examination using a scope
-eal	Pertaining to	-logy	The study of	-sepsis	Putrefaction
-ease	Condition	-lysis	Destruction of, decomposition	-some	Body
-ectasis	Dilation, stretching	-malacia	Softening	-stasis	Maintenance, maintaining a constant level
-ectomy	Excision, removal of	-megaly	Enlargement	-stenosis	Narrow, tighten, short, constrict
-ema	Swelling, distention	-oid	Form, like, resemble	-stomy, -ostomy	Creation of an opening
-emesis (one of the few suffixes that can stand alone)	Vomiting	-oma	Tumor	-thymia	Thymus gland, mind, soul, emotions
-emia	Blood condition	-opsy	View of	-tomy, -otomy	Incision, cutting into
-ferent	Bear, carry	-osis	Condition	-tonia	Stretching, putting under tension
-feron	To strike	-otomy	Cutting into	-trophic	Related to growth, development, or nutrition
-form	Shape, structure	-paresis	Paralysis	-ule	Little, small
-genesis	Development, production, creation	-pathy	Disease	-uria	Condition of the urine
-globin	Protein	-penia	Lack, deficiency	-version	To turn
-gram	Record	-phobia	An exaggerated fear	-vert	Turn

Modified from Fritz S: *Mosby's fundamentals of therapeutic massage*, ed 3, St Louis, 2004, Mosby.

ACTIVITY 3-1

The beauty of medical terminology is that it allows new words to be created as needed. From the lists of prefixes, root words, and suffixes, make up five silly words and define them.

Example
Oligorhinoscoliosis: oligo, small; rhino, nose; scoliosis, curve

Your Turn

A Analysis or assessment of the subjective and objective data and analysis of the effectiveness of the intervention, methods used, and action taken during the session

P Plan, including the methodology for future intervention and the progress of the sessions

S and *O* are the data-collecting (fact-gathering) parts of the SOAP method. The *A*, or analysis, part of the SOAP method is perhaps the most complex of the four parts. Detailed steps in that process are presented next.

Step 1

What are the facts gathered from the data collection from the client and research about the situation presented?

What is considered normal or balanced function?

What has happened? (Spell out the events.)

What caused the imbalance? (Can the cause be identified?)

What was done or is being done?

What has worked or not worked?

TABLE 3-4
Common Abbreviations and Their Meanings

Abbreviation	Meaning	Abbreviation	Meaning	Abbreviation	Meaning
ABD	Abdomen	Dx	Diagnosis	OTC	Over the counter
ADL	Activities of daily living	ext	Extract	P	Pulse
ad lib	As desired	ft	Foot (or feet)	PA	Postural analysis
alt dieb	Every other day	fx	Fracture	PM, pm	Afternoon
alt hor	Alternate hours	GI	Gastrointestinal	PT	Physical therapy
alt noct	Alternate nights	GU	Genitourinary	Px	Prognosis
AM, am	Morning	h, hr	Hour	R	Respiration, right
a.m.a.	Against medical advice	H_2O	Water	R/O	Rule out
ANS	Autonomic nervous system	Hx	History	ROM	Range of motion
approx	Approximately	IBW	Ideal body weight	Rx	Prescription
as tol	As tolerated	ICT	Inflammation of connective tissue	SOB	Shortness of breath
BM	Bowel movement	id	The same	SP, spir	Spirit
BP	Blood pressure	L	Left, length, lumbar	Sym	Symmetric
Ca	Cancer	lig	Ligament	T	Temperature
CC	Chief complaint	M	Muscle, meter, myopia	TLC	Tender loving care
c/o	Complains of	ML	Midline	Tx	Treatment
CPR	Cardiopulmonary resuscitation	meds	Medications	URI	Upper respiratory infection
CSF	Cerebrospinal fluid	n	Normal	WD	Well developed
CVA	Cerebrovascular accident, stroke	NA	Nonapplicable	WN	Well nourished
DJD	Degenerative joint disease	OB	Obstetrics		
DM	Diabetes mellitus				

ACTIVITY 3-2

Using the abbreviations in Table 3-4, decipher the message below. (The answers can be found on p. 94.)

Your Turn

In the am ________ evaluate Hx ________
and ADL ________. Use this information ad lib ________ to CC ________
of GI ________ and ABD ________
meds ________. Use ROM ________
as tol ________ on the h ________
as PT ________ on the ft ________
to assist R ________. Monitor T ________
and P ________ in the pm ________
and provide H_2O ________ and TLC ________
as requested for OB ________ clients.

Step 2
What are the possibilities? (What could all the information mean?)
What does my intuition suggest?
What are the possible patterns of dysfunction?
What are the possible contributing factors?
What are possible interventions?
What might work?
What are other ways to look at the situation?
What do the data suggest?
Step 3
What is the logical progression of the symptom pattern, contributing factors, and current behaviors?
What are the logical cause and effect of each intervention identified?
What are the pros and cons of each intervention suggested?
What are the consequences of not acting?
What are the consequences of acting?
Step 4
For each intervention under consideration, what would be the effect on the persons involved: the client, the practitioner, and other professionals working with the client?
How does each person involved feel about the possible interventions?
Is the practitioner within the scope of practice to work with such a situation?
Is the practitioner qualified to work with such a situation?
Does the practitioner feel confident to work with such a situation?
Does a feeling of cooperation and agreement exist among all parties involved?

The *P*, or plan, section of the SOAP method involves the development and implementation of a care or treatment plan. After the analysis has been completed, a decision must be made on what will be involved in the care or treatment plan. The plan is not an exact protocol set in stone but rather a guideline. After implementing the plan, the practitioner reevaluates and adjusts it as necessary.

SOAP may be summarized as follows:

S and *O* are the facts obtained during data collection and what was done during the session.
A is the analysis of the data from *S* and *O* and research in terms of possibilities, logical cause and effect, consequences, and effect on the persons involved.
P is the decision making and implementation structure.

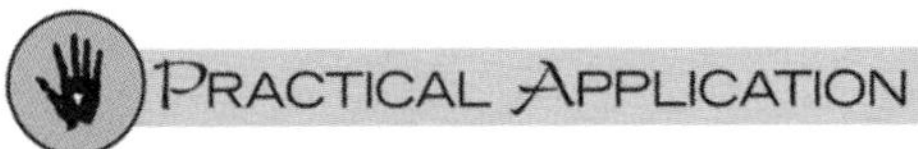

The ability to apply what is learned from the study of anatomy and physiology comes from the reasoning and problem-solving processes. With this skill the information acquired becomes alive and practical. Effective work with clients is a continual learning process of assessing, deciding on interventions, and analyzing effectiveness through evaluation of progress from session to session. Even in the most basic sessions, when the client's goals are pleasure and relaxation, the practitioner must decide on the best way to encourage the body to respond to meet the client's goals. ■

To use the information collected from the subjective and objective assessment, the practitioner must be able to collect data from client, history, assessment, and any necessary research; analyze the data; and make decisions about what the data mean and what patterns are represented in the whole person. Because of the amount of information involved and because most human difficulties are multidimensional, involving body, mind, and spirit, all areas must be addressed, although not necessarily by the same practitioner. Assessment and analysis may indicate a need to refer the client elsewhere or to use a team approach, working in a multidisciplinary cooperative effort to provide the best possible care for each client. Effective practice and ethical behavior require a practitioner to stay within the competencies of a professionally defined scope of practice and a personal level of training, expertise, and experience.

Effective communication among client, practitioner, and fellow professionals serving the client is essential. A continuing written record provides the means for sharing information. The use of a model for information gathering and decision making as found in various forms of POMR, SOAP, or a similar format is important. The terms of anatomy and physiology often become the common language base among health disciplines, and these terms also are relevant in cross-discipline and cross-cultural sharing of knowledge.

This textbook has been developed on a logical reasoning model. A model is a pattern to imitate. See if you can identify the reasoning model through the exercises and activities that

ACTIVITY 3-3

Using the list in Table 3-4, as well as lists from a medical dictionary and your own imagination, develop a key for abbreviations you plan to use the most.
Hint: Think in terms of symptoms, anatomic locations, methods and techniques, directional terms, body movement patterns, assessment, and referrals. As your learning progresses, you may want to expand this list.
Some examples have been provided to help you get started.

Example
Symptoms
ACP: Acupuncture point
CFS: Chronic fatigue syndrome
HA: Headache
TP: Trigger point

Your Turn

Example
Anatomic Locations
L-5: Fifth lumbar
LB: Low back
SI: Sacroiliac

Your Turn

Example
Methods and Techniques
CTM: Connective tissue massage
DP: Direct pressure
EB: Energy balance
MET: Muscle energy technique
MLD: Manual lymph drainage
SH: Self-help
STM: Soft tissue manipulation
XFF: Cross-fiber friction

Your Turn

Example
Directional Terms
ant: Anterior
L: Left
R: Right
sup: Superior

Your Turn

Example
Body Movement Patterns
flex: Flexion
ROM: Range of motion
SB: Side bending

Your Turn

Example
Assessment
inter: Intermittent
PB: Pain behavior
WNL: Within normal limits

Your Turn

Example
Referrals
AP: Acupuncturist
DC: Doctor of chiropractic
MD: Medical doctor

Your Turn

encourage analysis and reasoning. Imitating a model is a good way to begin a learning process. After the student understands the model and can use it effectively, the student can vary the model as necessary to provide the best response to each set of circumstances. A model is a tool, not an absolute (Activity 3-4).

GENERAL STRUCTURAL PLAN OF THE BODY

When you look at a map, you see that the layout of the map is fairly universal. North usually is placed at the top. A legend identifies how many miles are indicated per inch, and symbols indicate types of roads and landmarks. So the location of body areas is also universal. The map of the body begins with the body in the anatomic position (Figure 3-1).

The following information provides the basic knowledge needed to read the body map and give accurate descriptions to guide others around the body.

Regions of the Body and Surface Anatomy

Regional terms are used to designate specific areas of the body (Activity 3-5 on p. 71). The student should carefully study the diagram and chart shown in Figure 3-2, *A* on p. 72, and complete the exercise in Figure 3-2, *B* on p. 73.

Structural Plan

The structural organization of the body follows a clear plan. All human beings have a vertebral column that supports the trunk and determines the central axis of the body. The spine also supports two body cavities: the dorsal cavity, which holds the brain inside the skull and the spinal cord in the vertebral column, and the ventral cavities, which is the combined thoracic, abdominal, and pelvic cavity (sometimes referred to as the abdominopelvic cavity). Human beings are bilaterally symmetric beings with left and right mirror images. Also, the body is segmented; this is most obvious in the vertebral column, ribs, and spinal cord. The body is designed as a tube within a tube. The digestive system is a tube that lies within the greater tube of the trunk (Figures 3-3 and 3-4 on p. 74).

Terms Related to the Structural Plan

The following terms are used to describe the structural plan of the body:

Soma, somato: Root words that mean the body, as distinguished from the mind. Somatic organs and tissues are associated with the skin and skeleton (e.g., bone and skeletal muscles, extremities, and the body wall) and often can be controlled voluntarily.

Axial: Areas or organs along the central axis of the body, including the head, neck, trunk, brain, spinal cord, and abdominal organs.

Appendicular: The limbs, joined to the body as lateral appendages.

Torso, trunk: Structures related to the main part of the body, including the chest, abdomen, and vertebral cavity. The head and limbs are attached to the trunk.

Posterior Region of the Trunk

The two dorsal cavities are located toward the back of the body. They are as follows:

Cranial cavity: This cavity is found in the skull and contains the brain and related structures.

Vertebral cavity: The vertebral cavity extends from the base of the cranial cavity and contains the spinal cord.

The back or posterior surface of the trunk is divided into regions named for the corresponding vertebrae in the spinal column.

Cervical region: The neck (seven cervical vertebrae)

Thoracic region: The chest (twelve thoracic vertebrae)

Lumbar region: The loin (five lumbar vertebrae)

Sacral region: The sacrum (five sacral vertebrae fused into one bone)

Coccyx: The tailbone (four coccygeal vertebrae fused into one bone)

Anterior Region of the Trunk

Ventral cavities are located in the trunk. They include the following:

The *thoracic cavity,* also known as the chest, is found between the neck and the diaphragm and is surrounded by the ribs. The mediastinum is a part of the thoracic cavity in the middle of the thorax, between the pleural sacs containing the two lungs.

The *abdominal cavity*, or the belly, is located below the diaphragm and is enclosed within the abdominal muscles. This cavity contains the liver, kidneys, spleen, pancreas, stomach, and intestines.

The *pelvic cavity* is found inferior to the abdomen, inside the pelvic bones, and contains a portion of the large intestine, the bladder, and the internal reproductive organs.

The *viscera* are internal organs of the thoracic, abdominal, and pelvic cavities that are considered to be under involuntary control.

Two types of *membranes* are associated with the regions of the trunk: parietal membranes line the body cavities and visceral membranes cover the visceral organs.

Abdominal Quadrants and Regions

The abdomen is divided into four quadrants and nine regions, the names of which are used to describe the location of body structures, pain, or discomfort. The four quadrants are the right upper quadrant, left upper quadrant, right lower quadrant, and left lower quadrant (Figure 3-5, *A* on p. 74). The nine regions are the right hypochondriac, epigastric, left hypochondriac, right lumbar, umbilical, left lumbar, right iliac, hypogastric, and left iliac regions (Figure 3-5, *B* on p. 74).

ACTIVITY 3-4

Synthesize the section just completed on charting and clinical reasoning by answering the following questions. A shortened version of the analysis process is provided for this activity. There is no correct answer; rather the exercise is intended to assist the student in developing the analytical and decision-making skills necessary in a professional practice. Each section has an example to help you get started.

Step 1

1. What are the facts?
2. What has worked or not worked?

Example

1. Charting is written communication (fact).
2. To chart effectively, a practitioner needs a knowledge base of medical terms and abbreviations and of anatomy and physiology (fact).

Your Turn

Give three more facts about charting and clinical reasoning.

Step 2

1. What are the possibilities?
2. What does my intuition suggest?
3. What are other ways to look at the situation?
4. What does the data suggest?

Example

1. I may need to take a medical terminology class.
2. My instincts suggest that learning about assessment procedures is important.
3. I may need to be careful not to become too analytical.
4. The information suggests that further investigation of problem solving could be helpful.

Your Turn

Give three more possibilities.

Step 3

1. What are the pros and cons?
2. What are the consequences of acting or not acting?

Example

1. The pros of charting include having a continuous log of progress.
2. A consequence of not charting would be a lack of information for reference or for other professionals.

Your Turn

Give three more consequences.

Step 4

1. What would be the effect on the persons involved: client, practitioner, and other professionals working with the client? Does a feeling of cooperation and agreement exist among all parties?

Example

1. I would feel burdened with the paperwork and frustrated because of my spelling, but the client would feel a sense of caring.

Your Turn

Give three more effects on the persons involved.

Plan

Now that you have analyzed this information, write down your decisions on charting and problem solving and then develop an implementation plan based on that decision.

Example

I have come to the conclusion that charting is important and that I need to learn more about it. I want to explore methods other than SOAP. I will need to research charting procedures, and a logical place to begin would be nursing or psychologic charting systems. I will go to the library and check information on the computer about charting methods.

Your Turn

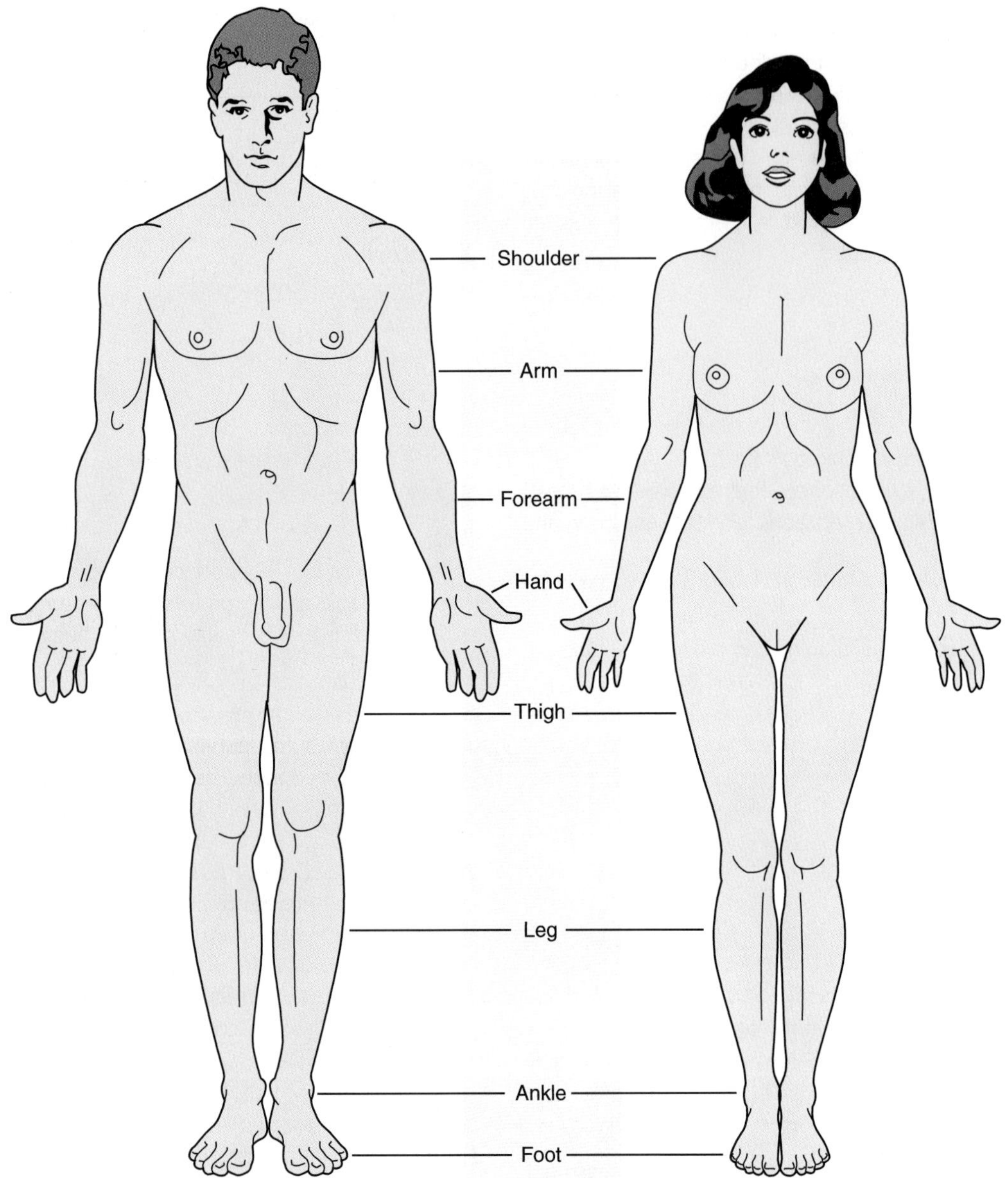

Figure 3-1
Anatomic position. The person is standing upright, facing forward, feet slightly separated, arms hanging at the sides with palms facing forward. Structures are named and their positions are described in this standard position.

Positions of the Body

Anatomic position is a term used in Western medicine to describe the position of the body and the location of its regions and parts. The central axis of the body passes through the head and trunk.

Terms related to the position of the body include the following:

Anatomic position: The body stands upright with the feet slightly apart, arms hanging at the sides, palms facing forward, thumbs outward (Figure 3-1).

Functional position: The body stands upright with the feet slightly apart, arms hanging at the sides, palms facing sides of body, thumbs forward.

Erect position: The body standing.

Supine position: The body lies horizontally with the face up (Figure 3-6, *A* on p. 75).

Prone position: The body lies horizontally with the face down (Figure 3-6, *B* on p. 75).

Lateral recumbent position: The body lies horizontally on the right or left side (Figure 3-6, *C* on p. 75).

Body Planes and Movements

The body can be divided into sections with imaginary lines and the various planes to identify the areas created (Figure 3-7 on p. 76).

Movements are described as beginning in or returning to the anatomic position. Movement terms define the action as the body part passes through the various planes.

ACTIVITY 3-5

Stand in front of a mirror and identify each landmark and point of surface anatomy and body region. Say the words out loud.

Write one sentence describing what it feels like to be your own anatomy model.

Example

I felt silly pointing at my body.

Your Turn

Repeat the exercise with a partner. Wearing a swimsuit or exercise wear that exposes more of the surface of the body is helpful.

Write one sentence about what it feels like to be an anatomy model.

Example

The same body parts can look somewhat different on two persons.

Your Turn

The sagittal plane is a vertical plane that divides the body into left and right. A midsagittal plane divides the body into equal left and right parts; a parasagittal plane divides it into unequal left and right parts.

The frontal (coronal) plane also runs vertically but divides the body into anterior and posterior (front and back) parts.

A transverse plane divides the body horizontally into two sections, described as superior (meaning above) and inferior (meaning below). The transverse plane runs perpendicular to the frontal and sagittal planes.

Movement

By definition, **kinesiology** is the study of movement. Kinesiology brings together the study of anatomy, physiology, physics, and geometry to understand human movement. Kinesiology uses principles of **mechanics,** musculoskeletal anatomy, and neuromuscular physiology. Mechanical principles that relate directly to the human body are used in the study of **biomechanics.** This may involve looking at the static (nonmoving) or dynamic (moving) systems associated with various activities. Dynamic systems can be divided into **kinetics** and **kinematics.** Kinetics are those forces causing movement, whereas kinematics are those time, space, and mass aspects of a moving system. A movement that takes a part of the body forward from the anatomic position within a sagittal plane is called flexion; movement backward is called extension.

Movements in a frontal plane that take a part of the body toward the midline are called adduction; movements away are called abduction. Lateral flexion or side bending of the head, neck or trunk also takes place in the frontal plane. A movement in a transverse plane that takes a part of the body away from the midline is called lateral rotation; movement inward is called medial rotation (Figure 3-8 beginning on p. 77).

Movement Terms

The following terms are commonly used to describe movement:

Flexion: A decrease in the angle between two bones as the body part moves out of the anatomic position; flexion is a sagittal plane movement.

Extension: An increase in the angle between two bones, usually moving the body part back toward the anatomic position; extension is a sagittal plane movement.

Hyperextension: The term may be defined two ways: (1) any extension beyond normal or healthy or (2) any extension that takes the part farther in the direction of the extension, farther out of the anatomic position.

Abduction: Movement of the appendicular body part away from the midline; abduction is a frontal plane movement.

Adduction: Movement of the appendicular body part toward the midline; adduction is a frontal plane movement.

Right lateral flexion: Movement of the axial body part to the right; right lateral flexion is a frontal plane movement.

Left lateral flexion: Movement of the axial body part to the left; left lateral flexion is a frontal plane movement.

Right rotation: Partially turning or pivoting the axial body part in an arc around a central axis to the right; right rotation is a transverse plane movement.

Left rotation: Partially turning or pivoting the axial body part in an arc around a central axis to the left; left rotation is a transverse plane movement.

Medial rotation: Partially turning or pivoting a body part of the appendicular body in an arc around a central axis toward the midline of the body; medial rotation is a transverse plane movement.

Lateral rotation: Partially turning or pivoting a body part of the appendicular body in an arc around a central axis away from the midline of the body; lateral rotation is a transverse plane movement.

Circumduction: Circumduction is not a movement, rather it is a sequence of movements that turn or pivot the part through an entire arc, making a complete circle. (Note: Circumduction involves no rotation and is a multiplanar movement.)

Protraction: Pushing of the part forward in a horizontal plane.

Retraction: Pulling of the part back in a horizontal plane.

Elevation: Moving the part upward (superiorly).

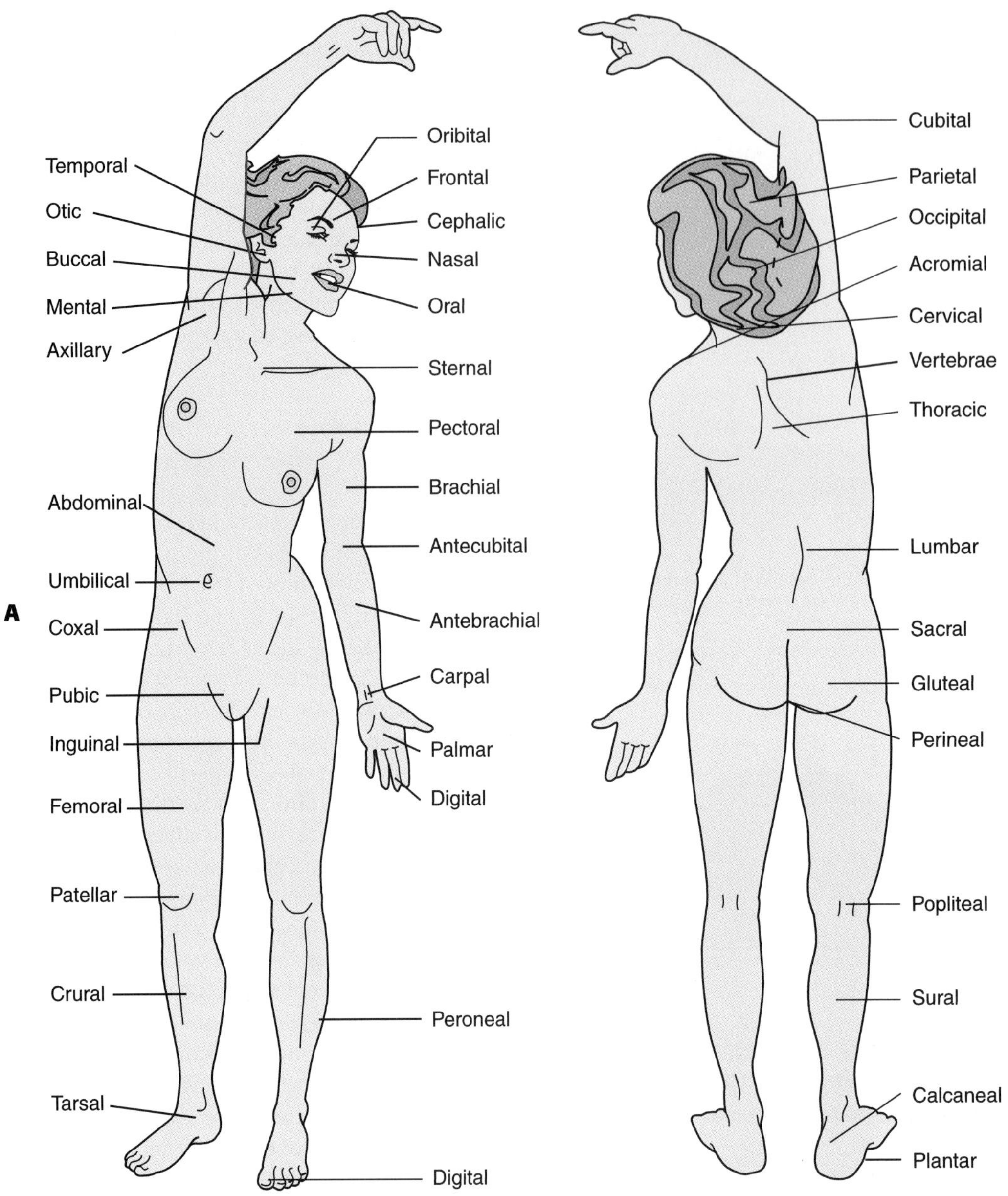

Figure 3-2
A, Anatomic regions and surface anatomy.

Depression: Moving the part downward (inferiorly).
Supination: Movement of the forearm (at the radioulnar joint, not the elbow joint) that turns the palm anteriorly (upward), as in cupping a bowl of soup.
Pronation: Movement of the forearm (at the radioulnar joint, not the elbow joint) that turns the palm posteriorly (downward).
Inversion: Movement of the sole of the foot inward, toward the midline.
Eversion: Movement of the sole of the foot outward, away from the midline.
Plantar flexion: Movement of the foot downward (may also be called flexion).
Dorsiflexion: Movement of the foot upward (may also be called extension).

Directional Terms

Certain terms are used to describe the relationship of one body position to another (Figure 3-9). The following directional terms, which are organized in pairs of opposites, are derived from some of the prefixes listed in this chapter:
Anterior (ventral): In front of or toward the front
Posterior (dorsal): Behind, in back, or in the rear
Proximal: Closer to the trunk or the point of origin (usually used on the appendicular body only)
Distal: Situated away from the trunk or midline of the body; away from the origin (usually used on the appendicular body only)
Lateral: On or to the side, outside, away from the midline
Medial: Relating to the middle, center, or midline
Ipsilateral: The same side

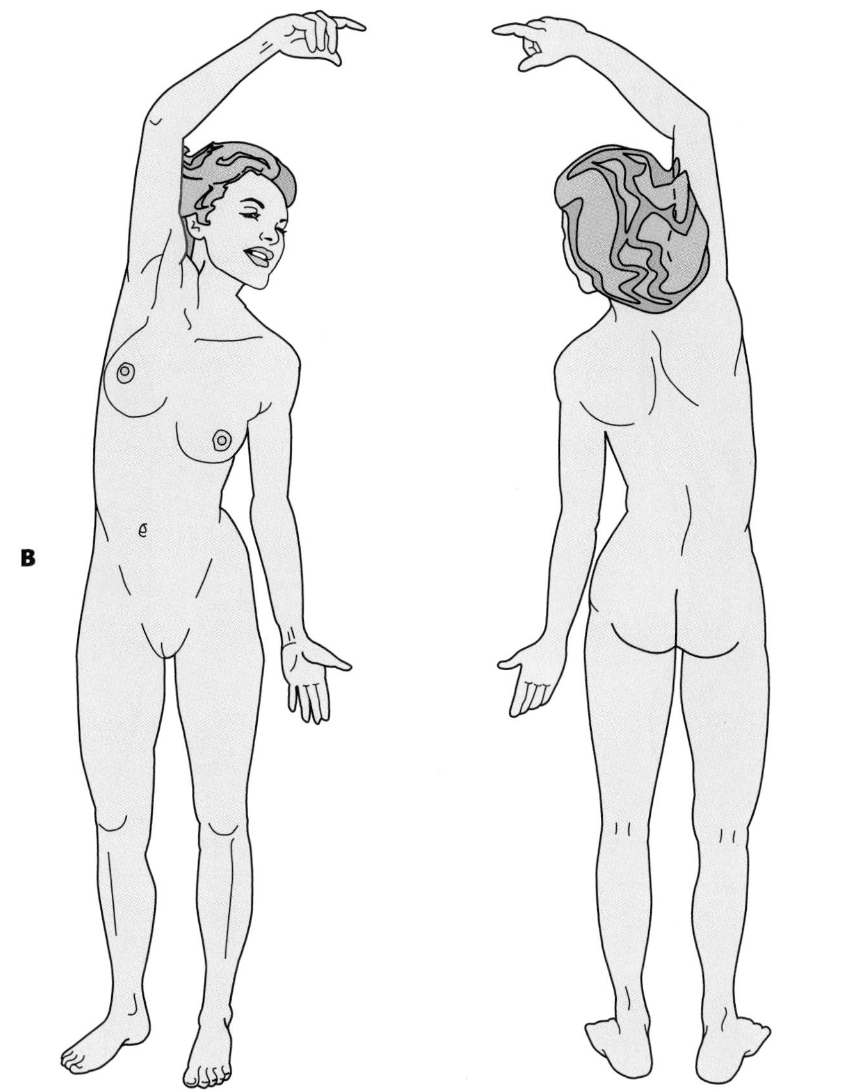

Figure 3-2, cont'd.
B, Anatomic region exercise.

Contralateral: The opposite side
Superior: Higher than or above (usually used on the axial body only)
Inferior: Lower than or below (usually used on the axial body only)
Volar (palmar): The palm side of the hand
Plantar: The sole side of the foot
Varus: Ends bent inward; angulation of a part of the body inward toward the midline: ><
Valgus: Ends bent outward; for example, bent toward the wall: <>
Internal: An inside surface or the inside part of the body
External: The outside surface of the body
Deep: Inside or away from the surface
Superficial: Toward or on the surface
Dextral (dextro): Right
Sinistral (sinistro): Left; levo also is used for left.

Ancient Healing Practices

Western science is a relatively new healing method, one that requires the practitioner to observe, measure concrete entities, accumulate data, and analyze findings in a clinical manner. Western science has a particular language. Medical terminology described in this chapter discusses the aspect of this language. Ancient approaches to healing also have a specific language and require observation, measurement, and accumulation and analysis of data, but in addition they validate the importance of intuition.

Intuition is defined as knowing something without going through a conscious, problem-solving, rational process of thinking. According to researcher and scientist Hans Selye, nothing can be investigated or validated scientifically unless

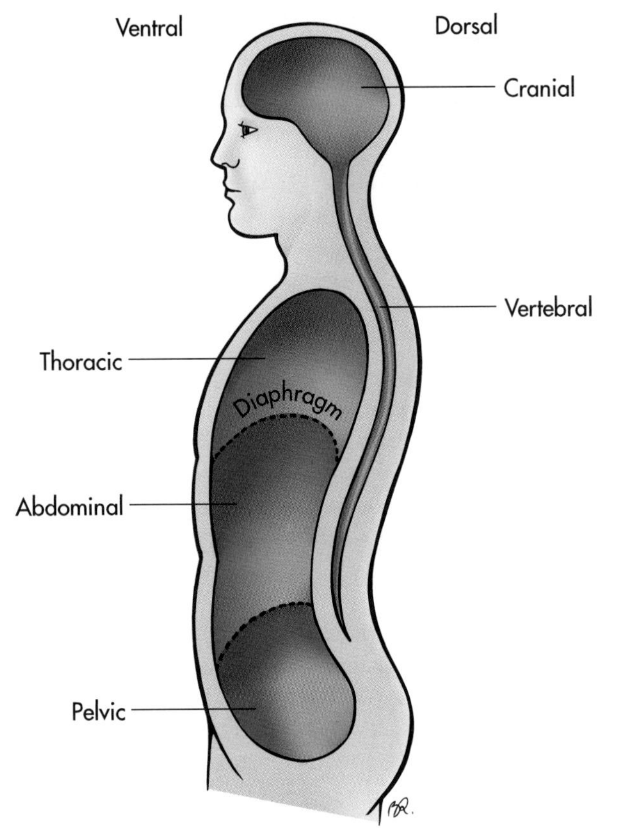

Figure 3-3
Body cavities. (From Fritz S: *Mosby's fundamentals of therapeutic massage,* ed 3, St Louis, 2004, Mosby.)

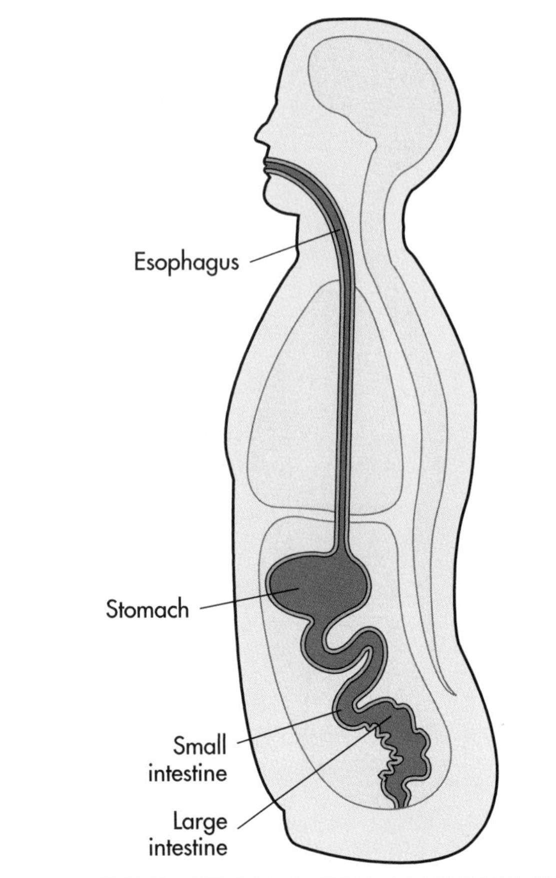

Figure 3-4
The body as a tube within a tube.

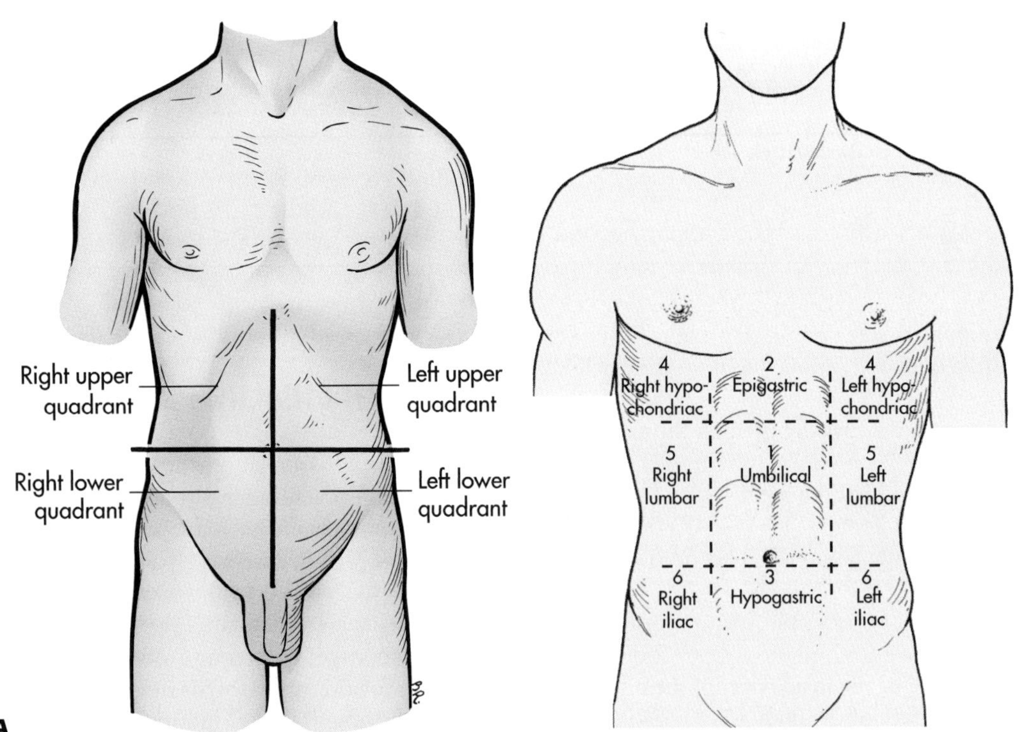

Figure 3-5
A, Quadrants of the abdomen. **B,** Anatomic abdominal regions. (**A** from Fritz S: *Mosby's fundamentals of therapeutic massage,* ed 3, St Louis, 2004, Mosby. **B** from LaFleur-Brooks M: *Exploring medical language: a student-directed approach,* ed 5, St Louis, 2002, Mosby.)

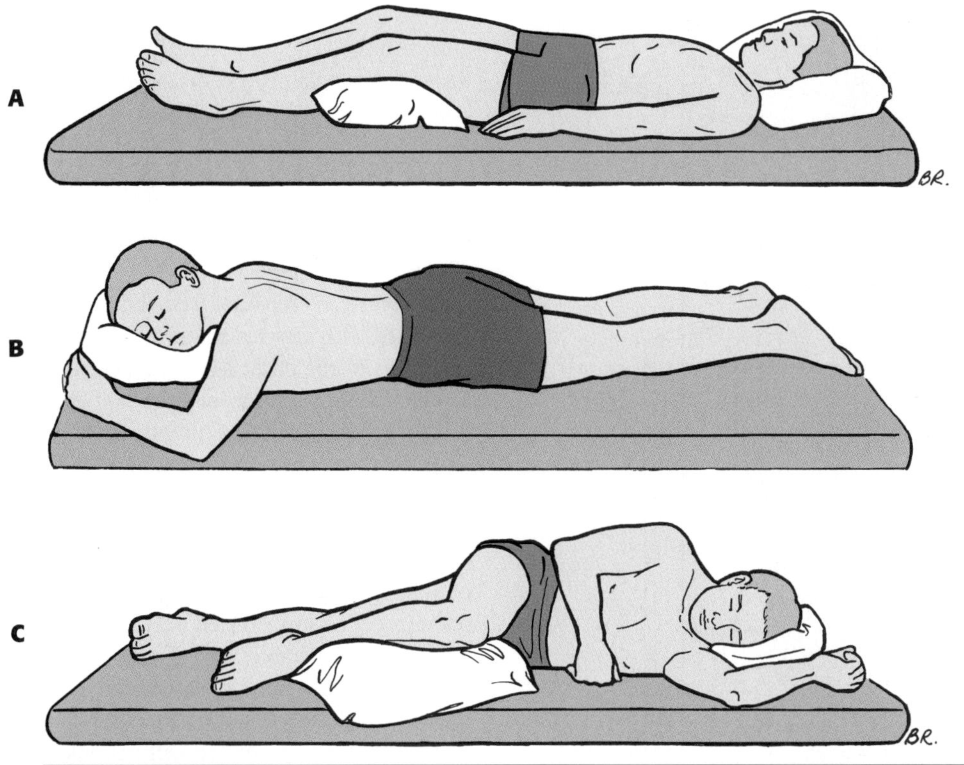

Figure 3-6
Positions of the body. **A,** Supine. **B,** Prone. **C,** Lateral recumbent. (From Fritz S: *Mosby's fundamentals of therapeutic massage,* ed 3, St Louis, 2004, Mosby.)

the researcher first has an idea, that is, uses intuition. Without validation the chances for practical application are limited. Ancient or indigenous healing practices do not separate the body, mind, and spirit as Western science does. Spiritual knowledge is knowledge based on intuition—that is, knowledge without material or concrete proof—and Western science until recently discounted anything that did not fit within the narrow boundaries of scientific validation. Today, technology and advances in research design are revealing the validity of the more subtle aspects of ancient healing wisdom. The gap between ancient and new knowledge is narrowing, and with this development comes the need to understand the terminologies involved in the different ways of describing the same thing.

As previously mentioned, the general structural plan of the body can be mapped out with standard descriptions and Western terminology. Each of the other healing systems also maps the body, using its own standards and terms, many of which are familiar to those who practice bodywork. These theories do not separate the body from the emotions or the mind. Western mind/body medicine is developing along similar lines.

The Chinese health system is one of the most ancient and is based on continual accumulation of knowledge through centuries of experiential observation. The system is similar to other cultural healing systems, which also endeavor to promote health by working toward homeostasis rather than by eliminating symptoms (a Western approach). Watching these older healing theories being "discovered" and explored and then become understood by Western science is exciting. As these systems move closer together in understanding, we all will benefit from the sharing and blending of all types of human knowledge.

The Asian perspective is based on the meridian system. **Acupuncture** points and the five-element relationship system are used to identify and explain anatomic and physiologic functions.

The **yin/yang** concept, which was discussed in the previous chapter, is an excellent example of the Asian perspective. In this chapter, we present more specific terminology for the meridian system and five-element theory (Activity 3-6).

In the past, treatments used to aid survival and recovery from trauma were mostly a matter of luck and chance. Some believe that before the advent of pain-relieving drugs or treatments, a person would press, rub, or hit an affected part of the body to alleviate pain. Sometimes when a person was burned, bruised by a stone, or cut, preexisting pain would dissipate and healing would occur. The earliest concept of acupuncture was to stimulate a painful point by pressing on it, puncturing it, or burning it. The point was referred to as an *Ah shi* point, which loosely translates to "Ah, yes, that's where it hurts." In Western science this method of treatment can be explained by the gate-control theory.

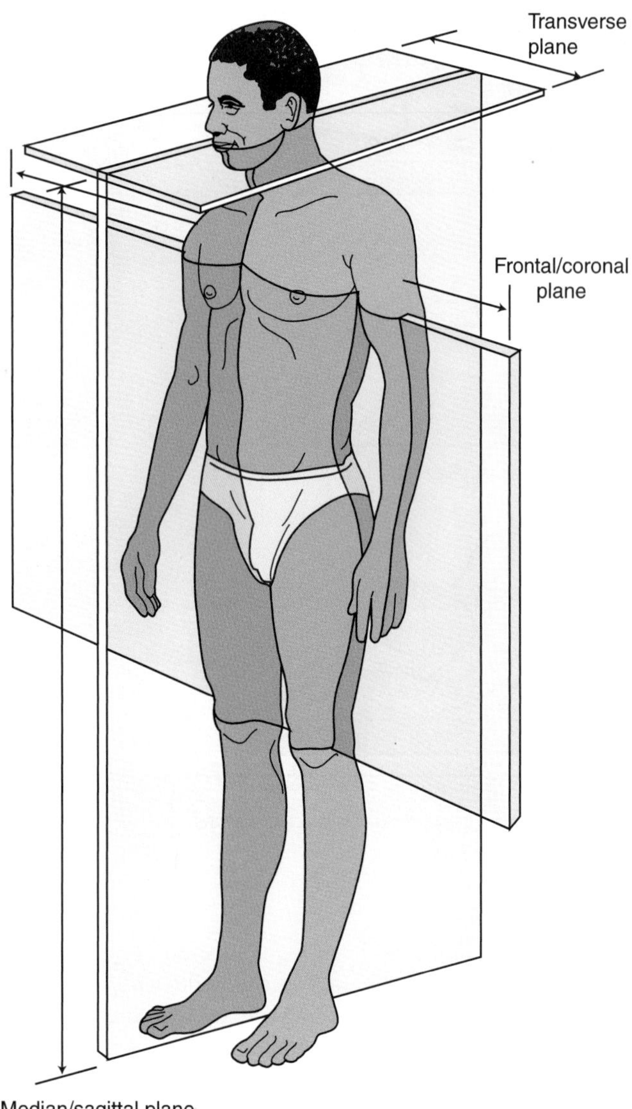

Figure 3-7
Anatomic planes.

ACTIVITY 3-6

List three areas in which ancient healing wisdom merges with current health practices.

Example
Breathing rhythm patterns with biofeedback and relaxation training

Your Turn

1. ______________________________

____

2. ______________________________

____

3. ______________________________

____

Healers identified specific points before they recognized any patterns. The mapping of points eventually developed into various healing systems. Meridians are then a system of connecting points that affect a particular physiologic function. The actual tracts of each meridian were determined by plotting the various sensations that radiate above or below a point when it is pressed (Figure 3-10 on p. 82). In the past the points used most were those located below the elbow and the knee.

In Western science, acupuncture points have been identified with various anatomic or physiologic locations or functions in the body. Many acupuncture points have been associated with the motor points of the nervous system. A motor point is the location where a nerve enters a muscle. Acupuncture points also correspond to Golgi tendon organs and muscle stretch receptors. These same acupuncture points have been shown to have a close correlation to the trigger points and corresponding pain patterns. A trigger point is a localized area of deep tenderness and increased tissue resistance. Pressure exerted on a trigger point causes referred pain in a predictable area (Figure 3-11 on p. 84). Ancient practitioners may have observed the referred pain pattern as they mapped the meridians. Pressure on acupuncture points also affects the levels of dynorphins, enkephalins, and endorphins (pain- and mood-modulating opiate-like chemicals in the body), which block transmission of pain signals along nerve fibers. Ayurveda also uses a point system. These points, called marmas, are clustered around joints and also have a high location correlation to meridians, acupuncture points, and trigger points.

Point phenomena in the ancient and Western scientific systems have many commonalities; for example, they all share the following characteristics:

1. They are located in a palpable depression.
2. They are associated with a neurovascular formation consisting of free nerve endings, Golgi tendon receptors, spindle cells, pacinian corpuscles, and lymph or blood vessels that pass through the fasciae.
3. They are located on the surface of alpha and delta fiber afferent fast-transmitting receptors sensitive to sharply pointed stimuli or heat. These points may correlate to the acupuncture points.
4. They are deep to the alpha and delta fibers in the same area; they have intramuscularly placed, C afferent slow-transmitting fibers, which are more sensitive to chemicals and may correlate to the trigger point.

Mapping of 100 acupuncture points showed them to be located over large nerve trunks and cutaneous neurovascular bundles.

In less technical terms, points stimulated to create a body change are located in the same area on top of nerves (Activity 3-7 on p. 85). The more superficial nerves may be the acupuncture points, and the deeper nerves may be the trigger points (Chaitow, 1997) (Figure 3-12).

Particular effects may be demonstrated following acupuncture treatment. Some of these effects involve the alteration of the function of organs or systems. An analgesic

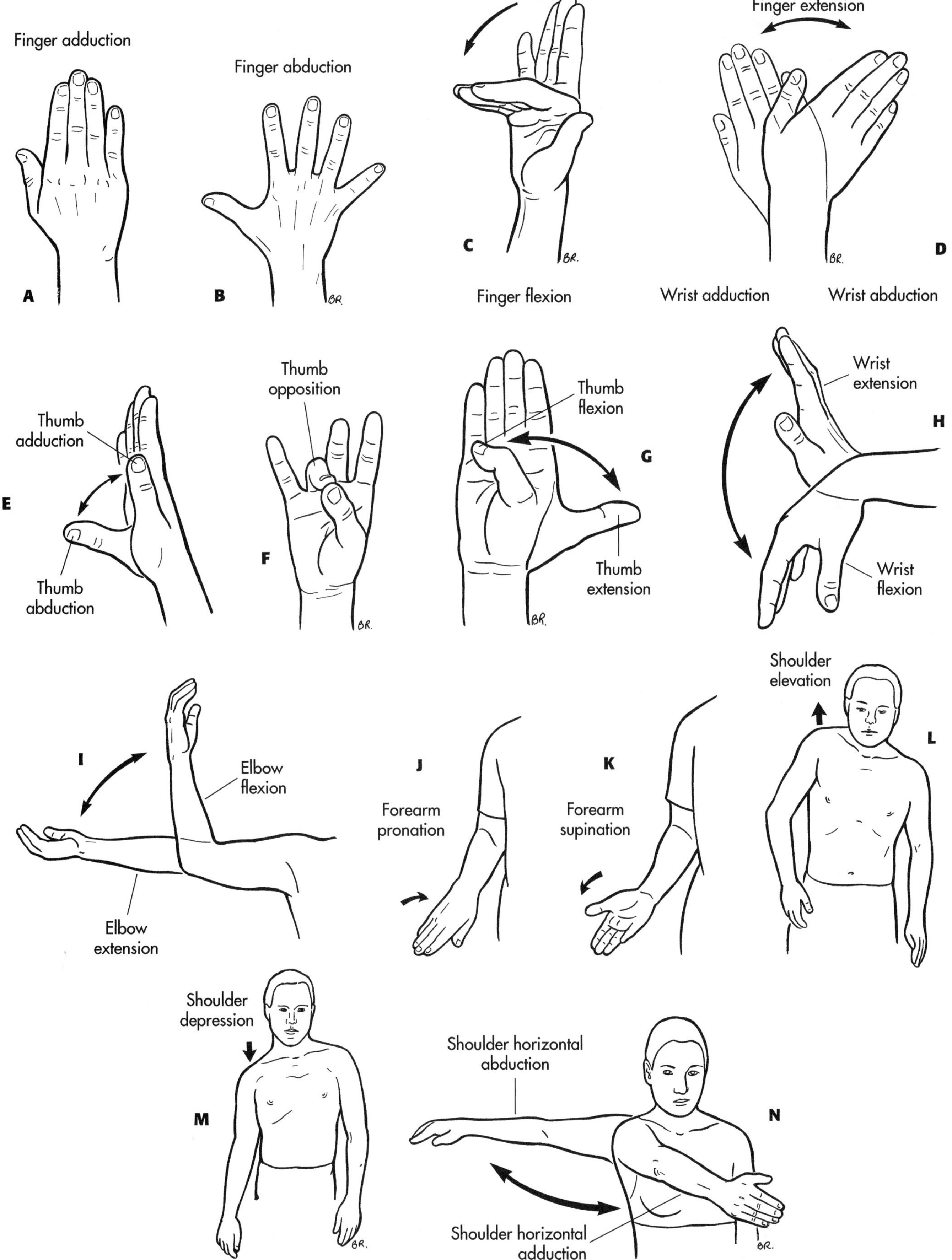

Figure 3-8
Body movements. (**A** through **GG** from Fritz S: *Mosby's fundamentals of therapeutic massage,* ed 3, St Louis, 2004, Mosby.)

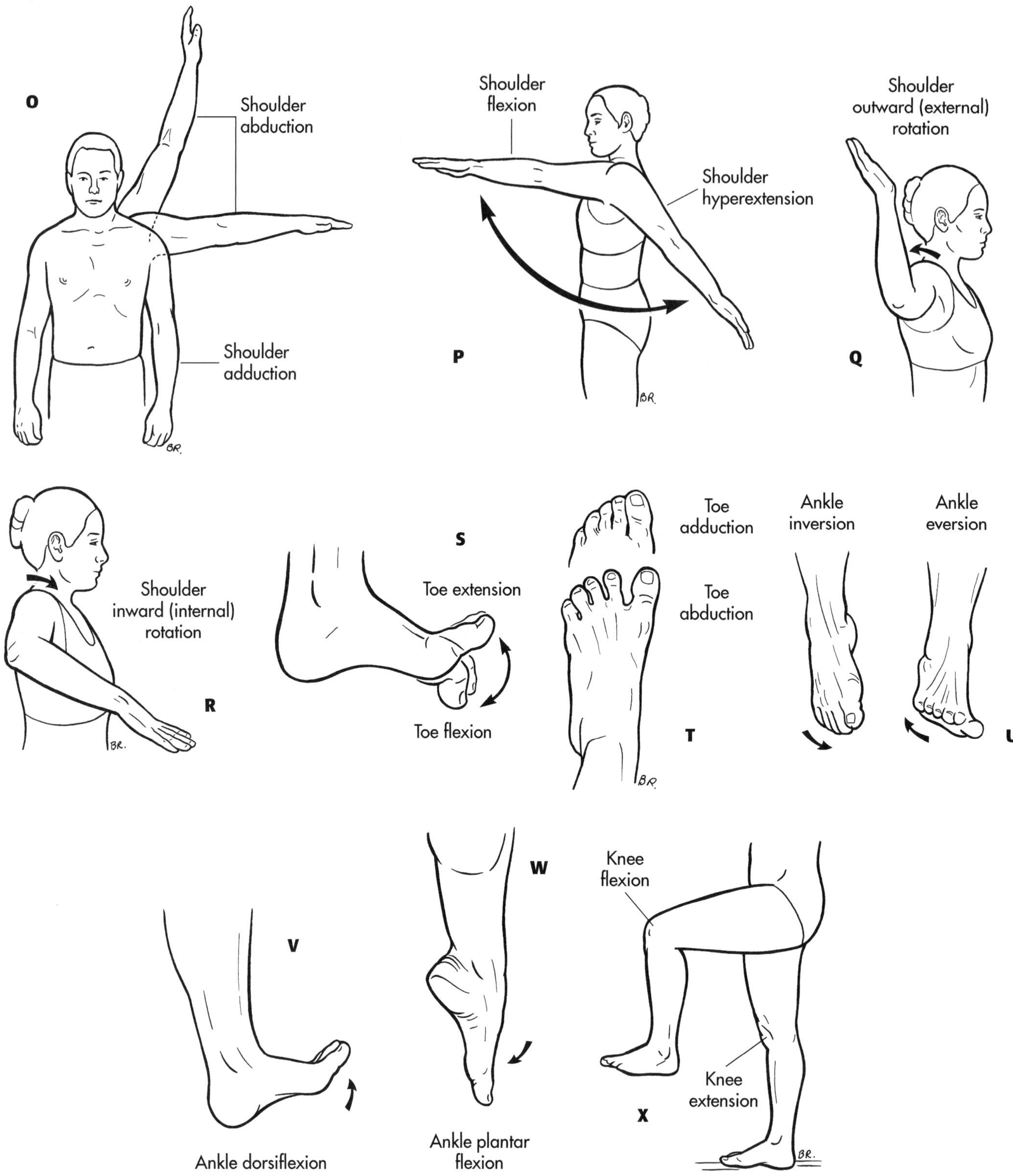

Figure 3-8, cont'd.

effect and also an anesthetic effect occur. The reflexes involved may not yet be explained fully. In China, acupuncture was used in combination with herbal medicine, dietetic regimens, and psychologic guidance. The use of finger-pressure on an acupuncture point has been demonstrated successfully to induce the desired feeling of soreness and fullness that is a forerunner of the anesthetic effect. Electrophysiologic studies showed that deep pressure applied to muscles and tendons had a definite inhibitory effect on the unit discharge of neurons in the nonspecific nucleus of the thalamus.

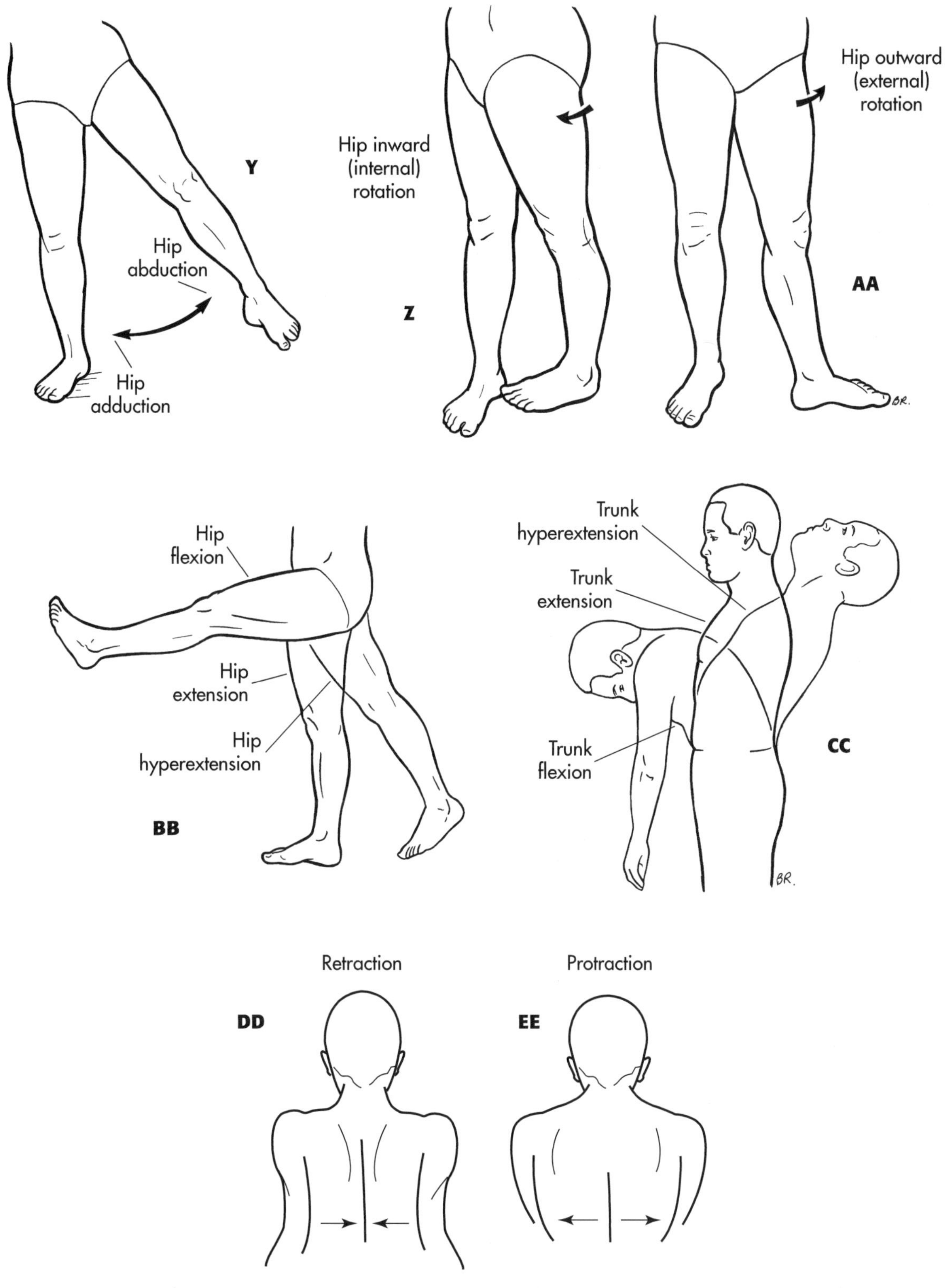

Figure 3-8, cont'd.

Because the body strives toward health, it uses all helpful stimuli to that goal. If through acupuncture or manual pressure (acupressure) this function can be assisted, the homeostatic interplay of organ systems will carry on the work to the extent possible at that time. By correcting the imbalance between yin and yang (the two equal and opposite forces of the universe which act through **Qi**), the homeostatic tendency of the body is supported, whereby a stable internal environment is maintained through the interaction of the various body processes and systems.

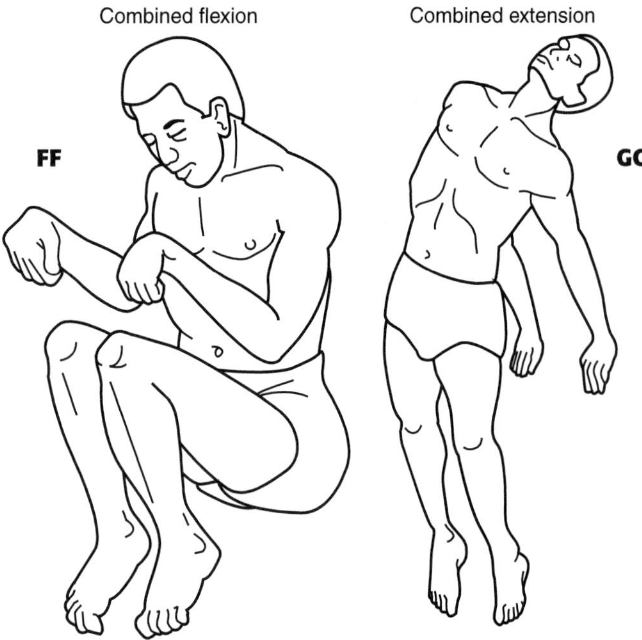

Figure 3-8, cont'd.

Points and Meridians

The patterns that acupuncture points make on the surface of the body have been charted by practitioners of acupuncture for centuries. They have been grouped together in lines (called channels or meridians) and have been allocated to the organs or functions on which they appear to act. In addition to the twelve pairs of bilateral meridians, two meridians lie on the anterior and posterior midline of the trunk and head, and various extrameridians also exist that appear to relate to the organs and functions of the body. Other points in the ear surfaces, the hands, and the face have specific reflex effects.

These 12 main meridians are bilateral, symmetrically distributed lines of acupuncture points with affinity for or effects on the functions or organs for which they are named (Figure 3-12 on p. 85). They are as follows:

1. The *lung meridian* (L; yin) begins on the lateral aspect of the chest, in the first intercostal space, and then passes down the anterolateral aspect of the arm to the root of the thumbnail.
   11 points
   Pathologic symptoms: Fullness in the chest, cough, asthma, sore throat, colds, chills, and aching of the shoulders and back.
2. The *large intestine* (LI; yang) meridian starts at the root of the fingernail of the first finger and passes up the posterolateral aspect of the arm over the shoulder to the face, ending at the side of the nostril.
   20 points
   Pathologic symptoms: Abdominal pain, diarrhea, constipation, nasal discharge, and pain along the course of the meridian.
3. The *stomach* (ST; yang) meridian starts below the orbital cavity; runs over the face and up to the forehead from where it passes down the throat, the thorax, and the abdomen; and continues down the anterior thigh and leg to end at the root of the second toenail (lateral side).
   45 points
   Pathologic symptoms: Bloat, edema, vomiting, sore throat, and pain along the course of the meridian.
4. The *spleen* (SP; yin) meridian originates at the medial aspect of the great toe and then travels up the internal aspect of the leg and thigh to the abdomen and thorax, where it finishes on the axillary line in the sixth intercostal space.
   21 points
   Pathologic symptoms: Gastric discomfort, bloat, vomiting, weakness, heaviness of the body, and pain along the course of the meridian.
5. The *heart* (H; yin) meridian begins in the axilla and runs down the anteromedial aspect of the arm to end at the root of the little fingernail (medial aspect).
   9 points
   Pathologic symptoms: dry throat, thirst, cardiac area pain, pain along the course of the meridian.
6. The *small intestine* (SI; yang) meridian starts at the root of the small fingernail (lateral aspect) and then travels up the posteromedial aspect of the arm and over the shoulder to the face, where it terminates in front of the ear.
   19 points
   Pathologic symptoms: Pain in lower abdomen, deafness, swelling in the face, sore throat, and pain along the course of the meridian.
7. The *bladder* (B; yang) meridian starts at the inner canthus and ascends and passes over the head and down the back and the leg to terminate at the root of the nail of the little toe (lateral aspect).
   67 points
   Pathologic symptoms: Urinary problems, mania, headaches, eye problems, and pain along the course of the meridian.
8. The *kidney* (K; yin) meridian starts on the sole of the foot and ascends the medial aspect of the leg and runs up the front of the abdomen to finish on the thorax, just below the clavicle.
   27 points
   Pathologic symptoms: Dyspnea, dry tongue, sore throat, edema, constipation, diarrhea, motor impairment and atrophy of the lower extremities, and pain along the course of the meridian.
9. The *circulation* (C; yin) meridian (also known as heart constrictor or pericardium) begins on the thorax lateral to the nipple, runs down the anterior surface of the arm, and terminates at the root of the nail of the middle finger.
   9 points

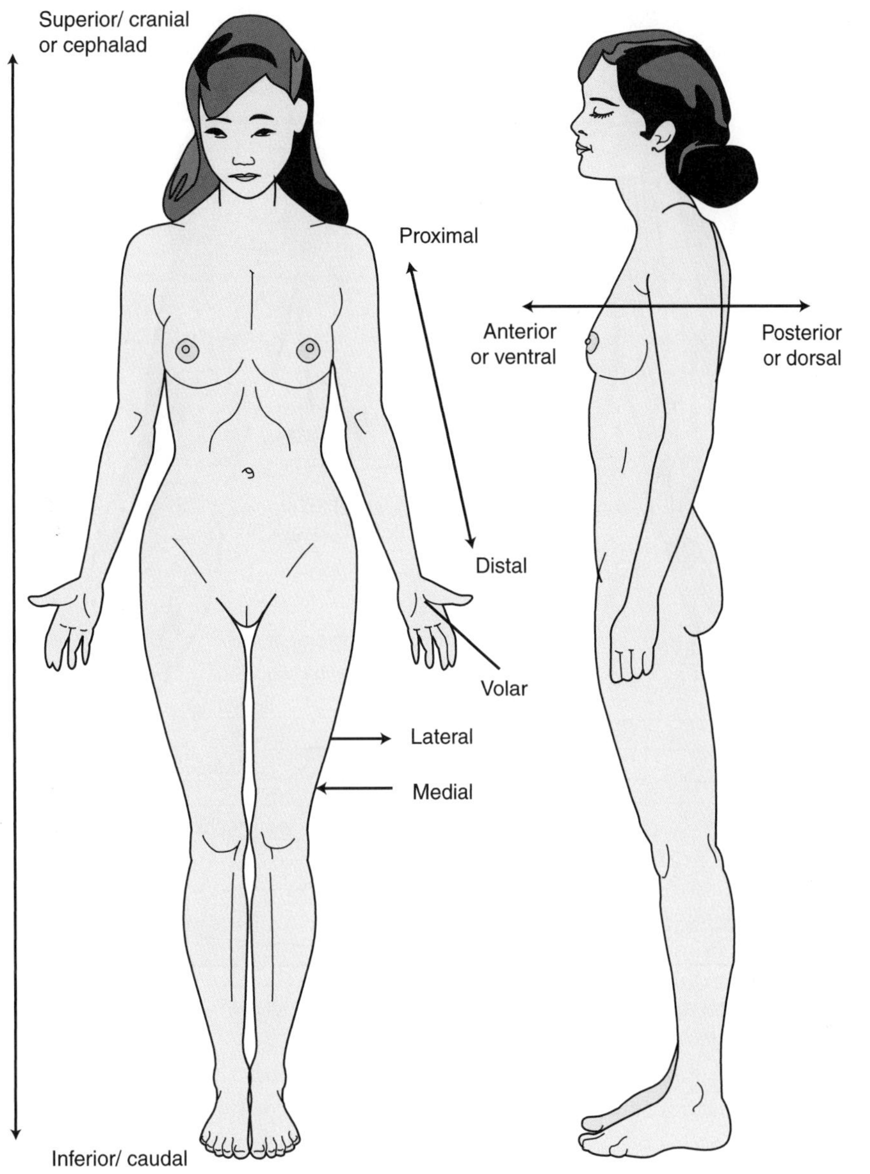

Figure 3-9
Directional terms.

Pathologic symptoms: Angina, chest pressure, heart palpitations, irritability, restlessness, pain along the course of the meridian.

10. The *triple-heater* (TH; yang) meridian begins at the nail root of the ring finger (ulnar side) and runs up the posteromedial aspect of the arm, over the back of the shoulder, and around the ear to finish at the outer aspect of the eyebrow.
    23 points
    Pathologic symptoms: Abdominal distortion, edema, deafness, tinnitus, sweating, sore throat, and pain along the course of the meridian.
11. The *gallbladder* (GB; yang) meridian starts at the outer canthus and runs backward and forward over the head, passing over the back of the shoulder and down the lateral aspect of the thorax and abdomen. The meridian passes to the hip area and then down the lateral aspect of the leg to terminate on the fourth toe.
    44 points
    Pathologic symptoms: Bitter taste in mouth, dizziness, headache, ear problems, and pain along the course of the meridian.
12. The *liver* (LIV; yin) meridian begins on the great toe, runs up the medial aspect of the leg and up the abdomen and terminates on the costal margin (vertically below the nipple).
    14 points
    Pathologic symptoms: Lumbago, digestive problems, retention of urine, pain in lower abdomen, and pain along the course of the meridian.

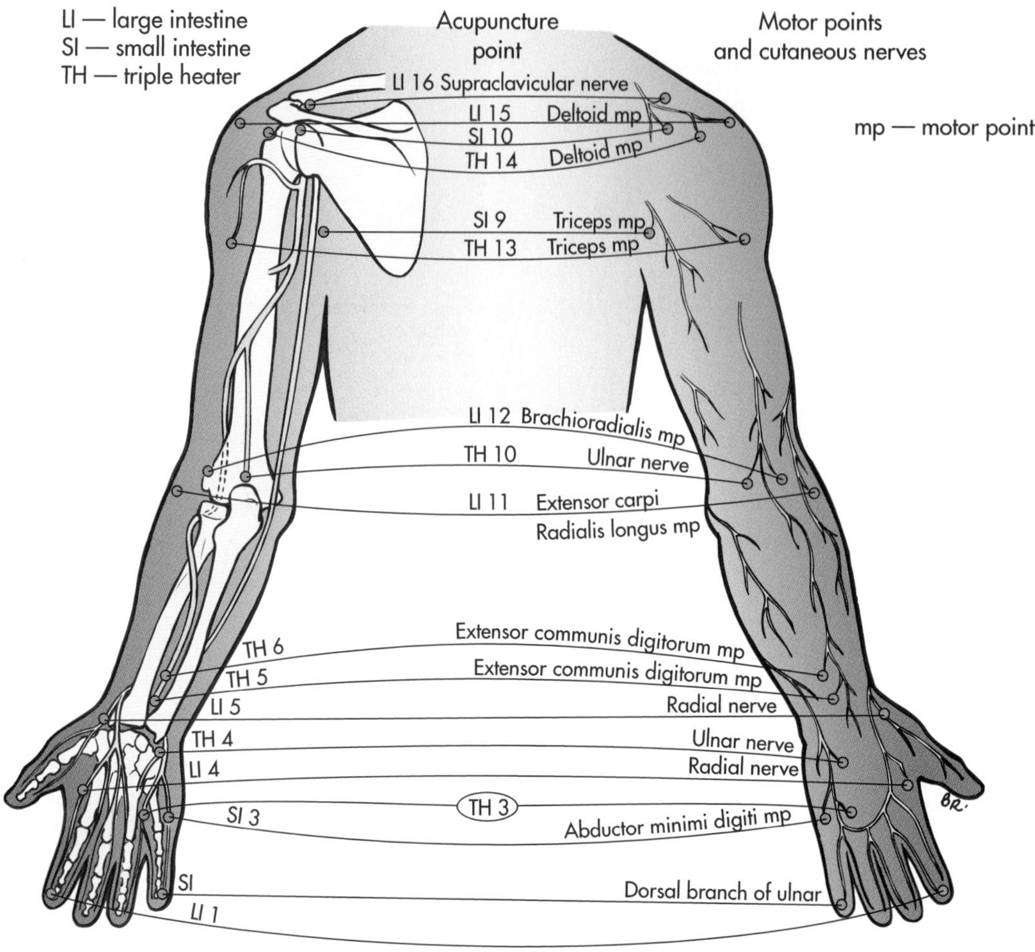

Figure 3-10
Comparison of traditional acupuncture points, median points, and cutaneous nerves of the arm and leg. (From Fritz S: *Mosby's fundamentals of therapeutic massage,* ed 3, St Louis, 2004, Mosby.)

Midline Meridians

The body has two midline meridians. The conception or central vessel (CV; yin) meridian starts in the center of the perineum and runs up the midline of the anterior aspect of the body to terminate just below the lower lip and is responsible for all yin meridians (24 points); the governing vessel (GV; yang) meridian starts at the coccyx and runs up the center of the spine and over the midline of the head and terminates on the front of the upper gum and is responsible for all yang meridians (28 points).

If we remove from the acupuncture/meridian phenomenon the concepts of yin and yang and of vital energy or life force (Qi), the explanation provided by neuroanatomy and neurophysiology remains partial. Western research has so far produced no great breakthrough in our understanding of acupuncture.

Sufficient evidence has been acquired regarding acupuncture to explain many of the effects as being neurohumoral chemical mechanisms.

For now, science is beginning to understand the basic concepts of Asian health practices: shu-xue, Qi, and yin-yang. Studying and understanding the Chinese system more fully is helpful for the therapeutic massage student because historic and current Chinese medicine has an important influence on massage practice.

In traditional Chinese medicine this system of points and meridians is known as jing luo, which usually is translated into English as either "meridians" or "channels and network vessels."

Jing Luo

The channels and network vessels or meridian system form an essential feature of the human body. The jing luo comprises the network of routes for the circulation of Qi and blood. Through this network the entire body is interconnected: the viscera, bowels, the extremities, upper and lower, interior and exterior, and all parts of the body are brought into communication with one another. The jing luo joins the tissues and organs of the body into an organic whole. The word *jing* means "warp; channels; longitude; manage; constant, regular; scripture, classic; pass through." The word *luo* means "something that resembles a net; the subsidiary channels; to hold something in place with a net; to wind or twine."

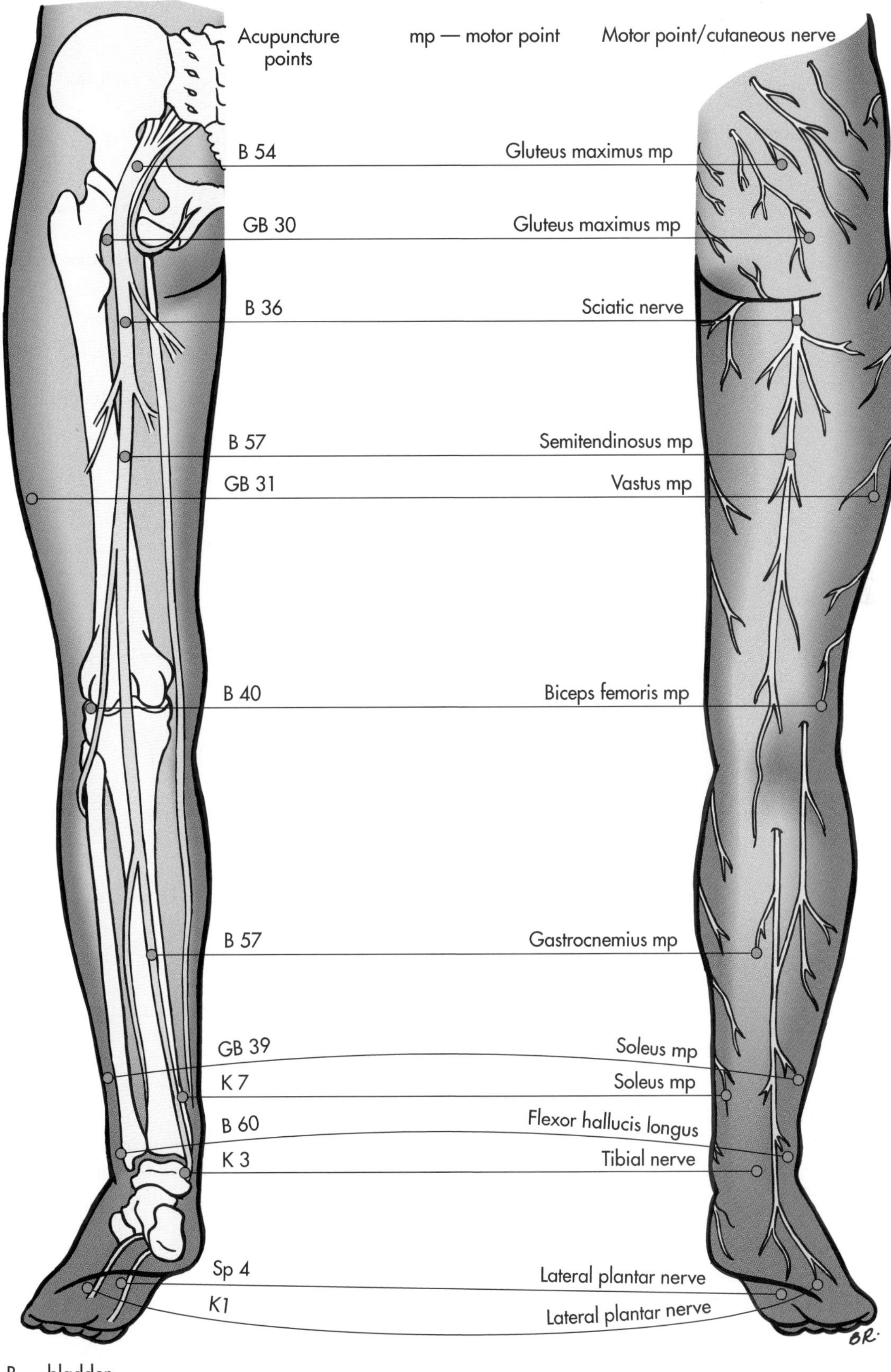

Figure 3-10, cont'd.

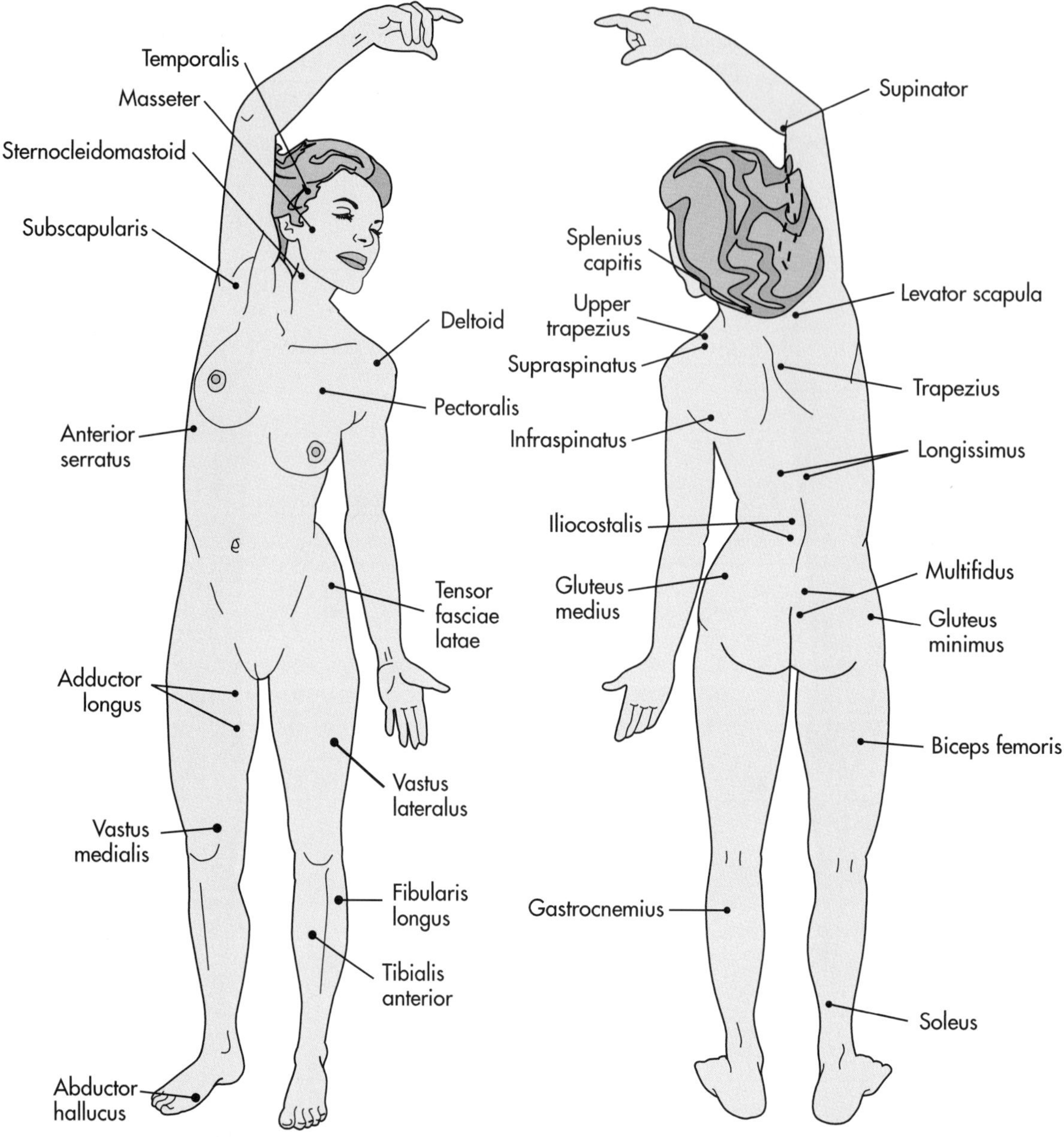

Figure 3-11
Common trigger points. (From Fritz S: *Mosby's fundamentals of therapeutic massage,* ed 3, St Louis, 2004, Mosby.)

Disturbances in the meridians are reflected in abnormalities along their course. Acupuncture, acupressure, and cupping are based largely on the theory of the channels and network vessels.

Thus the system of acupuncture points, organized as meridians, is the fundamental infrastructure of Chinese anatomy and physiology. The system is a comprehensive matrix that passes through the body, connecting all of its parts and serving as an energy/communications grid that generates, propagates, stores, and releases information and forces related to the body and its various components. Every place in the body is permeated by and connected with every other place in the body by means of the jing luo system. Interestingly, new information and understanding of the fascial network and concept of an interconnected fascial web is similar to the Chinese description of jing luo.

The Chinese word-concept that we translate into English as acupuncture point is composed of elements conveying the sense of body transport or communications hole.

Functionally, acupuncture points seem to have two basic actions: they open and they close. The names of the many points include words that mean gate, pass, or door. In opening, they release information and energy. In closing they store it.

In clinical use, the meridian point system is the thoroughfare through which the practices of Chinese medicine can influence the condition if the body is restoring the balance of fundamental processes.

ACTIVITY 3-7

Palpate one of your forearms and hands with moderate pressure, making sure you cover every inch. Whenever you find an Ah shi point, mark it with a washable marker. Compare the points you have identified on your arm and hand to the point charts in this chapter.

Draw a picture of your arm and the points located on it. Describe what you found.

Your Turn

Yin-yang theory

Yin-yang theory is one of the oldest doctrines in Chinese culture. The words *yin* and *yang* were originally representations of the shady and sunny sides, respectively, of a mountain or a hill. They came to represent two primordial forces that were the fundamental constituents of the universe and everything in it.

When yin and yang were separated from the singularity at the beginning of existence, the resulting potential gave rise to Qi. To the Chinese, Qi is a vital component of everything and is sensed or experienced in a manifestation of Qi.

Yin and yang frequently are described as opposites or complementary opposites. In terms of Western science, the notion of opposing forces is a powerful one, echoing in religious, moral, and ethical concepts of right and wrong, good and evil. However, in Chinese theory, yin and yang are conceived as being in opposition but not conflict. Yin and yang nourish and foster the growth of one another; they restrain each other; they support one another; they penetrate each other; they co-exist.

Traditional Terminology

The following words describe the additional aspects of Chinese medicine theory.

Cun: A method of measurement that uses a relative standard, usually the length of the second phalange of the second finger. Cun most often is applied in Asian bodywork forms.

Cupping: A method that uses suction to increase blood flow to an area or to remove ingestion.

Disharmony: Distortions in health that result when the functions or systems are neither balanced nor working at their optimum.

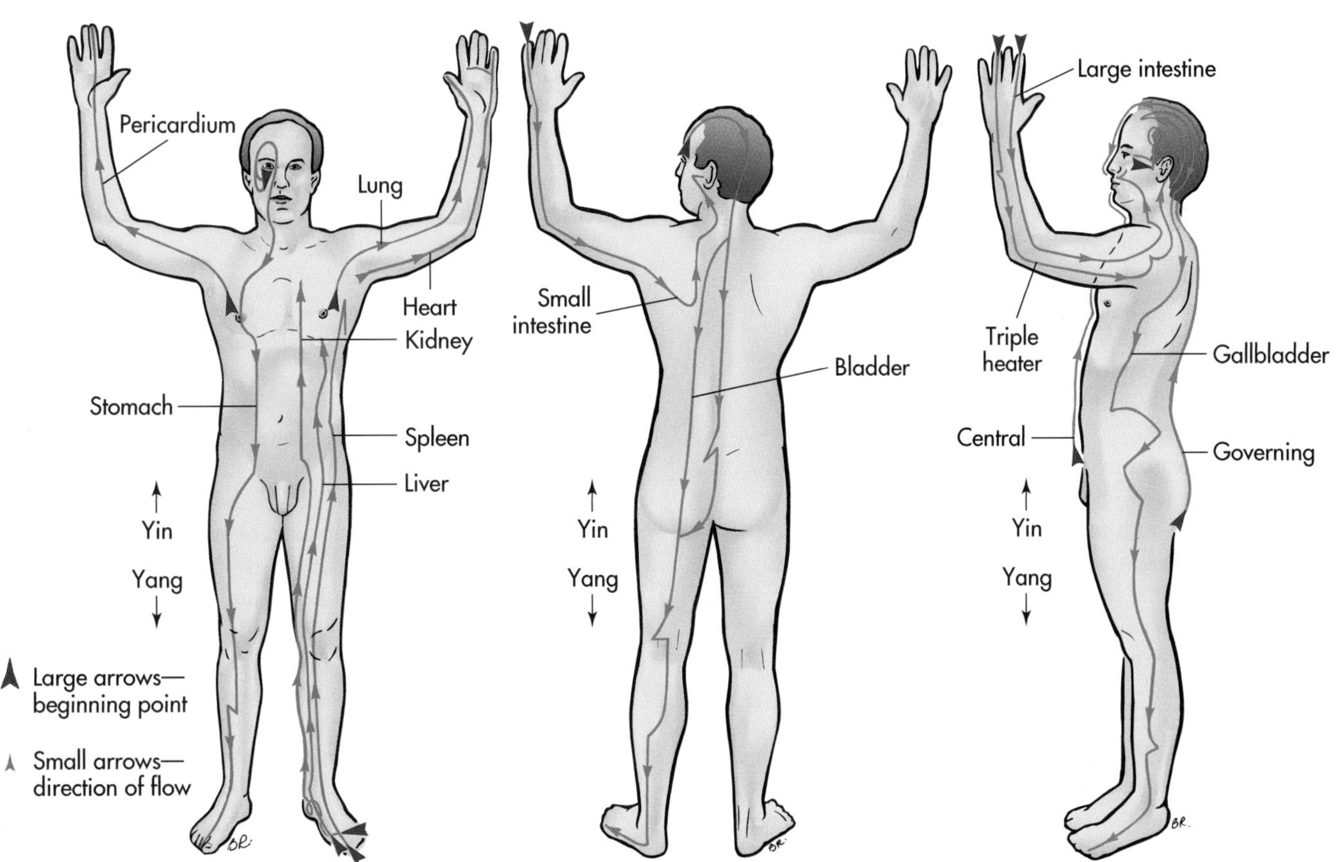

Figure 3-12
Typical location of meridians. Meridians tend to follow nerves. (From Fritz S: *Mosby's fundamentals of therapeutic massage,* ed 3, St Louis, 2004, Mosby.)

Essential substances: The fluids, essences, and energies that maintain balance in the body, mind, and spirit. They include the *Qi,* or life force; *shen,* or spirit; *jing,* or essence; *xue,* or blood fluids; and *jin ye,* or fluids.

Han re: Meaning cold and heat, this term refers to two of the eight principal syndromes in differential diagnosis, which are considered to be the primary manifestations of yin and yang, that is, symptoms that evidence predominance of cold or heat. These two signs of disease are considered of primary importance for herbal ingredients for prescriptions to treat illness. The word *han* means cold. The word *re* means heat.

Jin ye: Fluids; a general term for all the liquid components of the body other than the blood. Jin ye is one of the basic substances that transforms into blood. Jin ye exists extensively within the human body, between organs and tissues serving a nutritive function, and is composed of two categorically different substances that form a single entity and can transform one into the other.

Jing: The yin essence of life that nurtures growth, reproduction, and development.

Liu fu: The six bowels; the six hollow organs; a term given collectively to the gallbladder, stomach, large intestine, small intestine, urinary bladder, and the hard-to-define "triple-heater" (san jiao). In contrast to the five zang (wu zang) organs, the six fu organs are considered to be hollow and to be involved in the transportation of substances rather than the storing of essential substances and to decompose food and eliminate waste. The word *liu* means six. The word *fu* means bowel.

Liu Qi: This term describes the environmental conditions that ancient theorists identified as pathogenic factors. This concept also is called the *Six Pernicious Influences.* Liu Qi refers to the wind, cold, summer heat, dampness, dryness, and fire, or the six kinds of weather. When changes in weather exceed an individual's tolerance, disease may result. Identifying which of the six Qi are involved in the pathogenesis of a disease is an important step in the diagnosis of body substances, referring to essence, Qi, liquid, humor, blood, and vessels (or pulse).

Wind diseases are most common in spring, heat diseases in summer, damp diseases in long summer, dryness diseases in autumn, and cold diseases in winter.

Moxibustion: A form of heat therapy in which burning herbs are used to stimulate specific acupuncture points.

Qigong: An ancient Chinese art of exercise and meditation that encourages the flow of Qi and supports homeostasis.

Qi heng zhi fu: Literally, extraordinary organs; this is a designation given to a group of organs that resemble the fu organs in structure and the zang organs in function, including the bones, blood vessels, gallbladder, and uterus. They are different from the bowels because they do not decompose food or convey waste and different from the viscera because they do not produce and store excess. The gallbladder is an exception, because it is classed as a bowel and as an extraordinary organ. The gallbladder is considered a bowel because it plays a role in the processing and conveyance of food, and stands in interior-exterior relationship with its paired viscus, the liver. However, the bile the gallbladder produces is regarded as a "clear fluid" rather than as waste; hence it also is classed among the extraordinary organs.

The brain, marrow, bone, blood vessels, gallbladder, and womb are born of the Qi of the earth. They represent the nature of earth and belong to yin. Thus they can store essence and not release it.

Qi qing: The term describes seven affects, referring to emotional as well as mental activities in general and their potential as pathogenic factors in the onset and progress of disease. Ancient theorists recognized that intense or prolonged emotional disturbance can act as a pathogenic factor and identified seven such states: anger, melancholy, anxiety, sorrow, terror, fright, and excessive joy. Each of these can act to disturb the normal function of the Qi, blood, and viscera, resulting in disease.

Qi: Also known as Chi, Qi refers to the life force.

Shen: The word *shen* refers to the eternal dimension of life, to the magical or heavenly aspects of being alive. The term means "God, deity, divinity or divine nature; supernatural; magical expression, look, appearance; smart, clever."

Si shi: The four seasons; a general term for spring, summer, autumn, and winter in which the third month of summer (the sixth month of the Chinese lunar year) is termed long summer. The four seasons are correlated with the five phases thus: spring, wood; summer, fire; long summer, earth; autumn, metal; winter, water.

Wu xing: The five phases (elements): metal, water, wood, fire, and earth. They refer to a theoretic structure that supports much of traditional Chinese thought. Wu xing is as an extension or expression of yin-yang theory applied to the nature of material substance and to the various interrelationships that exist between matter in its different phases. These five phases function metaphorically, providing images that ancient theorists used to organize their thinking about the physical world. The five basic processes or phases describe a cycle that represents the inherent capabilities of change, which reflect yin and yang movements as observed in nature. The five-element phases, like yin and yang, are representatives of quality and relationship (Table 3-5). When combined with the principles of Chinese medicine, they are used to determine the diagnosis and treatment of a dysfunction (Figure 3-13).

Wu zang: The word *zang* means viscera, internal organ. This is a name given collectively to the solid organs: the heart, liver, spleen, lungs, and kidneys. These organs constitute one category that is distinguished from the six fu organs in structure and function. The zang organs are thought of as solid, essence-containing organs.

TABLE 3-5
Qualities of the Five Elements

PHASE	ELEMENT METAL	EARTH	FIRE	WATER	WOOD
Yin	Lung	Spleen	Heart	Kidney	Liver
Yang	Large intestine	Stomach	Triple-heater Small intestine	Bladder	Gallbladder
Sense	Smell	Taste	Speech	Hearing	Sight
Organ	Nose	Mouth, lips	Tongue	Ears	Eyes
Liquid	Mucus	Saliva	Sweat	Urine	Tears
Color	White	Yellow	Red	Blue/black	Green
Expression	Weeping	Singing	Laughing	Groaning	Shouting
Extreme emotion	Grief, anxiety	Worry, reminiscence	Shock, overjoy	Fear	Anger
Balanced emotion	Openness, receptivity	Sympathy, empathy	Joy, compassion	Resolution, trust	Assertion, motivation
Taste	Pungent, spicy	Sweet	Bitter, burned	Salty	Sour
Season	Fall	Indian summer	Summer	Winter	Spring
Related activity	Releasing	Thinking	Inspiration, intimacy	Willpower and vitality	Planning and decision making
Times	Lung, 3-5 AM Large intestine, 5-7 AM	Stomach, 7-9 AM Spleen, 9-11 AM	Heart, 11 AM-1 PM Small intestine, 1-3 PM	Bladder, 3-5 PM Kidney, 5-7 PM Triple-heater, 9-11 PM	Gallbladder, 11 PM-1 AM Pericardium, 7-9 PM Liver, 1-3 AM

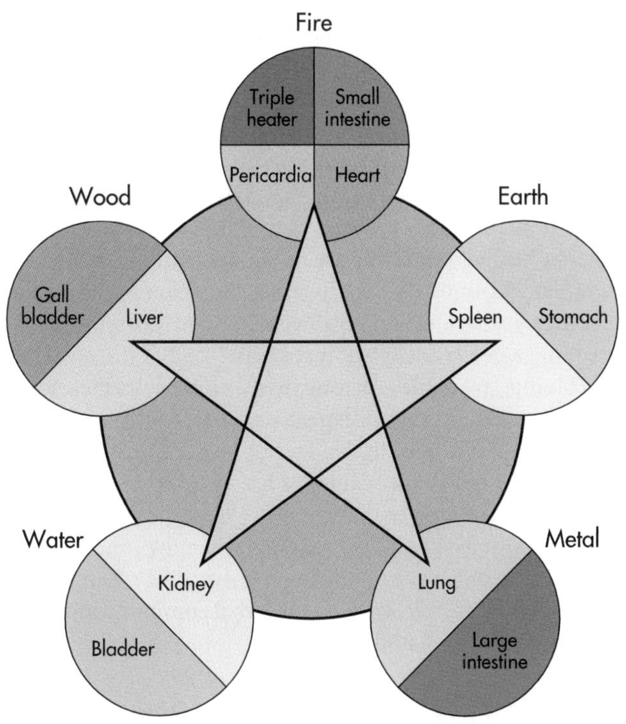

Figure 3-13
Five-element wheel showing the relationship between elements and organs. Circle relationship is a creation cycle. Star relationship is the control cycle.

Xu shi: This word is translated as deficiency and excess, insubstantial and substantial (particularly in the martial arts), replete and deplete, full and empty. Xu shi refers to two principles for estimating the condition of the patient's resistance and the pathogenic factors present.

Xue: The word *xue* is used to mean the blood itself in the same sense as it is understood in modern physiology. Xue also is used to mean something specific to Chinese medicine: the substantial fraction of the circulatory system in a unique relationship with the circulation of Qi.

Ying: Construction (Qi), construction nutriment; one of the essential substances for sustaining vital activities. Ying is derived from the digested food and absorbed by the internal organs. Ying circulates through the channels as a part of the blood to nourish all parts of the body, is the essential ingredient of the blood, and is responsible for the production of blood and the nourishment of body tissues. The blood (xue) and the ying are inseparable. Thus they often are referred to as ying xue.

Zheng xie: Righteous and evil, normal and pathogenic; this term refers to a distinction between the normal functions of the organism as contrasted to the pathogenic changes accompanying and characterizing disease.

Organ Relationships

Unlike the Western concept of organs, Chinese medicine thinks in terms of organ systems, which comprise an organ, essences, and fluids as they interact with the meridians. Ayurveda describes body functions in terms of doshas: Vata, Pitta, and Kapha (see Chapter 2). Randolph Stone integrated both systems coupled with other energetic methods to develop the polarity system. Ancient healing methods always have treated internal functions by external stimulation of the body, using methods such as acupuncture and massage. Practitioners have been using these techniques for centuries to help reestablish homeostasis within their bodies, adding to the belief that these practices must have some sort of consistent benefit to remain in existence. Current research has validated cutaneous/visceral connections as part of these processes.

As discussed in Chapter 2, nerve reflexes of internal organs manifest themselves in the surface areas of the body, showing up as referred pain patterns. The following are examples of other manifestations of nerve patterns that connect the internal organs with the surface:

- Pain sensations felt on the skin may be referred by internal organs.
- Muscular splinting may be noted over an area of internal disturbance.
- The autonomic nervous system influences surface areas of the body.
- Stimulus causes shifts in endogenous chemicals (those manufactured inside the body), which can affect organ function.

Theoretic discussion of using surface stimulation techniques to stimulate or balance internal organ function could explain the organ relationship of meridian and acupuncture points to specific internal physiologic features.

If the multitude of points described in the various health practices were mapped on the body, little space would be left. The case can be made that the entire body is a series of points. All this information can be used to reinforce the idea that events on the inside of the body affect the outside and vice versa.

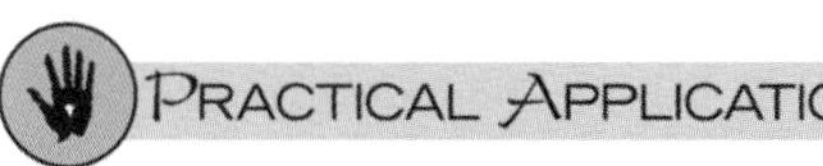

Because trigger points are located in shortened muscle fibers, these fibers must be lengthened to the normal resting length of the muscle, and any connective tissue shortening must be addressed with stretching methods. Often the type of point being addressed is not clear; therefore, unless contraindicated, the shortened muscles should be restored to an appropriate resting length through lengthening and stretching methods. Regardless of the classification or name of the tender point, methods of treatment include some sort of stimulation to the point, often in the form of pressure, to bring about a combined neurologic and chemical adjustment in the tissues of the area, as well as to the system as a whole. This method restores and adjusts the homeostatic mechanisms. Focusing massage applications over the meridians in the direction of their energy flow can be an effective approach for supporting the body's self-healing qualities. An awareness of Asian theory and practice helps the massage practitioner understand the complementary application of Asian disciplines. ■

SUMMARY

The competent massage therapist is able to understand the language of the scientific community as well as to understand the language and underlying philosophy of other healing practices such as the body therapies of Asia. Even though the main focus of this text is Western science, a tremendous overlap still exists between Western and Eastern methods, and therapeutic massage is influenced richly by ancient healing practices.

The ancient and indigenous healing traditions share a similar philosophy but use different terminology. Two additional examples are the chakra system (described in Chapter 6) and the dosha system (described in Chapter 2). Common to these healing traditions is the use of soft tissue methods; movement; meditation and inner reflection; exercise; dietary influences, including the use of naturally occurring substances for medicinal purposes; emotional influences; and spiritual connections that make human beings one with their environment and the universe. These ancient systems are often based on metaphor, describing naturally occurring, observable phenomena correlated to physical and psychologic function.

Western scientific study is no less colorful and weaves a tapestry of its own. Western science is a young discipline, which eventually will reach the harmony of approaches evident in ancient practices. Western methods, theories, and ancient healing traditions are not in opposition; rather, they complement one another. Together they blend the learning and application of ancient wisdom and current understanding as we strive for homeostasis.

Having available various texts that describe Asian, Eastern, and native perspectives on health would be beneficial. Those used in the development of this text, which are listed in the Works Consulted section at the end of this book, are a good place to begin.

Professional practices such as charting and writing reports mandate proficiency in language usage. Language is the basis for effective written and verbal communication and provides a point of understanding.

evolve

Log on to your student EVOLVE account and complete the medical terminology crossword puzzles under Chapter 3.

WORKBOOK SECTION

SHORT ANSWER

1. List and define the three word elements used in medical terms.

2. Break the following words into their word elements and give the meaning of each element. Then define the word.
   Antiseptic

   Contralateral

   Subaxillary

   Neurogenic

   Bradycardia

   Neuralgia

   Contraindication

   Periosteum

   Intracephalic

   Arthroplasty

3. Give the meanings of the following abbreviations:
   ADL

   ad lib

   a.m.a.

   ANS

   as tol

   BP

   CC

   c/o

   Dx

   h (hr)

   H_2O

   Hx

   IBW

   ICT

id

L

lig

M

ML

meds

n

NA

OTC

P

PA

PT

Px

R

R/O

ROM

Rx

SOB

SP, spir

Sym

T

TLC

Tx

WD

4. Define charting and explain the problem-solving model of charting.

5. In what ways do the Asian view and terminology act as a model for indigenous ancient healing practices? Compare the Asian discipline with Western theory and terminology.

6. Write the terms used to describe the position of the body in relation to other body parts.

   a. ________________ In front of or toward the front of the body or body part

   b. ________________ Behind, in back of, or in the rear of the body or body part

   c. ________________ Situated away from the trunk or midline of the body; away from the origin

   d. ________________ On or to the side, outside, away from the midline

   e. ________________ Relating to the middle, center, or midline of the body

   f. ________________ Closer to the trunk or to the point of origin

   g. ________________ The same side

h. ________________ The opposite side

i. ________________ Toward the head

j. ________________ Toward the tail

k. ________________ Higher than or above

l. ________________ Lower than or below

m. ________________ The circumference or an area away from the center

n. ________________ The palm side of the hand; also called palmar

o. ________________ The sole side of the foot

p. ________________ Bent inward; angulation of a part of the body inward toward the midline

q. ________________ Bent outward; bent toward the wall

r. ________________ Right

s. ________________ Left

t. ________________ The inside surface or the inside part of the body

u. ________________ The outside surface of the body

v. ________________ Far beneath the surface

w. ________________ Toward or on the surface

x. ________________ The wall of a part of the body

FILL IN THE BLANK

A (1) ____________ is part of a word. A (2) ____________ is placed at the beginning of a word to alter the meaning of the word. A vowel added between two roots or a root and a suffix to make pronunciation easier is a (3) ____________. The (4) ________________ word element contains the basic meaning of the word, and the (5) ______________ is placed at the end of a root to change the meaning of the word. A shortened form of a word or phrase is an (6) ________________. A (7) ________________ is a written record of professional interactions representing a clinical reasoning methodology emphasizing a (8) ____________ approach. The (9) ________________ is a problem-oriented medical record, and (10) ________________ is the acronym (subjective, objective, assessment/analysis, and plan) for the four parts of the written account of the health assessment.

(11) ______________ is an ancient philosophic concept and orientation that sees the universe and each individual as one and the same. By definition, (12) ______________ is the study of movement. Mechanical principles that relate directly to the human body are used in the study of (13) ________________. (14) ________________ is the dynamic balance between opposing forces and the continual process of creation and destruction within the natural order of the universe and of each person's inner being. (15) ____________ is the art and science of manipulating the flow of (16) ________________, the basic life force. The patterns that acupuncture points make on the surface of the body have been charted by practitioners of acupuncture for centuries and are grouped together in lines called (17) ________________ or (18) ________________. In traditional Chinese medicine this system of points and meridians is known as (19) ________________. (20) ________________ are the fluids, essences, and energies that keep the mind, body, and spirit in balance. (21) ________________ is the spirit. Moxibustion uses (22) ________________ herbs placed on or near the body to stimulate specific acupuncture points. Unlike the Western concept of organs, Chinese medicine thinks in terms of an (23) ________________, which comprises an organ, essences, and fluids as they interact with the meridians.

(24) ________________ is an ancient Chinese art of exercise and meditation that supports homeostasis. The Seven Emotions are (25) ____________, ____________, ______________, ____________, ______________, ________________, ________________. Heat, cold, wind, dampness, dryness, and summer heat are known as the (26) ________________. The Seven Emotions and the Six Pernicious Influences are internal triggers of disharmony in (27) ________________ .

The (28) ________________ are five basic processes or phases of a cycle that represent inherent capabilities of change. The Five Elements are (29) ______________, ______________, ______________, ______________, and ________________.

A (30) ________________ is a method of measurement using a relative standard of size and spacing on an individual, regardless of size or shape.

PROBLEM SOLVING

Analyze the following situation using the problem-solving model and complete the exercise at the end.

Agreement on terminology is an abiding issue in the sharing of information. Professionals often are speaking of the same process, methodology, or diagnosis but approaching it from a different cultural and language base. In one study, Mexican Americans refused medical treatment because their explanation of the disease process was discounted. If cultural differences were better understood, such problems might not arise. As researchers and health professionals take a serious look at ancient forms of healing and as more validity is given to noninvasive methods such as massage, some sort of common language base must be found or we will be unable to speak to one another. Consumers, meanwhile, will remain confused, unable to make informed decisions about the services they want to use. In all of these approaches, the body remains the same. Anatomy and physiology do not change.

In the following exercise, the first statement is provided as a guide. Fill in at least two more statements.

Facts

1. Terminology is an abiding issue in the sharing of information.
2. ____
3. ____

Possibilities

1. Schools could teach more cross-cultural terminology.
2. ____
3. ____

Logical Cause and Effect

1. If schools expanded their curricula, more teachers and textbooks would be needed and the cost of education would rise.
2. ____
3. ____

Effect

1. Persons may find their spiritual belief systems challenged in the study of healing disciplines in which a spiritual practice has an intrinsic part, and they may feel uncomfortable with these philosophies.
2. ____
3. ____

What can you do as a professional to bridge the communication gap?

____

____

____

____

____

____

____

____

____

____

____

____

____

____

____

FURTHER STUDY

1. Using additional resource material (see Works Consulted list at the end of this book), identify the chapters that pertain to the information presented in this chapter.
2. Do some research on one other ancient healing practice. Identify the major components of the discipline and correlate it to the Western model presented in this text. Pay particular attention to the following elements:

   Healing practice

   Soft tissue methods

   Movement and exercise

   Meditation and inner reflection

   Dietary influences

   Use of naturally occurring herbs for medicinal purposes

   Emotional influences

   Spiritual connections

   Metaphor based on naturally occurring phenomenon

   Correlation with Western scientific theories

Answer Key

1. Prefix: A word element added to the beginning of a root to change the meaning of the word.
   Suffix: A word element added to the end of a root to change the meaning of the word.
   Root: A word element that contains the basic meaning of the word.
2. Anti: against; septic: germs. Definition: Effective against germs.
   Contra: opposing; lateral: side. Definition: The opposite side.
   Sub: under; axilla: armpit. Definition: Under the armpit.
   Neur: nerve; genic: origin. Definition: Originating in the nerves.
   Brady: slow; card: heart; ia: a state or condition. Definition: Slow heartbeat.
   Neur: nerve; algia: pain. Definition: Nerve pain.
   Contra: opposing; indication: desired result. Definition: Opposite of the desired result.
   Peri: around; oste: bone. Definition: Around the bone. (Periosteum is a specialized membrane that surrounds bone.)
   Intra: within; cephal: head. Definition: Within the head.
   Arthro: joint; plasty: surgical repair. Definition: Reconstruction of a joint.
3. ADL: Activities of daily living
   ad lib: As desired
   a.m.a.: Against medical advice
   ANS: Autonomic nervous system
   as tol: As tolerated
   BP: Blood pressure
   CC: Chief complaint
   c/o: Complains of
   Dx: Diagnosis
   h (hr): Hour
   H_2O: Water
   Hx: History
   IBW: Ideal body weight
   ICT: Inflammation of connective tissue
   Id: The same
   L: Left; length; lumbar
   lig: Ligament
   M: Muscle; meter; myopia
   ML: Midline
   meds: Medications
   n: Normal
   NA: Nonapplicable
   OTC: Over the counter
   P: Pulse
   PA: Postural analysis
   PT: Physical therapy
   Px: Prognosis
   R: Respiration; right
   R/O: Rule out
   ROM: Range of motion
   Rx: Prescription
   SOB: Shortness of breath
   SP, spir: Spirit
   Sym: Symmetric
   T: Temperature
   TLC: Tender loving care
   Tx: Treatment
   WD: Well developed
4. Charting is the process of keeping a written record of professional interactions. SOAP (subjective, objective, assessment/analysis, and plan) is the mnemonic for the four parts of the written account of the health assessment. In a problem-solving model of charting, the practitioner collects a database before beginning the process of identifying the client's problems. The database contains all the subjective and objective information available that contributes to therapeutic intervention. Next, the information is analyzed. Each problem identified represents a conclusion or decision that arises from examination, investigation, and analysis of the data collected. A decision then is made about a plan of intervention. The plan needs to be implemented, reevaluated, and adjusted as necessary. The action taken, its effectiveness, and the outcome are recorded progressively from session to session.
5. Western science is a young discipline that uses the scientific methods of observation; it involves measuring concrete entities, accumulating data, and analyzing findings. Ancient approaches also require observation, measurement, and accumulation and analysis of data, but in addition, they have validated the importance of intuition. Ancient or indigenous healing practices do not separate the body, mind, and spirit as Western science does. Most ancient healing systems are grounded in concepts similar to those presented in the Asian model, mainly the idea of bringing the body into balance to promote health, rather than simply eliminating symptoms, as has been the method of the young Western scientific

approach. Western mind/body medicine is developing according to similar theories.

Ancient methods reflect a common belief that internal functions can be affected by surface stimulation, such as in the application and rubbing in of ointments, the use of various types of massage and acupuncture, and the laying on of hands. In light of the accumulation of knowledge over eons, if these practices had not shown some sort of consistent benefit, they would not still be in effect. We now know that nerve reflexes of internal organs manifest themselves in the surface areas of the body.

Common to these ancient and indigenous healing traditions is the use of soft tissue methods, movement, meditation and inner reflection, exercise, dietary influences and use of naturally occurring herbs for medicinal purposes, and emotional influences and spiritual connections to help make human beings one with their environment and the universe. Metaphor based on naturally occurring phenomena that can be observed often is correlated with physical and psychologic function. Western scientific theories are not in opposition to these practices; rather they actually are complementary.

6. a. Anterior or ventral
   b. Posterior or dorsal
   c. Distal
   d. Lateral
   e. Medial
   f. Proximal
   g. Ipsilateral
   h. Contralateral
   i. Cephalad
   j. Caudal
   k. Superior
   l. Inferior
   m. Peripheral
   n. Volar
   o. Plantar
   p. Varus
   q. Valgus
   r. Dextral
   s. Sinistral
   t. Internal
   u. External
   v. Deep
   w. Superficial
   x. Parietal

FILL IN THE BLANK

1. word element
2. prefix
3. combining vowel
4. root
5. suffix
6. abbreviation
7. chart
8. problem-solving
9. POMR
10. SOAP
11. Tao
12. kinesiology
13. biomechanics
14. Yin/yang
15. Acupuncture
16. Qi
17. channels
18. meridians
19. jing luo
20. Essential Substances
21. Shen
22. burning
23. organ system
24. Qigong
25. joy, anger, fear, fright, sadness, worry, grief
26. Six Pernicious Influences
27. mind/body/spirit
28. Five Elements
29. water, wood, fire, metal, earth
30. cun

ANSWERS TO ACTIVITY 3-2

am: morning
Hx: history
ADL: activities of daily living
ad lib: as desired
CC: chief complaint
GI: gastrointestinal
ABD: abdominal
meds: medications
ROM: range of motion
as tol: as tolerated
h: hour
PT: physical therapy
ft: foot (or feet)
R: respiration
T: temperature
P: pulse
pm: Afternoon
H_2O: water
TLC: tender loving care
OB: obstetrics

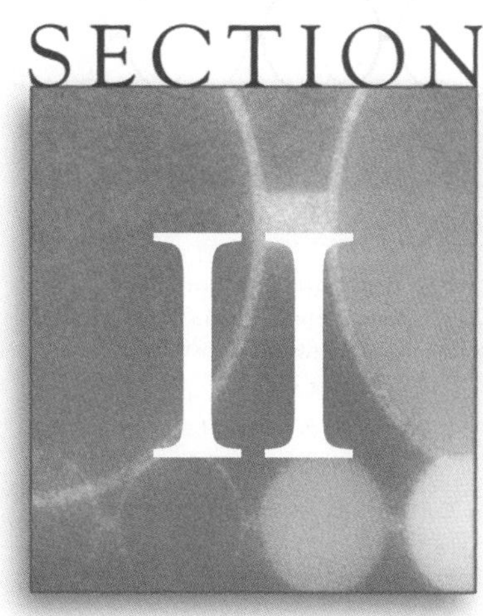

Systems of Control

The study of the way the body functions makes evident that two systems, the nervous system and endocrine system, share in the coordination of body activities. These two systems of control are interdependent and cannot function effectively without each other.

After the student understands the mechanisms of control, learning about the rest of the body becomes a matter of recognizing the structure of the pieces (anatomy) of each system functioning (physiology) under the direction of the control systems. Massage professionals often focus extensively on the musculoskeletal system. However, without the nervous system and endocrine system, the musculoskeletal system does not function. This section comes before the study of the skeleton, joints, and muscles to establish the larger picture of the way the body—including movement—functions.

The major benefits derived from massage and bodywork depend on reflex mechanisms and neurochemical feedback loops, all coordinated through the nervous system and endocrine system. Function and structure have a circular relationship, each influencing the other.

Physics is the study of the way things work. Physicists ask the question, "How does the world behave?" Newtonian principles were developed in a linear pathway (i.e., from an understanding that the world behaves in predictable ways of cause and effect). To believe that the nervous system and endocrine system tell the rest of the body what to do and that the parts respond in a predictable way would be Newtonian. Usually this assumption is accurate, but not always. Quantum principles look at the world more interactively. Instead of predictable outcomes, decisions—at a subatomic to cosmic level—are made constantly. Simply in the process of thinking, outcomes can be influenced in a multidimensional loop of events. Viewing the world linearly and thinking that a specific nerve pathway, neurotransmitter, or hormone always produces the same predictable response is much easier. However, the body does not always respond that way. Life is not always predictable and neither is physiology. Quantum theory exists from a basis of tendency to exist or happen. Nothing is for sure. The human potential to decide in terms of body, mind, and spirit is more circular and uncertain, harder to predict, and more elusive to learn. The student, then, should proceed with fascination focused on possibilities as well as facts in undertaking the study of the functional aspect of the body (see Table).

Even though these factors seem to be in opposition, they also reflect the duality of wholeness, which seems to be an accurate reflection of the way the body functions (Zukav, 1980; Dossy, 1982).

TABLE

Comparison of Newtonian Physics and Quantum Mechanics

NEWTONIAN PHYSICS	QUANTUM MECHANICS
Can be pictured	Cannot be pictured
Based on ordinary sense perceptions	Based on systems not directly observable
Describes things, individual objects in space, and their changes in time	Describes statistical behavior of systems and groups
Predicts events	Predicts possibilities
Holds that we can observe something without changing it	Holds that we cannot observe something without changing it

Certainly, as we explore each of the other body systems, reviewing again the effect of the control systems on specific structure and function will be important. These chapters lay the foundation so that future study will be more than memorizing body parts and functions in a piece-by-piece approach. Instead, what we hope to accomplish is an appreciation of innate body intelligence and the orchestrated synchronized symphony conducted by the nervous and endocrine systems.

During the process of researching these chapters, what became apparent is that the study of these important controlling mechanisms is a lifelong endeavor, and we concede that, particularly in this area, there is simply too much to know. Even the most comprehensive anatomy and physiology texts consulted resorted to choosing what to cover, recognizing that covering all the information in one general textbook was impossible. In addition, current research is concentrated on these control systems. The information base is being expanded and altered almost daily. Whereas the study of the musculoskeletal system, cardiovascular system, and so forth is more stable because the bulk of the information concerns the anatomy, which is relatively static, the study of the nervous and endocrine systems is focused mostly on the function of the body. This information is more likely to change and expand as researchers explore more deeply the subtleties of neuroendocrine influences. The student should keep in mind that factual structure changes.

The information presented in these chapters is by no means an exhaustive study, and much important and interesting information has not been addressed. However, the student must begin somewhere in the learning process. Reference texts are an invaluable resource. We hope that the material we have decided to discuss is of practical importance in understanding the mechanisms of effect for therapeutic massage approaches and in understanding function and associated behavior from neuroendocrine influences.

As you completed the activities in the previous section, did you notice the following in Chapter 1?

- The characteristics of life involve the movement of energy from one point to another.
- Subtle forms of energetic bodywork are based on electrical and chemical functions.
- Touch therapies stimulate sensory function of the skin.
- The storage and release of fat from adipose tissue is regulated by hormonal and nervous stimuli.
- Although not fully understood, the piezoelectric property of collagen produces some form of electrical influence.
- Nervous tissue is one of the four basic tissue types and is developed specifically to regulate and integrate body activity.

Did you notice the following in Chapter 2?

- The Vata dosha directs nerve impulses.
- The nervous system and endocrine system are the most important in maintaining homeostasis.

- Feedback loops are afferent and efferent information pathways traveled by nerve impulses or chemical hormone messengers. Each feedback loop consists of a sensory, integrating, and effector component from the nervous or endocrine system.
- Massage methods work through feedback loops.
- Body rhythms are influenced by the autonomic nervous system and endocrine system.
- Entrainment is coordinated by the nervous and endocrine systems.
- Pain and pain management are based on neurochemical mechanisms.
- The general adaptation syndrome response and effects of long-term stress are endocrine and autonomic nervous system events.
- Massage is a sensory stimulation approach that promotes mechanisms of health and stress management.

Did you notice the following in Chapter 3?

- The dorsal body cavity houses the central nervous system.
- The point phenomenon in ancient healing practices is correlated to the nervous and endocrine systems.

Overview of the Nervous System and Endocrine System

The nervous system is the most complex of the body systems and is composed of more than 110 billion nerve cells. The nervous system is divided into the central nervous system (CNS)—composed of the brain, spinal cord, and coverings—and the peripheral nervous system, which includes the cranial nerves, spinal nerves, and ganglia. The peripheral nervous system is divided further into autonomic and somatic divisions. These subdivisions combine and communicate to innervate the somatic and visceral parts of the body. The somatic division is associated with the bones, muscles, and skin. The visceral or autonomic division is associated with the internal glands, organs, blood vessels, and mucous membranes. The autonomic nervous system (ANS) is divided further into two divisions. The sympathetic nervous system activates arousal responses and expends body resources in such a way to respond to emergency situations or any activity of excitement or acceleration. The parasympathetic nervous system reverses the response of the sympathetic nervous system by returning the body to a nonalarm state and restoring body resources. The sympathetic division is considered the "flight, fight, fear" system. But any highly emotional state of joy, excitement, and elation is also sympathetic. The parasympathetic nervous system is associated with the "relaxation response." Much of the interaction between body and mind takes place through ANS activity. The concepts of yin and yang are reflected in the ANS, with parasympathetic functions relating to yin and sympathetic functions relating to yang.

The basic structure of the nervous system is the neuron, or nerve cell. The nerve cell is an impulse-transmitting fiber connecting the CNS with all parts of the body. Three basic types of neurons exist:

1. Afferent or sensory neurons that carry impulses to the CNS
2. Connecting or associative interneurons that transmit nerve impulses between neurons
3. Efferent or motor neurons that transmit impulses away from the CNS to the muscles, organs, and glands

The nervous and endocrine systems transmit information from one part of the body to another, but they do it in different ways. The nervous system transmits information rapidly with a short duration of action by nerve impulses conducted from one body area to another. The endocrine system is a network of ductless glands and other structures that secrete chemicals called hormones directly into the bloodstream, affecting the function of specific target organs. The action of hormones is slower and longer than that of nerve impulses. Often the nervous system initiates a response and the endocrine system sustains it.

Both systems use chemicals. The nervous system uses neurotransmitters, and the endocrine system uses hormones. Many times these are the same chemicals. If the chemical is found in the synapses, the space between nerve endings of the nervous system, it is a neurotransmitter. If the same chemical is found in the blood, it is a hormone. The influence of the nervous system regulates the endocrine system, and the endocrine system influences the nervous system, forming a feedback loop that increases or decreases activity for healthy function. The feedback system and autoregulation (maintenance of internal homeostasis) are interlinked in all body functions.

ACTIVITY

In Chapters 1 through 3, many references were made to the nervous system, in particular the autonomic nervous system, certain neurotransmitters, and the endocrine system. We have touched on the interaction of theory and application of therapeutic massage modalities. Review these three chapters and underline or highlight any references made to nerves, neurotransmitters, the autonomic nervous system (sympathetic and parasympathetic divisions), hormones, and chemicals of the body.

CHAPTER 4

Nervous System Basics and the Central Nervous System

CHAPTER OBJECTIVES

After completing this chapter, the student will be able to perform the following:

- List the parts of the neuron.
- Explain the function of the nerve cell.
- Describe neurotransmitter functions.
- Relate brain chemistry to behavior.
- Define the parts and functions of the central nervous system.
- Describe consciousness and altered states of consciousness.
- Explain the process of memory and learning.
- Describe common pathologic conditions of the central nervous system.
- List drugs that influence the central nervous system.
- Explain the influence of massage methods on the central nervous system.

CHAPTER OUTLINE

KEY TERMS

Amyotrophic lateral sclerosis (a-MI-o-TROF-ik) A progressive disease that begins in the central nervous system and involves the degeneration of motor neurons and the subsequent atrophy of voluntary muscle. Also called Lou Gehrig disease.

Ascending tracts Tracts that carry sensory information to the brain.

Axon (AK-son) A single elongated projection from the nerve cell body that transmits impulses away from the cell body.

Brain The largest and most complex unit of the nervous system, the brain is responsible for perception, sensation, emotion, intellect, and action.

Brainstem The primitive portion of the brain that contains centers for vital functions and reflex actions, such as vomiting, coughing, sneezing, posture, and basic movement patterns.

Central nervous system The brain and spinal cord and their coverings.

Cerebellum (sair-e-BELL-um) The second largest part of the brain, the cerebellum is involved with balance, posture, coordination, and movement.

Cerebrospinal fluid (sair-e-bro-SPY-nal) A clear, colorless fluid that flows throughout the brain and around the spinal cord, cushioning and protecting these structures and maintaining proper pH balance.

Cerebrum (se-REE-brum) The largest of the brain divisions, the cerebrum consists of two hemispheres that occupy the uppermost region of the cranium. The cerebrum receives, interprets, and associates incoming information with past memories and then transmits the appropriate motor response.

Dendrites (DEN-drites) Branching projections from the nerve cell body that carry signals to the cell body.

Continued

Descending tracts Tracts that carry motor information from the brain to the spinal cord.
Dorsal root One of two roots that attaches a spinal nerve to the spinal cord.
Epilepticus (ep-i-LEP-TIK-us) A continuous seizure.
Essential tremor A chronic tremor that does not proceed from any other pathologic condition.
Gray matter Unmyelinated nervous tissue, particularly that found in the central nervous system.
Monoplegia (mon-O-PLE-JE-a) Paralysis of a single limb or a single group of muscles.
Myelin (MY-e-lin) A white, fatty, insulating substance formed by the Schwann cells that surrounds some axons. Also produced in the central nervous system by oligodendrocytes.
Neurilemma (noo-ri-LEM-mah) The outer cell membrane of a Schwann cell that is essential in the regeneration of injured axons. The thin membrane spirally wraps the myelin layers of certain fibers, especially of peripheral nerves, or the axons of certain unmyelinated nerve fibers. Also called Schwann's membrane, sheath of Schwann, and endoneural membrane.
Neuroglia (noo-ro-Glee-ah) Specialized connective tissue cells that support, protect, and hold neurons together.
Neurons (NOO-ronz) Nerve cells that conduct impulses.
Neurotransmitters (noo-ro-TRANS-mit-erz) Chemical compounds that generate action potentials when released in the synapses from presynaptic cells.
Paraplegia (par-a-PLE-JE-a) Paralysis of the lower portion of the body and of both legs.
Quadriplegia (quad-ra-PLE-JE-a) Paralysis or loss of movement of all four limbs.
Schwann cell (shwon) A specialized cell that forms myelin.
Spinal cord Portion of the central nervous system that exits the skull into the vertebral column. The two major functions of the spinal cord are to conduct nerve impulses and to be a center for spinal reflexes.
Synapse (SIN-aps) Spaces between neurons or between a neuron and an effector organ.
Tracts Collections of nerve fibers in the brain and spinal cord with a common function.
Ventral root One of two roots that attaches a spinal nerve to the spinal cord.
White matter Myelinated nerve fibers, particularly those found in brain and spinal tissue.

NERVOUS SYSTEM BASICS

Nerve Cell Structure

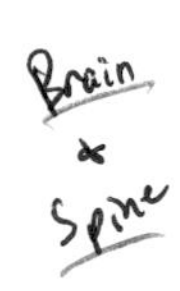

Two types of cells are found in the **central nervous system** (CNS): the **neurons,** or nerve cells that conduct impulses, and **neuroglia,** specialized connective tissue cells. The function of the neuron is to receive and transmit electrical signals to other neurons, muscles, or glands. The neuroglia (*glia* means glue) supports and protects neurons as it holds them together. In addition, neuroglia support the tiny blood vessels (capillaries) in the **brain.**

Nerve cells consist of a cell body and its nerve fibers, the **axons** and **dendrites.** The cell body contains a nucleus and its organelles. The dendrites, which look like small hairs, are extensions of the cytoplasm of the cell. Their job is to carry signals to the cell body. The axon is an elongated projection that carries signals away from the cell body. An axon may have branches known as *collaterals* that allow communication among neurons.

In the peripheral nervous system, the neuroglia forms a protective sheath around the axons. The neuroglia contains a fatty insulator called **myelin,** which is produced by **Schwann cells.** The outer membrane is called the **neurilemma** and also is formed by Schwann cells. Small gaps between segments of the myelin sheath are called *nodes of Ranvier* and help speed the nerve impulses.

Neurons are identified by their functions. A sensory neuron conducts sensory signals to the CNS, whereas motor neurons conduct motor signals away from the CNS. Association or interneurons act as bridges in the CNS to conduct signals from one neuron to another (Figure 4-1).

Nerve Functions

Let us examine a neuron to see the way nerve signals are sent through a healthy body.

When a neuron is at rest, the outside of its cell membrane is positively charged, whereas inside the cell is negatively charged. This difference is called the membrane potential and is created by the concentration of ions in the fluids in and around the cell. Excess sodium ions (Na^+) tend to concentrate in the extracellular fluid, and the cell membrane does not allow them to flow into the cell. Potassium ions (K^+) predominate inside the cell membrane. A stimulus such as a pressure, light, temperature, or chemical change results in a brief change in the charge of one segment of the neuron, which is called depolarization.

During depolarization, the permeability of the cell membrane changes and channels made of protein in the cell membrane are signaled to open by the change in voltage (voltage-gated channels) and the sodium ions are allowed into the neuron. The outside of that segment of the membrane becomes negatively charged as it depolarizes, whereas the inside becomes positively charged. This change is called the *action potential.* As this process continues along the nerve fiber, the nerve impulse depolarizes the next section, causing it to reverse its charges while the previous segment returns to its original polarity or is repolarized; as sodium channels close and potassium channels open, the outside again becomes positively charged and the inside becomes negatively charged. The term *excited* is used to describe the segment as it switches charges with the action potential, and the term *inhibited* describes the reversal of that action (Figure 4-2).

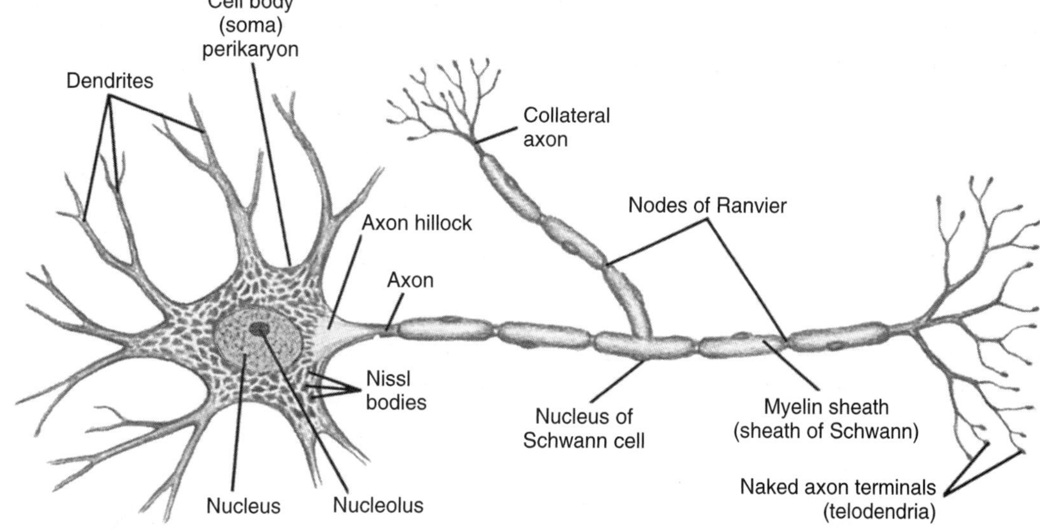

Figure 4-1
Neuron. (From Thompson et al: Mosby's clinical nursing, ed 5, St Louis, 2002, Mosby.)

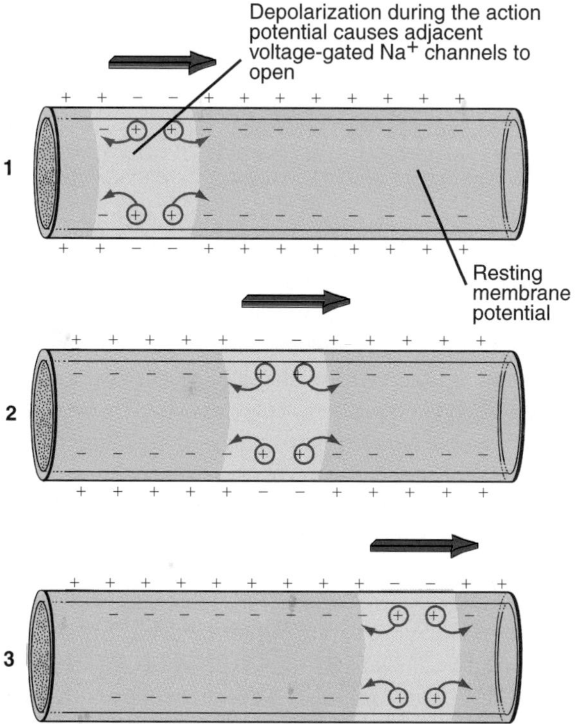

Figure 4-2
Conduction of the action potential. The reverse polarity characteristic of the peak of the action potential causes local current flow to adjacent regions of the membrane (*small arrows*). This stimulates voltage-gated Na^+ channels to open and thus creates a new action potential. This cycle continues, producing wavelike conduction of the action potential from point to point along a nerve fiber. Adjacent regions of membrane behind the action potential do not polarize again because they are still in their refractory period. (From Thibodeau GA, Patton KT: *Anatomy and physiology*, ed 5, St Louis, 2003, Mosby.)

The *refractory period* is the brief period after inhibition when the neuron recovers. The *absolute refractory period* is the time during which a neuron will not respond to any stimuli. This is followed by the *relative refractory period*, when the neuron will only respond to a strong stimulus.

The path of the nerve impulse is different in myelinated and unmyelinated nerve fibers. The nerve impulse travels over the surface of the cell membrane in unmyelinated nerves and excites one segment at a time. This process results in a slowly transmitted signal. With myelinated fibers, the impulse jumps from one node of Ranvier to the next node. During this *saltatory conduction*, the speed of the moving signal is much faster (The term *saltate* means to dance and is used to describe the way this signal moves from one place to the next) (Figure 4-3).

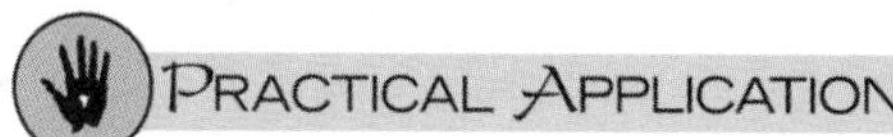

PRACTICAL APPLICATION

Therapeutic massage methods such as muscle energy techniques and proprioceptive neuromuscular facilitation use the refractory period to their advantage. Muscles often resist lengthening by initiating a protective spasm. If the muscle is first contracted and then lengthened, it is less likely to spasm during the refractory period, and the muscle can be restored more easily to a more normal resting length. Because these periods are short, gentle applications of lengthening procedures need to be used. Methods that generate any sort of strong stimuli, especially pain, must be avoided. If too strong a stimulus is introduced, instead of the muscle relaxing, it will generate nerve impulses and contract, thus resisting any sort of lengthening or stretching methods. ■

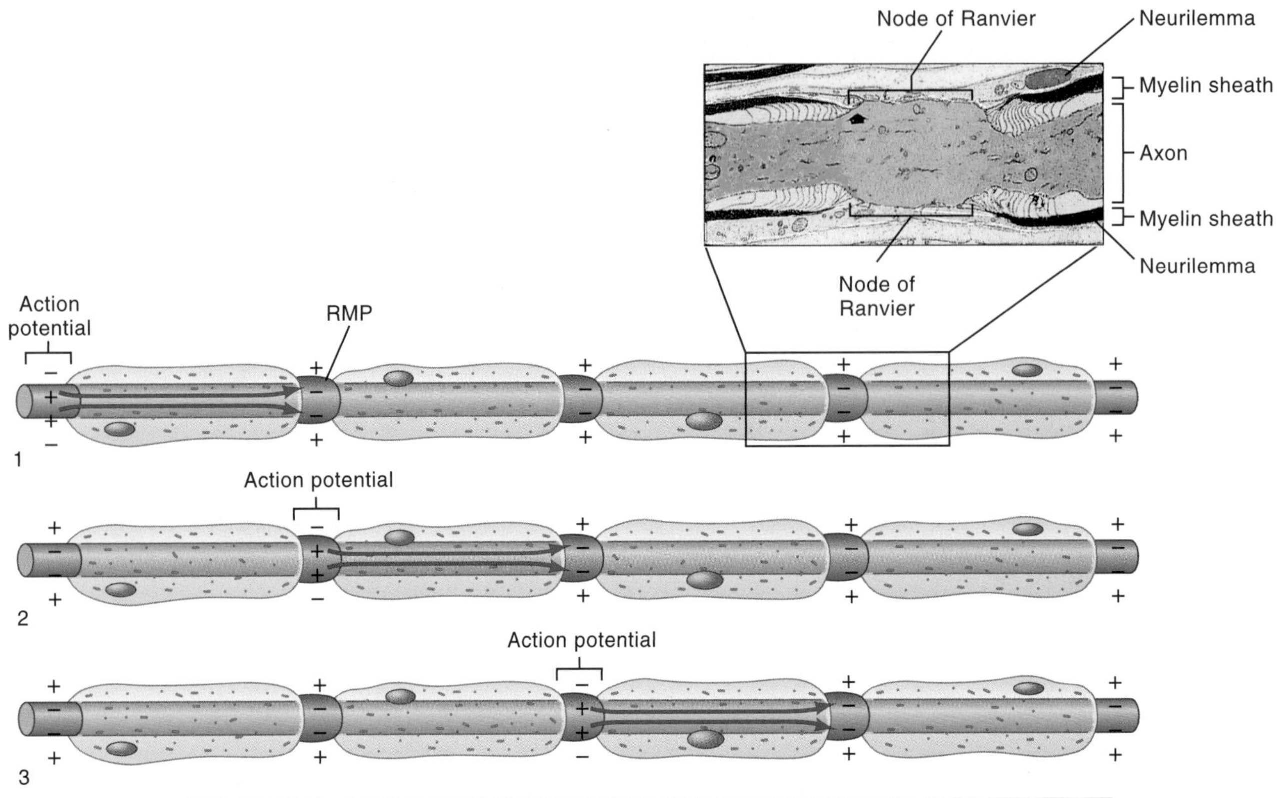

Figure 4-3
Saltatory conduction. This series of diagrams shows that the insulating nature of the myelin sheath prevents ion movement everywhere but at the nodes of Ranvier. The action potential at one node triggers current flow (*arrows*) across the myelin sheath to the next node, producing an action potential there. The action potential thus seems to leap rapidly from node to node. The inset is a transmission electron micrograph showing a node of Ranvier in a myelinated fiber. *RMP,* resting membrane potential. (From Thibodeau GA, Patton KT: *Anatomy and physiology,* ed 5, St Louis, 2003, Mosby; inset courtesy Georg Thieme Verlag.)

Synapses and Neurotransmitters

The space or junction between two neurons or a neuron and an effector organ is called a **synapse.** An electrical signal is transformed to a chemical signal to cross the junction. The neuron sending the signal is referred to as *presynaptic* because it is before the synapse, whereas the neuron or muscle fiber receiving the signal is *post-synaptic,* or after the synapse. The actual space in the synapse is called the *synaptic cleft* (Figure 4-4).

At the end of the axon of the presynaptic neuron, small sacs or vesicles are present that contain chemical compounds known as **neurotransmitters.** Once released, these chemicals cross the synaptic cleft and bind with or are absorbed by the post-synaptic neuron or muscle. This generates another action potential, and the nerve impulse continues to its destination.

As small as the vesicles are, they can store thousands of neurotransmitter molecules. After the neurotransmitters are released and their action is completed, they are broken down immediately by enzymes and diffuse out of the synaptic cleft or are reabsorbed by the axons. This ensures that only one action potential is transmitted by the release of one portion of neurotransmitters. In certain instances, medication may be used to interrupt the cycle by stopping the metabolism of the substance by preventing its binding to the post-synaptic membrane or slowing the reasbsorbtion of the neurotransmitter into the presynaptic vesicles.

Neurotransmitters regulate many of our body activities and senses. At present, more than 30 neurotransmitters have been identified, and many more are suspected to exist. When released into the bloodstream, many of these same chemicals are called hormones. Some of the known hormones are thought to work as neurotransmitters, implying a close link between the nervous system and endocrine activity.

To be classified as a neurotransmitter, a chemical must have certain characteristics. These characteristics include being found in presynaptic vesicles, having the ability to be removed from the synaptic cleft, and being capable of stimulating a nerve impulse. Neurotransmitters that cause the action potential to be transmitted across the synaptic cleft are considered stimulatory neurotransmitters. Those that slow or prevent the transmission of the action potential are inhibitory neurotransmitters. The two actions, stimulation and inhibition, support balance in nerves like the gas pedal and brakes in a car. The following is a list of some of the major neurotransmitters, their primary actions, and some of their locations:

Acetylcholine: Acetylcholine stimulates the skeletal muscles and primarily acts on the parasympathetic nervous

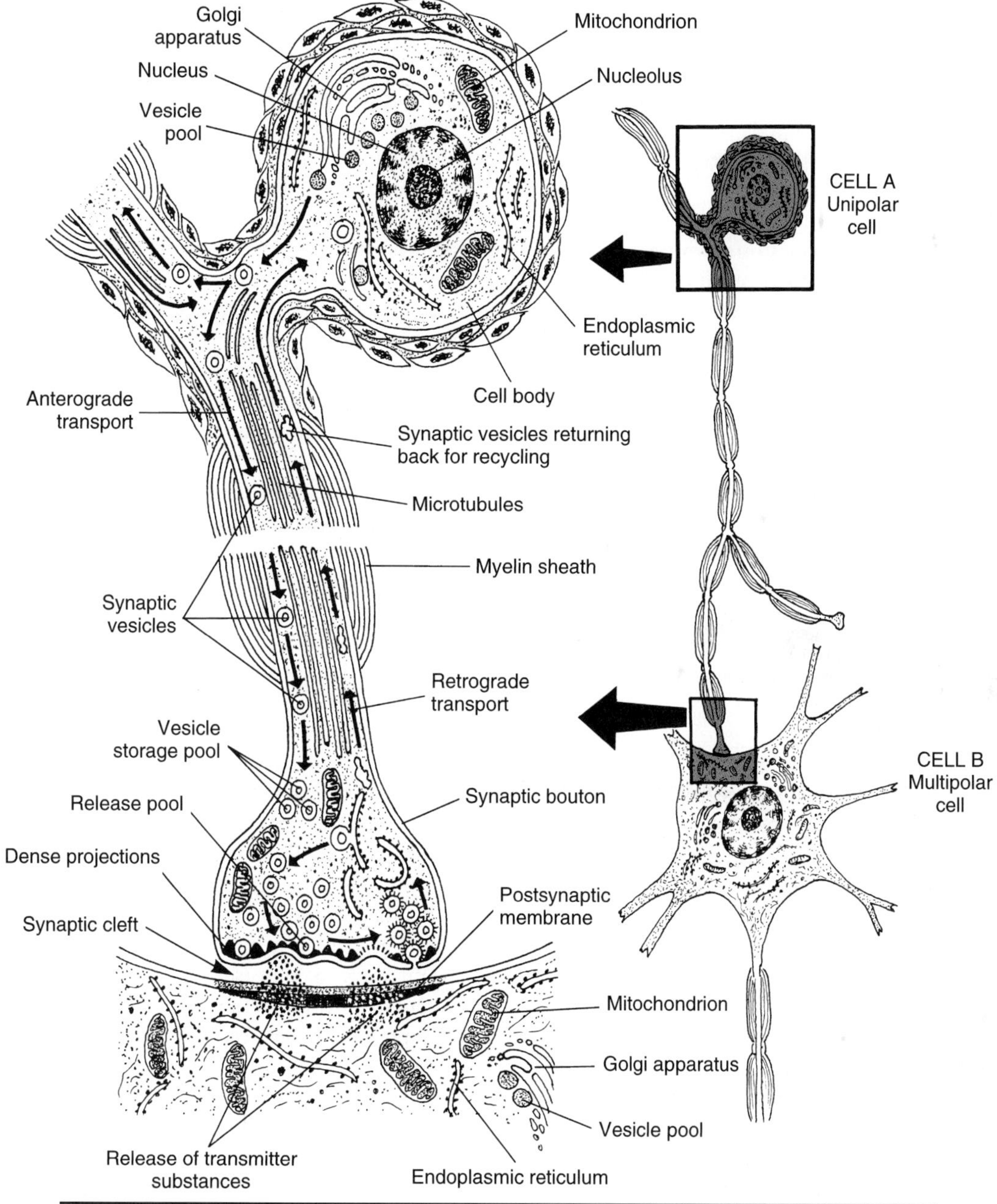

Figure 4-4
Functional relationship between two neurons in pathway. Electrical impulse travels along axon of first neuron to synapse. Chemical transmitter is secreted into synaptic cleft to depolarize membrane (dendrite or cell body) of the next neuron in pathway. (From Thompson JM et al: *Mosby's clinical nursing,* ed 5, St Louis, 2002, Mosby.)

system. Acetylcholine can stimulate or inhibit various organs, depending on the receptors to which it is bound. Plentiful in the brain, the chemical is involved in memory. A lack of acetylcholine has been found in many patients diagnosed with Alzheimer's disease, although a cause-and-effect relationship has not yet been established. Myasthenia gravis, which is a disease causing weakening of skeletal muscles, results from a reduction of acetylcholine receptors.

Catecholamines: Catecholamines are neurotransmitters involved in sleep, motor function, mood, and pleasure. Important endogenous (manufactured inside the body) catecholamines include the following:

Epinephrine: Epinephrine can be a stimulant or inhibitor, depending on the type of receptor bound. Epinephrine is found in several areas of the CNS and in the sympathetic divisions of the autonomic nervous system (ANS). Epinephrine also is involved in fight-or-flight responses such as dilation of blood vessels to the skeletal muscles and is classified as a hormone when secreted by the adrenal gland.

Norepinephrine: Like epinephrine, norepinephrine can excite or inhibit and is found in the CNS (especially the hypothalamus and limbic system) and the sympathetic division of the ANS. Norepinephrine causes constriction of skeletal blood vessels, is considered a "feel good" neurotransmitter, and is involved in emotional responses. The release of norepinephrine is enhanced by amphetamines. Cocaine stops the removal of norepinephrine from the synapses, so that stimulation of the synapses continues.

Neurotransmitters in the peptide group include the following:

Dopamine: Generally excitatory, dopamine is found in the brain and ANS. A feel-good neurotransmitter, dopamine is involved in emotions and moods and in the regulation of motor control and the executive functioning of the brain. Release is enhanced by L-dopa and amphetamines. Deficiencies occur in Parkinson's disease and possibly also in schizophrenia. Dopamine is part of the endogenous reward/pleasure, craving/seeking behavior system in the brain. Many addictive drugs stimulate dopamine activity, such as cocaine, narcotics, and alcohol.

Histamine: Considered a stimulant, histamine is released by the mast cells as part of the inflammatory process. Histamine causes itching at a cellular level and also works as a vasodilator. Also found in the hypothalamus, the chemical regulates body temperature and water balance and plays a role in our emotions. Histamine also stimulates pain receptors to sensitize against further stimulation, as during a sunburn.

Serotonin: Serotonin usually works as an inhibitor in the CNS and is synthesized into melatonin and affects our biologic cycles, sleep, and moods. Insufficient levels can result in anxiety or depression. Serotonin is described as one of the feel-good neurotransmitters.

Cholecystokinin: Found in the brain, retina, and gastrointestinal tract, the function of cholecystokinin in the nervous system is uncertain and may be related to feeding behavior. Cholecystokinin is a gut-brain peptide.

Endorphins and enkephalins: These endogenous morphines block the brain from feeling pain. Generally inhibitory, they are found in several regions of the CNS, retina, and intestinal tract. They inhibit pain by inhibiting substance P. Morphine and heroin mimic their effects. Endorphins and enkephalins seem to play a part in mood regulation, pain/pleasure cycles, and the internal reward system of the body.

Gamma-aminobutyric acid: Generally inhibitory and found in the brain, this acid is the most common inhibitory neurotransmitter in the brain.

Glutamate (glutamic acid): Generally excitatory and found in the CNS, glutamate is thought to be responsible for as much as 75% of the excitatory signals in the brain.

Somatostatin: Generally inhibitory, somatostatin inhibits the release of growth hormone and is a gut-brain peptide.

Substance P: Substance P is excitatory and is found in the brain, spinal cord, sensory pain pathways, and gastrointestinal tract. Substance P transmits pain information.

Vasoactive intestinal peptide: Found in the brain, some ANS and sensory fibers, retina, and gastrointestinal tract; the function of this peptide in the nervous system is uncertain.

Body Chemistry of Behavior and Pain

Behavior

Behavior is affected by the type and amount of neurotransmitters released at the synaptic junction. Our daily behaviors such as those involved in pleasure, pain, and survival are determined by our chemistry. A *pain behavior* refers to the way we act when under the influence of pain. Too little or too much of any one neurotransmitter results in a behavior that takes extra effort to manage.

Depression may follow a block of the release of catecholamines, whereas anxiety is aggravated by an increase in these neurotransmitters. Current research involves study of the effect of serotonin on migraine headaches. Too much dopamine in the brain may result in hallucinations and could cause mildly erratic behavior such as that displayed when we first fall in love or an extreme of schizophrenic behavior. Dopamine levels are thought to be involved in attention deficit hyperactivity disorders.

The presence of cholecystokinin and vasoactive intestinal peptide in the eye and the stomach indicates a connection between what we see and what we eat. These same neurotransmitters are in the brain. Could this suggest a connection between food, behavior, and emotions? Anyone who has emotional issues around food certainly would not deny that the food we eat changes the way we feel and influences the behavior connected with those emotions.

The matter, again, is of balance. Neurotransmitters balance one another. Those that excite are usually paired with those that inhibit. An ongoing dynamic balance exists in this chemical soup, allowing for behavior that is resourceful for each situation encountered. In addition, we behave in certain ways to increase or decrease levels of neurotransmitters or hormones (i.e., eating or not eating because we are depressed and exercising or not exercising because we are anxious). The television soap operas are good examples. Little program content tells about day-to-day life in the midrange of emotional or behavioral expression. Seldom do we find ourselves caught up in stories about making the bed, changing the oil in the car, or going to the market.

When medication is used to manage neurotransmitters, mood and behavior are affected. The natural functions of the body allow for a wide range of behavior by continually adjusting the neurotransmitter and hormone balance. When neurochemical levels are held in more static ratio by medication, feelings, mood, and resultant behavior are held within the expected parameters. Medication alters the ability to have the highs and lows of emotional expression appropriate to daily circumstances. Compliance with taking psychotropic or mood-altering medication often is affected because persons enjoy the edges of experiences where emotions are most intense. Persons sometimes miss the edges of their emotional selves and thus stop taking their medications, often with devastating results. Careful monitoring by the physician can minimize this situation, but recognizing that it exists is also important.

Behavior seems to be the outward manifestation of attempts at homeostasis, and we seek sensations that organize our brains. When behavior is effective in achieving some sort of balance, it will be reinforced. By observing behavior, we can make educated guesses at the neurotransmitters involved. If the behavior is destructive, possibly other forms of behavior that are less detrimental can be introduced that result in similar neurotransmitter activity. Recognizing that repeated behavior is in some way accomplishing the goal of a form of homeostasis is important—including destructive behavior such as drug addiction, excessive exercise, eating disorders, rage, thrill seeking, crisis orientation, and the deliberate creation of pain. An attempt to eliminate one form of behavior without replacing it with another way to achieve effective homeostasis almost always results in failure and reversion to old behaviors. For example, substituting binge eating with movement and aerobic exercise may work because they operate from a similar neurotransmitter base. Eliminating binge eating without a substitute behavior leaves the individual without a way to achieve chemical balance in the brain and body. Another common example is that eating chocolate affects serotonin (as does the consumption of potato chips, ice cream, and cookies), which is a feel-good neurotransmitter, but so do massage and exercise. However, chocolate is faster, takes less energy, and works. Although eating chocolate helps many persons feel good, if eating chocolate is the only way someone can feel good, other problems can occur. Changing a behavior from one that is quick and reliable to one that requires more effort is difficult.

The statements "moderation in all things" and "variety is the spice of life" are important and wise advice as far as brain chemistry is concerned. Sprinkled into this mix of expression are the highs and lows of ecstasy and despair because these feelings are important as well. This wisdom is found in most ancient healing practices. We will do best if we have many different ways to feel good. Understanding what is causing us to feel bad is also important. When we can respond deliberately with our behavior to generate appropriate feelings for the situation being faced, instead of reacting and relying on only one type of behavior to meet our needs and cope, our neurotransmitters work for us instead of against us (Activity 4-1).

Pain

Pain is a protective device for the body and therefore is important for survival. Pain is a complicated neurochemical event. Generally, the perception of pain occurs in the thalamus; interpretation of pain occurs in the cortex. A painful stimulus one day may not be painful the next. Pain results from a decision in the brain. Anesthetics, including alcohol and barbiturates, depress pain processing so that although the thalamus and other lower centers indicate pain, one "doesn't care" because pain perception is altered.

Drugs can interfere with the production of neurotransmitters or block the receptor sites of neurotransmitters. For example, aspirin interferes with the production of prostaglandin, which prevents it from sensitizing nerve endings to pain.

A pain-inhibiting system exists within the body. Receptors for opiates (e.g., morphine) are present along the pain pathway. Internal, or endogenous, opiates (e.g., endorphins and enkephalins) produced by the body block pain impulses in various portions of the pathway, probably as a protective device. The neurotransmitter substance P, secreted by pain fibers of the spinal cord, is blocked by enkephalins. During pregnancy, a woman's serotonin level gradually increases until it reaches its highest point at the time of delivery in preparation for birth pain. Serotonin modulates pain perception. Some of the food cravings experienced during pregnancy may be caused by the need of the body to increase serotonin levels.

Pain behavior results from pain or perpetuates pain. Pain behavior is a brain chemistry event. Endorphins and enkephalins affect mood. A runner's high is an endorphin experience. Paradoxically, behavior that causes pain sufficient to increase endorphin and enkephalin activity can result in a pleasant change in mood. Many forms of touch and movement modalities can "hurt good," and the deliberate use of controlled pain actually can be therapeutic. Such practice too can become out of balance when one continually creates or seeks pain for the secondary (gain) pleasure. This complex behavior pattern usually requires professional counseling and support to shift to a more appropriate coping style.

Nerve Repair or Regeneration

If the cell body is damaged or separated, the neuron dies. If damage is only done to the axon and the neurilemma is not destroyed, the nerve can repair itself. At the point of injury, the myelin sheath and the distal portion of the axon degenerate. A tunnel is formed by the neurilemma from the point of injury to the original axon destination—another axon, muscle, or gland. This tunnel provides a path for the axon to follow as it regenerates. Nerve regeneration can take a long time because of the length of the axon, location of the injury, inflammatory response, and scarring. This process occurs in the peripheral nervous system.

Oligodendrocytes are cells that produce myelin in the CNS. This myelin does not seem to form into the neurilemma needed to form the guiding tunnel from the area of injury. Therefore regeneration in the CNS is limited (Figure 4-5, *A* to *D*). Extensive and exciting research is occurring in the area of CNS regeneration and nerve growth factors. In the near future, nerve growth factors may be identified that can be used to assist those with spinal cord and brain injuries.

CENTRAL NERVOUS SYSTEM

Brain

The brain is the largest and most complex unit of the nervous system (Figure 4-6) and is composed of approximately 100 billion neurons packed together inside the skull.

ACTIVITY 4-1

Understanding the neurochemical influence of behavior is important to self-awareness and to clinical reasoning in the assessment and analysis process within the professional environment.

The following is an analysis of an event that resulted in a pattern of behavior.

1. Describe the event in factual terms.

Example

The hood on the car would not close, and I was late for an appointment.

2. Describe the emotions and feelings around the event.

Example

I became very frustrated and anxious because I could not drive the car with the hood unlatched.

3. Describe the behavior displayed.

Example

I tried to slam down the hood 3 or 4 times and then started to yell at the car.

4. Identify the possible neurotransmitters involved in the feelings and behavior.

Example

The catecholamines epinephrine and norepinephrine.

5. Indicate mode of action for the neurotransmitters (see pp. 102-104).

Example

Epinephrine and norepinephrine: mostly excitatory, activating sympathetic arousal.

6. Correlate neurotransmitters with the feelings and behavior.

Example

I was anxious because I was late. Stress levels that increase sympathetic activity were high before I noticed the problems with the car. The increase in the catecholamines would produce or perpetuate the fight-or-flight behavior, resulting in my hitting the car and yelling.

7. Propose a balancing behavior to reset homeostasis and identify possible neurochemical interaction.

Example

I could have tightened all my muscles for a few seconds and then relaxed them and repeated this 3 or 4 times. This would simulate the activity of fighting or fleeing and use up some of the epinephrine. The goal would be to calm down.

Choose an event from your life in which you were unable to alter an inappropriate behavior pattern.

1. Describe the event in factual terms.
2. Describe the emotions and feelings around the event.
3. Describe the behavior displayed.
4. Identify the possible neurotransmitters involved in the feelings and behavior.
5. Indicate mode of action for the neurotransmitters (see pp. 102-104).
6. Correlate the neurotransmitters with the feelings and behavior.
7. Propose a balancing behavior to reset homeostasis and identify possible neurochemical interaction.

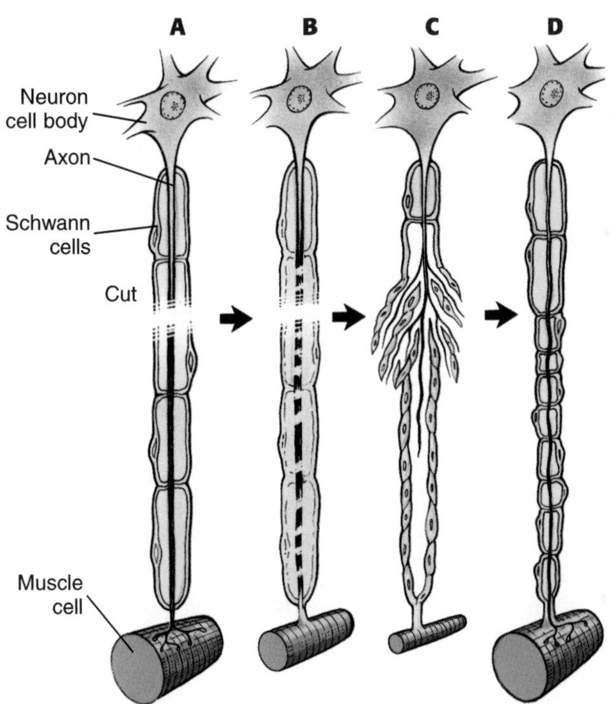

Figure 4-5
Repair of a peripheral nerve fiber. **A,** An injury results in a cut nerve. **B,** Immediately after the injury occurs, the distal portion of the axon degenerates, as does its myelin sheath. **C,** The remaining neurilemma tunnels from the point of injury to the effector. New Schwann cells grow within this tunnel, maintaining a path for regrowth of the axon. Meanwhile, several growing axon sprouts appear. When one of these growing fibers reaches the tunnel, it increases its growth rate, growing as much as 3 to 5 mm per day. (The other sprouts eventually disappear.) **D,** The connection of the neuron with the effector is reestablished. (From Thibodeau GA, Patton KT: *Anatomy and physiology,* ed 5, St Louis, 2003, Mosby.)

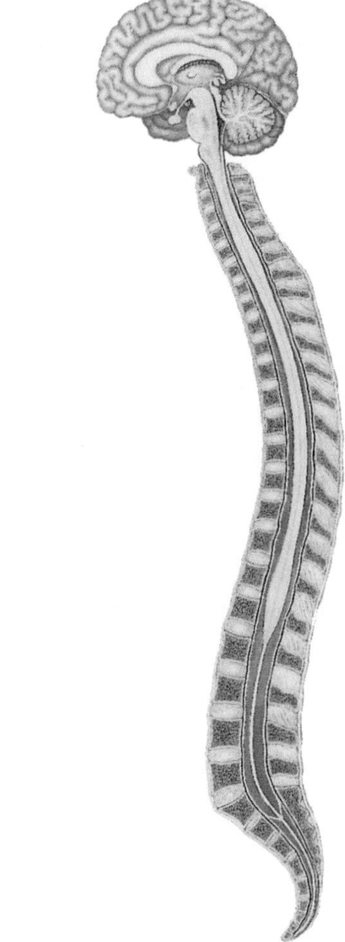

Figure 4-6
The central nervous system. (From Thibodeau GA, Patton KT: *Anatomy and physiology,* ed 5, St Louis, 2003, Mosby.)

Besides its responsibility for our intellect, emotions, and actions, the brain interprets, regulates, and coordinates physiologic activities. Although the brain weighs an average of only 3 pounds, it makes up more than 97% of the nervous system. More than half of its weight comes from the neuroglia. With a composition of more than 85% water, the brain contains a higher percentage of fluid than our blood. The brain is divided into the **cerebrum, cerebellum,** and **brainstem,** which includes the diencephalon.

Cerebrum

The cerebrum, also called the forebrain, is the largest portion of the brain. The major functions of the cerebrum are to receive sensory information, interpret it, associate it with past memories and experiences, and then transmit the most appropriate motor impulse in response to the input. The cerebrum also is involved in emotions and memories.

The cerebrum is divided into left and right hemispheres, each of which is divided further into five lobes. The surface of the cerebrum is covered by a thin layer of **gray matter** called the *cerebral cortex.* The gray color comes from the composition of dendrites and cell bodies. The cerebral cortex is formed into folds called convolutions or *gyri,* (*gyrus,* singular), which increase the available area of the cortex. These folds are separated by creases called *sulci.* The deepest sulci are called *fissures.* The fissures can be used as landmarks when identifying and locating certain areas of the brain.

The *longitudinal fissure* divides the cerebrum into the right and left hemispheres. The *central sulcus,* also known as the fissure of Rolando, separates the frontal and parietal lobes. The *lateral fissure,* the fissure of Sylvius, lies above the temporal lobe and below the frontal and parietal lobes. A fifth lobe, the *insula,* lies deep in the lateral fissure. The occipital and parietal lobes are separated by the *parietooccipital fissure.* The gyri are named for these fissures.

The left and right hemispheres each have motor control and receive sensory input from the opposite side of the body: the left hemisphere works with the right side of the body, and the right hemisphere works with the left side. A structure called the *corpus callosum* is located underneath the gray matter and functions to connect the left and right hemispheres. Because the corpus callosum is composed of myelinated axons, it is white. The corpus callosum is generally larger in women, which becomes clinically significant in the distribution of memory and functioning centers because women tend to be somewhat more random and less compartmentalized in brain function. Some types of brain injury to these memory and function centers can be compensated for far more easily by the female brain than by the more structured male brain (Figure 4-7).

Most of the cerebrum (Figure 4-8) is composed of **white matter.** Areas of nerve cell bodies found in the cerebrum and known as *basal ganglia* are small collections of gray matter that assist in coordination. The *limbic system* also is located on the interior of the cerebrum and is important in our emotional responses, including fear, rage, and pleasure. Therefore a built-in reward and avoidance process exists in the brain. The limbic system is connected to the hypothalamus by the fornix, a band of fibers.

Brain dominance refers to the primary functioning hemisphere that specializes in language functions and linear thought processing. Most right-handed persons have a dominant left hemisphere. More than 70% of left-handed persons are also left-hemisphere dominant. The right hemisphere, which is nondominant in most, concerns itself more with our creative and intuitive abilities and imagination. The left side of your brain works when you read this text, whereas the right side jumps in when you daydream or wonder what all the information means.

Each side of the cerebrum is divided into five lobes, four of which are named for the skull bone lying over them:

Frontal lobe: The anterior portion of the cerebrum, the frontal lobe is positioned behind the frontal bone and contains the prefrontal cortex (governing personality, intellect, and cognition), premotor cortex (directing learned motor skills), and the precentral gyrus (managing motor control of muscles). This lobe is primarily responsible for control of the voluntary skeletal muscles and is active in moods and activities of problem solving that involve concentration and planning. An area known as Broca's area is found in the dominant hemisphere and controls the muscle movements involved in speech.

Parietal lobe: Located next to the parietal bones, this lobe contains the post-central gyrus, which is the primary

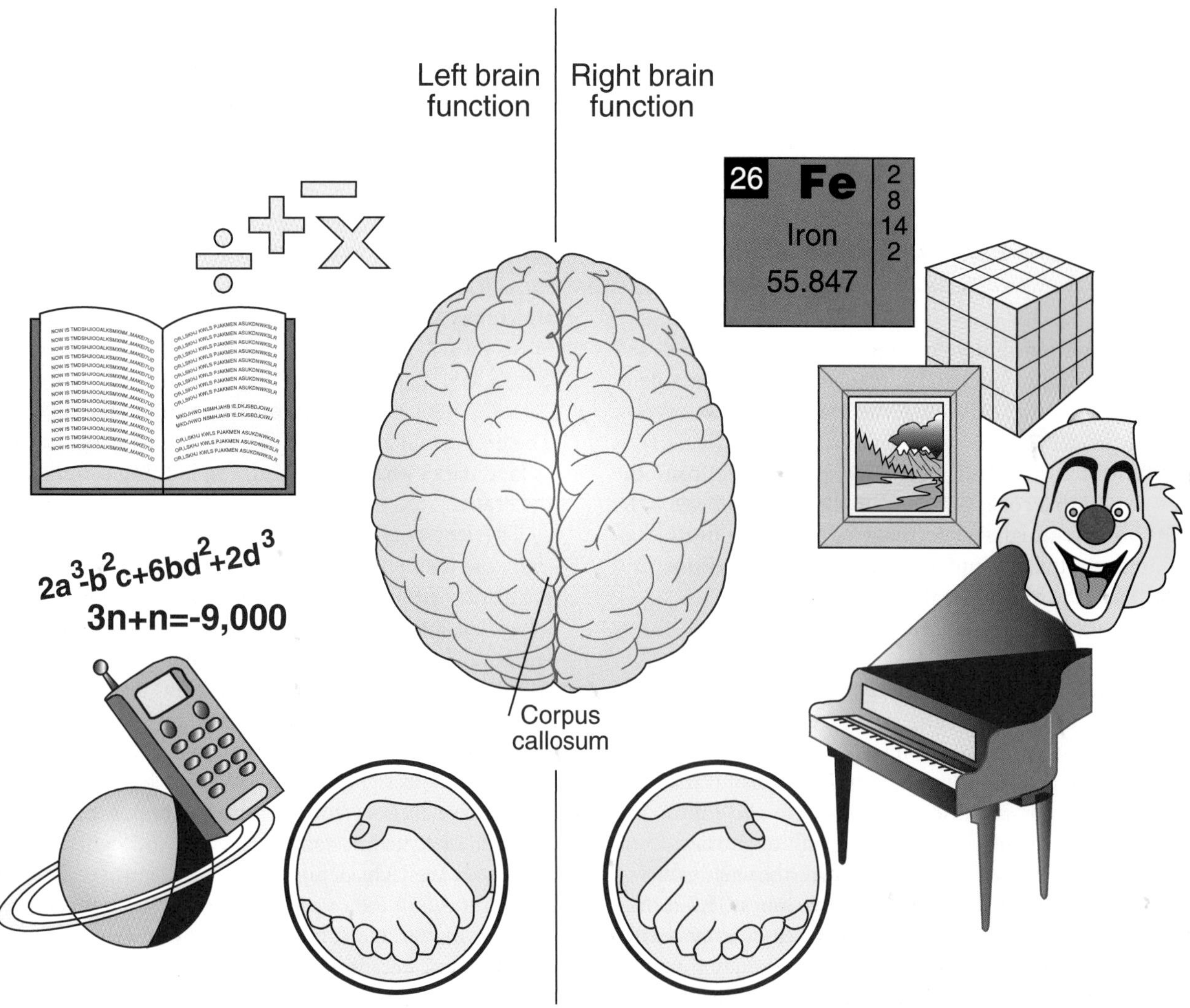

Figure 4-7
Left brain functions and right brain functions.

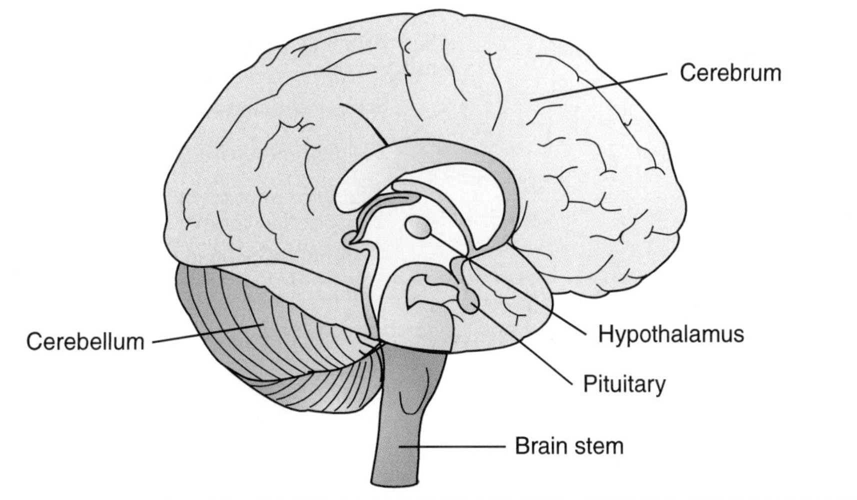

Figure 4-8
Location of brain structures.

sensory area of the brain. This lobe receives and evaluates the sensory information of temperature, pressure, touch, taste, and pain. Its areas of association include speech, thought, and emotions.

Temporal lobe: Found below the lateral fissure, this lobe is next to the temporal bones. The temporal lobe is responsible for the reception and evaluation involved in hearing and smell. *Wernicke's area,* which is located in the superior portion of the gyrus of the dominant hemisphere, is involved in understanding language and transmits information to the Broca's area of the frontal lobe. Broca's area processes language information comprehended by Wernicke's area and relays it to the precentral gyrus. The areas of association combine complex sensory data such as from music and visual scenes into comprehensive patterns that form our memories.

Occipital lobe: Located just anterior to the occipital bone of the skull, this lobe is not separated from the other lobes. The occipital lobe is responsible for the mechanical control of eyesight and integration of visual input with other sensory experiences.

Insula or island of Reil: This fifth lobe is located under the lateral fissure and is the part of the limbic system that gives us a feeling or impression of what is real, true, and important (Figure 4-9, *A* to *C,* and Table 4-1).

Integrative or associative functions of the cortex. Integrative or associative functions include all the activities that occur in the cerebrum after sensory signals are received and before motor responses are sent to where those signals originated. These responses include consciousness, emotions, memory, language, and learning mechanisms (Figure 4-10).

Consciousness is our awareness of the environment and our relationship to everyone and everything in that environment. Throughout the day, degrees of normal changes occur in the levels of consciousness, from sleeping to wide awake. Consciousness depends on excitation of cortical neurons by impulses conducted from the reticular activating system. The *reticular activating system* (described on p. 115) consists of centers in the brainstem that receive impulses from the spinal cord and relay them to the thalamus. The thalamus transmits the data to all parts of the cerebral cortex. Substances that stimulate the cerebrum, enhancing alertness, probably act by stimulating the reticular activating system.

Consciousness may be altered in many ways, including the use of medications or foods that change chemical processes, repetitive activities or sounds, and trance. For centuries, many cultures and religions have explored altered states of consciousness and have used them readily in defensive actions, healing, and pain control. Meditation, tai chi, and yoga are examples of ancient methods used to achieve altered consciousness. We can create the same result with gardening, drawing, knitting, or playing a musical instrument. Any activity that uses a repetitive motion or sound quiets or excites (depending on the speed of the rhythm) the nervous system through entrainment and alters the physiologic processes of the body. An altered state of consciousness also can be achieved during a massage session by the therapist and the client. When the altered state is achieved, it needs to be maintained for at least 15 minutes to achieve the best therapeutic benefit.

Because of religious and political overtones, many persons were hesitant in the past and still are hesitant to explore mystical imagery. Unconscious thought has been identified as a primary activity, whereas conscious thought is described as a secondary activity. States of higher consciousness refer to the primary activity that actually increases alertness and induces relaxation. Research has confirmed this to be a health-enhancing state.

Pleasure derived from the sense of well-being experienced by altered states of consciousness can be addictive. Various plants containing chemicals that alter consciousness

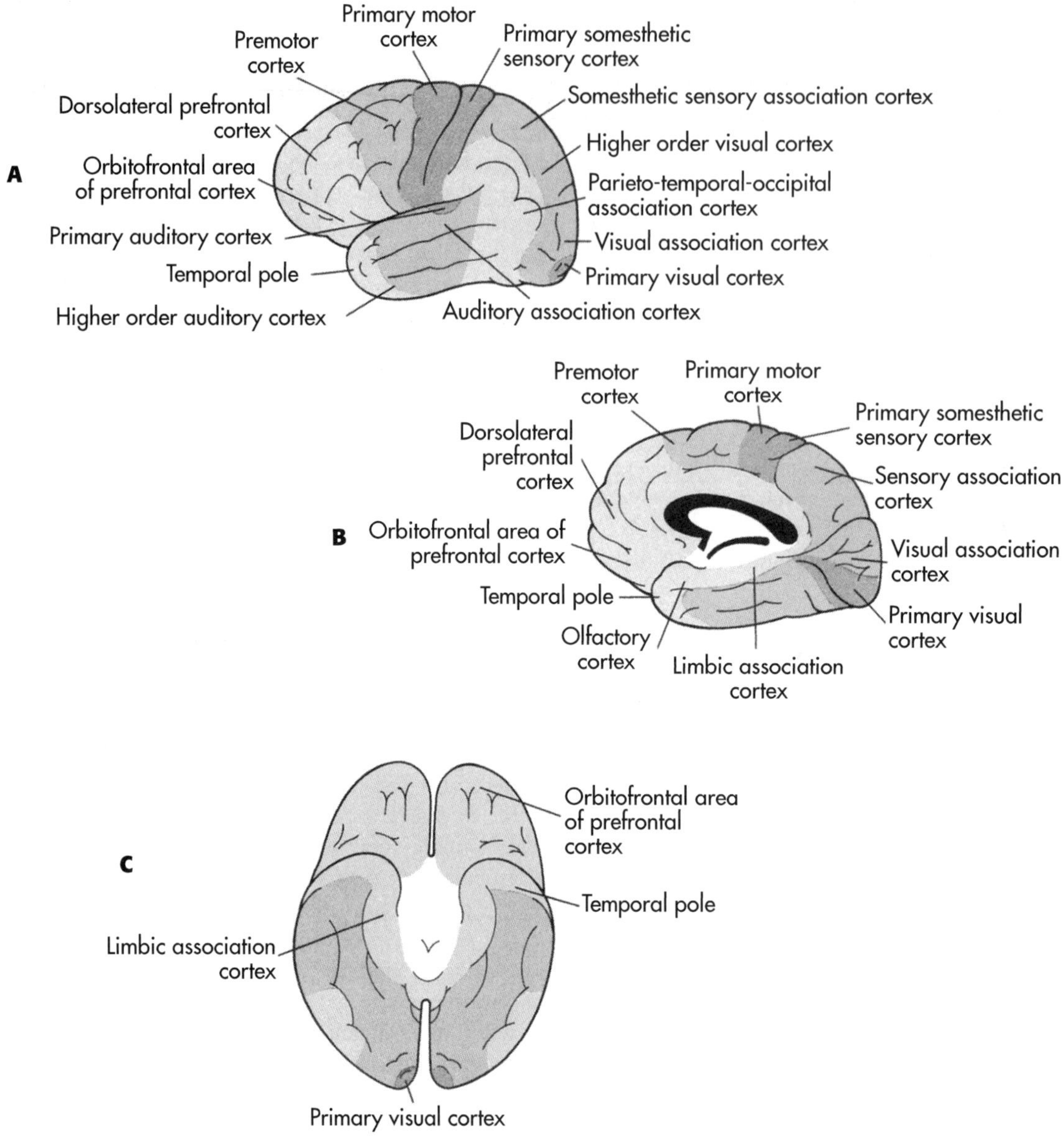

Figure 4-9
A to **C**, Functional organization of the cerebral cortex. (From Árnadóttir G: *The brain and behavior: assessing cortical dysfunction through activities of daily living,* St Louis, 1990, Mosby.)

have been used through the centuries in awareness rituals. Within the confines of cultural and religious ritual, the limited and judicial use of these plants was controlled. Today most, if not all, of the old discipline and structure is nonexistent, and drug abuse is contributing to the disempowerment of altered states of consciousness (Activity 4-2).

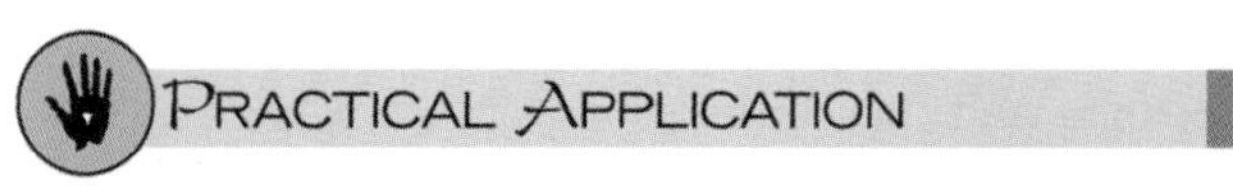

PRACTICAL APPLICATION

Massage therapy interacts with the cerebral cortex and reticular activating system, the same mechanisms involved in consciousness. Because of this, the sensations of altered states of consciousness often are generated by massage methods. Most of the major spiritual disciplines have a movement or positional aspect in their practices that contributes to the meditative states experienced by their participants. Some even incorporate touch, which enhances the experience. ■

Language. Language involves the perception of written and spoken words and the physical ability to speak and write. For 90% of the population, this takes place in the left hemisphere of the cerebrum in the frontal, parietal, and temporal lobes. The ability to apply labels to processes and subjects inside and outside the body also is tied to sensory systems.

TABLE 4-1
Functions of the Cerebral Cortex

Functional Area	Anatomic Area	Function and Performance Components
FRONTAL LOBES		
Primary motor area	Precentral gyrus	Execution of movement
Secondary association area	Premotor cortex	Planning and programming of movement
		Sequencing, timing, and organization of movement
	Frontal eye field	Voluntary eye movements
	Broca's area in the left inferior frontal gyrus	Programming of motor speech
	Supplementary motor area	Intention of movement
Tertiary association area	Orbitofrontal and dorsolateral prefrontal cortex	Ideation
		Concept formation
		Abstract thought
		Intellectual functions
		Sequencing, timing, and organization of action and behaviour
		Initiation and planning of action
		Judgment
		Insight
		Intention
		Attention
		Alertness
		Personality
		Working memory
		Emotion
PARIETAL LOBES		
Primary somesthetic sensory area	Postcentral gyrus	Fine touch sensation, proprioception, kinesthesia
Secondary somesthetic sensory association area	Superior parietal lobule	Coordination, integration, and refinement of sensory input
		Tactile localization and discrimination
		Stereognosis
Tertiary association area	Inferior parietal lobule	Gnosis: recognition of received tactile, visual, and auditory input
		Praxis: storage of programs or visuokinesthetic motor engrams necessary for motor sequences
		Body scheme: postural model of body, body parts, and their relation to the environment
		Spatial relations: processing related to depth, distance, spatial concepts, position in space, and differentiation of foreground from background

TABLE 4-1—cont'd
Functions of the Cerebral Cortex

FUNCTIONAL AREA	ANATOMIC AREA	FUNCTION AND PERFORMANCE COMPONENTS
OCCIPITAL LOBES		
Primary visual sensory area	Calcarine fissure	Visual reception (from the opposite visual field)
Visual association area	Brodmann's areas 18 and 19	Synthesis and integration of visual information
		Perception of visuospatial relationships
		Formation of visual memory traces
		Prepositional construction of language comprehension and speech
TEMPORAL LOBES		
Primary auditory sensory area	Superior temporal gyrus	Auditory reception
Secondary association area	Superior and middle temporal gyri (Wernicke's area)	Language comprehension
		Sound modulation
		Perception of music
		Auditory memory
Tertiary association area	Temporal pole, parahippocampus	Long-term memory
		Learning of higher-order visual tasks and auditory patterns
		Emotion
		Motivation
		Personality
LIMBIC LOBES		
Tertiary association area	Orbitofrontal cortex in frontal lobe, temporal pole, and parahippocampus in the temporal lobe	Attention
	Cingulate gyrus in frontal and parietal lobes	Motivation
		Emotions
		Long-term memory

Modified from Árnadóttir G: *The brain and behavior: assessing cortical dysfunction through activities of daily living,* St Louis, 1990, Mosby.

Emotions. We experience and express our feelings and emotions through the limbic system of the brain. Located inside the cerebrum, the limbic system works with other parts of the cerebral cortex. For most of us, the normal expressions of anger, pleasure, fear, and sorrow are under our control. Individuals whose limbic systems do not interact effectively with the cortex may have episodes of uncontrollable rage or other emotions. Motivation is driven by emotions, especially the pleasure sensations. They cause one to approach or move toward anticipated feelings of pleasure or move away from them to avoid situations remembered from past experiences of distress.

Memory. Memory is the storing of information in the brain and is one of our major mental activities. Two types of memory are short term (recent) and long term. Short-term memory is fragile, unstable, and disappears unless it is reinforced and transferred to long-term memory. The activities in this text are designed to assist in the transference of new data from short-term memory to long-term memory. Long-term memory can be retrieved days or even years after the initial event. The temporal lobes are involved with long-term memory. Long-term memory consists of some kind of structural traces called engrams in the cerebral cortex that involve protein synthesis and physical brain changes,

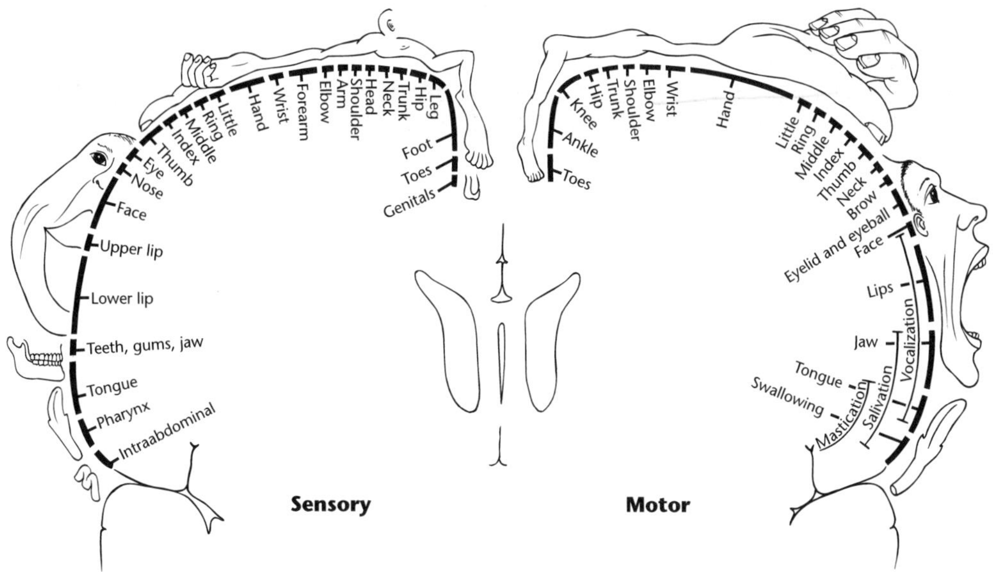

Figure 4-10
Sensory and motor area representations of the brain. Surface area is largest for sensory interpretation of the face, lips, and fingers. Motor surface area is largest for the hands and face. (From Greenstein GM: *Clinical assessment of neuromusculoskeletal disorders,* St Louis, 1997, Mosby.)

ACTIVITY 4-2

How could you alter your state of consciousness in a health-enhancing way? Write down two methods.

Example

Listen to gentle music for 15 minutes while rocking in a rocking chair.

Your Turn

____

____

____

____

resulting in permanent change in the synapses in a specific circuit of neurons. Repeated impulse conduction over a given neuronal circuit seems to produce the synaptic change. Many research findings indicate that the limbic system—the "emotional brain"—plays a key role in memory also. Personal experience substantiates a relationship between emotion and memory. Highly emotional events seem to become stored immediately in long-term memory, indicating neurotransmitter involvement in memory structures.

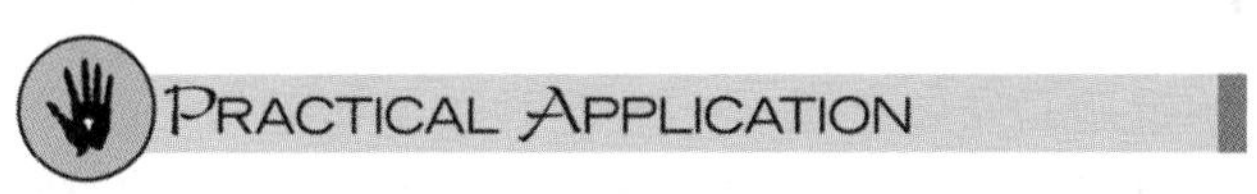

PRACTICAL APPLICATION

The key in long-term memory is repeated impulses. This text provides opportunities to review over and over in various forms the same information to assist in the process of developing long-term memory. Learning strategies often are focused around circular learning, in which information continues to reappear, reinforcing the neurocircuit storing the memory.

Learning that takes place with excitement and enthusiasm or even tears and sorrow is remembered better. Events that create tears of joy are some of the best remembered. Sometimes the memory takes the form of state-dependent memory. With *state-dependent memory* the engram cannot be accessed unless the consciousness state is similar to when the event occurred and was encoded originally. State-dependent memory can take many forms. Sometimes trauma beyond what the conscious centers can integrate is hidden in state-dependent memory. Any form of therapy that can engage the consciousness state, such as hypnosis, biofeedback, or various forms of bodywork, may recreate the sequence of the consciousness state that holds the key to the memory structure, allowing it to surface. Depending on the person's coping skills, resources, support systems, and professional services available, this awareness of past experience can be a time of conscious understanding and integration of a part of a person's life. However, without the proper resources, this type of resurfacing of state-dependent memory can be devastating and extremely harmful.

Pleasure states also are encoded in state-dependent memory. Warm feelings such as being held or the feelings of exhilaration such as running in the wind on a beautiful spring day can be remembered and in a sense recreated with various forms of bodywork. These are health-enhancing states that support homeostasis.

Learning can be thought of as the best and simplest way to solve a problem. Anatomically and physiologically, learning is the use of multiple synaptic pathways to process information. Advanced learning takes place in the association areas of the cerebral cortex (some learning also takes place in the brainstem). Learning involves memory because it is the development of neural structures that remember the way to solve a problem. This process supports survival. Learning can be thought of as conditioning. Pavlov's research identified some of the mechanisms of conditioning in which an external stimulus is connected to a natural occurrence in the body. With Pavlov, dogs were conditioned by a bell being rung at the same time as food was presented. Soon the dogs learned that the bell and food equaled the same thing. Then the sound of the bell alone stimulated digestion and eating behavior. This is behavioral conditioning. Conditioning also can be considered learned habit.

The process of learning is conscious, but after something has been integrated, it often becomes unconscious, a habit. Some habits are beneficial and others no longer serve their original purpose. Breaking a habit is hard. Learning a new way to do something involves making the thought process go down a different road to get to a result. The body and learned memory tend to resist change, especially because learned behavior has such a strong component of primitive survival connected with it. In addition, changing learned behavior takes tremendous energy, and the natural tendency of the body is to conserve energy. Unless the habit is causing us to expend resources in a detrimental way long enough to affect survival, rallying the resources of the body necessary to change the behavior is difficult. ■

Drugs affecting the cerebral cortex. Stimulants that affect the neurotransmitters and receptor sites of the cells in the cerebral cortex include caffeine, nicotine, amphetamines, and cocaine. Caffeine is a CNS stimulant that enhances the sense of alertness and diminishes the sense of fatigue and boredom. Nicotine first stimulates and then depresses the nervous system by affecting the release of norepinephrine and mimicking the action of acetylcholine. Amphetamines and cocaine stimulate the release of catecholamines (primarily norepinephrine and dopamine) from sympathetic neurons. Their effect on the CNS ranges from a feeling of well-being (euphoria) to psychosis.

Depressants (e.g., alcohol, narcotics, minor tranquilizers, and barbiturates) act on the cerebral cortex by blocking norepinephrine and dopamine. The paradoxical effect of alcohol as a "stimulant" results from inhibiting learned behavior and releasing primitive biologic impulses from inhibitory control. Depressants are also anesthetics. The chain of action is as follows: The cortex first is depressed, and then the more primitive centers (brainstem) are depressed as the dosage increases. Brainstem depression can result in death because respiration and cardiac function are slowed and eventually stop if the depression continues.

The hallucinogens include lysergic acid diethylamide (LSD), phencyclidine (PCP), peyote (mescaline), and marijuana (tetrahydrocannabinol). LSD blocks the neurotransmitter serotonin, and PCP blocks acetylcholine. These drugs seem to alter brain function by randomly stimulating and blocking neurotransmitters. A typical action would be that smell may be "seen," color may be "heard," and so forth. PCP is considered the most dangerous of the hallucinogens. PCP uncouples sensory pathways in the brain to produce a sensory deprivation syndrome, creating an increase in body strength accompanied by an acute schizophrenic reaction. Because of high fat solubility and the production of long-acting metabolites, PCP may remain in body tissues for months or even years, causing recurring episodes of violence and psychosis.

Physical dependency (addiction) means that when a drug is withdrawn, severe autonomic excitability occurs. The person thus requires the drug to feel normal. Time is required before the body reestablishes the ability to self-regulate without the drug.

Tolerance occurs with stimulants and depressants. Tolerance means that larger doses of the drug are required for the same effect because the body has adjusted to the current dose. This makes amphetamines dangerous because physical dependency does not exist (thus no warning system), but tolerance does. Consequently, the person may approach the lethal dose without being aware of it.

Brainstem

The brainstem is considered the primitive portion of the brain and is divided into three main parts: the midbrain, pons, and medulla oblongata. The diencephalon often is included as a fourth part. These areas are control centers for vital survival functions and reflex actions such as sneezing, coughing, vomiting, and balanced movements. Research shows that the brainstem likely processes much of the sensory data generated by massage modalities.

Midbrain

The midbrain, or mesencephalon, is located in the middle of the brain, below the cerebrum and between the thalamus and the pons. The midbrain contains reflex centers for visual and auditory stimuli and correlates information about muscle tone and posture. The midbrain contains an important part of the reticular activating system.

Pons

The pons (pons varolii) is in the middle of the brainstem between the midbrain and the medulla. The pons assists in the coordinated patterns of breathing, eye movement, and facial expressions and is involved in rapid eye movement (REM) sleep.

Medulla Oblongata

The medulla or medulla oblongata connects the pons with the spinal cord and is composed of white matter and the reticular formation, a network of white and gray matter. The fibers handle impulses to lower motor neurons. The fibers on one side of the medulla handle signals to the contralateral side. The medulla regulates the heartbeat, blood pressure, and breathing and reflex actions such as coughing or sneezing. Because the medulla controls vital life functions, an injury or disease of the medulla is often fatal.

Diencephalon

The diencephalon is found between the cerebrum and midbrain and contains the thalamus, hypothalamus, pineal body, and other small structures. These structures perform various functions.

Thalamus: The thalamus is created from the gray matter of nerve cell bodies deep in the white matter of the cortex. The thalamus is a relay station from the sense organs to the cerebrum for all sensory input except smell. Signals from the reticular activating system also are sent through the thalamus to the cerebral cortex. The thalamus is associated with pain, temperature, crude touch, and reflex muscle coordination. The thalamus associates pleasant and unpleasant feelings with sensory input and relays information to the limbic system. The thalamus may act as a biooscillator involved with internal biorhythm entrainment.

Hypothalamus: The hypothalamus lies below the thalamus and above the pituitary gland. The hypothalamus regulates and coordinates functions such as heart rate, blood pressure, peristaltic actions, appetite and satiety, pleasure, temperature, and general coordination of ANS functions. The hypothalamus produces releasing hormones that affect pituitary gland hormones, which in turn influence important activities such as hunger, appetite, sleep cycles, wakefulness, sexual arousal, and water balance. The hypothalamus is associated closely with the limbic system and is an important link between the nervous and endocrine systems, which allows the mind to affect the body—the mind-body connection.

PRACTICAL APPLICATION

The pleasure center deep inside the hypothalamus involves feel-good neurotransmitters and predisposes one to addictive behavior to feel good, alter mood, and so forth. Romantic love is a brain bath of norepinephrine and dopamine—feel-good chemicals. Therapeutic massage stimulation also influences the feel-good neurotransmitters. Substance abuse, including nicotine, alcohol, and caffeine, and behaviors such as extremes of eating, sex, gambling, exercise, thrill seeking, pain, violence, and crisis creating are feel-good chemical substitutes. They have a potential for addictive behavior because they interact with feel-good neurotransmitters as well. Many psychotropic or mood-regulating medications act on the feel-good neurotransmitters. The use of chemicals or extreme behaviors to produce pleasure often depletes or inhibits the natural production of the chemicals, resulting in a big downslide after a big high. The extremes of pleasure and discomfort create craving and seeking behaviors that support addictive behavior.

Because therapeutic massage stimulates the release of the feel-good neurotransmitters and hormones, inclusion of these therapies has been shown to support the treatment of addictive behavior by replacing a destructive manner of mood alteration with a constructive, more moderate way to feel good. That the treatment of complex factors such as those found in addiction be monitored and dealt with in a multidisciplinary team approach is essential. ■

Pineal body: The pineal body or gland is found on the dorsal side of the diencephalon. The pineal gland and its hormone melatonin are still a mystery. Approximately 30% of the pineal cells are magnetically sensitive and responsive to external magnetic patterns. The gland functions as an internal biologic clock that regulates daily activities (circadian rhythms), as well as yearly rhythms (circannual rhythms). Exposure to natural sunlight assists these functions. The pineal body needs darkness to convert serotonin to melatonin. Melatonin seems to be involved with sexual activity. Melatonin also triggers the pituitary gland to release luteinizing hormone, which affects sexual maturity and may be involved in puberty and menopause. Melatonin is involved in the sleep pattern.

Two of the best known sleep stages are slow wave sleep and REM sleep. Sleep has stages from 1 through 4, with 4 being the deepest sleep. Slow wave sleep produces slow-frequency, high-voltage brain waves and is associated with stages 2 and 3. Such sleep is almost entirely a dreamless part of the sleep pattern. At the deeper levels, the reticular activating system activity is depressed in the pons and medulla. REM sleep, however, is associated with dreaming. At intervals of 90 minutes or so, the closed eyes begin to move rapidly. Repeatedly waking a person at the beginning of REM sleep produces anxiety and irritability. If the person then is allowed to sleep, more than the usual REM sleep and dreaming occurs for a few nights to catch up. This process is called *REM rebound.* Many medications, particularly sleeping pills and tranquilizers, suppress REM and stage 4 sleep. Stopping the drug may result in REM rebound, sometimes associated with nightmares. Therefore using medicines with minimal REM rebound when medication is necessary is important.

Reticular Activating System

The reticular activating system is a structural and functional part of the reticular formation in the brainstem and maintains arousal levels in the cerebral cortex and alerts it to changes in homeostasis, thus keeping us awake and alert. The importance of this system in consciousness and the sleep state already has been discussed. The reticular activating system also helps regulate respiration, blood pressure, heart rate, endocrine secretion, and conditioned reflexes. Incoming stimuli are integrated by the reticular formation. Epinephrine and amphetamines stimulate reticular activating system conduction, whereas anesthesia and barbiturates depress conduction. Trauma or damage to the reticular activating system can cause a person to become comatose.

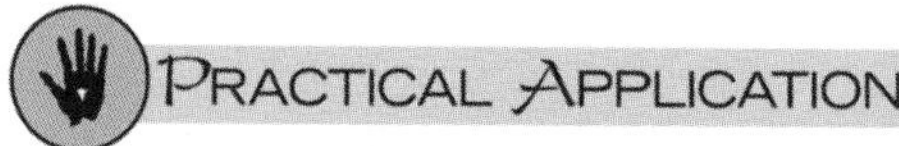

To maintain homeostasis, we need sufficient sleep for health and well-being. During this time of rest, most growth and repair of the body takes place. Disrupted sleep patterns are found in many chronic diseases. If sleep possibly can be restored to an effective pattern without the use of medications, often the body can better cope or even begin to heal a chronic problem over time. Massage is relaxing and conducive to supporting effective sleep patterns, providing benefit to the client and thus decreasing the effects of the chronic problem. ■

Cerebellum

The cerebellum is located in the posterior cranial fossa beneath the posterior portion of the cerebrum. The cerebellum is the second largest part of the brain and consists of a cortex composed of gray matter and an inner portion composed of white matter. Like the cerebrum, the cerebellum has sulci and gyri and contains two lateral hemispheres that are connected by the vermis. The cerebellum maintains balance and posture and, with proprioceptive input, coordinates everything from normal movements to the complex activities involved in dancing, gymnastics, and doing massage. The cerebellum, limbic system, and other relay centers of the brain have been shown to work on the same circuit (Hooper, 1986).

Vestibular Apparatus

This paired organ is part of the inner ear. Sensations produced in this organ are conveyed to the brain along with that of hearing via the vestibulocochlear nerve and are related directly to equilibrium, balance, and functions of the cerebellum.

The vestibular apparatus, on each side, consists of three circular canals that are interconnected and filled with fluid. The canal expands to form fluid-filled structures called *utricles* and *saccules.* The canals and the utricle and saccule have receptors that respond to movement, especially when the head is rotated and when the head moves forward or backward.

Every time the head is moved, the fluid in the semicircular canals is set in motion, generating nerve impulses. The impulses travel to the brainstem and to the cerebellum to give information about body and head movement, and neurons also provide information to the cranial nerves supplying the eye and adjust eye position according to the movement and direction. The motor cortex is stimulated and the body is able to increase and decrease tone and maintain balance and equilibrium.

The vestibular apparatus is important for spatial orientation. Spatial orientation, which is our sense of position in gravity, is aided by vision proprioceptors and by touch and pressure receptor input.

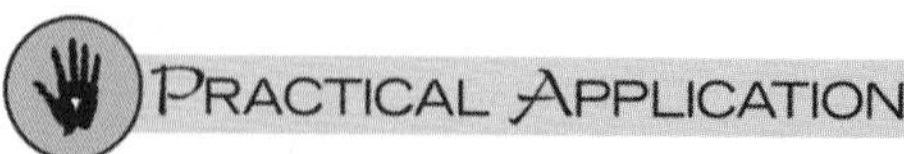

Massage techniques that stimulate the cerebellum, such as rhythmic rocking, have a widespread influence. Rocking produces movement at the neck and head that influences our sense of equilibrium. Rocking stimulates the balance mechanisms of the inner ear (vestibular balancing mechanisms), including the vestibular complex and the labyrinthine righting reflexes, which work to keep our head level. Rocking affects the whole body, stimulating muscle contraction patterns that pass throughout the body. Pressure on the side of the body may stimulate the righting reflexes. A close relationship exists between the vestibular nerves and the cerebellum. This feedback information, which adjusts and coordinates movement, is relayed directly to the motor cortex and to the cerebellum. Methods that alter body positional sense and initiate specific movement patterns change sensory input from muscles, tendons, joints, and the skin. The output from the cerebellum goes to the motor cortex and brainstem. Stimulation of the cerebellum by altering muscle tone, position, and vestibular balance also stimulates the hypothalamus to adjust ANS functions and thus restore homeostasis. ■

Ventricles

Four fluid-filled chambers called ventricles are found within the brain, one in each of the cerebral hemispheres, one positioned just below and between them, and one at the attachment of the cerebrum and the brainstem. **Cerebrospinal fluid** (CSF) fills these ventricles and then passes through several small openings to the subarachnoid space. CSF circulates through the brain and around the spinal cord and is returned to the venous system at the dural sinuses. CSF is replenished continuously from the fluid filtering out of the choroid plexus, a network of brain capillaries.

Classified as one of the circulating fluids of the body, CSF is a colorless, watery substance that flows throughout the brain and around the spinal cord, providing cushioning and protection. CSF maintains homeostasis of the brain environment, including pH balance (acid-base) (Figure 4-11).

Meninges

The brain and spinal cord are protected by the skull and spinal column. They also are surrounded by three membranes called the meninges (Figure 4-12). The dura mater is the outermost layer and is made up of a tough, white fibrous connective tissue membrane. The dura mater lines the cranial bones and covers the brain and spinal cord. Portions of the dura mater line the fissures between the left and right hemispheres of the cerebrum and cerebellum and cover the spinal nerve roots. Nerves and blood vessels run through the epidural space next to the dura mater.

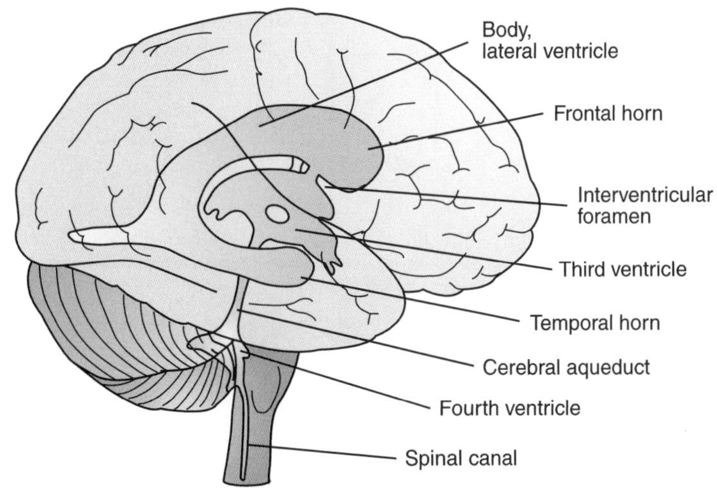

Figure 4-11
Ventricular system, lateral view.

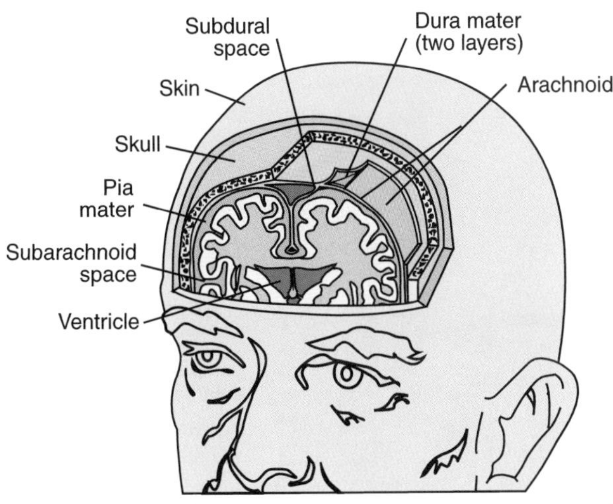

Figure 4-12
Meninges of the brain.

The second layer is the arachnoid mater, a cobweblike membrane containing many blood vessels. The third layer, the pia mater, is thin and adheres directly to the brain and spinal cord. The meninges form three spaces that add additional cushioning and protection to the CNS. They are the following:

Epidural space: Found between the skull and dura mater, this space contains connective tissue, including fat.

Subdural space: Found between the dura mater and arachnoid membrane, this space is filled with a cushioning serous fluid.

Subarachnoid space: Found between the arachnoid and pia mater, this space contains the CSF.

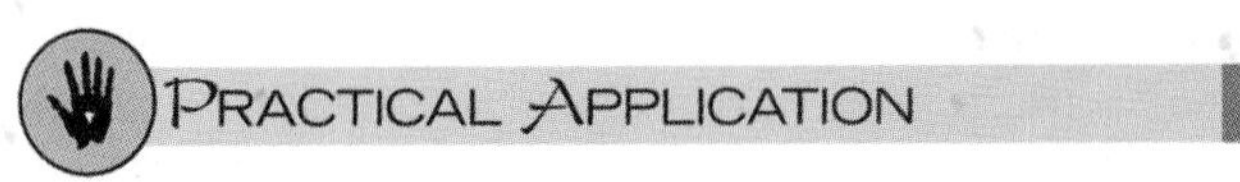

Some methods of bodywork, such as cranial sacral therapy, are thought to interact with the movement of the meninges, especially the dura mater, and to affect the flow of CSF. In the CNS a rhythm known as the cranial sacral impulse can be observed and palpated.

The effect of bodywork on this rhythm is still under investigation, although entrainment methods that synchronize the motions and rhythms of the body are credited with providing the most benefits. The application is to be done in a quiet, rhythmic manner by a quiet and focused practitioner who adds an additional external influence that allows the body rhythms to synchronize. When synchronization is achieved, homeostatic mechanisms seem to operate more efficiently. ■

Vessels of the Brain

Blood is supplied to the brain through the middle cerebral arteries, which are a continuation of the internal carotid arteries, and the basilar artery. These are created from the two vertebrobasilar arteries. These three brain arteries are connected at the midbrain in the *circle of Willis,* which is a check-and-balance system that provides blood flow to the brain in case of blockage or damage to any of the three arteries (Figure 4-13). Blood is transported out of the brain by several veins and the dural sinuses, which drain into the internal jugular veins.

Spinal Cord

The spinal cord is made of white and gray matter and is about 17 to 18 inches long in the average person. The spinal cord begins at the base of the brainstem, exiting through an opening in the skull called the foramen magnum, and continues through the vertebral column to the first and second lumbar vertebrae. At this point, the pia mater continues on as the *filum terminale* and connects to the dura mater at the second sacral vertebra, and they both end at the coccyx. Thirty-one pairs of spinal nerves connect the spinal cord and brain with the rest of the body as the peripheral nervous system.

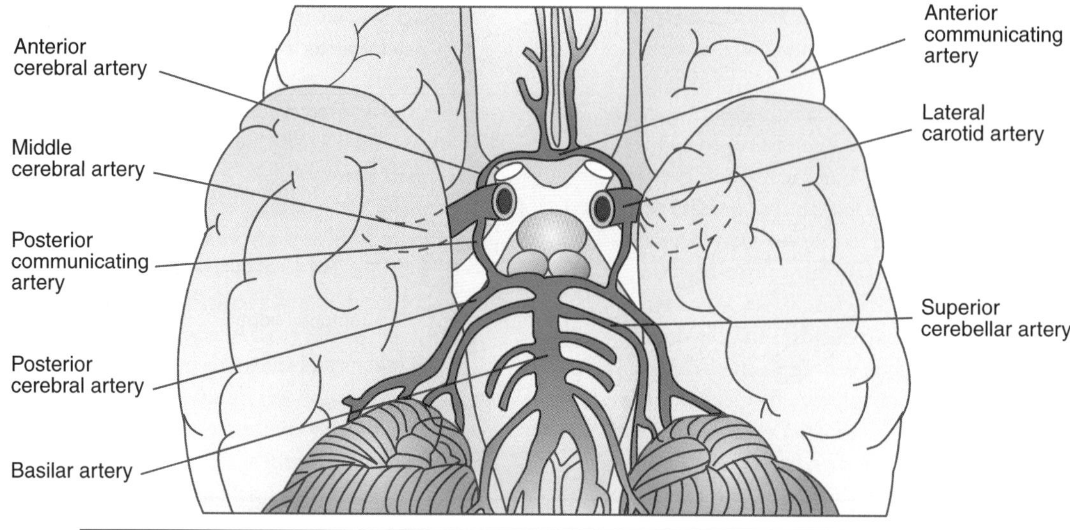

Figure 4-13
Anatomic diagram of circle of Willis.

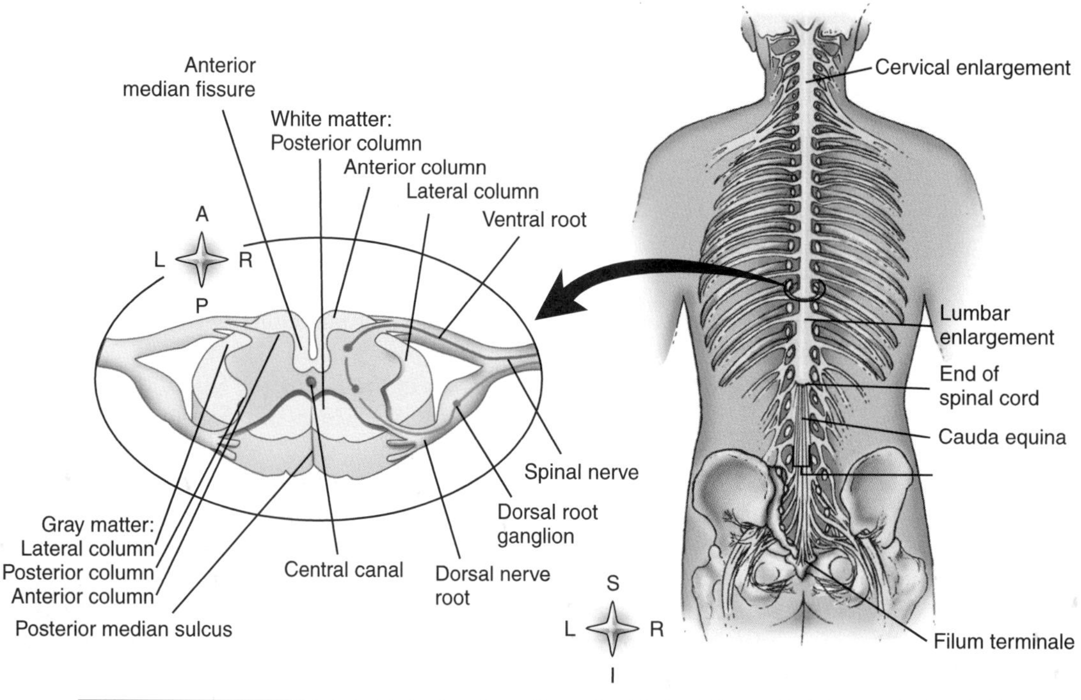

Figure 4-14
Spinal cord. The inset illustrates a transverse section of the spinal cord shown in the broader view. (From Thibodeau GA, Patton KT: *Anatomy and physiology*, ed 5, St Louis, 2003, Mosby.)

The section of the spinal cord that corresponds to a single pair of spinal nerves is known as a segment, and the spinal cord has 31 segments: 8 cervical, 12 thoracic, 5 lumbar, 5 sacral, and 1 coccygeal. Because the spinal cord is shorter than the vertebral column (ending at the second lumbar vertebra), the spinal nerves from the lower lumbar and sacral regions extend to and exit through the intervertebral foramen. The spinal and lower lumbar nerves, which are referred to as *cauda equina*, make the lower end of the spinal cord look like the tail of a horse. The spinal nerves are indicated easily in relation to the vertebra. For example, the nerve between the first and second thoracic vertebrae is T1.

Each spinal nerve is attached to the spinal cord by two roots: the **dorsal root** (sensory root) and the **ventral root** (motor root). The dorsal root is enlarged to form the dorsal root ganglion. Distal to the dorsal root ganglion, the sensory and motor roots are bound together to form a spinal nerve, making spinal nerves mixed nerves. Figure 4-14 shows the sectional anatomy of the spinal cord.

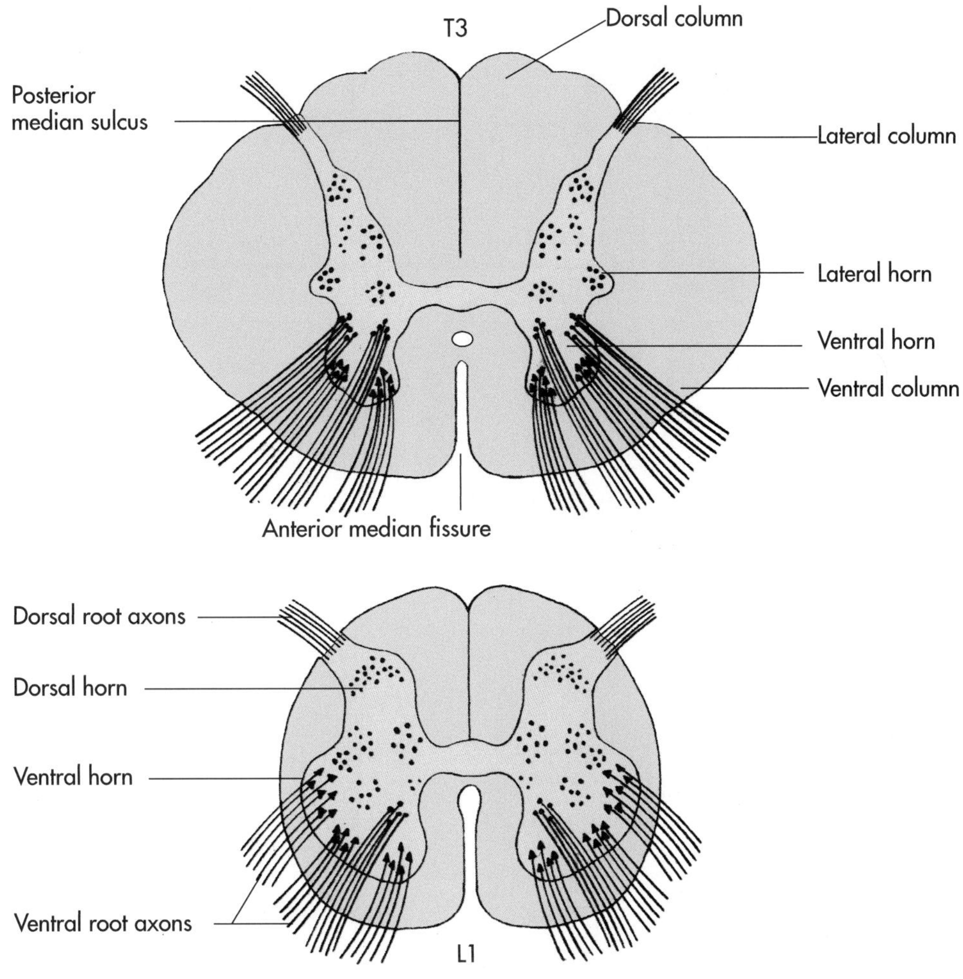

Figure 4-15
Inner structure of the spinal cord. (From Mathers LH et al: *Clinical anatomy principles,* St. Louis, 1995, Mosby.)

The two main functions of the spinal cord are to conduct nerve impulses and to be a center for spinal reflexes. The spinal cord is oval and, like the brain, has fissures. The anterior median fissure is deeper and wider than the posterior median sulcus (Figure 4-15). On the outside of the spinal cord are pathways of white matter called **tracts,** created from the myelinated nerve fibers. They ascend to and descend from the brain. The **ascending tracts** conduct sensory impulses such as pain, touch, and temperature up from the spinal nerves through the spinal cord to the brain, whereas **descending tracts** conduct motor impulses from the brain down the cord to the spinal nerves. The functions of the axons in each tract are limited to one action such as transmitting specific touch and pain sensations.

The gray matter in the inside extends the length of the spinal cord. A cross section shows that the gray matter forms an H pattern. The dorsal portion of the H forms the dorsal horns and is composed of the cell bodies of association, or interneurons. The anterior portion of the H forms the ventral horns, consisting of the cell bodies of motor nerves. The center of the gray matter is the central canal containing cerebrospinal fluid (Figure 4-16, *A* to *C*).

white matter -outside

Sensory Ascending Tracts

Sensory receptors are found in the skin, muscles, and all organs. When stimulated by touch, pain, and muscle action, they excite in response and initiate neural processes. The signals follow the nerve fibers from these receptors to the spinal cord, where they cross to the other side and ascend one of the sensory pathways or tracts to the thalamus, medulla, or cerebellum. In the brain the sensations are integrated into perceptions or filtered as unimportant. This sensory information is needed to help us maintain homeostasis.

Some of the most important sensory information supplied to the client's body during massage comes from sensory receptors and specifically proprioceptors that sense data concerning position and movement. Sensory fibers transmit signals about body position, deep touch or pressure, two-point discrimination (the ability to differentiate between two stimuli applied close to each other), and vibration. The proprioceptors are located in muscles, tendons, ligaments, and joints.

Some proprioceptive signals initiate a response in the spinal cord; these are called deep tendon reflex arcs. Other fibers ascend the dorsal portion of the spinal cord, cross over

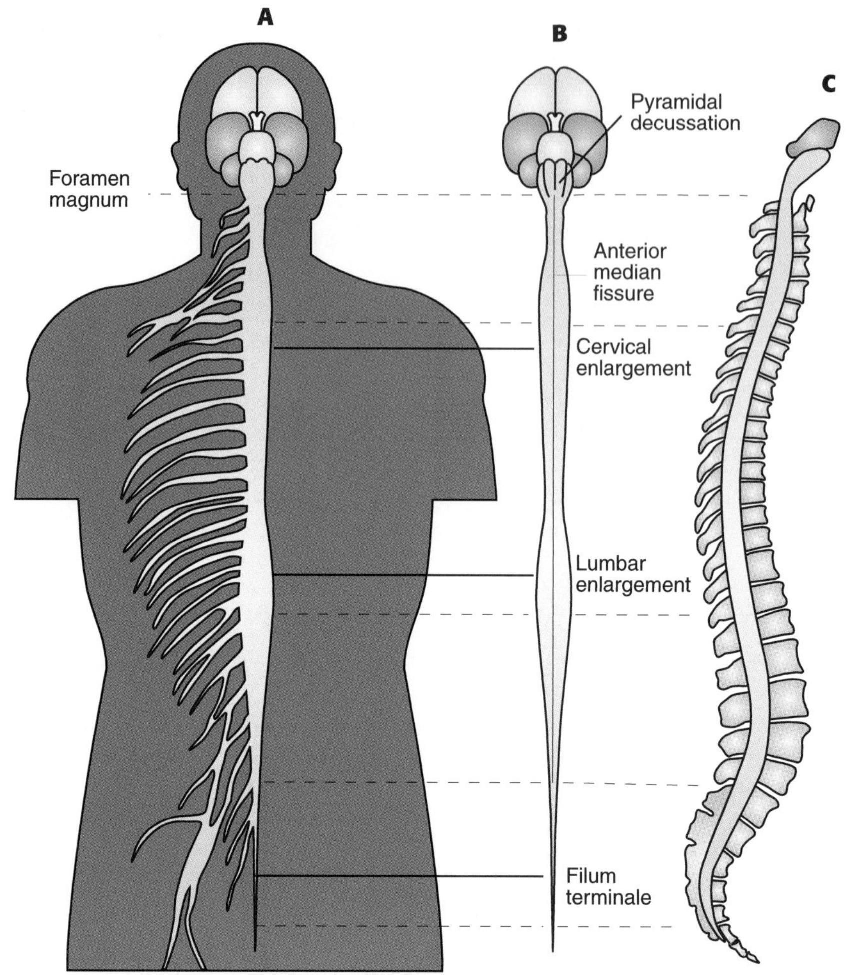

Figure 4-16
A, Posterior surface of a spinal cord within a vertebral canal dissected from the back. **B,** The way the anterior surface of the same spinal cord would look after removal of dura, arachnoid, and spinal nerves. **C,** Spinal cord exposed from the lateral direction.

in the medulla, and ascend to the thalamus and post-central gyrus.

For a sensory signal to get from a sensory receptor to the brain, it passes through three different neurons. The first one, referred to as the primary, is a relay from the receptor to the brainstem or the spinal cord. This is part of the peripheral nervous system and is discussed in detail in the next chapter.

The second neuron extends from the brainstem or spinal cord to the thalamus. The secondary neuron synapses with the tertiary (or third) neuron in the thalamus and ends in the post-central gyrus of the parietal lobe of the cortex. The axons of these third neurons make up the white matter of the cerebrum, referred to as the internal capsule, whereas the dendrites and cell bodies make up the gray matter of the cerebral cortex. The actual crossing of sensory signals from the left to the right side takes place mostly in the secondary neurons before they enter the thalamus (Figure 4-17).

Motor Descending Tracts

Motor tracts transmit information regarding adaptive responses and sensory experiences concerned with gross movements, posture, and fine motor skills. One of the main motor tracts is the pyramidal or corticospinal tract, which ties in to the voluntary motor system. The fibers begin in the cortex at the precentral gyrus and descend to the medulla, where they cross to the opposite side of the spinal cord. From that point they descend through the lateral corticospinal tract to the motor neurons of the skeletal muscles. The pyramidal fibers handle voluntary and reflex signals to the muscles.

For signals to get from the CNS to the muscles, they use the somatic motor pathways. For signals that begin in the brain, following the wiring of the somatic motor pathway may be difficult. Identifying the pathways for reflex signals that begin in the spinal cord is much simpler. Spinal reflexes are centered in the gray matter of the spinal cord; these

ACTIVITY 4-3

Summarize the ascending and descending functions of the spinal cord.

Ascending	***Descending***
Example	*Example*
Sends information to CNS regarding pain	Delivers information to muscles

actions are discussed in Chapter 5 because they directly involve the peripheral nervous system. We limit our exploration here to the nonreflex actions.

One important rule to remember is the *final common path principle.* Each motor unit within a muscle receives impulses that are conducted along a single motor neuron that begins in the anterior gray horn of the spinal cord. This principle is important to health care providers who are exploring muscle dysfunction and its relationship to spinal cord injuries. By identifying a muscle dysfunction, common relationship to the spinal nerve also can be surmised. The common path principle does not hold for the neurons from the cerebrum to the motor neurons in the spinal cord.

The spinal cord has five main motor tracts:

1. *Lateral corticospinal tracts:* These tracts handle our voluntary movements, especially the contraction of small groups of muscles such as those in the hands and feet. They affect muscles on the side of the body opposite from the cerebral cortex.
2. *Anterior or ventral corticospinal tracts:* These tracts handle the same lateral tracts, but the muscles are on the same side of the body as the cortex.
3. *Lateral reticulospinal tracts:* These tracts transmit facilitatory impulses from the medulla through the anterior horn motor neurons to skeletal muscles that handle muscle tone and extensor reflexes.
4. *Medial reticulospinal tracts:* These tracts carry mainly inhibitory impulses from the pons through the anterior horn motor neurons to skeletal muscles that deal with muscle tone and extensor reflexes.
5. *Rubrospinal tracts:* These tracts transmit impulses that coordinate body movements and maintain posture.

The term *pyramidal tracts* refers to the *lateral* and *anterior corticospinal tracts.* The neurons from the cerebral cortex cross through the pyramid areas of the medulla. From the medulla most of them cross to the other side and descend the spinal cord. The rest of the neurons extend through the pyramid areas and continue down the same side of the spinal cord. The pyramidal neurons are referred to as the upper motor neurons. When they reach their termination points in the gray matter of the spinal cord, they connect to lower motor neurons, which innervate the muscles. Most of these connections involve an additional synapse with an interneuron.

The *extrapyramidal tracts* are composed of the *lateral* and *medial reticulospinal* and *rubrospinal tracts,* none of which enter the medullar pyramid areas. They relay motor signals through the cerebrum, thalamus, brainstem, and cerebellum to the gray matter of the spinal cord. At this point, most synapse with interneurons, which then synapse with the lower motor neurons. One should note that facilitating and inhibiting signals are sent through these motor neurons.

Injuries to the upper and lower motor neurons result in different responses in the skeletal muscles. When upper motor neurons are damaged or destroyed through trauma or disease, the result is usually an increase in rigidity and an exaggerated response to reflexes. This is referred to as spastic paralysis. Injuries to the lower motor neurons result in a lack of signal to the muscles, causing absence of movement. This is known as flaccid paralysis (Figure 4-17).

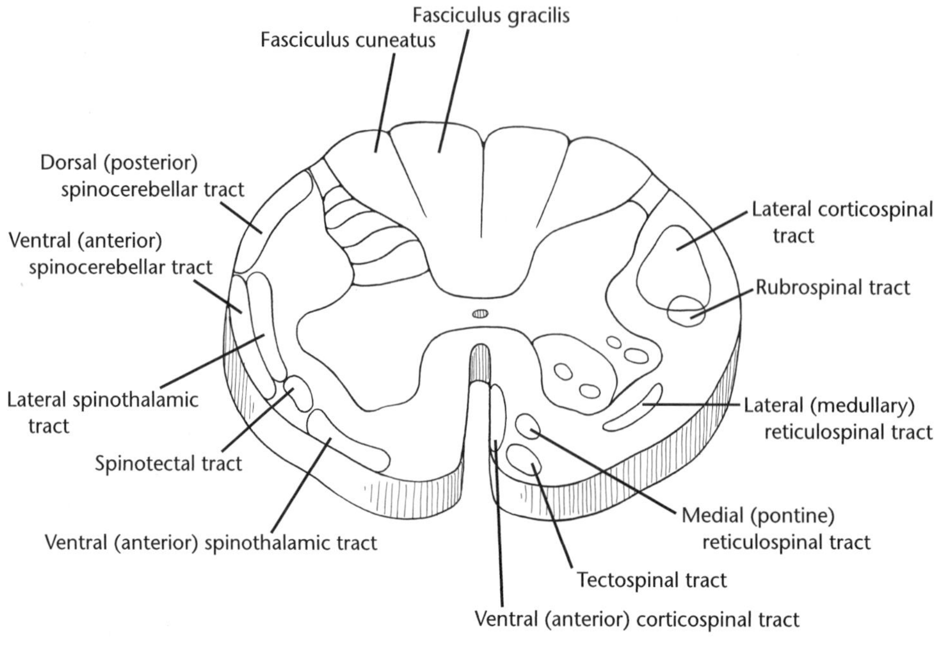

Figure 4-17
Ascending and descending tracts. (From Greenstein GM: *Clinical assessment of neuromusculoskeletal disorders,* St Louis, 1997, Mosby.)

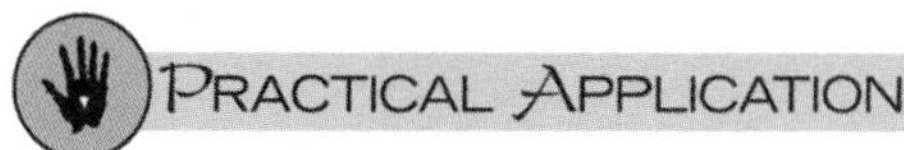

PRACTICAL APPLICATION

The disability or dysfunction caused by brain and spinal cord injuries is determined by the region and function of the area affected. The prognosis for trauma to the motor neurons is often difficult to identify. The use of soft tissue work and other forms of movement therapies seems to be most beneficial as part of the whole health care picture. Specific recommendations regarding massage are difficult to make based solely on the location of damage because of the compensation of the body through rerouting of the interrupted signals. This is why clinical reasoning methods are so important. The ability to process a situation and determine the best intervention methods to be used is essential to the successful therapeutic massage professional.

For example, spastic paralysis results from upper motor neuron injuries. A client with upper motor neuron injuries will have spastic paralysis of the muscles in the affected region. Voluntary control over movements is lost, and limbs may need to be restrained to prevent involuntary movement at inappropriate times. Usually less muscle atrophy is present, and lymph and blood flow continues because of the working of the muscles. The preferred modalities, when applied to each individual, can moderate some of the random spasms and keep the soft tissues more supple and the joints more mobile, resulting in less rigidity in the muscles. With lower motor neuron difficulties, the muscles atrophy and actions and reflexes are slow, limited, or nonexistent. Massage and joint movement may be able to replace the mechanical pumping action of normal muscle contraction and assist in moving the blood and lymph. In addition, keeping the soft tissue pliable may lessen any contractures. ■

PATHOLOGY

Cerebrovascular Accidents/Strokes

Cerebrovascular accident (CVA) or stroke is an umbrella term that covers disorders such as aneurysms and hemorrhages that damage brain tissue. Thrombosis is a common cause of blood vessel structure damage.

Ulcerated plaque from arteriosclerosis or a portion of a blood clot may break away from a different part of the body and form an embolus that travels to the brain. Any of these conditions deprives the brain of oxygen. Because brain cells consume large quantities of oxygen, any deficit can cause damage quickly.

A transient ischemic attack (TIA) is a prestroke condition that mimics a stroke. TIA resolves in less than 24 hours. In some cases when the deficit lasts longer than 24 hours and then clears completely, the condition is called a reversible neurologic deficit or a residual ischemic neurologic deficit.

The signs of a TIA are transient blindness in one eye, aphasia, numbness or weakness of the hand or foot, slurred speech, dizziness, ataxia, syncope, and numbness around the lips. The signs may last only a few minutes and then disappear. They often are ignored. Knowing the basic signs of TIA and referring the client immediately is important, because a TIA is frequently a warning of a major stroke.

When a stroke occurs, an artery in the brain is occluded or closed off from a blood clot called a thrombus. A stroke lasts longer than 24 hours. The location and duration that the blood flow is cut off determines the damage caused by the stroke. The following deficits may occur:

Hemiparesis: Partial motor deficit on one side of the body

Quadriplegia: Total motor deficit of both arms and legs (usually seen in trauma)

Sensory losses: Pain, temperature, vibration, and so forth

The limbs are initially flaccid (relaxed). Later they become spastic (contracted). The forearm in flexion and the leg in extension are common sights because of the unequal innervation of extensors and flexors. The cause of the spasticity is thought to be loss of control of lower motor neurons.

Behavioral changes caused by damage in the association areas of the cortex often are present. If the left hemisphere is involved, language difficulties (such as aphasia) occur. A stroke in the right hemisphere produces inattention and lack of concern. Confusion may be present if either hemisphere is affected.

Cerebrovascular Disease

Cerebrovascular disease is a gradual buildup of arteriosclerotic (thickened, hardened areas of reduced elasticity) lesions in arteries of the neck and brain. Hypertension is a strong predisposing factor. Arteries commonly affected are the common carotid, internal carotid, and middle cerebral arteries. Complications of cerebrovascular disease are blood clots and hemorrhage.

Aneurysm

An aneurysm is a weakening and bulging of any artery, including those in the brain. If the artery breaks, bleeding and complications can be fatal. Sometimes the rupture is preceded by a series of small leaks producing transient headache and neck stiffness. These symptoms are common in many other conditions, as well as with normal stress. These symptoms are why having a qualified medical professional rule out more serious conditions is important before one assumes that symptoms are minor or only stress related.

INDICATIONS/CONTRAINDICATIONS

For Therapeutic Massage

Therapeutic massage in a supervised setting can be supportive during rehabilitation. These methods are effective for managing discomfort caused by the functioning portions of the body working extra hard to compensate for nonfunctioning areas. Stress management is an important part of the long-term management of these conditions. Because anticoagulants often are used to prevent further CVAs or TIAs, care needs to be taken with soft tissue methods used so that bruising does not occur during therapy. Careful attention needs to be paid to any symptom of thrombosis, and the type of massage application used should not place heavy pressure over vulnerable vessels to avoid the possible movement of an embolism.

Central Nervous System Trauma

A sudden blow to the head or intense shaking of the head may or may not involve a fracture. The fracture itself is usually not important; more significant is the possibility of intracranial bleeding or brain swelling (edema). Trauma to the tissues of the brain and surrounding structures and a change in pressure or fluid concentration is of significance to any trauma regarding the CNS.

A concussion is brain trauma that may be mild, moderate, or severe. Symptoms of mild concussions include brief loss of consciousness or a state of confusion. A headache and vomiting may follow the episode. In most cases, complete recovery occurs in a matter of a few days to a week, although in rare cases recovery may be lengthier.

With moderate to severe concussions a brain contusion, or bruise, may cause swelling of the brain tissues. This is common in trauma known as closed head injuries. Prolonged unconsciousness and problems with vasomotor and respiratory functions may be present. On waking, the person may exhibit behavioral and personality changes, amnesia, and motor and sensory disturbances. The prognosis can range from complete recovery to continued deterioration. Because the amount of internal injury may not be immediately recognizable, any person with head injury should be watched carefully and referred to a medical professional if any loss of consciousness takes place or any of the aforementioned symptoms appear.

Intracranial bleeding, called intracerebral hemorrhage, may occur within brain tissue. When the bleeding occurs between the dura and arachnoid, it is called a subdural hematoma; when the bleeding is located between the skull and dura, it is referred to as an epidural hematoma.

Cerebral palsy is a general term for brain damage that takes place before, during, or shortly after birth. Damage may involve the whole brain but usually is limited to the pyramidal tracts, which results in motor function disturbance. The most common symptoms include muscle spasticity (especially in the feet, legs, and hands); impaired speech, vision, hearing, and tactile sensations; and seizures. Impaired intellectual function may or may not result.

INDICATIONS/CONTRAINDICATIONS

For Therapeutic Massage

Therapeutic massage is an effective part of a supervised comprehensive care program. Massage and other forms of bodywork can help manage secondary muscle tension resulting from the alteration of posture and the use of equipment such as wheelchairs, braces, and crutches.

Seizure

Seizures or convulsions are defined as a sudden involuntary series of muscle contractions. The most common group of seizure disorders is referred to as epilepsy, which occurs when the nerve cells of the cerebral cortex send out uncontrolled signals. In many cases the cause of the neuron stimulation is unknown, but known precipitating factors include hereditary factors, trauma to the head, stroke, brain tumor, and infections.

Minor seizures are known as petit mal and may not include actual spasms of the skeletal muscles. Usually seen in children, these seizures are typified by a moment of blankness. Major seizures, known as grand mal, begin with an aura or sensation such as a taste, smell, or feeling. The person usually has involuntary spasms or continuous tension in the skeletal muscles and loss of consciousness. A sense of confusion and a desire to sleep are common aftereffects.

Most forms of epilepsy can be controlled by antiseizure medication, most commonly phenobarbital and phenytoin (Dilantin). The side effects of the medications can include headache, muscle tension, nervousness, joint pain, and sleeping difficulties. A continuous seizure is called status **epilepticus** and is a medical emergency.

INDICATIONS CONTRAINDICATIONS

For Therapeutic Massage

The side effects of medications may be decreased by the application of massage techniques. Massage therapists must remember that any exaggerated or increased symptoms should be referred to the prescribing physician.

Tumors

A brain tumor rarely develops from a neuron because neurons do not divide. Most tumors are formed from the neuroglia, tissues of the membranes, and the blood vessels found in and around the brain. The tumors usually are started by the cells of malignant tumors that begin elsewhere in the body, often in the breasts of women and the lungs of men.

Most tumors that develop in the brain are benign. Because no space is available for them to expand, they compress the brain and its supporting tissues, sometimes with fatal results. For this reason surgical removal is indicated whenever possible.

Signs and symptoms of tumor-caused compression are as follows:

- The loss of sensory or motor function, mainly on one side of the body
- Personality changes, behavior changes, or both
- Headaches
- Awkward movement or gait (ataxia)

INDICATIONS CONTRAINDICATIONS

For Therapeutic Massage

Recognizing the signs and symptoms of a possible brain compression and referring the client for diagnosis are important. During rehabilitation from surgery, massage can be used as supportive care and in any compensation patterns from brain damage that results from surgery.

Degenerative Disorders

A variety of degenerative diseases referred to as dementia are organic mental disorders caused by things such as chemical imbalance, endocrine dysfunctions, and trauma to the brain, which can result in the destruction of brain neurons. As the degeneration progresses, symptoms such as memory loss, decreased attention span, diminished intellectual capacity, and loss of control of personality or behavior often are observed.

Alzheimer's disease is a type of dementia in which the brain degenerates, resulting in judgment errors, memory difficulties, and a tendency to become confused. Neuronal tangles and plaque found in brain tissue contain amyloid, a pathologic insoluble starchlike protein. Neurons essential for memory are particularly vulnerable to this degenerative process. The current theory is that Alzheimer's disease somehow is determined genetically by amyloid B, which is regulated by a gene located in chromosome 21.

Deficiencies in neurotransmitters also are implicated in dementia.

INDICATIONS CONTRAINDICATIONS

For Therapeutic Massage

The degeneration of Alzheimer's disease may be slowed with therapeutic intervention and medication. Studies indicate that sensory stimulation modalities such as rhythmic massage and movement may provide calming and orienting influences.

Amyotrophic Lateral Sclerosis

Also known as Lou Gehrig's disease, **amyotrophic lateral sclerosis** is a progressive disease beginning in the central nervous system, involves the degeneration of motor neurons, and eventually results in the atrophy of voluntary muscle.

Symptoms of amyotrophic lateral sclerosis include weakness, fatigue, and muscle spasms. The disease is most common in men between 40 and 70 years of age.

INDICATIONS CONTRAINDICATIONS

For Therapeutic Massage

Massage is indicated for amyotrophic lateral sclerosis, with caution and under a doctor's supervision. The degrees of pressure and intensity need to be adjusted as the disease progresses.

Schizophrenia

Schizophrenia is the most common mental disorder and includes a large group of psychotic disorders characterized by gross distortion of reality; disturbances of language and communication; withdrawal from social interaction; and disorganization and fragmentation of thought, perception, and emotional reaction. No single cause has been identified, but increased dopamine activity in parts of the brain is strongly indicated. A diagnosis of schizophrenia requires the exclusion of other disorders. Management of chronic schizophrenia requires expert multidisciplinary support along with psychopharmacologic and long-term psychosocial intervention.

As previously stated, schizophrenia is associated with increased dopamine levels in the brain. The symptoms are helped with medications that block or reduce the release of dopamine at the synapses. Large amounts of cocaine and some amphetamines associated with the increase of dopamine often mimic schizophrenic behaviors in otherwise normally behaved persons.

Depression

Depression is associated with a decrease in the neurotransmitters norepinephrine, serotonin, and dopamine. Affected persons often can be helped with medications such as amphetamines that inhibit the reuptake of norepinephrine and monoamine oxidase inhibitors that reduce the breakdown of norepinephrine. A class of medications known as serotonin uptake inhibitors is often helpful in managing depression.

Tremors

Tremors are involuntary muscle twitches. They may be minor and occur in a tired muscle or may be exaggerated in conditions such as St. Vitus' dance, Huntington's chorea, or Parkinson's disease. They are not a form of epilepsy, although they originate in the CNS.

Essential tremor is a chronic tremor that does not result from any other pathologic condition. The condition is slowly progressive but usually not debilitating. Onset can occur as early as adolescence but usually occurs in midlife. Essential tremor may be an inherited disorder.

Parkinson's Disease

In Parkinson's disease the neurons that release the neurotransmitter dopamine in the brain degenerate, thus slowing or stopping its release. Parkinson's disease occurs mainly in the elderly; the symptoms include rigidity of the muscles of the limbs, tremors while the person is at rest, a shuffling gait, and a masklike face.

Pharmacologic intervention includes the use of L-dopa (levodopa), the precursor of dopamine; amantadine (Symmetrel), which releases dopamine at the synapse; and benztropine (Cogentin) and trihexyphenidyl (Artane), both of which are anticholinergic drugs.

Chorea

Chorea results from the degeneration of neurons in the basal ganglia. The affected person's normal voluntary movements are replaced with involuntary dancelike motions. The most common forms are St. Vitus' dance and Huntington's chorea, a hereditary disease that also includes a form of dementia.

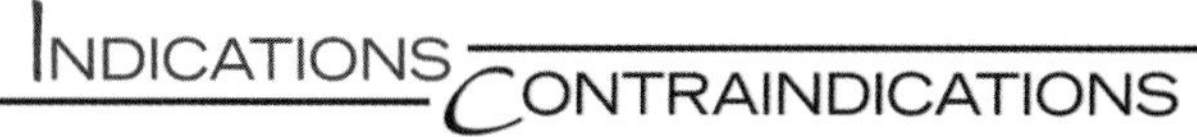

For Therapeutic Massage

Therapeutic massage is supportive in a multidisciplinary treatment of depression because serotonin, among other neurotransmitters, is influenced by such methods. Because massage has been shown to increase dopamine activity, its use is indicated in managing Parkinson's disease and tremor. In addition, secondary muscle tension can be managed effectively with methods such as massage therapy and other forms of soft tissue manipulation. ■

Infectious Disease

Most CNS infections are bacterial or viral. Infections of the brain are called encephalitis. Infection of the meninges is called meningitis. The two diseases may appear separately or together. Both have symptoms of fever, nausea, and vomiting. Encephalitis may affect motor function, cause seizures, and cause behavioral and mood changes. Meningitis, found mainly in the subarachnoid fluid, adds stiffness of the neck to its symptom list. As with other infections, the primary treatment for viral infection is support for general immune function, with antibiotics given for a bacterial infection.

Myelitis is an infection of the spinal cord or brainstem. In the past the poliomyelitis virus was the most common infection. Its symptoms affect motor and sensory functions. Because most forms of myelitis result from viruses, treatment supports the body while the immune functions resolve the infection.

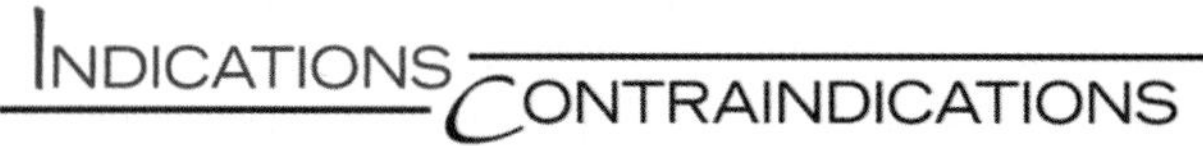

For Therapeutic Massage

Infectious processes are contraindicated for massage intervention unless closely supervised by appropriate medical personnel. A person with an unusual or unexplained stiff neck should be referred for diagnosis. ■

Headache

Headaches can be caused by stress, muscle tension, chemical imbalance, circulatory and sinus disorders, or tumors.

Migraine headache pain is believed to be caused by dilation of the cranial vessels. The pain is knifelike, throbbing, and unilateral. Any visual distortion (e.g., flashing lights) is believed to be caused by vasoconstriction preceding the vasodilation and pain.

Cluster headaches occur on one side of the head, with remissions and recurrence lasting for long periods. They usually occur at night and are associated with other symptoms, such as red eyes and sinus drainage.

Medications used to treat headaches are usually non-steroidal analgesics such as aspirin, but migraines may not respond to medication after the headache begins. Migraines sometimes may be prevented by the medication ergotamine (a vasoconstrictor) or other vasoconstricting medication. The judicious use of caffeine may reduce migraine symptoms.

INDICATIONS CONTRAINDICATIONS

For Therapeutic Massage

Massage and other forms of soft tissue therapy are effective in treating muscle tension headache but much less so with migraine or cluster headaches. Soft tissue therapy can relieve secondary muscle tension headache caused by the pain of the primary headache. Headache is often stress induced. Stress management in all forms usually is indicated in chronic headache conditions.

Spinal Cord Injury

Injuries to the spinal cord can result in a number of neurologic problems. Studies of blood flow and metabolism indicate that spinal cord injury involves not only direct neuronal trauma but also direct and delayed vascular trauma. The most frequently injured sites are at the most mobile segments of the spine such as the cervicothoracic (C7 to T1) and the thoracolumbar junctions (T12 to L1–L4). About 40% of spinal cord injuries result in complete function interruption. The rest of the injuries result in the impairment or destruction of certain sensory and motor functions.

Injury or cutting of the spinal cord is followed by a 2- to 3-week period of spinal shock when all spinal reflex responses are depressed. The spinal reflexes below the cut become exaggerated and hyperactive. The neurons become hypersensitive to the excitatory neurotransmitters and the spinal neurons may sprout collaterals that synapse with excitatory input. The stretch reflexes are exaggerated and the tone of the muscle increases.

If spinal cord injury occurs above the third cervical spinal nerve, a loss of voluntary movements of all the limbs occurs, and respiratory movements are affected if the phrenic nerve arising from the third, fourth, or fifth cervical nerve to supply the diaphragm is affected. Loss of movement of all four limbs is known as **quadriplegia.** If the lesion is lower, only the lower limbs are affected and the condition is called **paraplegia.** Should the nerves to only one limb be affected, the condition is referred to as **monoplegia.**

One of the complications common among persons with spinal cord injuries is decubitus ulcer. Because voluntary shifting of weight does not occur, the weight of the body compresses the circulation to the skin over bony prominences and produces ulcers.

Because of disuse, calcium from bones is reabsorbed and excreted in the urine, increasing the incidence of calcium stones in the urinary tract. Paralysis of the muscles of the urinary bladder results in stagnation of urine and urinary tract infection.

Connective tissue changes occur in the muscles and joints. The function of the autonomic system below the level of the lesion also is affected. Voluntary control of the bladder and rectum is lost if the lesion is above the sacral segments; reflex contractions of the bladder and rectum occur as soon as they become full, resulting in incontinence; and inconsistency of blood pressure can occur.

The mass reflex occurs when a slight stimulus to the skin triggers many reflexes such as emptying the bladder and rectum, sweating, and blood pressure changes. Persons with chronic spinal injuries can be trained to initiate these reflexes by stroking or pinching the thigh, triggering the mass reflex and intentionally giving them some control over urination and defecation.

INDICATIONS CONTRAINDICATIONS

For Therapeutic Massage

Massage is an effective part of a comprehensive, supervised rehabilitation and long-term care program. Massage and other forms of bodywork can help manage secondary muscle tension resulting from the alteration of posture and the use of equipment such as wheelchairs, braces, and crutches. Specifically focused massage can help manage difficulties with bowel paralysis. The circulation enhancement of massage can assist in the management of a decubitus ulcer.

SUMMARY

Many physiologic effects of therapeutic massage are caused by interaction with the functions of the central nervous system. Research has shown that applying massage effectively has beneficial influence on the central nervous system and the associated neurotransmitters.

Competence in the interpretation of symptoms and behaviors related to the central nervous system is necessary to determine the factors that are causing the distressing symptoms. Competency also is displayed by choosing the appropriate methods to encourage a return to effective functioning in the system or to create outcomes of relaxation and well-being. Therapeutic benefit is measured by achievable outcomes from massage and is related directly to the ability to use clinical reasoning skills and to solve problems. The basic massage methods and adjunct therapies such as hydrotherapy then are modified as necessary to meet the goals of the client.

Knowledge of the central nervous system also helps the massage professional to practice safely and to refer clients with conditions contraindicated for massage.

This chapter has focused on nervous system basics and

the components and functions of the CNS. Behavior and the nervous system are linked in the feedback loop pattern. Consciousness is a function of the CNS. Soft tissue and movement modalities are supportive, maintaining health of the CNS. Pathologic conditions of the CNS disrupt many types of body functions, and massage methods can provide support in coping with many of these dysfunctions.

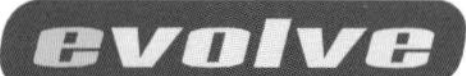

Log on to your student EVOLVE account, and complete the labeling activity for the central nervous system. Click on the link to review your answers. Feel free to print out the labeling activity to complete for further review when you are not at your computer.

WORKBOOK SECTION

SHORT ANSWER

1. List the parts of the neuron.

2. Explain the function of the nerve cell.

3. Describe neurotransmitter functions and list the major neurotransmitters.

4. Relate brain chemistry to behavior.

5. Define the major parts and functions of the CNS.

6. Describe consciousness and altered states of consciousness.

7. Explain the process of memory and learning.

8. Describe common pathologic conditions of the CNS.

9. List the drugs that influence the CNS.

10. Explain the influence of therapeutic massage on the CNS.

FILL IN THE BLANK

The central nervous system consists of the brain and (1) ____________. (2) ____________ are nerve cells that conduct impulses. Neuroglia are specialized (3) ____________ cells that support, protect, and hold neurons together. (4) ____________ are branching projections from the nerve cell body. Axons are (5) ____________ elongated projections from the nerve cell body. An axon may have branches known as (6) ____________, allowing communication among neurons.

(7) ____________ is the outer cell membrane of a Schwann cell that plays an essential part in the (8) ____________ of injured axons.

White matter is (9) ____________ nerve fibers. Gray matter is formed by nerve cell bodies in the CNS that are (10) ____________. (11) ____________ is a disease that causes weakening of skeletal muscles and results from a reduction of acetylcholine receptors.

Neurotransmitters are chemical transmitters released in the (12) ____________ from presynaptic cells. A synapse is a (13) ____________ between neurons. (14) ____________ modulates pain perception, and insufficient levels can result in anxiety or depression.

The (15) ____________ is the largest and most complex unit of the nervous system and is responsible for perception, sensation, emotion, and intellect. The (16) ____________ is the largest of the brain divisions and occupies the uppermost region of the cranium. It consists of two (17) ____________. The cerebrum is covered by a thin layer of gray matter called the (18) ____________ that is formed into folds called convolutions or (19) ____________. These folds are separated by creases called (20) ____________. Underneath the gray matter is the (21) ____________, which is made up of complicated pathways of myelinated axons called white matter that connect the gray matter of the left and right hemispheres.

The (22) ____________ of the cerebral cortex is the anterior area positioned behind the frontal bone. Its major function is to control the voluntary skeletal muscles in an area called the (23) ____________ and is active in functions of problem solving involving concentration and planning. The (24) ____________ is located next to the parietal bones of the skull and contains the (25) ____________, which is the sensory area of the brain and which functions with the sensory data reporting of temperature, pressure, touch, and pain. The (26) ____________ is positioned next to the temporal bones. The temporal lobe is responsible for the sensory functions of (27) ____________ and (28) ____________. The occipital lobe is located just anterior to the occipital bone of the skull and is responsible for the control of (29) ____________.

The (30) ____________ is a group of structures located on the interior of the cerebrum that plays an important role in arousal and emotional responses, endocrine and autonomic responses, and sexual behavior. Every time the head is moved, the fluid in the semicircular canals is set in motion, generating (31) ____________ impulses. The impulses travel to the (32) ____________ and to the (33) ____________ to give information. The cerebellum is the second largest part of the (34) ____________ and is involved with (35) ____________. The brainstem contains centers for (36) ____________ function connected with (37) ____________, as well as vomiting, coughing, and sneezing; posture; and basic movement patterns. Located in the (38) ____________ are the thalamus, hypothalamus, and pineal gland. The (39) ____________ is associated with pain, temperature, touch sensations, crude sensation, and muscular coordination. The (40) ____________ is stimulated, and the

WORKBOOK SECTION

body is able to increase and decrease tone and maintain balance and equilibrium.

The (41) hypothalamus controls the pituitary gland by producing releasing hormones and is the temperature center, the sexual center, the thirst and hunger center, and the rage and fear center. The pineal gland appears to act as a (42) biologic clock, regulating circadian rhythms. The midbrain or (43) mesencephalon is located between the thalamus and the pons and contains centers for visual and auditory reflexes and for correlating information about muscle tone and posture, as well as visual reflexes. Nerve fibers entering on one side of the (44) pons cross and exit the other side; therefore one side of the brain controls the opposite side of the body. The (45) medulla regulates heartbeat, blood pressure, breathing, coughing, sneezing, swallowing, and vomiting.

The CNS is surrounded by three membranes called the (46) menings. (47) Cerebrospinal fluid is a clear, colorless fluid that flows throughout the brain and around the (48) spinal cord, cushioning and protecting these structures.

The spinal cord is the portion of the CNS that exits the skull into the (49) vertebral column. The two major functions of the spinal cord are to conduct nerve impulses and to be a center for (50) spinal reflexes. (51) Tracts are collections of nerve fibers in the CNS having a common function.

EXERCISE

For the illustration of a neuron pictured below, fill in the blanks for each part indicated by a letter, and then color each part.

A. ____________________

B. ____________________

C. ____________________

D. ____________________

E. ____________________

F. ____________________

G. ____________________

H. ____________________

I. ____________________

J. ____________________

K. ____________________

L. ____________________

M. ____________________

N. ____________________

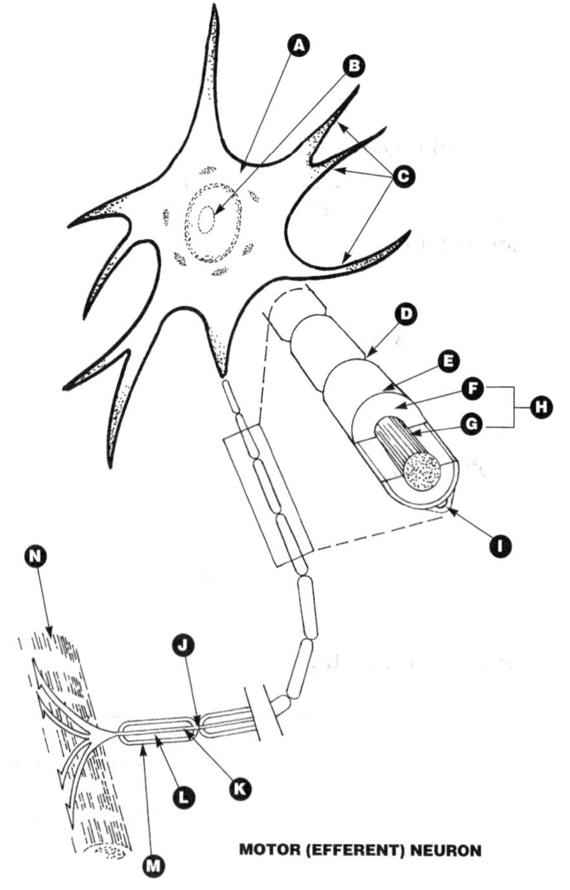

MOTOR (EFFERENT) NEURON

PROBLEM SOLVING

Read the problem presented. There is no correct answer; rather the exercise is intended to assist the student in developing analytic and decision-making skills necessary in a professional practice.

1. Identify the facts presented in the information.
2. Identify the possibilities ("what if" statements) presented, or develop your own possibilities that relate to the facts.
3. Evaluate each possibility in terms of the logical cause and effect and pros and cons.
4. Consider the feelings of those involved.
5. Write each answer in the space provided.
6. Develop your solution by answering the question posed.

Problem

Obviously behavior influences the CNS. For a person to engage in pleasure-seeking activity that stimulates the feel-good neurotransmitters seems important. Connected with this process is the drive for altered states of consciousness. Today's world places many demands on individuals. Most of these demands are performance based. Time becomes a rare commodity. When this is the case for an individual, the structure for satisfying pleasure needs decreases. Could this situation support the search for quick methods to affect neurotransmitters? Ancient meditative processes and touch and movement therapies, including exercise, are time consuming. Maybe individuals do not do what they know is beneficial because these methods are cumbersome to integrate into a busy lifestyle. How does one balance the need for pleasure, excitement, calm, joy, sadness, love, companionship, and so forth with the time necessary to procure such experiences? One wonders if this current situation is not responsible, at least in part, for extreme behavior and the use of chemicals to create the internal chemical response that satisfies these needs in a fast and reliable way, regardless of how destructive the long-term consequences may be.

Question

What do therapeutic massage and movement therapies have to offer to satisfy pleasure needs, and how does one efficiently integrate these methods into a busy schedule or begin to justify the time necessary to use the important approaches to CNS health?

Facts

1. Behavior influences the CNS.
2. ____
3. ____

Possibilities

1. Individuals may not take the time to fulfill pleasure needs.
2. ____
3. ____

Logical Cause and Effect

1. Not taking time to fulfill pleasure needs would seem to produce extreme behavior resulting in addictive actions.
2. ____
3. ____

Effect

1. Persons may feel helpless because they do not understand why they do something that initially felt good but ultimately hurts them.
2. ____
3. ____

What do therapeutic massage and movement therapies have to offer to satisfy pleasure needs, and how does one efficiently integrate these methods into a busy schedule or begin to justify the time necessary to use the important approaches to CNS health?

____

____

____

____

____

Professional Application

What additional knowledge base would one need to work in CVA rehabilitation and long-term care using therapeutic massage and movement therapies? Where might a practitioner find this information and get additional training?

____

____

____

____

____

Workbook Section

FURTHER STUDY

Using additional resource material (see Works Consulted list at the back of this book), identify chapters pertaining to the information presented in this chapter. Locate the information presented in this text and then elaborate by writing a paragraph of additional information on each of the following.

Nerve cell regeneration

Neurotransmitters

Memory

Difference in the male and female brain

Differences in dominant and nondominant cerebral hemisphere functions

Brainstem function in relationship to survival behavior

Reticular activating system

Spinal cord tracts

Answer Key

Short Answer

1. Neuroglia, dendrites, axon, neurilemma
2. A nerve impulse is a self-perpetuating wave of electrical energy that travels along the surface of the plasma membrane of the neuron. Nerve impulses have to be initiated by a stimulus that changes the environment of the neuron. A neuron is said to be excited when a stimulus triggers the opening of additional Na^+ channels, allowing the membrane potential to move toward zero. Inhibition occurs when the stimulus triggers the opening of additional K^+ channels, increasing the membrane potential. The electrical disturbance stimulates a similar change in the next section of membrane, resulting in a nerve impulse traveling in one direction along the surface of the neuron.

   After a local area of a neuron membrane has been stimulated and a nerve impulse has been generated, the neuron resists restimulation and will not respond to a stimulus, no matter how strong. This is called the refractory period.

   In myelinated fibers, action potentials in the membrane only occur at the nodes of Ranvier. If the traveling impulse encounters a section of membrane covered with insulating myelin, it jumps over the myelin, resulting in faster transmission than is possible in nonmyelinated sections.
3. Neurotransmitters are chemical compounds that regulate many body activities and states. Neurotransmitter effects may be excitatory, by increasing activity, or inhibitory, by decreasing an activity.

   Chemical synapses occur at presynaptic cells that release chemical transmitters called neurotransmitters across a tiny gap to the post-synaptic cell. The plasma membrane of a post-synaptic neuron has protein molecules that serve as receptors for the neurotransmitters. When a nerve impulse reaches a synaptic knob, thousands of neurotransmitter molecules flow into the synaptic cleft and bind to specific receptors, generating an action potential. The action of the neurotransmitter is terminated quickly by neurotransmitter molecules being transported back into the synaptic knob or being metabolized into inactive compounds. Many drugs act by disturbing the termination phase.

The major neurotransmitters are acetylcholine, serotonin, histamine, epinephrine, norepinephrine, and dopamine (endorphins); and glutamate (or glutamic acid), gamma-aminobutyric acid, substance P, somatostatin, cholecystokinin, and vasoactive intestinal peptide (enkephalins).

4. A change in neurotransmitter concentrations at various synapses causes a change in behavior. Mental illness behaviors and much of our daily behavior, especially pain, pleasure, and survival behavior, are determined by brain chemistry. An ongoing dynamic balance in this chemical soup allows for resourceful behavior for each situation we encounter. In addition, we behave in certain ways to increase or decrease levels of neurotransmitters or hormones.

   When medication is used to manage neurotransmitters, mood and behavior are affected. Repeated behavior is in some way accomplishing the goal of a form of homeostasis —even bizarre behavior such as drug addiction, excessive exercise, eating disorders, rage, thrill seeking, crisis orientation, and pain behavior. Pain behavior is also a brain chemistry event. Pain becomes a decision in the brain. A pain-inhibiting system exists in the body. Internal, or endogenous, opiates (endorphins and enkephalins) produced by the body block pain impulses in various portions of the pathway, probably as a protective device. The neurotransmitter substance P is blocked by enkephalins. Endorphins and enkephalins also affect mood.

5. The brain is the center for interpreting, regulating, integrating, and coordinating physiologic functions and is divided into the following major segments.

   The major functions of the *cerebrum* are as follows:
   - Interpretation of sensory information received from the eyes, ears, nose, taste, tactile, and other sensory structures of the body
   - Transmitting motor impulses that initiate voluntary movements and some involuntary movements in response to sensory data
   - Association functions that allow learning, reasoning, recall, language, and consciousness

   The *brainstem* contains centers for vital functions connected with survival; vomiting, coughing, and sneezing; posture; and basic movement patterns and houses cranial nerves. Located in the brainstem are the thalamus, hypothalamus, and pineal gland.

   The *midbrain* or mesencephalon contains centers for visual and auditory reflexes and correlating information about muscle tone, posture, and visual reflexes and contains cranial nerve nuclei, an important part of the reticular activating system.

   The *pons* (pons varolii), located between the midbrain and the medulla, functions in the rhythmic discharge of the respiratory center of the medulla, chewing, facial expressions, and eye movement and contains cranial nerve nuclei and important centers for REM sleep.

   The *medulla* or medulla oblongata connects the pons and spinal cord. The functions of the medulla include the following:
   - Cardiac center: regulates heartbeat
   - Vasomotor center: regulates blood pressure
   - Respiratory center: regulates breathing

   Other functions include controlling coughing, sneezing, swallowing, and vomiting.

   The *cerebellum,* located in the posterior cranial fossa of the skull, is the second largest segment of the brain; contains centers for balance, equilibrium, muscular coordination, posture, and balance; controls subconscious movements of skeletal muscle, input from proprioceptors, feedback loops, posture, and future positioning; and regulates sensations of anger and pleasure.

   The *reticular formation* and the *reticular activating system* are the primitive inner core of the spinal cord and brainstem involved in the regulation of respiration, blood pressure, heart rate, endocrine secretion, conditioned reflexes, learning, and consciousness

   The *meninges,* or membranes, are the dura mater, arachnoid mater, and pia mater. The three spaces created by the meninges are as follows:
   - Epidural space between skull and dura mater
   - Subdural space between dura and arachnoid mater
   - Subarachnoid space between arachnoid and pia mater that ends at the vertebral level

   Vessels of the brain include the internal carotid system and the vertebrobasilar artery, which connect (anastomose) at the midbrain as the circle of Willis, ensuring blood flow to the brain despite occlusion of the carotid or basilar arteries. Venous drainage from the brain occurs by several veins, as well as the dural sinuses, spaces in the dura that drain to the internal jugular veins.

   The *spinal cord* conducts nerve impulses and is a center for spinal reflexes; 31 pairs of peripheral spinal nerves connect the spinal cord and brain with all areas of the body.

   The *white matter* on the outside of the spinal cord is made up of myelinated nerve fibers, called tracts, that ascend to and descend from the brain. Ascending tracts conduct impulses up the spinal cord to the brain, transmitting pain, temperature, and positional information. Descending tracts conduct impulses from the brain down the cord, sending effector information to muscles and glands. The gray matter on the inside of the spinal cord forms an H pattern.

6. Consciousness is the awareness of the environment and the relationship of ourselves to those in that environment. Consciousness depends on excitation of cortical neurons by impulses conducted from the reticular activating system, which relays them to the thalamus. The thalamus transmits the data to all parts of the cerebral cortex. Drugs that stimulate the cerebrum, enhancing alertness, probably act by stimulating the reticular activating system.

   Persons of various cultures have explored altered states of consciousness for centuries. Many ways of altering consciousness exist. Meditation produces a state of higher consciousness typified by relaxation and alertness. Meditation is simply a highly focused peaceful state, usually in a calm environment, produced by synchronizing the breath and other body rhythms. Pleasure behavior derived from the sense of well-being experienced by altered states of consciousness can be addictive, and the associated behavior to achieve the pleasure state can be detrimental if excessive.

WORKBOOK SECTION

7. Memory is the storing of information in the brain and is one of our major mental activities. Two types of memory are short term (recent) and long term. Highly emotional events seem immediately to become stored in long-term memory, indicating neurotransmitter involvement in memory structures.

   The key in long-term memory is repeated impulses. Learning strategies often are focused on circular learning in which information continues to reappear, reinforcing the neurocircuit storing the memory.

   Learning in a basic and primitive sense can be thought of as the best and simplest way to solve a problem. Anatomically and physiologically, learning is the use of multiple synaptic pathways to solve problems. Advanced learning takes place in the association areas of the cerebral cortex (some learning also takes place in the brainstem). Learning requires memory and is the development of neural structures that remember the way to solve a problem. Solving problems supports survival. Learning can be thought of as conditioning. Conditioning also can be considered learned habit. The process of learning is conscious, but after something has been integrated, often it becomes unconscious.
8. CVA, or stroke, is an umbrella term that covers disorders such as aneurysms and blood clots and hemorrhages. When a stroke occurs, an artery in the brain is occluded or closed off from a blood clot called a thrombus.

   An aneurysm is a weakening and bulging of an artery.

   A blood clot may break away from a different part of the body and travel to the brain.

   CNS trauma may occur when a concussion causes a brief loss of consciousness or a state of confusion after a head injury. A contusion is a bruise of the brain. Intracranial bleeding is called intracerebral hemorrhage or hematoma.

   Cerebral palsy is a general term for brain damage before, during, or shortly after birth.

   Seizure in epilepsy is characterized by an abrupt alteration in brain function, ranging from a mild behavior change to a general convulsion.

   Primary tumors form from the neuroglia, membrane tissues, and blood vessels associated with the neuron. Most brain tumors do not originate in the brain. They are metastatic from malignant tumors elsewhere in the body.

   Spinal cord injury can result in a number of neurologic deficits.
9. The stimulants are caffeine, nicotine, the amphetamines, and cocaine. The depressants are alcohol, narcotics, minor tranquilizers, and barbiturates. The hallucinogens are LSD, PCP, peyote, and marijuana.
10. Therapeutic massage and movement therapies provide stimulation to the CNS, causing the brain and spinal cord to respond. Neurotransmitters also are affected.

FILL IN THE BLANK

1. spinal cord
2. Neurons
3. connective tissue
4. Dendrites
5. single
6. collaterals
7. Neurilemma
8. regeneration
9. myelinated
10. unmyelinated
11. Myasthenia gravis
12. synapses
13. junction
14. Serotonin
15. brain
16. cerebrum
17. hemispheres
18. cerebral cortex
19. gyri
20. sulci
21. corpus callosum
22. frontal lobe
23. precentral gyrus
24. parietal lobe
25. postcentral gyrus
26. temporal lobe
27. hearing
28. smell
29. eyesight
30. limbic system
31. nerve
32. brainstem
33. cerebellum
34. brain
35. movement
36. vital
37. survival
38. brainstem
39. thalamus
40. motor cortex
41. hypothalamus
42. biologic clock
43. mesencephalon
44. pons
45. medulla
46. meninges
47. Cerebrospinal fluid
48. spinal cord
49. vertebral column
50. spinal reflexes
51. Tracts

EXERCISE

A. Cell body
B. Nucleus
C. Dendrites
D. Node of Ranvier
E. Neurilemma
F. Myelin sheath
G. Axon
H. Nerve fiber
I. Nucleus of Schwann cell
J. Node of Ranvier
K. Axon
L. Myelin sheath
M. Neurilemma
N. Neuromuscular junction

CHAPTER 5

Peripheral Nervous System

CHAPTER OBJECTIVES

After completing this chapter, the student will be able to perform the following:

- Describe the peripheral nervous system.
- List the components of the peripheral nervous system.
- List the cranial nerves and describe the general function of each.
- Explain the function of spinal nerves.
- Identify the four nerve plexuses.
- Compare and contrast dermatomes and myotomes.
- Explain reflex mechanisms, sensory receptors, and reflex arcs and their relationship to massage and bodywork.
- Name the two divisions of the autonomic nervous system.
- List and compare the functions of the sympathetic and parasympathetic nervous systems.
- List the major medications that affect the autonomic nervous system.
- Describe the Eastern/Western connection as it relates to the functions of the autonomic nervous system.
- Describe four of the five basic senses.
- Explain the way therapeutic massage supports health in the peripheral nervous system.
- List pathologic conditions of the peripheral nervous system.

CHAPTER OUTLINE

KEY TERMS

Afferent nerves (AF-fer-ent) Sensory nerves that link sensory receptors with the central nervous system and transmit sensory information.

Autonomic nervous system (aw-toe-NOM-ik) A division of the peripheral nervous system composed of nerves that connect

Continued

the central nervous system to the glands, heart, and smooth muscles to maintain the internal body environment.

Cranial nerves Twelve pairs of nerves that originate from the olfactory bulbs, thalamus, visual cortex, and brainstem. They transmit information to and from the sensory organs of the face and the muscles of the face, neck, and upper shoulders.

Dermatome (DER-mah-tohm) A cutaneous (skin) section supplied by a single spinal nerve.

Efferent nerves (EF-fer-ent) Motor nerves that link the central nervous system to the effectors outside it and transmit motor impulses.

Free nerve endings Sensory receptors that detect itch and tickle sensations.

Mechanical receptors Sensory receptors that detect changes in pressure, movement, temperature, or other mechanical forces.

Mixed nerves Nerves that contain sensory and motor axons.

Myasthenia gravis A disease that usually affects muscles in the face, lips, tongue, neck, and throat, which are innervated by the cranial nerves, but that can affect any muscle group.

Myotome (MY-o-tohm) A skeletal muscle or group of skeletal muscles that receives motor axons from a particular spinal nerve.

Nerve A bundle of axons or dendrites or both.

Nociceptors (no-se-SEP-tors) Sensory receptors that detect painful or intense stimuli.

Parasympathetic nervous system The energy conservation and restorative system associated with what commonly is called the relaxation response.

Peripheral nervous system (pe-RIF-er-al) The system of somatic and autonomic neurons outside the central nervous system. The peripheral nervous system comprises the afferent (sensory) division and the efferent (motor) division.

Plexus (PLEK-sus) A network of intertwining nerves that innervates a particular region of the body.

Polio A viral infection first of the intestines and then (for about 1% of exposed persons) the anterior horn cells of the spinal cord.

Proprioceptors (pro-pree-o-SEP-tors) Sensory receptors that provide the body with information about position, movement, muscle tension, joint activity, and equilibrium.

Reflex An automatic, involuntary reaction to a stimulus.

Somatic nervous system (so-MA-tik) A system of nerves that keeps the body in balance with its external environment by transmitting impulses between the central nervous system, skeletal muscles, and skin.

Spinal nerves Thirty-one pairs of mixed nerves, originating in the spinal cord and emerging from the vertebral column, that make sensation and movement possible.

Sympathetic nervous system The part of the autonomic nervous system that provides for most of the active function of the body; when the body is under stress, the sympathetic nervous system predominates with fight-or-flight responses.

Thermal receptors Sensory receptors that detect changes in temperature.

Basics of the Peripheral Nervous System

The **peripheral nervous system** is comprised of the motor nerves, sensory nerves, and ganglia outside the brain and spinal cord. The system consists of 12 pairs of **cranial nerves** and 31 pairs of **spinal nerves,** as well as their various branches in the body.

Sensory, or **afferent,** peripheral nerves transmit information to the central nervous system; motor, or **efferent,** peripheral nerves carry impulses from the brain back to the body. The two signals usually travel together in one nerve, with some fibers serving as sensory transmitters and others as motor transmitters. At the spinal cord the fibers separate into a posterior (dorsal) sensory root and an anterior (ventral) motor root.

Fibers that innervate the body wall are called *somatic* fibers. Those that supply the internal organs are called *visceral* fibers.

The **autonomic nervous system** consists of the peripheral nerves involved in regulating cardiovascular, respiratory, endocrine, and other automatic body functions.

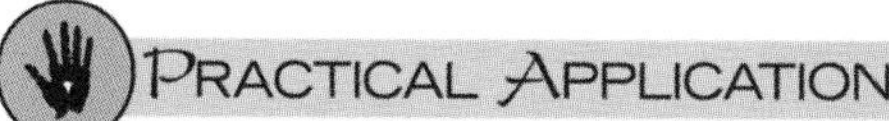

Stimulation of the peripheral nervous system (PNS) and the responses elicited by this stimulation constitute one of the main physiologic modes by which massage and bodywork benefit the client. Those who practice these therapies must understand thoroughly the anatomy and physiology of the PNS and comprehend the way soft tissue and movement methods interact with the PNS. ■

Nerves

A **nerve** is a bundle of axons or dendrites or both. Nerves may be of the motor, sensory, or mixed type. *Motor nerves* innervate or provide action, whereas *sensory nerves* transmit input from sensory receptors. **Mixed nerves** contain sensory and motor fibers. A delicate connective tissue covering known as the *endoneurium* surrounds and holds each nerve fiber. A group of nerve fibers is called a *fasciculus,* and each fasciculus is surrounded by a sheath of connective tissue called the *perineurium* (Figure 5-1). The entire nerve is surrounded by a connective tissue covering called the *epineurium.*

Cranial Nerves

Twelve pairs of cranial nerves enter (sensory) or leave (motor) the olfactory bulbs, thalamus, visual cortex, and brainstem. They are identified by roman numerals (according to their order from the front to the back of the brain) and by names (which refer to their function or distribution) (Figure 5-2; Table 5-1).

Disorders of the cranial nerves can arise from a stroke or tumor or from trauma. A lack of function may indicate damage to a nerve associated with a certain function. The resulting change in action may help locate the lesion. For example, the accessory nerves (XI) affect the trapezius and sternocleidomastoid muscles. Dysfunction in either of these muscles may indicate involvement of this nerve.

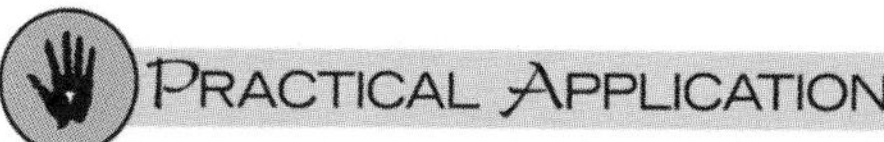

The distribution of the vagus nerve affects many visceral functions. Massage has been shown to support vagus nerve function, especially in premature babies, resulting in better development (particularly in weight gain) and fewer developmental problems. ■

Spinal Nerves

Thirty-one pairs of spinal nerves originate in the spinal cord and emerge from the vertebral column. All contain sensory and motor fibers in the same nerve (forming a mixed nerve), making sensation and movement possible. The nerve path generally follows the path of the arteries. Each nerve attaches to the spinal cord by way of two short roots on each side, one in front and one in back. The anterior, or ventral, root is motor; the fibers originate in the ventral horn cells and innervate skeletal muscles. The posterior, or dorsal, root is sensory; the fibers originate in the sensory receptors and travel to the dorsal roots of the spinal cord. The dorsal root of each spinal nerve is recognized by a swelling, known as the dorsal root ganglion, that contains the cell bodies of the sensory neurons.

Spinal nerves are identified by a letter and a number, which refer to their segment of attachment to the spinal cord (Figure 5-3; Table 5-2).

Nerve Plexuses

Most of the spinal nerves, except those that emerge from the second to twelfth thoracic vertebral spaces, converge in small groups to form an intersecting network known as a nerve **plexus.** Each plexus contains fibers that innervate a specific region of the body. Overlap of nerve function prevents total loss of function if just one of the nerves in the group is damaged. The four major plexuses are the cervical, brachial, lumbar, and sacral plexuses.

Cervical Plexus

The cervical plexus, formed from nerves C1 to C4 and part of C5, consists of sensory distribution from the head, front of the neck, and upper part of the shoulders, as well as motor impulses to many neck and shoulder muscles and the diaphragm (Figure 5-4).

Nerve	*Innervation*
Ansa cervicalis	Hyoid muscles
Lesser occipital	Skin behind and above the ear

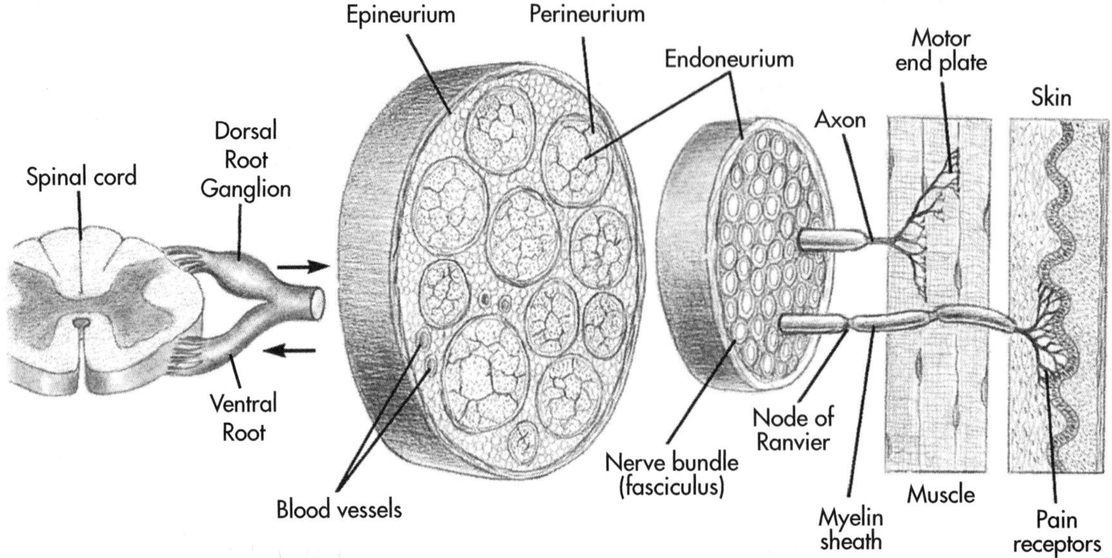

Figure 5-1
Peripheral nerve trunk and coverings. (From Thompson JM, et al: *Mosby's clinical nursing,* ed 5, St Louis, 2002, Mosby.)

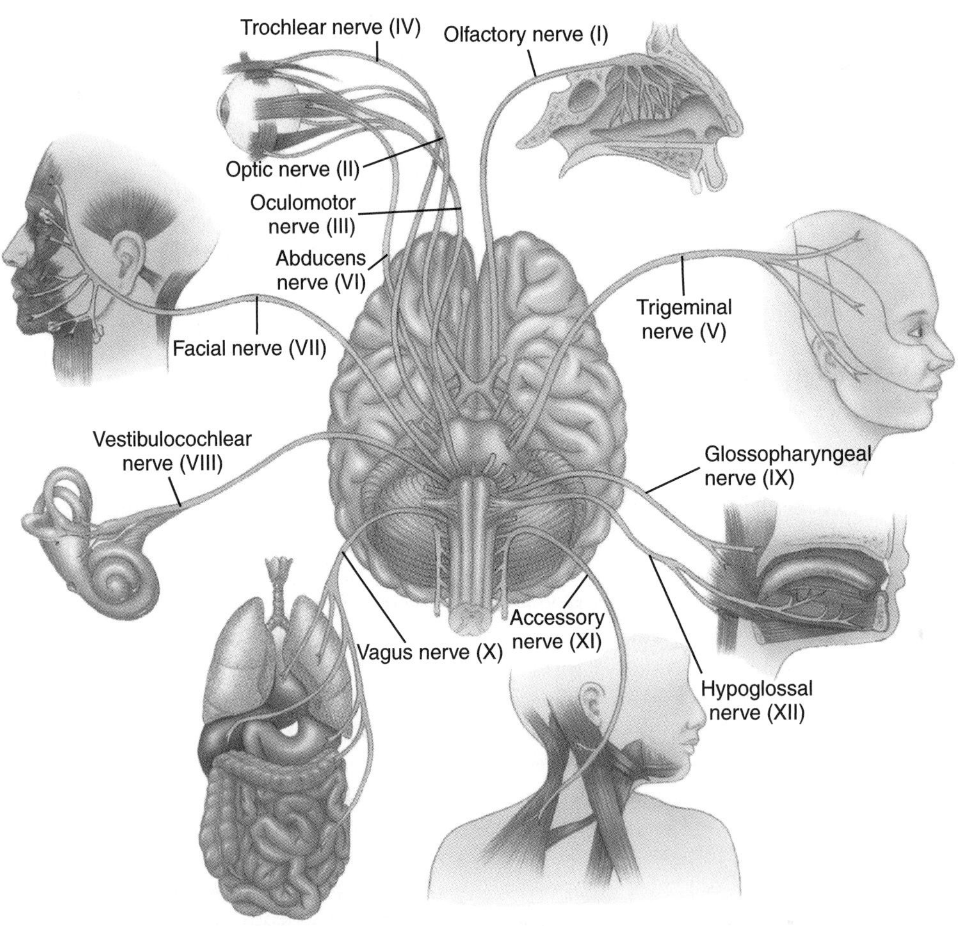

Figure 5-2
Cranial nerves. Ventral surface of the brain, showing the attachments of the cranial nerves. (From Thibodeau GA, Patton KT: *Anatomy and physiology,* ed 5, St Louis, 2003, Mosby.)

TABLE 5-1
Cranial Nerves

Cranial Nerve	Description
I	The olfactory nerves are sensory and transmit information about taste and smell from the nasal cavity to the cerebrum (into the olfactory bulb of the forebrain).
II	The optic nerves are sensory and transmit information about clarity and field of vision from the retina to the midbrain of the cerebrum via the thalamus.
III	The oculomotor nerves are sensory and motor. The sensory portion transmits information about eye movement. The motor portion originates in the midbrain and controls all external eye muscles (except the superior oblique and lateral rectus muscles) and pupil contraction and relaxation.
IV	The trochlear nerves comprise mainly motor nerves, which begin in the midbrain. They innervate the superior oblique eye muscles. The few sensory neurons provide proprioceptive information about eye movement.
V	The trigeminal nerves arise in the pons. The motor neurons innervate the muscles involved in chewing. The sensory neurons carry information about sensations and proprioception for the head, face, skin of the face and mucosal linings, eyelids, and tongue. The trigeminal nerves are the largest of the cranial nerves.
VI	The abducens nerves arise in the pons. The motor neurons innervate the lateral rectus eye muscle (an eye abductor). The sensory neurons provide proprioceptive information about eye movement.
VII	The facial nerves have motor fibers that arise in the pons and innervate the muscles that produce facial expression and the glands that release tears and saliva. The sensory fibers carry information about taste to the cerebral cortex. Some of the fibers also relay proprioceptive information about the face and scalp.
VIII	The vestibulocochlear nerves are sensory and are divided into two branches. The vestibular branch begins in the semicircular canals of the ear and carries signals for equilibrium to the pons, medulla, and cerebellum. The cochlear branch arises in the organ of Corti and carries impulses for hearing to the pons and medulla.
IX	The glossopharyngeal nerves contain sensory and motor neurons. The sensory fibers extend to the medulla from the pharynx and the tongue; they are concerned primarily with taste. Another sensory fiber extends from the carotid sinus in the internal carotid artery and aids in the control of respiration and blood pressure. The motor neurons arise in the medulla and affect saliva production, swallowing, and the gag reflex.
X	The vagus nerves contain sensory and motor neurons. The motor fibers originate in the medulla and carry signals that control the muscles involved in swallowing and speaking. Other motor fibers terminate in the muscles of the digestive and respiratory tracts and in the heart. The sensory fibers arise from the same structures that the motor fibers innervate and carry information about sensations and proprioception of these organs.
XI	The accessory nerves arise in the medulla and are primarily motor neurons for speaking, turning the head, and moving the shoulders. The few sensory neurons relay proprioceptive information from these muscles.
XII	The hypoglossal nerves originate in the medulla and contain mostly motor neurons, which innervate the tongue and throat. A few sensory neurons carry proprioceptive information from the tongue.

Greater auricular	Skin in front of, below, and over the ear and parotid glands
Transverse cervical	Skin on the anterior portion of the neck
Phrenic	Diaphragm
Supraclavicular	Skin on the shoulders and upper portion of the chest
Segmental branches	Deep neck muscles, midscalenes, and levator scapula muscle

Brachial Plexus

The brachial plexus, formed from nerves C5 through T1, is organized into three divisions: the superior, middle, and inferior trunk. These divisions supply the skin and muscles of the upper limbs (Figure 5-5).

Nerve	*Innervation*
Dorsoscapular	Superficial muscles of the scapula
Long thoracic	Serratus anterior muscle
Subclavian	Subclavius muscle
Suprascapular	Infraspinatus and supraspinatus muscles
Musculocutaneous	Biceps, brachialis, and coracobrachialis muscles, and skin
Subscapular	Subscapularis and teres major muscles
Median	Forearm flexors and palmar surface of the skin of the thumb, index, and middle fingers

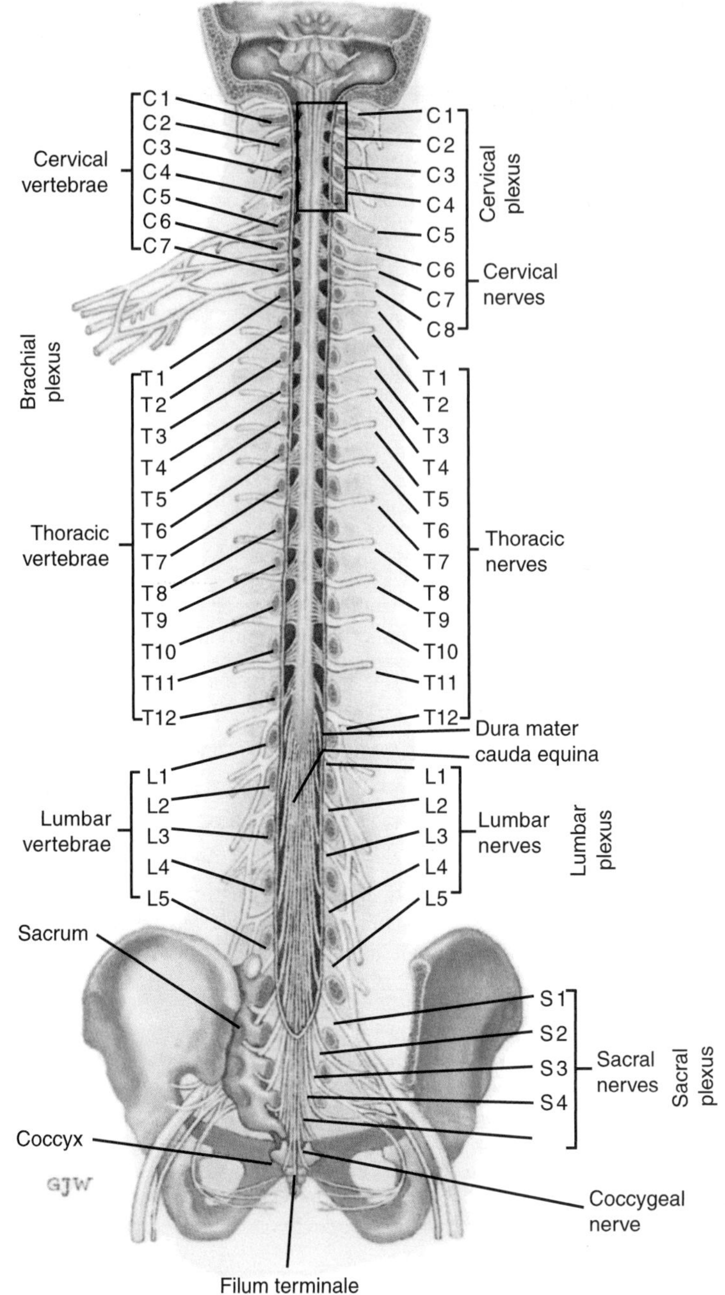

Figure 5-3
Spinal nerves. (Each of 31 pairs of spinal nerves exits the spinal cavity from the intervertebral foramina. Notice that after leaving the spinal cavity, many of the spinal nerves interconnect to form networks, called *plexuses*. (From Chipps EM, Clanin JJ, Campbell VG: *Neurologic disorders*, St. Louis, 1992, Mosby.)

Thoracodorsal	Latissimus dorsi muscle
Pectorals	Pectoralis major and minor muscles
Axillary	Deltoid and teres minor muscles and skin
Radial	Triceps and forearm extensors, skin of the forearm and hand, and dorsal surface of the thumb, index, and middle fingers
Medial cutaneous	Skin of the arm
Ulnar	Muscles of the hand and skin of the ring and baby fingers

Thoracic nerves that are not part of the brachial plexus are the motor nerves to the intercostal muscles and sensory nerves from the skin of the thorax.

The lumbar and sacral nerves combine to form the lumbosacral plexus (Figure 5-6). We present them separately.

TABLE 5-2
Spinal Nerves

Nerve	Number and Location
Cervical (neck)	8 pairs: C1 to C8
Thoracic (chest)	12 pairs: T1 to T12
Lumbar	5 pairs: L1 to L5
Sacral	5 pairs: S1 to S5 (These exit through the sacral foramina.)
Coccygeal	1 pair: Long thoracic nerve

C, Cervical; *T,* thoracic; *L,* lumbar; *S,* sacral.

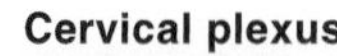

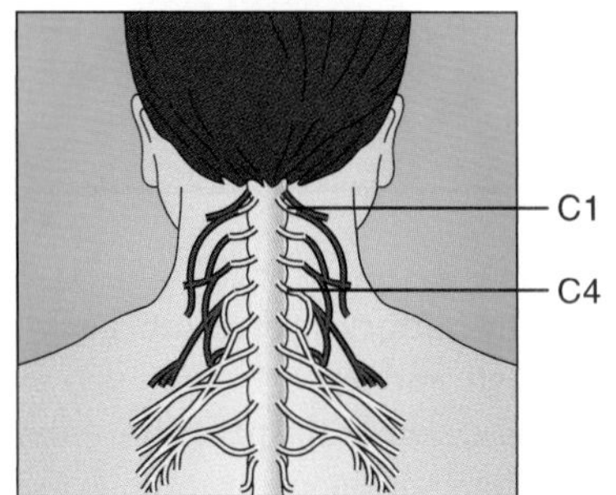

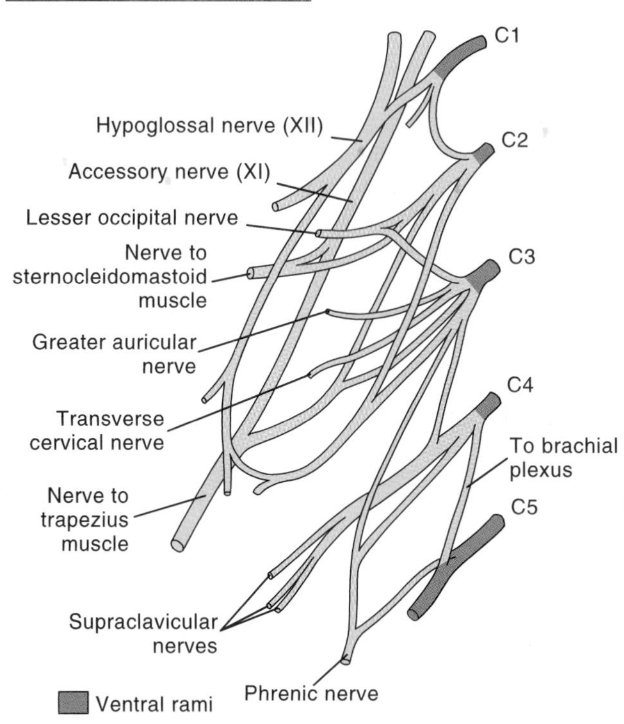

Figure 5-4
Cervical plexus. Ventral rami of the first four cervical spinal nerves (C1 through C4) exchange fibers in this plexus found deep within the neck. Some fibers from C5 also enter this plexus to form a portion of the phrenic nerve. (From Thibodeau GA, Patton KT: *Anatomy and physiology,* ed 5, St Louis, 2003, Mosby.)

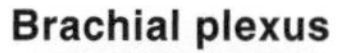

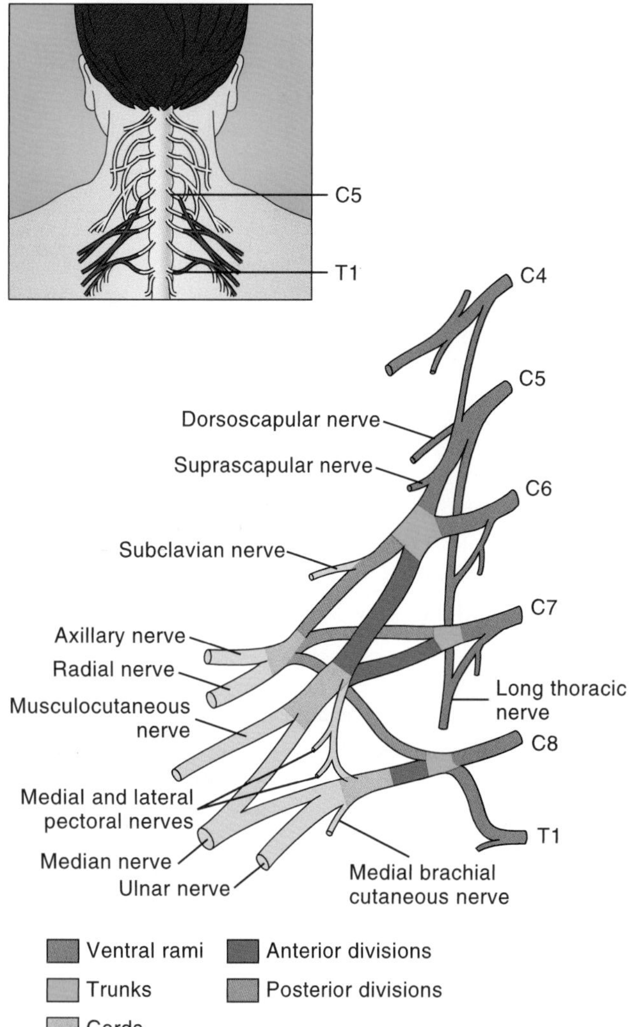

Figure 5-5
Brachial plexus. From the five rami, C5 through T1, the plexus forms three trunks. Each trunk subdivides into an anterior and a posterior division. The divisional branches reorganize into three cords, and the cords give rise to the individual nerves that exit this plexus. (From Thibodeau GA, Patton KT: *Anatomy and physiology,* ed 5, St Louis, 2003, Mosby.)

Lumbar Plexus

The lumbar plexus is composed of nerves L1 to L4.

Nerve	*Innervation*
Iliohypogastric	Abdominal muscles and skin of the abdomen and buttocks
Ilioinguinal	Abdominal muscles and skin of the external genitalia
Genitofemoral	Skin of the external genitalia and inguinal region
Lateral femoral cutaneous	Skin of the thigh (except the medial portion)
Femoral	Hip flexors and extensors and skin of the medial and anterior thigh and medial leg and foot
Obturator	Adductor muscles and skin of the medial thigh

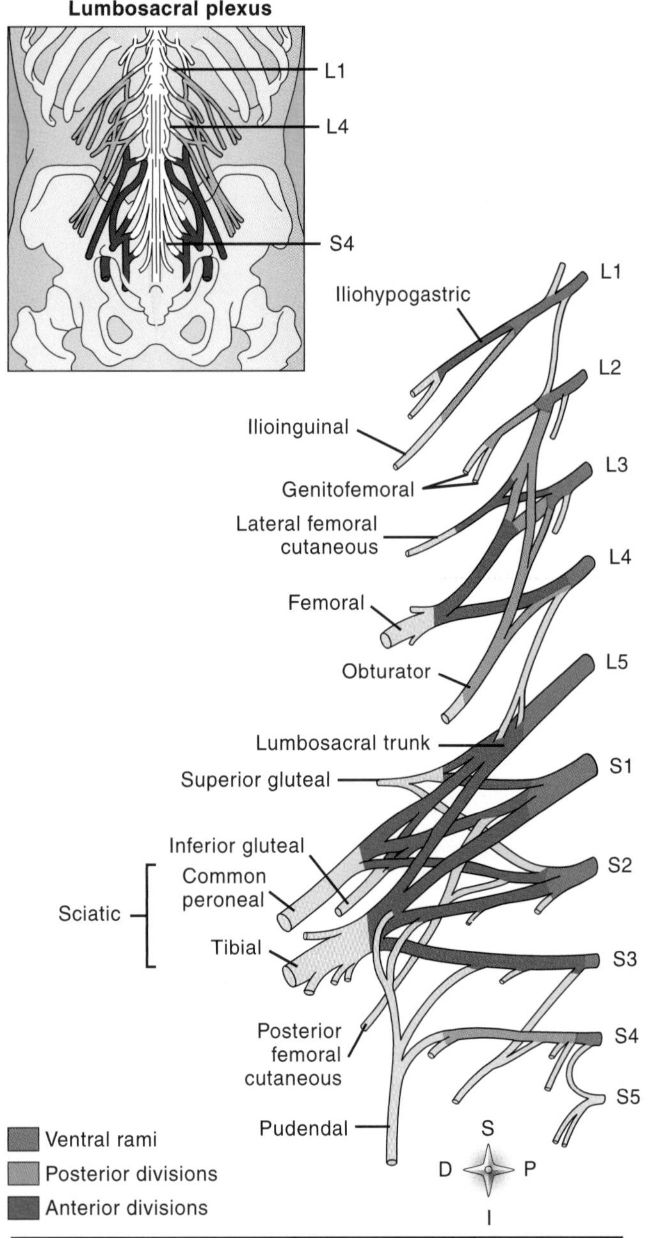

Figure 5-6
Lumbosacral plexus. The lumbosacral plexus is formed by the combination of the lumbar and the sacral plexuses, as shown in the inset. The ventral rami split into anterior and posterior divisions before reorganizing into the individual nerves that exit this plexus. (From Thibodeau GA, Patton KT: *Anatomy and physiology,* ed 5, St Louis, 2003, Mosby.)

Sacral Plexus

The sacral plexus is created from nerves L5 to S3.

Nerve	*Innervation*
Sciatic	Leg and foot muscles; the skin of the foot, which divides into the tibial and peroneal nerves at the popliteal fossa
Gluteal	Buttocks and tensor fasciae latae muscle
Nerves to hip rotators	Piriformis, quadratus femoris, obturator internus, and superior and inferior gemellus
Posterior femoral cutaneous	Skin of the buttocks, perineum, back of the thigh, and leg
Pudendal	Muscles and skin of the perineum (may be considered in the coccygeal plexus)

ACTIVITY 5-1

What could happen if each of the following nerves was damaged?

Phrenic nerve

Thoracodorsal nerve

Radial nerve

Lateral femoral cutaneous nerve

Posterior femoral cutaneous nerve

Injury

Injury to the sensory portion of any spinal nerve causes loss of sensation (anesthesia) in the innervated area; injury to the motor portion results in flaccid paralysis of the muscles of that area (Activity 5-1). For example, damage to the radial nerve (C5 to C8) at the forearm results in anesthesia of the dorsal portion of the first three fingers and paralysis of the hand and finger extensors. This causes a condition known as wrist drop.

Dermatomes

A **dermatome** is a section of skin supplied by a single spinal nerve. Dermatomes are identified by the number of the nerve. Although Figure 5-7 shows a clear boundary for each cutaneous segment, the nerve supplies in adjoining dermatomal segments overlap. Knowing the dermatome pattern enables a clinician to locate injuries in the spinal cord and spinal nerves. A correlation can be seen between dermatome patterns and the pathway of Chinese meridians.

Myotomes

A skeletal muscle or group of muscles that receives motor axons from a single spinal nerve is known as a **myotome.**

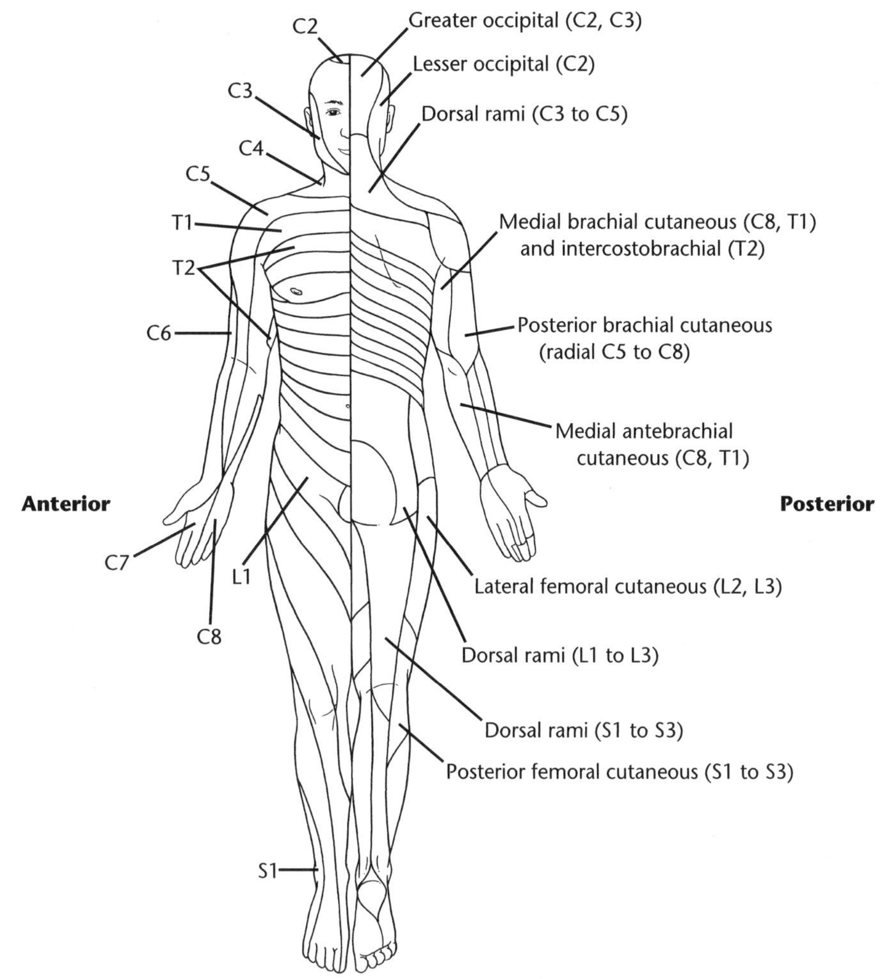

Figure 5-7
Dermatomal map (*anterior view*) and cutaneous nerve distribution (*posterior view*) of the human body. (From Greenstein GM: *Clinical assessment of neuromusculoskeletal disorders,* St Louis, 1997, Mosby.)

As with dermatomes, the boundaries of myotomes are not always exact; some muscle groups may be innervated by motor axons from more than one spinal nerve. Figure 5-8 shows which spinal nerves innervate the skeletal muscles that produce the movements indicated by arrows.

Reflex Mechanisms

A nerve **reflex** is an involuntary action. Because of the "wiring" of the body, a simple activity that stimulates a few receptors can involve many neurons going to and from muscles and glands. A brief action such as bumping the funny bone (the ulnar nerve) requires many neurons. Some conduct signals to and from the spinal cord to prompt withdrawal of the arm; others carry signals to and from the brain, letting us know when to yell "Ow!" and to stimulate tears.

Involuntary reflexes involve receptors, neurons, interneurons, and the spinal cord. Conditioned learned reflexes also involve the brain. Almost every reflex is polysynaptic, meaning that internal reflex signals cross many synapses. Breaking down these complex patterns is often difficult but can be a clinical necessity if we are to understand the automatic and sometimes perpetuating responses of functional and dysfunctional reflex patterns that interact in the continual attempt of the body to maintain homeostasis.

Somatosomatic reflexes involve stimulus of sensory receptors in the skin, subcutaneous tissue, fascia, striated muscle, tendon, ligament, or joints producing a reflex response in segmentally related somatic structures; for example, from one such site on the body to another segmentally related site on the body. Massage therapy and hydrotherapy commonly evoke such reflexes.

Somatovisceral reflexes occur where a localized somatic stimulation (from cutaneous, subcutaneous, or musculoskeletal sites) produces a reflex response in a segmentally related visceral structure (internal organ or gland). Massage and hydrotherapy commonly affect these reflexes.

Viscerosomatic reflexes occur when a localized visceral (internal organ or gland) stimulus produces a reflex response in a segmentally related somatic structure (cutaneous, subcutaneous, or musculoskeletal). Viscerosomatic reflexes occur when organ dysfunction produces superficial effects

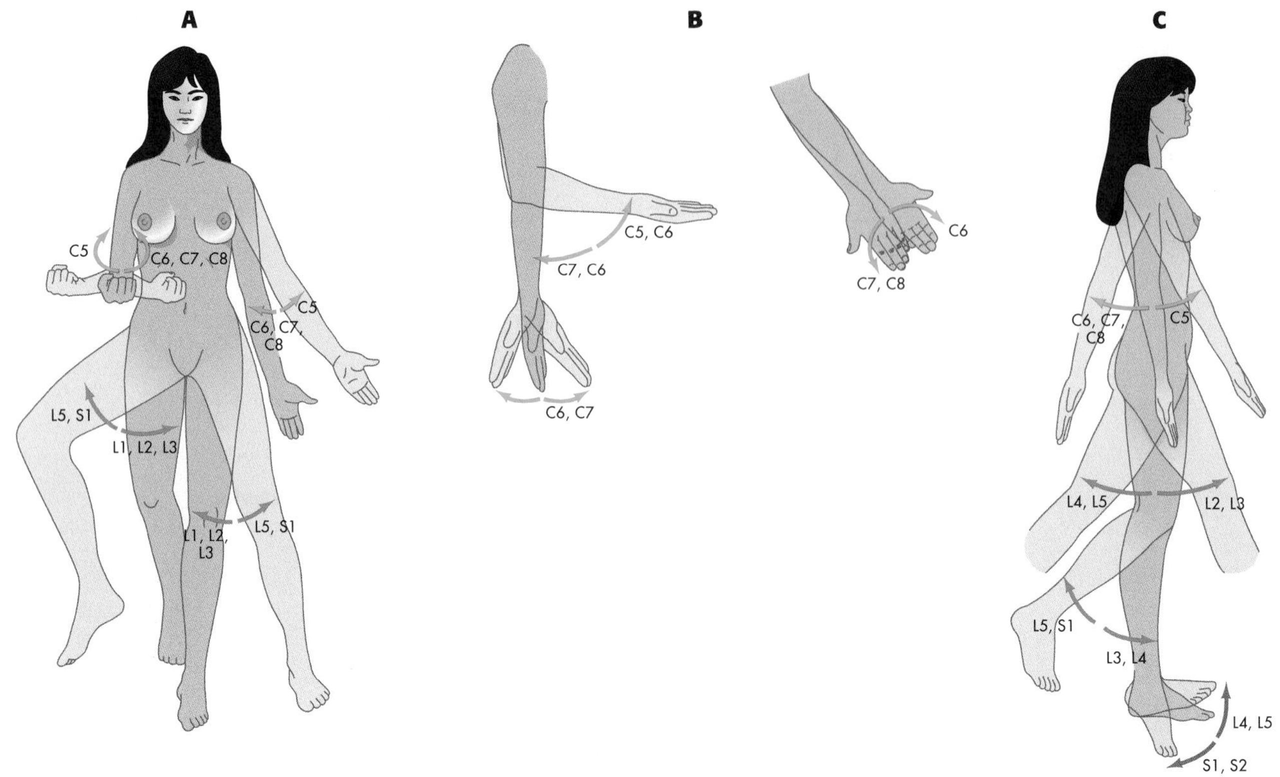

Figure 5-8
Myotomes and body movement. Myotomes are skeletal muscles innervated by one or more given spinal nerves. These examples show which spinal nerves innervate the skeletal muscles that produce the movements indicated by the arrows. **A,** Rotation and abduction/adduction of the arm and hip. **B,** Flexion/extension of the hand and wrist; pronation/supination of the hand. **C,** Flexion/extension/hyperextension of the arm, hip, and knee; dorsiflexion and plantar flexion of the foot. *C,* Cervical spinal nerves; *L,* lumbar spinal nerves; *S,* sacral spinal nerves; *T,* thoracic spinal nerves. (From Thibodeau GA, Patton KT: *Anatomy and physiology,* ed 5, St Louis, 2003, Mosby.)

involving the skin (including pain and tenderness). Examples include right shoulder pain in gallbladder disease and cardiac ischemia producing the typical angina distribution of right arm and thoracic pain.

Viscerovisceral reflexes occur when a stimulus in an internal organ or gland produces a reflex response in another segmentally related internal organ or gland.

Sensory Receptors

Our bodies contain many types of receptors located in various areas. Receptors on the outside of our bodies are called exteroceptors and are stimulated by actions or changes in our external environment. Two examples are our eyes and ears. Changes in our internal environment stimulate the visceroceptors, or interoceptors. These receptors receive signals monitoring factors such as blood pressure and hunger. In and around the muscles and joints of our body are the **proprioceptors,** which are affected by changes in position, movement, and tension (Figure 5-9).

Most of the time we are not aware of the subtle changes that stimulate sensory receptors or of the adaptations that result from these changes. These natural reflexes, processed in the brainstem or portions of the spinal cord, affect not only our physical response but also the behavior that may result. We can train ourselves to be aware of the stimuli and purposefully adapt our responses; this is called a conditioned reflex. These learned behaviors are present in our daily actions, such as tying our shoes, and are highlighted in forms of sports training and conditioning. We can learn to shoot a basketball or throw a baseball or swing a golf club. After the basic skills have been mastered, we do not have to think about most of the actions; these are conditioned reflexive patterns. Personal habits such as nail biting or eating while watching television also are conditioned reflexive patterns, and these habits may be hard to break after they become reflexive.

When an appropriate stimulus stimulates a sensory receptor, the receptor sends an impulse to the central nervous system, where the information is processed. Sensory receptors adapt by becoming less sensitive to a stimulus, and they reduce the number of signals sent, or stop altogether, even if the stimulus is still present. If this did not happen, we would never get used to things such as clothing because the nervous system constantly would be aware of the sensations and would be unable to sort through what is important to respond to and what is not. Some forms of minimal brain damage or learning difficulties that involve difficulty

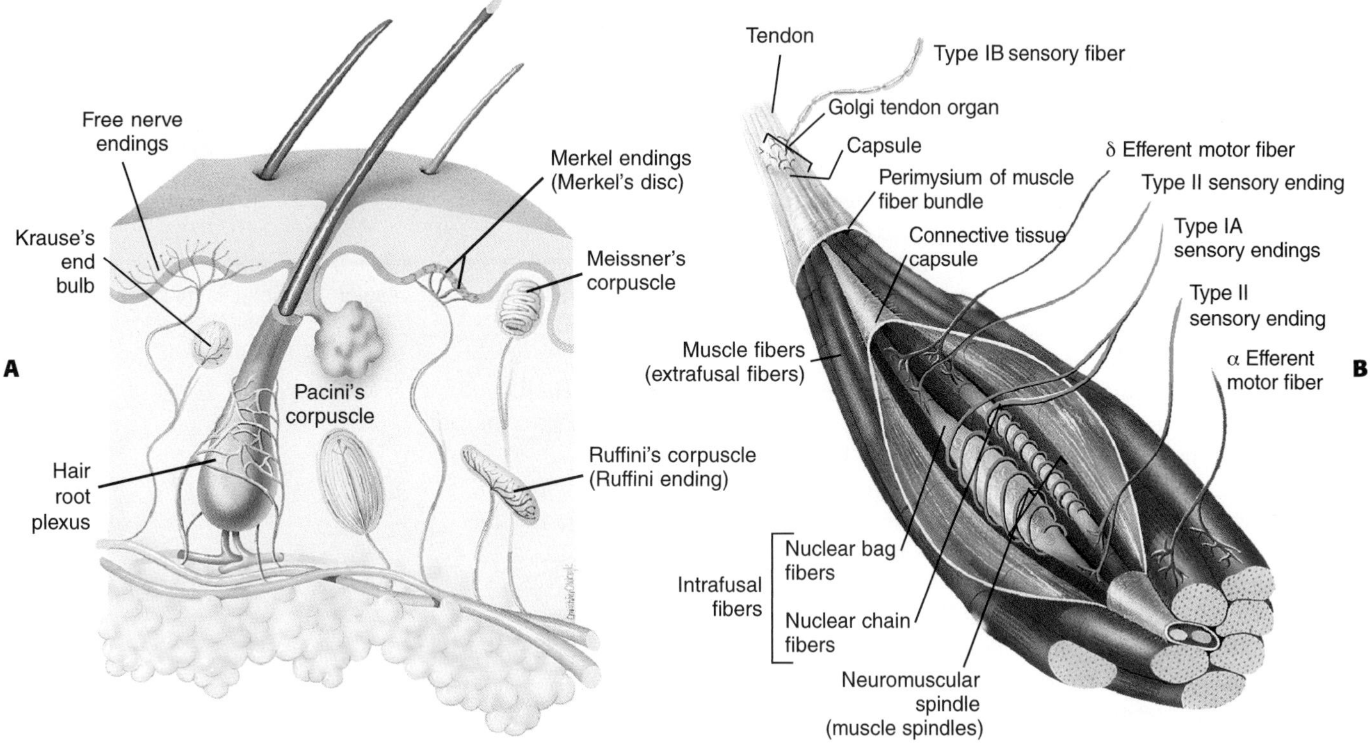

Figure 5-9
Somatic sensory receptors. **A,** Exteroceptors. **B,** Proprioceptors. (From Thibodeau GA, Patton KT: *Anatomy and physiology,* ed 5, St Louis, 2003, Mosby.)

focusing or attending to sensory input seem to be perpetuated by a diminished capacity for sensory adaptation. Some of the receptors, especially those associated with pressure and touch, adapt quickly; such receptors play a major role in signaling changes in a particular sensation. Other receptors, such as those that detect pain and body position, adapt slowly and signal information about steady states of the body.

Each sensory receptor is specialized to convert one form of stimulus into action potentials in the sensory nerves. The sensation perceived and the ability to localize the part of the body from which it originated is determined by the particular part of the sensory cortex activated by the impulse. Changes in the frequency of action potentials and the number of receptors stimulated determines the intensity of sensation.

Numerous sensory structures are classified as **mechanical receptors.** Some of them are listed below:

Mechanoreceptors: These structures detect changes in pressure, movement, temperature, or other mechanical forces. Massage stimulates these sensory receptors.

Pacinian (lamellated) corpuscles: This type of corpuscle senses brief touch, pressure, and high-frequency vibrations. Located in the submucosal, subcutaneous, and connective tissue of the hands, feet, genitals, joints, and other structures, pacinian corpuscles respond to most forms of rapidly changing mechanical stimulation.

Meissner's corpuscles: These corpuscles are touch receptors found in the hairless portions of the skin, mainly on the palms, fingertips, and soles of the feet, as well as on the eyelids, lips, tongue, and genitals. They can identify the exact location of touch (known as discriminative touch), the initial onset of touch, and low-frequency vibration, and they adapt quickly.

Hair root (root hair) plexuses: This type of plexus is a network of dendrites that surrounds hair follicles. Subtle hair movements such as those caused by light touch or a soft breeze stimulate hair root plexuses. They respond and adapt quickly.

Ruffini's end organs: These structures are touch and pressure receptors located in the deeper areas of hairy portions of our skin and in our joints. They recognize heavy and continuous touch, pressure, steady position, and direction of movement.

Merkel's disks: These disks are a type of mechanoreceptor and can be found in hairless portions of the skin. They function in discriminative touch.

Free nerve endings: These structures detect temperature and are known as **thermal receptors** (thermoreceptors). One type detects warmth, and another type senses the lack of warmth, or coolness. The brain compares this information to help identify what we would perceive as hot, warm, cool, or cold. The dorsal side of the hand has many thermal receptors, is suited ideally for identifying temperature, and is used commonly by caregivers to check a child for fever. A clinician can use the dorsal side of the hand to assess for warm areas on the body. Free nerve endings also detect itch and tickle sensations.

Nociceptors: These are specific free nerve endings that detect painful stimuli. Overstimulation of any of the thermal receptors can signal pain as a protective response.

Mechanical receptors that provide us with information about position and movement are called proprioceptors. We achieve balance with input from muscle tension, joint position, and the relative movement of each of our parts as well as movement of the whole body. Because proprioceptors adapt slowly to sensations, they tend to signal the central nervous system (CNS) over longer periods. The motor control centers in the brain receive these signals and coordinate normal muscle actions and patterns of movement. Some signals elicit a response when the signal reaches the spinal cord; these are called *reflexes.* Reflexes have a faster response time and allow the body to prevent injury by withdrawing or changing position to compensate for the additional stress. Some of these reflexes persist even when injury or disease affects the spinal cord.

Some mechanical receptors also work as joint proprioceptors. Ruffini's end organs (referred to as type II cutaneous mechanoreceptors) are located in the joint capsule and monitor joint pressure. Pacinian corpuscles, also found in the joint capsule and surrounding connective tissue, respond to pressure in and to the muscles and to pain in the joint itself. Pacinian corpuscles also monitor joint acceleration.

The following are proprioceptors:

Muscle spindles (neuromuscular spindles): Muscle spindles are located primarily in the belly of the muscle. They are stretch receptors that monitor and respond to sudden and excessive lengthening. These same fibers send signals via the spinal cord to inhibit actions in the antagonist muscle (the muscle that creates the opposite movement of an action).

Golgi tendon organs: These fibers, which are found in the tendons and musculotendinous junctions, respond to increases in tension. The signals they send out produce a slight stimulation to the antagonist muscle, which prevents return responses from reaching the signaling muscle, causing it to relax.

The ligaments have receptors called *joint kinesthetic receptors* that work in a similar manner. To prevent injury when excessive strain or tension is applied to a joint, they initiate a signal that results in inhibition of the adjacent muscle or muscles.

When proprioceptors are stimulated, the somatic reflex arcs process and interpret the signal as a spinal reflex (Activity 5-2). A feedback loop works to protect the muscles and joints from injury. If the demand on either could cause injury, the result often is pain, weakness, or muscle relaxation.

ACTIVITY 5-2

Depending on the modality being studied, highly successful soft tissue and movement treatments in some way stimulate many if not all of the various sensory receptors. For each receptor given, identify a technique and explain the way it stimulates the receptor. An example is given to get you started.

Example: Pacinian (lamellated) corpuscles
Use of a mechanical vibrator to stimulate high-frequency vibrations

Your Turn

Meissner's corpuscles

Hair root plexuses

Ruffini's end organs

Merkel's disks

Thermal receptors

Nociceptors or free nerve endings

Muscle spindles

Golgi tendon organs

Joint kinesthetic receptors

PRACTICAL APPLICATION

Massage and bodywork introduce stimulation through touch, pressure, vibration, and movement, causing sensory receptors to respond. Input from the sensory systems plays a role in controlling motor functions by stimulating spinal reflex mechanisms. Almost all forms of bodywork use some aspect of touch that stimulates the various touch receptors found in the skin. Methods that use light touch stimulate root hair plexuses, free nerve endings, Merkel's disks, Meissner's corpuscles, and Ruffini's end organs. Techniques such as compression; deep, gliding strokes; and joint movement stimulate the pressure receptors such as the pacinian corpuscles. The rapid, repetitive sensory signals of vibration and percussion techniques directly influence the pacinian corpuscles. Movement affects all the proprioceptors. ■

Reflex Arc

A reflex is a fast automatic response to a stimulus that helps maintain homeostasis. A reflex arc is the pathway that the nerve impulse follows from the receptor through sensory neurons to the spinal cord (or brain), back through motor neurons to the effector of the action. Association neurons between the sensory and motor neurons help connect the signal pathway for its most efficient routing. The effector is a muscle that contracts or a gland that secretes. The response is classified as somatic with a skeletal muscle contraction and autonomic (visceral) with a glandular secretion or contraction of a smooth or cardiac muscle.

The somatic reflexes most often stimulated by massage and bodywork are the stretch reflex, tendon reflex, flexor reflex, and crossed extensor reflex. We discuss autonomic reflexes later.

The simplest form of reflex results from a monosynaptic (one synapse) and ipsilateral (one-sided) reflex arc. The reflex begins with the stimulation of a receptor, which sends out a nerve impulse via an afferent (sensory) neuron. The signal travels to the brain or spinal cord and synapses with an efferent (motor) neuron. The only true monosynaptic reflex is a deep tendon reflex, which involves just sensory and motor neurons. Deep tendon reflexes are important because they can be used to evaluate the sensory nerve, a portion of the spinal cord, the motor nerve, and the muscle or muscles supplied by the nerve. To evaluate the reflex, a physician or trained medical professional uses a device to tap the tendon, which stimulates the receptor in the tendon. The impulse travels along the sensory nerve to the spinal cord, where it synapses with motor neurons and continues along the motor axon, signaling the muscle to contract. A defect at any point in this arc interferes with the reflex contraction of the muscle.

The following are important deep tendon reflexes:

- The *biceps* and *triceps* reflexes help one to evaluate spinal cord levels C5 and C6, the brachial plexus, and the biceps and triceps muscles.
- The *patellar reflex* (the knee-jerk reflex) helps one evaluate spinal cord level L4, the lumbar plexus, the femoral nerve, and the quadriceps muscle.
- The *Achilles tendon reflex* (the ankle-jerk reflex) helps one evaluate spinal cord level S1, the sacral plexus, and the gastrocnemius and soleus muscles. The result of such an evaluation would be abnormal, for example, if low back pain that radiated to the leg and foot accompanied the stimulus (tendon tapping); this could indicate a slipped disk at the level of L5 to S1.

PRACTICAL APPLICATION

Reflex patterns can be used during bodywork to make muscles contract. This could be done to stimulate a weakened muscle or assist lengthening and stretching by stimulating a muscle to contract, which would inhibit any action in its antagonist and thus allow the antagonist muscle to relax. ■

Stretch Reflex

The stretch reflex is a protective contraction that results when a muscle is stretched suddenly or intensely. Not to be confused with the action of slow stretching or lengthening, the stretch reflex is a homeostatic mechanism that prevents muscle trauma in response to a stretch. The muscle spindles initiate a nerve impulse that travels to the posterior root of the spinal nerve and into the spinal cord. A nerve impulse then conducts back to the same muscle. The impulse reaches the muscle, generating the action potential and causing the muscle to contract. This contraction prevents the muscle spindle from initiating any more nerve impulses. The stretch reflex itself is monosynaptic (one synapse). However, the response becomes a polysynaptic (many synapses) reflex arc. Association neurons in the spinal cord cause synergist muscles to contract and relay impulses. Other association neurons interrupt the signal to the antagonist muscles or muscle, allowing it to relax.

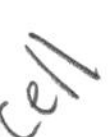

Reciprocal innervation is the wiring of our circuitry that prevents injury and allows for coordinated actions by allowing the signal for contraction of one muscle to continue while interrupting the signal to its opposing muscle. Reciprocal inhibition is the action or lack of action that results from this process. During a massage, the practitioner often uses reciprocal inhibition as preparation for stretching to avoid stimulating the stretch reflex and thus prevent muscle spasm. Because muscles operate in groups, this stretch reflex coordinates the various contractions and relaxation and the stabilization and balance we need to move effectively, if not always gracefully.

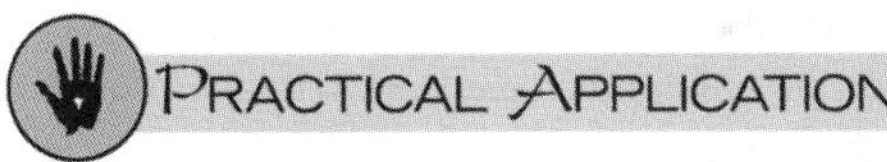

Massage methods can use the stretch reflex to normalize weakened muscle patterns by stretching the muscles just to the point of initiating the reflex. The response would be for the muscle to begin contracting. The result is restoration of a more normal strength pattern in the muscle. An awareness of this reflex response is important in all methods intended to lengthen and relax the muscles to their more normal resting length. In these instances one must avoid the stretch reflex. As a caution, for stretch reflexes to become hyperactive is not uncommon, resulting in increased muscle tension. Such hyperactivity may occur in the leg muscles after a fall when the muscles were quickly and extensively stretched. The stretch reflex may become more sensitive, and in affected muscles, cramping may be more common. ■

Tendon Reflex

Also known as the *inverse stretch reflex,* the tendon reflex is a feedback mechanism that controls muscle tension by allowing for muscle relaxation. Golgi tendon organs detect and respond to changes in muscle tension. As the tension increases, often because of an increase in a muscle contraction, these sensors initiate a signal that follows the sensory neuron to the spinal cord. Association neurons inhibit any signal from returning to the same muscle, while other neurons continue allowing a signal to reach the antagonist via motor neurons. This causes a slight contraction in the antagonist, which allows the prime mover to relax because no impulse is available to generate the action potential.

In some medical texts the term *tendon reflex* is used to describe a reflex action initiated by tapping a tendon rather than by stretching the muscle belly (which may be called a *muscle reflex* even if the result is the same for both). The student needs to be aware that such references describe the stimulus and not the resulting reflex action.

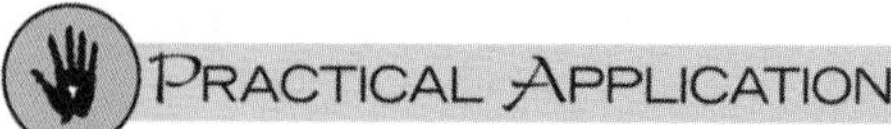

The most common massage technique used to stimulate the tendon reflex is postisometric relaxation. A muscle is contracted against a resisting force, which increases the tension in the tendon. If the load or stimulation is sufficiently strong, initiating the tendon reflex results in relaxation of the muscle. During the relaxation phase, one can lengthen or stretch the muscle or both more easily. This technique increases tension at the tendon by introducing contraction in the muscle, usually the result of active participation of the client. ■

The stretch reflex and tendon reflex are simple examples of the way our bodies are programmed to maintain homeostasis. In our normal actions, these reflexes usually are activated for full-body responses instead of isolated muscle groups. The *flexor (withdrawal) reflex* and the *crossed extensor reflex* are polysynaptic reflex arcs that work with larger areas and the whole body.

Flexor Reflex

The flexor reflex begins with stimulation of the sensory receptor, often by something painful such as stepping on a pin or contact with a noxious stimulus such as a hot flame. The signal travels to the spinal cord, crosses association neurons (as in the tendon reflex), and returns to the muscles involved. This muscle contracts to withdraw; simultaneously, signals have been sent to other muscles on the same limb to do likewise. For example, if you step on a pin with your left foot, your left anterior tibialis muscle, quadriceps (rectus femoris), and psoas contract. The antagonist muscles, including the gastrocnemius, soleus, hamstrings, and gluteus maximus, are inhibited from acting (remember the way in which the association neurons can block signals), thus allowing the entire leg to remove itself from the stimuli. The withdrawal reflexes are powerful, taking precedence over all other concurrent reflex actions.

Crossed Extensor Reflex

The crossed extensor reflex works in coordination with the flexor reflex. When the initial signal reaches the spinal cord, not only does it travel to the flexor muscles on the same side of the body to allow the limb to withdraw, but it also crosses the spinal cord and travels to the extensor muscles to maintain balance. This action starts contraction of the right gastrocnemius, soleus, hamstrings, and gluteus maximus while inhibiting the action of the right anterior tibialis, quadriceps, and psoas. The muscles of the torso and arms also can be stimulated or inhibited through this reflex for complete balance if needed.

This reflex action explains why a tension pattern in one part of our body can be seen in other areas. The extensive pathways that the signals follow are called contralateral reflex arcs. The initial stimulus given in the previous example was pain, but the body can respond similarly to other stimuli. If you are standing and begin to walk by lifting your right foot off the floor, the signal of loss of balance begins this process, allowing the right leg and left arm to swing forward (flexing), and the left leg and right arm to keep the body steady (extending). This reflex interaction is known as gait.

Proprioception: Gamma Motor Neurons and Muscle Tone

Gamma motor neurons innervate muscle spindles. If the gamma motor neuron is stimulated, contraction occurs at both ends of the spindles, resulting in stretching of the middle region of the spindle where the sensory nerves are located. The sensory nerve endings detect the stretch and produce action potentials that cause the muscle to be more sensitive to stretch. Gamma motor neurons are then responsible for the muscle tone.

A muscle that offers little resistance to stretch is said to be *flaccid*. Flaccidity occurs if the nerve to the muscle is cut. A muscle that offers great resistance to stretch is said to be hypertonic or spastic. Spasticity occurs when hyperactive stretch reflexes exist and may be seen in individuals with spinal cord injury or stroke, in whom the inhibitory impulses to the gamma motor neurons from the brain have been removed. A muscle is hypotonic when the gamma motor neuron discharge is low.

Control of Gamma Motor Neuron Discharge

The gamma motor neurons regulate the sensitivity of the muscle spindles, and hence the stretch reflexes and tone of the muscle can be altered according to the change in posture. Many factors affect the gamma motor neuron discharge. For example, anxiety and stress increase its discharge, resulting in tensing of muscles and hyperactive tendon reflexes. If the skin of the hand on one side is stimulated by a painful stimulus, the result is increased discharge to the flexors and decreased discharge to the extensors of the same side, facilitating flexion and quick removal. At the same time, the opposite happens in the other side, adjusting posture and weight distribution.

The clasp-knife effect or lengthening reaction can occur while one treats individuals with spastic muscles. Stretching the muscle results in the muscle seeming to resist and give alternately. For example, if the elbows are flexed passively, immediately resistance occurs because of the stretch reflex in the triceps muscle. Further stretch activates and causes the triceps to relax suddenly, reducing the resistance.

Sometimes spastic muscles respond to a sudden stretch by a regular, rhythmic contraction. This reaction is known as *clonus* and is caused partly by the hyperactive muscles being subjected to alternating activity of stretch reflex and tendon reflex.

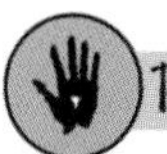

PRACTICAL APPLICATION

Most benefits derived from massage therapies result from resetting tension patterns caused by reflex actions, especially those that begin as a result of a fall or trauma, repetitive movement, or maintenance of a fixed position. The practitioner who understands the interactive patterns can use corrective bodywork procedures to resolve or support these actions. Because of the crossed extensor reflex, the practitioner can deliberately stimulate limbs on one side of the body to affect the limbs on the opposite side of the body. For example, if the goal is relaxation of the flexors of a lower limb, stimulating the extensors of the upper limb on the opposite side produces reciprocal innervation in the thigh flexors, resulting in this relaxation response.

One can puzzle out many of these patterns by thinking in terms of reflex patterns. By effective application of these reflex arcs, a therapist can affect any neuromuscular area of the somatic system without even touching that area; this is beneficial for sensitive areas that are in pain or areas that are difficult to reach, such as the deep muscles of the axilla or groin (Activity 5-3). Reflex patterns are also responsible for many compensatory body patterns found in relation to posture. Imagine that a person suddenly stumbles when walking. The crossed extensor reflexes, via

ACTIVITY 5-3

Try to determine three upper and lower body interactions based on the withdrawal and contralateral reflex arc. An example is provided to get you started. Pay attention to the patterns and movements, not the specific names and functions of muscles.

Example:

Lower body situation: Tight calf on the left

Possible interactions:

Weak dorsiflexors on the left; tight dorsiflexors on the right

Weak calf on the right

Weak hip flexors on the left; tight hip flexors on the right

Tight hip extensors on the left; weak hip extensors on the right

Weak arm flexors on the left; tight arm flexors on the right

Tight arm extensors on the left; weak arm extensors on the right

Weak neck extensors; tight neck flexors

Weak abdominal muscles

Tight back extensors

Your Turn

1. ____________________

2. ____________________

3. ____________________

contralateral reflex arcs, respond to restore balance. The attempt by the body to stay upright by avoiding the fall may result in a chain reaction of muscle tension and relaxation adjustments throughout the body, which can develop into postural distortion over time if the situation continues. The body may readjust muscle tension patterns, and neuromuscular feedback loops may become confused. The resulting skeletal muscle pathologic conditions can lead to discomfort and postural distortion from uneven muscle contraction and relaxation patterns. Therapeutic massage often resets these unproductive reflex patterns. Resetting of reflex communication patterns may result in a return of more efficient and coordinated movement patterns. ■

The effects produced by massage depend heavily on the reflex mechanism. The effectiveness of the particular techniques depends on how efficiently one stimulates the receptors for these reflexes. The practitioner must reach the targeted receptor with the appropriate technique and level of intensity so that the reflex stimulated is allowed to function in the appropriate manner. Fast- and slow-acting receptors, light- and deep-touch receptors, and so on are stimulated by different durations and levels of intensity of touch and movement. The massage practitioner must understand what type of message to send to the CNS to be processed. Treatment methods do not produce the desired benefit if the wrong signal is sent.

Touch and movement are considered stimuli because they constitute a change in the environment. When the body is called on to restore homeostasis, problematic nerve transmission pathways often can be overridden and a more effective pattern can be established. The student will find learning the receptor language of the body and exploring the reflex patterns initiated by the various forms of stimuli worthwhile so as to override these nonproductive transmissions. The more this information is incorporated into practical applications, the more effective the therapeutic massage intervention will be.

Autonomic Nervous System

We have been discussing the somatic division of the peripheral nervous system and its feedback loops that provide for voluntary and reflexive control of our skeletal muscles. Maintenance of the internal environment of the body is the responsibility of the autonomic nervous system. The autonomic nervous system (ANS) controls the actions of the smooth muscles and glands and is another division of the PNS. As in the somatic PNS, ANS information from sensory receptors goes to the brain, which in turn relays the most effective effector response to maintain homeostasis. The sensors are located in areas such as the smooth muscles, blood vessels, lungs, and glands. Motor neurons carry the signals to these same organs to prompt an increase or decrease in the rate of our heartbeat, breathing, or digestive processes or to initiate glandular secretion. The system is called involuntary because its actions normally are outside conscious control.

The ANS is divided into the sympathetic and parasympathetic divisions. In general, the **sympathetic nervous system** tends to stimulate and functions primarily when the body is under stress (Figure 5-10). The **parasympathetic nervous system,** which usually diminishes or inhibits actions, tends to work most often under normal body conditions or to conserve energy (Figure 5-11).

Our skeletal muscles are innervated by neurons that carry a signal to contract or carry no signal at all, which causes the muscles to relax. The ANS has a different form of control. Most of the organs contain neurons from the sympathetic and parasympathetic divisions; this is called *dual innervation.* By constantly receiving signals from both divisions, the body can maintain or quickly restore homeostasis because the organs can be stimulated or inhibited rapidly. This form of autonomic antagonism is another example of the duality of wholeness discussed previously in this text. If sympathetic impulses tend to stimulate an effector, parasympathetic impulses tend to inhibit it. This type of antagonistic activity gives precise control, just like having accelerator and brake pedals on a car.

For example, moment-to-moment regulation of blood pressure involves continuously changing sympathetic and parasympathetic signals to the heart. The regulation comes from centers in the brainstem that "turn up" or "turn down" each type of input to keep blood pressure constant as the body changes position or activity.

Another major difference is that in the ANS, two neurons relay the signal from the brainstem or spinal cord to the organ, gland, or smooth muscle innervated. The first neuron synapses with the second, and the second synapses with the receptor. In the sympathetic nervous system, the synapse, or ganglion, is located near the spinal cord. In the parasympathetic system the ganglion is near or at the receptor organ, gland, or muscle. The neurotransmitter released at the ganglion synapse near the spinal cord is acetylcholine, just as in the **somatic nervous system.** At the postganglionic synapse to the organs, different neurotransmitters are involved. The sympathetic postganglionic synapse releases noradrenaline (norepinephrine), except in the adrenal medulla, which releases adrenaline (epinephrine) and only some noradrenaline. The benefit of adrenaline in the blood is that it reinforces and prolongs the effect of noradrenaline. Acetylcholine is found in the parasympathetic postganglionic synapse. Based on the neurotransmitter secreted, the autonomic nervous system can be divided into cholinergic (acetylcholine-secreting) and adrenergic (adrenaline-secreting) divisions. All preganglionic and postganglionic fibers of the parasympathetic system belong to the cholinergic division. Postganglionic sympathetic fibers that supply sweat glands and blood vessels of skeletal muscles produce vasodilation and are cholinergic. The postganglionic fibers of the sympathetic system are adrenergic. Other neurotransmitters such as dopamine are secreted by interneurons located in the ganglia. Stimulation of the sympathetic

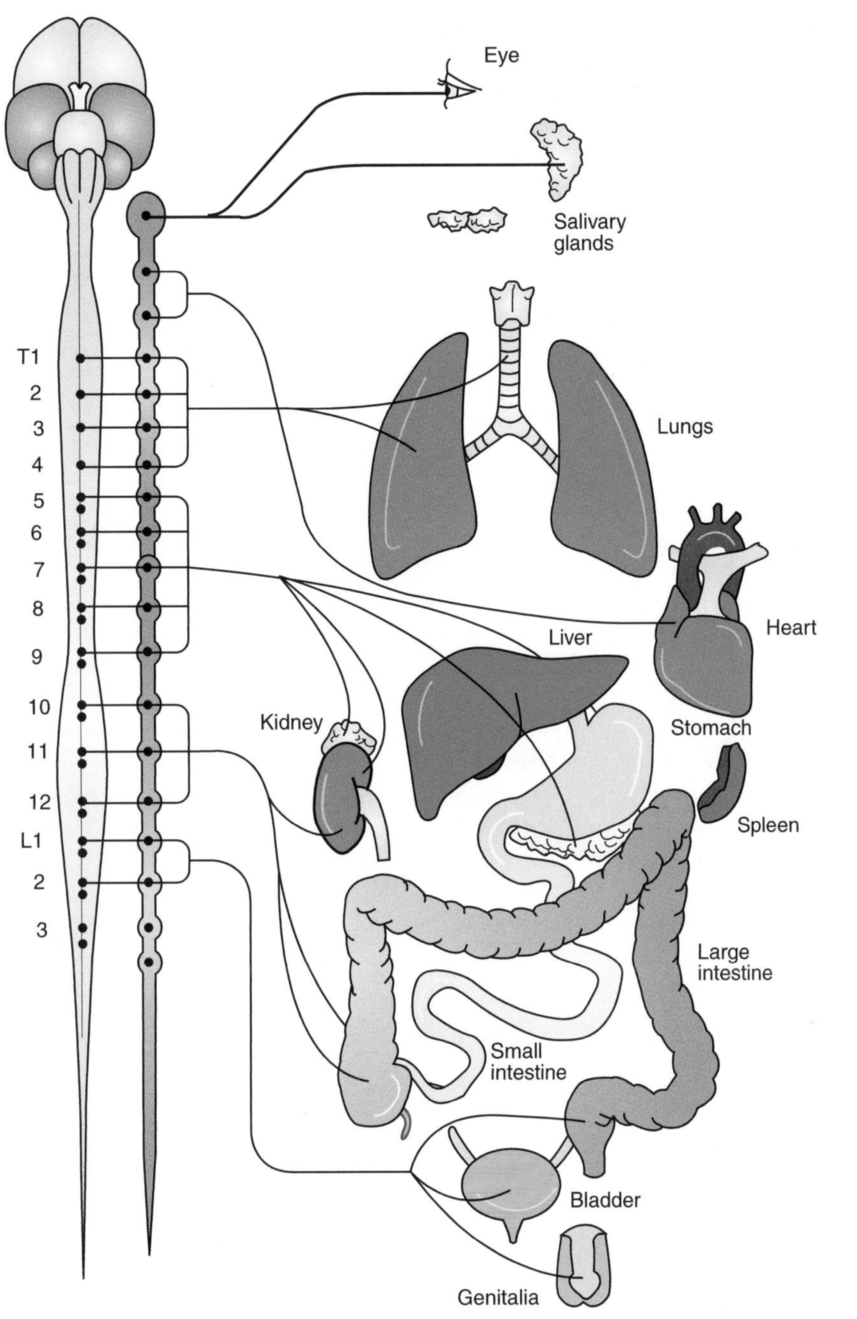

Figure 5-10
The sympathetic portions of the autonomic nervous system.

nervous system can excite or inhibit the smooth muscles, depending on the receptors in the organ involved. Receptors are divided into two major groups: alpha-receptors, which respond to norepinephrine (noradrenaline) and certain blocking substances, and beta-receptors, which respond to epinephrine (adrenaline) and similar blocking substances. Each of these groups can be divided again, into alpha-1 and alpha-2 and beta-1 and beta-2, which better classifies the generalized responses they produce.

When alpha-receptors are stimulated, they cause dilation of the pupils and constriction of the smooth muscles and blood vessels. Stimulation of beta-1-receptors, which are found mainly in the heart, results in an increase in the force and rate of heart muscle contraction; beta-2-receptors, located in the lungs, cause relaxation of the bronchial muscles, resulting in bronchodilation.

As with sympathetic nerve fibers, the effect of the parasympathetic postganglionic fibers on a target organ

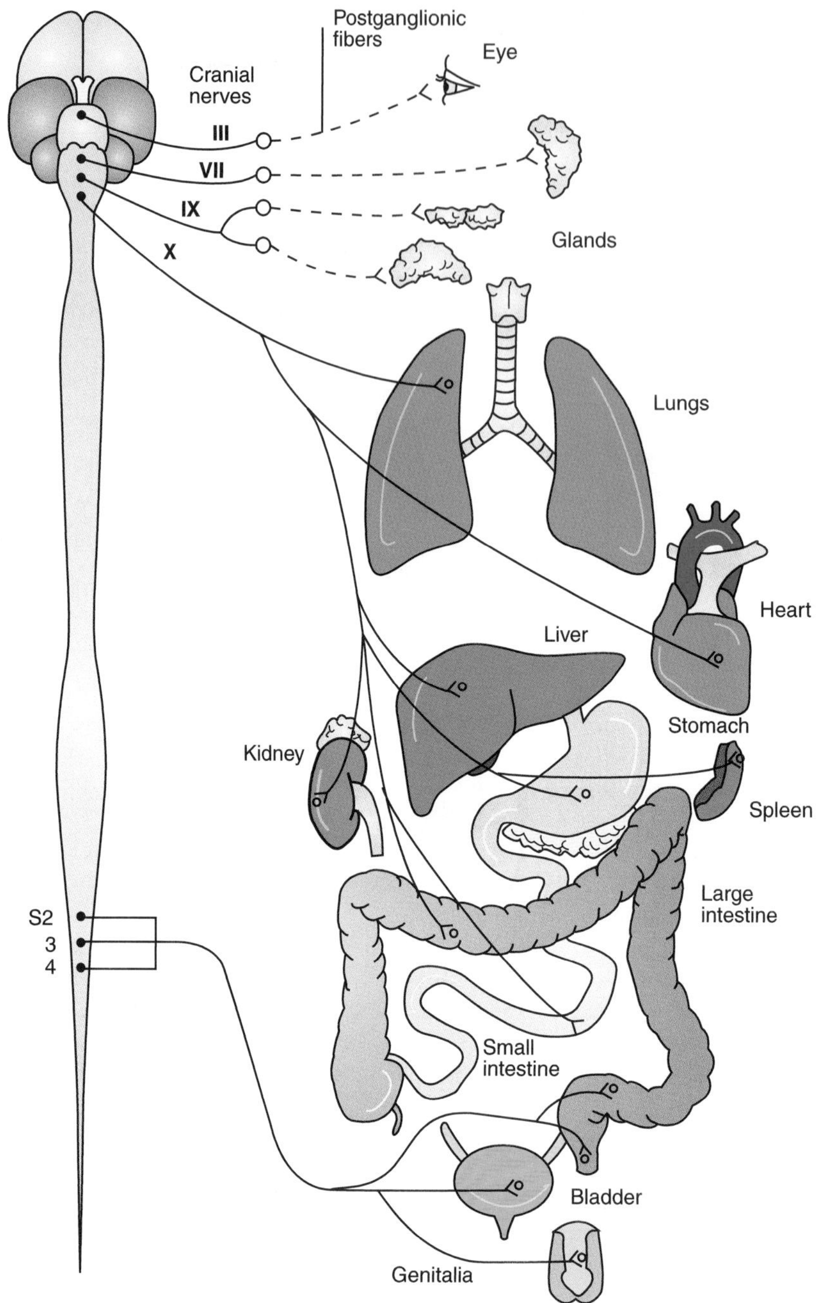

Figure 5-11
The parasympathetic portions of the autonomic nervous system.

depends on the type of receptors present in the cells. Two types of receptors, nicotinic and muscarinic, have been identified. The nicotinic receptors are present in the parasympathetic and sympathetic ganglions and in the neuromuscular junction. The muscarinic receptors are located in target organs supplied by postganglionic parasympathetic fibers. The terms *nicotinic* and *muscarinic* are based on the effects of nicotine, a powerful toxin that can be obtained from a variety of sources including tobacco, and muscarine, a toxin present in poisonous mushrooms. So, if one ingests a large quantity of nicotine, it produces symptoms according to the presence of nicotinic receptors such as vomiting, diarrhea, sweating (parasympathetic effects), high blood pressure, rapid heart rate, and sweating. By stimulating skeletal muscles, convulsion also may occur.

The symptoms muscarine poisoning produces are almost all caused by parasympathetic effects and include vomiting,

ACTIVITY 5-4

Identify a control process you use to influence the sympathetic and parasympathetic divisions of the autonomic nervous system and explain the way it works. An example is provided to get you started.

Example

Sympathetic: Brisk walking for 30 minutes in the morning. The fast pace activates the sympathetic functions and helps wake me up and give me energy for the day.

Parasympathetic: Eating a bowl of cereal before bed. Eating signals digestion and also helps make me sleepy.

Your Turn

diarrhea, constriction of bronchi, low blood pressure, and slow heart rate.

Knowledge of the receptors, actions, and distribution of parasympathetic and sympathetic nervous systems is important to all health professionals. Almost all drugs used in conditions such as asthma, hypertension, the common cold, constipation, diarrhea, and many other conditions have been developed and are being used based on this knowledge. Side effects of all these drugs can be derived logically if one knows which receptors they affect and whether the drug imitates or opposes the sympathetic and parasympathetic systems.

The effect the neurotransmitter has on a target organ depends on the type of receptor for the neurotransmitter the cells of the organ possess. For example, the effect of postganglionic parasympathetic fibers may be stimulatory or inhibitory depending on the receptor. In general, postganglionic sympathetic fibers are excitatory (Activity 5-4).

Sympathetic Structure and Function

The sympathetic nervous system begins in the spinal cord, where the neurons exit between the first thoracic vertebra and second lumbar vertebra. Because of the location the system often is referred to as the *thoracolumbar division.* The sympathetic ganglia found near the spinal cord are connected by collateral tissues and form a chain. This interconnected chain allows for many different sources of input of sympathetic activity to each of the effectors, thus producing more sympathetic activity with little input. The preganglionic neurons are short and end in this chain; the postganglionic neurons are much longer and end at the effector organs.

The major function of the sympathetic nervous system involves the emergency response. The signals sent out allow the body to be more prepared for an increase in the intensity of activities that require increased metabolism, higher blood sugar levels, a stronger heartbeat, and dilated bronchi, allowing for more oxygen to the lungs and faster exhalation of carbon dioxide. During this function, the blood is rerouted from the digestive system to the muscles so that they can respond to the increased stress.

Whether the stimulus is physical or psychologic or whether the threat is real or imagined, all our responses are set into action immediately. Walter B. Cannon described this group of sympathetic responses as the fight-or-flight reaction. These responses are normal and healthy in times of stress. However, chronic exposure to stress or perceived threats to our well-being can affect our health adversely, leading to dysfunction of sympathetic effectors and perhaps even to the dysfunction of the ANS itself. Excessive sympathetic output causes most of the stress-related diseases physicians encounter. Problems with headaches, gastrointestinal difficulties, high blood pressure, anxiety, muscle tension and aches, and sexual dysfunction can be related to excessive sympathetic stimulation.

We think of the aforementioned functions as life preserving because they can be used to remove us from dangerous situations and keep us active in self-preservation. However, the sympathetic system also is active during many of our normal daily functions. Dual innervation allows the sympathetic system to oppose the effects of the parasympathetic system, providing balance and maintaining homeostasis.

The fact that smooth muscles in the walls of the blood vessels are innervated only by sympathetic fibers is also important. The fibers maintain the tone of the muscles of the arteries, resulting in proper blood pressure whether we are active or at rest. This is another example of general homeostatic balance.

Parasympathetic Structure and Function

The parasympathetic nervous system is referred to as the craniosacral division because of the location of its nerves. Parasympathetic fibers leave the CNS through cranial nerves, including the oculomotor, facial, glossopharyngeal, and vagus nerves and at the sacrum and some pelvic nerves. The three long preganglionic neurons that innervate the pupil and the salivary and lacrimal glands end outside the actual organs. The rest of the preganglionic neurons end at the walls of the organs, with the short postganglionic fibers entering the organs. This configuration is the opposite of the sympathetic division, in which the neurons end just before the organ.

The parasympathetic system generally functions as the energy conservation system, which allows our body to rest and restore itself after emergency responses. The result is a relaxation response. To maintain balance with the sympathetic division, the parasympathetic system is dominant under nonstressful conditions; this means that during nonstressful times, more impulses to the effectors are received by parasympathetic fibers than by sympathetic fibers.

The parasympathetic system is active in regulating digestive processes, slowing the heart rate, and constricting eye muscles to focus on near vision. In addition, the parasympathetic system increases glandular secretions, constricts the bronchioles in the lungs, and slows breathing. Parasympathetic stimulation of the nerves to the internal and external genitalia in males and females causes vasodilation in the clitoris and labia minora and erection in the penis.

Reactions to parasympathetic stimulation are highly localized and tend to counteract the adrenergic effects of the sympathetic system (Activity 5-5, Table 5-3). Learning one system usually is simpler, because the other is the opposite. Memorizing the fight-or-flight response seems to be the more practical way. These responses make fighting or fleeing possible; for example, pupillary dilation improves vision, faster heart rate increases cardiac output to supply muscles with blood, bronchodilation improves breathing, and slowing of digestive responses reduces interference with fight or flight.

Medications That Affect the Autonomic Nervous System

Certain groups of medications bind to or join with alpha- and beta-receptors, thereby enhancing or blocking the receptor sites for the binding of norepinephrine (noradrenaline), acetylcholine, or other neurotransmitters and hormones. The effects determine the medication used to modify ANS function. The major problem with many of these medications is the side effects, which range from tachycardia to constipation.

Alpha-Adrenergic Blockers

Alpha-adrenergic blockers (alpha-blockers) bind to receptors and thus prevent norepinephrine from binding, causing a decrease in blood vessel tone; this lowers blood pressure and increases circulation. Ergotamine (Cafergot, Ercaf, Wigrane) diminishes the intensity of blood vessel contraction in the cranial arteries and can relieve migraine headaches. Hydralazine (Apresoline, Unipres) dilates blood vessels, which reduces blood pressure. Nitroglycerin, one of the most widely known alpha-blockers, rapidly dilates arteries and veins, reduces blood pressure, and increases blood flow to the heart muscles. Nitroglycerin is used primarily for patients with angina and coronary artery disease. Alpha-blockers used to treat hypertension include doxazosin (Cardura), terazosin (Hytrin), and prazosin (Minipress).

Beta-Adrenergic Medications

Medications that include epinephrine (adrenaline) (which is a beta-1- or beta-2-agonist) or that affect beta-2-receptors by enhancing the uptake of epinephrine (adrenaline) are used most commonly to treat respiratory disorders such as asthma, chronic bronchitis, and emphysema. Epinephrine-adrenaline inhalers (Bronkaid Mist, Primatene Mist) dilate bronchial tubes while causing the walls of the blood vessels to contract, increasing blood flow to the lungs. Other forms of this medication are used as eye drops for glaucoma to reduce internal eye pressure. Drugs that enhance epinephrine uptake without causing as many cardiac side effects include pirbuterol (Maxair), metaproterenol (Alupent, Metaprel), and albuterol (Proventil, Ventolin).

Beta-Adrenergic Blockers

Beta-adrenergic-blockers (beta-blockers) diminish the force and rate of heart muscle contractions and are used to treat hypertension, irregular heart rhythms, and angina. Commonly prescribed medications include metoprolol (Lopressor), penbutolol (Levatol), and atenolol (Tenormin). Propranolol (Inderal) and nadolol (Corgard) are beta-blockers commonly used to treat hypertension and migraines.

Chemical substances that mimic the effect of or increase the uptake of norepinephrine (noradrenaline) are called sympathomimetic, because they imitate sympathetic stimulation. Besides the bronchodilators used to treat asthma, bronchitis, and emphysema, these drugs include medications used during surgery to counteract the parasympathetic effects of anesthetics and maintain normal blood pressure. Ephedrine is used in many over-the-counter preparations for colds and sinus congestion.

Monoamine oxidase inhibitors are medications that reduce or stop the breakdown of norepinephrine and serotonin; they commonly are used to treat phobias, depression,

ACTIVITY 5-5

After reviewing the effects of sympathetic and parasympathetic stimulation, identify a sensation, body function, daily activity, or behavior influenced by the autonomic nervous system. An example is given to get you started.
Cardiovascular System
Cardiac muscle
Sympathetic: Increased rate and strength of contraction (beta-receptors)

Example
Feeling that the heart is pounding

Your Turn
Parasympathetic: Decreased rate of strength of contraction

Example: Possible lower blood pressure; may feel washed out or fatigued.

Your Turn
Smooth muscle of blood vessels
Sympathetic: Skin, blood vessels: constriction (alpha-receptors)

Example
Hands and feet get cold.

Your Turn
Parasympathetic: No effect

Example
Hands and feet get warmer.

Your Turn
Skeletal muscle blood vessels
Sympathetic: Dilation (beta-receptors)

Example
Feels as if the body wants to move and is restless.

Your Turn
Parasympathetic: No effect

Example
Increased ability to sit still

Your Turn
Abdominal blood vessels
Sympathetic: Constriction (alpha-receptors)

Example
Stomach seems in a knot.

Your Turn
Parasympathetic: No effect

Example
Stomach seems relaxed.

Your Turn
Blood vessels of external genitals
Sympathetic: Constriction (alpha-receptors)

Example
May not feel sexual.

Your Turn
Parasympathetic: Dilation of blood vessels, causing erectile tissues to engorge

Example
May have sexual thoughts.

Your Turn
Smooth muscle of hollow organs and sphincters
Bronchioles
Sympathetic: Dilation (beta-receptors)

Example
May feel like can't get enough air.

Your Turn
Parasympathetic: Constriction

Example
Breathing may get slower.

Your Turn
Digestive tract, except sphincters
Sympathetic: Decreased peristalsis (beta-receptors)

Example
May be constipated.

Your Turn
Parasympathetic: Increased peristalsis

Example
May digest food better.

Your Turn
Digestive tract sphincters
Sympathetic: Constriction (beta-receptors)

Example
May be constipated.

Your Turn
Parasympathetic: Relaxation

Example
May have more frequent bowel movements.

Your Turn
Urinary bladder
Sympathetic: Relaxation (beta-receptors)

Example: Can go long periods without urinating.

Your Turn
Parasympathetic: Contraction

Example: May need to urinate after a period of relaxation.

ACTIVITY 5-5—cont'd

Your Turn
Urinary sphincters
Sympathetic: Constriction (alpha-receptors)

Example: May have difficulty urinating.

Your Turn
Parasympathetic: Relaxation

Example: May leak urine when coughing.

Your Turn
Eye
Iris
Sympathetic: Contraction of radial muscle; dilated pupil

Example: May need sunglasses even in moderate lighting.

Your Turn
Parasympathetic: Contraction of circular muscle; constricted pupil

Example: Frequently finds lighting too dim.

Your Turn
Ciliary body
Sympathetic: Relaxation; accommodation for far vision

Example: May find newspaper harder to read.

Your Turn
Parasympathetic: Contraction; accommodation for near vision

Example: May not be able to read road signs.

Your Turn
Glands
Sweat glands
Sympathetic: Increased sweat (neurotransmitter: acetylcholine)

Example: Get sweaty palms when nervous.

Your Turn
Parasympathetic: No effect

Example: Palms are dry when relaxed.

Your Turn
Lacrimal glands
Sympathetic: No effect

Example: Have difficulty crying when anxious.

Your Turn
Parasympathetic: Increased secretion of tears

Example: May cry more easily at a heart-warming movie.

Your Turn
Digestive (e.g., salivary and gastric)
Sympathetic: Decreased secretion of saliva and gastric secretions

Example: Finds food harder to swallow when anxious.

Your Turn
Parasympathetic: Increased secretion of saliva

Example: May drool when relaxed.

Your Turn
Pancreas (including islets)
Sympathetic: Decreased secretion

Example: May have indigestion.

Your Turn
Parasympathetic: Increased secretion of pancreatic juice and insulin

Example: May be prone to hypoglycemia.

Your Turn
Liver
Sympathetic: Increased glycogenolysis or conversion of glycogen to glucose (beta-receptors); increased blood sugar level

Example: May feel a sugar high when excited.

Your Turn
Parasympathetic: No effect

Example: Mood stays more even.

Your Turn
Adrenal medulla
Sympathetic: Increased epinephrine secretion

Example: May have exaggerated response to conflict.

Your Turn
Parasympathetic: No effect

Example: Stays calm in confused environment.

Your Turn
Hairs (pilomotor muscles)
Sympathetic: Contraction produces goose pimples, or piloerection (alpha-receptors).

Example: May become more aware of the movement of persons because of increased sensitivity to air movement.

Your Turn
Parasympathetic: No effect

Example: Are less aware of persons entering a room.

TABLE 5-3
How Sympathetic and Parasympathetic Divisions Affect Organs of the Body

Target Organ	Parasympathetic System Response	Sympathetic System Response
Skin		
Sweat glands	None identified	Secretion increased
Arrector pili muscle	None identified	Contraction, erection of hairs
Skeletal Muscles	None identified	Contraction force increased
Eye		
Radial muscle of iris	None identified	Contraction (pupils dilate)
Sphincter muscles of iris	Contraction (pupils constrict)	None identified
Ciliary muscle	Contraction (lenses bulge for near vision)	Reflex (lenses become thinner for far vision)
Lacrimal (tear) glands	Secretion	None identified
Cardiovascular System		
Heart	Heart rate and contraction force decreased	Heart rate and contraction force increased; vasodilation of coronary vessels
Blood vessels to the following:	None identified	Constriction
Skin		Dilation
Skeletal muscle		Dilation
Heart (coronary)		Constriction
Intestines (gut)		Constriction
Veins		
Respiratory System		
Bronchial muscles	Contraction	Relaxation
Bronchial glands	Secretion stimulation	Possible inhibition
Digestive System		
Salivary glands	Mucus secretion	Watery, serous secretion
Motility and tone	Increased	Decreased
Sphincters	Relaxation	Contraction
Secretions	Stimulation	Possible inhibition
Liver	Glycogen synthesis	Glycogen breakdown; glucose synthesis and release
Pancreas	Increased secretion of exocrine and endocrine (insulin)	Exocrine secretion decreased
Adipose Tissue	None identified	Breakdown and release of fatty acid
Urinary System		
Kidney	Urine production increased	Urine production decreased
Urinary bladder	None identified	None identified
Detrusor muscle	Contraction	Relaxation
Sphincter	Relaxation	Contraction
Reproductive Systems		
Male sex organs	Erection	Ejaculation
Uterus	Varies	Varies
Blood Coagulation	None identified	Coagulation increased
Mental Activity	None identified	Alertness increased

Adapted from Premkumar K: *The massage connection: anatomy, physiology & pathology*, Calgary, Alberta, 1997, VanPub Books.

migraines, and hypertension. The monoamine oxidase inhibitors interact with many other drugs, foods, and herbs, especially those containing the amino acid tyrosine.

Other medications or recreational drugs such as codeine and opium also affect norepinephrine use by mimicking the sympathetic effect. A side effect is constipation.

Parasympathetic Blockers

Many of the alkaloid medications are anticholinergic and block the uptake of acetylcholine. Because of its bronchodilatory effect, atropine (Atrovent) is used to treat chronic bronchitis and emphysema, as well as some forms of asthma.

Withdrawal from medications or other substances that affect the ANS produces a variety of sympathetic effects (e.g., tachycardia and pupillary dilation) and parasympathetic effects (e.g., increased tearing and diarrhea). The distress of withdrawal symptoms continues until the body is able to restore homeostatic balance without the substance.

Eastern/Western Connection

The ganglia of the parasympathetic system tend to occupy the same areas traditionally identified as chakras, or energy centers, by Eastern meridian systems (Figure 5-12). The sympathetic chain ganglia follow one of the paths of the bladder meridian, located on either side of the vertebral column. Specific acupuncture points on this meridian, called back-shu points, are considered to be the locations where Qi of the respective yin or yang organs is assimilated (Figure 5-13). Practitioners use techniques for stimulating these points to relieve dysfunctions of the corresponding organs. One can see a correlation between sympathetic ANS function and these important organ points in the Asian meridian system (Table 5-4).

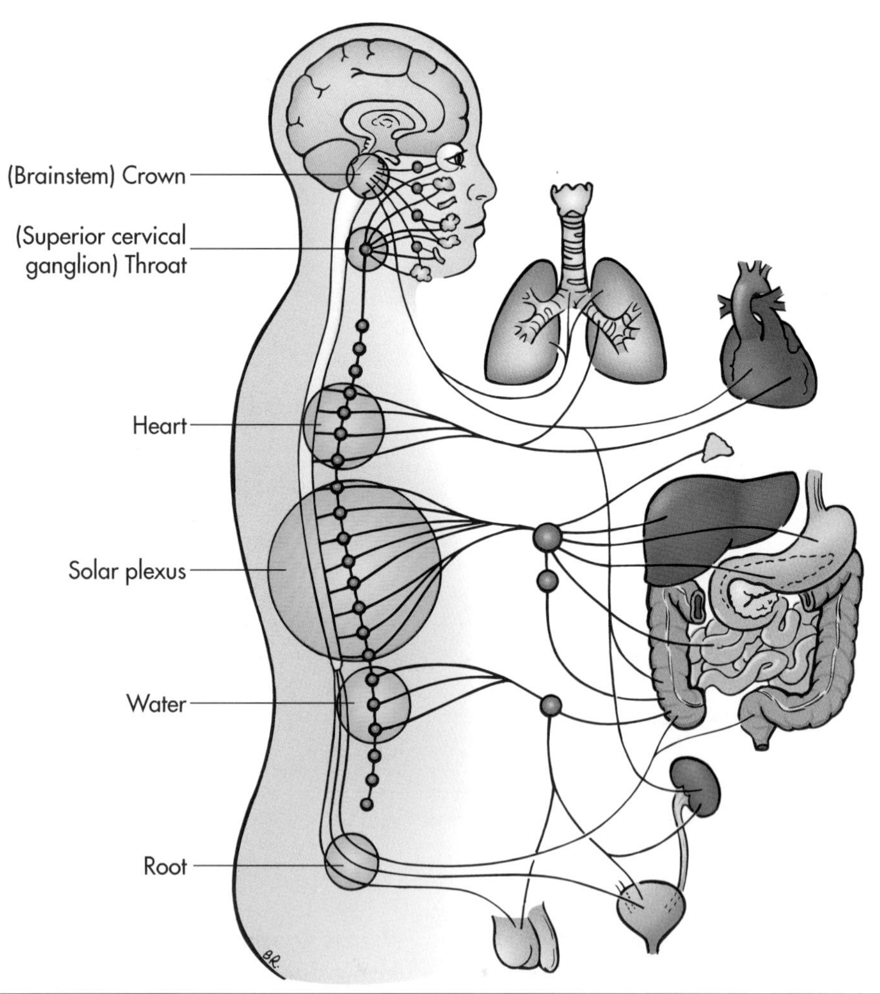

Figure 5-12
Comparison of the ANS and traditional energy centers. (From Fritz S: *Mosby's fundamentals of therapeutic massage*, ed 3, St Louis, 2004, Mosby.)

ACTIVITY 5-6

Using basic massage methods, describe how you would design and implement a 45-minute massage that would result in:

A. Sympathetic dominance

B. Parasympathetic dominance

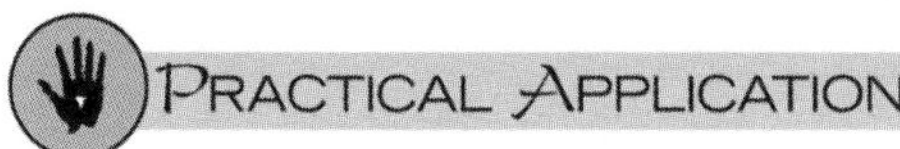

Massage modalities seem initially to stimulate sympathetic functions. Homeostatic mechanisms then work to increase restorative parasympathetic functions as needed. Point holding methods such as acupressure, reflexology, or the dry needling of acupuncture release the body's own pain killers and mood-altering chemicals from the entire endorphin class. These chemicals stimulate the parasympathetic responses of relaxation and contentment. Acupressure is a specific pinpoint compression over motor points and other areas of neurovascular concentration. These specific points and areas are the focal meeting of superficial nerves in the sagittal plane, superficial nerves or plexuses, and muscle tendon junctions at the Golgi tendons. These areas, where nerves are close to the surface of the body, correspond with many of the traditional acupuncture points. Acupressure produces sympathetic inhibition. Acupuncture probably works by taking advantage of the natural inhibitory influences in the body such as endorphins and enkephalins that normally block pain pathways. For example, researchers have established that sensory pain fibers release the neurotransmitter known as substance P, which increases the transmission of pain impulses. Endorphins and enkephalins block the release of substance P, inhibiting pain transmission to the brain. The effects of these and other neurotransmitters may validate the use of sensory stimulation methods to treat pain and anxiety. ■

Research over the past 20 years has identified the crucial role the ANS plays in stress-related disorders. This research also has validated the effectiveness of many ancient healing, cultural, and spiritual practices that serve to bring the ANS under voluntary control, bringing conscious control to homeostatic processes (Activity 5-6).

FIVE BASIC SENSES

With all the possibilities of sensory stimulation, compartmentalizing the types of stimuli and our responses makes studying and understanding the phenomena easier. More than 20 different senses have been identified. For our purposes, we will focus our study on the basic five special

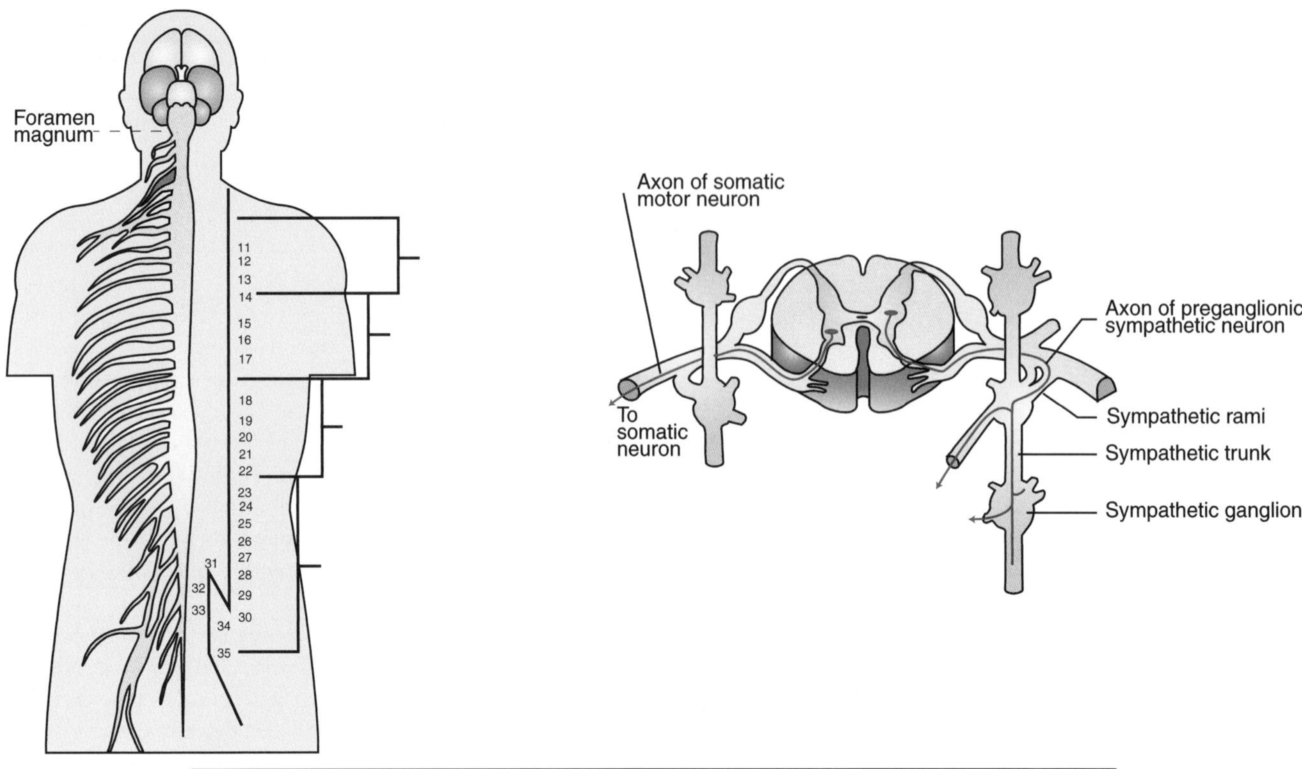

Figure 5-13
Comparison of sympathetic chain ganglia and back-shu points. See Table 5-4 below.

TABLE 5-4
Back-Shu Points of Internal Organs

Zangfu Organs	Back-Shu Points	Locations
Lung	Feishu (U.B. 13)	1.5 Cun* lateral to lower border of T3
Pericardium	Jueyinshu (U.B. 14)	1.5 Cun lateral to lower border of T4
Heart	Xinshu (U.B. 15)	1.5 Cun lateral to lower border of T5
Liver	Ganshu (U.B. 18)	1.5 Cun lateral to lower border of T9
Gallbladder	Danshu (U.B. 19)	1.5 Cun lateral to lower border of T10
Spleen	Pishu (U.B. 20)	1.5 Cun lateral to lower border of T11
Stomach	Weishu (U.B. 21)	1.5 Cun lateral to lower border of T12
Sanjiao	Sanjiaoshu (U.B. 22)	1.5 Cun lateral to lower border of L1
Kidney	Shenshu (U.B. 23)	1.5 Cun lateral to lower border of L2
Large intestine	Dachangshu (U.B. 25)	1.5 Cun lateral to lower border of L3
Small intestine	Xiaochangshu (U.B. 27)	1.5 Cun lateral to lower border of L4
Urinary bladder	Pangguangshu (U.B. 28)	1.5 Cun lateral to lower border of L5

*Cun is a method of measurement that uses a relative standard, usually the length of the second phalange of the second finger.
Modified from Ding L: *Acupuncture meridian theory and acupuncture points,* San Francisco, 1990, China Books and Periodicals.

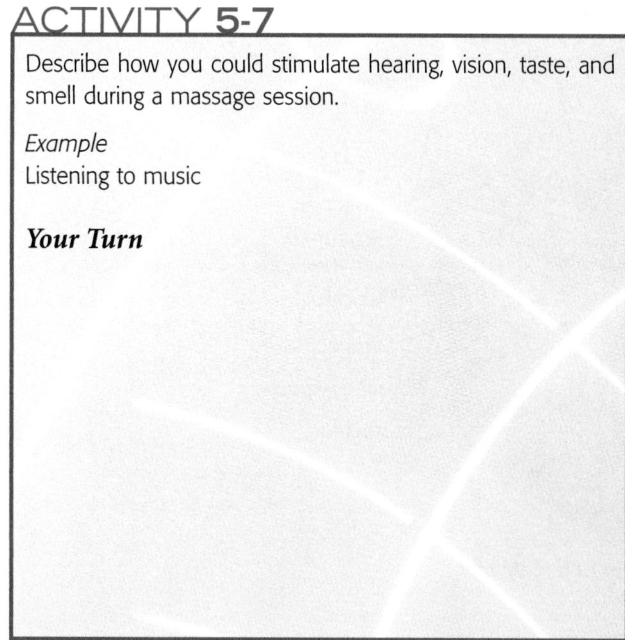

ACTIVITY 5-7

Describe how you could stimulate hearing, vision, taste, and smell during a massage session.

Example
Listening to music

Your Turn

senses we encounter and use daily. The five basic senses are touch, hearing, vision, taste and smell. We cover touch in detail in the discussion of the integumentary system in Chapter 11. Research brings more new information about the way senses work, the way they are processed in our brains, and the way they interact to enhance our lives.

The processes of sensation involve taking in the constantly received mechanical, chemical, and thermal energy forms with our sensory receptors, modifying or enhancing them, transforming them into electrical signals, and sending that information to the brain to be processed and associated with previous experiences (Activity 5-7).

Hearing

Sounds are vibrations created by mechanical methods that are turned into recognizable patterns of electrical energy in our nervous system. These vibrations can travel through air, water, or solid substances.

The brain can recognize immense variations in pitch, volume, and tone. When several sounds reach the ear, they are transferred to the hair cells in the ear. The lower-frequency signals are given priority when transmitted as electrical signals to the brain; thus a slow, deep, even voice is the best one to use when we really want to be heard.

Our sense of hearing is well-developed even at birth. Newborns can identify the direction of a voice and turn in response. Only in the past decade has investigation been conducted into the ability of the fetus to hear or sense sound carried through the amniotic fluid. Research indicates that the fetus does respond to sound.

Vibrations in the air are taken in by the external ear, called the auricle or pinna, and funneled into the external auditory meatus, which leads to the middle ear (Figure 5-14). Inside the middle ear, the sounds reach the tympanic membrane, or eardrum. As the eardrum vibrates in response, it pulls on the tiny bones called ossicles to amplify the sounds. These three bones of the middle ear work together. The motion transfers to the hammer (malleus), which hits the anvil (incus), which pulls on the stapes, or stirrup. This bone rests on the oval window, a membrane at the beginning of the inner ear. The eustachian (auditory) tube connects the middle ear with the throat and equalizes pressure between the middle ear and the outside air. Any imbalance in pressure can cause pain and distort or muffle sounds. Activities that open this tube (e.g., yawning, swallowing, or chewing) often can relieve the pressure.

Sound waves leave the middle ear and travel to the inner ear, where the *cochlea,* named for its shape as a spiral shell, is the center of our hearing. The inner ear has three canals. The outer two carry the amplified vibrations. The sound waves travel through a thin membrane to the middle canal, the organ of Corti. In this region, fluid-filled circular ducts are positioned at right angles to each other, and each duct contains hair cells embedded in a gelatinous substance. These specialized receptor cells respond to vibrations and motion. As we move, the directional hair cells transfer information about our head position and speed of movement. All this sensory information is transformed into electrical signals, which the auditory nerve conducts to the brain.

If this proprioceptive mechanism is disrupted, the result often is vertigo, or balance problems. If the disruption goes undetected or untreated, the erroneous sensory information can contribute to anxiety and panic disorders.

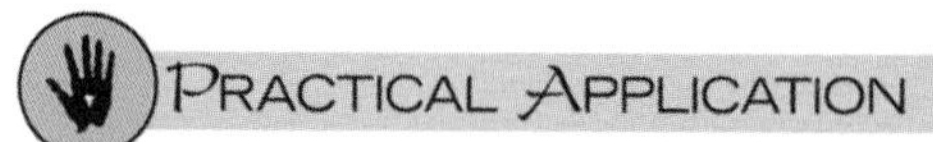

PRACTICAL APPLICATION

Any movement activity, especially those that cause head movements that affect the inner ear, shifts the perception of balance in the somatic system, thus altering muscle tension patterns. Many of the benefits of massage therapy are derived indirectly through the effect on the inner ear balance system.

Rhythmic rocking is used universally to calm infants, children, and adults because it interacts with balance mechanisms that influence the ANS to initiate parasympathetic functions. The rocking chair can be a lifelong calming companion in our hectic world. ■

Vision

The eyeball is a fluid-filled sphere composed of three layers of tissue (Figure 5-15). The outer layer comprises the sclera and the cornea. The sclera is a white, fibrous structure that maintains the shape of the eye and protects the inner structures. The cornea is the clear portion in the front that allows light to enter the eye.

In the middle layer of the eyeball are the ciliary body, choroid, and iris. The ciliary body, on the anterior portion, contains smooth muscles attached to the lens by ligaments. The choroid, which covers the posterior of the sclera, is filled

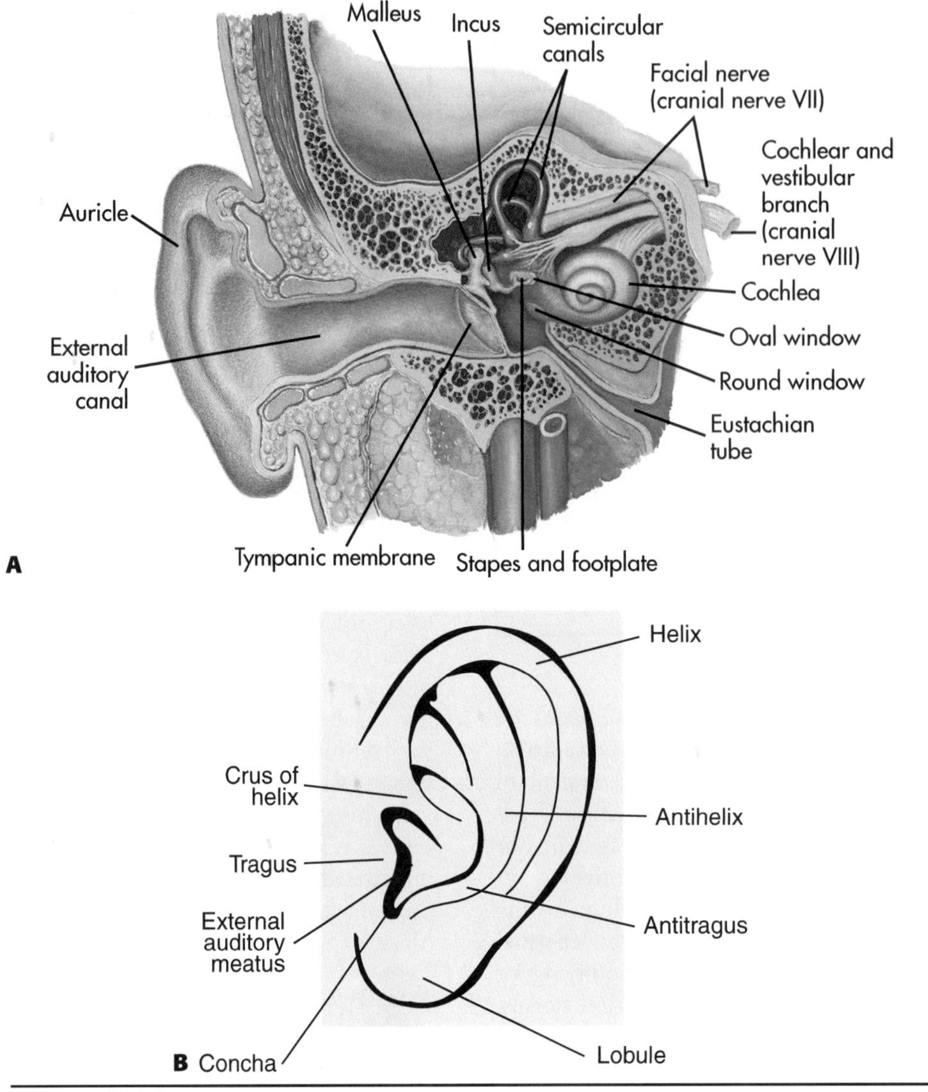

Figure 5-14
A, External auditory canal, middle ear, and inner ear. **B,** Structures of the external ear (pinna). (**A** from Barkauskas VH et al: *Health and physical assessment,* ed 3, St Louis, 2002, Mosby.)

with capillaries that nourish the eye. The cells of the choroid contain melanin and absorb light as it enters the eye. The iris, the colored portion of the eye, contains smooth muscles and controls the size of the pupil, which increases or decreases the amount of light allowed to enter the eye. Vision occurs when light rays enter through the lens and are focused onto the retina.

The inner layer of the eyeball is the retina, which contains photoreceptor cells and neurons. The rods, which are concentrated on the outer edges of the retina, take in information about the levels of lightness and darkness. The rods are responsible for recognizing shapes and patterns and providing contrast. Cones, which are concentrated at the fovea, or center, of the retina, help us identify color and brightness. We can see colors that range from red to purple. Rods and cones receive the mechanical signals, transform them into chemical substances, and create an electrical signal that is sent to the brain via the optic nerve. The optic nerve is created from association neurons in the retina. The point where the nerves exit the eye is called the optic disk, or blind spot, because it has no photoreceptors.

Vision signals are organized and processed in our cerebral cortex. Information received from the left and right eyes stays separate until it converges in the visual cortex. Signals received when we are not paying attention to any specific item are sent to the posterior parietal cortex for processing. Anything we focus on is sent to the visual cortex. Items that reflect a change in the environment cause a signal to be sent

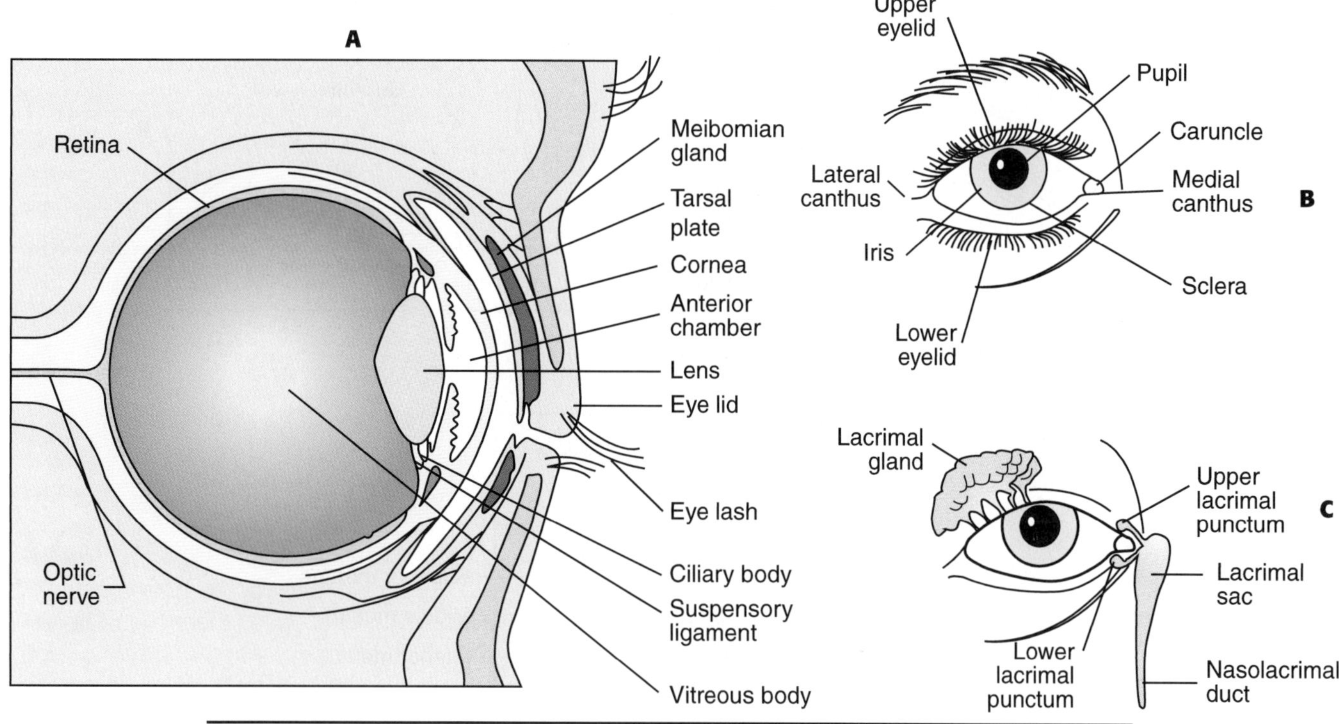

Figure 5-15
A, Structures of the eyelid and globe of the eye. **B,** Anterior view of the eye. **C,** Lacrimal system.

to the frontal lobe. These three areas of the brain (cerebral cortex, visual cortex, and parietal cortex) work to process and coordinate visual information.

The eyeball is protected by the skull within cavities known as orbits. Six muscles control movement of the eyeball. These muscles are highly sensitive and coordinate to control the position of the eye. Eyelids and eyelashes close over the eyes for protection, to block light, and to maintain distribution of fluid. The lacrimal glands produce the fluids known as tears that keep our eyes moist, fight infections, and remove foreign particles. These glands, which are located supralaterally, release their product into the eye, where it evaporates or drains into the nasolacrimal duct alongside the nose, thus explaining why the nose becomes stuffed up and runs when we cry.

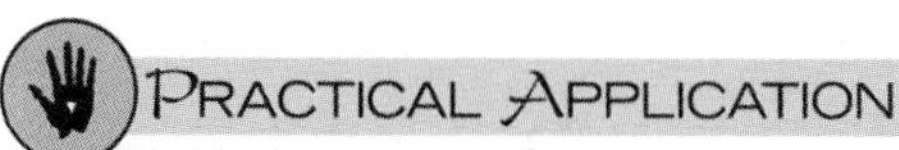

Visual orientation and eye movement are important in posture mechanisms. Visual orientation aids in posture by confirming sensations coming from proprioceptive senses in the muscles and joints. The body shifts positions as necessary to keep the eyes level with the horizontal plane. Position of the eyes is involved in righting reflexes that orient the body in gravity. The combination of proprioceptive, visual, and inner ear (vestibular) information activates various posture or righting reflexes that activate muscular responses to regain balance. Disturbance of the vestibular, visual, or proprioceptive impulses that initiate these reflexes may cause equilibrium disturbances, nausea, vomiting, muscle tension, and other symptoms. Some forms of movement methods use various eye positions as part of the intervention protocol. The effectiveness of these methods depends partly on the visual orientation aspects of posture. Because of the number of sensory receptors involved with the muscles of the eyes, coupled with the various posture reflexes, subtle movement activates muscle facilitation and inhibition of skeletal muscles especially in the neck and shoulder area. A simple way to use this response therapeutically during massage is to have the client roll the eyes in slow circles as various massage methods are applied. Muscle groups that would turn the body in the direction of the eye position tense in preparation for movement while antagonist muscles begin to relax. ■

Taste

Taste is one of the more complex of our senses. Separating taste from smell is difficult. Specific areas on the tongue correspond to four distinct tastes: sweet, sour, salty, and bitter. Molecules of food bind to receptor sites on the tongue, cheeks, and floor of the mouth. The rest of our tasting

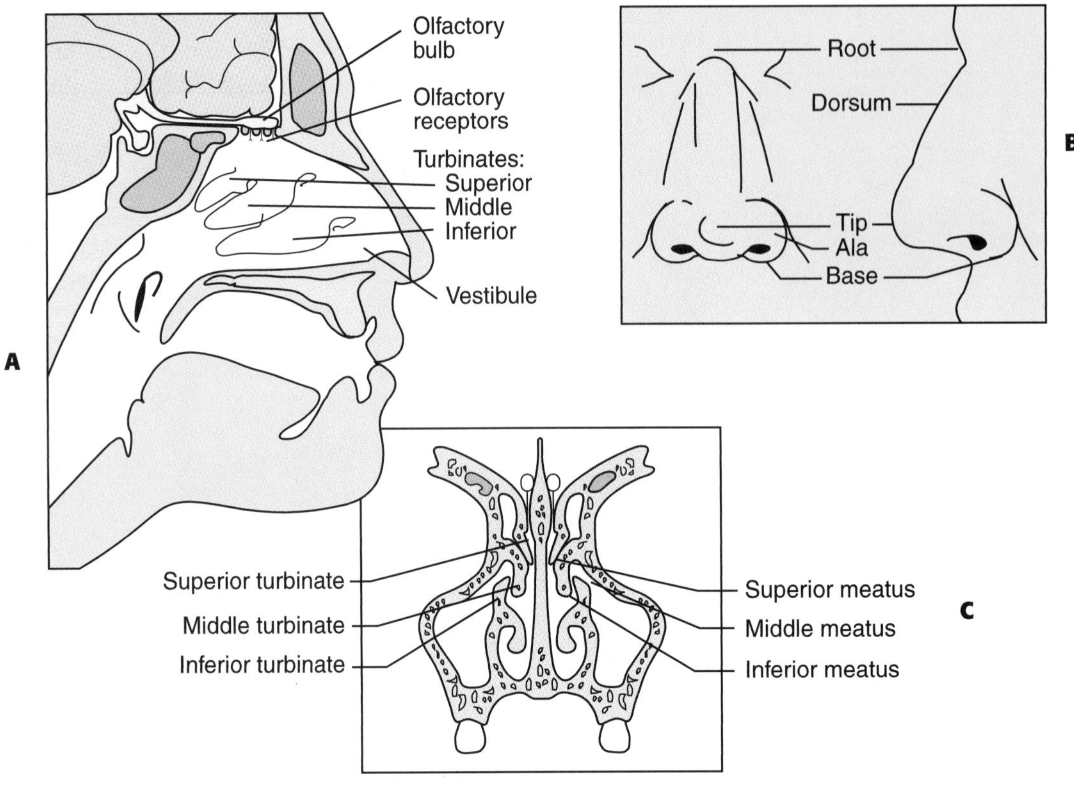

Figure 5-16
A, Lateral view of the left nasal cavity. **B,** External structure of the nose. **C,** Internal structure of the nose.

is done through our nose and combines with the sense of smell. (You can confirm this by holding your nose and tasting something.)

On average, an adult has more than 10,000 taste buds; but as we age our taste buds, which usually last about 10 days, are not replaced as frequently, which may explain why older adults are much less sensitive to taste than younger persons. Most of the nerve fibers that carry taste information to the brain can carry information about more than one taste, although they are mainly sensitive to just one and usually are classified as such.

Our individual preferences for certain tastes may be because of cultural differences or genetics. We can be much more or much less sensitive to certain tastes, making them something we love or something unpleasant. For most of us, bitter tastes are the most easily identified, which may be because most of the poisonous substances around us are bitter.

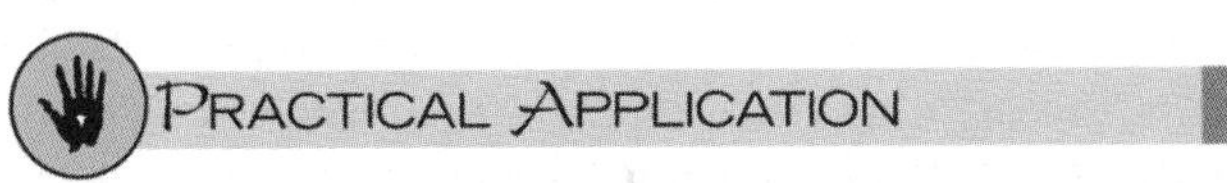

Many ancient healing practices use taste as part of their diagnostic and treatment criteria. During the assessment process, the practitioner gathers information on the foods eaten and what types of taste predominates as an indication of the imbalance. The practitioner also considers the taste of a person's secretions, such as sweat. Current medical practice considers this criterion a possible indicator of a pathologic condition. ■

Smell

The actual activity of olfaction, or smell, involves chemical receptors found in the roof of the nasal cavity. Figure 5-16 shows the structure of the nose. As an odor makes contact with the receptors, they transform chemical signals into electrical signals and transmit them to the temporal lobes of the brain. The smell centers in the brain are connected with the limbic system and thus have an emotional and a behavioral effect. Blocked nasal passages affect the senses of smell and taste.

Unlike with our other senses, smells are hard to imagine. We can picture a scene, remember a soothing voice, and conjure up a taste that makes our mouth water. But most of us have difficulty imagining a smell. Smell also is the hardest sense to describe to another person.

The sense of smell is a primitive sense that does not translate well to methods of human communication. For our ancestors, smell was a main lifesaving sense. Today smell still alerts us to dangers. The sense of smell is considered primitive because it deals with our unconscious, animal-like behaviors and experiences and elicits gut-level emotions. The nerves from the nose end in the olfactory bulb in the limbic area of the brain, the portion of the brain that also controls much of our autonomic, involuntary actions. The more civilized we become, the more we attempt to cover up our body smells and what they mean. Each of us has a unique body odor that changes in response to our emotions. That we can smell fear, danger, anger, and sexual arousal and that we can smell a friend is true. Past memories, associated with déjà vu, are elicited most with our sense of smell. Much of the information we receive from smells helps integrate other information being processed at the same time.

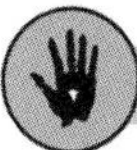

PRACTICAL APPLICATION

We can use smell therapies, such as aromatherapy, deliberately to influence our physiology and moods. Scents used as the trigger for conditioned learning can be helpful in establishing a method of reaching a more desirable state of homeostatic balance. Application involves connecting a smell to a particular state of consciousness, be it a relaxed state or a state of focused arousal. While the person is in the conscious state, he or she smells a chosen scent. If this is done consistently, the two become connected in the body. Eventually the smell alone elicits the state of consciousness. This type of conditioned behavior is beneficial for managing pain and anxiety. With conditioning, one can use a pleasant scent to trigger responses such as reduced pain or increased activity. The scent lavender has been shown to be calming. A person can carry drops of lavender or other pleasant aromas on a cotton ball and smell them as needed to support a calming affect. ■

PATHOLOGIC CONDITIONS OF THE PERIPHERAL NERVOUS SYSTEM

Entrapment and Compression

Technically, entrapment and compression are different. Entrapment results when soft tissue (e.g., muscles and ligaments) exerts inappropriate pressure on nerves; compression occurs when hard tissue (e.g., bone) exerts inappropriate pressure on nerves. Regardless of what is impinging (pressing) on the nerve, the symptoms are similar; however, the therapeutic intervention is different. Soft tissue approaches are beneficial in entrapment but are less so with compression.

Tissues that can bind and impinge on nerves are the skin, fasciae, muscles, ligaments, and bones. Shortened muscles and connective tissue (fasciae) often impinge on major and minor nerves, causing discomfort. Because of the structural arrangement of the body, these impingements often occur at major nerve plexuses. The specific nerve root, trunk, or division affected determines the condition, producing disorders such as thoracic outlet syndrome, sciatica, and carpal tunnel syndrome.

If the *cervical plexus* is impinged, the person most likely will have headaches, neck pain, and breathing difficulties. The muscles most responsible for pressure on the cervical plexus are the suboccipital and sternocleidomastoid muscles. Shortened connective tissue at the cranial base also presses on these nerves. The cervical plexus is formed by the ventral rami of the upper four cervical nerves. The phrenic nerve is part of this plexus and innervates the diaphragm. Any disruption to this nerve affects breathing. Many cutaneous (skin) branches of the cervical plexus transmit sensory impulses from the skin of the neck, ear area, and shoulder. The motor branches innervate muscles of the anterior neck. Impingement causes pain in these areas.

The *brachial plexus* is situated partly in the neck and partly in the axilla and consists of virtually all the nerves that innervate the upper limb. Any imbalance that increases pressure on this complex of nerves can result in pain in the shoulder, chest, arm, wrist, and hand. The muscles most often responsible for impingement on the brachial plexus are the scalenes, pectoralis minor, and subclavius muscles. The muscles of the arm also occasionally impinge on branches of the brachial plexus. Brachial plexus impingement is responsible for *thoracic outlet symptoms,* which often are misdiagnosed as carpal tunnel syndrome. Whiplash injury often causes impingement on the brachial plexus.

Carpal tunnel syndrome is caused by compression of the median nerve as it passes under the transverse carpal ligament at the palmar aspect of the wrist. The condition often occurs in postmenopausal women but also occurs in conditions in which fluid retention causes swelling of the hand and wrist. The syndrome is common in workers who use their hands in repetitive movements, usually because of inflammation that results in compression on the nerve. The symptoms are palmar pain and numbness in the first three digits. Sometimes surgically opening the transverse carpal ligament can help relieve the pain.

Impingment on the *lumbar plexus* gives rise to low back discomfort, which is marked by a beltlike distribution of pain and pain in the lower abdomen, genitals, thigh, and medial lower leg. The main muscles that impinge on the lumbar plexus are the quadratus lumborum and the psoas muscles. Shortening of the lumbar dorsal fascia exaggerates a lordosis and can cause vertebral impingement on the lumbar plexus.

The *sacral plexus* has about a dozen named branches. About half of these serve the buttock and lower limb; the others innervate pelvic structures. The main branch is the sciatic nerve. Impingement on this nerve by the piriformis muscle gives rise to *sciatica.* Shortened ligaments that stabilize the sacroiliac joint can affect the sacral plexus. Pressure on the sacral plexus can cause pain in the gluteal muscles, leg, genitals, and foot.

INDICATIONS/CONTRAINDICATIONS

For Therapeutic Massage

Various forms of massage reduce muscle spasm, lengthen shortened muscles, and soften and stretch connective tissue, restoring a more normal space around the nerve and alleviating impingement. When massage is combined with other appropriate methods, surgery is seldom necessary. If surgery is performed, the practitioner must manage adhesions appropriately to prevent reentrapment of the nerve in the future by maintaining soft tissue suppleness around the healing surgical area and, as healing progresses, extending the therapeutic massage to deal with the forming scar more directly. Before doing any work near the site of a recent incision, the practitioner must obtain the physician's approval. In general, work close to the surgical area can begin after the stitches have been removed and all inflammation abates. Direct work on a new scar usually is safe 8 to 12 weeks into healing. ■

Nerve Root Compression

Many different conditions can result in compression of the nerve root, including tumors, subluxation of vertebrae, and muscle spasms (entrapment) and shortening. Disk degeneration is a common cause. As the degeneration progresses and the fluid content of the disk decreases, the disk becomes narrower. As a result, the amount of space between vertebrae declines. Because spinal nerves exit and enter in the spaces between the vertebrae, this situation increases the likelihood of nerve root compression. The condition most commonly occurs in the areas where the spine moves the most: C6 to C7, T12 to L1, L3 to L4, and L5 to S1 (*C*, cervical; *T*, thoracic; *L*, lumbar; *S*, sacral). The result is radiating nerve pain, often associated with protective and stabilizing muscle spasm or weakness or both.

Disk Herniation

Disk herniation occurs when the fibrocartilage surrounding the intervertebral disk ruptures, releasing the nucleus pulposus, which cushions the vertebrae above and below. The resultant pressure on spinal nerve roots may cause pain and damage the surrounding nerves. This condition most often occurs in the lumbar region and involves the L4 or L5 disk and L5 or S1 nerve roots. This particular back pain radiates from the gluteal area down the lateral side or back of the thigh to the leg or foot. Back strain or injury often causes disk herniation, but occasionally coughing and sneezing may precipitate the condition.

The symptoms of herniation are similar to those produced by a compressed disk but often are more severe. In extreme cases, surgical intervention may be necessary; however, more conservative measures usually are attempted first. Conservative treatment consists of rest, exercise, and other methods, including massage to reduce spasm. Traction can be beneficial.

INDICATIONS/CONTRAINDICATIONS

For Therapeutic Massage

Various forms of massage are important for managing the muscle spasm and pain associated with the aforementioned conditions. The student must remember that the muscle spasms serve a stabilizing and protective function called guarding. Without some protective spasm, the nerve could be damaged further, but too much muscle spasm increases the discomfort. Therapeutic intervention seeks to reduce pain and excessive tension and restore moderate mobility while allowing for the resourceful compensation produced by the muscle tension pattern. Because low back pain is a common disorder, the massage practitioner must be familiar with its causes and treatment protocols. ■

Bell's Palsy

Bell's palsy causes partial or total paralysis of the facial muscles on one side as the result of inflammation or injury to the seventh cranial nerve. The exact cause of the inflammation is unknown, but current research suggests a reactivation of the herpes simplex virus as one of the probable causes. Mechanical causes include bone spurs, tumors, or temporomandibular joint disorders. Bell's palsy also occurs in persons affected by diabetes and Lyme disease. The facial nerve swells and is compressed in its narrow course through the temporal bone. The primary method of treatment is oral administration of steroids. The condition usually resolves and normal functioning returns within 6 weeks.

Guillain-Barré Syndrome

Guillain-Barré syndrome, or infectious polyneuritis, may occur 1 or 2 months after a viral infection. Lymphocytes and macrophages invade the myelin sheath, causing partial demyelination. The person develops tingling in the hands or feet, and motor weakness, and a decrease in deep tendon reflexes (DTRs); mild sensory loss ensues. Paralysis usually begins in the legs and moves upward. Facial weakness is common and may appear as Bell's palsy. Sometimes respiratory support must be given. Most individuals recover in a few weeks.

Herpes

Herpes zoster, or shingles, is a self-limiting viral disease in which groups of vesicles (fluid-filled blisters) appear along a cutaneous nerve distribution, usually on one side of the trunk. Pain occurs before the rash is visible. The varicella-zoster virus, a member of the Herpesviridae family, is the same virus that causes chickenpox. Some researchers believe that after infection, the virus remains in the body in an inactive state in dorsal root ganglia. Primary treatment consists of administration of an analgesic and the antiviral medication acyclovir (Zovirax).

The herpes simplex virus, which is categorized as type 1 or type 2, causes contagious, chronic viral infections that produce painful, fluid-filled blisters on the skin and mucous membranes. Outbreaks seem to be related to stress. Acyclovir can control the symptoms and accelerate healing but does not destroy the virus or cure the infection. Herpesvirus lies dormant in the nerve between outbreaks.

INDICATIONS/CONTRAINDICATIONS

For Therapeutic Massage

Massage approaches for infectious disease can be supportive and can reduce stress. Massage can help control the number of recurrent outbreaks by managing stress, especially in recurring viral conditions. The practitioner must follow universal precautions with any contagious disease. The patient's total stress load is an important factor. When a person is immunocompromised to the extent that he or she is susceptible to viral and bacterial disease, the stress load is greater. The practitioner should keep in mind that many forms of massage produce stress in a therapeutic sense. One must gauge the intensity and duration of any therapeutic intervention so that the demand on the body to adapt does not overtax an already stressed system, aggravating the condition. The less-is-more philosophy of intervention, which calls for shorter, more frequent interventions, often is indicated. ■

Demyelination Disease

Multiple sclerosis is a disease of autoimmune or viral cause (or both) in which myelin degenerates in random areas of the central nervous system. Hard, plaquelike lesions replace the destroyed myelin, and inflammatory cells invade affected areas. The myelin around the axons is lost, impairing nerve conduction, and weakness, diminished coordination, gait difficulties, incontinence, vision problems, and speech disturbances occur. Multiple sclerosis is a chronic condition with periodic remissions, because the axon is preserved even though the myelin degenerates. Relapse shows some indication of the condition being responsive to stress. One should not confuse multiple sclerosis with amyotrophic lateral sclerosis, which involves degeneration of motor neurons.

Myasthenia Gravis

Myasthenia gravis is a disorder of neuromuscular transmission that usually affects muscles in the face, lips, tongue, neck, and throat, which are innervated by the cranial nerves, but the condition can affect any muscle group. Eventually, muscle fibers may degenerate, and weakness, especially of the head, neck, trunk, and limb muscles, may become irreversible. When the disease involves the respiratory system, it may be life-threatening.

The disease follows an unpredictable course with periodic exacerbations and remissions. Spontaneous remissions occur in about 25% of patients. No cure exists, but thanks to drug therapy, patients may lead relatively normal lives except during exacerbations.

The cause of myasthenia gravis is unknown. The condition commonly accompanies autoimmune and thyroid disorders. In fact, 15% of patients with myasthenia gravis have thymoma.

INDICATIONS/CONTRAINDICATIONS

For Therapeutic Massage

Massage can be an effective part of a comprehensive, long-term care program. Stress management also is an important component of an overall care program for any chronic disease. Massage and other forms of bodywork can help manage secondary muscle tension caused by the alteration of posture and the use of equipment such as wheelchairs, braces, and crutches. As previously mentioned, because therapeutic massage produces some stress, the practitioner must gauge the intensity and duration of any therapeutic intervention so as not to aggravate the condition. ■

Neurotransmitter-Based Disorders

Depression

Depression is one of the more common causes of physical complaints that are a manifestation of underlying psychiatric illness. Many forms of depression respond to medications that increase norepinephrine, dopamine, or serotonin in certain synapses in particular areas of the brain. Imipramine (Tofranil), amitriptyline (Elavil), fluoxetine (Prozac), and phenelzine (Nardil) are examples of these types of medications. Although primarily considered a CNS disease, dysfunction can be linked to synaptic transmission as the peripheral nervous system delivers information to the CNS.

INDICATIONS/CONTRAINDICATIONS

For Therapeutic Massage

Massage has the effect of increasing the availability of the aforementioned neurotransmitters and as such can play an important part in the care program for depression. Aerobic exercise is another important component in depression management. These methods use the peripheral nervous system as the point of access. ■

Anxiety States

Anxiety states are classified into two basic types. The first type, endogenous anxiety, is a biochemical phenomenon usually unrelated to environmental stimuli. Panic disorder, involving hyperventilation syndrome and other breathing difficulties, heart palpitations, chest pain, dizziness, sweating, and feelings of impending doom, is an example of this type. An increase in the activity of the neurotransmitters gamma-aminobutyric acid, epinephrine, and norepinephrine is implicated. The medications imipramine, monoamine oxidase inhibitors, and alprazolam have proved moderately effective in treating panic disorder.

Breathing pattern disorder may be an underlying factor in anxiety, resulting in a change in body chemistry that alters the feedback loop mechanisms. Restrictions in the soft tissue or the bony structures of the thorax may interfere with appropriate breathing, predisposing a person to breathing in excess of physical need. Massage can be effective in restoring more balanced function and supporting appropriate breathing. Thus breathing restraint may be an important factor in managing anxiety. Chapter 12 presents additional information on hyperventilation syndrome.

The second basic anxiety type is reactive, or exogenous, anxiety, which is prompted by anxiety-provoking stimuli such as specific events, situations, relationships, or conflicts. Management of this type of anxiety requires dealing with the precipitating difficulties directly or improving mechanisms and skills for coping with environmental or social problems. Making changes in the stressful situation, resolving smoldering conflicts, using relaxation methods, and cognitive restructuring of the client's views of the situation are helpful. Professional counseling often is beneficial. Other helpful measures include avoiding caffeine, exercising regularly, eating a healthful diet, and generally gaining control of those things we can control ourselves. Diazepam-type medications such as Valium are useful in short-term management of this type of anxiety.

Both types of anxiety can be thought of as activation of the sympathetic autonomic nervous system. With endogenous anxiety, a faulty internal feedback system results in panic. With exogenous anxiety, the tendency for responding with fight-or-flight behavior is present, but some sort of inhibition of those feelings is in place. What occurs is a fight-or-flight response without the appropriate expression; it therefore internalizes as anxiety.

INDICATIONS CONTRAINDICATIONS

For Therapeutic Massage

Massage and exercise are often effective as part of a comprehensive management strategy dealing with anxiety symptoms. ■

Neuropathy

Neuropathy is the inflammation or degeneration of the peripheral nerves. *Neuralgia* is severe nerve pain caused by a variety of noninflammatory disorders of the nervous system. *Neuritis* is the inflammation of a nerve. Reflex sympathetic dystrophy is also called causalgia syndrome. The situation causes pain following soft tissue or bone injury that does not follow a normal healing course. Instead, pain continues after the healing process is complete for no known reason.

Ketoacidosis and hypoglycemic reaction of diabetes cause diabetic neuropathy because they affect the myelin covering of the neuron. The condition is a painful and severe complication of diabetes for which effective control measures are limited. One such pain-control measure is hyperstimulation analgesia, which interrupts the pain for a short period.

Trigeminal neuralgia (tic douloureux) causes sudden, severe pain in the jaw area on one side of the face. Often the pain is caused by chewing or simply by touching the face. The cause is unknown. One hypothesis is that the condition is related to a viral infection of the upper portion of the trigeminal nerve. The analgesic carbamazepine (Tegretol) can be effective in some cases, although surgical intervention sometimes is necessary. One should exercise extreme caution if any form of therapy is to be performed in this area.

INDICATIONS CONTRAINDICATIONS

For Therapeutic Massage

Nerve pain is difficult to manage, does not respond well to analgesics, and often is intractable. Massage, because of its interface with the nervous system, may provide short-term, symptomatic pain relief through shifts in neurotransmitters and stimulation of alternate nerve pathways, resulting in hyperstimulation analgesia and counterirritation. Any therapy that increases mood-elevating and pain-modulating mechanisms makes coping with nerve pain somewhat easier for short periods. ■

Polio

Polio is a viral infection first of the intestines and then (for about 1% of exposed persons) the anterior horn cells of the spinal cord. The destruction of CNS motor neurons leads to degeneration, atrophy, and finally paralysis of skeletal muscles.

INDICATIONS CONTRAINDICATIONS

For Therapeutic Massage

Massage is beneficial for postacute polio syndrome but only under a doctor's supervision. ■

Headache

Headache is a common symptom with a multitude of causes. Because the brain has no sensory innervation, headaches do not originate in the brain. The pain of a headache is produced by pressure on the sensory nerves, vessels, meninges, or the muscle-tendon-bone unit.

A tension or muscle contraction headache is the most common type. Tension headaches are believed to be caused by a muscle-tendon strain at the origin of the trapezius and deep neck muscles at the occipital bone or at the origin of the frontalis muscle on the frontal bone (occipital or frontal headaches). Tension headache also can originate in the temporomandibular joint muscle complex. Connective tissue structures that support the head may be implicated in headache if they are shortened and pull the head into nerves, creating pain. Conversely, if connective tissue support structures are lax and fail to support the neck and head, nerve structures may be compressed as well.

The treatment for most headaches is nonsteroidal antiinflammatory drugs such as aspirin or ibuprofen.

Indications/Contraindications

For Therapeutic Massage

Massage and other forms of soft tissue therapy are effective in treating muscle tension headaches. Because stress often induces headaches, stress management in all forms usually is indicated in chronic headache conditions. ■

Vertigo

Vertigo is the sensation that the body or environment is spinning or swaying and can occur when disturbances occur in the inner ear balance mechanism or between the visual-vestibular balance mechanisms. The most common type of vertigo is called benign paroxysmal positional vertigo. This condition occurs when otolith particles stimulate movement sensations that do not actually exist. Muscle tension, nausea, and mood disturbances, particularly anxiety, can result.

Indications/Contraindications

For Therapeutic Massage

Movement therapies can help or aggravate vertigo; therefore one must take care to design an individual therapeutic program based on the client's history. Massage methods can deal effectively with muscle tension and diminish anxiety and nausea, but the benefit is temporary because the symptoms return with a recurrence of vertigo. ■

Summary

Understanding how the peripheral nervous system works specifically influences the massage practitioner's ability to plan and arrange an effective massage session. Massage applications and outcomes experienced by the client from the massage session depend on the practitioner's knowledge of the physiologic effects of the massage manipulations and techniques. Understanding normal function and pathology of the peripheral nervous system helps the massage professional make good decisions regarding indications and contraindications for massage.

In this chapter, we studied the peripheral nervous system, its components, and the names of its many parts. We presented important information about reflexes and sensory receptors because these portions of the peripheral nervous system function directly with massage.

We reinforced the role of the autonomic nervous system, the body/mind connection, and the perspectives of Eastern and Western thought as well.

We discussed four of the five basic senses briefly and related massage to specific functions of the peripheral nervous system. A student of massage would do well to learn this particular material thoroughly, because massage therapy works closely with the peripheral nervous system. Such an understanding can only benefit the clients we strive to serve.

evolve

Log on to your student EVOLVE account, and complete the labeling activities for the various parts of the peripheral nervous system. Click on the links to review your answers. Feel free to print out the labeling activity to complete for further review when you are not at your computer.

WORKBOOK SECTION

SHORT ANSWER

1. Define the peripheral nervous system.

2. List the components of the peripheral nervous system.

3. List the cranial nerves and describe the general function of each.

4. List and describe the spinal nerves.

5. Identify the four nerve plexuses.

6. Compare and contrast a dermatome and a myotome.

7. Explain reflex mechanisms and sensory receptor reflex arcs and their relationship to therapeutic massage and movement therapies.

8. Identify the two divisions of the autonomic nervous system.

9. List and compare the functions of the sympathetic and parasympathetic nervous systems.

10. List the major drugs that affect the autonomic nervous system.

11. Describe the Eastern/Western connection as it relates to autonomic nervous system functions.

12. Describe the four basic senses discussed in this chapter.

13. List at least 12 of the various pathologic conditions of the peripheral nervous system.

1.
2.
3.
4.
5.
6.
7.
8.
9.
10.
11.
12.

14. Explain the way therapeutic massage supports health in the peripheral nervous system.

FILL IN THE BLANK

The (1) Peripheral nervous system consists of neurons outside the central nervous system. The (2) afferent (sensory) division consists of nerves that link sensory receptors with the CNS. The efferent, or (3) motor, division consists of nerves that link the CNS to the effectors outside the CNS. The (4) somatic nervous system is made up of nerves that act to keep the body in balance with its external environment by transmitting impulses between the CNS and the skeletal muscles and skin. The (5) autonamic nervous system connects the CNS to the glands, heart, and smooth muscles to maintain the (6) internal body environment. The (7) sympathetic nervous system functions when the body is under stress, producing fight-or-flight responses. The (8) parasympathic nervous system functions under normal body conditions and is the energy conservation and restorative system, associated with what commonly is called the (9) relaxation response.

A nerve is a group of (10) pheripheral nerve fibers, or axons, wrapped together. Twelve pairs of (11) cranial nerves originate from the olfactory bulbs, thalamus, visual cortex, and brainstem. Thirty-one pairs of (12) spinal nerves originate in the spinal cord and emerge from the vertebral column. (13) Mixed nerves make sensation and movement possible.

WORKBOOK SECTION

Workbook Section • Workbook Section • Workbook Section • Workbook Section • Workbook Section • Workbo

A (14) plexus is a network of intertwining nerves that innervates a particular region of the body. The four nerve plexuses are the (15) cranial plexus, the (16) brachial plexus, the (17) Lumbar plexus, and the (18) Sacral plexus.

A (19) dermatome is a cutaneous (skin) section supplied by a single spinal nerve. A (20) myotome is a skeletal muscle or group of muscles that receives motor axons from a given spinal nerve. (21) Mechanical receptors are sensory receptors that detect changes in pressure, movement, or temperature or other mechanical forces.

(22) Thermal receptors are sensory receptors that detect changes in temperature. (23) Nociceptors are sensory receptors that detect painful stimuli. (24) Proprioceptors are sensory receptors that provide the body with information about position, movement, muscle tension, joint activity, and equilibrium.

A reflex in the physiologic or functional unit of nerve function is a (an) (25) involuntary action. The (26) stretch reflex results when stretching of a muscle elicits a protective contraction of that same muscle. The tendon reflex operates as a feedback mechanism to control muscle (27) tension by causing muscle relaxation. The flexor (withdrawal) and crossed extensor reflexes are (28) polysynaptic reflex arcs. When these reflexes are stimulated, an entire area on one side of the body (29) (withdrawal reflex) or specific areas on both sides of the body (30) (crossed extensor reflex) are affected.

The four basic senses discussed are (31) taste, (32) smell, (33) hearing, and (34), vision.

PROBLEM SOLVING

Read the problem presented. There is no correct answer; rather the exercise is intended to assist the student in developing the analytic and decision-making skills necessary in a professional practice. After reading the problem, follow the next six steps:

1. Identify the facts presented in the information.
2. Identify the possibilities presented ("what if" statements) or develop your own possibilities.
3. Evaluate each possibility in terms of the logical cause and effect and pros and cons.
4. Consider the effect on the persons involved.
5. Write each answer in the space provided.
6. Develop your solution by answering the question posed.

Problem

Most soft tissue and movement therapies are beneficial because of a direct interaction with the peripheral nervous system. The sensory mechanisms of the peripheral nervous system are the communication link with the rest of the systems and functions of the body. Research is demonstrating the beneficial effects of these therapies on the somatic nervous system, primarily through reflex arcs and dermatome and myotome patterns, coupled with the interaction with the autonomic nervous system. Some difficulty may arise because various approaches have emerged within therapeutic massage and movement therapy based on specific protocols developed by gifted practitioners and teachers over the course of centuries. At the time the particular approach developed, science may not yet have been able to identify the underlying physiology. Consequently, many forms of therapeutic massage and movement therapy have developed along individual paths, and they work for the same physiologic reasons. This does not discount the uniqueness and value of any one particular approach. However, confusion results with many different methods working through the same basic anatomy and physiology with slight variations in style and different terminology bases. Professionals in therapeutic massage and movement therapies often may not realize that they are talking about the same thing. If we have some difficulty understanding each other, then how much more confusing is it for professionals outside the touch and movement therapy discipline? Explaining treatment methods in terms of anatomy and physiology may help, because this language base is understood more universally. Such an effort could give rise to an agreement and understanding of the overlap of methods, especially in terms of the peripheral nervous system interaction.

WORKBOOK SECTION

Question

How would you explain the benefit of therapeutic massage and movement therapy in terms of the peripheral nervous system? Examples are provided to get you started. Fill in at least two more statements.

Facts

1. Touch and movement therapies are not always explained in terms of anatomy and physiology.
2. ______________________________
3. ______________________________

Possibilities

1. Professionals may not be able to share information effectively.
2. ______________________________
3. ______________________________

Logical Cause and Effect

1. Appropriate referral between professionals would not happen for lack of information.
2. ______________________________
3. ______________________________

Effect

1. Professionals may feel frustrated when they discover that they were talking about the same thing all along.
2. ______________________________
3. ______________________________

How would you explain the benefit of touch and movement therapies in terms of the peripheral nervous system?

FURTHER STUDY

Using additional resource material (see the Works Consulted list at the back of this book), identify chapters that pertain to the information presented in this chapter. Locate the information presented in this text and then elaborate on it by writing a paragraph of additional information on each of the following topics.

Nerve distribution patterns for the four nerve plexuses

Reflex mechanisms

Autonomic nervous system and the body/mind influence

Taste

Smell

Hearing

Vision

PROFESSIONAL APPLICATION

Groups of individuals with a common need or interest sometimes are referred to as populations. When one considers touch and movement therapies, certain populations need different types of approaches. Working with an athlete on balancing reflex patterns is somewhat different from working with a person who has cerebral palsy who wants a similar outcome. Nerve entrapment in the elderly is common, but this condition also is common in repetitive work environments. Interaction with anxious clients is different from interaction with someone who is depressed, even though therapeutic intervention focuses on the autonomic nervous system. The approaches are similar, yet different. Identify a pathologic condition listed in this chapter and develop two hypothetical treatment plans for the condition with two different populations. After you have done this, identify the differences and similarities in theories and the practical applications of the methods.

Answer Key

SHORT ANSWER

1. The peripheral nervous system is made up of neurons outside the central nervous system.
2. Nerves are peripheral nerve fibers or axons wrapped together. They include afferent or sensory nerves, efferent or motor nerves, and the somatic and autonomic nervous system.
3. Cranial nerve I: The olfactory nerves are sensory and transmit taste and smell information directly to the cerebrum.
   Cranial nerve II: The optic nerves are sensory and transmit visual information (e.g., visual acuity, pupillary reaction, and visual fields) to the thalamus.
   Cranial nerve III: The oculomotor nerves are sensory and motor nerves; they originate in the midbrain and transmit information about eye movement.
   Cranial nerve IV: The trochlear nerves arise in the midbrain and are composed primarily of motor nerves that contain few sensory neurons. These nerves innervate the muscles of the eyeball.
   Cranial nerve V: The trigeminal nerves arise in the pons and contain sensory neurons for the head, face, skin of the face, and corneas; they also contain motor neurons for mastication (chewing).
   Cranial nerve VI: The abducens nerves arise in the pons and contain numerous motor neurons that innervate eye muscles; they also have sensory neurons that provide information about eye movement.
   Cranial nerve VII: The facial nerves arise in the pons and contain sensory neurons for taste and motor neurons for facial expression, tear production, and salivation.
   Cranial nerve VIII: The vestibulocochlear (acoustic or auditory) nerves arise in the pons and are sensory nerves for hearing and equilibrium.
   Cranial nerve IX: The glossopharyngeal nerves arise in the medulla; they contain sensory neurons for taste and motor neurons for saliva production, swallowing, and the gag reflex.
   Cranial nerve X: The vagus nerves arise in the medulla, with some motor axons originating in the pons. They contain sensory neurons for the pharynx, larynx, trachea, heart, carotid body, lungs, bronchi, esophagus, stomach, small intestine, and gallbladder. Motor neurons carry impulses to the pharyngeal and laryngeal muscles, where they control swallowing and thoracic and abdominal viscera; they also carry impulses to the heart and other body organs, where they control the heart rate and other visceral activities. Most motor fibers of the vagus nerves are autonomic (parasympathetic) fibers.
   Cranial nerve XI: The accessory nerves arise in the medulla and contain mainly motor neurons for speaking, turning the head, and moving the shoulders (they supply the larynx, pharynx, trapezius muscles, and sternocleidomastoid muscles).
   Cranial nerve XII: The hypoglossal nerves arise in the medulla and contain mostly motor neurons, which innervate the tongue and throat.
4. Thirty-one pairs of mixed spinal nerves originate in the spinal cord and emerge from the vertebral column, making sensation and movement possible. Each spinal nerve attaches to the spinal cord by means of two short roots. The dorsal root is sensory, and the ventral root is motor.
5. The cervical plexus, brachial plexus, lumbar plexus, and sacral plexus; nerves T2 through T12 do not form a plexus
6. A dermatome is a cutaneous (skin) section supplied by a single spinal nerve. A myotome is a skeletal muscle or group of skeletal muscles that receives motor axons from a particular spinal nerve. The dermatomes and myotomes are distributions of spinal nerves; however, dermatomes relate to skin function, and myotomes relate to muscle function.
7. Input from sensory systems plays a role in the control of motor functions by stimulating spinal reflex mechanisms. Therapeutic massage and movement therapies introduce touch, pressure, vibration, and positional stimuli, causing sensory neurons to respond. Most benefits derived from movement therapies result from a resetting of reflex patterns that may be disrupted by a fall, trauma, repetitive movement, or fixed position. Because of the crossed extensor reflex, the limbs on one side of the body can be stimulated deliberately to affect the limbs on the opposite side. Reflex patterns are also responsible for many compensatory body patterns found in relation to posture. Therapeutic massage and movement therapies depend heavily on the reflex mechanism; the effectiveness of the techniques depends on how efficiently the receptors for these reflexes are stimulated. The practitioner must reach the target receptor with the appropriate technique and intensity so that the reflex stimulated can function in the appropriate manner. The practitioner must understand the type of message to be sent to the central nervous system for processing.
8. Sympathetic and parasympathetic
9. Sympathetic stimulation; neurotransmitter is usually norepinephrine; adrenergic
   Parasympathetic stimulation; neurotransmitter is acetylcholine; cholinergic
   Cardiovascular System
   Cardiac muscle
   Sympathetic: Increased rate and strength of contraction (beta-receptors)
   Parasympathetic: Decreased rate and strength of contraction
   Smooth muscle of blood vessels
   Sympathetic: Skin blood vessels—constriction (alpha-receptors)
   Parasympathetic: No effect
   Skeletal muscle blood vessels
   Sympathetic: Dilation (beta-receptors)
   Parasympathetic: No effect
   Abdominal blood vessels
   Sympathetic: Constriction (alpha-receptors)
   Parasympathetic: No effect
   Blood vessels of external genitals
   Sympathetic: Constriction (alpha-receptors)
   Parasympathetic: Dilation of blood vessels, causing erectile tissues to engorge

WORKBOOK SECTION

Smooth Muscle of Hollow Organs and Sphincters
Bronchioles
Sympathetic: Dilation (beta-receptors)
Parasympathetic: Constriction
Digestive tract (except sphincters)
Sympathetic: Decreased peristalsis (beta-receptors)
Parasympathetic: Increased peristalsis
Sphincters of digestive tract
Sympathetic: Constriction (alpha-receptors)
Parasympathetic: Relaxation
Urinary bladder
Sympathetic: Relaxation (beta-receptors)
Parasympathetic: Contraction
Urinary sphincters
Sympathetic: Constriction (alpha-receptors)
Parasympathetic: Relaxation
Eye
Iris
Sympathetic: Contraction of radial muscle; dilated pupil
Parasympathetic: Contraction of circular muscle; constricted pupil
Ciliary body
Sympathetic: Relaxation; accommodates for far vision
Parasympathetic: Contraction; accommodates for near vision
Glands
Sweat glands
Sympathetic: Increased sweat (neurotransmitter: acetylcholine)
Parasympathetic: No effect
Lacrimal glands
Sympathetic: No effect
Parasympathetic: Increased secretion of tears
Digestive (e.g., salivary and gastric)
Sympathetic: Decreased secretion of saliva and gastric secretions
Parasympathetic: Increased secretion of saliva
Pancreas (including islets)
Sympathetic: Decreased secretion
Parasympathetic: Increased secretion of pancreatic juice and insulin
Liver
Sympathetic: Increased glycogenolysis (conversion of glycogen to glucose) (beta-receptors); increased blood sugar level
Parasympathetic: No effect
Adrenal medulla
Sympathetic: Increased epinephrine secretion
Parasympathetic: No effect
Hairs (Pilomotor Muscles)
Sympathetic: Contraction produces goose pimples, or piloerection (alpha-receptors)
Parasympathetic: No effect

10. Epinephrine is a beta-1- and beta-2-agonist; examples are metaproterenol (Metaprel, Alupent), pirbuterol (Maxair), and albuterol (Ventolin). Beta-blocking agents such as propranolol (Inderal), metoprolol (Lopressor), and nadolol (Corgard) are useful for treating cardiac arrhythmias, angina, and hypertension. Opiates have a sympathetic effect (sympathomimetic action) on the gastrointestinal tract and cause constipation.
11. Autonomic parasympathetic ganglia tend to occupy the same areas traditionally identified as chakras, or energy centers. The sympathetic chain ganglia follow one of the paths of the bladder meridian.
    Point holding, such as acupressure, reflexology, or dry needling of acupuncture, releases the body's own pain killers and mood-altering chemicals from the entire endorphin class. These chemicals stimulate the parasympathetic responses of relaxation and contentment. Acupressure is a specific pinpoint compression over motor points of the body at the focal meeting of superficial nerves in the sagittal plane, superficial nerves or plexuses, and the muscle-tendon junction at the Golgi tendons. These areas where nerves are close to the surface of the body correspond to the traditional acupuncture points. Acupressure produces sympathetic inhibition. Acupuncture probably works by taking advantage of the natural inhibitory influences of the body that normally block pain pathways. Research over the past 20 years has identified the crucial role the autonomic nervous system plays in stress-related disorders. This research has validated ancient healing, cultural, and spiritual practices that bring the autonomic nervous system under voluntary control and as such bring conscious control to homeostatic processes.
12. Taste: The four primary taste sensations are sweet, sour, salty, and bitter. Most chemical receptors for the sense of taste are located on the tongue; a few are located in the cheeks and on the floor of the mouth.
    Smell: Also called olfaction, this sense relies on chemical receptors located in the roof of the nasal cavity. Smell centers are interconnected with the limbic system and therefore have emotional and behavioral implications.
    Hearing: The ear is a complex of three structures, all of which are necessary to effect the process of hearing.
    Vision: The eyes, the organs of vision, are contained within protective bony cavities of the skull called orbits. The eye perceives light in the form of colors ranging from violet to red. Six small muscles attached to each eye effect movement.
13. Nerve root compression, disk herniation, Bell's palsy, Guillain-Barré syndrome (infectious polyneuritis), herpes zoster (shingles), herpes type 1 and 2, multiple sclerosis, depression, anxiety, entrapment and compression, neuropathy, trigeminal neuralgia (tic douloureux), headache from muscle tension, and vertigo
14. All bodywork methods are based on the peripheral nervous system. The effects on the autonomic nervous system relate directly to stress, as do the effects on the somatic nervous system function of posture and movement. By encouraging balance in this system, the practitioner supports health.

Workbook Section

Fill in the Blank

1. peripheral nervous system
2. afferent
3. motor
4. somatic
5. autonomic
6. internal
7. sympathetic
8. parasympathetic
9. relaxation
10. peripheral
11. cranial nerves
12. spinal nerves
13. Mixed
14. plexus
15. cervical
16. brachial
17. lumbar
18. sacral
19. dermatome
20. myotome
21. Mechanical
22. Thermal
23. Nociceptors
24. Proprioceptors
25. involuntary
26. stretch
27. tension
28. polysynaptic
29. withdrawal reflex
30. crossed extensor reflex
31. taste
32. smell
33. hearing
34. vision

CHAPTER 6

Endocrine System

▼ CHAPTER OBJECTIVES

After completing this chapter, the student will be able to perform the following:

- List the traditional endocrine glands.
- Define endocrine tissues and give examples.
- Describe the functions of hormones.
- Explain the difference between hormones and neurotransmitters.
- Describe hypersecretion and hyposecretion pathologic conditions of the endocrine system.

▼ CHAPTER OUTLINE

▼ KEY TERMS

Endocrine gland (EN-doe-krin) A ductless gland that secretes hormones directly into the bloodstream.

Endorphins (en-DOR-finz) Peptide hormones that mainly work like morphine to suppress pain. They influence mood, producing a mild euphoric feeling such as is seen in runner's high.

Exocrine gland (EK-so-krin) A gland that secretes hormones through ducts directly into specific areas. Exocrine glands are part of the endocrine system.

Half-life The amount of time required for half of a hormone to be eliminated from the bloodstream.

Hypersecretion The excessive release of a hormone.

Hyposecretion The insufficient release of a hormone.

Negative feedback system A control mechanism that provides a stimulus to decrease a function, such as a fire alarm, that causes a series of reactions that work to reduce the fire.

Tropic (or trophic) hormones Hormones produced by the endocrine glands that affect other endocrine glands.

The endocrine system works in partnership with the nervous system to maintain homeostasis in the body. In this capacity the endocrine system is involved primarily with physiologic function. Functional aspects of hormone molecules include the mobilization of body defenses against stressors; maintenance of electrolyte, water, and nutrient balance of the blood; and regulation of cellular metabolism and energy balance. Not only are hormones of the endocrine system involved with maintaining homeostasis, but also they direct the creation of our very form (such as our size, shape, and sexual characteristics). The major form processes controlled and integrated by hormones are reproduction, growth, and development. Therefore hormonal pathologic conditions affect function, as does the nervous system, and can also affect form.

The **endocrine glands** are ductless glands that secrete hormones directly into the bloodstream or diffuse into nearby tissues (Figure 6-1). In contrast, **exocrine glands**, or glands with ducts, such as salivary and sweat glands, secrete their products directly into ducts that open to specific areas.

The endocrine glands of the body include the pituitary, thyroid, parathyroid, adrenal, pineal, and thymus glands. In addition, several organs of the body such as the pancreas, ovaries, and testes contain areas of endocrine tissues that produce hormones and exocrine products. The hypothalamus, considered part of the nervous system, also produces and releases hormones and thus can be considered a neuroendocrine organ.

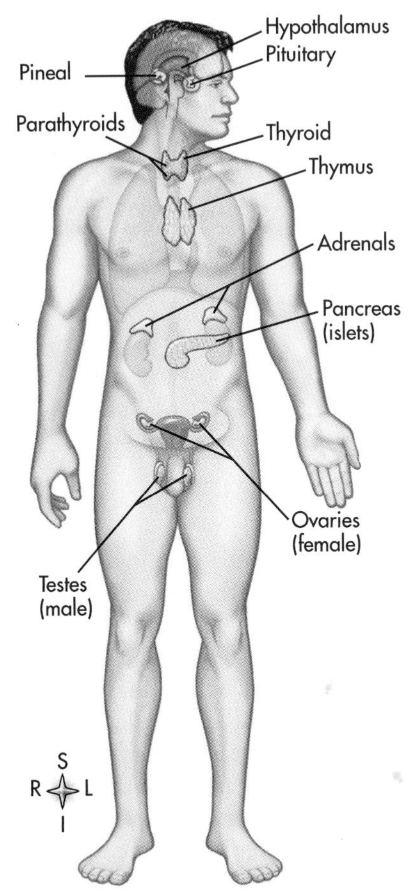

Figure 6-1
Locations of the major endocrine glands.

The endocrine glands have important implications in the *Eastern chakra system.* The chakra system is a mapping of energy centers with interesting anatomic correlations to the autonomic nervous system plexus and functional aspects interrelated with the endocrine gland functions. Many Eastern healing traditions (e.g., Ayurvedic and Tibetan) work from this knowledge base, just as many Asian healing philosophies were developed around the meridian system.

The body of knowledge of the chakra system is expansive and consistent with Western scientific thought. Just as the meridian system sees anatomy and physiology as an interrelated system encompassing emotional and spiritual energy conjoined with the major organs, the chakra system represents similar patterns in relationship to the endocrine functions. As we describe various endocrine functions, we also present the related chakra pattern (Leadbetter, 1927) (Figure 6-2).

New research in endocrinology continues to discover endocrine tissues that are separate from the traditional endocrine glands. The heart and intestinal mucous membranes are now known to secrete hormones. The concept of tissue hormones or hormonelike substances such as the prostaglandins has altered and expanded the idea of hormones being carried throughout the blood to distant sites in the body. Not only do prostaglandins have a local effect in surrounding tissue, but also because they are carried by blood, they affect distant sites in the body.

Endocrine functions typically are regulated by **negative feedback systems.** Pathologic conditions are found mainly with **hyposecretion** (not enough) and **hypersecretion** (too much). This pattern now should seem familiar as the elegance of the body shows itself in repetition of basic patterns (Figure 6-3).

In the previous chapters, we learned that a chemical found in the synapse is called a neurotransmitter. When the same chemical is found in the bloodstream or tissue, it is a hormone. Neurotransmitters act on adjacent cells, whereas hormones may travel long distances in the body before they reach their target cells. The main differences between the endocrine system and the nervous system control are speed and duration of effect. The nervous system is fast acting with a short duration of effect, whereas the endocrine system is slow acting with a long duration of effect. This offers a balance of control, with the nervous system responding quickly and the endocrine system taking over to sustain a response (Activity 6-1 on p. 182).

HORMONES

Hormones are derived from amino acids or steroids (Table 6-1 on p. 183). Hormones exert their effect on target organs and cells at low blood concentrations. The concentration of

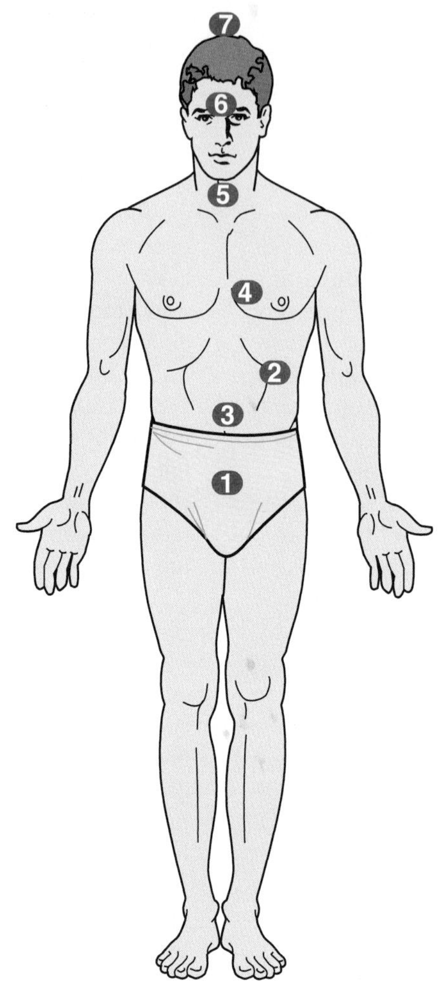

	English Name	Situation
1	Root or basic chakra	At the base of the spine
2	Spleen or splenic chakra	Over the spleen
3	Navel or umbilical chakra	At the navel, over the solar plexus
4	Heart or cardiac chakra	Over the heart
5	Throat or laryngeal chakra	At the front of the throat
6	Brow or frontal chakra	In the space between the eyebrows
7	Crown or coronal chakra	On the top of the head

Figure 6-2
Name and location of major chakras.

a hormone in the blood is determined by the rate of release and the speed of inactivation and removal from the body. The influence of a hormone in the blood can range from seconds to 30 minutes. The term ***half-life*** describes the time required for half of the hormone to be eliminated from the bloodstream. After this occurs, the effect is slowed. Hormones require various amounts of time to generate noticeable influences in the body or on behavior. Some hormones promote target organ responses almost immediately, such as the effect of epinephrine on the heart. In contrast, steroid hormones such as testosterone and estrogen may require hours or days for their effects to be seen. Endocrine glands release hormones in response to three types of stimuli. Some hormones are released when a shift occurs in the concentration of a specific substance in the body fluids, such as when the parathyroid gland responds to a rise and fall in calcium levels in the blood.

Other hormones are released when the larger endocrine gland receives instructions from another endocrine organ. For example, the ovaries secrete estrogen under the influence of **trophic hormones** from the pituitary. Some hormones are secreted when the nerves stimulate the gland, as when the adrenal gland releases adrenaline when stimulated by sympathetic nerves.

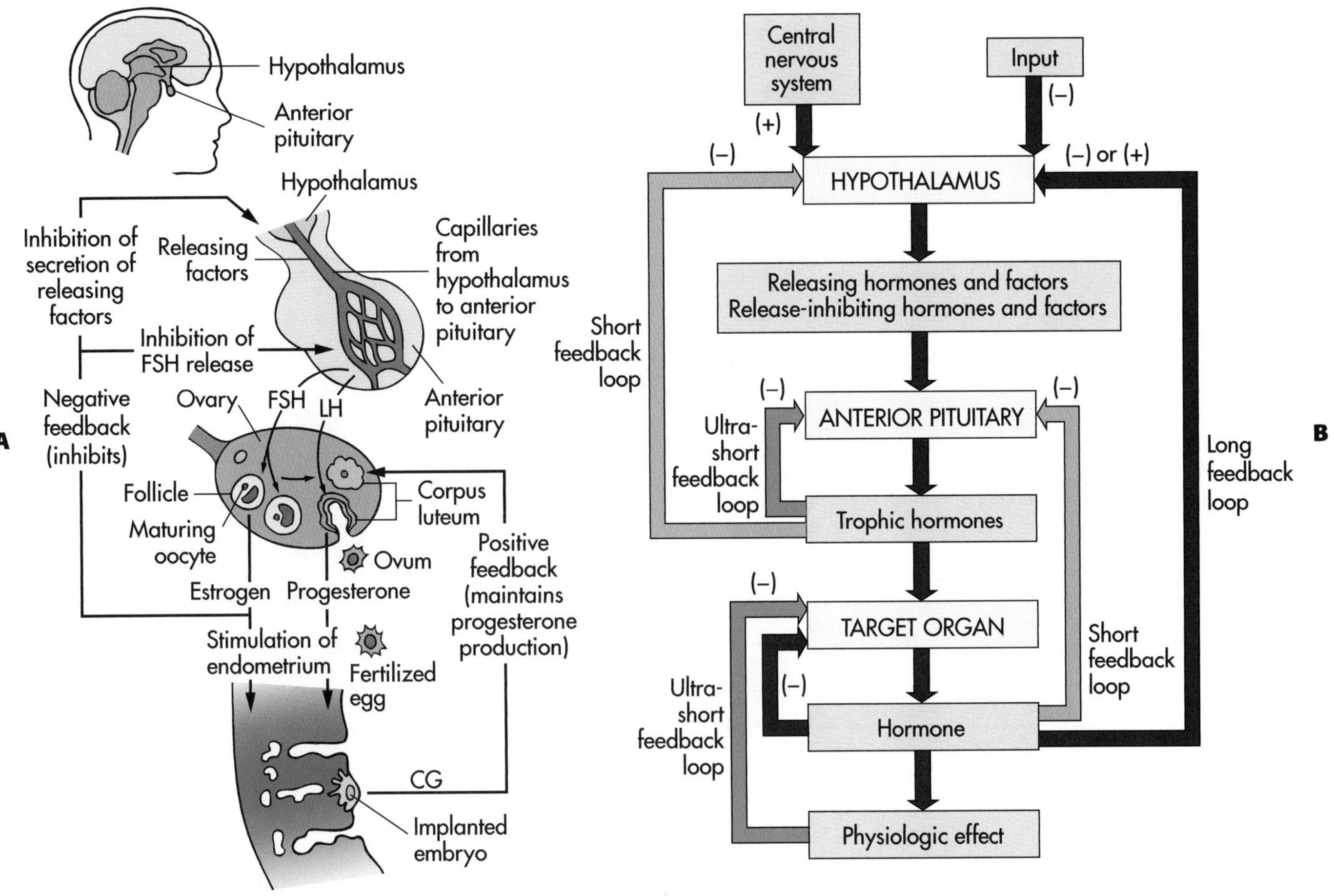

Figure 6-3
Feedback loops. **A**, Endocrine feedback loops involving the hypothalamus-pituitary gland and end organs (endocrine regulation). **B**, General model for control and negative feedback to hypothalamic-pituitary target organ systems. Negative-feedback regulation is possible at three levels: target organ (ultrashort feedback), anterior pituitary (short feedback), and hypothalamus (long feedback). (From McCance KL, Huether SE: *Pathophysiology: the biologic basis for disease in adults and children,* St Louis, 2002, Mosby.)

Endocrine glands and other specialized cells secrete hormones into the bloodstream to bind to specific receptors on or in their target cells. In a lock-and-key mechanism, hormones bind only to receptor molecules that "fit" them exactly. Any cell with one or more receptors for a particular hormone is said to be a target of that hormone. Cells usually have many different receptors, so they can be target cells for many different hormones (Figure 6-4). A new concept of the lock-and-key mechanism is that molecular chains that form the various hormones actually change shape as necessary to stimulate the cell receptors. This theory represents a more dynamic quantum view of neurohormonal function than the more static newtonian lock-and-key systems. As with most understanding, as knowledge evolves, the answer is most likely a combination of both ideas instead of an either/or pattern.

Each hormone-receptor interaction produces different regulatory changes within the target cell. Hormones bring about their characteristic effects on the normal cellular processes of target cells by increasing or decreasing the rate of those cell processes.

Even though the diffusion of a hormone is usually systemwide through the blood, the effects are more specific because of the specificity of the target cells in organs and tissues. Ancient healing practices speak often of internal communication mechanisms and identify the blood as an important life-giving force. Today, what science calls hormones seem representative of this ancient wisdom (Activity 6-2).

Primary Mechanisms of Endocrine Disease

Diseases of the endocrine system are numerous. They generally take the form of tumors or other abnormalities and frequently are caused when the glands secrete too much or too little of their hormones. Production of too much hormone by a diseased gland is called hypersecretion. If too

ACTIVITY 6-1

List three situations in which you believe that nervous system control is most effective and explain why. An example is given.

Example
While we are driving, a car stops suddenly in front of us. Normal reflexes activate our muscles to step on the brake. The quick response of the nervous system and short duration of response is sufficient to handle this situation.

1. ______________________________

____

____

2. ______________________________

____

____

3. ______________________________

____

____

List three situations in which you believe endocrine system control would be most effective and explain why. An example is given.

Example
Sledding in the cold for a couple of hours. The longer effect of hormones better supports the increase in heat production required to maintain body temperature.

1. ______________________________

____

____

2. ______________________________

____

____

3. ______________________________

____

____

little hormone is produced, the condition is called hyposecretion.

Hypersecretion

Any of several different mechanisms may be responsible for a given case of hypersecretion. Tumors are often responsible for an abnormal proliferation of endocrine cells and the resulting increase in hormone secretion. Another cause of hypersecretion is autoimmunity caused by the immune system functioning abnormally. Another possible cause of hypersecretion of a hormone is a failure of the feedback mechanisms that regulate secretion of a particular hormone.

Hyposecretion

Various mechanisms have been shown to cause hyposecretion of hormones. Although most tumors cause oversecretion of a hormone, they can cause a gland to undersecrete its hormone(s). Tissue death, caused by a blockage or failure of blood supply, also can cause a gland to reduce its hormonal output. Still another way in which a gland may reduce its secretion below normal levels is through abnormal operation of regulatory feedback loops. An example of this is hyposecretion of testosterone and gonadotropic hormones in men who abuse anabolic steroids. Men who take testosterone steroids increase their blood concentration of this hormone above set-point levels. The body responds to this high concentration by reducing its own output of testosterone and gonadotropins, which may lead to sterility and other complications.

Abnormalities of immune function also may cause hyposecretion. An autoimmune attack on glandular tissue sometimes has the effect of reducing hormone output. Some endocrinologists theorize that autoimmune destruction of pancreatic islet cells, perhaps in combination with viral and genetic mechanisms, is a culprit in many cases of diabetes mellitus (type I, insulin-dependent).

Recent research has shown many types of hyposecretion disorders to be caused by insensitivity of the target cells to pituitary tropic hormones rather than from actual hyposecretion. Tropic hormones target other endocrine glands, stimulate their growth, and promote their function (Activity 6-3).

Three Additional Types of Disorders of the Endocrine System

Some endocrine disorders are not caused by the glands themselves. The following are other possible causes of endocrine disorders:

1. Some cancers can produce hormonelike substances that cause endocrine syndromes.
2. An abnormal decrease in the number of hormone receptors on target cells can occur, thus blocking hormonal action.
3. Target cells may have abnormal metabolic responses to the hormone-receptor complex.

TABLE 6-1
Categories of Hormones

STRUCTURAL CATEGORY	EXAMPLES
Peptides	Growth hormone Insulin Parathyroid hormone Prolactin
Glycoproteins	Follicle-stimulating hormone Luteinizing hormone Thyroid-stimulating hormone
Polypeptides	Adrenocorticotropic hormone Antidiuretic hormone Calcitonin Endorphins Glucagon Hypothalamic hormones Lipotropins Melanocyte-stimulating hormone Oxytocin Somatostatin Thymosin Thyrotropin-releasing hormone
Amines	Epinephrine Norepinephrine Thyroxine (both thyroxine [T_4] and triiodothyronine [T_3])
Lipids Steroids (cholesterol is a precursor for all steroids)	Estrogens Glucocorticoids (cortisol) Mineralocorticoids (aldosterone) Progestins (progesterone) Testosterone
Derivatives of arachidonic acid	Leukotrienes Prostacyclins Prostaglandins Thromboxanes

Data from Seeley RR, Stephens TD, Tate P: *Anatomy & physiology,* ed 6, New York, 2003, McGraw-Hill.

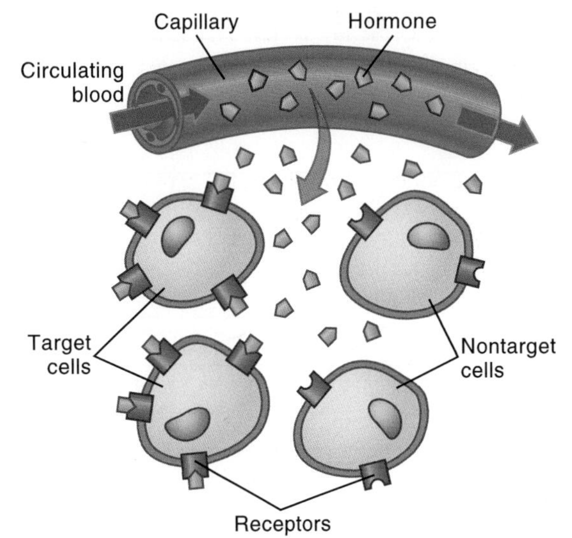

Figure 6-4
The target cell concept. A hormone acts only on cells that have receptors specific to that hormone because the shape of the receptor determines which hormones can react with it. This is an example of the lock-and-key model of biochemical reactions. (From Thibodeau GA, Patton KT: *Anatomy and physiology,* ed 5, St Louis, 2003, Mosby.)

ACTIVITY 6-2

Before we go any further in this chapter, do the following. In 1 minute, list as many physiologic processes influenced by hormones as you can. Come back at the end of the chapter and compare your before and after knowledge.

Example
Pregnancy

Your Turn

HYPOTHALAMUS

The hypothalamus is the link in the body/mind and nerve/endocrine function. The main purpose of the hypothalamus is homeostasis; for example, its effects on blood pressure, body temperature, and fluid and electrolyte balance. During stress, the hypothalamus translates nerve impulses into hormone secretions by endocrine glands. The hypothalamus exerts its primary influence over the pituitary gland, which in turn controls other endocrine glands with tropic hormones. The hypothalamus secretes releasing or inhibiting hormones that affect the secretion of pituitary hormones. Psychosocial dwarfism, failure-to-thrive syndrome, and delayed tissue healing, which result from stress, emotional disorders, and deprivation, result from suppression of the hypothalamic release of growth hormone-releasing hormone. This hormone signals the secretion of growth hormone from the pituitary gland (Table 6-2).

ACTIVITY 6-3

List three causes of hypersecretion.

1. ______________________________

2. ______________________________

3. ______________________________

List three causes of hyposecretion.

1. ______________________________

2. ______________________________

3. ______________________________

PRACTICAL APPLICATION

Therapeutic massage provides the hypothalamus with the stimulation needed to function efficiently, as if a touch hunger needs to be fed to maintain homeostasis. It is important for the body to be able to deal with its individual stress load systems. That is why stress management systems are so important. If we analyze ancient healing practices and spiritual wisdom made concrete through ritual practices, we easily can see similarities to current recommendations for stress management programs.

Because isolation is a recognized problem with many, even within social groups (lonely in a crowd?), many types of professionals are concerned about the quality of physical, emotional, and spiritual health for those without touch interactions. Psychosocial influences on hypothalamic function reflect the importance of resourceful contact with fellow human beings or loving pets. Even caring for plants has been shown to increase the sense of well-being for some. We seem to be preconditioned to need others to be healthy. On a professional level, practitioners using a primary modality of touch can offer important health-restoring interventions and act in a preventive mode for those at risk from touch deprivation (Activity 6-4). ■

ENDOCRINE GLANDS, TISSUES, AND HORMONES

Pituitary Gland

The pituitary gland, or hypophysis, is located in the head at about eye level (Figure 6-5). The gland hangs down from the hypothalamus and sits in the sella turcica, a recessed area in the sphenoid bone. About the size of a peanut, the pituitary gland has an anterior lobe and a posterior lobe. The posterior lobe is not a true endocrine gland because it only stores and releases hormones but does not synthesize them. According to tradition, the pituitary gland and its regulating counterpart the hypothalamus are related to the crown or brow chakra, with primary functions of integration of energetic patterns and realization of the total self.

The pituitary gland secretes hormones that regulate growth, fluid balance, lactation, and childbirth. The gland is the main source of tropic hormones, hormones that have a

TABLE 6-2
Hypothalamic Hormones (Hypophysiotropic Hormones)

HORMONE	TARGET TISSUE	ACTION
Thyrotropin-releasing hormone (TRH)	Anterior pituitary	Stimulates release of thyroid-stimulating hormone (TSH) Modulates prolactin secretion
Gonadotropin-releasing hormone (GnRH)	Anterior pituitary	Stimulates release of follicle-stimulating hormone (FSH) and luteinizing hormone (LH)
Somatostatin	Anterior pituitary Gastrointestinal tract	Inhibits release of growth hormone (GH) Decreases gastric motility, intestinal secretion, and secretion of TSH, parathyroid hormone, renin, glucagon, and insulin
Growth hormone-releasing factor (GRF)	Anterior pituitary	Stimulates release of GH
Corticotropin-releasing hormone (CRH)	Anterior pituitary	Stimulates release of adrenocorticotropic hormone (ACTH) and β-endorphin
Substance P	Anterior pituitary	Inhibits synthesis and release of ACTH Stimulates secretion of GH, FSH, LH, and prolactin
Prolactin-inhibiting factor (PIF; possibly dopamine)	Anterior pituitary	Inhibits secretion of prolactin
Prolactin-releasing hormone (PRH)	Anterior pituitary	Stimulates secretion of prolactin

From McCance KL, Huether SE: *Pathophysiology: the biologic basis for disease in adults and children*, ed 4, St Louis, 2002, Mosby.

ACTIVITY 6-4

First, identify a current stress management program and briefly describe the process. Then describe a ritual process with which you are familiar. Compare the two processes. Two examples are provided to get you started.

Example

1. Current stress management programs often use a combined method of sitting quietly and concentrating on the number 1 while repeating the word one slowly over and over.
   Ancient meditative practices used seated positions while chanting a mantra, sound, or phrase slowly over and over.

Comparison

Both use repetitive patterns and static positions to reduce stress responses.

2. Current practices of therapeutic massage use oil lubricants to rub the soft tissues of the body.
   Many ancient religious practices use anointing or rubbing with oil as part of a healing or purification ritual.

Comparison

Both use the application of oil and rubbing.

Your Turn

Current practice

Ancient practice

Comparison

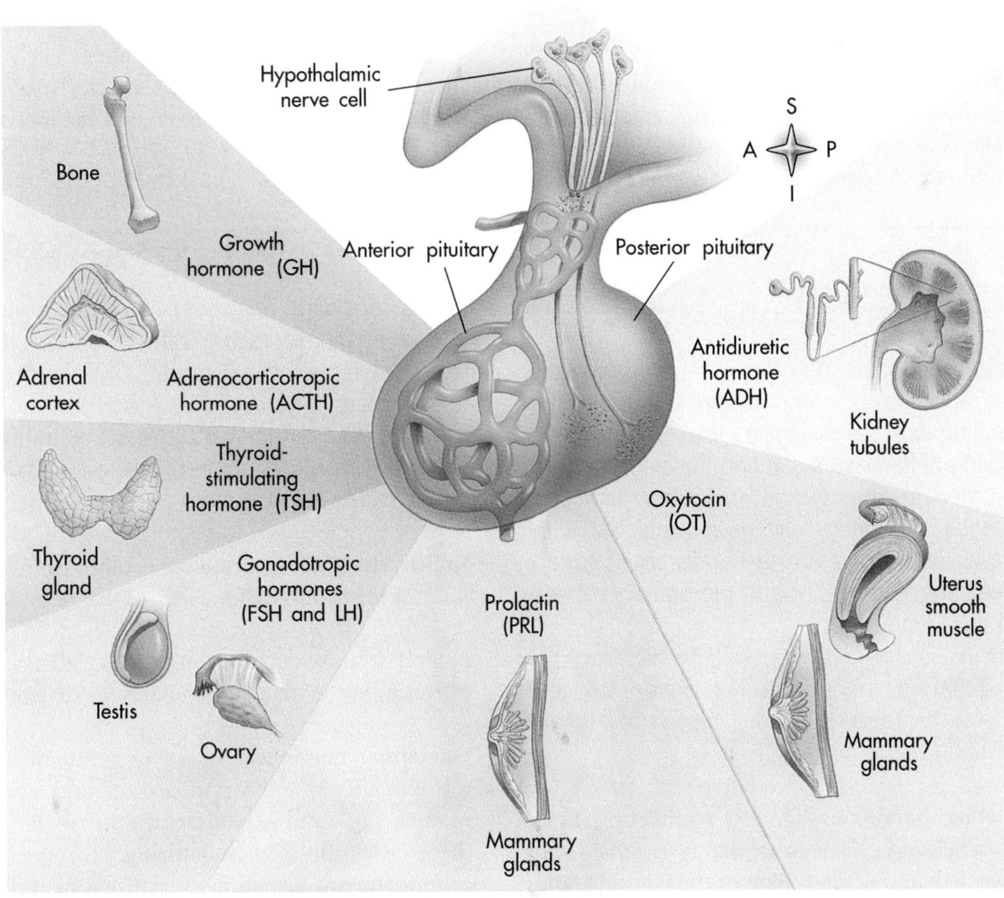

Figure 6-5
Anterior pituitary hormones and their target organs. (Modified from Thibodeau GA, Patton KT: *Anatomy and physiology,* ed 5, St. Louis, 2003, Mosby.)

stimulating effect on other endocrine glands. The hypothalamus regulates the pituitary gland through releasing and inhibiting hormones. The negative feedback mechanism affects the pituitary gland by acting on the hypothalamus. (A negative feedback system provides a stimulus to decrease a function.) The terms *primary* and *secondary* refer to target organ problems versus problems in other organs that affect the target gland. For example, primary hyperthyroidism means that the cause is in the thyroid gland. Secondary hyperthyroidism refers to the pituitary gland and its influence on the thyroid gland.

The larger anterior lobe secretes seven major hormones, and the posterior lobe secretes two major hormones.

Anterior Pituitary Hormones

Growth hormone or somatotropin. Growth hormone, or somatotropin, stimulates most body cells to increase in size and divide. The major target organs are bones and muscles. In the adult the response of growth hormone is the repair and rebuilding of tissues. Growth hormone follows a circadian cycle, with the highest levels occurring during evening sleep, primarily delta-level sleep. Growth hormone releases stored fat and raises blood glucose concentrations to provide us with energy. Growth hormone also is triggered for release during exercise and periods of hurt, tension, and stress. As we age, the total amount of growth hormone secreted declines.

Growth hormone release can be inhibited by emotional deprivation, excessive blood sugar, and high blood fat levels. Disruption in the sleep pattern interferes with growth hormone functions as well. Growth hormone disturbances often are implicated in chronic pain disorders such as fibromyalgia.

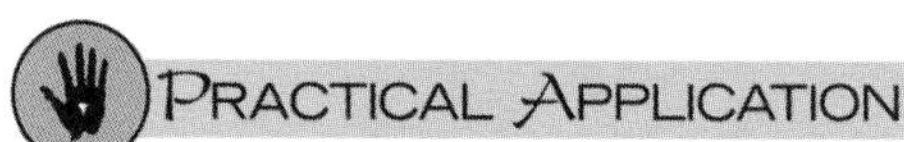

PRACTICAL APPLICATION

Growth hormone stimulates the production of fibroblasts, mast cells, ground substance, and collagen fibers and is essential in healing wounds. Because growth hormone is most active during delta-wave sleep and the sleep pattern usually is disrupted in fibromyalgia and other pain and fatigue syndromes, the body may have problems with cellular repair. Given this premise, a disrupted sleep pattern has been suggested as one of the primary causes of fatigue and pain syndromes.

Therapeutic massage has been shown through research to have a beneficial influence on the development of a restful sleep pattern, thus enabling the body to better restore and heal itself. ■

Thyroid-stimulating hormone. Thyroid-stimulating hormone (TSH) is a tropic hormone that promotes and maintains the growth and development of the thyroid gland and controls the release of thyroid hormones in a negative feedback system. Production of TSH often increases in response to cold temperature.

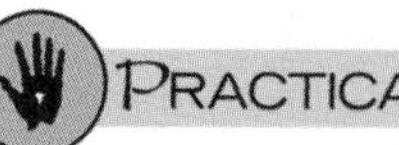

PRACTICAL APPLICATION

A licensed medical professional may recommend hydrotherapy (the use of water) for therapeutic intervention to encourage the production of TSH, if hyposecretion is a concern. Cold has an effect on the hypothalamus, resulting in the release of TSH. Typical applications include standing in cold water or alternating hot and cold water baths or showers. Whenever one uses cold therapeutically, the client's body needs to be warm first. Before the client stands in cold water, the person should warm the feet in a warm foot bath. The client then alternates hot and cold baths or showers, beginning with a warm water application for 5 to 15 minutes, then adding cold applications, starting with 15 to 30 seconds, gradually increasing to up to 5 minutes. The entire cold process starts with tepid water and gradually, over days or even weeks, the practitioner reduces the temperature and increases the duration of the cold water application. These methods are contraindicated in conditions in which a hypersensitivity to cold such as Raynaud's disease exists. ■

Adrenocorticotropic hormone. Adrenocorticotropic hormone (ACTH) is a tropic hormone that promotes and maintains normal growth and development of the adrenal cortex by stimulating the release of glucocorticoids and androgens. Androgens are hormones such as testosterone that produce secondary male characteristics. Stress, mild-to-moderate fevers, and hypoglycemia can increase the amount of ACTH secreted.

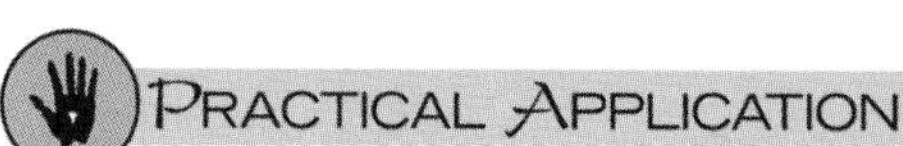

PRACTICAL APPLICATION

Stress encountered over a long period generates abnormal glucocorticoid effects on the body that are responsible for some diseases. Glucocorticoids are known to suppress the immune system. Any modality that reduces the effects of stress, including therapeutic massage, promotes appropriate levels of ACTH and thus brings the immune system back in balance. ■

Follicle-stimulating hormone. Follicle-stimulating hormone is a tropic hormone in the female that stimulates the growth and maturation of ovarian follicles, which contain eggs. Follicle-stimulating hormone also stimulates the secretion of estrogen; in the male it stimulates sperm production.

Luteinizing hormone. In women, luteinizing hormone is a tropic hormone that causes ovulation (the release of the mature egg) and stimulates progesterone production in the ovaries. In men, luteinizing hormone stimulates the production and secretion of testosterone in the testes.

Prolactin. Although found in men and women, prolactin primarily works in two areas of a woman's body. First, in combination with other hormones, prolactin plays a part in breast development. Second, prolactin initiates milk production when stimulated by the central nervous system. Receptors for prolactin in lymphocytes suggest that prolactin is involved in immune function.

Melanocyte-stimulating hormone. Melanocyte-stimulating hormone acts on the pigment cells in the skin and the adrenal glands. The exact function is uncertain. One theory suggests that melanocyte-stimulating hormone, ACTH, and other hormones that darken the skin control pigmentation of normal skin.

Posterior Pituitary Hormones

Posterior pituitary hormones are made by hypothalamic neurons and stored in the posterior pituitary gland.

Oxytocin. Oxytocin stimulates smooth muscle contraction, especially in the uterus. Oxytocin is released in large quantities just before a woman gives birth. This is part of a positive feedback cycle that ends when the child is born. Pitocin is synthetic oxytocin used mainly to induce labor in women. Oxytocin stimulates the milk letdown response, which causes the breast ducts to contract and release milk. Oxytocin also may be implicated in bonding behavior or feelings of belonging to another as occurs between a parent and child. When increased sympathetic activity releases epinephrine, which inhibits oxytocin, problems in lactation and bonding may occur. Oxytocin is found in men and nonpregnant women and pregnant and postpartal women. The role of this hormone in men has been suggested to be to support pair bonding between couples and to enhance parental behavior.

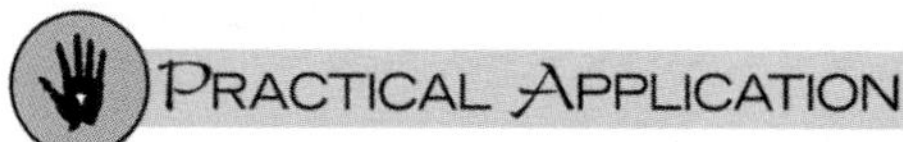

Research has shown that giving and receiving massage reduces sympathetic arousal. This enhances the effects of oxytocin, supporting lactation and bonding between infants and parents. Research also has shown that pleasurable rhythmic skin stimulation increases levels of oxytocin. This could explain some of the feelings of connectedness that occur between the client and massage practitioner when these types of methods are used. ■

Antidiuretic hormone. Also known as vasopressin, antidiuretic hormone (ADH) stimulates the kidneys to remove water from urine and release it into the bloodstream. Release of ADH is stimulated by pain, anxiety, nicotine, tranquilizers, and low blood pressure. Release of ADH is inhibited by alcohol, so the amount of urine produced increases. Because ADH can cause arterioles to contract, it increases blood pressure, which is beneficial during hemorrhaging due to the rerouting of blood to the internal organs. ADH can decrease the rate of perspiration, thus helping a person who is dehydrated (Figure 6-6).

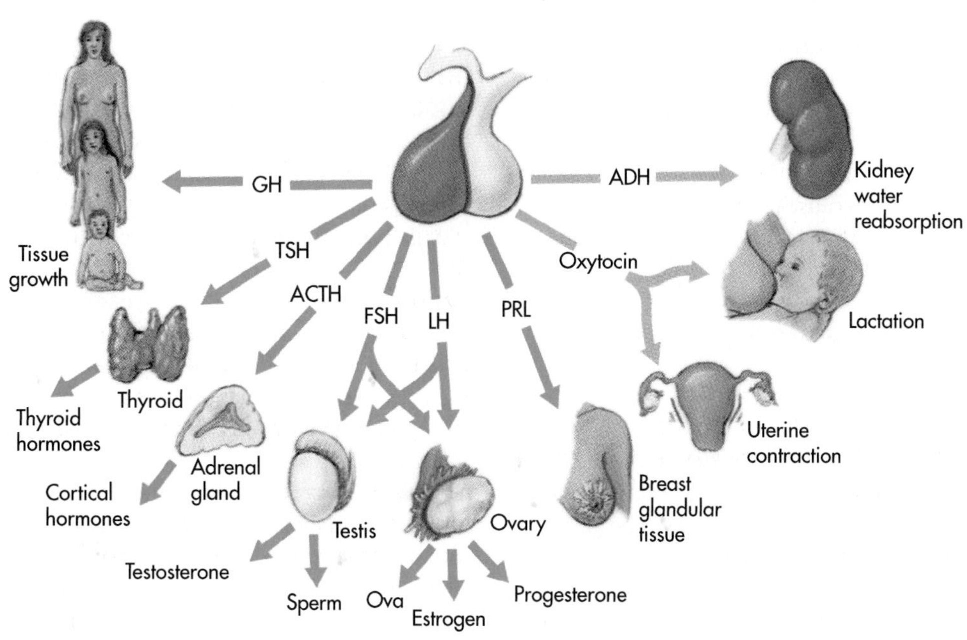

Figure 6-6
The effect of pituitary hormones on target tissues. (From Applegate EJ: *The anatomy and physiology learning system,* Philadelphia, 1995, Saunders.)

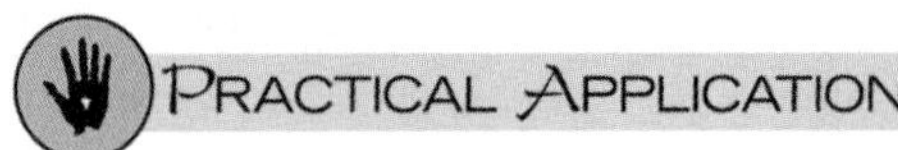

Therapeutic massage reduces the perception of pain and anxiety and indirectly interacts with the release of ADH, possibly supporting a more effective homeostatic function. ■

Pathologic Conditions

In gigantism and acromegaly, the pituitary gland produces excessive growth hormone. The term *gigantism* refers to the condition if it begins in infancy or early childhood. The condition results in excessive growth of the entire body. *Acromegaly* is an abnormal condition that occurs in adults, in whom the excess hormone thickens bones and enlarges organs. In secondary *Cushing's disease* the pituitary gland produces excessive ACTH, resulting in increased production of steroids by the adrenal gland. The symptoms include increased fat on the face and between the shoulder blades, thinning of bones and skin, and bruising. Treatment of gigantism, acromegaly, and secondary Cushing's disease includes surgery or radiation therapy. If a pituitary tumor is present, drug therapy with somatostatin is usually the treatment of choice.

Decreased growth hormone production and insufficient tropic hormones may cause height deficiencies. In pituitary deficiency a decrease exists in all pituitary hormones, which results in the loss of target organ hormones, specifically adrenal steroids, thyroxine, and the gonadotropins. *Dwarfism* can be the result. Dwarfism in children is treated by administration of synthetic growth hormone and, if necessary, replacement of thyroid, adrenal, and sex steroid hormones.

In *diabetes insipidus* (not to be confused with diabetes mellitus) the pituitary gland releases less vasopressin. Scarring or damage from head injuries often causes the condition. The ability of the water in urine to be reabsorbed decreases, and urine output increases, sometimes up to 20 L per day. Maintaining an adequate fluid intake may control mild cases, but in others treatment with a synthetic form of vasopressin has proved effective. If the inability of the kidney to respond to vasopressin causes diabetes insipidus, the normal treatment is reducing salt intake and taking medications focused on kidney function. Radiation therapy, surgery, or both are indicated in rare cases in which a tumor causes diabetes insipidus (Activity 6-5).

Thyroid Gland

The thyroid gland lies on the trachea below the thyroid cartilage and consists of a right and left lobe connected by a bridge (isthmus), resulting in a butterfly shape. The gland is heavier in women than in men. The thyroid and parathyroid glands are related to the Eastern energy chakra of the throat, the function of which is communication and creativity in a balanced function.

The thyroid gland regulates metabolism in the body by maintaining an adequate amount of oxygen consumption at the cellular level. The two principal hormones are thyroxine and triiodothyronine. TSH from the pituitary gland stimulates these hormones, and iodine is necessary for their synthesis. A third hormone, calcitonin, inhibits bone reabsorption by limiting the rate at which bone tissue releases calcium to plasma. This in turn reduces the blood calcium level and counters the effect of the parathyroid hormones.

Pathologic Conditions

Hyperthyroidism. *Hyperthyroidism,* or thyrotoxicosis, is the second most common endocrine disorder after diabetes mellitus and mostly affects women. The most common cause is autoimmune dysfunction. Symptoms include increased metabolic rate, excessive sweating, weight loss even with increased food intake, fatigue, nervousness, loose stools, tachycardia, warm moist skin, hand tremor, and hyperactivity. Hyperthyroidism mimics manic-depressive psychosis and almost always is accompanied by a goiter. (A goiter, which is an enlarged thyroid gland, may be found in hyperfunction, hypofunction, or normal thyroid function.) Plummer's disease, or toxic nodular goiter, is another form of hyperthyroidism.

The symptoms of *Graves' disease,* also a form of hyperthyroidism, include an enlarged thyroid gland and abnormal eyeball protrusion, called *exophthalmos,* which results from excess fluid behind the eye and may not diminish even after treatment. Graves' disease runs in families, is associated with autoimmune problems, and is most common in women between the ages of 20 and 40. Treatments include thyroidectomy, the use of antithyroid medications such as propylthiouracil (blocks iodine from being incorporated into thyroxine), or the use of radioactive iodine, which shrinks (destroys) the thyroid gland without affecting other tissues (Figure 6-7).

Hypothyroidism. *Hypothyroidism* can result from treatment for hyperthyroidism by radioactive iodine, overdose of antithyroid medication, or partial or complete thyroidectomy. The next most common causes are autoimmune dysfunction and a decrease in thyroid-releasing hormone from the hypothalamus. Symptoms include weakness, fatigue, lower metabolic rate, constipation, hoarseness, bradycardia, skin dryness, weight gain (often resulting in obesity), sluggishness, and slowed mental function sometimes with psychotic behavior. Again, a goiter is often present. Mild hypothyroidism is common in perimenopausal women between the ages of 35 and 45. Because of this, thyroid function should be checked as part of the routine health care of women. Hypothyroidism responds well to oral medication.

If thyroid hormones are absent in the fetus or during infancy, the result can be *cretinism,* a condition that results in mental retardation and dwarfism. *Hashimoto's disease* is an autoimmune hypothyroid disorder that is hereditary, found mainly in women ages 30 to 50, and causes tissue changes in the thyroid gland itself. *Myxedema* is the most severe form of hypothyroidism, causing many of the

ACTIVITY 6-5

If the pituitary hormones were represented by cartoon characters, what would each one be? Create and draw a cartoon character or other figure in the appropriate space or find a picture of one and paste it in the space to represent each pituitary hormone.

Growth hormone

Thyroid-stimulating hormone

Adrenocorticotropic hormone

Follicle-stimulating hormone

Luteinizing hormone

Prolactin

Oxytocin

Antidiuretic hormone

previously mentioned symptoms as well as swelling of the face, hands, and feet (Figure 6-7).

Table 6-3 gives a summary of the major effects and disturbances of triiodothyronine and thyroxine on the body.

INDICATIONS CONTRAINDICATIONS

For Therapeutic Massage

Some studies suggest that mild cases of hypothyroidism respond to cold water hydrotherapy and moderate aerobic exercise. Exposure to cold triggers release of TSH. ■

Therapeutic massage may be beneficial in managing symptoms of hyperthyroidism and hypothyroidism. Because thyroid conditions can go undiagnosed as a result of the symptoms being common to many stress-related conditions, referring clients for medical assessment to rule out thyroid dysfunction is important when they have any hyperthyroid or hypothyroid symptom patterns (Activity 6-6 on p. 192).

Parathyroid Glands

The parathyroid glands are made up of four round, pea-sized bodies located on the posterior surface of the thyroid lobes. Their hormone, parathormone, when combined with vitamin D decreases the amount of calcium excreted, causes the release of calcium from bone, and absorbs more calcium from the gastrointestinal tract, resulting in an increase in blood levels of calcium and phosphorus.

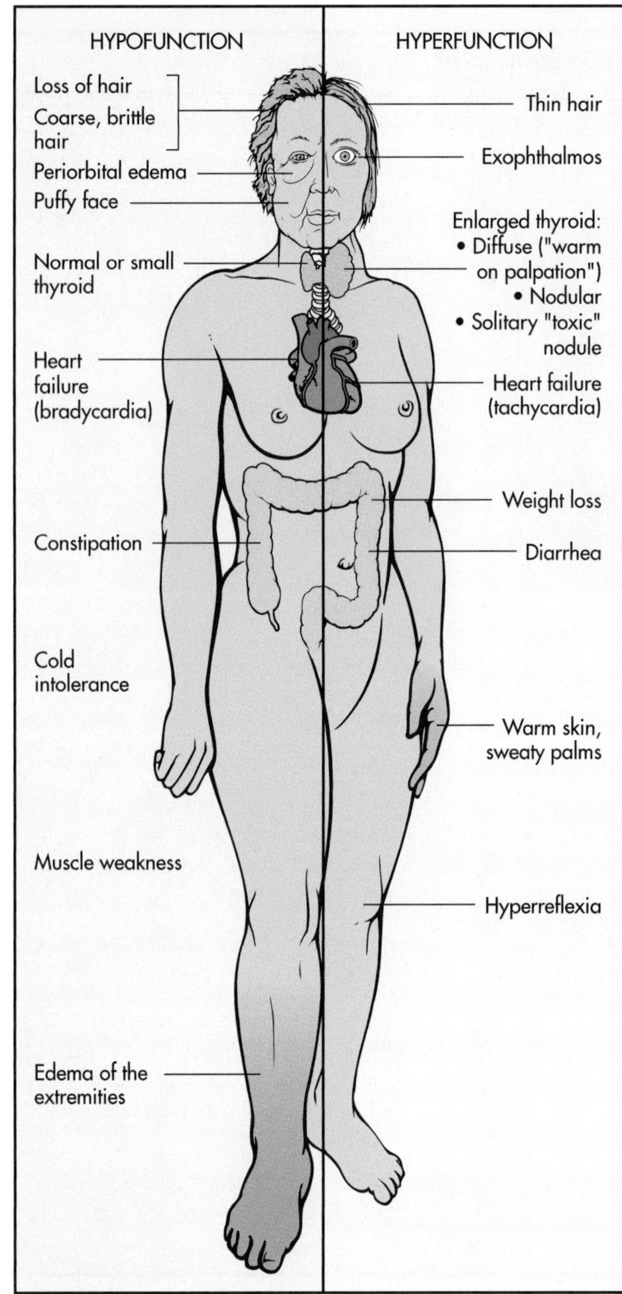

Figure 6-7
Comparison of hyperthyroidism and hypothyroidism. (From Damjanov I: *Pathology for the health-related professions,* ed 2, Philadelphia, 2000, Saunders.)

Pathologic Conditions

An excess of parathormone causes too much calcium to be removed from bone, resulting in weak bones. A deficiency of parathormone can cause hypocalcemic tetany, the symptoms of which include loss of sensation, muscle twitches, uncontrolled spasm, and convulsion.

In hypoparathyroidism the levels of calcium in blood and urine are less than normal, frequently resulting in spasms of skeletal muscles. Moderate-to-mild deficiency can result in neuromuscular excitability that could be misdiagnosed as simple muscle tension. Anxiety may result as well. Ruling out hypoparathyroidism in cases of unresolved anxiety and muscle tension is important. Emergency treatment of tetany caused by hypoparathyroidism is an injection of calcium chloride. For maintenance therapy, calcium and vitamin D supplements are used.

In primary hyperparathyroidism, usually resulting from a benign tumor, levels of calcium increase in blood and urine. In secondary hyperparathyroidism, resulting mostly from kidney disease, blood calcium decreases and urine calcium increases. The frequency of hyperparathyroidism is much more common than hypoparathyroidism and is increasing.

INDICATIONS/CONTRAINDICATIONS

For Therapeutic Massage

The symptoms of hyperparathyroidism include mild to severe skeletal pain and possibly osteoporosis. The client may seek body therapies for these conditions, and the massage therapist must take care to provide the appropriate referral to determine the underlying cause of the problem.

Pancreas

The pancreas is a long, slender gland located behind the stomach. In Eastern philosophies, the pancreas is related to the solar plexus chakra located at the thoracolumbar junction and navel. This chakra functions with willpower and awareness of emotion.

The pancreas is an exocrine and endocrine gland. Although its enzymes aid in digestion, our focus is on its hormone production. Islands of cells called the islets of Langerhans are interspersed within the exocrine gland tissues. These islets produce the hormones insulin and glucagon. The pancreas secretes two other hormones in small amounts: somatostatin inhibits the release of all islet hormones, and amylin acts as an antagonist to insulin.

The beta cells of the islets of Langerhans secrete the hormone insulin, which lowers blood glucose levels by transporting glucose into cells to be used for energy. Insulin binds to the cells and allows glucose and potassium to be transported across the cell membrane. Although insulin receptors are present on most cell membranes, only our muscle, connective tissue, and white blood cells need it for glucose transport. However, glucose is readily available to the liver, brain, and kidneys no matter what our blood insulin levels. Insulin removes glucose from blood, making it available for cellular activity.

Insulin

The pancreas releases insulin when levels of blood sugar, amino acids, and fatty acids rise. Other hormones, including ACTH, growth hormone, epinephrine, thyroxine, and glucocorticoids also affect insulin secretion. Because these hormones necessitate response from muscles, the demand for energy increases, thus insulin secretion supplies energy. Fluctuations in blood sugar during experiences of stress put additional strain on the body because the body often actually does not need increased amounts of energy.

TABLE 6-3
Normal Versus Major Effects and Disturbances of Triiodothyronine and Thyroxine on the Body

Normal Function	Hyposecretion	Hypersecretion
Maintains basal metabolic rate (BMR) and temperature regulation to promote appropriate oxygen consumption and production of heat and energy; enhances effects of catecholamines and sympathetic nervous system activity.	Can result in BMR less than normal with a decreased body temperature, cold intolerance, decreased appetite, weight gain, muscle and joint pain, decreased sensitivity to catecholamines, and general slowed state; low thyroid function mimics many disease symptoms and should be checked when any of the above symptoms are present.	Can result in BMR greater than normal with an increase in body temperature; heat intolerance; appetite; weight loss; sensitivity to catecholamines, which may lead to hypertension (high blood pressure); mood changes; and anxiety-type symptoms.
Thyroid hormones also promote appropriate carbohydrate/lipid/protein metabolism and glucose catabolism, mobilize fats. Thyroid hormones also are essential for protein synthesis and enhance liver secretion of cholesterol.	Can result in decreased glucose metabolism, elevated cholesterol and triglyceride levels in the blood, decreased protein synthesis, and edema.	Can result in enhanced catabolism of glucose and fats, weight loss, increased protein catabolism, and loss of muscle mass.
Promotes development of the nervous system in the fetus and infant, as well as normal adult nervous system function.	Can result in slowed brain development in the infant with retardation and mental dulling, and depression, paresthesias, memory impairment, listlessness, and hypoactive reflexes in the adult.	Can result in irritability, restlessness, insomnia, overresponsiveness to environmental stimuli, bulging eyes (exophthalmos), and personality changes.
Promotes functioning of the heart	Can result in decreased efficiency of the pumping action of the heart, slow heart rate, and lower blood pressure.	Can result in rapid heart rate and high blood pressure and, if prolonged, can lead to heart failure.
Promotes normal muscular development, tone, and function.	Can result in sluggish muscle action, muscle cramps, and myalgia.	Can result in muscle atrophy and weakness.
Promotes growth and maturation of the skeleton.	Can result in growth retardation, skeletal malabsorption, retention of child's body proportions in adults, and joint pain in the adult.	Can result in excessive skeletal growth initially, followed by early epiphyseal closure and short stature in children; adults experience demineralization of skeleton.
Promotes gastrointestinal (GI) motility and tone and increases secretion of digestive juices.	Can result in depressed GI motility and tone and increased secretion of digestive juices.	Can result in excessive GI motility, diarrhea, and loss of appetite.
Promotes female reproductive ability and normal lactation	Can result in depressed ovarian function, sterility, and depressed lactation.	Can result in depressed ovarian function in females and impotence in males.
Promotes secretory activity of skin.	Can result in skin that is pale, thick, and dry; facial edema; coarse and thin hair; and hard, thick nails.	Can result in skin that is flushed, thin, and moist; may produce thin and soft hair and nails.

Glucagon

Alpha cells of the islets of Langerhans secrete the hormone glucagon, which increases blood glucose, the opposite of the insulin response. Growth hormone stimulates these cells, which are a part of the feedback loop in hypoglycemia. High protein intake and exercise raise the amount of amino acids in the blood, which also increases glucagon secretion. This happens by requiring the liver to speed up the conversion of glycogen to glucose, as well as creating glucose from fatty acids, lactic acid, and amino acids. Blood levels of glucose increase but do not enter the cells, so cellular levels of glucose decrease.

Pathologic Conditions

Hyperfunction. A benign tumor occasionally causes high insulin levels. More commonly, high insulin levels occur in diabetic clients who take insulin without eating properly. The result is what is known as an insulin reaction, which

ACTIVITY 6-6

List three thyroid dysfunction symptoms that may cause a client to seek bodywork modalities. Examples are provided to get you started.

Examples
Nervousness, fatigue, constipation

Your Turn
1. ______
2. ______
3. ______

means the body is flooded with insulin. Glucose enters the cells at an increased rate and the blood glucose level falls, causing hypoglycemia (low blood sugar). When the brain is deprived of glucose, confusion and weakness result. A deficient production of glucagon may cause hypoglycemia.

True hypoglycemia is rare. More common is reactive hypoglycemia, a diet-induced condition that can be corrected by eating a balanced diet on a regular schedule.

Hypofunction. The disorder known as *diabetes mellitus* results from the pancreas not producing enough insulin or totally stopping insulin production. Because cells do not absorb glucose, the amount in the bloodstream increases (hyperglycemia). Glucose is a powerful diuretic, so glucose entering the urine is accompanied by water. As glucose flows through the kidneys, some of the excess is released in the urine (glycosuria). This causes many of the first symptoms of diabetes, such as dehydration, increased thirst (polydipsia), increased urination (polyuria), and an increased appetite (polyphagia).

When the body is unable to use glucose, it uses fats for energy. The breakdown in fats results in the formation of ketones (ketoacids) as by-products, increasing body acidity and causing ketoacidosis. In severe instances the combination of dehydration, high blood sugar, and acidosis may depress the cerebral cortex to the point of coma. This metabolic acidosis stimulates the respiratory center to increase the breathing rate.

Two types of diabetes mellitus exist. Type I, or insulin-dependent diabetes, is usually severe and occurs at a young age. Symptoms develop quickly, with ketoacidosis often being the first manifestation. Ketoacidosis is treatable with saline, bicarbonate, potassium, and insulin. A controlled diet and the daily use of insulin are the most common long-term treatments.

Type II, or non–insulin-dependent diabetes, is usually milder and in most cases begins in adults. However, type II diabetes is occurring in younger persons. Heredity and obesity are important contributing factors. Symptoms include dehydration, increased thirst and appetite, frequent urination, reduced resistance to infection, blurred vision, and fatigue. These symptoms most often develop over a period of years. Treatment usually begins with dietary changes, such as those recommended by the American Diabetes Association. An exercise program is implemented to control weight and increase general fitness. Weight loss is an important first step because fewer insulin receptors are present and they become less sensitive to insulin in an overweight person. Oral medications, including chlorpropamide (Diabinese) or tolbutamide (Orinase), reduce blood sugar levels. Insulin may be used if blood sugar levels remain high but is not necessarily a permanent form of treatment.

Complications of diabetes can include vascular disease because diabetes increases the development of arteriosclerosis. High glucose levels also raise the chances of infection because they provide a good medium for bacterial growth. Other complications include kidney disease, heart attacks (diabetics have twice the average), eye problems (diabetic retinopathy), impotence in men, and loss of menstrual cycles in women. Gangrene of the feet in diabetic clients accounts for more amputations of the feet than any other condition, including trauma. Treatment for the complications of diabetes includes meticulous attention to the hygiene of the feet and an exercise program for weight loss and fitness. Diabetic neuropathy, a painful and difficult-to-manage condition resulting from peripheral nerve damage, is more severe with type I diabetes because nerve damage results from the ketoacidosis (ketoacidosis is not seen as often in those with type II diabetes) (Figure 6-8).

INDICATIONS CONTRAINDICATIONS

For Therapeutic Massage

A general stress management program supports the management of diabetes. Therapeutic massage can be an integral part of such a program. An important part of working with the diabetic client is that bodywork be a part of an overall treatment program with medical supervision. Careful observation of the feet during massage supports a hygiene program. The practitioner should refer the client for immediate medical care for any noted tissue changes. In pain management of diabetic neuropathy, using massage approaches as part of a supervised program can prove beneficial for short-term reduction of pain symptoms (Activity 6-7). ■

Adrenal Glands

We have two adrenal glands, one on top of each of our kidneys. Each gland consists of an inner portion called the medulla and an outer layer called the cortex. The adrenal glands are related to the root or basic chakra center located at the base of the spine and focused on functions of survival and grounding.

Adrenal Medulla

The tissue structure of the adrenal medulla is similar to nerve tissue and functions as part of the sympathetic nervous system. The adrenal medulla secretes two catecholamines,

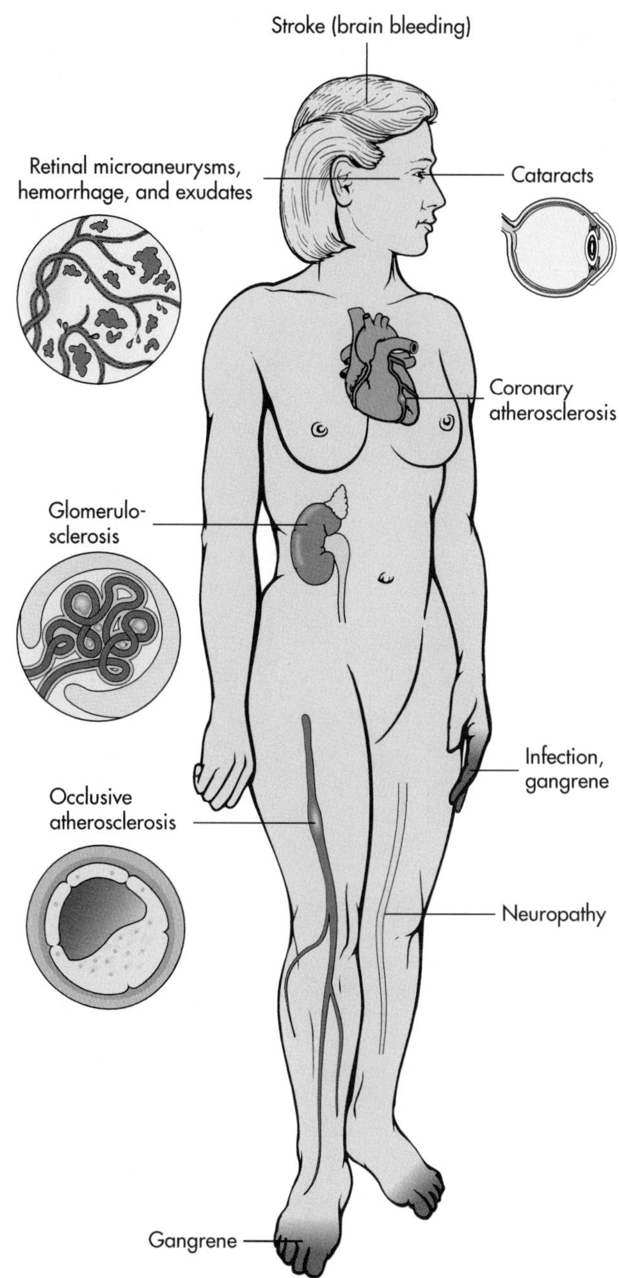

Figure 6-8
Complications of diabetes mellitus. (From Damjanov I: *Pathology for the health-related professions,* ed 2, Philadelphia, 2000, Saunders.)

epinephrine (sometimes called adrenaline) and norepinephrine (or noradrenaline). They are the hormones active in the sympathetic fight-or-flight or alarm response to stress. Epinephrine has its primary influence on the heart, causing an increase in heart rate, whereas norepinephrine has a greater effect on peripheral vasoconstriction, which raises blood pressure. The hormones produced by the adrenal medulla prolong and intensify the activity begun by the sympathetic nervous system neurons. The hypothalamus, the adrenal medulla, and the adrenal cortex are linked and interdependent in the management of the stress response. When stress-producing events are unresolved within about 15 minutes (Selye's alarm phase), these symptoms activate a more prolonged stress-coping pattern of the adrenocortical responses (Selye's resistance phase). Over the long term, if epinephrine and norepinephrine remain elevated, they perpetuate predisposing factors for stress-related disease.

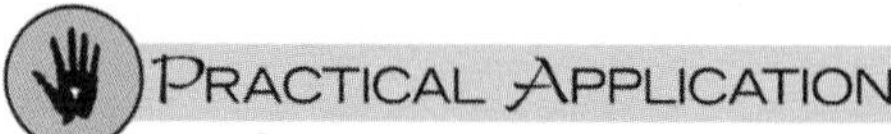

Therapeutic massage methods have been shown to help dissipate the concentration of adrenal medulla hormones, reducing their detrimental effects in the body. Because the effects of catecholamines dissipate within a short time, the usual goal for therapeutic massage is to support the body in a return to homeostasis and to prevent a recurrence of the excessive alarm response so that the body can remain in a state of homeostasis. The general application in a typical 1-hour session is to work with more vigorous methods for the first 15 minutes to use up the catecholamines and then to begin the transition to trigger and support the relaxation response of parasympathetic function over the next 45 minutes.

Because the major repair and energy-restoring mechanisms of the body are supported most effectively in the parasympathetic pattern and because most energy is expended and tissue damage created during fight-or-flight activity, we can begin to see the wisdom in supporting parasympathetic function to allow sufficient time for restoration and repair of the body. A general rule of thumb is that for every 15 minutes of catecholamine-generated sympathetic activity, the body requires about 45 minutes of parasympathetic balancing time. In a healthy, well-balanced person, sympathetic activities account for 25% of daily actions, with parasympathetic restorative actions making up another 25%. The other 50% of the time is taken up with activities that use sympathetic and parasympathetic functions together. One suggestion is that this seldom happens, and the ratio often is reversed. Dysfunction occurs when sympathetic activity dominates, often because of lifestyle demands. Over time the body cannot provide enough restorative action, and homeostatic balance is disrupted. Again, many of the healing rituals of old seem to be based on supporting parasympathetic activity and providing effective outlets for the fight-or-flight hormones of the adrenal glands. The use of sweat lodges, ceremonial bathing, quiet reflection, chanting, dancing, feasting, and other such activities are seen as effective ways to dissipate the fight-or-flight hormones while promoting restorative functions (Activity 6-8). ■

Adrenal Cortex

The adrenal cortex secretes three major glucocorticoid (glucose-producing steroid) hormones that are derived from cholesterol. ACTH from the pituitary gland, which receives its messages from the hypothalamus, stimulates the release of these hormones—cortisol, aldosterone, and the gonadocorticoids. The adrenal cortex hormones are involved with

ACTIVITY 6-7

Identify a reason why therapeutic massage can be beneficial as part of a total diabetes management program. Justify your position using the clinical reasoning model.

Example

Statement: Therapeutic massage supports weight loss programs.

1. What are the facts?
   Weight loss and changes in diet result in chemical changes in the body. Mood-elevating chemicals that are generated from high-sugar, high-fat foods are reduced substantially in a diabetic diet.
   Therapeutic massage increases the feel-good chemicals in the body.
2. What are the possibilities?
   Therapeutic massage can act as a substitute for food to provide stimulation for mood elevation.
3. What are the pros and cons? What are the consequences of not acting (not doing bodywork)? What are the consequences of acting (doing bodywork)?
   Positive consequences include pleasure sensations that do not contribute to the diabetic problem. Negative consequences include the cost and inconvenience that may prevent easy implementation of these methods into a person's lifestyle.
4. What would be the effect on the persons involved: client, practitioner, and other professionals working with the client?
   The person would feel cared for and supported during the weight loss program by receiving the personal attention from a professional during a time in which he or she may feel deprived.

Your Turn

Statement:

1. What are the facts?

2. What are the possibilities?

3. What are the pros and cons? What are the consequences of not acting? What are the consequences of acting?

4. What would be the effect on the persons involved: client, practitioner, and other professionals working with the client?

metabolism of most body cells. Without a functioning adrenal cortex, a person could die from excessive stress and its effects.

Cortisol. Cortisol is secreted in minute amounts. If the body does not have sufficient supplies of fat or glycogen stored to use for energy, cortisol synthesizes certain amino acids into glucose (gluconeogenesis), causing a rise in blood sugar. Cortisol also converts starches into glycogen in the liver if the body does not acquire enough carbohydrates to use.

Eating and activity stimulate cortisol secretion, which seems to follow daily biologic rhythms. Peak cortisol levels occur shortly after waking, whereas the lowest levels are reached just as the sleep cycle begins. High levels of cortisol in the blood may disrupt the sleep cycle. Any situation that produces acute stress increases blood levels of cortisol, and the sympathetic nervous system overrides any inhibitory effects in feedback loop regulation. This results in a rise in blood levels of glucose, fatty acids, and amino acids, all because of cortisol. Levels of stress often are measured by cortisol levels, and research in stress-management methods

ACTIVITY 6-8

Design a personal 15-minute sympathetic activity sequence. Then design a personal 45-minute parasympathetic relaxation sequence.

Example

15-minute sympathetic activity sequence: I will go to the recreation center and spend 5 minutes on the track and 10 minutes on the stair-climbing machine.

45-minute parasympathetic relaxation sequence: I will spend 15 minutes doing slow stretching combined with coordinated breathing. I will take a 15-minute hot bath, and I will read inspirational and heart-warming stories for 15 minutes.

Your Turn

Design a personal 15-minute sympathetic activity sequence.

Design a personal 45-minute parasympathetic relaxation sequence.

often uses cortisol as a measurement criterion, with a drop indicating a reduction in the stress response. Cortisol contains antiinflammatory agents that limit the amount of substances released during the inflammatory response. Cortisol slows wound healing because of a decreased rate of connective tissue regeneration. Excessively high levels of cortisol, especially over a long period, can cause symptoms such as a decrease in cartilage and bone formation; inhibition of the inflammatory response, which reduces normal signals for tissue repair; depression of the activity of the immune system; increase in fat storage in adipose tissue; depression of brain activity; and promotion of detrimental changes in cardiovascular, neural, and gastrointestinal function.

Remember the idea of balance is important. The body needs glucocorticoids for normal function to achieve homeostasis. Excessive stress and use of steroids, such as pharmacologic agents, may lead to the disruption of this homeostasis.

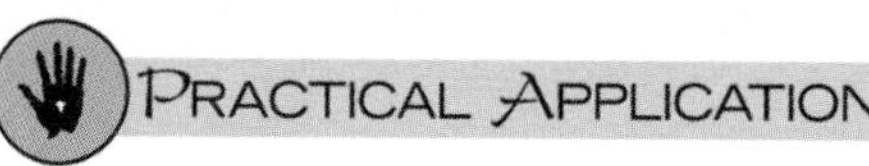

Studies show that massage reduces cortisol levels and therefore promotes activities such as improved sleep, better digestion, increased immune function, and improved tissue repair. Other forms of relaxation, including moderate aerobic exercise and slow stretching methods such as yoga, show similar results. The most effective interventions seem to be rhythmic, with a duration of 15 to 60 minutes producing the best results. Because the effects wear off within a 24-hour period, some sort of relaxation method needs to be done every day to support well-being best. ■

Aldosterone. Aldosterone is a mineralocorticoid, a sodium- and potassium-regulating steroid. Aldosterone causes the kidneys to reabsorb more sodium and water and excrete more potassium and hydrogen. Although aldosterone is necessary for our survival, excessive amounts of the hormone lead to sodium and water retention accompanied by elevation of potassium ions and in some instances alteration of the acid-base balance of blood. Under excessive stress the hypothalamus secretes corticotropin-releasing hormone. ACTH blood levels rise and trigger an increase in aldosterone secretion. The resulting increase in blood volume and blood pressure helps ensure adequate delivery of nutrients and respiratory gases during the stressful period.

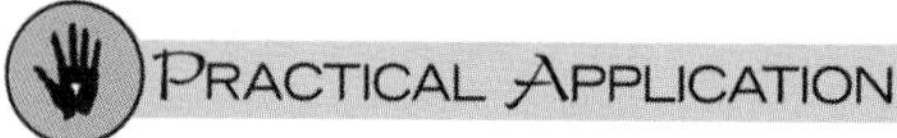

The release of aldosterone, although effective when the body is expending physical energy such as required in actual fighting behavior, increases the likelihood of stress-induced disease such as high blood pressure when the energy expenditure is less than the physiologic response. This happens often as persons try to deal with increased emotional and mental stress without physical activity. Aerobic activity and moderate weight-resistance exercises are helpful in managing this situation, balancing emotional and mental activity (Activity 6-9). ■

Gonadocorticoids. Although the ovaries and testes produce most of the sex hormones, the adrenal glands also produce similar male and female sex steroids called gonadocorticoids. Both sexes secrete estrogen, progesterone, and the male androgens, with androgens predominating. This hormone secretion is significant in the fetus and during early puberty. The effect of the adrenal sex hormones increases as we age and hormone production in the gonads decreases. For this reason, postmenopausal women may use adrenal estrogen when ovarian function decreases.

ACTIVITY 6-9

Outline the progression of the adrenal hormone patterns in response to a stress that lasts 24 hours. Identify the stressor, the hormones involved, the possible duration of effect, and the possible results.

Example
Situation: Parent worried about adolescent child who comes home 2 hours late.

1. Anger; first 15 minutes; epinephrine and norepinephrine; results in increase in fight-or-flight response and increased sympathetic activity.
2. Worry; next 30 minutes; with increase in anxiety, still supporting continuance of catecholamine response.
3. Increased worry; next 60 minutes; shift to cortisol release, resulting in inability to sleep.
4. Recurring anger; 15 minutes; epinephrine and norepinephrine with aldosterone increase; results in increased fight-or-flight response and increased sympathetic activity with rise in blood pressure because of increasing fluid levels of blood.
5. Child comes home and is met by an angry and worried parent.
6. Inability of parent to sleep the rest of the night because of increased cortisol levels.
7. Fatigue the next day with irritability and a dull headache caused by effects of increased cortisol and aldosterone levels.
8. Because of increased cortisol and aldosterone levels, parent has suppressed immune function and catches a cold 3 days later.

Your Turn
Situation:

Response pattern:

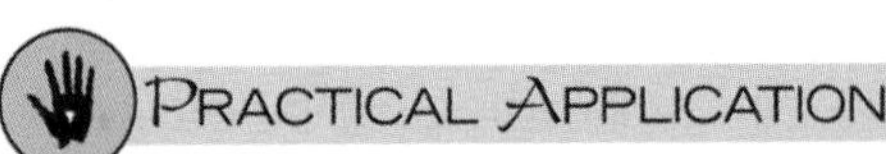

PRACTICAL APPLICATION

Healthy, functioning adrenal glands support successful aging. As gonadocorticoids secreted by the gonads decline, the secretion of these hormones form strong and healthy adrenal glands, which supports the body in vitality well into the aging process.

Care of the adrenal glands is the same as care for the whole body. Effective stress management, adequate exercise and rest, fresh air, sunshine, proper nutrition, good social support, and a feeling of purpose in life all contribute to this care. Is it possible that the ageless quality of sages, elders, gurus, and others considered as the old ones of wisdom is due in part to the care they took of their adrenal glands? ■

Pathologic Conditions

In *Cushing's syndrome,* corticosteroid levels in the blood and urine are elevated, specifically cortisol and urinary 17-hydroxycorticosteroid, both of which are excretory products of cortisol. The usual cause of Cushing's disease is taking large doses of corticosteroid drugs for long periods. ACTH is low in primary Cushing's disease. ACTH is high in secondary Cushing's disease. Usually caused by a pituitary tumor, the secondary condition is referred to as Cushing's disease instead of syndrome. In both cases, symptoms include fat accumulation, edema, hyperglycemia, muscle weakness, suppressed immunity, osteoporosis, acne, and increased facial hair. Diabetes mellitus can be brought on during Cushing's disease and can develop into a chronic condition.

Conn's syndrome, caused by an adrenal tumor, is primary hyperaldosteronism. In rare cases, if caused by a nonspecific enlargement of the adrenal glands, the syndrome is referred to as aldosteronism. Levels of aldosterone and sodium are elevated in plasma and urine, and potassium is decreased. Symptoms include headache, tingling and weakness in the limbs, increased thirst, fatigue, hypertension, and increase in urine volume, especially at night.

Addison's disease shows low plasma cortisol, low sodium, and high potassium levels (all opposite of Cushing's disease). Urinary 17-hydroxycorticosteroid and blood glucose levels are low. Primary Addison's disease shows a high ACTH level (with no cortisol to oppose ACTH). Secondary Addison's disease shows a low ACTH level because of nonstimulation of the adrenal gland by the pituitary gland. Symptoms include weakness, decreased endurance, increased pigmentation of the skin and mucous membranes, anorexia, dehydration, weight loss, intestinal disturbances, anxiety, depression (or similar emotional distress), and decreased tolerance to cold. The onset is usually gradual and may be mistaken as general stress symptoms. The condition can be life-threatening, and proper diagnosis is essential for appropriate treatment.

INDICATIONS / CONTRAINDICATIONS

For Therapeutic Massage
After these conditions are diagnosed, stress management can be an important part of ongoing therapeutic management. ■

Pharmacologic Use of Synthetic Adrenocorticosteroids

Synthetic steroids (corticosteroids and steroids) are used primarily to decrease the effects of inflammation by reducing capillary dilation and permeability. Steroids also prevent the release of vasoactive substances such as histamine and kinins. Allergic disorders such as asthma, reactions to bee stings, contact dermatitis, drug reactions, hay fever, and hives are treated with steroids. Steroids also are used to treat arthritis, bursitis, and autoimmune disorders, including lupus erythematosus and rheumatoid arthritis. Steroids have been shown to be useful in treating leukemia, multiple myeloma, Crohn's disease, ulcerative colitis, kidney failure, infections, and skin disorders.

Common side effects of synthetic steroid use include symptoms as diverse as mood changes, insomnia, high blood pressure, increased susceptibility to infection, glaucoma, headache, reduced wound healing, sweating, fragile skin, vertigo, stunted growth in children, osteoporosis, and an increased risk of bone breakage.

Using steroids for extended periods without reevaluation is dangerous. Periodic decreases in dosage are often necessary, but dosages must never be altered or stopped except by licensed medical practitioners. Weaning gradually from large doses of steroids is necessary because they suppress the pituitary gland and ACTH by negative feedback. When ACTH is suppressed, the adrenal glands do not function. When steroid treatment stops, sometimes the adrenal glands do not rebound to a functioning mode, and the person may lapse into Addison's disease. A side effect of oral steroid therapy is gastrointestinal bleeding. Protection of the stomach lining with cimetidine (Tagamet) is often necessary when one uses oral steroids.

INDICATIONS/CONTRAINDICATIONS

For Therapeutic Massage

Some forms of massage may be used to manage some of the side effects of synthetic steroids. However, the practitioner should avoid massage methods such as frictioning that may cause inflammation when a person is taking synthetic adrenocorticosteroids. Massage also is contraindicated directly over areas of injected steroids used to treat localized inflammation such as bursitis because it is important for the steroid to remain in the localized tissues (Activity 6-10).

ACTIVITY 6-10

Develop a list of at least three indications and contraindications for integrating therapeutic massage in combination with synthetic pharmacologic steroid use.

Example
Indications: Beneficial to sleep
Contraindications: Heavy compressive force on bones

Your Turn
Indications:
1. ____________________
2. ____________________
3. ____________________

Contraindications:
1. ____________________
2. ____________________
3. ____________________

Testes and Ovaries

The male and female gonads are located in the pelvic cavity and produce sex hormones identical to those of the adrenal cortex. Because this is their primary function, they secrete larger amounts than the adrenal cortex and, in the female, secrete them in a cyclic manner to regulate the menstrual cycle, support pregnancy, and prepare for lactation.

The testes and ovaries are related to the root chakra located at the base of the lumbar vertebrae in the lower abdomen near the genitals and womb. The function of this chakra is desire, pleasure, sexuality, and procreation, with the attraction of opposites.

The two primary female sex hormones are estrogen and progesterone. Male sex hormones are called androgens. The main male sex hormone is testosterone. These hormones help develop and maintain primary sexual characteristics. Sexual behavior, male and female brain development, and gender behavior have been linked directly to concentrations of these hormones. Testosterone has an effect on the sex drive (libido) for men and women. Sex hormones influence biologic function and behavior throughout life. Males and females are most similar in the beginning and end of life, with the greatest differences from puberty to midlife (the reproductive years), when these hormones are more active.

These sex hormones have other effects on the body. Estrogen, progesterone, and androgens affect epithelial and connective tissue and circulation. Continuing research concerning the sex hormones secreted by the adrenal glands indicates functions of these hormones other than reproduction. Testosterone, along with other androgens, is known to influence hair growth and distribution of hair in men and women. Androgens also affect the skin and are a factor in acne development.

Androgens and estrogens exert their major influence at puberty. Androgens in particular stimulate growth and maturation of bone, cartilage, and muscle. Low levels of estrogens promote growth, whereas high levels inhibit growth. Beyond puberty, androgens increase hemoglobin levels, whereas estrogen protects against bone loss and epidermal tissue atrophy. Estrogen also can be synthesized by adipose tissue, which converts naturally occurring androgens.

Besides the primary sex hormones, the ovaries produce relaxin, a hormone that relaxes and dilates the cervix near the end of pregnancy and relaxes pelvic and pubic ligaments to prepare for delivery. The ovaries also produce inhibin, the hormone that inhibits FSH and luteinizing hormone after ovulation and during pregnancy. The testes produce inhibin, which controls sperm production.

Pineal Gland

The pineal is a tiny gland inside the brain within the diencephalon and surrounded by pia mater. All the functions of this gland have not been identified. To add to the mystery of the gland, it is located in the position of the third eye in many Eastern philosophies and is related to the crown or brow chakra, depending on the Eastern discipline. The functions of this chakra area concern inner sight or awareness.

Serotonin, norepinephrine, dopamine, histamine, and other neurotransmitters and hormones have been identified from this gland, but its major function seems to be to secrete melatonin. The gland is light sensitive and is involved with regulating the rhythmic patterns of the body. The pineal gland also produces a hormone that stimulates secretion of aldosterone by the adrenal cortex.

Many body rhythms have long been known to move in step with one another or to be entrained. Body temperature, pulse, hormone concentrations, and the sleep-wake cycles seem to follow the same beat over a 24-hour period. The influences of light on the biologic clock of the hypothalamus activate many of these rhythms. Melatonin secretion is inhibited when light reaches the eyes and is enhanced during darkness. Light produces melatonin-mediated effects on reproductive, eating, and sleeping patterns. Light intensity, spectrum (color mixture), and timing (day/night or seasonal changes) influence individuals.

Conditions such as illness, drug use, jet travel, alteration of eating pattern, weather changes, changing to the night shift, or other disruptions in the sleep-wake cycle can throw these rhythms out of synchronization. Disruptions in these rhythms cause mood changes, affect the immune function, alter digestion, and unsettle the entire homeostatic balance. Researchers have identified a common emotional disorder called *seasonal affective disorder* in which mood swings are exaggerated grossly. As the days grow shorter each fall, persons with seasonal affective disorder become irritable, anxious, sleepy, and socially withdrawn. Their appetite becomes insatiable; they crave carbohydrates and gain weight readily. Phototherapy, the use of bright lights, for up to 2 hours daily reversed these symptoms in nearly 90% of persons studied and was more effective than the use of antidepressant drugs in the research. When persons stopped receiving phototherapy or were given melatonin, their symptoms returned as quickly as they had lifted, indicating that melatonin may be a key to seasonal mood changes also.

Symptoms of seasonal affective disorder are virtually identical to those of individuals with *carbohydrate-craving obesity* and *premenstrual syndrome*, except that carbohydrate-craving obesity affects sufferers daily and premenstrual syndrome affects sufferers monthly. Phototherapy relieves premenstrual syndrome symptoms in some women according to some research.

Persons who work all night exhibit reversed melatonin secretion patterns. When it is exposed to light during the night, the pineal gland releases no hormone; during daytime sleeping hours, the gland releases high levels of melatonin. If these persons are awakened from sleep and exposed to bright light, their melatonin levels drop. The same sort of melatonin inversion occurs in those who fly from coast to coast. The reversal disrupts sleep patterns. Anything that disrupts sleep eventually causes widespread stress in the body.

Peoples have worshipped the sun since the earliest times. Many ancient healing rituals were timed with the rising or setting of the sun. The cycles of the moon are also important in biologic rhythm regulation. Some native traditions refer to the menstrual cycle as the moon time because women would usually menstruate during the full moon. The word *lunatic* is derived from lunar or the moon because tradition has attributed increased emotional behavior to the full moon.

Not only are we deficient in natural light, but also we are starved of dark. Exposure to artificial light well beyond the natural cycle has influenced the drastic increase in insomnia and disruptive sleep patterns. Our bodies are out of touch with the natural rhythms they were designed to follow, which places more stress on our systems. Artificial lights do not provide the full spectrum of sunlight. Incandescent bulbs used in homes primarily provide red wavelengths, whereas fluorescent bulbs used in many businesses and schools provide yellow-green wavelengths. Animals exposed for long periods to artificial lighting exhibit reproductive abnormalities and an enhanced susceptibility to cancer. Could it be that some of us are unknowingly experiencing the same effects?

Scientists are just now beginning to understand the reasons for these effects, and as they do, they increasingly are distressed about windowless offices, restricted and artificial illumination of work areas, and the growing number of institutionalized and isolated individuals who rarely feel the energy of the sun, the natural rhythm of the moon, or the quieting enveloping of the dark.

INDICATIONS CONTRAINDICATIONS

For Therapeutic Massage

Relaxation methods, including therapeutic massage, can support effective sleep patterns. Adhering to a bedtime and wake-time schedule can reestablish sleep patterns. Sleeping in the dark and experiencing adequate natural light during the day seems to be important. Moderate exercise during the day and a gentle stretching program before retiring is beneficial. Eating on a regular schedule also reinforces the rhythm (Activity 6-11). ■

Thymus

The thymus gland is located deep to the sternum and mediastinum of the thorax and between the lungs at the level of the fourth and fifth thoracic vertebrae. Often considered part of the lymphatic system and identified as the master gland of the immune system, the thymus does have endocrine secretions. Thymus hormones are thymopoietin,

ACTIVITY 6-11

Develop a daily schedule that supports biologic rhythms, particularly those mediated by the pineal gland. Carry this schedule from awakening to bedtime.

Example
5:30 am: Wake up
5:45 am: Quiet meditation
6:00 am: Exercise outside in rising sun
7:30 am: Breakfast

Your Turn

thymic humoral factor, thymic factor, and thymosin. These hormones function in the growth and development of T cell lymphocytes of the immune system. The thymus is large in children, providing some evidence that its production of hormones may slow down with aging.

The thymus is located in the general region of the heart and is related to the heart and spleen chakras with the functions of love, compassion, and transformation in Eastern doctrine.

Other Endocrine Tissues

Endocrine glands are not the only tissues that secrete hormones. Numerous cells and tissues throughout the brain, gut, and cardiovascular system produce hormones as well. As an example, the placenta is an endocrine gland. The following are a few of the major hormones produced throughout the body.

Endorphins

Endorphins belong to a family of peptide hormones that have many different effects but that especially work like morphine to suppress pain. They are synthesized in the brain, primarily in the anterior lobe of the pituitary, and bind to receptors in the brain that increase pain thresholds. Endorphins appear to enhance the release of thyroid-releasing hormone from the hypothalamus and also influence the neurosecretion of vasopressin, ACTH, and growth hormone. Endorphins influence mood, producing a mild euphoric feeling such as that seen in runner's high. They also help control body temperature; assist with memory and learning; and help regulate sex hormones that control puberty, sex drive, and reproduction. Endorphins are a factor in mental illness, especially schizophrenia and depression.

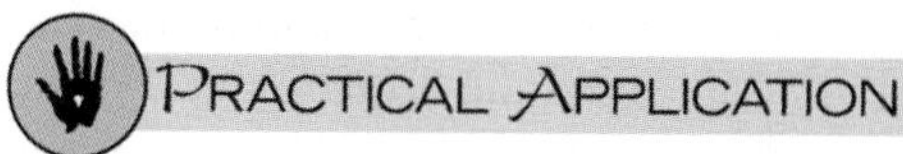

Research has shown that massage and acupuncture stimulate the release of endorphins, supporting the use of these methods in pain management. ■

Atrial Natriuretic Factor

Besides its obvious function, the heart is part of the endocrine system. Specific cells located in the right atrium produce atrial natriuretic hormone. As the fibers stretch when blood returns to the heart, the cells release the hormone. Atrial natriuretic hormone works like a calcium channel blocker, inhibiting aldosterone secretion, thus lowering blood pressure by increasing the amount of water excreted, and also inhibits the release of ADH, resulting in the same effect.

Erythropoietin

If oxygen levels in the body decrease, the kidneys produce erythropoietin to stimulate the production of red blood cells in the bone marrow.

Insulin-Like Growth Factor

Insulin-like growth factor is produced primarily in the liver and looks like the insulin molecule. The factor is released in response to growth hormone and stimulates the growth in target cells of insulin, matrix production in cartilage, and growth of fibroblasts in connective tissue. Insulin-like growth factor also synthesizes lipids and glycogen in adipose tissue.

Gastrointestinal Hormones

Gastrointestinal hormones were the first hormones discovered. The mucosa of the gastrointestinal tract produces these hormones and releases them when food is present to help regulate digestion. Although many types of gastrointestinal hormones are produced, we give only a brief overview of three of the most prominent.

Gastrin is produced in the mucosal cells of the stomach and duodenum and stimulates the release of hydrochloric acid and pepsin from the stomach. *Secretin,* produced by the small intestine, stimulates the release of pancreatic digestive enzymes. *Cholecystokinin* is produced in the mucosa of the intestine and secreted into the bloodstream. Cholecystokinin controls digestion based on the amount of food located in the gastrointestinal tract. Cholecystokinin causes the release of bile from the gallbladder, stimulates the pancreas to release its digestive enzymes, and inhibits the secretion of stomach enzymes.

Tissue Hormones

Unlike most hormones that travel to distant target cells, most of the tissue hormones work in the vicinity of or on the exact organs where they are found. These local hormones are called *prostaglandins* and are a group of about 14 unsaturated fatty acid hormones. Prostaglandins are important and powerful substances found in a variety of tissues. They play an important role in communication and control of many body functions but do not meet the definition of a typical hormone. Prostaglandins are specific, highly concentrated, and the shortest acting of the naturally occurring biologic compounds. They are important in overall endocrine regulation and vascular, metabolic, gastrointestinal, reproductive, respiratory, and inflammatory functions.

Inflammation causes release of prostaglandins and histamines, resulting in vasodilation and pain. Aspirin and other antiinflammatory agents act as analgesics by inhibiting the synthesis of prostaglandins. Aspirin also acts as an anticoagulant by preventing the release of the prostaglandins that cause platelet clumping (Activity 6-12).

SUMMARY

The ability to integrate knowledge into practical application, including effective clinical reasoning and decision making, is the foundation of competent practice. Regardless of whether we provide informed consent, the foundation of the work is taking a history, doing a physical assessment, determining outcome goals for the client, charting, maintaining appropriate scope of practice, supporting interdisciplinary teams, and understanding anatomy and physiology. The endocrine system may seem removed from the therapeutic application of massage but it is not. Massage powerfully interacts with the endocrine system, a major system of control.

Endocrine functions coordinate most body functions with the nervous system. The nervous system functions as the yang portion, working quickly, expending energy, and responding to demand, whereas the endocrine system functions as the yin, sustaining, coordinating, and restoring physiologic function. The wisdom of ancient healing arts combines with the concreteness of scientific understanding to validate the wonder of human form and function. These two systems of control (the nervous system and the endocrine system) provide the organic basis for the healing mysteries. As our understanding increases, more of the knowledge found in Eastern and Western healing traditions, ancient and future thought, and body, mind, and spirit likely will blend into our understanding.

evolve

On the Fritz EVOLVE site under Course Materials Chapter 6 are several critical thinking multiple choice questions related to how therapeutic massage affects the endocrine system. Read through these and take the quiz, and then review your answers.

ACTIVITY 6-12

Review all the hormone functions described in this chapter and make an intuitive choice by picking the one gland you believe needs the most consideration in support of your personal homeostasis and endocrine health. Justify the choice. After this choice, design a support program for yourself that includes a form of therapeutic massage and movement therapy.

Example

Thyroid: The idea that the thyroid is linked to communication and creativity intrigues me because a large part of my day is involved in communicating to teach others. Also, the link to metabolism and oxygen consumption seems relevant to my busy lifestyle. Because osteoporosis is a concern and healthy thyroid function supports proper bone density, it would serve me to support my thyroid function.

Program: The hypothalamus stimulates thyroid function in response to cold. As a program to support thyroid function, I could first take a warm shower in the morning and then turn the water to a cold shower. I could seek out a polarity practitioner and work on balancing my throat chakra. I could also increase my exercise walking pace to support oxygen delivery to the cells. Investigation of nutritional support for the thyroid along with a sound diet would be appropriate.

Your Turn

Gland:

Program:

WORKBOOK SECTION

SHORT ANSWER

1. What are the traditional endocrine glands?

____
____
____
____

2. What are endocrine tissues? Give examples.

____
____
____
____

3. What are the functions of hormones?

____
____
____
____
____

4. What is the difference between hormones and neurotransmitters?

____
____
____
____

5. Briefly describe hypersecretion and its causes.

____
____
____
____

6. Briefly describe hyposecretion and its causes.

____
____
____
____

FILL IN THE BLANK

The main differences between endocrine system and nervous system control are speed and duration of effect. The nervous system is (1) fast acting with a (2) short duration of effect, whereas the endocrine system is (3) slow acting with a (4) long duration of effect.

The concentration of a (5) hormone in the blood is determined by the rate of release and the speed of inactivation and removal from the body. The term (6) half-life describes the time required for half of the hormone to be eliminated from the bloodstream. Hormones are secreted by endocrine glands and other specialized cells into the bloodstream to bind to specific (7) receptors on or in their (8) target cells. In a (9) lock-and-key mechanism, hormones bind only to receptor molecules that fit them exactly.

The (10) hypothalamus is the link between the body/mind and the nerve/endocrine function. During stress, it translates nerve impulses into hormone secretions by endocrine glands. The (11) pituitary, or hypophysis, is located in the head at about eye level. It sits in a recessed area in the sphenoid bone and secretes hormones that regulate growth, fluid balance, lactation, and childbirth.

The (12) thyroid gland lies on the trachea below the thyroid cartilage. It consists of a right and left lobe connected by a bridge (isthmus), resulting in a butterfly shape. It regulates metabolism in the body by maintaining an adequate amount of oxygen consumption at the cellular level.

The (13) parathyroid glands are made up of four round, pea-sized bodies located on the posterior surface of the thyroid lobes. Their hormone, parathormone, when combined with vitamin D, decreases the amount of calcium excreted, causes the release of calcium from bone, and absorbs more calcium from the gastrointestinal tract,

Workbook Section

resulting in an increase in blood levels of calcium and phosphorus.

The (14) pancreas is a long, slender gland located behind the stomach. It is both an exocrine and endocrine gland.

We have two (15) ~~pituitary~~ adrenal glands, one on top of each of our kidneys. Each gland consists of an outer layer called the cortex and inner portion called the medulla.

The (16) testes + ovaries are the male and female gonads. They are located in the pelvic cavity and produce sex hormones identical to those of the adrenal cortex.

The (17) pineal gland is a tiny gland inside the brain within the diencephalon and is surrounded by pia mater. The complete functions of this gland have not been identified. Serotonin, norepinephrine, dopamine, histamine, and other neurotransmitters and hormones have been identified from this gland, but its major function seems to be to secrete melatonin. The gland is light sensitive and is involved with regulating the rhythmic patterns of the body.

The (18) thymus gland is located deep to the sternum and mediastinum of the thorax and between the lungs at the level of the fourth and fifth thoracic vertebrae. Often considered part of the lymphatic system and identified as the master gland of the immune system, it does have endocrine secretions.

PROBLEM SOLVING

Read the problem presented. There is no correct answer; rather the exercise is intended to assist the student in developing the analytic and decision-making skills necessary in professional practice. After reading the problem, follow the next six steps:

1. Identify the facts presented in the information.
2. Identify the possibilities ("what if" statements) presented or develop your own possibilities that relate to the facts.
3. Evaluate each possibility in terms of the logical cause and effect and pros and cons.
4. Consider the effect on the persons involved.
5. Write each answer in the space provided.
6. Develop your solution by answering the question posed.

Problem

In the subclinical or early onset stages of many endocrine dysfunctions the symptoms are vague and may be mistaken easily for stress-related disease. More than in any area of pathology, persons may seek therapeutic massage and movement therapists to deal with what seem to be simple stress-related symptoms. In reality, many forms of stress-induced disease are endocrine related and actually can be managed by stress management lifestyle changes. Who is to know that a heavy stress load is not causing a substantial amount of endocrine dysfunction? Could it be possible that some early stage endocrine dysfunction resolves itself when the body is better able to handle the stress load? Would the client be best served if stress management and a healthful lifestyle were the first intervention?

Of concern is the need to refer those with endocrine symptoms for proper diagnosis and the willingness of the medical community to take a look at symptoms of early onset endocrine dysfunction. Changes in lifestyle and more generalized health approaches that support homeostasis can be used successfully after a thorough medical workup.

On the other side of this issue, even if a referral for diagnosis is made, we sometimes feel that we have to be really sick before the condition can be identified by standard laboratory tests. What do low or high normals mean? Are these ends of the normal spectrum the beginning of dysfunction? What is normal anyway? Endocrine function is so variable, depending on so many physiologic factors, that the result of medical tests could be questioned easily. Maybe running the same test on different days would give a more reliable norm for a particular person. Therapeutic massage therapists need to observe subtle symptoms that could indicate endocrine dysfunction and refer clients to other health care professionals.

Question

What is the responsibility for referral by the massage therapist and what type of education is necessary to support educated decisions in these matters? Analyze the information to formulate your response to the question posed. An example is provided as a guide to get you started. You fill in at least two more statements.

Facts

1. In the subclinical or early onset stages of many endocrine dysfunctions, the symptoms are vague and may be mistaken easily for stress-related disease.

2. ______________________________

____

3. ______________________________

____

Possibilities

1. Bodywork therapists may not be trained adequately to recognize these symptoms.
2. ____

____
3. ____

____

Logical Cause and Effect

1. Because the symptoms are not recognized, the massage practitioner may not refer clients.
2. ____

____
3. ____

____

Effect

1. Individuals may be confused by the symptoms and not understand the referral.
2. ____

____
3. ____

____

What is the responsibility for referral of the massage therapist and what type of education is necessary to support educated decisions in these matters?

____

____

____

____

____

____

____

____

____

____

FURTHER STUDY

Using additional resource material, (see Works Consulted list at the back of this book), identify chapters pertaining to the information presented in this chapter. Locate the information presented in this text and then elaborate by writing a paragraph of additional information on each of the following:

Hypothalamus

____

____

____

____

____

____

____

____

Growth hormone

____

____

____

____

____

____

____

____

Type II, or non–insulin-dependent, diabetes

____

____

____

____

____

____

____

____

Workbook Section

Aldosterone

Pineal gland

Thymus

Prostaglandins

Professional Application

Refer to Chapter 2 of this text to review negative feedback loops. Remember, if a stimulus (stress) disrupts homeostasis in a controlled condition monitored by receptors, afferent receptors send input to a control center. The signal is interpreted and output responses to effectors are sent to bring about a change or response that alters the controlled condition, returning it to balance.

If the response reverses the original stimulus, the system is a negative feedback system. Negative feedback systems stabilize physiologic function and are responsible for maintaining a constant internal environment. Most feedback systems are of this type.

Identify a hyposecretion and hypersecretion pathologic condition resulting from a failure of the negative feedback loop control. Then develop a plan for using therapeutic massage and movement therapy to support the care received by the primary physician. Justify each recommendation.

Complete the following:

1. Identify the hormone and gland.
2. Identify the pathologic condition.
3. List possible medical interventions.
4. Develop the support care plan.
5. Justify the plan.

Hypersecretion

1.
2.
3.
4.
5.

Hyposecretion

1.
2.
3.
4.
5.

Answer Key

Short Answer

1. Pituitary, thyroid, parathyroid, adrenal, pineal, and thymus; also the pancreas, ovaries, testes, and hypothalamus
2. They are separate tissues in the body that secrete hormones. They include the heart and intestinal mucus membranes.
3. They mobilize the defenses of the body against stressors; maintain electrolyte, water, and nutrient balance in the blood; and regulate cellular metabolism and energy balance. They direct the creation of our form, especially during reproduction, growth, and development.
4. The main difference is location. When they are found in the bloodstream or in a tissue, they are called hormones. When found in the synapses, they are neurotransmitters.
5. Hypersecretion is the release of too much hormone and often is caused by tumors, immune system dysfunction (autoimmunity), and failure of the feedback mechanisms to regulate secretion.
6. Many factors can cause a gland to reduce its hormonal output. Hyposecretion may be caused by tumors, tissue death, or abnormal operation of the regulatory feedback loops. Abnormal immune function also can reduce hormonal output, as well as insensitivity of the target cells to tropic hormones.

Fill in the Blank

1. fast acting
2. short
3. slow acting
4. long
5. hormone
6. half-life
7. receptors
8. target cells
9. lock-and-key
10. hypothalamus
11. pituitary
12. thyroid
13. parathyroid
14. pancreas
15. adrenal
16. testes and ovaries
17. pineal
18. thymus

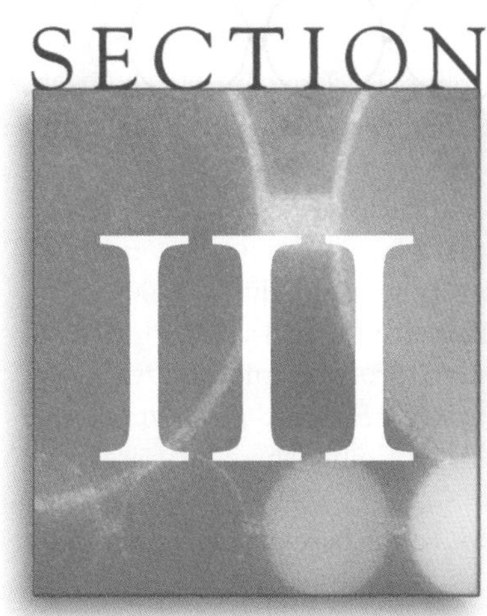

Support, Movement, and Biomechanics

Massage professionals directly interact with the musculoskeletal system more than with any other body system. Because the musculoskeletal system and the rest of the body are interdependent, through the anatomy of this system we are able to influence the physiology of the entire body, supporting the maintenance of homeostasis.

A major portion of this text is devoted to the study of the anatomy of bones, joints, and muscles; the parts, we might say—and the body has a lot of parts. Through an understanding of the design of movement, we can appreciate the physiology (function) of movement. This information will benefit the student in two ways:

- First, this knowledge is the foundation for the primary technical requirements of the therapeutic massage discipline.
- Second, the student will be better able to work with other health care and service professionals as part of an interdisciplinary team, sharing information and treatments so as to best serve each client.

This unit begins with the study of the bones and ends with lessons in developing skills in assessment procedures used to evaluate human movement, or biomechanics. The successive chapters build on each other, so that when the student reaches Chapter 10, *Biomechanics Basics*, he or she will be familiar with the terminology that describes biomechanics. With a solid foundation, the student will be able to predict the movement pattern of a particular bone, joint, or muscle unit.

Students should set themselves the following goals for this section:

1. Learn the names and landmarks of the bones and muscles.
2. Identify the attachment points of a muscle or group of muscles (the bones to which the ends of the muscle or muscles attach).
3. Identify the bones that move when the muscles contract and shorten. Usually one bone remains still while the other bone or bones are pulled toward or away from it. The point of motion is the joint.
4. Identify the types of action; for example, flexion, extension, and rotation.

Throughout the study of this section, the student will find it beneficial to refer to previous chapters to reinforce the knowledge and terminology needed to understand how we move.

Many references were consulted in the development of this section. Not all authorities agree on the specifics of the anatomy or the function of the musculoskeletal system. The most commonly accepted information has been adapted for use in this text.

Important clinicians, researchers, and teachers have been major influences in the development of this section; they include Dr. Joseph Muscolino, Dr. Janet Travell, Dr. David Simons, Dr. John Mennell, Dr. Philip Greenman, Dr. Leon Chaitow, Dr. David Gurevich, and Dr. John Warfel, to name a few.

The major resource for the activities in Chapter 10 was the classic text by Helen Hislop and Jacqueline Montgomery, *Daniels and Worthingham's Muscle Testing Techniques of Manual Examination*, first published in 1946 and now in its seventh edition (2002). The methods have been adapted and simplified for this text. Florence Kendall's "Muscle Testing Video Library" was a valuable tool in this simplification process. Another text used extensively in the development of Chapter 10 was *Therapeutic Exercise: Foundations and Techniques* (fourth edition), by Carolyn Kisner and Lynn Allen Colby. These texts are listed in the Works Consulted section of this book.

All of these individuals, as well as countless others, supplied the base of information that has been organized for presentation in this section.

CHAPTER 7

Skeletal System

▼ CHAPTER OBJECTIVES

After completing this chapter, the student will be able to perform the following:

- List the seven main functions of the skeletal system.
- Describe the structure and development of bone.
- List and describe the six shapes of bone.
- Identify bony landmarks.
- Describe the two divisions of the skeleton and list the bones in each.
- List and describe the individual bones of the body by region.

▼ CHAPTER OUTLINE

▼ KEY TERMS

Appendicular skeleton (ap-en-DIK-u-lar) The part of the skeleton composed of the limbs and their attachments.

Articulation (ar-tik-u-LAY-shun) Another word for joint, the structure created when bones connect to each other.

Axial skeleton (AK-see-al) The axis of the body; the axial skeleton consists of the head, vertebral column (the spine), and the ribs and sternum and provides the body with form and protection.

Compact (dense) bone The hard portion of bone that protects spongy bone and provides the firm framework of the bone and the body. The osteocytes in this type of bone are located in concentric rings around a central haversian canal, through which nerves and blood vessels pass.

Endoskeleton The bony support structure found inside the human body that accommodates growth.

Endosteum (en-DOSS-tee-um) A thin membrane of connective tissue that lines the marrow cavity of a bone.

Periosteum (PAIR-ee-OSS-tee-um) The thin membrane of connective tissue that covers bones except at articulations.

Piezoelectric (PIE-eh-zoh-EE-lek-trik) The quality of bones that allows them to deform slightly and vibrate when electrical currents pass through them and to produce minute electric current when deformed or compressed. Bone formation patterns follow lines of stress load directed by the piezoelectric currents.

Sesamoid bones (SES-ah-moyd) Round bones that often are embedded in tendons and joint capsules. The largest of these is the patella.

Spongy (cancellous) bone The lighter weight portion of bone that is made up of trabeculae.

Trabeculae (tra-BEK-u-lee) An irregular meshing of small, bony plates that makes up spongy bone; its spaces are filled with red marrow.

What would we look like if we did not have bones? Picture yourself as a mass of soft tissue with little form. Managing the forces of gravity would be almost impossible without the structure supplied by our skeletons. Getting from one place to another would be difficult. We would certainly be more susceptible to injury as we slithered around. Have we possibly taken our skeletons for granted? As we explore the most concrete aspect of our anatomy—the skeletal system—the knowledge we acquire will make us appreciate its functions even more, considering what life would be like without it (Activity 7-1).

Human beings have an **endoskeleton,** which means that our support structure is inside us and we grow around it. Some animals, such as lobsters, have an exoskeleton, a support structure that is on the outside of the body. Although an exoskeleton is appropriate for a lobster, it is not for a human being. Because an exoskeleton does not grow at the same rate as the rest of the body, it can become too small; also, an exoskeleton needs to be shed as a new one is grown. An endoskeleton accommodates growth easily.

In this section we will study the bones first. Because muscles attach to bones, learning the names, functions, and various landmarks of the bones helps in locating the muscles studied later in this section. Other chapters focus on the joints, on biomechanics, and on kinesiology (the action of muscles on joints in movement patterns). This chapter contains many illustrations. Studying each one carefully is important. The labeling of the illustrations is often more specific than the major features of the bones discussed in the text.

SKELETAL SYSTEM BASICS

The skeletal system comprises the bones, joints, and related connective tissues. The connective tissue component is important to the functioning of the system. Because the bones do not have enough room for all the muscles to attach, the membranes between the bones and the ligaments at the joints function to expand the skeletal structure, allowing adequate space for muscle attachments. When the structures of the muscles and bones are combined, they form the functional unit known as the musculoskeletal system.

ACTIVITY 7-1

Draw a picture of a human being without bones.

Bones connect at a joint, which is also known as an **articulation.** Ligaments and other connective tissues hold bones together at the joints. Muscle contractions produce the actions that move the joints. The actions of skeletal muscles are voluntary, coordinated by the nervous system.

Main Functions of the Skeletal System

Besides the obvious functions of support and motion, bones have other important roles, including the following:

- Supporting soft tissues and serving as a framework for the entire body
- Providing attachment points for muscles and ligaments
- Protecting delicate internal organs such as the brain, spinal cord, heart, and lungs
- Serving as levers to provide movement begun by the attached muscles
- Storing calcium, phosphorus, and other minerals for release to the body as needed
- Storing lipids in bone marrow for use as energy
- Producing blood cells (hematopoiesis) in the red marrow

Bones

No matter their size, shape, or location, all bones are made of the same fundamental cells and matrix, are covered with the same sheets of connective tissue, and are nourished and stimulated by the same variety of vessels and nerves. Bones develop into different shapes, which serve specific functions.

The protective bones of the skull differ in shape from the supportive and lengthening bones of the limbs. Disease, injury, and aging affect the structure and function of bones. The location and shape of a bone determine its function. The function of a bone can change its structure through a remodeling process, supporting once again the theme of interacting structure and function in a continuous, interdependent cycle.

Bones are hard, dense, and slightly elastic organs of the skeleton. They have their own system of blood, lymphatic vessels, and nerves. The body has 206 bones, with some individual variations; for example, some persons have more or fewer **sesamoid bones** (a type of bone that develops within a tendon or joint capsule) and others may have an extra rib. Although all bones support the body, store calcium and other minerals, and house marrow for the production of red blood cells, some bones play more specific roles. The skull and the vertebral column protect the brain and spinal cord, and the bones of the limbs allow motion.

Bones are composed chiefly of bone tissue, called osseous tissue. Bones are not lifeless, but rather ever changing. The spaces between the cells of bone tissue are permeated with stony deposits of inorganic mineral salts of calcium and phosphorus, along with small amounts of magnesium, potassium, sodium, and carbonate ions. The cells dispersed among these mineral deposits are very much alive.

Two thirds of bone tissue is made up of inorganic minerals, which provide rigidity, and one third of bone tissue is composed of organic material, which provides elasticity. We all understand the need for bone to be rigid, but few of us realize that bone is also somewhat flexible. Without this elasticity, bone would break readily.

Bones are subject to mechanical strain. They must support the weight of the body; disperse the impact shock of activities such as walking, running, and jumping; and withstand the force of muscle contractions.

Bones have a **piezoelectric** quality. Piezoelectric substances such as the collagen in bones deform slightly and vibrate when electric currents pass through them. In reverse, when stretched, twisted, or compressed, bone produces minute electric currents; the strength and direction of these currents change with the direction of the stress load. Bone formation patterns follow lines of stress load directed by these piezoelectric currents. Exactly how this happens is not yet fully understood.

Many cultural and healing traditions assert that certain kinds of stones and other crystalline substances, in particular quartz, have healing qualities. Some spiritual places reputed to have healing qualities are located in areas of stony form, particularly granite, or structures constructed of stone (often granite), or contain statues made of stone. Quartz is considered a piezoelectric material, and granite, often used in building and sculpture, has a high concentration of quartz. We do know that small electric currents can accelerate the healing of broken bones. Does this show a connection? In what way do the small electric currents generated by bone affect homeostasis? Could a physiologic connection exist between the healing disciplines that use stones and these qualities of bone? These traditions are cross-cultural, suggesting the existence of some underlying, physiologically unified thread. The questions are interesting; the connection is plausible (Activity 7-2).

Bone Structure

Bones share four features that allow them to work together as parts of the skeleton. Despite the different shapes of bones, they have these attributes in common:

1. Hard cells and a rigid matrix give bones strength and shape to sustain weight and movement.
2. Bones usually articulate with other bones, thereby transferring forces and movement through the skeleton.
3. A connective tissue structure, called the **periosteum,** covers every bone and provides vessels for nutrition, bone cells for growth, and attachments for tendons and ligaments.

ACTIVITY 7-2

If you were to speculate about the piezoelectric quality of bones and other collagen connective tissues, what do you think would be the effects of the compressive, stretching, and twisting action of massage? List three. An example is provided to get you started.

Example

The electric current produced by compression against bone during massage methods may stimulate the so-called energetic mechanism of meridians, because these Asian energy lines generally follow bones.

Your Turn

1. ______________________________

____

____

2. ______________________________

____

____

3. ______________________________

____

____

4. Oppositional growth of new bone matrix and remodeling of existing bone matrix are responsible for shaping bones.

The structure and function of bones are connected intrinsically. Bones remodel themselves constantly, depending on the functional demand. Although it may seem static, the skeletal system is one of the more dynamic systems of the body.

Bone Development

In the embryo, bone development begins near the end of the second month. The process that creates our skeleton is called ossification. Ossification is a two-part process: first, chondroblasts, or cartilage-forming cells, create the cartilage model of bones. Then, osteoblasts, or bone-building cells, develop the bone tissue from the cartilage model. This process does not create the hard bones with which we are familiar. Instead, these cells remain soft and pliable, allowing the fetus to remain flexible to exit the body more easily during birth.

Shortly after birth, calcification takes place. This hardening of the bones, called osteogenesis, occurs as calcium salts are deposited in the gel-like matrix of the forming bones. Osteocytes are mature bone cells, which maintain the bone during our lifetimes.

The different areas of a bone contain one of two types of tissue, compact bone or spongy bone. **Compact (dense) bone** has little space between its tissues. This hard portion of the bone makes up the main shaft of the long bones and the outer layer of other bones. Compact bone protects spongy bone and provides the firm framework of the bone and the body. The osteocytes in this type of bone are located in concentric rings called lamellae around a central haversian canal, through which nerves and blood vessels pass. Within the hard layers of lamellea, lacunae or small pools of tissue fluid exist. These cylinder-shaped units are called osteons.

The second type, **spongy (cancellous) bone,** has larger spaces between cells than does compact bone, which makes the bones lighter in weight. Cancellous bone is made of an irregular meshing of small, bony plates called **trabeculae** and is found at the ends of the long bones or at the center of other bones. In some bones the trabecular spaces are filled with red marrow, which produces blood cells. Spongy bone tissue forms a supporting grid that can be altered mechanically by construction, destruction, or reorganization of the trabecular network. Piezoelectric current seems to be responsible for guiding these changes, which occur in response to postural change, muscle tension, and the stresses of weight.

Bones contain two kinds of marrow, red and yellow. Red marrow, which manufactures red blood cells, is found at the end of long bones and at the center of other bones of the thorax and pelvis. Yellow marrow of the soup bone type, which is largely fat, is found chiefly in the central cavities of the long bones.

Except for the ends that form joints, bones are covered with a thin membrane of connective tissue, which is called periosteum. On the inside of this membrane are osteoblasts, which are essential to bone formation during periods of growth and in the repair of bones. Blood and lymph vessels in the periosteum play an important role in the nourishment of bone tissue. Nerve fibers in the periosteum make their presence known when they are traumatized, such as a blow to the shin or a fractured arm.

A thinner membrane of connective tissue, called the **endosteum,** lines the marrow cavity of a bone; the endosteum also contains cells that aid in the growth and repair of bone tissue (Figure 7-1).

Articular Cartilage

Bones of synovial or movable joints make physical contact at their cartilaginous ends. The only remaining cartilage in bone is called articular (or hyaline) cartilage; articular cartilage is massaged by joint movement, which aids the absorption of synovial fluid, oxygen, and nutrition. The degenerative process of arthritis involves the breakdown of articular cartilage. Cartilage is a form of connective tissue; it is smooth, slippery, porous, malleable, insensitive, and bloodless and is found wherever bones come together at synovial or freely movable joints. Because cartilage is an integral component of the synovial joint, we discuss it in more detail in Chapter 8.

Ligaments

Ligaments are dense bundles of parallel connective tissue fibers, primarily collagen. Ligaments connect bones and strengthen and stabilize the joints. They are not typically elastic nor do they have much stretch. Some joint positions place ligaments under tension, whereas other positions slacken them. We make only a general mention of ligaments in this chapter. Because ligaments are specific to joint function, we also discuss them in more detail in Chapter 8.

Classification of Bones

The bones of the skeleton are identified by their many different shapes. The customary classifications are as follows:

Flat bones: These generally are more flat than round. Examples: the ribs and skull bones

Irregular bones: These have complex shapes that occur as two or more forms within the same bone structure. Examples: the vertebrae and scapula

Long bones: These bones are longer in one axis than another. Bones of this type are characterized by a medullary cavity, a hollow diaphysis, or shaft, of compact bone, and at least two epiphyses, which are active in the growth of long bones. Most of the bones of the arms and legs are long bones. The hollow structure of the diaphysis gives strength with light weight. Examples: the femur and ulna

Short bones: These are shaped like long bones but are much smaller. These bones make up the structures of the hands, fingers, feet, and toes. This shape of bone also can be classified as long bones. Example: the metacarpals

Cube-shaped bones (sometimes classified as short bones): These are predominately cancellous bone with a thin cortex of compact bone and no cavity. Examples: the wrist bones (carpals) and ankle bones (tarsals)

Sesamoid bones: These are round bones often embedded in tendons and joint capsules. Example: the patella

Bone Growth and Repair

In a long bone the transformation of cartilage into bone begins at the center of the shaft. Later, secondary bone-forming centers develop across the ends of the bones at the epiphyses. The long bones continue to grow in length at these centers through childhood and into the late teens.

A growth spurt often occurs during puberty through the influence of the sex hormones estrogen and testosterone. Both hormones promote the growth of long bones; testosterone also increases bone density. At higher levels of estrogen, long bone growth stops; for this reason, women generally are shorter and have bones that are less dense than those of men (Activity 7-3).

By the late teens or early twenties, again through the influence of the sex hormones, the epiphyses of the long bones close and the bones stop growing in length. Each

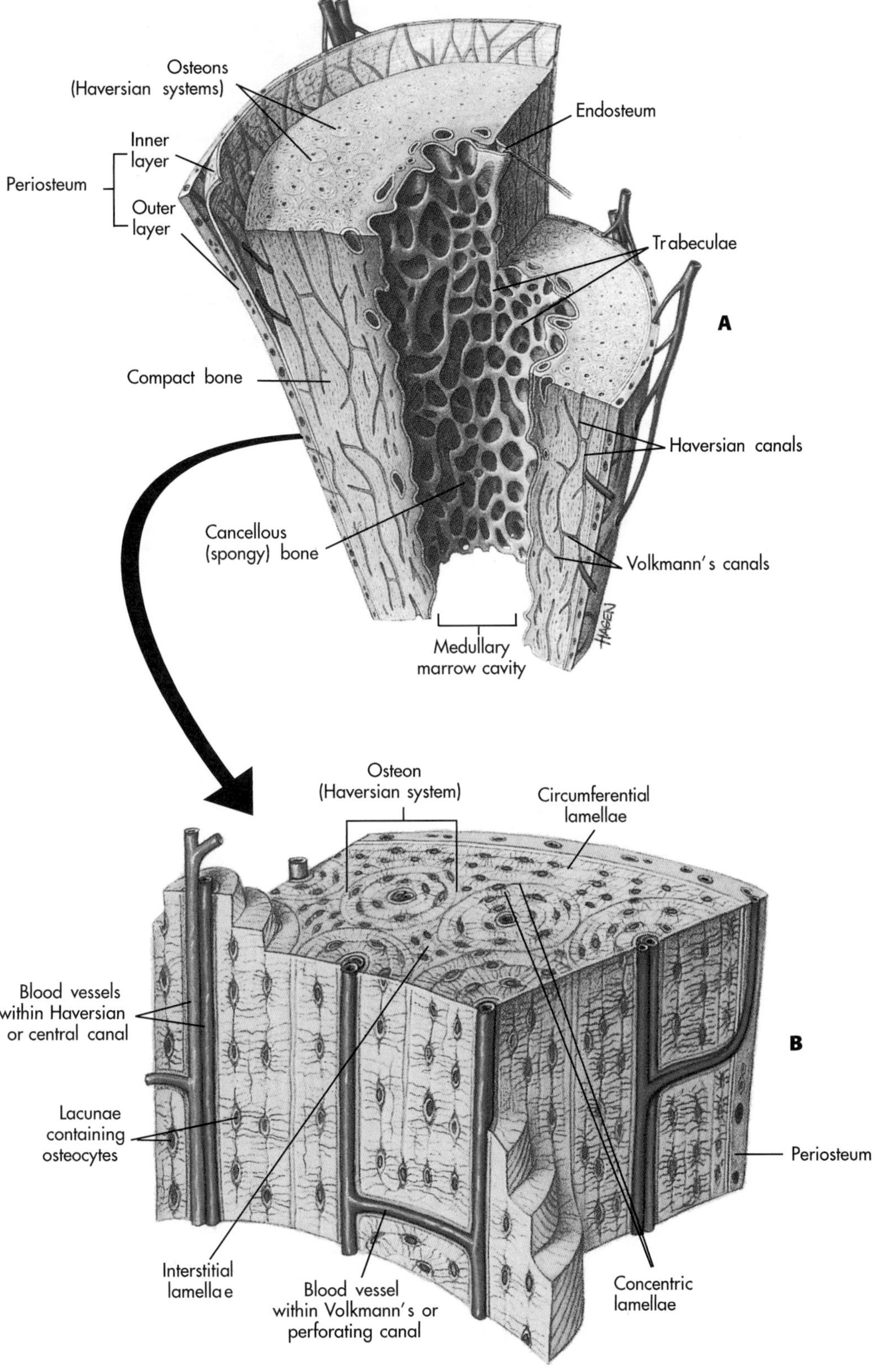

Figure 7-1

Structure of compact and cancellous bone. **A,** Longitudinal section of long bone showing cancellous and compact bone. **B,** Magnified view of compact bone.

Continued

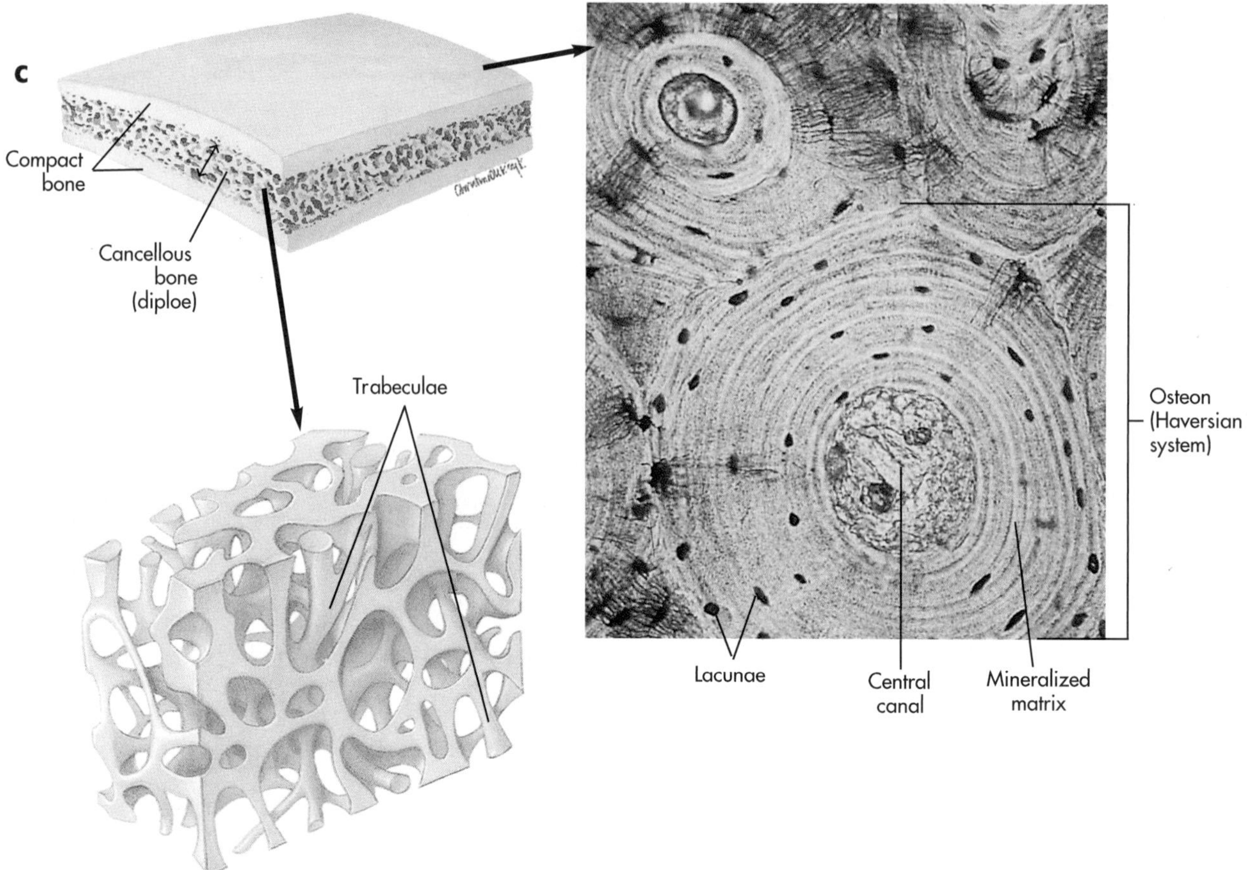

Figure 7-1, cont'd.
Structure of compact and cancellous bone. **C,** Section of flat bone. Outer layers of compact bone surround cancellous bone. The fine structure of compact bone and cancellous bone is shown to the right. (From Thibodeau GA, Patton KT: *Anatomy and physiology,* ed 5, St Louis, 2003, Mosby.)

ACTIVITY 7-3

Refer to Chapter 6 and explain the influence of the sex hormones on bone. Include the page number where you found the information.
An example is provided to get you started.

Example
High estrogen levels slow the growth of girls, including the bones, at puberty (p. 197).
Provide two more explanatory statements.

Your Turn
1. ______________________________
2. ______________________________

Identify two other hormones that affect bone formation. (Hint: See the sections in Chapter 6 on the thyroid and parathyroid glands.)
1. ______________________________
2. ______________________________

bone-forming region hardens and can be seen in radiographic films as a thin line across the end of the bone. Physicians can judge the future growth of the bone by the appearance of these lines on the radiographic film.

As we grow, our bones widen and lengthen, and the central cavity follows this change in size. This all takes place because osteocytes are added in some areas of bone and reabsorbed in others.

As mentioned previously, children are more flexible because their bodies contain more cartilage and soft bone cells; complete calcification has not taken place yet. In older adults, the situation is reversed; bone cells outnumber cartilage cells, and the bone is more brittle because it contains more minerals and fewer blood vessels. This makes the bones prone to fracture and slower to heal.

Physicians treat fractures by reduction, which means that the physician pulls the broken ends into alignment to establish the continuity of the bone so that healing can take place. The process of fracture healing is truly one of regeneration. Fractures heal with normal bone, not with scar tissue. Physicians perform closed reduction by manual manipulation of the fractured bone so that the fragments are brought into proper alignment and make no surgical incision. Open fractures are highly contaminated and must be debrided and cleaned in the operating room. A fracture also may require internal fixation with pins, nails, metal.

Once the physician accomplishes closed reduction, he or she immobilizes the bone by application of a cast or by an apparatus exerting traction on the distal end of the bone.

Acute fracture healing follows the same three phases that soft tissue does but is more complex. In general, acute fracture healing has five stages: hematoma formation, cellular proliferation, callus formation, ossification, and remodeling.

Acute inflammation usually lasts approximately 4 days. When a bone fractures, trauma to the periosteum and surrounding soft tissue occurs. A hematoma accumulates in the medullary canal and surrounds soft tissue in the first 48 to 72 hours. The exposed ends of vascular channels become occluded with clotted blood accompanied by death of the osteocytes, disrupting the intact blood supply. The dead bone and related soft tissue begin to elicit a typical inflammatory reaction. The hematoma in a bone fracture gradually forms a fibrous junction between the fractured ends, which becomes a fibrous callus, and then cartilage, and finally a woven bone. With adequate immobilization and compression, the bone ends become crossed with a new haversian system that eventually leads to the laying down of primary bone. The ossification stage is the completion of the laying down of bone. The fracture is bridged and firmly united. Osteoclasts resorb excess callus.

Remodeling occurs after resorption of the callus and laying down of trabecular bone along the lines of stress. Complete remodeling may take many years. The influence of bioelectrical stimulation (piezoelectric effect) is the basis for development of new trabecular bone to be laid down at the point of greatest stress.

Skeletal Changes Caused by Aging

As we age, various changes occur in the skeleton. Loss of calcium begins earlier in women than in men. The bone matrix is not replaced as quickly because the body produces less protein; this may lead to a problem with brittle bones. Bone fractures also heal more slowly in elderly persons. Beginning about age 40, the intervertebral disks begin to thin, and the average person loses a half inch of height every 20 years. The vertebral bodies specifically lose height in our later years. The cartilage on the ribs calcifies, leading to a decrease in the diameter of the rib cage and a more barrel-shaped chest, caused by the lack of flexibility.

Bony Landmarks

The contour of bones varies and includes configurations such as flat areas, knobs, projections, spikes, dents, holes, and ridges. These landmarks often serve as regions for muscle attachment or provide passage or space for nerves and vessels. The student learns the bony landmarks because this knowledge will assist him or her in learning muscle attachments later in this study (Activity 7-4).

Depressions and Openings

The following are the types of depressions and openings found in bones:

Canal: A tunnel or tube in bone. Example: the carotid canal in the temporal bone

Fissure: A groove or slit between two bones. Example: the orbital fissure of the sphenoid bone

Foramen: An opening in a bone. Example: the vertebral foramen of the spinal column (through which the nerves pass)

Fossa: A shallow depression in the surface or at the end of a bone. Example: the infraspinous and supraspinous fossae of the scapula

ACTIVITY 7-4

For each of the landmarks listed, identify a metaphor that will help you remember what each represents. A few examples are provided to get you started.

Examples

Foramen: hula hoop
Groove: ditch
Sinus: cave
Now, make up some of your own.

Your Turn

Canal:
Fissure:
Foramen:
Fossa:
Groove:
Meatus:
Notch:
Sinus:
Sulcus:
Condyle:
Head:
Facet:
Process:
Trochlea:
Crest:
Epicondyle:
Spinous process or spine:
Trochanter:
Tubercle:
Tuberosity:

Groove: A depression in the bone that holds blood vessels, nerves, or tendons. Example: the radial groove of the humerus

Meatus: A tunnel or canal found in a bone. Example: the canal in the skull that extends from the external ear to the eardrum

Notch: An indentation or large groove. Example: the greater and lesser sciatic notches of the ilium

Sinus: An air cavity within a bone. Example: the frontal sinuses

Processes That Form Joints

The following are types of processes that form joints:

Condyle: A rounded projection at the end of a bone that articulates with other bones to form a joint. Example: the medial condyle of the femur

Head: A rounded projection atop the neck of a bone. Example: the head of the femur

Facet: A smooth, flat surface. Example: the facet of a rib or vertebra

Process: Any prominent, bony growth that projects. Example: the olecranon process of the ulna

Trochlea: A pulley-shaped structure. Example: the trochlea of the humerus

Processes to Which Tendons and Ligaments Attach

The following are types of bony processes to which tendons and ligaments attach:

Crest: A ridge on a bone. Example: the iliac crest

Epicondyle: A projection above a condyle. Example: the medial epicondyle of the femur

Line: A ridge that is smaller than a crest. Example: the linea aspera of the femur

Spinous process, spine, or spina: A sharp, bony, or slender projection. Example: the spinous process of the vertebral column or scapular spine

Trochanter: One of two large, bony processes found only on the femur. Example: the greater or lesser trochanter

Tubercle: A small, rounded process. Example: the adductor tubercle of the femur

Tuberosity: A large, rounded protuberance. Example: the tibial tuberosity

Divisions of the Skeleton

The skeleton is divided into two groups of bones: the **axial skeleton** and the **appendicular skeleton.**

The axial skeleton, which forms the axis of the body, consists of the head, vertebral column (spine), ribs, and sternum. The axial skeleton provides the body with form and protection. The appendicular skeleton is composed of the limbs of the body and their attachments (Activity 7-5). The shoulder and hip girdles, which have similar structures, connect the appendicular skeleton to the axial skeleton.

The long bones of the upper and lower limbs, in combination with the muscles, provide our fine and gross motor movements. Similar in design, these long bones are the humerus, radius, and ulna in the upper limbs and the femur, tibia, and fibula in the lower limbs. In the same manner, the short carpals of the wrist and the tarsals of the ankle allow for the flexibility needed in the hands and feet.

The six bones of the ear make up a third group of bones.

The more we study the basic construction of the skeletal system, the more we notice the elegant and simple pattern. Simplicity and repetition of form reflect this effective biomechanical design (Figure 7-2).

ACTIVITY 7-5

Match six similar sets of bones of the upper and lower appendicular skeleton. An example is provided.

Example

Femur/humerus

Your Turn

1. ______________________
2. ______________________
3. ______________________
4. ______________________
5. ______________________
6. ______________________

INDIVIDUAL BONY FRAMEWORK BY REGION

The skeletal system, just as the whole body, functions as a unit. To support learning, information about the skeletal system will be described in sections, according to regions of the body.

Bones of the Axial Skeleton

Framework of the Head

The bony framework of the head, or skull, is made up of the cranial bones and the facial bones (Figure 7-3).

Eight cranial bones enclose and protect the brain:

- The frontal bone forms the forehead, the anterior portion of the roof of the skull, the top of the eye sockets, and part of the floor of the cranium. The frontal sinuses (air spaces) are within the frontal bone and open into the nasal cavities.
- Two parietal bones form most of the sides and top of the cranium.

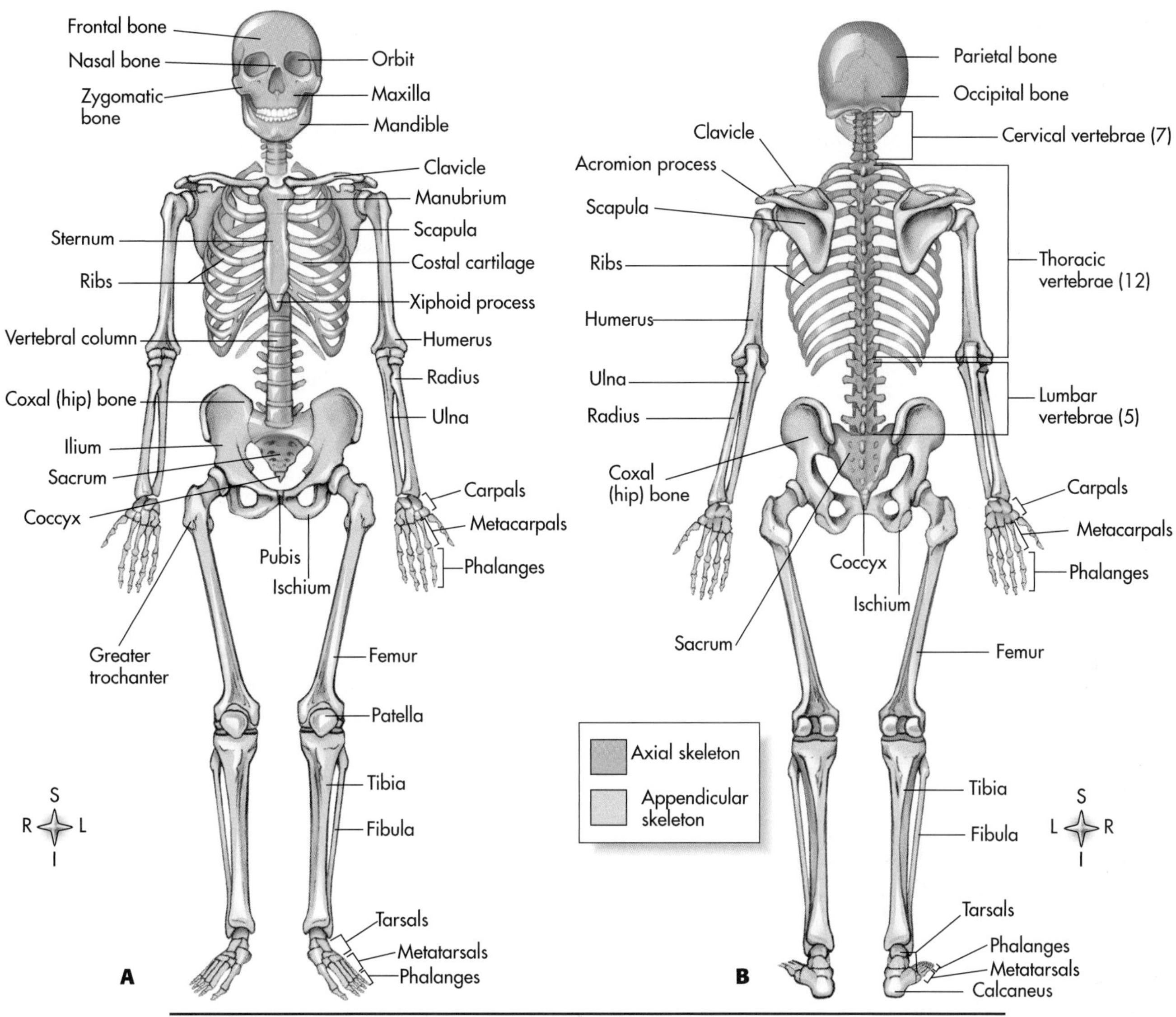

Figure 7-2
Skeleton. **A,** Anterior view. **B,** Posterior view. (From Thibodeau GA, Patton KT: *Anatomy and physiology,* ed 5, St Louis, 2003, Mosby.)

- Two temporal bones form part of the side and part of the floor of the skull. Each temporal bone contains mastoid sinuses, an ear canal, an eardrum, and the middle and inner ears.
- The ethmoid bone, which is part of the anterior portion of the cranial floor, is a light, spongy bone located between the eyes. The ethmoid bone forms part of the medial wall of the eye sockets and most of the nasal roof and contains some of the paranasal sinuses. An extension of the ethmoid bone forms most of the superior portion of the nasal septum. If this bone is fractured, its proximity to the brain means that cerebrospinal fluid could leak into the nasal cavity. A runny nose that develops after a head injury could be the result of trauma to the sinuses or an indication of a serious condition.
- The sphenoid bone is in the middle of the base of the skull in front of the temporal bones. When viewed from above, the bone looks like a bat with its wings extended. The sphenoid sinuses are located within this bone. The sella turcica, or Turkish saddle, is a cavity on the superior surface of the body of the sphenoid that supports the pituitary gland.
- The occipital bone forms the posterior portion and a large part of the base of the cranium. This large, curved bone provides attachments for muscles of the neck and trunk.

Fourteen facial bones form the front of the skull:

- The mandible, or lower jawbone, is the only voluntarily movable bone of the skull. The largest of the facial bones, the mandible forms the chin, which is classified as a mental prominence.

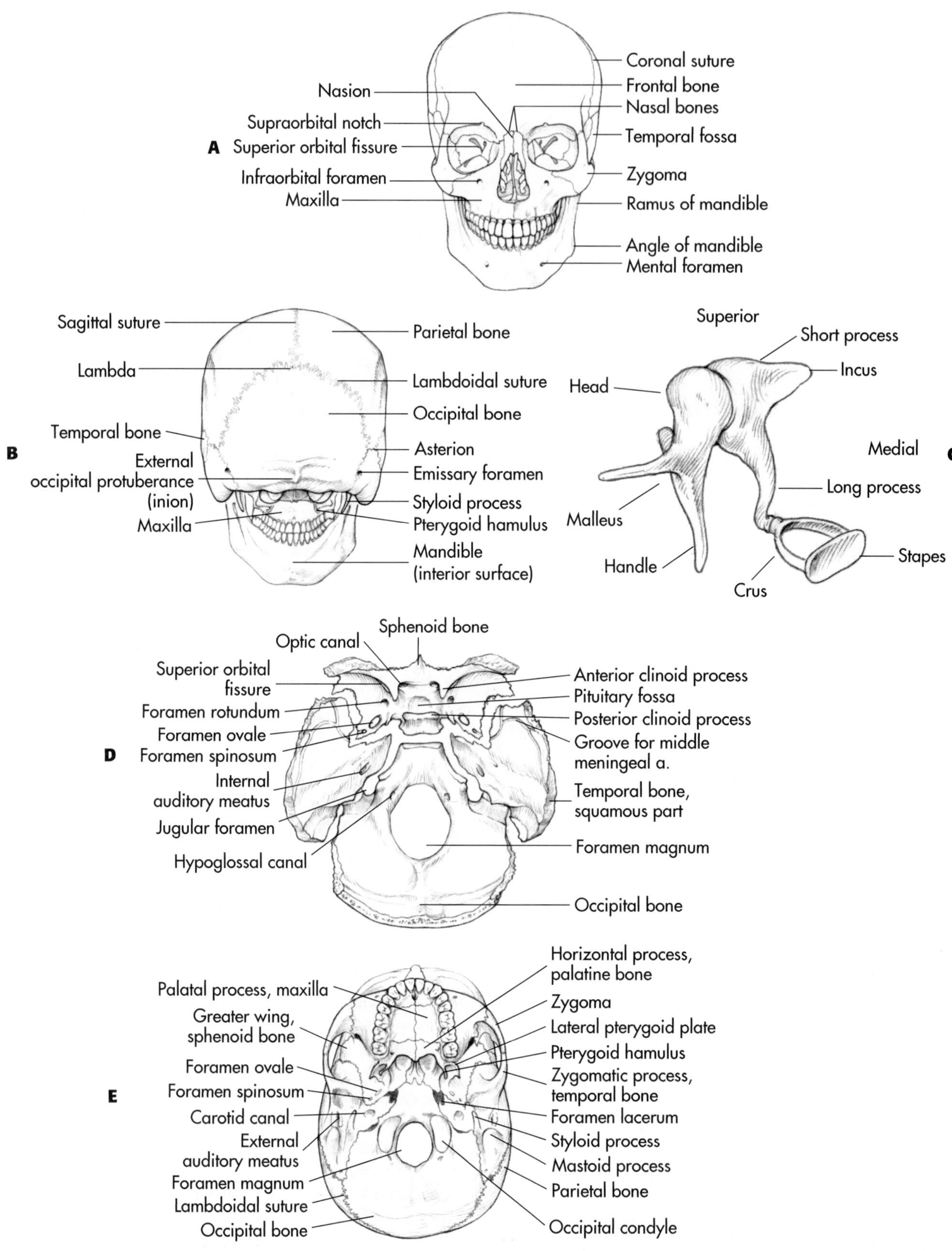

Figure 7-3

A, Anterior (frontal) view of the skull. **B,** Posterior view of the skull. **C,** The three ossicles. The malleus attaches to the inner surface of the tympanic membrane. The incus links the malleus to the stapes. The stapes is attached to the wall of the inner ear. **D,** Detailed view of the base of the skull. The sphenoid, occipital, and temporal bones are presented as slightly separated to show that many of the important apertures traversing the floor of the skull are found within one of these bones or along their mutual borders. **E,** Basal view of the skull, showing several of the important foramina that convey nerves and vessels in and out of the cranial cavity. (From Mathers LH et al: *Clinical anatomy principles,* St. Louis, 1996, Mosby.)

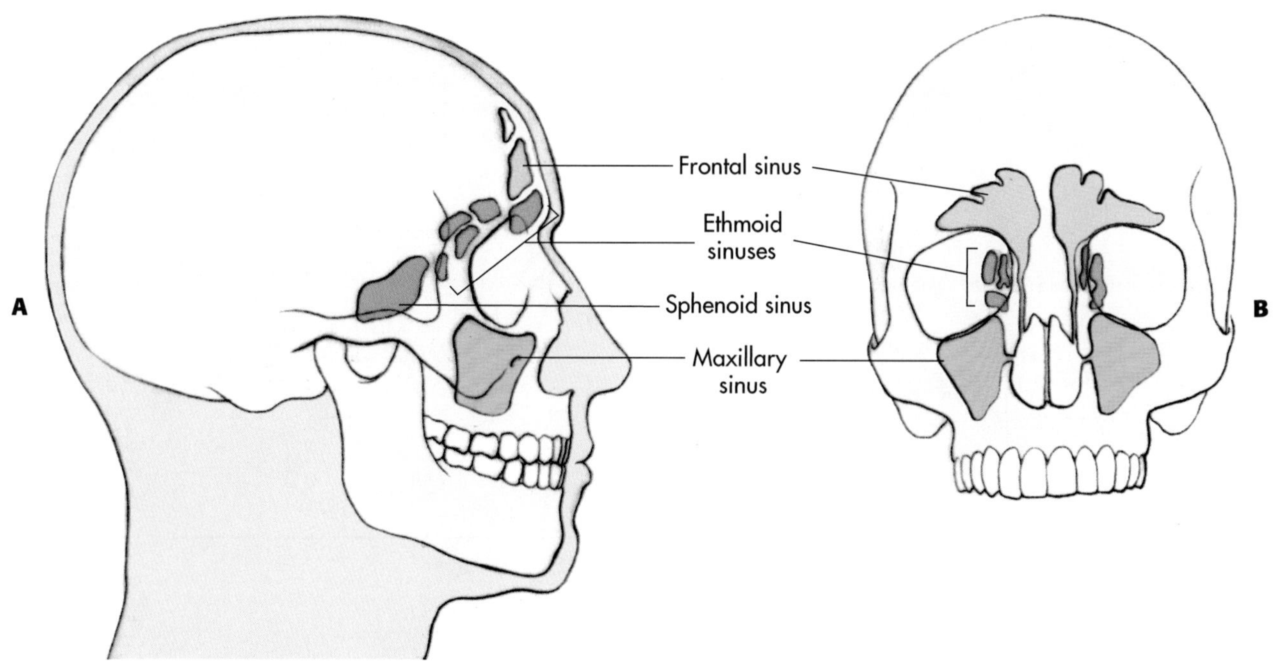

Figure 7-4
Air sinuses in the nose. **A,** Lateral view. **B,** Anterior view.
(From Mathers LH et al: *Clinical anatomy principles,* St. Louis, 1996, Mosby.)

- Two maxilla bones unite to form the upper jawbone, part of the floor of the eye sockets, part of the roof of the mouth, including the front of the hard palate, and the outer walls and floor of the nasal cavity. Each maxilla contains a maxillary sinus, a large air space that empties into the nasal cavity.
- Two zygomatic bones, or cheekbones, form the prominences of the cheeks and a portion of the floor and outer wall of the eye sockets.
- Two small, oblong nasal bones, in the superior middle of the face, form the bridge of the nose.
- Two lacrimal bones, each about the size and shape of a fingernail, are posterior and lateral to the nasal bone. They form part of the medial wall of the eye sockets.
- The vomer is a triangular bone that forms the inferior and posterior nasal septum.
- Two L-shaped palatine bones form the posterior portion of the hard palate and part of the floor of the nasal cavity.
- Two inferior nasal concha bones form a portion of the lateral wall of the nasal cavities. They work with the superior and middle conchae of the ethmoid bone to circulate and filter air that enters the nose.

In addition to the cranial and facial bones, other bones of the axial skeleton are found in the neck and head. The six ossicles, three in each middle ear, are discussed in Chapter 5. The hyoid bone is a U-shaped bone. Although the bone is attached to the temporal bone by muscles and ligaments, it does not form an articulation with any other bones and supports tongue function.

The structure of the skull is important to the function of other systems. Nerves and blood vessels enter and exit the skull through spaces, or foramina, in the base. Muscles attach to the various projections and prominences on the outside of the skull. The sinuses are air spaces that resonate the voice and remove some of the weight of the bones, making the head lighter (Figure 7-4).

Between the bones of the skull are specialized joints called sutures. The four most prominent sutures are the sagittal suture, between the parietal bones; the lambdoidal suture, between the parietal bones and the occipital bone; the coronal suture, between the parietal bones and the frontal bones; and the squamous suture, between the temporal and parietal bones.

In the skull of an infant, bone formation is incomplete in some areas; these soft spots are called fontanelles. Found between the cranial bones, fontanelles are formed from dense connective tissue, which is replaced with bone as the infant grows. The fontanelles allow for compression of the skull as the infant travels through the birth canal and for expansion of the skull as the brain grows. They close when the child is 18 to 24 months old. The largest of the fontanelles is the anterior fontanelle, found near the front of the head at the junction between the two parietal bones and the frontal bone (Figure 7-5; Activity 7-6).

Framework of the Trunk

The skeletal structure of the trunk is made up of the vertebral column and the bones of the chest. A child's vertebral column has 33 (or sometimes 34) irregularly shaped bones,

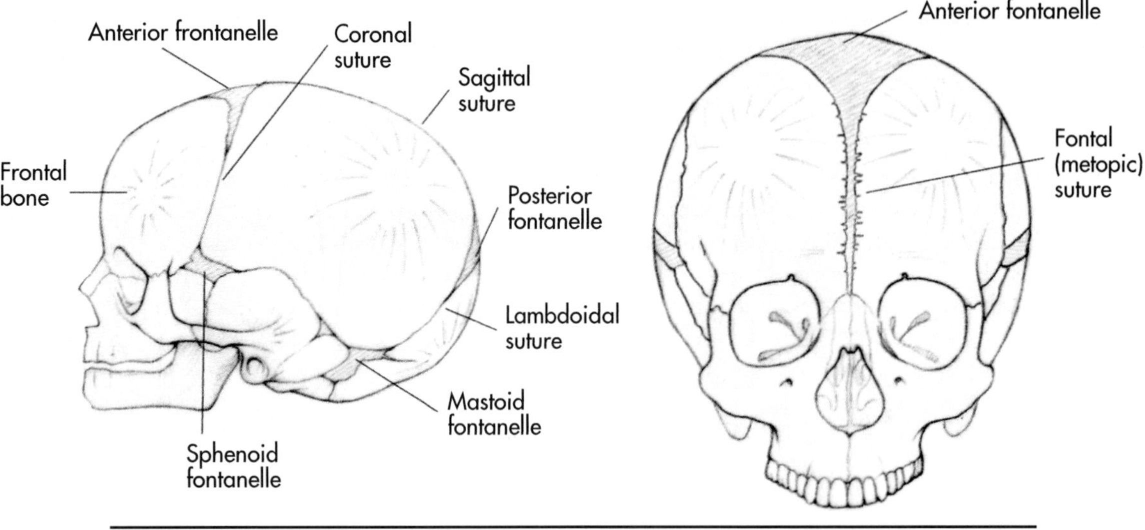

Figure 7-5
Infant skull.
(From Mathers LH et al: *Clinical anatomy principles,* St. Louis, 1996, Mosby.)

ACTIVITY 7-6

The names of the eight cranial bones start with various letters. To help you remember them, make up a sentence that uses the first letter of each in whatever order works for you. Get creative!

Occipital
Parietal
Frontal
Temporal
Ethmoid
Sphenoid

Example
Please Stop The Flying Ostrich Egg.

Your Turn

The facial bones are the following:

Nasal
Vomer
Lacrimal
Zygomatic
Palatine
Maxilla
Mandible
Inferior nasal concha

Make up a creative sentence that uses the first letter of each.

which fuse in the lower portion to become 26 bones in the adult. Each of the vertebrae has two main sections, the anterior body and the posterior arch. All vertebrae, except the atlas and the axis, have the following features:

1. A drum-shaped body, or centrum, located toward the front (anterior), which serves as the weight-bearing portion of the bone.
2. A vertebral arch, which is connected to the body by two pedicles. Two laminae unite posteriorly to form the bony arch that encircles the spinal cord, called the spinous process. The spinous process usually can be felt just under the skin of the back. The thickened junctions between the pedicles and the laminae have superior and inferior cartilaginous articular facets and a laterally projecting transverse process.
3. The bones of the spine are stacked one on the other: each vertebra has a joint surface, called an articular facet, which provides the articulating surface for this stacking arrangement.
4. A large hole, or foramen, in the center of each vertebra. All vertebrae are linked in a series by strong bands of connective tissue (ligaments), and these spaces form the

spinal canal, a bony cylinder that protects the spinal cord. As the vertebrae stack, they form the intervertebral foramina, which allow passage of the spinal nerves.

Although not technically a part of the vertebrae, the intervertebral disks (or discs; both spellings are correct) between the vertebral bodies act as shock absorbers and spacers and provide flexibility. The disk consists of two components. The outer edge, or anulus fibrosus, is composed of concentric rings of fibrocartilage arranged like the layers of an onion. Internally, the center, or nucleus pulposus, is made of a gelatinous substance. If a disk ruptures, the fibrocartilage splits and the nucleus pulposus leaks. The disk becomes smaller and is less able to disperse pressure and maintain space between the vertebrae. In severe cases the vertebrae can impinge on nerves (Figure 7-6). Again, the student should study all illustrations carefully because they provide more detail in labeling than the text.

Ligaments. Three ligaments extend the length of the vertebral column. The anterior longitudinal ligament attaches to the front of the vertebral bodies and acts as a resistance to extension. The posterior longitudinal ligament attaches to the back of the bodies and stabilizes flexion. The supraspinous ligament runs along the tips of the spinous processes and restrains flexion.

Other vertebral ligaments are between individual vertebra. The ligamenta flava connect the laminae of each adjacent vertebra. The interspinous ligaments connect the spinous processes, and the intertransverse ligaments connect the transverse processes. Right-side bending stretches the left intertransverse ligaments; left-side bending stretches the right intertransverse ligaments (Figure 7-7). Chapter 8 discusses vertebral movement patterns (Activity 7-7).

The bones of the vertebral column are named and numbered on the basis of location from the neck downward.

The seven cervical vertebrae (C1 to C7) are located in the neck. The first vertebra (C1), called the atlas, supports the head. When you nod your head "yes," the skull rocks on the atlas at the occipital condyles of the occipital bone. The atlas is modified greatly for articulation within the occipital region of the skull. The atlas does not have a body or spinous process; rather, it essentially is a bony ring consisting of anterior and posterior arches and two lateral masses. The second cervical vertebra (C2), called the axis, serves as a pivot when the head is turned from side to side (as in the gesture "no"). The axis has a peglike dens, or odontoid process, projecting superiorly from its anterior side. The pivot joint of C1 to C2 consists of a ringlike structure that rotates around the dens. Considerable movement, especially in rotation, is possible because of the design of this joint.

A strong, fibrous band called the nuchal ligament runs along the notched spinous processes of C2 to C6 and helps support the weight of the head. The vertebral arteries heading toward the brainstem pass through the foramina of the transverse processes of the upper six cervical vertebrae. These vessels are subject to stretching injuries with extreme cervical rotation of the hyperextended neck.

The 12 thoracic vertebrae (T1 to T12) are located in the thorax (the body area between the neck and diaphragm). The posterior ends of the 12 pairs of ribs are attached to these vertebrae at posterior demifacets (thought of as one half of a facet). T1 has a whole facet joint space for the first rib articulation and an inferior demifacet, which works with the corresponding superior demifacet of T2 for articulation with the second rib. T2 to T8 each have superior and inferior demifacets, which together form the vertebral portion of the articulation with the ribs. T9 has one superior demifacet, and T10 to T12 each have a whole facet to articulate with the ribs. The arrangement of the vertebrae in the thorax allows for a certain amount of flexion, extension, and side bending, but movements generally are limited, with most movement occurring at the thoracic-lumbar junction at T11, T12, and L1. The main functions of the thoracic vertebrae are to provide spaces on which to build the rib cage, which protects the heart and lungs, and to house the spinal cord.

The five lumbar vertebrae (L1 to L5) are located in the lower back. They are larger and heavier than the other vertebrae, which allows them to support more weight. The interlocking shape of the vertebrae makes rotation difficult but facilitates flexion, extension, and side bending. L4 and L5 allow the most motion. Most disk injuries occur at L4 to L5 and S1, the area of the lumbar-sacral junction.

The sacral vertebrae are five separate bones in a child; however, they eventually fuse to form a single bone, the sacrum, in an adult. Wedged between the two hipbones, the sacrum completes the posterior part of the bony pelvis. Four transverse ridges are the remnants of intervertebral disks. At the ends of each ridge are paired sacral foramina, through which the branches of the sacral nerves pass.

The coccyx, or tailbone, consists of four or five tiny bones in a child. As we develop, they fuse to form a single bone in an adult (Figure 7-8).

Vertebral curves. When viewed from the side, the vertebral column has curves that correspond to the groups of vertebrae. In a newborn, the entire column is a concave forward shape; this is the primary curve. When the infant begins to assume an erect posture, secondary curves, which are convex, form. For example, the cervical curve appears when infants begin to hold up their heads at about 3 months of age; the lumbar curve appears when they begin to walk. The curves of the vertebral column provide some of the resilience and spring so essential to walking and running.

The cervical region is concave, or has a lordosis. The thoracic region is convex, called a kyphosis; an abnormal lateral curvature of the thoracic region is called scoliosis. The lumbar region is concave again (lordosis can refer to an exaggeration of the curvature or to the normal condition). The sacrum is convex toward the back.

Vertebral curvatures develop dysfunction generally from exaggerated posture, activity, obesity, pregnancy, trauma, and disease. These conditions have the same name as the normal curves but are considered abnormal if they are exaggerated enough to cause problems. For example, osteo-

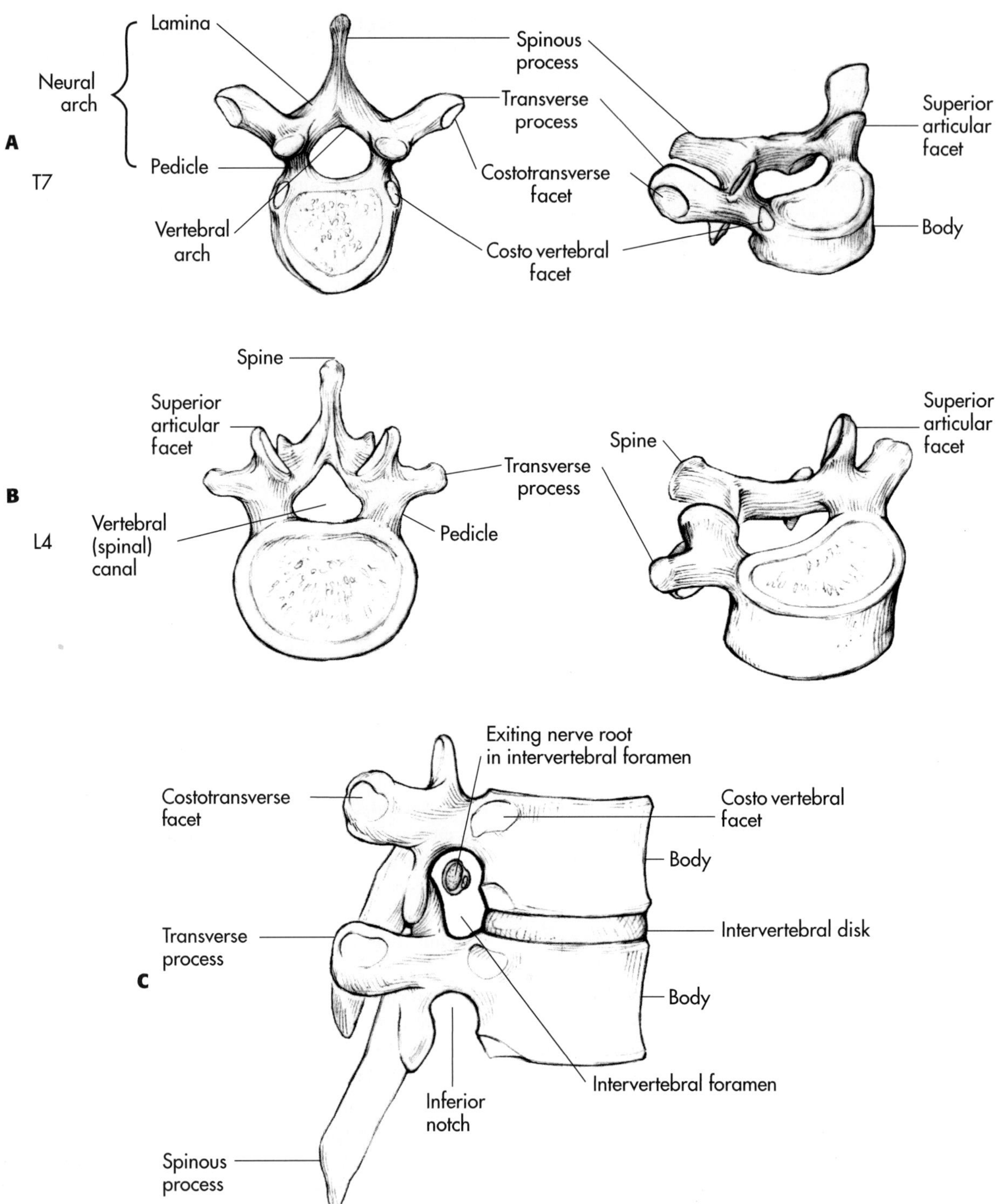

Figure 7-6
Common types of vertebrae (two views of T7 and L4 vertebrae). **A,** Superoinferior views. **B,** Right anterior oblique views. **C,** Intervertebral foramen. Vertebrae T5 and T6 have been articulated, showing the resulting intervertebral foramen with a segmental nerve in place. Blood vessels (not shown) enter and leave the interior of the vertebral canal through the intervertebral foramen. (From Mathers LH et al: *Clinical anatomy principles,* St. Louis, 1996, Mosby.)

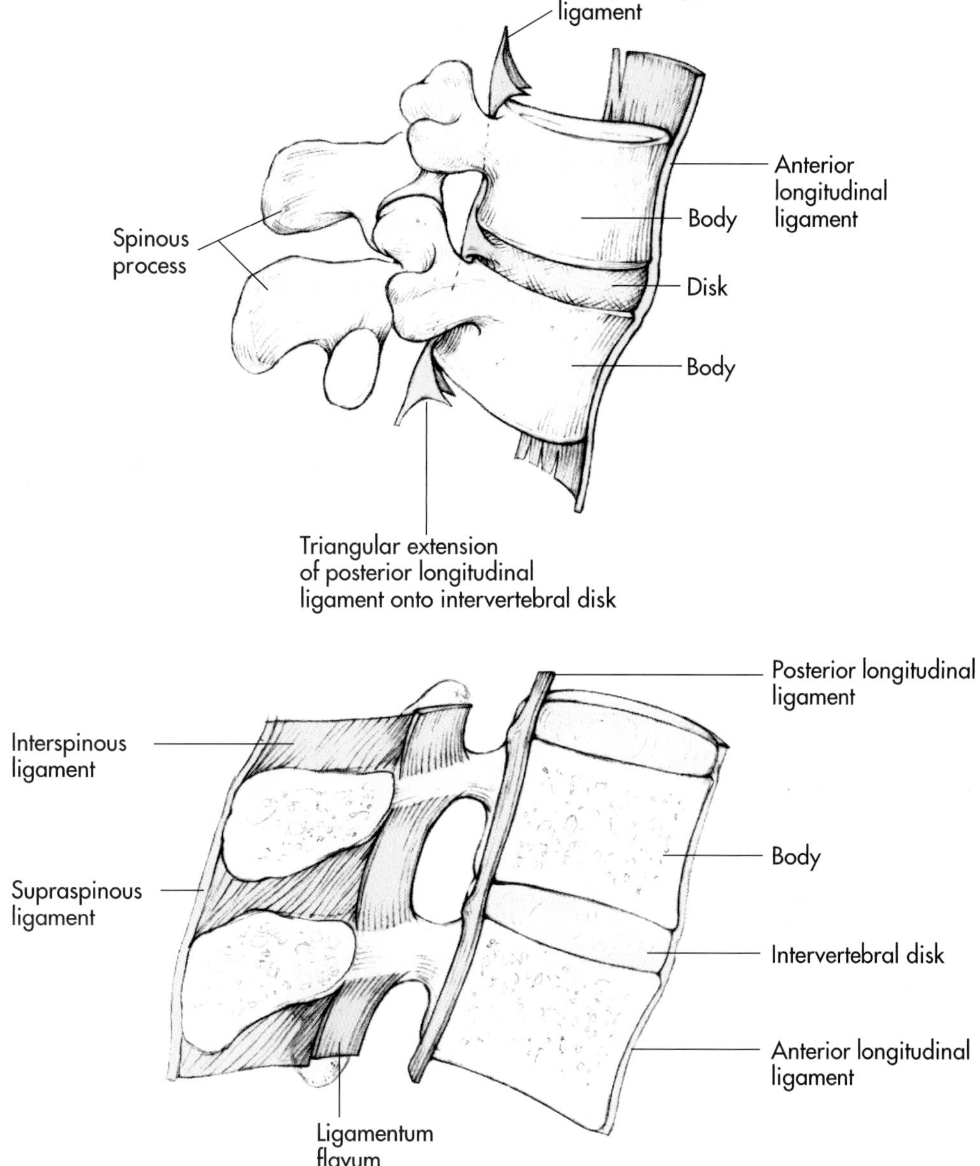

Figure 7-7
Vertebral ligament. (From Mathers LH et al: *Clinical anatomy principles,* St. Louis, 1996, Mosby.)

porosis can lead to the development of a hump in the thoracic vertebrae, called kyphosis or dowager's hump. A swayback of the lower back is a lordosis. As mentioned earlier, abnormal lateral bending is called scoliosis. Any exaggerated curve puts a strain on the musculoskeletal posture mechanisms and may predispose a person to pain and impaired movement (Figure 7-9; Activity 7-8).

Bones of the Thorax

The thorax is the body area between the base of the neck and the diaphragm muscle. The bones of the thorax form a cone-shaped cage. Twelve pairs of ribs form the bars of the cage, attaching to the sternum, or breastbone, anteriorly. The thorax protects the heart, the lungs, and other organs.

The sternum is fairly flat and consists of three parts: the manubrium at the top, the body in the middle, and the xiphoid process at the lower end. The xiphoid process is used as a landmark in cardiopulmonary resuscitation to locate the region for chest compression. One performs chest compressions above the xiphoid process to avoid breaking it off the sternum (Figure 7-10; Activity 7-9).

The ribs are elongated, flattened, and twisted bones. At the posterior end of each rib is a head, which has two facets for articulation with the bodies of the thoracic vertebrae. The neck of the rib is a constricted portion next to the head. The tubercle has an articular part, which is connected to the transverse process of a thoracic vertebra, and a nonarticular part for ligament attachment. The body, or shaft, is long and curved. The shaft also has a sharp bend, called the costal

ACTIVITY 7-7

Draw a thoracic or lumbar vertebra from the superior view and label the following areas. Be as accurate as you can without worrying about artistic ability. Looking at an anatomy picture or diagram will help (Figure 7-6).

Body (centrum) (Place drawing here.)
Vertebral arch
Vertebral foramen (canal)
Pedicle
Lamina
Spinous process
Transverse process
Articular facet
Demifacets for ribs

Now draw two stacked vertebrae and label the following:

Intervertebral disk (Place drawing here.)
Intervertebral foramen
Anterior longitudinal ligament
Posterior longitudinal ligament
Supraspinous ligament
Ligamenta flava
Interspinous ligaments
Intertransverse ligaments

angle. The anterior end is joined to the costal cartilage. Most ribs articulate with two thoracic vertebrae at three points. As mentioned before, the two facets on the head of the rib contact the demifacets of the vertebral bodies, and the tubercle contacts the transverse process (Activity 7-10; Figure 7-10).

The 12 pairs of ribs are classified by their anterior attachments. The first seven pairs are the true ribs; they attach directly to the sternum via the costal cartilages. The next five pairs of ribs are known as the false ribs. The first three (or the eighth, ninth, and tenth ribs) attach to the cartilage of the rib above. The eleventh and twelfth pairs are referred to as floating ribs because they have no anterior attachment. Each of our ribs attaches to the posterior vertebrae. The intercostal spaces, between the ribs, contain muscles, blood vessels, and nerves.

Bones of the Appendicular Skeleton

The appendicular skeleton may be considered as having two divisions: upper and lower.

The upper division includes the shoulders (or pectoral girdle); the arms between the shoulders and the elbows; the forearms between the elbows and the wrists; and the wrists, hands, and fingers. In everyday conversation we refer to the arm as the whole appendage from the shoulder to the wrist. In anatomic terms, the arm is the portion from shoulder to elbow. The only bony attachment of the pectoral girdle to the axial skeleton occurs at the sternoclavicular joint, the articulation of the clavicle and the manubrium.

The lower division includes the hips (or pelvic girdle); the thighs between the hips and knees; the legs between the knees and ankles; and the ankles, feet, and toes. The student should note that in anatomic terms, the leg is the portion from the knee to the ankle.

Upper Division

The bones of the upper division can be divided into two groups. One group comprises the bones of the pectoral girdle, the clavicle, and the scapula (some references include the manubrium, upper thoracic vertebrae, and first two ribs as functional units of the pectoral girdle). The other group includes the bones of the upper extremity.

Clavicle. The clavicle, or collar bone (Figure 7-11), is long and flat and has two bends that give it an S shape (Activity 7-11). The lateral clavicle articulates with the acromion, and together they form the upper portion of the shoulder. This structure functions as a strut by keeping the scapula posterior, which maintains the position of the glenoid fossa (the point of articulation of the humerus on the scapula). The clavicle articulates medially with the manubrium and

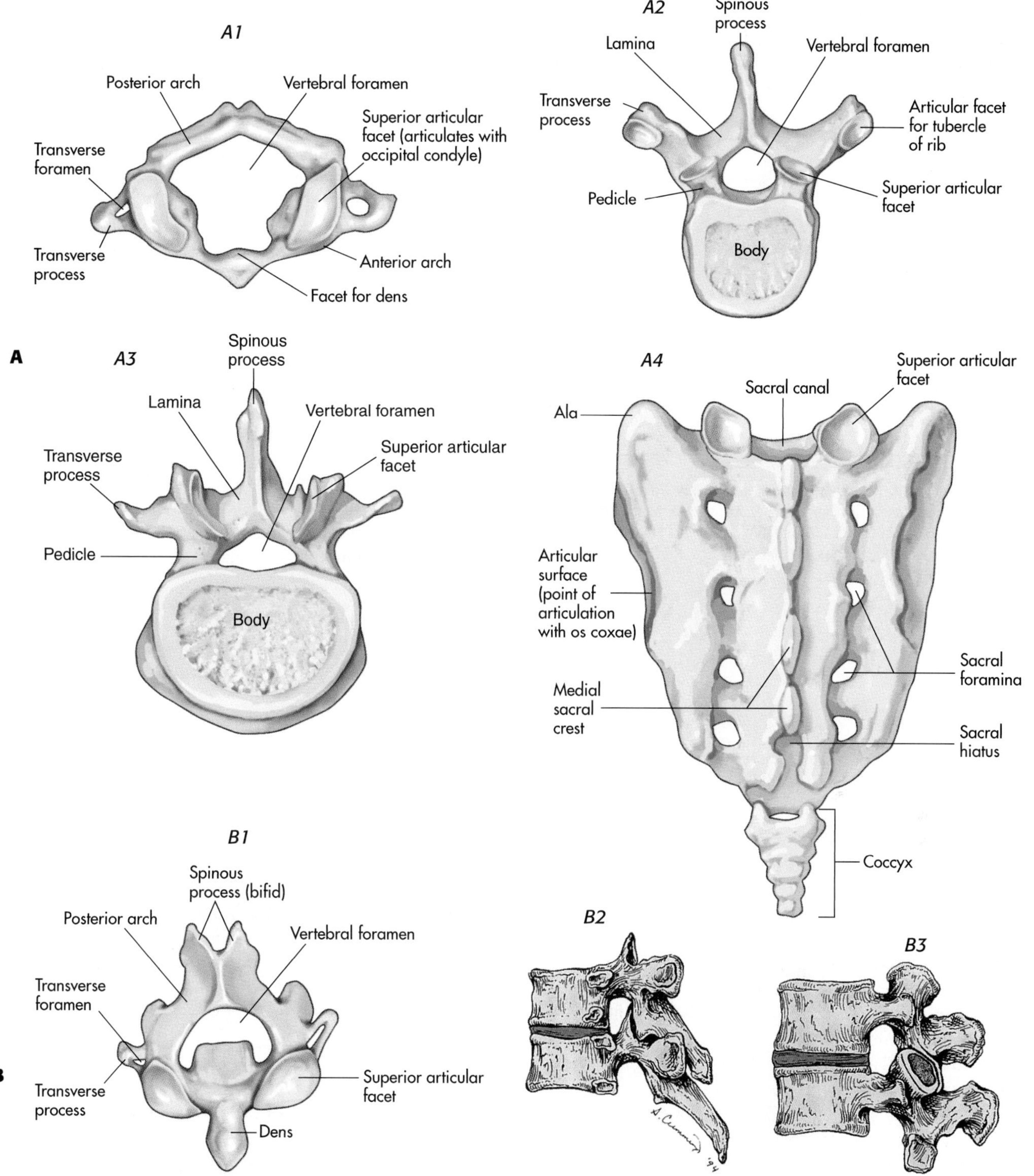

Figure 7-8

Six types of vertebrae. **A**: *A1*, Atlas (first cervical vertebra), superior view. *A2*, Thoracic vertebra, superior view. *A3*, Lumbar vertebra, superior view. *A4*, Sacrum and coccyx, posterior view. (From Thibodeau GA, Patton KT: *Anatomy and physiology*, ed. 5, St. Louis, 2003, Mosby). **B**: *B1*, Axis (second cervical vertebra), slightly posterior and superior view. (From Thibodeau GA, Patton KT: *Anatomy and physiology*, ed. 5, St. Louis, 2003, Mosby). *B2*, Thoracic vertebrae. *B3*, Lumbar vertebrae. (Modified from Cramer GD, Darby SA: *Basic and clinical anatomy of the spine, spinal cord, and ANS*, St. Louis, 1995, Mosby.)

Continued

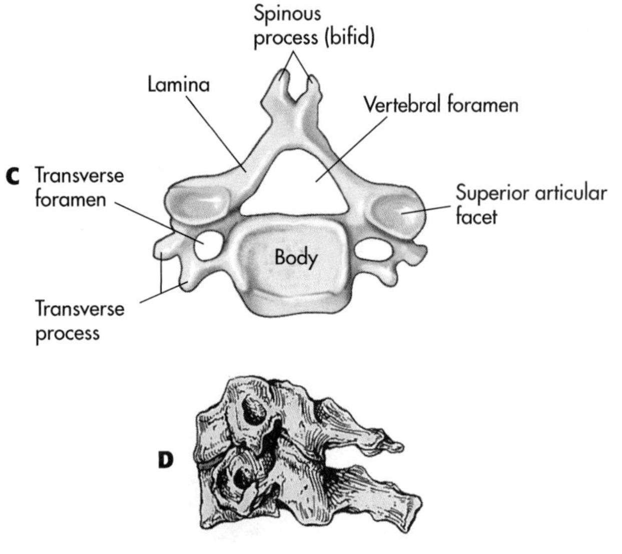

Figure 7-8, cont'd.
Six types of vertebrae. **C**, Fifth cervical vertebra, superior view. (From Thibodeau GA, Patton KT: *Anatomy and physiology*, ed. 5, St. Louis, 2003, Mosby.) **D**, Cervical vertebrae. (Modified from Cramer GD, Darby SA: *Basic and clinical anatomy of the spine, spinal cord, and ANS*, St. Louis, 1995, Mosby.)

the superior edges of the cartilage of the first rib to form the sternoclavicular joint. This fragile bone transmits force from the arms to the thorax. For this reason, when a person falls with arms outstretched, this bone often breaks or the joint separates when the clavicle hits the acromion.

Scapula. The scapula, or shoulder blade (Figure 7-12), is an irregular, triangular bone with a flat anterior surface. The posterior surface has a large spine and two major processes, all easy to palpate. At the lateral end of the scapular spine is the acromion process, the highest point of the bony portion of the shoulder. The coracoid process is a fingerlike projection from the anterior portion of the superior border.

The three corners of this triangular bone are referred to as the inferior, superior, and lateral angles. The edges of the bone are also landmarks and attachment points for muscles; these are the medial, superior, and lateral borders. The medial border also is known as the vertebral border. The superior border is the hardest to palpate because it lies under the shoulder muscles. The lateral (or axillary) border is the thickest of the three and contains the glenoid cavity, a shallow depression that articulates with the head of the

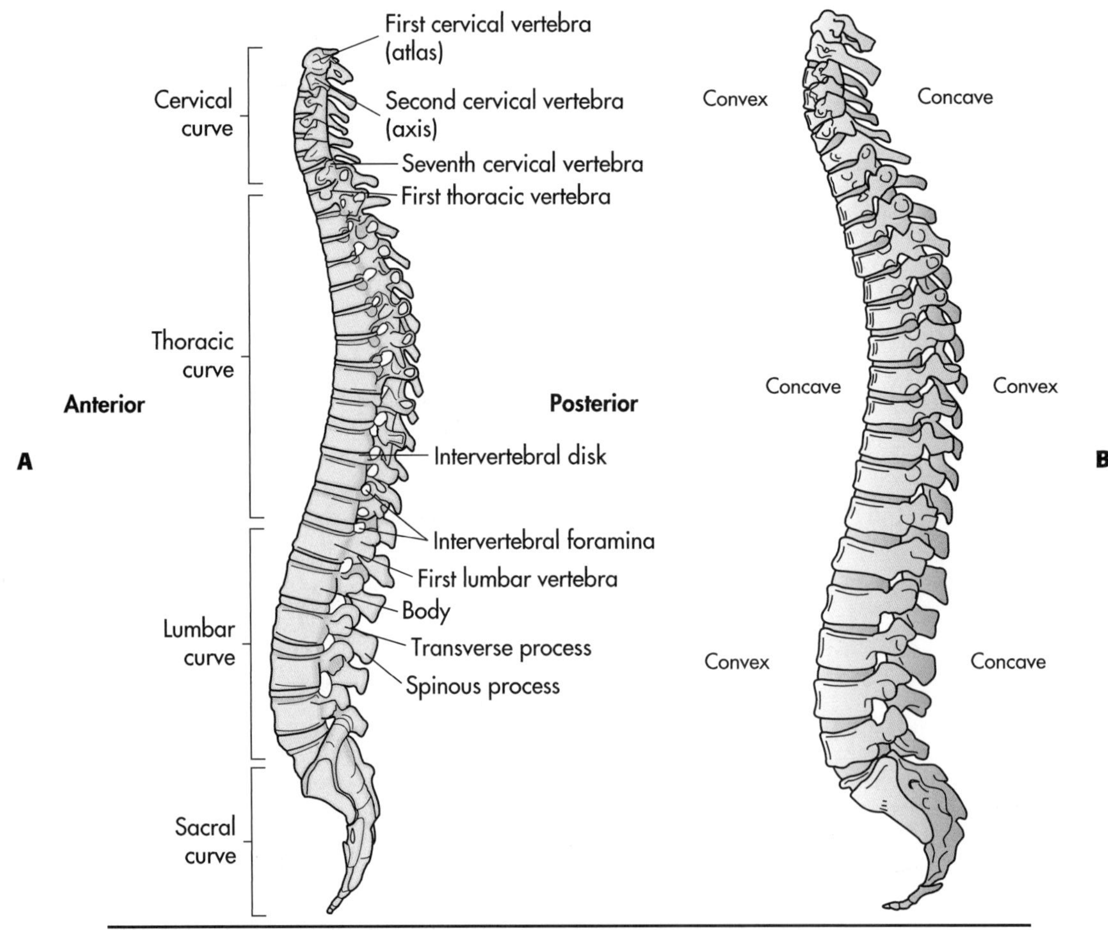

Figure 7-9
A, Vertebral column. **B,** The convex and concave curves of the vertebral column.

ACTIVITY 7-8

Draw the vertebral column and label the structures in the list below. Include the vertebral curve pattern and label the curves. Again, be accurate in your drawing but do not worry about artistic ability. Using diagrams or pictures from this text is helpful.

(Place drawing here.)

Atlas
Axis
Cervical vertebrae (C1 to C7)
Nuchal ligament
Thoracic vertebrae (T1 to T12)
Thoracic-lumbar junction at T11, T12, and L1
Lumbar vertebrae (L1 to L5)
Lumbar-sacral junction at L4 to L5 and S1
Sacrum
Coccyx

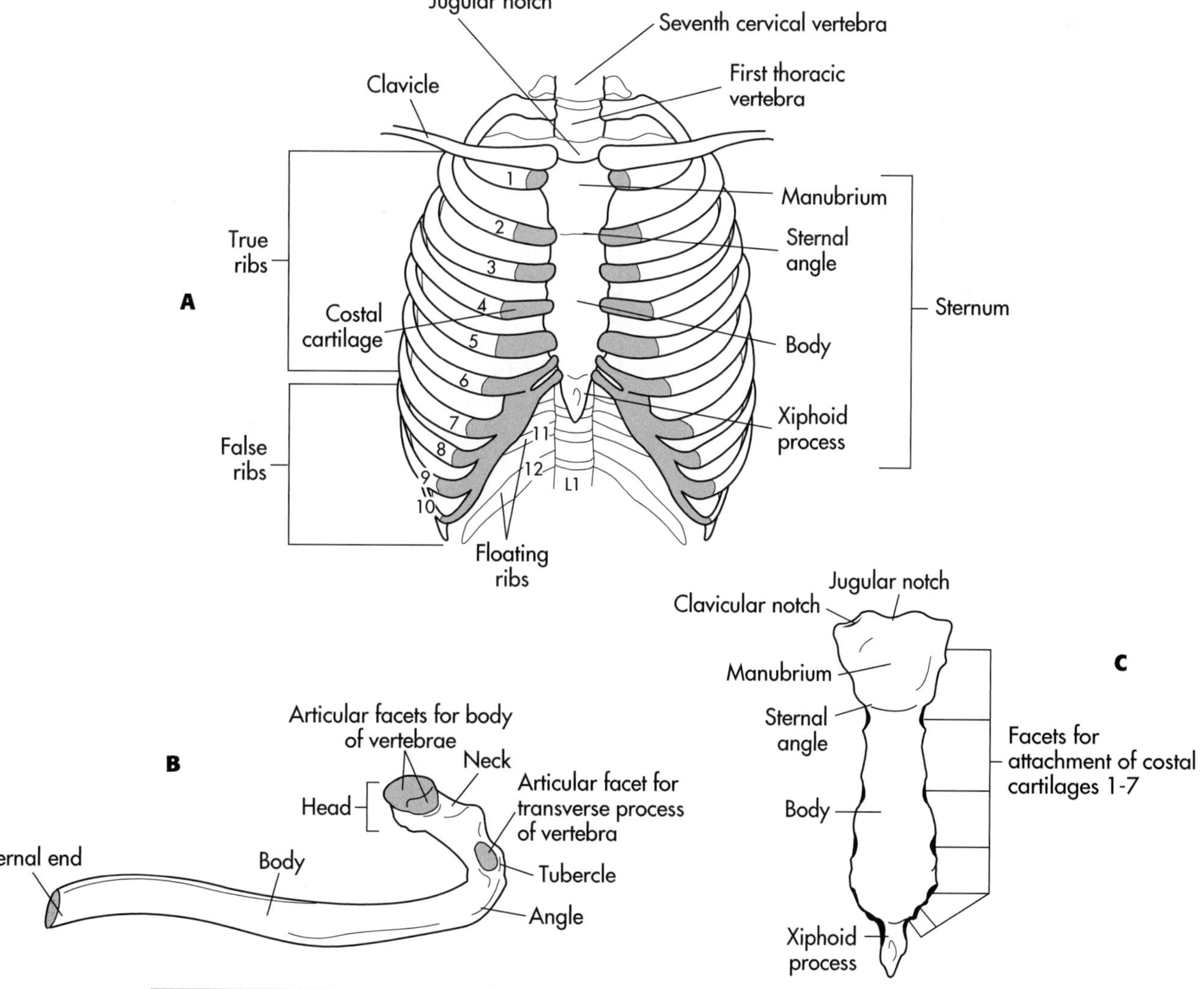

Figure 7-10
A, Rib cage. **B,** Typical rib. **C,** Sternum.

ACTIVITY 7-9

Draw the sternum and label the following:

Manubrium (Place drawing here.)
Body
Xiphoid process

ACTIVITY 7-11

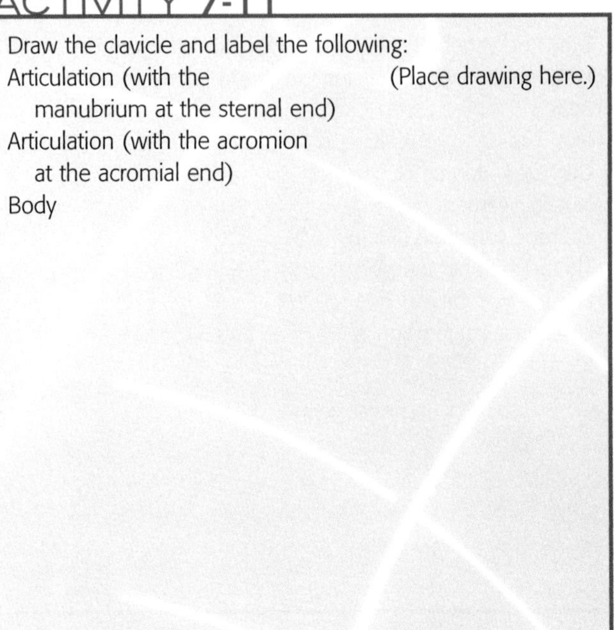

Draw the clavicle and label the following:

Articulation (with the manubrium at the sternal end) (Place drawing here.)
Articulation (with the acromion at the acromial end)
Body

ACTIVITY 7-10

Draw a typical rib and label the following:

Head (with two facets for articulation) (Place drawing here.)
Neck
Tubercle
Body (shaft)
Costal angle

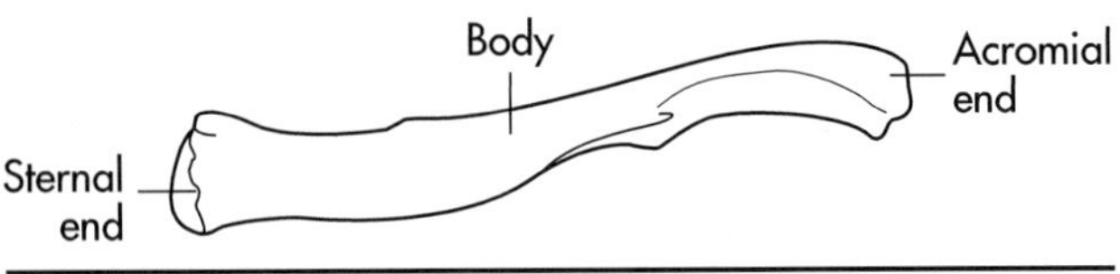

Figure 7-11
Clavicle.

humerus to form the shoulder joint. The supraspinous and infraspinous fossae and the fossa on the anterior portion of the scapula are attachment points for muscles that connect the shoulder to the thorax (Activity 7-12).

The second group of bones of the upper division comprises the bones of the upper extremity, which are the humerus, radius, ulna, and the bones of the wrist and hand.

Humerus. The humerus, or arm bone (Figure 7-13), is a long bone. The head of the humerus, at the proximal end, forms the glenohumeral joint, which articulates with the glenoid fossa of the scapula.

The distal end of the humerus articulates with the radius and ulna to form the elbow joint. On the lateral edge of the distal end of the humerus is a rounded surface, called the capitulum. The medial edge of the distal end of the humerus forms a pulley-shaped surface, the *trochlea.*

Just above these projections on the anterior surface are the radial and coronoid (ulnar) fossae. The *olecranon fossa* is on the posterior surface. During flexion and extension, the radial head slides on the capitulum, and the trochlear notch of the ulna slides over the trochlea of the humerus.

In full flexion, the radial head and the ulnar coronoid process fit into the radial and coronoid fossae of the humerus. At full extension, the olecranon process of the ulna moves into the olecranon fossa of the humerus, which prevents extension beyond 180 degrees.

The medial and lateral epicondyles of the humerus are attachment points for muscles and are prone to problems from repetitive use (Activity 7-13).

Bones of the forearm. The *radius,* which is on the lateral side of the forearm, is narrow at the elbow and widens just above the wrist (Figure 7-14). The head of the radius, at the proximal end, articulates with the capitulum during flexion and extension. During full flexion, the radius slides into the radial fossa of the humerus. At the distal end of the radius

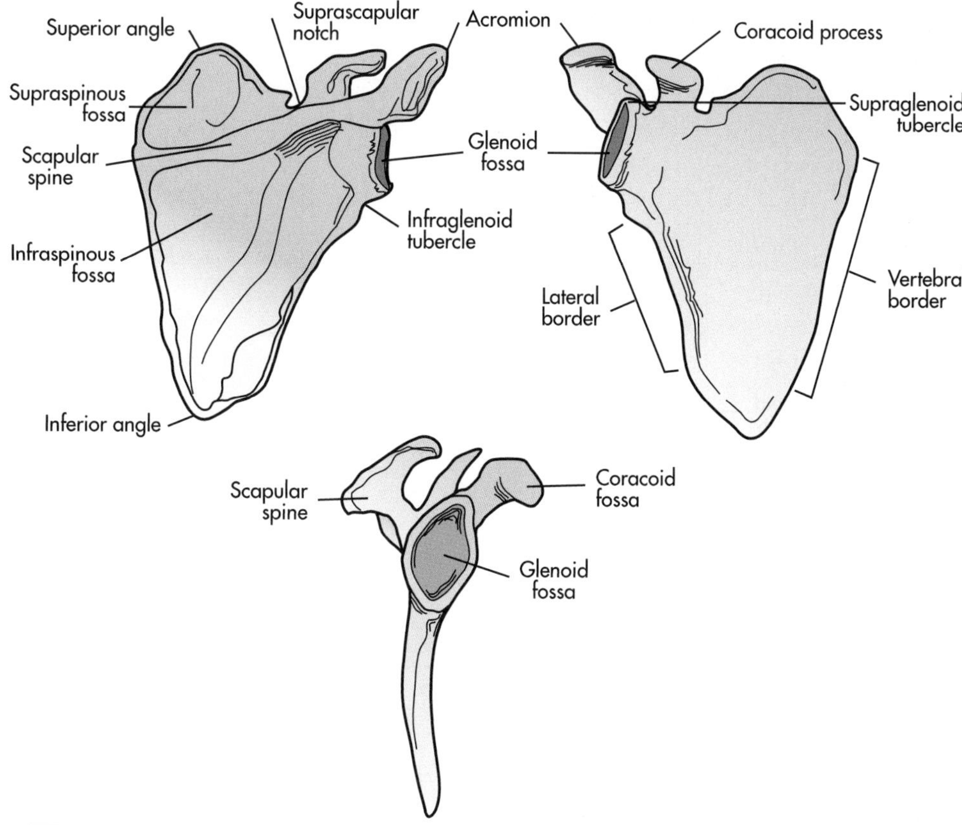

Figure 7-12
Scapula (three views).

ACTIVITY 7-12

Draw the posterior view of the scapula and label the following:

Acromion (Place drawing here.)
Scapular spine
Inferior angle
Superior angle
Lateral border
Vertebral border
Glenoid fossa
Supraspinous fossa
Infraspinous fossa

the articular surface combines with the carpals to form the wrist joint. The styloid process of the radius is a bony projection at the distal end, just above the thumb.

The *ulna,* which provides most of the stability of the forearm, lies on the medial side. Opposite in shape to the radius, the ulna is wider at the elbow and narrower at the wrist. At its proximal end is the trochlear notch, which articulates with the trochlea of the humerus. The olecranon process is the large projection that most persons refer to as their elbow. The olecranon process slides into the olecranon fossa of the humerus during extension. On the anteroproximal surface of the ulna is the coronoid process, which moves into the coronoid fossa of the humerus during full flexion. At the distal end of the ulna is the head. The head of a bone usually is at the proximal end, so the student should not become confused. The styloid process of the ulna is a bony landmark found above the wrist. Just beyond the proximal end is an articular disk, which articulates with the carpals to provide some of the movements of the wrist.

Between the radius and ulna lies the interosseous membrane, made of flexible connective tissue, which provides strength, support, and additional movement capabilities. The radius and ulna work together to produce many diverse, well-coordinated actions, at the elbow and in the hand and wrist (Activity 7-14). Chapter 8 discusses the actions of the joint in more detail.

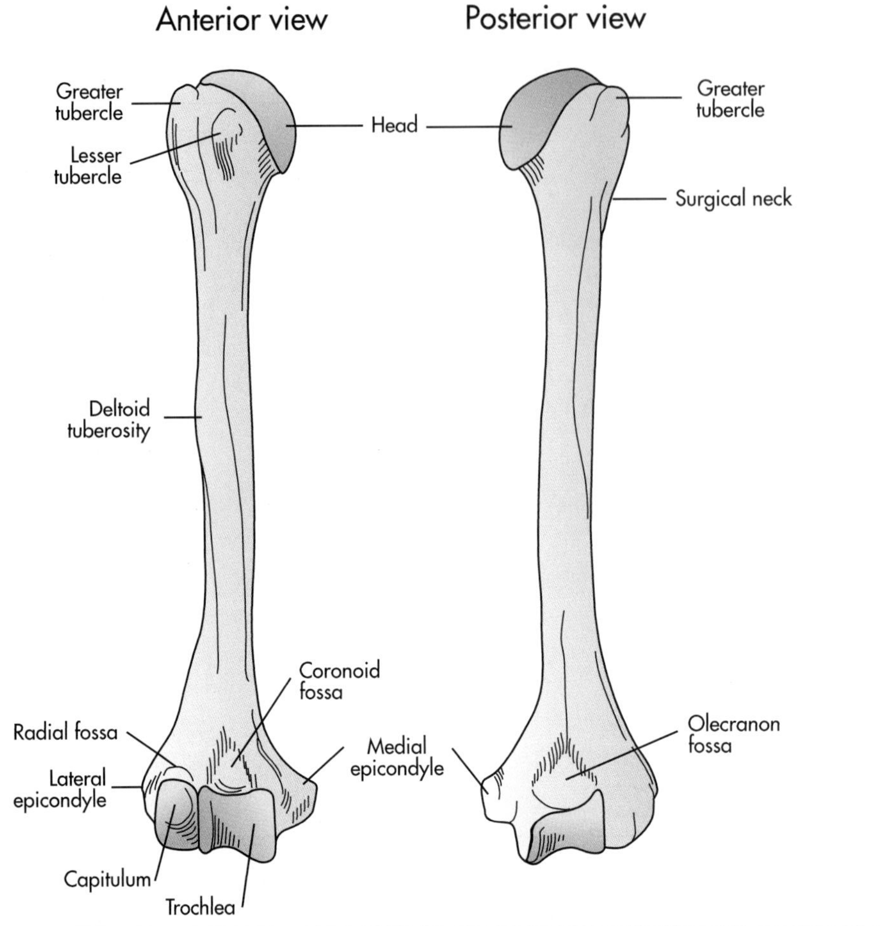

Figure 7-13
Humerus (anterior and posterior views).

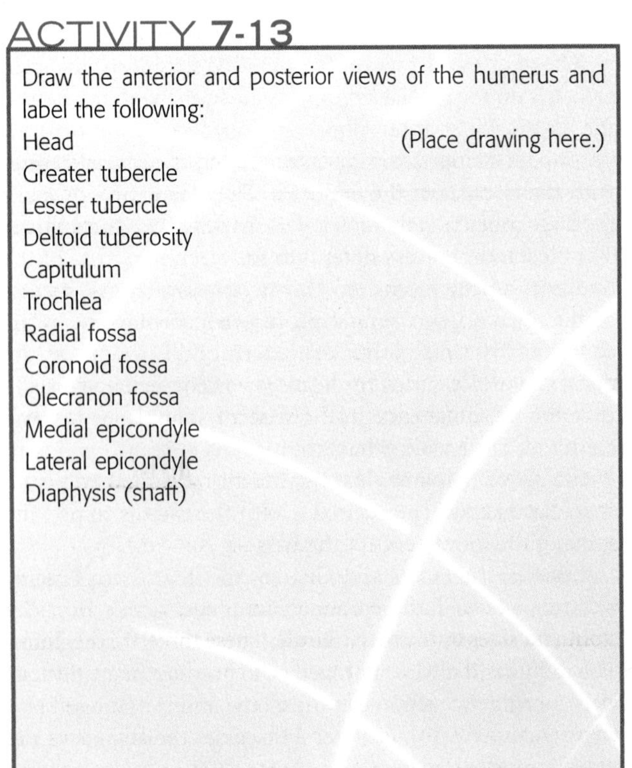

ACTIVITY 7-13

Draw the anterior and posterior views of the humerus and label the following:

(Place drawing here.)

Head
Greater tubercle
Lesser tubercle
Deltoid tuberosity
Capitulum
Trochlea
Radial fossa
Coronoid fossa
Olecranon fossa
Medial epicondyle
Lateral epicondyle
Diaphysis (shaft)

Bones of the wrist and hand. The wrist contains the carpals: eight small, cube-shaped bones arranged in two rows of four. In the proximal row are the scaphoid, lunate, and triquetrum, which articulate with the radius to form the wrist joint. The pisiform is also in the first row but does not articulate with the radius. The distal row contains the trapezium, trapezoid, capitate, and hamate. Many skeletal injuries occur with falls on the hand, especially when the hand is forced into extreme hyperextension. Fractures of the scaphoid and radius are common because forces produced by a fall on the hand are transmitted through the scaphoid and lunate and are absorbed by the radius.

The transverse arch of the wrist, formed by the carpals, is anteriorly concave. A wide, thick ligament, the flexor retinaculum, connects the pisiform and hamate to the scaphoid and trapezium. The dorsal side of the wrist has six tunnels for the extensor tendons, and the palmar side has two tunnels to carry nerves, arteries, and flexor tendons. The carpal tunnel, one of the palmar tunnels, is the most commonly traumatized and contains the median nerve, which can become compressed, especially when repetitive movements of the fingers cause friction and inflammation.

In the palm of the hand are five metacarpal bones, short bones that form the framework of each hand. Knuckles are the rounded distal ends of the metacarpals.

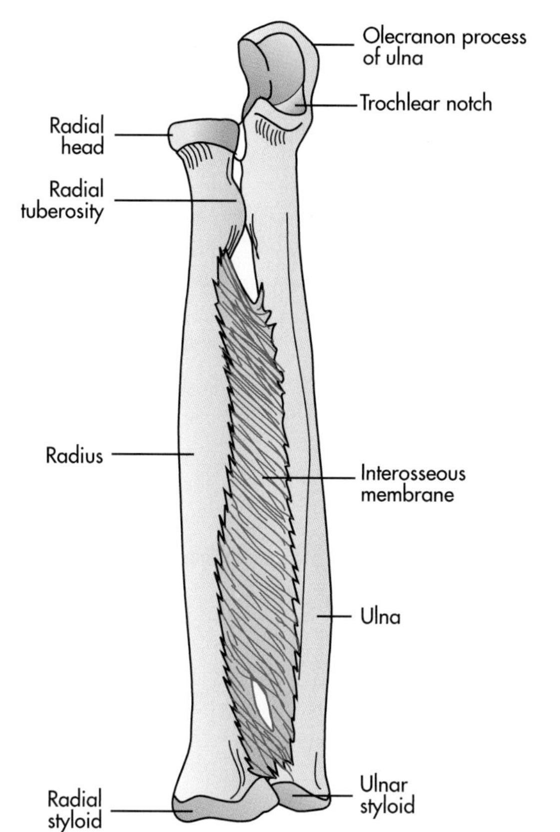

Figure 7-14
Forearm bones.

ACTIVITY 7-14

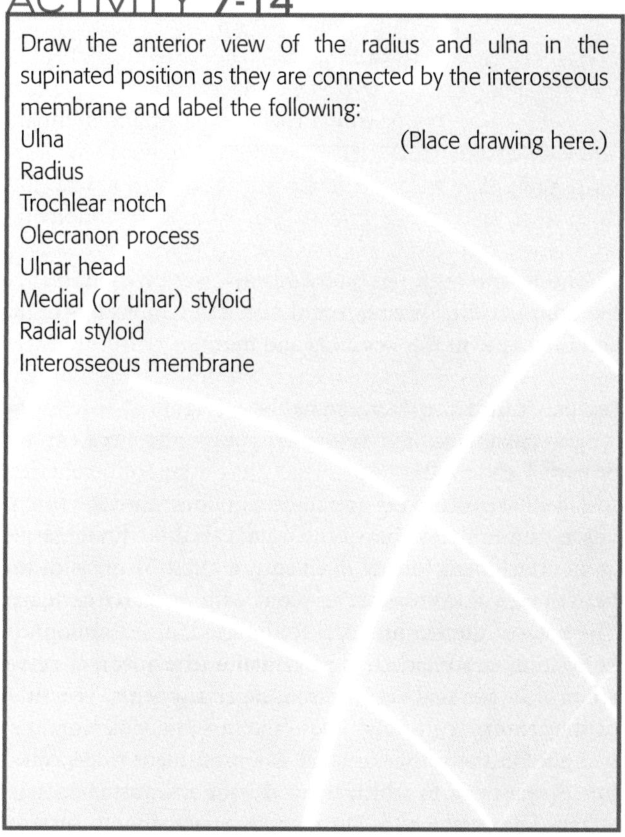

Draw the anterior view of the radius and ulna in the supinated position as they are connected by the interosseous membrane and label the following:

(Place drawing here.)

Ulna
Radius
Trochlear notch
Olecranon process
Ulnar head
Medial (or ulnar) styloid
Radial styloid
Interosseous membrane

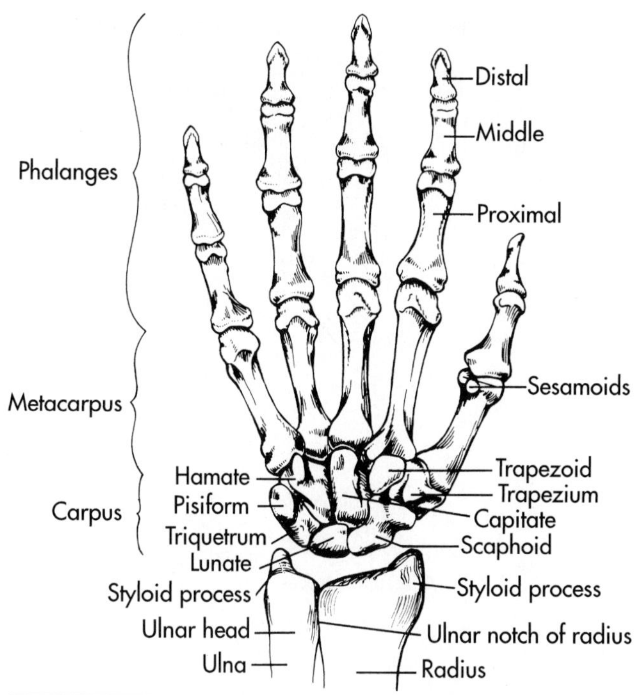

Figure 7-15
Volar view of the bones of the hand. (From Malone TR, McPoil T, Nitz AJ: *Orthopedic and sports physical therapy*, ed 3, St Louis, 1996, Mosby.)

Each hand has fourteen phalanges, or finger bones, two for the thumb and three for each finger. Each of these short bones is called a phalanx. The first, or proximal phalanx, articulates with a metacarpal. The second and third, in the supine position, are referred to as the middle and distal phalanges. The student should note that the thumb has only a proximal phalanx and a distal phalanx (Figures 7-15 and 7-16; Activities 7-15 and 7-16).

Lower Division

The bones of the lower division are grouped in a manner similar to that of the upper division. The two primary groups of the lower division are the bones of the pelvic girdle and the bones of the lower extremity.

The bony pelvis (Figure 7-17) supports the trunk and the organs in the lower abdomen, or pelvic cavity. The pelvis also absorbs stress from the lower limbs when we are moving, whether walking or jumping. The female pelvis is adapted for pregnancy and childbirth and is wider and lighter than the male pelvis.

The pelvic girdle is a strong, bony ring composed of the coxal bones and the sacrum. Unlike the shoulder girdle, the pelvic girdle is attached anteriorly at the symphysis pubis and posteriorly at the sacroiliac joint. Three bones fuse as we grow to create the coxae, or hipbones, which form the front and sides of the pelvic girdle. These three are the ilium, which forms the superior flared portion and is important for muscle attachments; the ischium, which is the inferior portion, and the strongest; and the pubis, which forms the anterior portion of the pelvis. In the middle of the pubis is

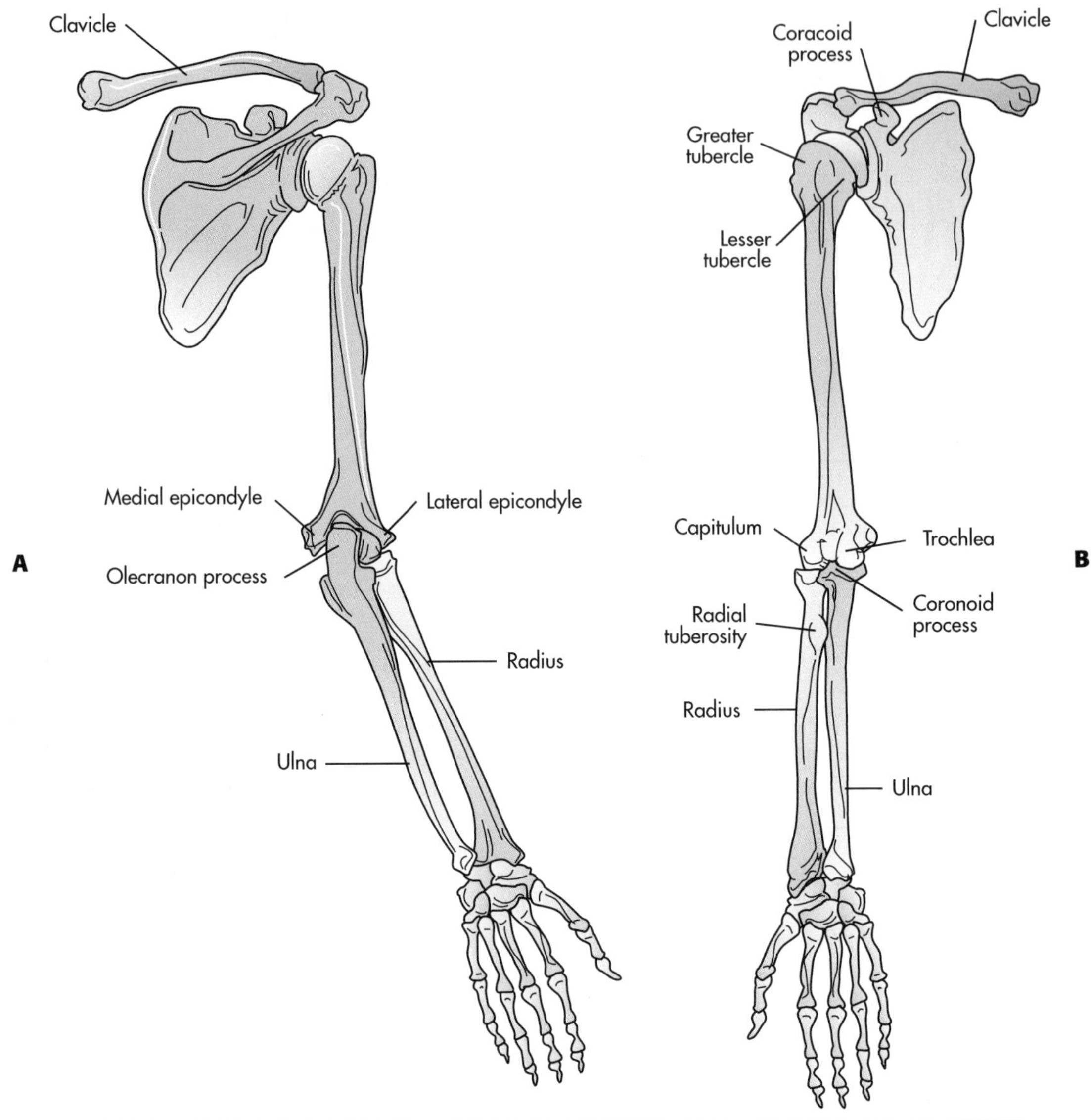

Figure 7-16
A, Bones of the upper limb (posterior view). **B,** Bones of the upper limb (anterior view).

the symphysis pubis, which is the anterior connection of the pelvis. The fibrocartilaginous disk at the symphysis pubis allows this joint to function as a shock absorber.

The posterior portion of the pelvic girdle is created from the sacrum, which we discuss with the spine.

The lateral portion of the pelvis, where the ilium, ischium, and pubis fuse, creates a deep socket called the acetabulum, which articulates with the head of the femur to form the coxal (hip) joint.

At the superior portion is the iliac crest. On the anterior end of the crest is the anterior superior iliac spine, which often is used as a bony landmark, especially in assessment and treatment. The posterior superior iliac spine is a bony prominence at the posterior end of the iliac crest. Just below the posterior superior iliac spine is the posterior joint of the pelvis, the sacroiliac joint. On the surface of the body is a small dimple or depression over the sacroiliac joint; the posterior superior iliac spine lies just above it (Activity 7-17).

The second group of bones of the lower division, that is, the bones of the lower extremity, are the femur and patella and the bones of the lower leg and foot.

Femur. The femur, or thigh bone (Figure 7-18), is the longest, strongest, and heaviest bone in the body. At the proximal end is the head, which has a smooth, spherical surface that fits into the acetabulum to form the hip joint. A depression in the center of the head, called the fovea, serves as an attachment for the ligamentum teres. All areas of the head except the fovea are covered with articular cartilage. The neck of the femur, distal to the head, is a common site of fracture in the elderly. The greater and lesser trochanters are projections that serve as muscle attachments. The shaft of the femur, as in most long bones, is triangular in cross section. On the posterior shaft is a prominent ridge, called the linea aspera, to which the adductor and vastus muscles attach. The lateral and medial condyles are smooth surfaces

ACTIVITY 7-15

Draw the wrist and hand and label the following:

Scaphoid (Place drawing here.)
Lunate
Triquetrum
Pisiform
Trapezium
Trapezoid
Capitate
Hamate
Five metacarpal (metacarpus) bones
Fourteen phalanges

ACTIVITY 7-16

The following list names the bones of the upper limb:

Clavicle
Scapula
Humerus
Radius
Ulna
Carpals
Metacarpals
Phalanges

Make up a silly sentence to help you remember these bones by using the first letter of each name.

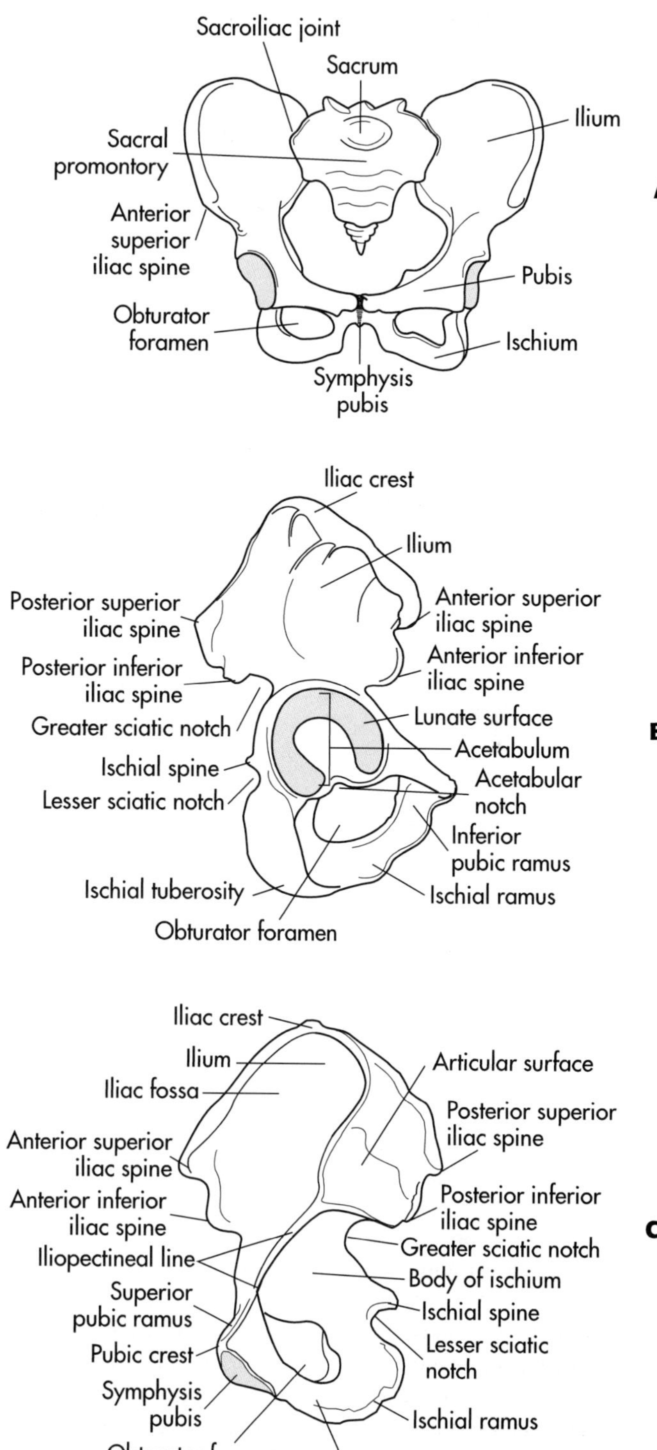

Figure 7-17
Pelvis. **A,** Anterior view. **B,** Lateral view. **C,** Medial view.

that articulate with the proximal tibia. Between the condyles is the anterior patellar surface. The lateral and medial epicondyles, which are above the condyles, are points of muscle attachment. The intercondylar fossa is a depression on the posterior surface between the condyles that articulates with the intercondylar eminence of the tibia. The menisci are cartilaginous cushions (lateral and medial) that lie between the femur and tibia (Activity 7-18).

Patella. The patella, or kneecap (Figure 7-19), is a sesamoid bone encased within the tendons of the quadriceps femoris, where it crosses the knee joint. The patella is

ACTIVITY 7-17

Draw anterior and lateral views of the pelvis and label the following:

(Place drawing here.)

Sacrum
Sacroiliac joint
Ilium
Ischium
Pubis
Symphysis pubis
Acetabulum
Iliac crest
Obturator foramen
Anterior superior iliac spine
Anterior inferior iliac spine
Posterior superior iliac spine
Posterior inferior iliac spine
Ischial tuberosity
Greater sciatic notch

triangular; the broad superior edge is called the base, and the more pointed inferior edge is called the apex. The patella sits in the trochlear groove of the femur. The two articular facets on its posterior surface fit against the medial and lateral condyles of the femur.

Bones of the lower leg. The lower leg comprises two bones, the tibia and the fibula (Figure 7-20). The tibia, or shinbone, is on the medial, big toe side. The shinbone is the longer and stronger of the two bones and is a weight-bearing bone. At the proximal end are the *lateral* and *medial condyles,* which fit against the identically named surface of the femur. The medial condyle is larger than the lateral condyle. The *intercondylar eminence,* a ridge that separates the two condyles, moves into the intercondylar fossa of the femur during knee flexion. The *tibial tuberosity,* at the proximal anterior superior tibia, is the attachment point for the patellar ligament. The distal end forms the *medial malleolus,* a bony landmark of the ankle. The tibia articulates with the fibula at the proximal end (the superior tibiofibular joint) and at the distal end (the distal tibiofibular joint). The tibia also articulates with the ankle bones.

The fibula is on the lateral side of the leg. This slender bone does not reach the knee joint and so does not bear weight. The main function of the fibula is as an attachment for muscles and fasciae. The head of the fibula articulates with the tibia. The distal end of the fibula, which forms the *lateral malleolus,* articulates with the talus. Despite its small size, the fibula can withstand more tensile pull and strain than any other bone in the body. As with the forearm, an interosseous membrane connects the tibia and fibula (Activity 7-19).

Bones of the foot. The structure of the foot (Figure 7-21) is similar to that of the hand. The difference lies in the fact that, because the foot supports the weight of the body, it must be stronger and does not have to be as mobile as the hand. The foot has 26 bones, 31 joints, and more than 20 intrinsic (inside the structure) muscles. Seven *tarsal bones* connect the foot to the leg. The largest is the *calcaneus,* or heel bone. The *talus* is the major weight-bearing bone of the foot during upright motions; it is next in size to the calcaneus.

The talus and calcaneus are the most posterior of the tarsal bones. They articulate anteriorly with the other tarsals. The talus articulates with the tibia and fibula on its superior side and with the calcaneus inferiorly. Because no muscles insert on the talus, motion occurs by the movement of the bone and soft tissue structures around it. The other tarsals are cube-shaped and lie between the talus, calcaneus, and the metatarsals; they are the anterior tarsals. The *navicular bone* articulates with the talus and *cuneiform bones.* The *cuboid* articulates with the calcaneus. Together they form the *transverse arch* of the foot, also known as the instep. These gliding joints have less flexibility than the corresponding wrist bones.

The transverse arch is concave from the medial to lateral aspect of the foot. The medial longitudinal arch is the longest and highest arch and is made up of the calcaneus, talus, and navicular, medial cuneiform, and first metatarsal bones. The lateral longitudinal arch is made up of the calcaneus, cuboids, and fifth metatarsal bones (Figure 7-22).

Five short metatarsal bones form the instep, and the heads of these bones form the ball of the foot. They articulate proximally with the three cuneiforms and the cuboid and distally with the phalanges. Each of the metatarsals begins the actual formation of an individual toe. The phalanges are organized in the same way as in the hand. Each toe has three phalanges, except the great toe, which has two. The phalanges are identified in the same manner as in the hand (i.e., the first phalanx is known as the proximal phalanx) (Activities 7-20 and 7-21).

The *plantar aponeurosis* is a large band of connective tissue that begins at the inferior calcaneus and runs along the plantar surface of the foot, attaching at the toes. This tissue adds stability to the arch of the foot but can shorten if the person often wears improperly fitting shoes. Plantar fasciitis is a painful condition caused by this shortening. Inflammation from repetitive use is common in track

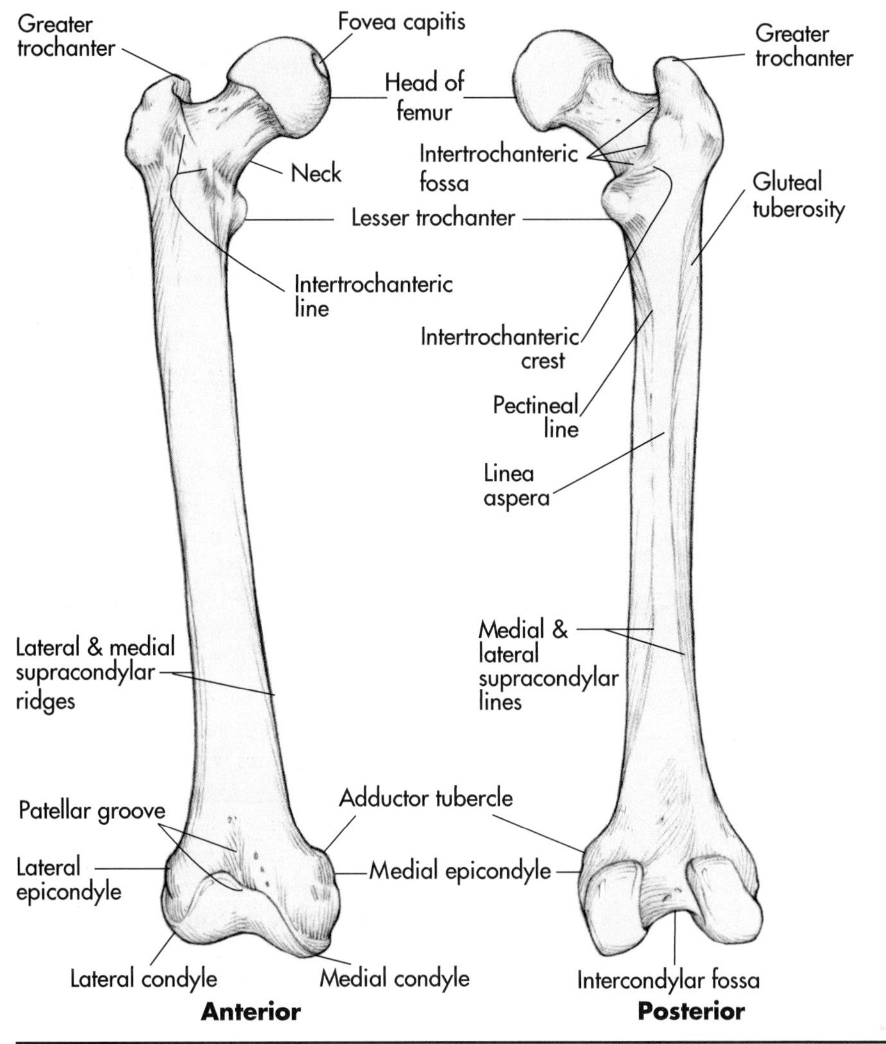

Figure 7-18
Femur (anterior and posterior views of the right femur). (From Mathers LH et al: *Clinical anatomy principles,* St. Louis, 1996, Mosby.)

ACTIVITY 7-18

Draw the anterior and posterior views of the femur and label the following:

Head of the femur
Fovea (fovea capitis)
Neck
Greater trochanter
Lesser trochanter
Lateral condyle

(Place drawing here.)

Medial condyle
Lateral epicondyle
Medial epicondyle
Linea aspera
Intercondylar fossa

(Place drawing here.)

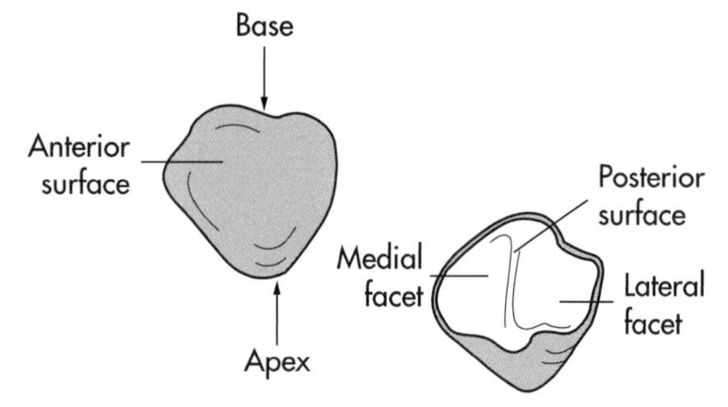

Figure 7-19
Patella.

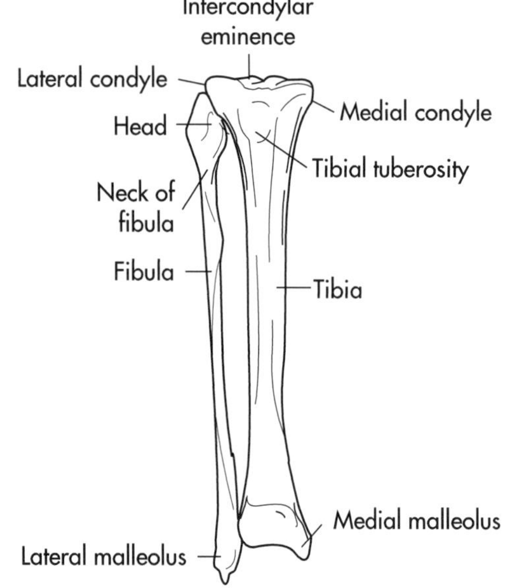

Figure 7-20
Tibia and fibula.

ACTIVITY 7-19

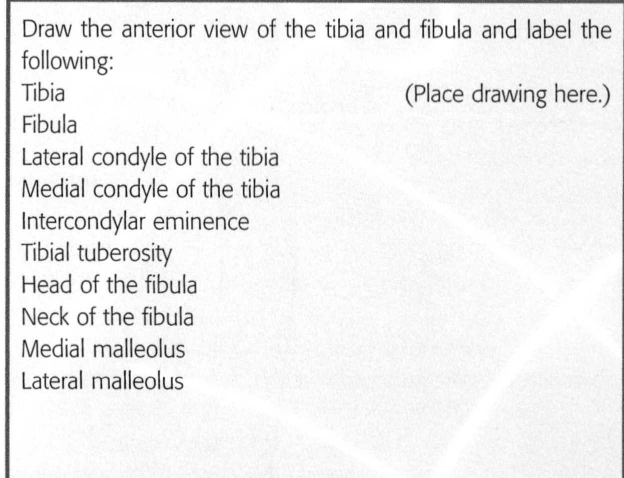

Draw the anterior view of the tibia and fibula and label the following:

(Place drawing here.)

Tibia
Fibula
Lateral condyle of the tibia
Medial condyle of the tibia
Intercondylar eminence
Tibial tuberosity
Head of the fibula
Neck of the fibula
Medial malleolus
Lateral malleolus

athletes (Figure 7-23). (For review of the bones, complete Activity 7-22.)

PATHOLOGIC CONDITIONS

Skeletal pathologies are not typically addressed by the massage therapist, but she should be able to recognize skeletal conditions and alter massage application to protect clients and/or to refer them to the appropriate health care professional. Pathologic conditions are divided into developmental problems, tumors, nutritional disorders, and disorders caused by trauma.

Developmental Problems

Spina Bifida

If the vertebral arches in a growing fetus do not fuse into the spinous processes, the result is spina bifida. Instead of being protected by bone, the nerves of the dorsal spinal cord may be covered by a thin membrane of skin, muscle, or spinal meninges. This condition may range from a mild case, with the child showing no symptoms, to severe spinal cord damage and paraplegia. The most common site of the defect is the lumbosacral region.

Cleft Palate

Cleft palate is a congenital deformity involving a gap in the roof of the mouth from behind the teeth to the back of the mouth. Newborns with this defect may have difficulty nursing or swallowing because their mouths are open to the nasal cavities above. They suck in air rather than milk, or the milk may enter the nose instead of the esophagus. The condition usually is corrected surgically.

Osteogenesis Imperfecta

Osteogenesis imperfecta is a group of hereditary disorders that appear in newborns or young children. The bones are deformed and fragile as a result of demineralization and defective formation of connective tissue.

Clubfoot (Talipes)

Clubfoot is the most common of the lower extremity congenital deformities. In most cases one or both feet are bent downward and adducted; in other cases the feet are pointed upward and abducted. Mild cases respond to splinting and stretching, but severe cases require surgical correction. Clubfoot is more prominent in boys and may result from genetic predisposition or the position of the fetus in the womb.

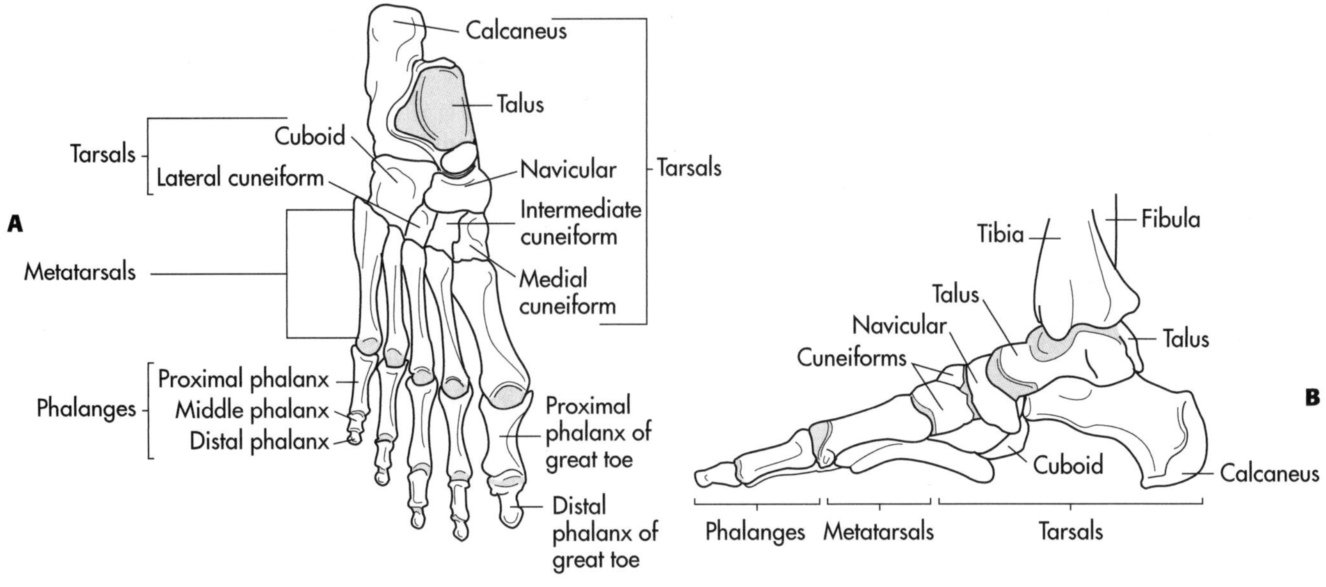

Figure 7-21
A, Dorsal view of the bones of the foot. **B,** Medial view of the bones of the foot and ankle.

ACTIVITY 7-20

Draw the dorsal view of the bones of the foot and label the following:

(Place drawing here.)

Calcaneus
Talus
Cuboid
Navicular
Cuneiform bones
Metatarsals
Phalanges

ACTIVITY 7-21

The list below names the bones of the lower limb:
Ilium
Ischium
Pubis
Femur
Patella
Tibia
Fibula
Tarsals
Metatarsals
Phalanges
Make up a silly sentence to help you remember these bones by using the first letter of each name.

Spinal Curve Abnormalities

Abnormal curvatures of the spine (Figure 7-24) may be congenital; may result from paralysis, weakness, or tension in spinal muscles; or may result from rapid growth of the body, especially after puberty. Bad posture habits, especially during periods of accelerated growth, can contribute to the problem. Scoliosis, a lateral curvature, is most often found in young girls, especially during or just after puberty, because of the rapid growth of the body. When discovered and treated early, the results are often good. As discussed previously, exaggeration of the thoracic curve is known as *kyphosis* (or hunchback), and excessive lumbar curvature is referred to as *lordosis.* One of the major problems caused by any extreme spinal curve is compression of the internal organs.

INDICATIONS/CONTRAINDICATIONS

For Therapeutic Massage

If skeletal problems create or are part of a permanent condition, supportive care is required. Massage methods are helpful in managing compensatory muscle spasms and connective tissue changes. Any type of compressive force or joint movement methods are contraindicated for a fragile skeletal structure,

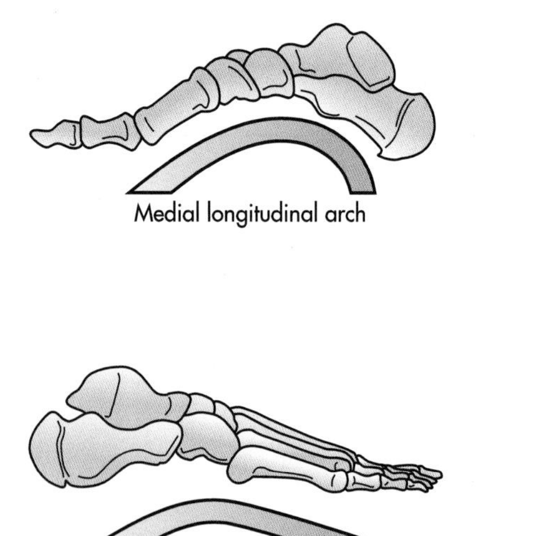

Figure 7-22
Medial and lateral arches of the foot.

regardless of the cause, unless appropriate medical professionals carefully supervise the massage. Light, superficial methods, such as the gentle laying on of hands used in some forms of touch systems, might be indicated, again with supervision.

Bone Demineralization Disorders

Osteoporosis

Osteoporosis is a disorder of the bone in which calcium and other minerals are lacking and bone protein is diminished. Under normal conditions, bone replaces itself with osteoblasts (bone-forming cells); with osteoporosis, this happens much more slowly, leaving the bones soft, fragile, and more likely to break. The condition occurs most often in postmenopausal women as a result of the decrease in hormone levels. Osteoporosis primarily affects the spine and pelvis. Other causes include deficiencies in the nutritional intake, absorption, or assimilation of protein and minerals, cigarette smoking, and inactivity. Treatments include hormone

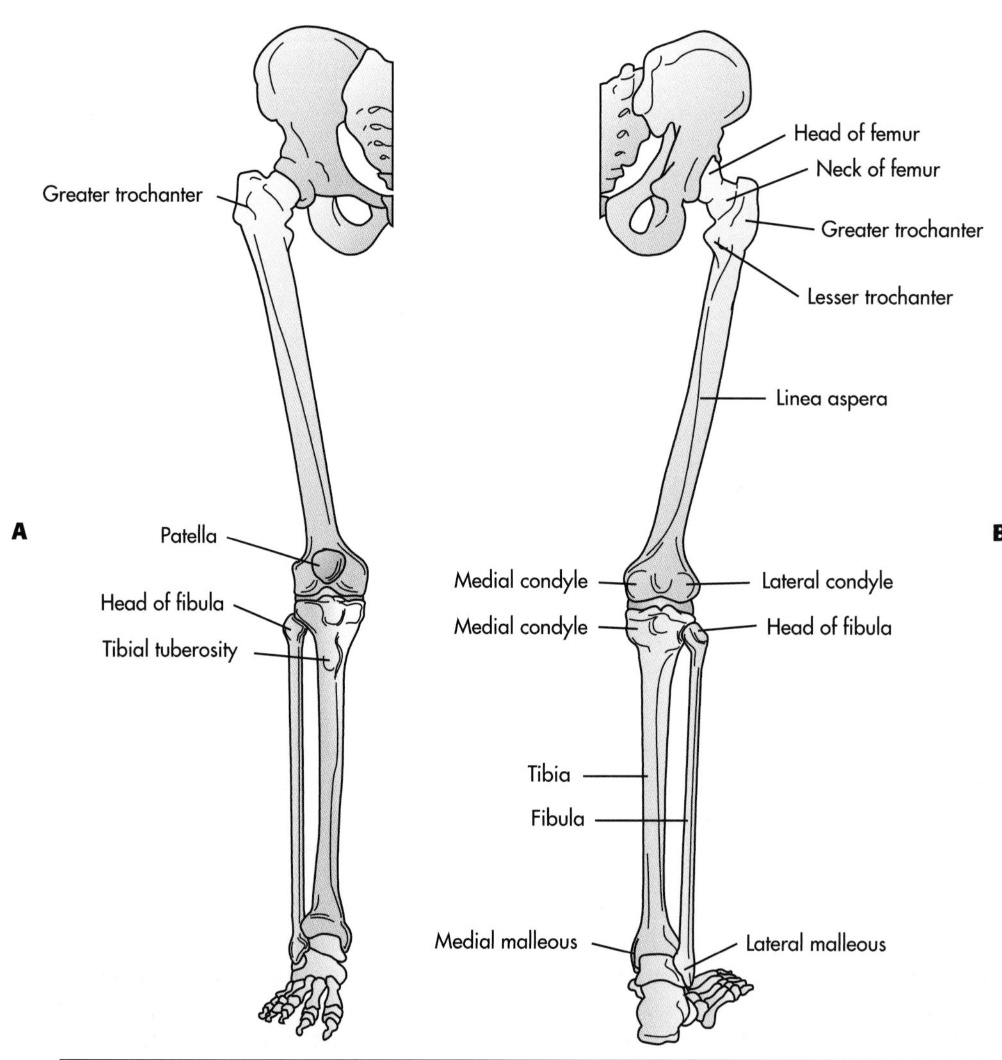

Figure 7-23
A, Bones of the lower limb (anterior view). **B,** Bones of the lower limb (posterior view).

ACTIVITY 7-22

Locate each of the following bony landmarks on yourself. You may need to refer to the illustrations in this chapter.

Zygomatic bone (cheekbone)

Seventh cervical vertebra (the most pronounced of the cervical vertebrae, especially with the neck flexed)

Mastoid process of the temporal bones

Clavicle (collar bone)

Coracoid process of the scapula

Sternum (breastbone) between the ribs

Sternal notch of the manubrium

Xiphoid process (at the inferior end of the sternum; it has a pointed tip)

Scapula

- Acromion of the scapula (the highest point of the shoulder)
- Spine of the scapula
- Medial or vertebral border
- Lateral or axillary border
- Inferior angle
- Superior angle
- Lateral angle

Humerus

- Greater and lesser tubercles
- Bicipital or intertubercular groove (runs between the two tubercles)
- Anatomic neck (just below the head of the humerus)
- Deltoid tuberosity (the insertion point for deltoid muscle)
- Lateral epicondyle (the bump at the distal end)
- Medial epicondyle (the bump at the distal end)
- Olecranon process (the point of the elbow)
- Head of the radius (the bony knob just distal to the lateral epicondyle; you can feel it rolling during supination and pronation)

Pisiform bone (the medial carpal bone on the anterior wrist)

Iliac crest (near the level of the waist)

Anterior superior iliac spine

Posterior superior iliac spine

Sacrum (the curved, triangular bone beneath the lumbar spine)

Coccyx (the caudal tip of the vertebral column, deep between the gluteal muscle masses)

Ischial tuberosity (the "sit bones" in the middle of the lower gluteals)

Pubic symphysis (the anterior midline joint of the pelvic girdle)

Femur

- Greater trochanter (large protuberance on the lateral side)
- Lesser trochanter (small elevation; on the medial side near top of inner thigh)
- Medial epicondyle
- Lateral epicondyle

Patella

Head of the fibula (bump on the lateral side of leg just distal to the knee)

Tibial tuberosity (the large bump just inferior to the patella)

Lateral malleolus

Medial malleolus

Calcaneus

therapy (primarily estrogen, progesterone, and calcitonin), increasing exercise, and including more sources of calcium, magnesium, boron, and vitamin D in the daily diet.

Paget's Disease

Paget's disease, or osteitis deformans, occurs when the bones undergo normal periods of calcium loss followed by periods of excessive new cell growth. Bone cells are replaced with fibrous tissue and blood vessels. As a result, the bones harden, deform, and become susceptible to fracture. Currently, we know neither the cause nor a cure. The condition is found most commonly in men over 40 years of age.

Osteitis Fibrosa Cystica

In osteitis fibrosa cystica, fibrous tissue and cysts replace bone tissue, making the bones weak and prone to fracture. This disorder occurs in long-standing hyperparathyroidism.

Disorders Caused by Radiation Therapy

When radiation is used to treat a bone disorder or is given as part of the treatment of a malignancy, bone may become brittle and fragile because of the changes in its structure. This happens if the bone is treated directly or if the treatment site involves bony structures.

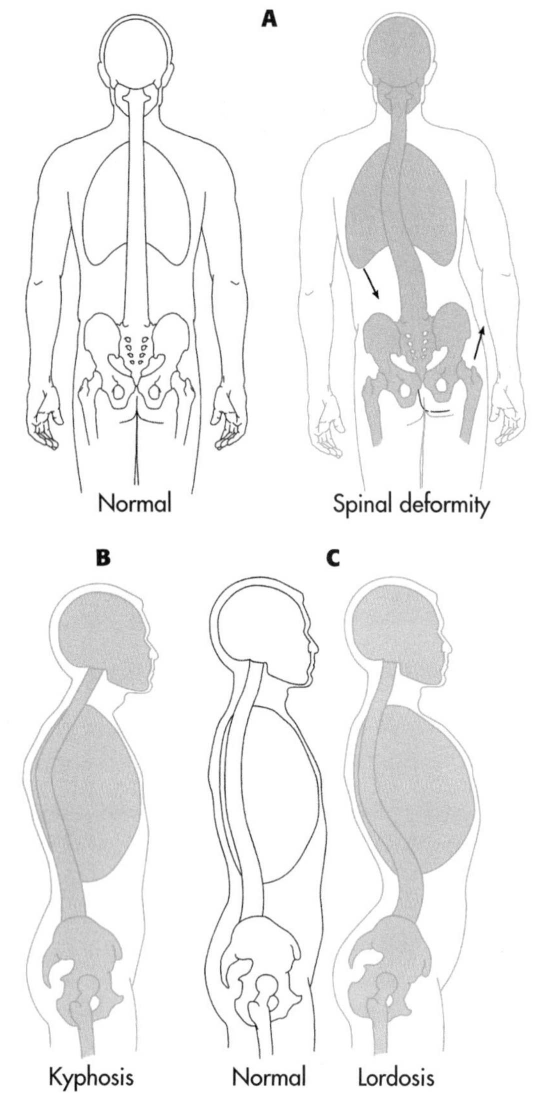

Figure 7-24
A, Deformity of the spine. Scoliosis is a lateral deviation of the spine. Arrows indicate the direction of the thoracic and pelvic tilt. **B,** Kyphosis, a flexion deformity of the spine. **C,** Lordosis, an extension deformity of the spine. (Modified from Barkauskas VH, et al: *Health and physical assessment,* ed 3, St Louis, 2002, Mosby.)

INDICATIONS CONTRAINDICATIONS

For Therapeutic Massage

Caution is required before the practitioner uses any massage requiring any amount of compressive force on a client with a condition that causes demineralization of bone or that results in brittle, fragile bones. A fragile skeletal structure, regardless of the cause, is a contraindication for any type of compressive force or joint movement methods unless appropriate medical professionals supervise these methods carefully. Light, superficial methods, such as the gentle laying on of hands used in some forms of touch systems, might be indicated with supervision. Bone involvement may be localized, such as with radiation treatment. In these cases, massage therapy methods can be used on the unaffected areas and avoided over the involved area.

Necrosis - cell or tissue death

Osteonecrosis (Ischemic Necrosis)

Various pathologic changes occur in the bone when its blood supply is diminished or cut off, or when infection, malignancy, or trauma occur. These conditions are among the common causes of hip pain and disability. The changes usually occur following a primary disease such as lupus, especially when the disease is treated with glucocorticoids. Symptoms include pain during active motion and at night. Because of its slow, progressive deterioration, necrosis may go undiagnosed.

Legg-Calvé-Perthes Disease

More commonly known as Perthes disease, Legg-Calvé-Perthes disease involves degeneration and necrosis at the head of the femur, followed by recalcification. The disorder, most often seen in young boys, occurs when the vascular supply to the head of the femur is compromised, resulting in developmental deformity. The condition lasts about 3 years and may predispose the child to arthritis in the area as an adult. Symptoms include hip pain and gait abnormalities.

Scheuermann's Disease

Scheuermann's disease is caused most commonly by necrosis or inflammation in bone or in a disk of the thoracic vertebrae. The disease begins during puberty, results from a genetic predisposition or trauma (or both), and leads to back pain and kyphosis. The excessive curvature is caused by the changes in the structure of the vertebrae, from columnar to wedge shaped.

Osteochondritis Dissecans

In osteochondritis dissecans the cartilage and adjacent bone separate from the bone itself. This disorder is most common in adults and is caused by inflammation and necrosis of the particular area. At the affected joint, portions of dead tissue may break away and lodge in the joint capsule, restricting movement and causing pain. The condition most often occurs in the knee joint.

INDICATIONS CONTRAINDICATIONS

For Therapeutic Massage

Necrosis usually is a localized condition that requires regional avoidance of the involved bone area. Because massage provides the generalized effect of enhanced circulation, indirect benefits might be realized with careful use of these methods. However, because these disorders are pathologic conditions, the practitioner must do massage with the permission and supervision of the primary health care provider.

Growth-Related Diseases

Osgood-Schlatter Disease

Osgood-Schlatter disease, which affects the tibial tuberosity, most often occurs in boys between 10 and 15 years of age. The tuberosity becomes inflamed or separates from the tibia because of irritation caused when the patellar tendon pulls on the tuberosity during periods of rapid growth or overuse of the quadriceps.

General Growing Pains

One of the many causes of growing pains occurs during growth spurts in children and adolescents when the bone grows faster than the attached muscles. The pain results when the muscle pulls on the pain-sensitive periosteum.

INDICATIONS CONTRAINDICATIONS

For Therapeutic Massage

Treatment of local areas may be contraindicated if inflammation or necrosis is present. General growing pains often are soothed by methods that do not introduce any sort of therapeutic inflammation, such as intense stretching and frictioning methods, which one should avoid. Methods that relax and lengthen the muscle and soften the connective tissue are appropriate. ■

Infectious Diseases

Osteomyelitis

Osteomyelitis is an inflammation in the bone, bone marrow, or periosteum, usually caused by pyogenic (pus-producing) bacteria. The bacteria reach the bone through the bloodstream or by way of an injury in which the skin is broken. Osteomyelitis most often occurs in children near the joints in the legs or arms. When promptly treated medically, the chance of a full recovery is excellent.

Tuberculosis

Tuberculosis is a systemic disease caused by the tubercular bacillus. Involvement in the skeletal system causes destruction of the bone tissue and necrosis. Tuberculosis of the spine, known as Pott's disease, affects mostly children. The onset of skeletal tuberculosis is insidious, usually marked by vague complaints of pain.

INDICATIONS CONTRAINDICATIONS

For Therapeutic Massage

Massage is contraindicated in infectious diseases unless carefully supervised by medical personnel. The therapist must always refer clients with vague pain symptoms for proper diagnosis. ■

Tumors

Tumors in the skeletal system can be primary or secondary. Primary tumors such as cysts or osteomatas (bony knobs in or on a bone) are rare and usually benign. Some tumors are malignant such as *osteosarcomatas,* which often arise in the femur or tibia of a young person. Some of the signs of malignancy are pain, unexplained swelling over a bone, a feeling of warmth on the skin, and prominent veins over the area.

Secondary tumors develop from primary sites, most often in the breast, lungs, or prostate. In older individuals, metastases from epithelial tumors or carcinomatas of various organs can spread to the bones.

Tumors also can be found in cartilage. Osteochondroma is a benign tumor of the cartilage and bone tissue of long bones. *Chondrosarcomatas* are malignant tumors of the cartilage.

INDICATIONS CONTRAINDICATIONS

For Therapeutic Massage

Prompt referral for diagnosis is a must for any sign that may indicate the growth of a tumor. Benign tumors are a local contraindication for massage. These therapies are contraindicated for individuals with malignant tumors unless the medical team directly and carefully supervises the therapist. ■

Nutritional Disorders

Rickets

Rickets is a childhood disease that is rare in the Western world yet that still occurs with conditions of extreme nutritional deficiency. Rickets is characterized by numerous bone deformities. Deficiency of the active form of vitamin D prevents the absorption of calcium and phosphorus through the intestine; these minerals, then, are not available for deposit in the bones, which remain soft and become distorted. The deformity patterns may be noticeable in older clients who had rickets as children.

Osteoporosis

Osteoporosis, discussed in more detail previously, also can be considered a nutritional disorder.

Scurvy

Scurvy is a vitamin C deficiency. Vitamin C is necessary for the production of collagen of the fibrous tissue and bone matrix. With scurvy, bone density is lost. Treatment involves increasing the vitamin intake, but some damage may be permanent. As with rickets, this disease is rare in the Western world but can occur under conditions of inadequate nutrition, such as with eating disorders.

INDICATIONS CONTRAINDICATIONS

For Therapeutic Massage

Regardless of the cause, a fragile skeletal structure is a contraindication for any type of compressive force or joint movement methods unless appropriate medical professionals supervise these methods carefully. Light, superficial methods such as the gentle laying on of hands used in some forms of touch systems might be indicated with supervision. ■

Disorders Caused By Trauma and Repetitive Use (Microtrauma)

Whiplash

In whiplash the anterior longitudinal ligament and cervical disks sometimes are injured.

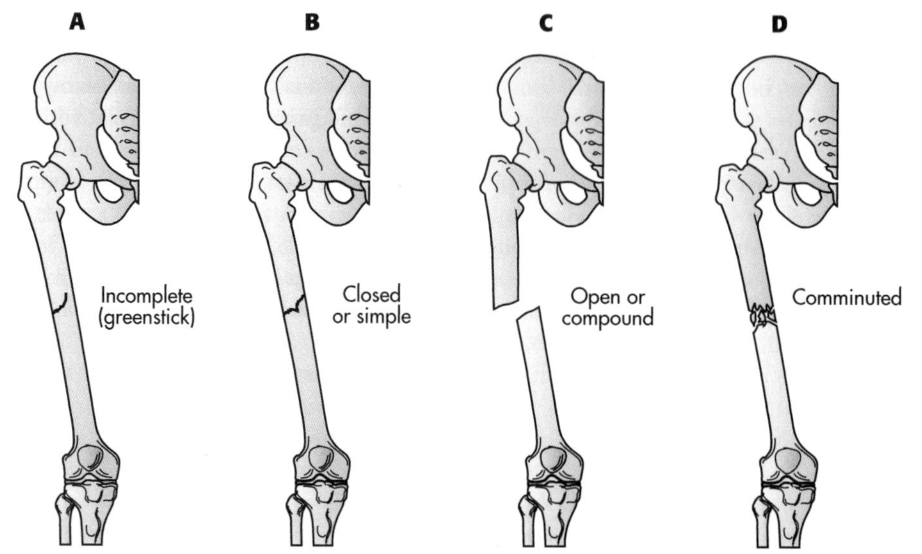

Figure 7-25
Types of fractures. **A,** Incomplete. **B,** Closed or simple. **C,** Open or compound. **D,** Comminuted.

Dislocation

A dislocation is the displacement of the bones of a joint; a subluxation is a partial dislocation.

Fractures

Severe force can fracture almost any bone. The term *fracture* means a break or rupture in a bone (Figure 7-25). Fractures may be classified as follows:

- Compound (open) fracture: The skin and other soft tissues are torn, and the bone protrudes through the skin.
- Simple (closed) fracture: The break in the bone does not break the skin or injure soft tissue.
- Greenstick fracture: The break in the bone is incomplete, producing a split such as might occur in a green piece of wood. This type is most common in children.
- Impacted fracture: The broken ends of the bones are jammed into each other.
- Comminuted fracture: The break involves more than one fracture line, with several fragments resulting, often with much soft tissue damage.
- Complete fracture: The break goes across the entire bone.
- Incomplete fracture: The break does not go across the entire bone.
- Compression fracture: The bone is squeezed or crushed (this type most often occurs in the spinal column).
- Depressed fracture: Bone in the skull is driven inward.
- Stress fracture: This type of fracture actually is a crack in the bone, often caused by repeated mechanical stress and strain.
- Spiral fracture: A break in which the bone is twisted apart. These fractures are common in skiing accidents.

The signs and symptoms of fractures include local swelling, pain, loss of function or abnormal movement of the affected part, and deformities such as angulation, shortening, or rotation. Crepitation, a grating sound produced when bone fragments rub together, also may be heard. Pain may not occur immediately because of temporary loss of nerve function and shock.

The most important step in first aid for a fracture is to prevent movement of the affected parts. One should summon expert help immediately and should protect the area to prevent movement, leaving the area as is if possible.

When a bone fractures, blood vessels and periosteum rupture and blood seeps into the fracture site; this is called the *fracture hematoma,* which develops 48 to 72 hours after injury. The hematoma surrounding the fracture site provides a loose fibrin mesh in which fibroblasts and capillaries form granulation tissues that replace the blood clot. Osteoblasts and chondroblasts become active in forming new bone and cartilage, and within approximately 7 days are dispersed throughout the soft tissue callus. This temporary bony union is called a *procallus.* Eventually bone replaces the procallus, forming a rigid, bony callus.

The healing process for a fractured bone usually takes 6 weeks, and it is essential that this process not be interrupted. Fractures often require immobilization and casting. Extensive soft tissue damage, including nerve damage and infection, can result following the fracture. These conditions can continue to cause difficulties long after the bone itself has healed.

Plantar Fasciitis

Plantar fasciitis develops from strain or injury to the plantar fascia of the foot. The signs and symptoms include acute pain when assuming activity after a period of rest. The pain improves (lessens) as the tissue warms and then begins to hurt again with use. A deep sharp and bruised sensation occurs at the arch and at the attachment at the heel.

Shin Splints

Shin splints involve muscle strain and potential hairline fractures of the tibia.

Indications/Contraindications

For Therapeutic Massage

Massage therapy is contraindicated locally over a trauma area until healing is complete. Light, subtle methods of touch therapies (e.g., a gentle laying on of hands) may be beneficial in diminishing pain. The process usually calms and soothes, which encourages healing through stress management. Massage therapy methods are beneficial in supporting the rest of the body during the healing process, especially in managing compensation patterns caused by immobilization of an area, and in helping the client learn the use of crutches and canes.

Stress fractures may not be readily detectable. Referral is indicated if the history points toward a mechanical stress condition such as a participation in a recent athletic event (Activity 7-23).

Massage is beneficial for plantar fasciitis and shin splints so long as it does not cause an increase in pain and inflammation. Massage is contraindicated for tibial fractures, which must be ruled out before one applies massage. ■

Activity 7-23

List three benefits of massage in dealing with pathologic conditions of the skeletal system.

Example

Stress management promotes healing.

Your Turn

1. ______________________________

2. ______________________________

3. ______________________________

List three contraindications for the use of massage in dealing with pathologic conditions of the skeletal system.

Example

Necrosis is locally contraindicated.

Your Turn

1. ______________________________

2. ______________________________

3. ______________________________

Summary

This chapter focuses on the general structure of the skeletal system and the specific anatomy of the bones of the body. The various activities review and integrate the data so that the names, shapes, and functions of bones are familiar. Information about the skeleton is important to our study of the way the body moves, which continues in later chapters.

evolve

Complete the crossword puzzle under Course Materials Chapter 7 on the EVOLVE site accompanying this book to form a better understanding of the skeletal system of the human body.

Workbook Section

1. List the seven main functions of the skeletal system.

2. Describe the structure and development of bone.

3. List and describe the six shapes of bone.

4. List and describe bony landmarks and give an example of each type.

WORKBOOK SECTION

5. Describe the two divisions of the skeleton and list the bones in each division.

____

____

____

____

____

____

____

____

____

____

FILL IN THE BLANK

The appendicular skeleton is composed of the (1) __limbs__ of the body and their attachments. Another name for a joint is a (an) (2) __articulation__.

The (3) __axial__ skeleton consists of the head, the vertebral column (spine), and the ribs and sternum. It provides the body with form and protection.

Compact bone is the (4) ______________ portion of bone that protects spongy bone and provides the firm framework of the bone and the body. The osteocytes in this type of bone are located in concentric rings called (5) ______________ around a central (6) ______________ canal, through which nerves and blood vessels pass.

The (7) ______________ is a thin membrane of connective tissue that lines the marrow cavity of a bone.

An endoskeleton is found (8) ______________ the human body; it accommodates growth.

The (9) ______________ is a thin membrane of connective tissue that covers bones except at the articulations.

The (10) ______________ quality of bones allows them to deform slightly and vibrate when electrical currents pass through them.

Sesamoid bones are round bones that often are embedded in tendons and joint capsules. The largest of these is the (11) ______________.

Spongy bone is also known as (12) ______________ bone.

(13) ______________ are an irregular meshing of small, bony plates that make up spongy bone. Its spaces are filled with (14) ______________ marrow.

A bone fracture is treated by (15) ______________, which means that the broken ends are pulled into alignment. In general, acute fracture healing has five stages: hematoma formation, (16) ______________ proliferation, callus formation, ossification, and remodeling. A (17) ______________ accumulates in the (18) ______________ canal and surrounds soft tissue in the first 48 to 72 hours.

WORKBOOK SECTION

EXERCISE

Identify each bone in the figure shown on p. 247 by filling in the blanks with the appropriate name.

A. ______

B. ______

C. ______

D. ______

E. ______

F. ______

G. ______

H. ______

I. ______

J. ______

K. ______

L. ______

M. ______

N. ______

O. ______

P. ______

Q. ______

R. ______

S. ______

T. ______

U. ______

V. ______

W. ______

X. ______

Y. ______

Z. ______

AA. ______

WORKBOOK SECTION

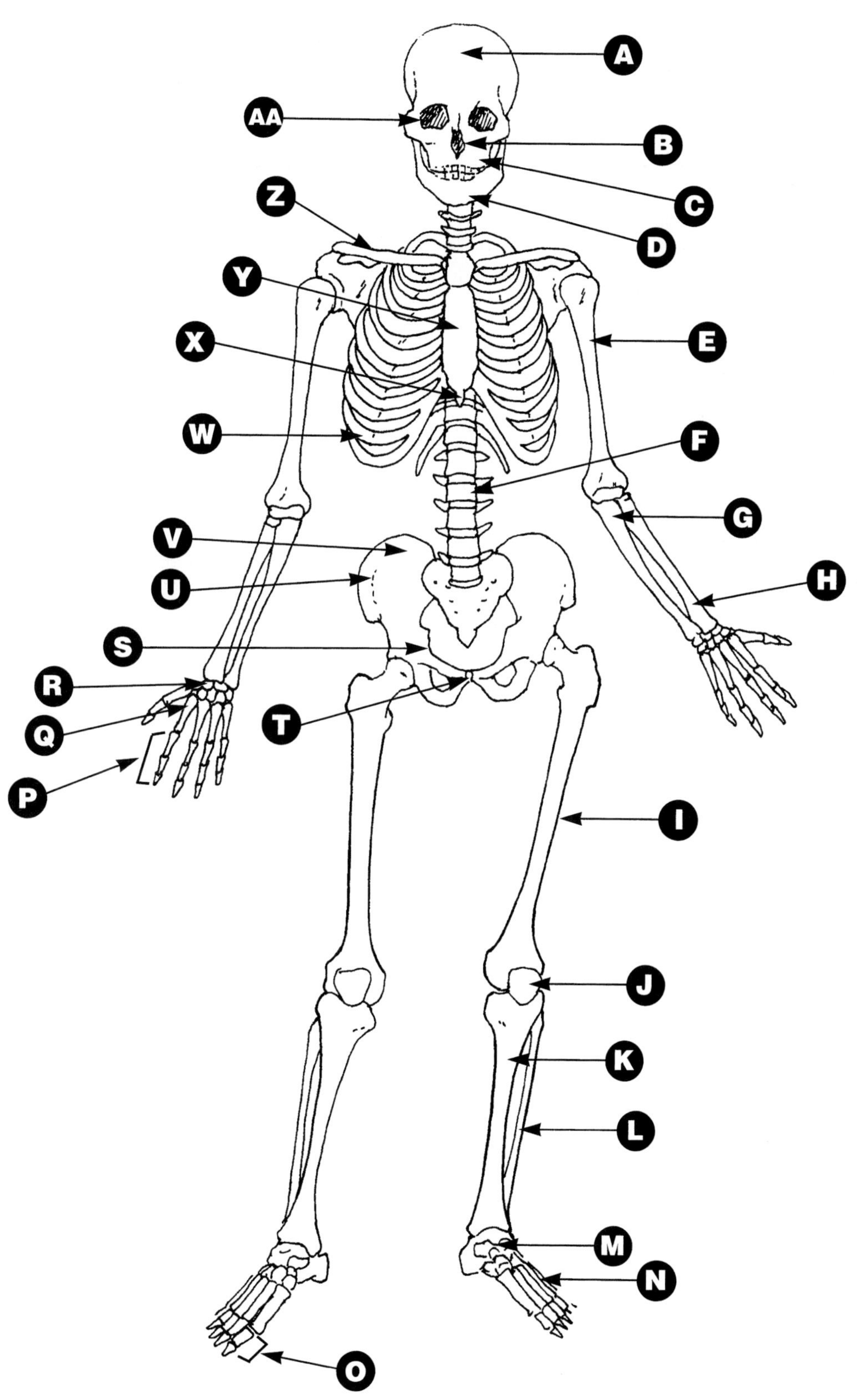

WORKBOOK SECTION

Now identify each part of the vertebral column, shown on p. 249 by filling in the blanks with the appropriate name.

A. ______________________________

B. ______________________________

C. ______________________________

D. ______________________________

E. ______________________________

F. ______________________________

G. ______________________________

H. ______________________________

I. ______________________________

J. ______________________________

K. ______________________________

L. ______________________________

Individual Vertebra

A. ______________________________

B. ______________________________

C. ______________________________

D. ______________________________

E. ______________________________

F. ______________________________

WORKBOOK SECTION

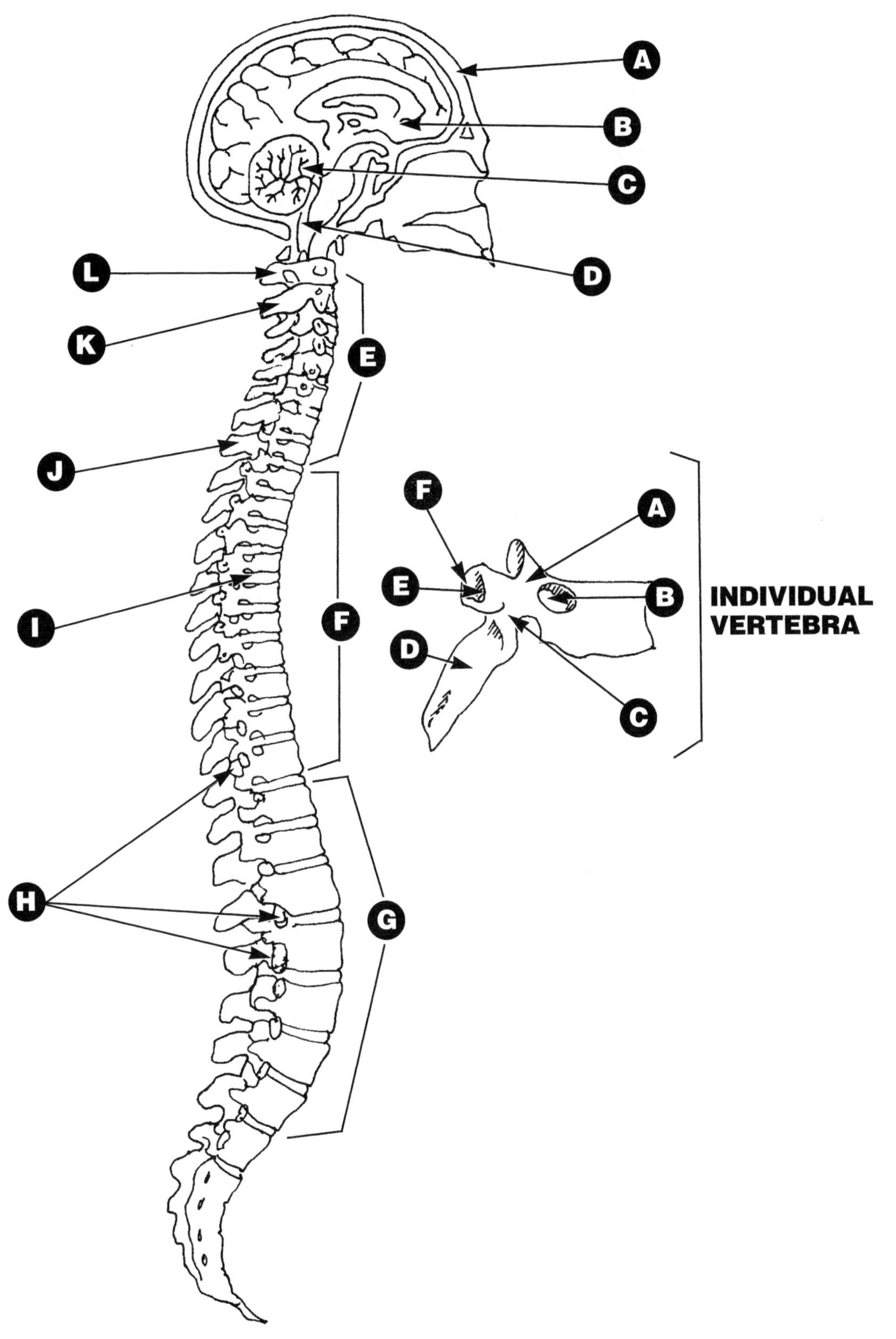

WORKBOOK SECTION

PROBLEM SOLVING

Read the problem presented. There is no correct answer; rather the exercise is intended to assist the student in developing the analytic and decision-making skills necessary in a professional practice. After reading the problem, follow the next six steps:

1. Identify the facts presented in the information.
2. Identify the possibilities ("what if" statements) or develop your own possibilities that relate to the facts.
3. Evaluate each possibility in terms of the logical cause and effect and pros and cons.
4. Consider the effect on the persons involved.
5. Write each answer in the space provided.
6. Develop your solution by answering the question posed.

Problem

The bones are not necessarily thought of as soft tissue. For this reason, direct work with the bones could be considered outside the scope of practice of the soft tissue or movement therapist. However, because muscles attach to bone and movement is related directly to bones, the bones logically would seem to be part of the anatomy and physiology affected by massage. Any approach that promotes general well-being affects the entire body, including the bones.

Question

In what way would you justify a scope of practice that included the bones as part of the body affected by therapeutic massage and movement therapy?

The first response is provided as a guide to get you started.

Fill in at least two more statements.

Facts

1. Muscles attach to bones.
2. ______________________________
3. ______________________________

Possibilities

1. Direct work with bones could be considered outside the scope of practice for therapeutic massage and movement therapists.
2. ______________________________
3. ______________________________

Logical Cause and Effect

1. Logically, therapeutic massage and movement therapy affect bone; therefore bones should be part of the scope of practice.
2. ______________________________
3. ______________________________

Effect

1. Clients may be uncertain as to who can address certain situations if the scope of practice lines are not clear.
2. ______________________________
3. ______________________________

How would you justify a scope of practice that includes the bones as part of the body affected by therapeutic massage and movement therapy?

____

____

____

____

____

____

____

____

____

____

____

FURTHER STUDY

Using additional resource material (see the Recommended Reading section of the list of Works Consulted), identify the chapters that pertain to the information presented in this chapter. Locate the information presented in this text and then elaborate by writing a paragraph of additional information on each of the following topics.

Piezoelectric quality of bones

____

____

____

____

____

____

____

____

____

____

____

Remodeling process of bone

Degenerative process of articular cartilage

Bone growth and repair

Skeletal changes caused by aging

Sinuses

The foot

WORKBOOK SECTION

Spinal curve abnormalities

____

____

____

____

____

____

____

____

____

____

Osteoporosis

____

____

____

____

____

____

____

____

____

____

Answer Key

1. (1) Supports soft tissues and serves as a framework for the entire body.
   (2) Provides attachment points for muscles and ligaments.
   (3) Protects delicate internal organs such as the brain, spinal cord, heart, and lungs.
   (4) Bones work as levers to provide movement begun by the attached muscles.
   (5) Stores calcium, phosphorus, and other minerals for release to the body as needed.
   (6) Stores lipids in bone marrow for use as energy.
   (7) Serves as production site for blood cells (hematopoiesis) in the red marrow.
2. Bones are hard, dense, and slightly elastic organs of the skeleton. They have their own system of blood, lymphatic vessels, and nerves.

   The process that creates our skeleton is called ossification. Ossification is a two-part process: chondroblasts, or cartilage-forming cells, create the cartilage model of bones. Bone-building cells, called osteoblasts, develop the bone tissue from the cartilage model.

   Shortly after birth, calcification takes place. This hardening of the bones, called osteogenesis, occurs as calcium salts are deposited in the gel-like matrix of the forming bones.

   Osteocytes are mature bone cells, which maintain the bone during the lifetime.

   Bones are composed chiefly of bone tissue, called osseous tissue. Two thirds of bone tissue is composed of inorganic mineral, which gives rigidity, and one third is composed of organic components, which provide elasticity. Bones have a piezoelectric quality. The structure and function of bones are connected intrinsically. Bones remodel themselves constantly, depending on the functional demand.

   Compact (dense) bone has little space between its tissues. This hard portion of the bone makes up the main shaft of the long bones and the outer layer of other bones. The osteocytes in this type of bone are located in concentric rings around a central haversian canal, through which nerves and blood vessels pass.

   Spongy (cancellous) bone has larger spaces between cells than compact bone, which makes cancellous bones lighter. This type of bone is made of an irregular meshing of small, bony plates, called trabeculae, and is found at the ends of the long bones or at the center of other bones. In some bones the trabecular spaces are filled with red marrow, which produces blood cells. Bones contain red marrow and yellow marrow.

   Except for the ends that form joints, bones are covered with a thin membrane of connective tissue, called periosteum. A thinner membrane, the endosteum, lines the marrow cavity of a bone; it too contains cells that aid in the growth and repair of bone tissue. Bones of a synovial or movable joint make physical contact at their cartilaginous ends. The only remaining cartilage in bone is called articular (or hyaline) cartilage.
3. (1) Flat bones: Generally these bones are more flat than round. Examples: Ribs and skull bones.
   (2) Irregular bones: These bones have two or more complex shapes within the same bone structure. Examples: Vertebrae and scapula.
   (3) Long bones: Longer in one axis than another, these bones are characterized by a medullary cavity, a hollow diaphysis (shaft) of compact bone, and at least two epiphyses, which are active in the growth of long bones. Most of the bones of the arms and legs are long bones; the hollow structure of the diaphysis has the advantages of strength and light weight. Examples: Femur and ulna.
   (4) Short bones: Shaped like long bones but much smaller, these bones make up the structures of the hands and fingers and the feet and toes. This shape of bone also can be classified as a long bone. Example: Metacarpals.
   (5) Cube-shaped bones (sometimes classified as short bones): These bones are predominantly cancellous, with a thin cortex of compact bone and no cavity. Examples: Wrist and ankle bones.
   (6) Sesamoid bones: Round bones that often are embedded in tendons and joint capsules. Example: Patella.
4. (a) Depressions and openings

   Canal: A tunnel or tube in bone. Example: Carotid canal in the temporal bone.

   Fissure: A groove or slit between two bones. Example: Orbital fissure of the sphenoid bone.

Foramen: An opening in a bone. Example: Vertebral foramen of the spinal column, through which the nerves pass.
Fossa: A shallow depression in the surface or at the end of a bone. Example: Infraspinous and supraspinous fossae of the scapula.
Groove: A depression in the bone that holds blood vessels, nerves, or tendons. Example: Radial groove of the humerus.
Meatus: A tunnel or canal found in a bone. Example: Canal in the skull from the external ear to the eardrum.
Notch: An indentation or large groove. Example: Greater and lesser sciatic notches of the ilium.
Sinus: Air cavity within a bone. Example: Frontal sinuses.

(b) Processes that form joints
Condyle: A rounded projection at the end of a bone that articulates with other bones to form a joint. Example: Medial condyle of the femur.
Head: A rounded projection found on top of the neck of a bone. Example: Head of the femur.
Facet: A smooth, flat surface. Example: Facet of a rib or vertebra.
Process: Any prominent, bony growth that projects. Example: Olecranon process of the ulna.
Trochlea: A pulley-shaped structure. Example: Trochlea of the humerus.

(c) Processes to which tendons and ligaments attach
Crest: A ridge on a bone. Example: Iliac crest.
Epicondyle: A projection above a condyle. Example: Medial epicondyle of the femur.
Line: A ridge that is smaller than a crest. Example: Linea aspera of the femur.
Spinous process, spine, or spina: A sharp, bony or slender projection. Example: Spinous process of the vertebral column or scapular spine.
Trochanter: One of two large, bony processes found only on the femur. Example: Greater or lesser trochanter.
Tubercle: A small, rounded process. Example: Adductor tubercle of the femur.
Tuberosity: A large, rounded protuberance. Example: Tibial tuberosity.

5. The two divisions of the skeleton are the axial skeleton and appendicular skeleton.

The axial skeleton, which forms the axis of the body, consists of the head, vertebral column (spine), and the ribs and sternum and provides the body with form and protection. The shoulder and hip girdles, which have similar structures, are the connectors to the axial skeleton.

The appendicular skeleton is composed of the limbs of the body and their attachments. The long bones of the upper and lower limbs, in combination with the muscles, provide fine and gross motor movements. Similar in design, these long bones are the humerus, radius, and ulna, and the femur, tibia, and fibula. In the same manner, the short carpals of the wrist and the tarsals of the ankle provide the flexibility needed in the hands and feet.

Fill in the Blank

1. limbs
2. articulation
3. axial
4. hard
5. lamellae
6. haversian
7. endosteum
8. inside
9. periosteum
10. piezoelectric
11. patella
12. cancellous
13. Trabeculae
14. red
15. reduction
16. cellular
17. hematoma
18. medullary

Exercise

Answers for figure on p. 247.

A. Cranium
B. Nasal bone
C. Maxilla
D. Mandible
E. Humerus
F. Vertebral column
G. Ulna
H. Radius
I. Femur
J. Patella
K. Tibia
L. Fibula
M. Tarsals
N. Metatarsals
O. Phalanges
P. Phalanges
Q. Metacarpals
R. Carpals
S. Ischium
T. Pubis
U. Ilium
V. Innominate bone
W. Costal cartilage
X. Xiphoid process
Y. Sternum
Z. Clavicle
AA. Orbit

Answers for figure on p. 249.

A. Skull
B. Brain
C. Cerebellum
D. Brainstem
E. Cervical curve
F. Thoracic curve
G. Lumbar curve
H. Intervertebral foramina
I. Intervertebral disk
J. Seventh cervical vertebra
K. Second cervical vertebra (axis)
L. First cervical vertebra (atlas)

CHAPTER 8

Joints

▼ Chapter Objectives

After completing this chapter, the student will be able to perform the following:

- Describe the elementary principles of joint design.
- Define the two main types of joints.
- Define arthrokinematics and osteokinematics.
- Describe joint play.
- Describe the structures that contribute to joint stability.
- Identify and palpate individual joints of the body.
- Identify pathologic conditions of joints and describe general treatment protocols used for intervention.
- Design a joint movement sequence for the body.

▼ Chapter Outline

▼ Key Terms

Anatomic range of motion The amount of motion available to a joint based on the structure of the joint and determined by the shape of the joint surfaces, joint capsule, ligaments, muscle bulk, and surrounding musculotendinous and bony structures.

Arthrocentesis (ar-THRO-sen-te-sis) Puncture of a joint space with a needle to remove accumulated fluid from the joint.

Arthrokinematics (ar-THRO-ki-ne-ma-tiks) Movement of bone surface in the joint capsule including role, spin, and slide.

Articulation (ar-tik-yoo-LAY-shun) A joint in which two or more bones meet to connect parts and allow for movement in the body.

Ball-and-socket joint Joint that allows movement in many directions around a central point. Ball-and-socket joints are ball-shaped convex surfaces fitted into concave sockets. This type of joint gives the greatest freedom of movement but also is the most easily dislocated.

Bursa (BER-sah) A flat sac of synovial membrane in which the inner sides of the sac are separated by a fluid film. Bursae are located where moving structures are apt to rub.

Closed kinematic chain The positioning of joints in such a way that motion at one of the joints is accompanied by motion at an adjacent joint.

Close-packed position The position of a synovial joint in which the surfaces fit precisely together and maximal contact between the opposing surfaces occurs. The compression of joint surfaces permits no movement, and the joint possesses its greatest stability.

Collagen (KOL-ah-jen) A fibrous tissue that provides stability to connective tissue structures of fasciae, tendons, and ligaments. Collagen makes up one fourth of the protein in the body.

Condyloid (condylar) joint Joint that allows movement in two directions, but one motion predominates. The joint resembles a condyle, which is a rounded protuberance at the end of a bone forming an articulation.

Continued

Diarthrosis (dye-ar-THRO-sis) A freely movable synovial joint.

Elastin (e-LAS-tin) A connective tissue fiber type that has elastic properties and allows flexibility of connective tissue structures.

Fibrocartilage (fye-bro-KAR-ti-lij) A connective tissue that permits little motion in joints and structures. It is found in places such as the intervertebral disks, and forms our ears.

Gliding joints Known also as synovial plane, gliding joints allow only a gliding motion in various planes.

Hinge joint Joint that allows flexion and extension in one direction, changing the angle of the bones at the joint, like a door hinge.

Hyaline cartilage (HYE-ah-lin) The thin covering of articular connective tissue on the ends of the bones in freely movable joints in the adult skeleton. Hyaline cartilage forms a smooth, resilient, low-friction surface for the articulation of one bone with another, distributes forces, and helps absorb some of the pressure imposed on the joint surfaces.

Hypermobility A range of motion of a joint greater than would be permitted normally by the structure. Hypermobility results in instability.

Hypomobility A range of motion of a joint less than what would be permitted normally by the structure. Hypomobility results in restricted range of motion.

Joint capsule A connective tissue structure that indirectly connects the bony components of a joint.

Joint play The involuntary movement that occurs between articular surfaces that is separate from the range of motion of a joint produced by muscles. Joint play is an essential component of joint motion and must occur for normal functioning of the joint.

Loose-packed position The position of a synovial joint in which the joint capsule is most lax. Joints tend to assume this position when inflammation occurs to accommodate the increased volume of synovial fluid.

Open kinematic chain A position in which the ends of the limbs or parts of the body are free to move without causing motion at another joint.

Pathologic range of motion The amount of motion at a joint that fails to reach the normal physiologic range or exceeds normal anatomic limits of motion of that joint.

Physiologic range of motion The amount of motion available to a joint determined by the nervous system from information provided by joint sensory receptors. This information usually prevents a joint from being positioned so that injury could occur.

Pivot joint A bony projection from one bone fits into a ring formed by another bone and ligament structure to allow rotation around its own axis.

Saddle joint Joint that is convex in one plane and concave in the other with the surfaces fitting together like a rider on a saddle.

Suture A synarthrotic joint in which two bony components are united by a thin layer of dense fibrous tissue.

Symphysis (SIM-fi-sis) A cartilaginous joint in which the two bony components are joined directly by fibrocartilage in the form of a disk or plate.

Synarthrosis (sin-ar-THRO-sis) A limited-movement, nonsynovial joint.

Synchondrosis (SIN-kond-ROE-sis) A joint in which the material used for connecting the two components is hyaline growth cartilage.

Syndesmosis (SIN-dez-mo-sis) A fibrous joint in which two bony components are joined directly by a ligament, cord, or aponeurotic membrane.

Synovial fluid (si-NO-vee-al) A thick, colorless, lubricating fluid secreted by the joint cavity membrane.

Synovial joint A freely moving joint allowing motion in one or more planes of action.

Viscoelasticity The combination of resistance offered by a fluid to a change of form and the ability of material to return to its original state after deformation. This term describes connective tissue.

Yellow elastic cartilage Cartilage that is more opaque, flexible, and elastic than hyaline cartilage and is distinguished further by its yellow color. The ground substance is penetrated in all directions by frequently branching fibers.

JOINT OVERVIEW

Move. Wiggle. Put on some music and dance. Hug someone. Scratch your nose. Touch your toes. Joints are where we bend and twist. Body movement depends on joints. Many systemic body functions such as respiration and movement of blood and lymph depend on the mechanical pumping action of joint movement. For example, lymph nodes often are located at jointed areas so that with every movement, the body massages the lymph system. The mechanical actions of breathing in and out depend on movement of the ribs. A firm understanding of the anatomy and physiology of jointed areas is necessary because massage therapists interact most directly with the somatic structures of the body wall (i.e., the muscles, connective tissue, joint structure, and bones) as the entry point to the entire body.

Metaphorically, joints are interdependent relationships. A joint cannot exist with only one bone; at least two must work together. Joints seldom operate independently of other joints, but instead an orchestrated, synchronized network of links develops similar to relationships within a family. Joints are passive and unable to function without the muscles. They can do nothing alone but depend on others to get the job done, just as do families, friends, and work teams. Joints and muscles need each other. Joints must move to be healthy and can only function best in the way they are designed to move.

So it is with us. Persons need to be active and do best when they work with their unique structure of personal gifts. A knee would not make a good shoulder joint nor would the elbow be able to operate as a knee, but an elbow is designed to be a good elbow and is essential and equal to the knee in the function of the body.

A joint or **articulation** connects parts of a structure. In the body the structures joined are the bones. Joints illustrate the strong relationship that exists between structure and function. The design of a joint depends on its function and vice versa. Joints that provide stability or static support are different from joints that provide mobility. In the body, structure such as bone shape and the way the bones attach at the joint determines joint function.

Each part of a joint has one or more specific functions essential for the overall performance of the joint. Any disruption or change in any of the parts affects the function of the joint.

Joints connect approximately 200 bones of various sizes and shapes in the human skeleton. Effective functioning of the total structure depends on the integrated action of many joints, some providing stability and some providing mobility. Generally, stability must be achieved before mobility. **Joint capsules,** ligaments, and tendons stabilize joints. Most joints serve a dual function of mobility and stability.

Joint designs in the human body vary from simple to complex. The simplest human joints usually have stability as a primary function, whereas the more complex joints usually have mobility as a primary function. Joints serving a single function are less complex than joints serving multiple functions. Complex joints are more likely to be affected by injury, disease, or aging than are simple joints because the complex joints have more parts and are subject to more wear and tear than stability joints (Activity 8-1).

Connective Tissue and Joint Structure

Chapter 1 first discussed connective tissue. This chapter provides more specific detail relating to joint function. Chapter 9 provides additional information relating to muscle structure and function.

Connective tissue is used in the construction of human joints in the form of bones, ligaments, tendons, bursae, disks, plates, menisci, fat pads, and membranes.

As discussed in Chapter 1, the structure of the connective tissue is characterized by a large extracellular matrix and a wide dispersion of cells. The extracellular matrix has a nonfibrous component, referred to as the *ground substance,* and a fibrous component.

The ground substance consists of proteins responsible for attracting and binding water. The concentration of these proteins in the extracellular matrix of bone, cartilage, membranes, tendons, or ligaments affects the water content and therefore pliability of these structures. The nonfibrous component also plays an important role in protecting the connective tissue structure and strengthening it.

The fibrous component of the extracellular matrix contains two types of fibers: **collagen** and **elastin.**

Collagen

The primary fibrous component of the intercellular substance in dense fibrous tissue is collagen (white fibrous tissue). Collagen has a tensile strength similar to steel and is responsible for the functional stability of connective tissue structures.

Collagen fibers are nonelastic but still provide limited mobility. In the relaxed position of some structures, collagen fibers assume a wavy configuration called crimp. The crimp or wave can be straightened out, allowing for some flexibility in the structure.

Collagen has piezoelectric properties that generate small electric currents when it is deformed, and collagen oscillates or vibrates if electric currents travel through it (Figure 8-1, *A*).

Elastin

Elastin, or yellow fibrous tissue, has elastic properties that allow fibers to return to their original condition after a deforming force has been applied (Figure 8-1, *B*). The arrangement of the collagen fibers along with the collagen-to-elastin fiber ratio in various ligaments and tendons determines the ability of these structures to provide stability and mobility for a particular joint.

The fibrous component of the extracellular matrix in ligaments and tendons contains a greater collagen content

ACTIVITY 8-1

Consider the following principles and characteristics of joint design. Write down a social interaction that is similar. Some examples are provided to get you started.

Example
Some joints provide stability.
Having my grandmother over to talk stabilizes my connection with my family and my past.
Some joints provide mobility.
Relationships with my teachers move my knowledge forward.
The structure of the joint determines the function of the joint.
The relationship I have with my dog is one of companionship, and the relationship I have with my chickens is one of a caretaker.
A breakdown or change of any joint structure affects the entire joint function.
My son's divorce affected our entire immediate family, and the holidays were particularly difficult the first year.

Your Turn

Joints connect two or more bones together.

The design of a joint depends on its function.

Some joints provide stability.

Some joints provide mobility.

The structure of the joint determines the function of the joint.

Each part of the joint has a specific function that is essential to the whole function of the joint.

The breakdown of any joint structure affects the entire joint function.

Complex joints are more likely to malfunction than simple joints.

Effective functioning of the whole body depends on the integrated action of many joints working together.

Generally, stability must be achieved before mobility.

Most joints serve a dual function of mobility and stability.

Simple joints provide more stability.

Complex joints provide more mobility.

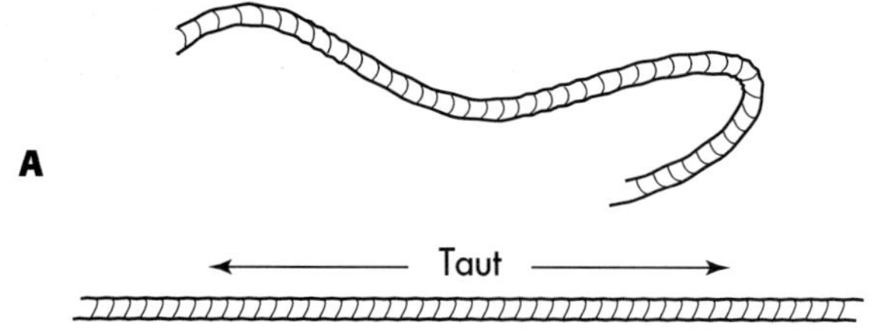

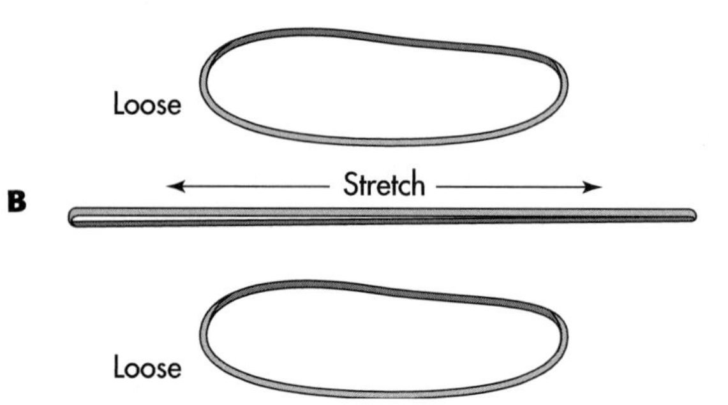

Figure 8-1
A, Collagen–like a rope. **B,** Elastin–like a rubber band.

than elastin content. However, the ratio of collagen to elastin fibers and their arrangement varies considerably among different ligaments. Generally, the collagen fibers in tendons are arranged in a parallel configuration to handle pulling forces, whereas the collagen fibers in ligaments have a more varied arrangement, depending on the function of the ligament.

In addition to their usual connective tissue components, tendons and ligaments are surrounded by loose areolar connective tissue that forms complete or partial sheaths around these structures. Double layers of connective tissue around the tendons at the wrist and hand form complete sheaths. These tendons sometimes are called *sheathed tendons.* The sheath protects the tendon and produces **synovial fluid,** which helps reduce friction.

Bursae

Bursae are flat sacs of synovial membrane in which the inner sides of the sacs are separated by a fluid film. Bursae are located where moving structures are apt to rub. Subcutaneous bursae are located between the skin and bones. Subtendinous bursae are located between tendons and bones. Submuscular bursae are located between muscles and bones. Although most of us have bursae in the same places, bursae can form from demand if the body needs additional cushioning.

Cartilage

Cartilage is usually divided into three types: **fibrocartilage, yellow elastic cartilage,** and **hyaline cartilage.**

Fibrocartilage. Fibrocartilage is subdivided into white and yellow elastic types.

White fibrocartilage consists primarily of collagen fibers and forms the cement in joints that permit little motion. This type of cartilage also forms the intervertebral disks and the menisci in the knees.

Yellow elastic cartilage is found in the ears and epiglottis and differs from white fibrocartilage in that it has a higher ratio of elastin to collagen fibers. It is more opaque, flexible, and elastic than hyaline cartilage and is distinguished further by its yellow color. The ground substance is penetrated in all directions by frequently branching fibers.

Hyaline cartilage. Hyaline cartilage forms a thin covering of articular cartilage on the ends of the bones in freely movable joints in the adult skeleton. It forms a smooth, resilient, low-friction surface for the articulation of one bone with another; and disperses joint pressure over a wider area. Hyaline cartilage distributes any additional stresses applied to a joint and helps absorb some of the pressure imposed on the joint surfaces. These cartilaginous surfaces are capable of bearing and distributing weight over the lifetime of a person. Water is the most abundant component of hyaline cartilage and, when combined with protein substances in the ground substance, forms a stiff gel (Figure 8-2).

Synovial fluid is distributed during joint motion or when the cartilage is compressed. The fluid flows back into the cartilage after motion or compression stops. Because hyaline cartilage is devoid of blood vessels and nerves in the adult, its nourishment is derived solely from this back-and-forth flow of fluid. The free flow of fluid is essential for the survival of cartilage and as an aid to reducing friction. The effects of immobilization, in which compression of joint surfaces is absent or diminished, can cause hyaline cartilage to degenerate.

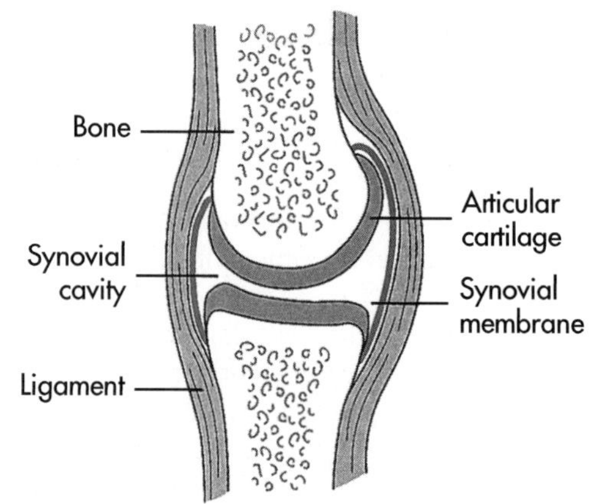

Figure 8-2
Articular cartilage in the joint capsule. (From Barkauskas VH et al: *Health and physical assessment*, ed 3, St Louis, 2002, Mosby.)

Bone

Bone is the hardest of all connective tissues found in the body. As with other forms of connective tissue, bone consists of a cellular component, a ground substance, and a fibrous component.

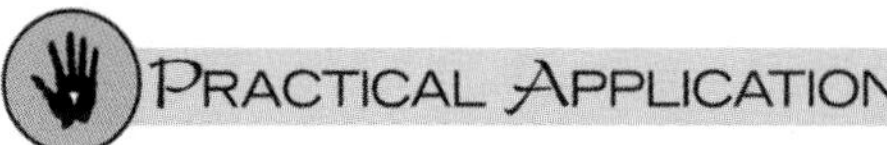

The availability of adequate water in the body is important to the function of connective tissue and cartilage. Studies have shown that an increase in water intake can reduce certain types of disk and joint pain. The connective tissues rehydrate whenever possible, and as they do, intervertebral disks expand somewhat, increasing the space between the vertebrae and reducing pressure on the nerves. In **synovial joints** a similar process takes place with a rehydration of the articular cartilage, as well as all of the connective tissue structures.

The benefit of most connective tissue modalities results from an increase in the pliability of the connective tissue. Because this pliability also depends on the water content of the tissue, unless adequate fluid is available to which the protein can bind, the connective tissue is unable to change structure readily. Therefore an increase in water intake, along with connective tissue modalities, seems to be a logical approach when working with joints. Drinking adequate amounts of water seems to be a simple thing to do, and the benefits are certainly demonstrable.

Movement is also essential to joint health. Therapeutic massage can support joint function and in some instances replace movement to encourage the production and distribution of synovial fluid in the joint. Methods that use passive and active forms of movement are the modalities of choice in these instances. ■

Viscoelasticity of Connective Tissue

Although connective tissue appears in many forms throughout the body, all connective tissue exhibits the common property of **viscoelasticity.** The behavior of viscoelastic materials is a combination of the properties of elasticity and viscosity.

Elasticity refers to the ability of a material to return to its original state after deformation (pulling). *Viscosity* refers to the resistance to a change of form offered by a fluid. When a constant compressive or tensile force deforms connective tissue, the tissue moves in the direction of the force and then attempts to return to its original state. Under normal conditions, viscoelastic materials initially modify in the direction of the force applied and then slowly return to their original state (called creep). If a connective tissue structure is held in a deformed position for an extended period of time, over days or weeks, the viscous creep pattern may become permanent, thus altering the structure and therefore the function of a joint.

Connective tissue subjected to sudden, prolonged, or excessive forces may exceed its elastic limits, and the tissue may enter the *plastic range.* In the plastic range the tissue is permanently deformed and is no longer able to return to its original state after the removal of the deforming force. This situation is similar to what happens when ligaments are overstretched and become lax. The ligaments are no longer capable of returning to their original length after being elongated and remain in a partial state of elongation. Ligament laxity places a joint at risk for injury because it compromises an important source of joint support and protection.

When the plastic range of connective tissue is exceeded, a failure (break or tear) of the tissue occurs. In the case of a ligament or tendon, the failure may occur in the middle of the structures, through tearing and disruption of the connective tissue fibers and is called a *rupture.* Failure that occurs through a tearing off of the bony attachment of the ligament or tendon is called an *avulsion.* Failure that occurs in bony tissue is called a *fracture.*

Each type of connective tissue can undergo a certain percentage of deformation before failure. This percentage varies not only among the types of connective tissue but also within the various types. Generally, tendons can deform more than ligaments, ligaments can deform more than cartilage, and cartilage can deform more than bone.

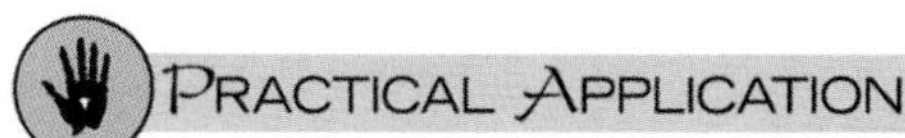

Two types of general pathologic conditions develop with changes in elasticity and viscosity of connective tissue: laxity and shortening. Laxity occurs when connective tissue is too long, as previously described, and most often happens with prolonged overstretching of joint structures or with a sudden trauma. Gymnastics, dancing, figure skating, and excessive use of stretching systems such as yoga can produce this condition. Too much flexibility results in instability. One must remember that stability is established before mobility. When connective tissue is unstable around a joint, the muscles of the jointed area increase contraction to provide the necessary joint stability. This action pulls the bones of a joint together, decreasing joint space, which may result in increased friction in the joint capsule. Although this is a good short-term strategy, other problems with joint function, such as predisposition to osteoarthritis, develop over the long term.

One can use massage approaches to manage the muscle contractions around the joint and support the compensation pattern by keeping the muscle contractions appropriate to the need for stabilization and minimizing the excessive pulling together of the bones of the joint. The use of certain types of frictioning techniques on individual connective tissue structures such as ligaments can create a therapeutic inflammation process. Because inflammation triggers the formation of connective tissue, the massage practitioner possibly can encourage the development of additional ligament structure. One combines this procedure with moderate immobilization necessary to allow the connective tissues to form and rehabilitative exercise to prevent adhesions from developing during the restructuring process. Therefore a combination of purposeful therapeutic inflammation, external stability in the form of moderate immobilization such as wrapping the area with elastic bandages or soft supports, and appropriate rehabilitative exercise that includes range of motion without resistance creates a broadening of the muscles or connective tissue structures of the area. A series of pulsing activities that do not stretch the tissues but instead mobilize the area through a gentle range of motion also increase stability in lax ligaments. This form of intervention for lax ligaments is a slow and deliberate process.

Connective tissue also tends to shorten and dehydrate, pulling structures together and stiffening the area, thus decreasing mobility. This situation provides too much stability and tends to develop to compensate for form alteration in response to a change in function. Should the body need to alter position for an extended period of time such as static positions from working at a computer daily for hours at a time, connective tissue slowly alters to support that position. Connective tissue can thicken and shorten if any inflammatory process does not resolve itself effectively. In these situations the plastic component of connective tissue must be elongated in the direction of the shortening to restore the pliability and redirect the creep pattern.

When one stretches a shortened connective tissue structure to elongate it, the tissue should be warm. One then applies an appropriately intense but slow pulling or pushing force to the connective tissue area and sustains it to produce creep and increase pliability. The goal is to extend the elastic range of connective tissue structures by altering the plastic range of shortened connective tissue. Myofascial massage therapy methods incorporate these principles. Movement methods such as yoga and other forms of slow, sustained stretching are based on similar principles. To access the plastic range of connective tissue, one must avoid the protective muscle contraction initiated by the stretch-reflex response. Lengthening all muscle components to their available resting length is important before increasing the force to stretch beyond the elastic range to elongate the plastic component of connective tissue. As already mentioned, an adequate intake of water is essential for the success of these methods.

Some restricted joint function develops from the tissues surrounding the joint instead of within the capsule itself. Because of this, one must assess the entire area for shortening. For example, shortening in the lumbodorsal fascia or pectoral fascia can limit the range of motion of the shoulder joint. Over time the reduction in movement causes pathologic immobilization in the joint. Therefore any therapeutic massage or movement methods affecting joint function should address the entire body broadly. Working with connective tissue is a slow process. Allowing time for the form to change gently and integrate effectively into the entire function of the jointed area and surrounding tissue is essential (Activities 8-2 and 8-3). ■

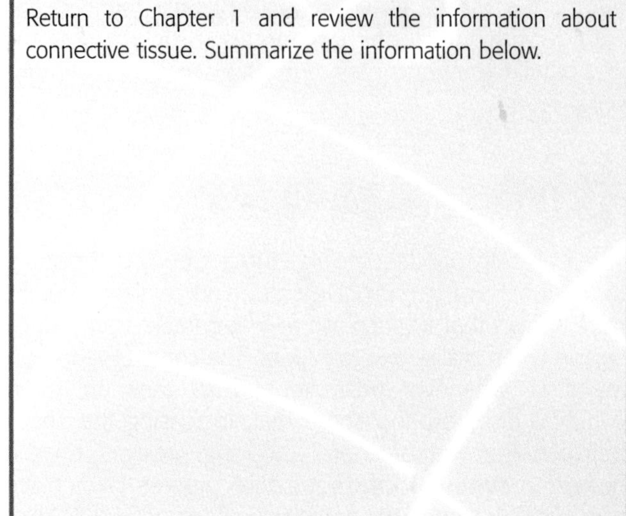

ACTIVITY 8-2

Return to Chapter 1 and review the information about connective tissue. Summarize the information below.

Joint Categories

The joints of the human body are divided into three categories based on the type of motion allowed at the joint. The three categories of joints (arthroses) are these:

Synarthroses: nonsynovial fibrous limited-movement joints
Amphiarthroses: cartilaginous joints that are slightly movable
Diarthroses: synovial, freely movable joints

Synarthroses (Fibrous Joints)

In fibrous joints the fibrous tissue directly connects bone to bone (Figure 8-3). The material used to connect the bony components in synarthrodial joints is interosseus fibrous and cartilaginous connective tissues. The connective tissue directly unites one bone to another in a bone–solid connective tissue–bone configuration.

Three different types of fibrous joints are found in the human body: sutures, gomphoses, and syndesmoses.

A **suture** is a joint in which two articulating bones are held together by a thin layer of dense fibrous tissue that is continuous with the periosteum. The ends of the bony components are grooved so that the edges interlock or overlap. This type of joint is found only in the skull. Early in life these sutures allow a small amount of movement. In adulthood

ACTIVITY 8-3

Develop a therapeutic intervention for a hypothetical connective tissue dysfunction. First, define and describe the assessment procedures you would use. Then develop a therapeutic goal for the area. Finally, develop treatments on the basis of the listed principles. Do plans for a hypermobile and hypomobile situation. Use therapy modalities you are studying presently in your technique classes. Remember that the actual implementation of such a plan often would be supervised by the appropriate health care professional, who would approve the plan before it is implemented. The principles are listed next, followed by an example.

Principles

Assessment Principles

Hypermobility: connective tissue becomes lax

- Too much flexibility results in instability.
- Muscle splinting develops to stabilize the area.

Hypomobility

- The entire area must be assessed for shortening.
- Over time, the reduction in movement causes pathologic immobilization in the joint itself.
- Any therapeutic massage methods affecting joint function need to address the body broadly.

Therapeutic Goals

Hypermobility

- Restore stability to connective tissue structures.
- Reduce muscle spasms surrounding the jointed area.

Hypomobility

- Extend the elastic range of connective tissue structures by altering the plastic range.
- Elongate the plastic component of connective tissue in the direction of the shortening.
- Restore pliability.
- Redirect the creep pattern.

Treatment Principles

Hypermobility

- Manage the muscle contraction around the joint to support the compensation pattern by keeping the muscle contraction appropriate to the need for stabilization and minimizing the excessive pulling of the joint cavity together.
- Apply frictioning techniques to individual connective tissue structures such as ligaments to create a therapeutic inflammation process.
- Combine this procedure with moderate immobilization.
- Use rehabilitative exercise to prevent adhesions from developing.

Hypomobility

- Avoid the protective muscle contraction initiated by the stretch reflex response to access the plastic range of connective tissue.
- Lengthen all muscle components to their available resting length before increasing the force to stretch beyond the elastic range to elongate the plastic component of shortened connective tissue.

To stretch out (elongate) a connective tissue structure:

1. Warm the tissue.
2. Use appropriately intense but slow pulling or pushing force.
3. Sustain the force for a period of time to produce creep and increase pliability.
4. Work toward the goal of extending the elastic range of connective tissue by altering the plastic range.
5. Make sure the person has an adequate intake of water.

Example

Situation: Hypermobile ankle from a bad sprain 3 years ago.

Assessment:

- Assess ankle for laxity in ligaments and other connective tissue structures by studying range of motion.
- Assess for muscle splinting and spasm with palpation.

Therapeutic goal:

- Increase stability of the ankle to prevent future ankle sprains.

Treatment principles:

- Manage the muscle contraction around the joint with therapeutic massage.
- Create a therapeutic inflammation process by use of frictioning on the appropriate lax ligaments.
- Suggest the client wrap the ankle for moderate immobilization.
- Teach client ways to move the frictioned area through a series of pulsing activities that do not stretch the tissues but instead mobilize the area through a gentle range of motion to prevent adhesions from developing.

Your Turn

Hypermobility

Situation:

Assessment:

Therapeutic goal:

Treatment principles:

Continued

ACTIVITY 8-3—cont'd

Hypomobility

Therapeutic goal:

Situation:

Treatment principles:

Assessment:

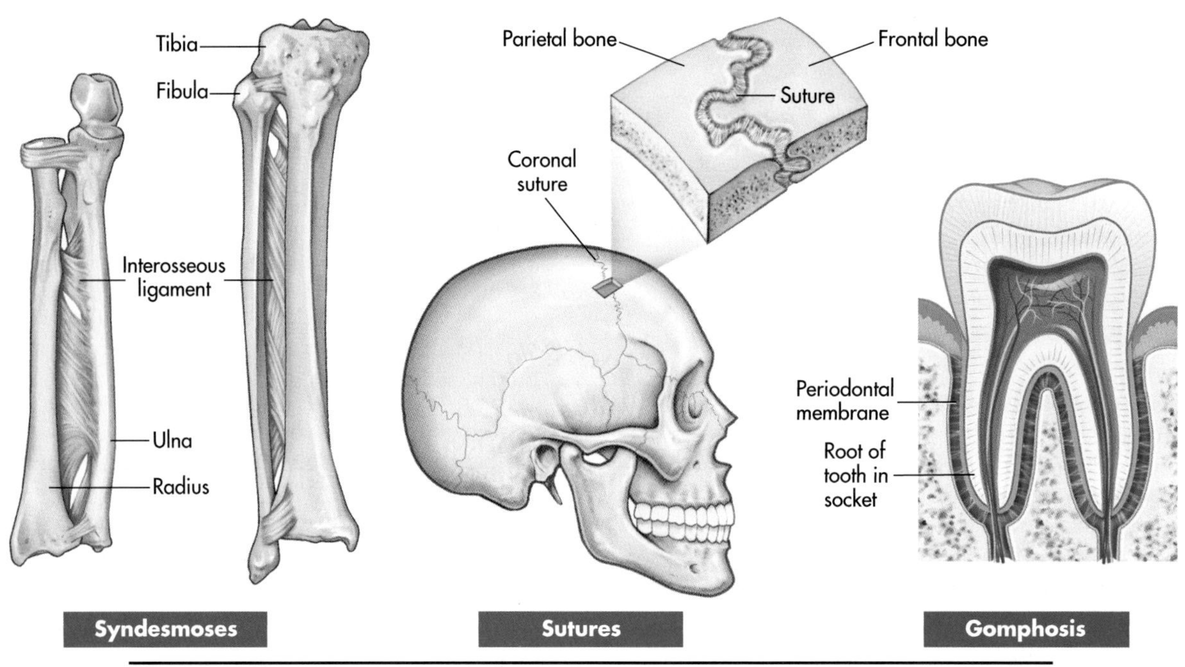

Figure 8-3
Examples of the types of fibrous joints. (From Thibodeau GA, Patton KT: *Anatomy and physiology*, ed 5, St Louis, 2003, Mosby.)

the bones slowly grow together to form a *synostosis*, or bony union, in which little or no motion is possible. The sagittal suture is an example of a suture.

A **gomphosis** is a joint in which the bony components fit together like a peg in a hole. The only gomphosis joint that exists in the human body is found between a tooth and the mandible or maxilla. In most adults the loss of teeth mainly results from disease processes that affect the connective tissue cementing or holding the teeth. Under normal conditions in the adult, these joints do not permit motion.

A **syndesmosis** is a fibrous joint in a ligament, cord, or aponeurotic membrane that joins the articulating bones. For example, a membrane joins the shaft of the tibia directly to the shaft of the fibula. A slight amount of motion at this joint accompanies movement at the knee and ankle joints.

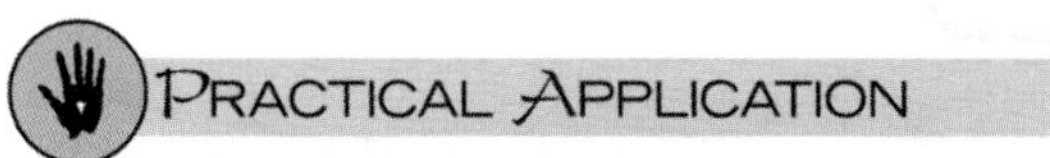

PRACTICAL APPLICATION

One particular method of therapeutic massage deals with the slight movements of the cranial sutures and works to normalize the gentle cranial/sacral rhythm, of which movement of the cranial sutures is a part. Experts disagree about the mechanisms involved in the cranial rhythm and whether the cranial sutures do indeed move in the adult skull. Many theories exist, none of which has solid validation. The methods that work with the cranial sutures seem to have clinical validity, even if not agreed on scientific justification. The massage practitioner uses gentle pressure, and the client experiences more of an intent or thought of movement. ■

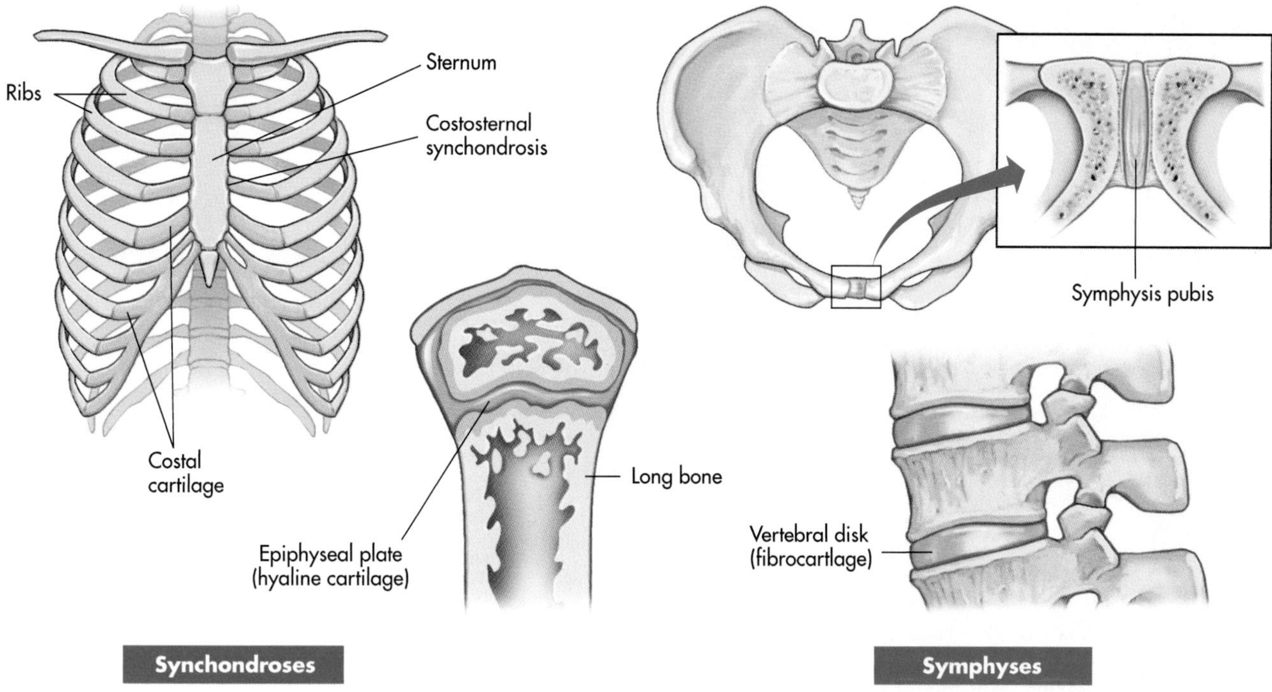

Figure 8-4
Examples of the types of cartilaginous joints. The epiphyseal plate between the epiphysis and diaphyses of a long bone is a temporary synchondrosis that does not move. The plate of hyaline cartilage is totally replaced by bone at skeletal maturity. (Most cartilaginous joints are amphiarthroses, or slightly moveable joints.) (From Thibodeau GA, Patton KT: *Anatomy and physiology*, ed 5, St Louis, 2003, Mosby.)

Amphiarthroses (Cartilaginous Joints)

An amphiarthrosis is slightly movable (Figure 8-4). Fibrocartilage or hyaline growth cartilage holds one bony surface to another in a bone-cartilage-bone configuration. The two types of cartilaginous joints are symphyses and synchondroses.

A **symphysis** is a joint in which thin layers of hyaline cartilage over each bone are separated from each other by fibrocartilage in the form of disks or plates. The symphysis pubis is the articulation of the two pubic bones. Its structure allows for good stability, with the thick fibrocartilage providing a stable union between the two bones.

A **synchondrosis** is a joint in which a thin layer of hyaline growth cartilage connects the two bones. The cartilage forms a bond between the two ossifying centers of bone. This type of joint permits bone growth while providing stability and allowing a small amount of movement. When bone growth is complete, these joints ossify and convert to bony unions. The first sternocostal joint is a synchondrosis. Articular cartilage directly connects the adjacent surfaces of the first rib and sternum.

Diarthroses (Synovial Joints)

Most of our joints are synovial joints, which are freely movable (Figure 8-5). All synovial joints are constructed similarly with the following features:

- A joint capsule formed of fibrous tissue surrounds the joint.
- A joint capsule encloses a joint cavity.
- Synovial fluid forms a lubricating film over the joint surfaces.
- A synovial membrane lines the inner surface of the capsule.
- Hyaline cartilage covers the joint surfaces.

In synovial joints the ends of the bony components move freely in relation to one another because no cartilaginous tissue directly connects the bones, as in fibrous and cartilaginous joints. Instead, the bony components connect indirectly to one another by means of a joint capsule, ligaments, and tendons.

The joint capsule consists of two layers, an outer layer called the *stratum fibrosum* and an inner layer called the *stratum synovium.*

The stratum fibrosum, composed of dense fibrous tissue, completely surrounds the joint and is continuous with the periosteum of the adjoining bones. This outer layer is poorly vascularized but richly innervated by joint receptors. The receptors located in and around the joint capsule can detect the rate and direction of motion, compression, tension, vibration, and pain. Hilton's law states that a nerve trunk that supplies a joint also supplies the muscles of the joint and the skin over the insertion of the

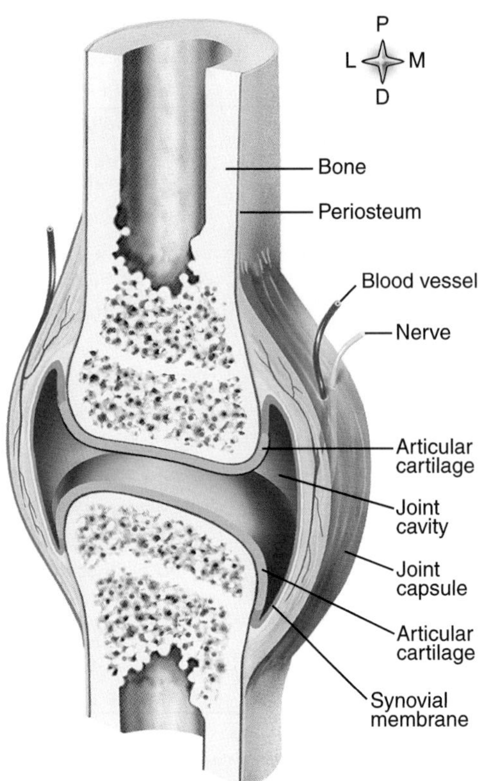

Figure 8-5
Structures of a synovial joint (the knee). (From Thibodeau GA, Patton KT: *Anatomy and physiology,* ed 5, St Louis, 2003, Mosby.)

muscles. Therefore the stratum fibrosum is the source for extensive sensory data that affect the joint, muscles, and skin in the area.

The inner layer or stratum synovium of the joint capsule is highly vascularized but poorly innervated and is insensitive to pain but undergoes vasodilation in response to heat and vasoconstriction in response to cold. The stratum synovium produces matrix collagen and serves as an entry point for nutrients and an exit point for waste materials.

Ligaments and tendons play an important role in keeping joint surfaces connected and often assist in guiding motion. Separation of joint surfaces is limited by passive tension in ligaments, the joint capsule, and tendons. Active tension in muscles also limits the separation of joint surfaces.

A smooth layer of articular cartilage protects the bone surfaces in freely movable joints. The bones in this type of joint have a space between them called the joint cavity, which contains a small amount of thick, colorless fluid that resembles uncooked egg white. This lubricant, called synovial fluid, is secreted by the membrane that lines the joint cavity. Small sacs called bursae are filled with synovial fluid and are located near some joints. As discussed earlier, bursae lie in areas subject to stress and help ease movement over and around the joints. Such a design not only helps to provide stability for the joint but also permits motion.

The same structures that hold joints together also serve to maintain joint space or hold joints apart. When these structures weaken and become worn, the joint cavity is not maintained as effectively, and the ends of bone begin to contact each other and rub together. Friction develops and production of synovial fluid increases in an attempt to reduce friction and maintain joint space. The end result of the deterioration most often is called arthritis but more accurately is called degenerative joint disease. In response to the pain, protective muscle spasms develop. Instead of increasing the joint space, which would alleviate the problem, the contraction of the muscles that surround the joint actually pull the ends of the bone together, which further decreases the space between the bones.

In addition, synovial joints often have accessory structures such as fibrocartilaginous disks and plates or menisci. Menisci, disks, and the synovial fluid help prevent excessive compression of opposing joint surfaces.

Forces and Stress

Every time we take a step, push against an object with our arms, or bend and twist, our bones and joints have to dissipate the forces of stress imposed on them. When forces meet an obstacle such as a bend or curve in a bone, the bone absorbs some forces and reflects others. Absorbed forces are transmitted to the soft tissues outside the bone, which helps dissipate excessive stress forces on joint surfaces. One can use these same forces therapeutically during massage application.

Mechanical forces are actions that involve pushing, pulling, friction, or sudden loading, such as a direct blow. Mechanical forces act on the body in many different ways. Five different kinds of force act on the body tissues. Tissue types respond differently to different forces. Bending forces seldom harm the soft tissues but will break bone. Tensile forces seldom injure bone but often damage soft tissues. The following describes the types of forces and the potential injury and therapeutic application pertinent to therapeutic massage.

Compression (Figure 8-6)

Compression forces occur when two structures are pressed together. Compression is a common way that tissues become injured. Compression can be sudden and strong, such as a direct blow, or sustained, such as found in nerve impingement. Ligaments and tendons resist compressive injury. Muscle tissue, because of its extensive vascular structure, is not as resistant to compressive forces. Excessive compression force ruptures or tears the integrity of the muscle tissue, causing bruising and connective tissue damage. Compression is a major force used in the application of massage to support circulation, stimulate nerve function, and restore connective tissue pliability. One applies compression in such a way to achieve benefits without damaging tissue. One most often uses broad-based application of compressive force.

Tension (Figure 8-7)

Tension forces, also called tensile forces, occur when two ends of a structure are pulled away from each other. Bone resists tensile forces. Tensile stress injuries are the most common way soft tissues are damaged. Examples of tensile stress injuries include muscle strains, ligament sprains, tendonitis, fascial pulling or tearing, and nerve traction injuries (sudden nerve stretching such as that which occurs in whiplash). Tensile stress injuries are described as first degree (mild), second degree (moderate), and third degree (severe). One applies tensile force during massage particularly during gliding and traction. Therapeutically, tensile force supports proper alignment of fiber structures and response of muscles and can increase pliability in connective tissue.

Bending (Figure 8-8)

Bending forces are a combination of compression and tension. One side of a structure is exposed to compressive forces, while the other side is exposed to tensile forces. Bending forces are a common cause of bone fractures and ligament injuries but seldom harm other soft tissues. One uses bending during massage when applying kneading methods. The proprioceptors in muscles and tendons respond to these forces. Bending forces also affect connective tissues, especially the viscosity of the ground substance.

Shear (Figure 8-9)

Shear is a sliding force with friction created between structures that are sliding against each other. Excessive shearing force at a tendon creates an inflammatory irritation that leads to adhesion and fibrosis. Shear and friction, called cross-fiber friction, is a massage method that uses specific force to create therapeutic inflammation to reverse fibrotic connective tissue changes.

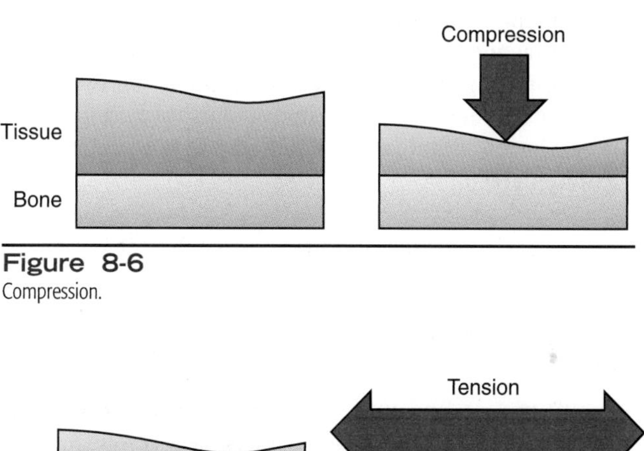

Figure 8-6
Compression.

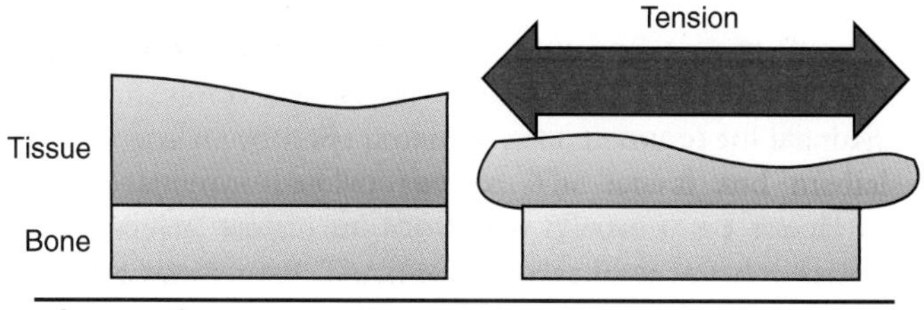

Figure 8-7
Tension.

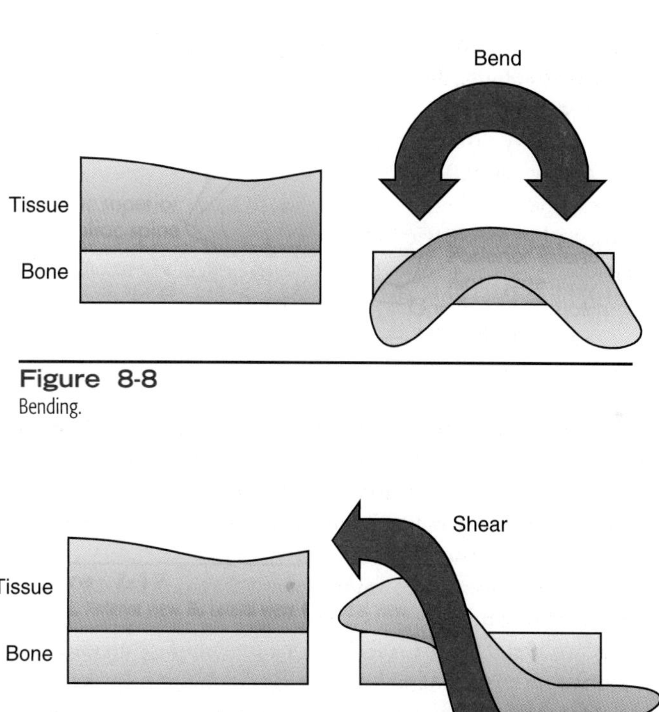

Figure 8-8
Bending.

Figure 8-9
Shear.

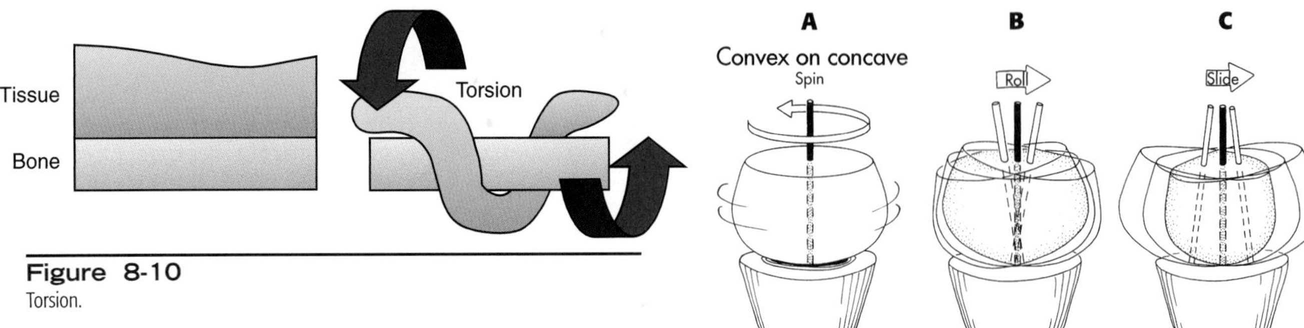

Figure 8-10
Torsion.

Torsion (Figure 8-10)
Torsion forces are twisting forces. Torsion occurs with other forces such as tension and shear. Torsion stress as applied to a joint is likely to cause significant injury. Kneading massage methods introduce torsion force into tissue and are especially effective in increasing pliability of connective tissue.

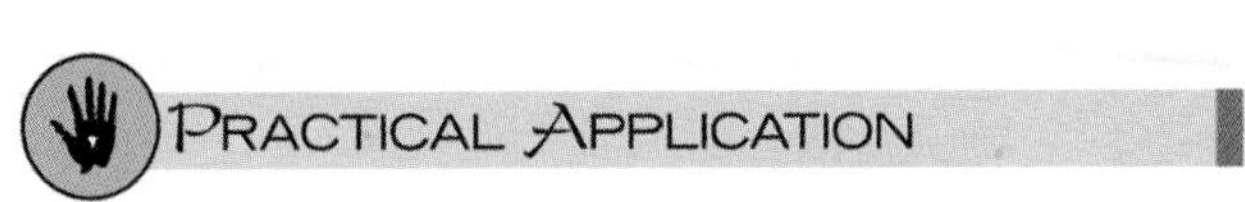

Massage can decrease the protective muscle spasm, which in turn allows some separation of bony structures in the joint and results in a small increase in the joint cavity space. Because the muscle spasms are often protective, one needs to decide how much reduction in spasm is desirable to increase space in the joint without totally eliminating the protective stability provided by the muscle splinting. The application of various forces singly or in combination is the basis of therapeutic application of massage methods. Instead of causing injury to the body, one achieves a benefit by choosing the correct force type and application method. ■

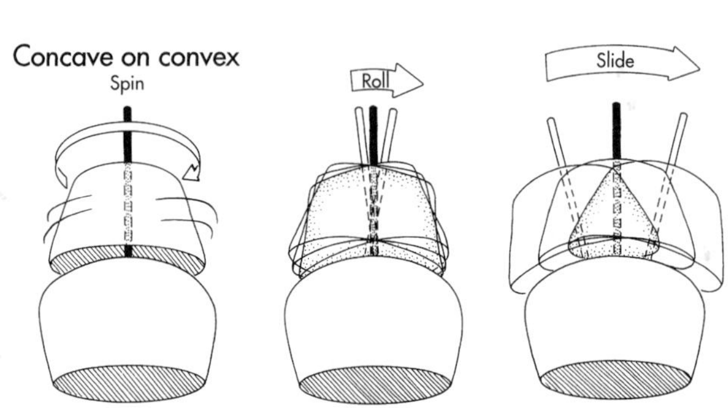

Figure 8-11
Accessory movements. **A,** Spin. **B,** Roll. **C,** Slide. (From Malone TR, McPoil T, Nitz AJ: *Orthopedic and sports physical therapy*, ed 3, St Louis, 1997, Mosby.)

JOINT MOTION

Arthrokinematics

The term ***arthrokinematics*** refers to *accessory movements* of the articulating surfaces of the bones at joint surfaces. Most often, one of the joint surfaces is more stable than the other and serves as a base for the motion, whereas the other surface moves on this relatively fixed base.

The terms *roll, slide,* and *spin* describe the type of motion that the moving part performs (Figure 8-11).

A roll refers to the rolling of one joint surface on another, similar to a bowling ball rolling down an alley. In the knee the femoral condyles roll on the fixed tibial surface.

Sliding refers to the gliding of one component over another, as when you slide on ice. In the hand the proximal phalanx slides over the fixed end of the metacarpal.

Spin refers to a rotation of the movable component, as when a top spins. The head of the radius spins on the capitulum of the humerus during supination and pronation of the forearm.

Combinations of rolling, sliding, and spinning occur during the process of joint motion. A large amount of motion can occur in a confined space by combining motions. When a moving component in a joint alternately rolls in one direction while sliding in the opposite direction, the range of motion available to the joint increases and opposing joint surfaces remain in contact with each other. Another method of increasing the range of available motion is by permitting both components to move at the same time. The humerus and the scapula move together during flexion and extension and during abduction and adduction at the glenohumeral joint.

Joint Play

The involuntary movements that occur between articular surfaces, which have nothing to do with the range of motion of a joint produced by muscles, are an essential component of joint motion and must occur for the joint to function normally. Called **joint play,** these small movements are essential for proper joint function.

The rolling and sliding movements of the articular surfaces are not usually visible or under voluntary control. An externally applied force, such as that applied by a therapist or physician, can produce movement of one articular surface on another, and one can assess the amount

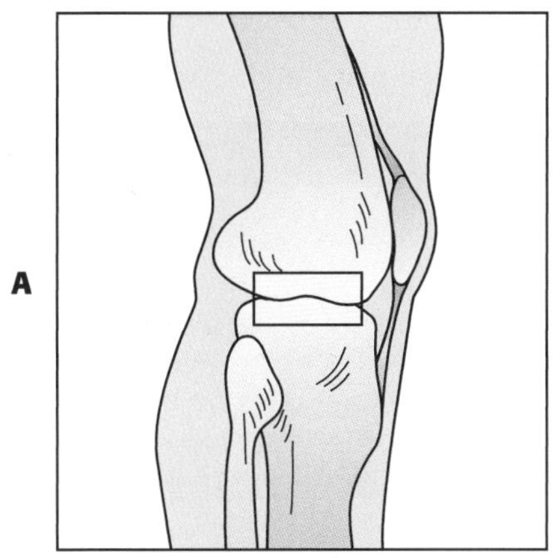

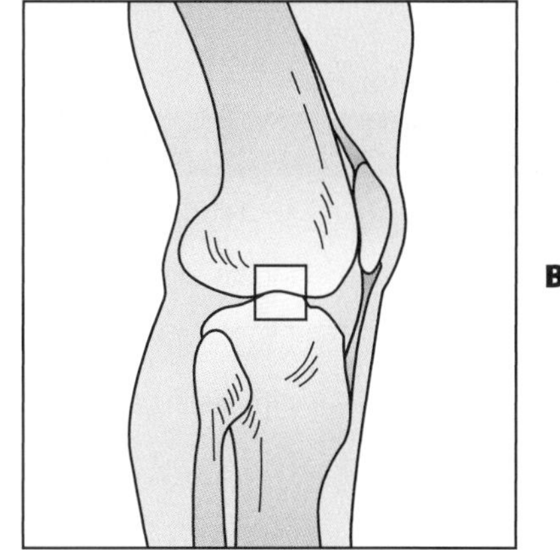

Figure 8-12
The congruence of articular surfaces. **A,** Close-packed position. **B,** Loose-packed position.

of joint play present. A door hinge is an excellent example. If you examine a door hinge, you will find that there are two plates, one attached to the door frame and one attached to the door. Between the two plates is a cylinder and inside the cylinder is a pin. The pin fits inside the cylinder with just enough space around it so that the pin is free to rotate in the cylinder, allowing the door to swing. The distance the door swings is comparable to the range of motion of a joint, whereas the amount of space in the cylinder that allows the pin to roll is comparable to joint play.

In an optimal situation a joint has a sufficient amount of play to allow normal motion. For the human body the amount of joint play is almost always approximately $^1/_8$ inch, no matter which synovial joint one examines or the amount of range of motion of that joint. If the supporting joint structures are lax, the joint may have too much play and become unstable. If the joint structures are tight or inflammation or degeneration is present, the joint has too little movement between the articular surfaces, the amount of joint play is reduced, and range of motion may be restricted.

Joint Positions and Stability

In most of our synovial joints the ends of the articulating surfaces of the bones are opposite in shape to each other, usually convex and concave. All synovial joints have only one position where the surfaces fit together and in which maximal contact between the opposing surfaces occurs. This is called the **close-packed position,** or locked position, and it allows no movement. The close-packed position is usually at the extreme end of the range of motion where the joint surfaces are compressed and the joint exhibits its greatest stability. The position of extension is the close-packed position for the elbow, knee, and interphalangeal joints. When not in this position, the joint is said to be in the **loose-packed position,** or unlocked, where the amount of contact is reduced and movements of spin, roll, and glide may occur (Figure 8-12, *A* and *B*). Each joint also has a *least-packed position* in which the capsule is at its most lax. Joints tend to assume this position when inflammation occurs to accommodate the increased volume of synovial fluid. In an injured joint that has swelling, the close-packed position is a position of discomfort. In the least-packed position the joint cavity has a greater volume and therefore the position is one of comfort.

Movement in and out of the close-packed position is likely to have a beneficial effect on joint nutrition because the movement squeezes out the synovial fluid during each compression against the cartilage, and the fluid is reabsorbed when the compression is removed (Tables 8-1 and 8-2).

Osteokinematics: Range of Motion

Osteokinematics refers to the movement of the bones by action of the muscles, rather than the movement of the articular surfaces. Three categories of range of motion (ROM) are anatomic, physiologic, and pathologic.

The **anatomic range of motion** refers to the amount of motion available to a joint within its structural limits. A number of factors determine the extent of the anatomic range, including the shape of the joint surfaces, the joint capsule, ligaments, muscle bulk, and surrounding musculotendinous and bony structures. Some joints have no bony joint limitations to motion, and the ROM is limited only by soft tissue structures. For example, the knee joint has no bony limitations to motion. Flexion is limited by soft tissues, often muscles, whereas extension stops with ligament stretch. Other joints have definite bony restrictions to motion in addition to soft tissue limitations. The elbow joint is limited in extension (close-packed position) by bony contact of the ulna with the olecranon fossa of the humerus.

The anatomic ROM may extend the limits of available movement to a point where joint injury can occur. Therefore many joints have an established **physiologic range of motion**

TABLE 8-1
Least-Packed Positions of Joints

JOINT(S)	POSITION
Spine	Midway between flexion and extension
Temporomandibular	Mouth slightly open
Glenohumeral	55° abduction, 30° horizontal adduction
Acromioclavicular	Arm resting by side in normal physiologic position
Sternoclavicular	Arm resting by side in normal physiologic position
Elbow	70° flexion, 10° supination
Radiohumeral	Full extension and full supination
Proximal radioulnar	70° flexion, 35° supination
Distal radioulnar	10° supination
Wrist	Neutral with slight ulnar deviation
Carpometacarpal	Midway between abduction/adduction and flexion/extension
Thumb	Slight flexion
Interphalangeal	Slight flexion
Hip	30° flexion, 30° abduction and slight lateral rotation
Knee	25° flexion
Ankle	10° plantar flexion, midway between maximum inversion or eversion
Subtalar	Midway between extremes of range of movement
Midtarsal	Midway between extremes of range of movement
Tarsometatarsal	Midway between extremes of range of movement
Metatarsophalangeal	Neutral
Interphalangeal	Slight flexion

(From Magee DJ: *Orthopedic physical assessment,* ed 4 Philadelphia, 2002, Saunders.)

set by the nervous system from information provided by joint sensory receptors. Usually this physiologic ROM is somewhat less than the anatomic ROM, preventing a joint from being positioned where injury could occur.

Pathologic range of motion occurs when motion at a joint fails to reach the normal physiologic range or exceeds normal anatomic limits of motion. The limits may be structural or functional. Two main pathologic conditions exist: **hypomobility** and **hypermobility.**

End Feel

The ability to palpate normal end feel and to distinguish changes from normal end feel is important in protecting joints during ROM assessment and massage application. The four major types of end feel are soft, hard or bony, and capsular. *Soft end feel* of a joint is the normal sensation for most physiologic limits of range of motion. The joint moves in a normal arc and when one reaches the range limit, a small, pliable give remains if slightly more pressure is given. The space identified is the range between the physiologic and anatomic barriers. *Bony* or *hard end feel* is characterized by a hard and abrupt limit to joint movement. This occurs when bone contacts bone at the end of the ROM. An example would be normal elbow extension. Usually a hard end feel indicates a pathologic condition. *Capsular end feel* is characterized by a hard, leatherlike limitation of motion that has a slight give and occurs in full normal joint motion of the shoulder; otherwise, this type of end feel indicates dysfunction and is related to capsular restriction.

One can use two additional characteristics to quantify the limitation of joint motion. One can feel a rebound, or spring back, movement at the end of the ROM characteristic of *springy block.* This sensation occurs with internal derangement of a joint, such as torn cartilage or if connective tissue

TABLE 8-2
Close-Packed Positions of Joints

Joint(s)	Position
Spine	Extension
Temporomandibular	Clenched teeth
Glenohumeral	Abduction and lateral rotation
Acromioclavicular	Arm abducted to 30°
Sternoclavicular	Maximum shoulder elevation
Elbow	Extension
Radiohumeral	Elbow flexed 90°, forearm supinated 5°
Proximal radioulnar	5° supination
Distal radioulnar	5° supination
Wrist	Extension with ulnar deviation
Carpometacarpal	Full flexion
Thumb	Full opposition
Interphalangeal	Full extension
Hip	Full extension and medial rotation*
Knee	Full extension and lateral rotation of tibia
Ankle	Maximum dorsiflexion
Subtalar	Supination
Midtarsal	Supination
Tarsometatarsal	Supination
Metatarsophalangeal	Full extension
Interphalangeal	Full extension

*Some authors include abduction. (From Magee DJ: *Orthopedic physical assessment,* ed 4, Philadelphia, 2002, Saunders.)

structures are binding. *Asymptomatic limited ROM* results from soft tissue approximation and occurs when the soft tissue of body segments prevents further motion such as at normal terminal elbow flexion when the upper and lower arm meet and the muscles touch together.

Hypomobility

When the ROM is less than what normally would be permitted by the structure, the joint is hypomobile. Hypomobility may be caused by bony or cartilaginous blocks to motion or by the inability of the capsule, ligaments, or surrounding tissues to elongate sufficiently to allow a normal ROM. A contracture, which is a term that describes the shortening of soft tissue structures around a joint, is one cause of hypomobility.

An increased sensitivity and reactivity of joint receptors can cause the nervous system to increase muscle tension patterns, which in turn would limit ROM because muscles would not relax to their normal resting length. The result would be hypomobility of joint movement even though nothing is dysfunctional in the joint itself. If this limited range is maintained, the joint capsule often alters tissue structure and becomes dysfunctional itself. These conditions are much more difficult to manage because of the complexities of dysfunctional patterns and compensation throughout the body.

Hypermobility

Hypermobility may be caused by a failure to limit motion by the bony or soft tissues and results in instability. Weak or flaccid muscles can contribute to hypermobility because the muscles provide a stabilizing force to the joints. The joint may be subject to more trauma or damage because of excessive ROM, instability of the surrounding structures, or inability to withstand stresses.

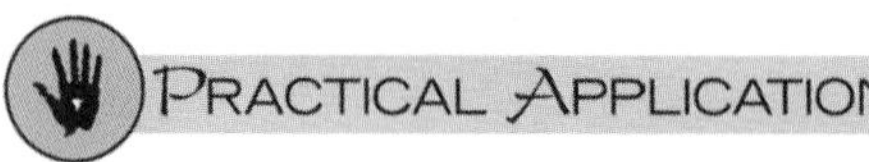

PRACTICAL APPLICATION

Hypermobility and hypomobility of a joint may have undesirable effects, not only at the affected joint but also at adjacent joint structures, because the body develops compensation patterns to deal with the dysfunction.

One can use therapeutic massage methods to increase or decrease the ROM of a joint by helping to return it to normal from a pathologic condition. By providing sensory stimulation to the joint nerve receptors, one can disrupt abnormal tension patterns of surrounding muscles and restore homeostasis, thus restoring ROM. Using methods that elongate connective tissue structures, one can reverse some forms of hypomobility. Methods that create therapeutic inflammation, combined with appropriate rehabilitation, sometimes can increase stability in lax joint structures. Methods that strengthen surrounding muscles can provide alternative stabilizing forces when the joint is lax. The practitioner can manage the splinting action of the muscle with therapeutic massage so that spasm does not cause pain and pull the joint capsule together.

Finding the right combination of therapeutic care is not a precise protocol but more often an experimental decision-making process. The student should remember that any disruption to a part of the joint structure affects the entire joint function. When one joint is affected, the whole body must use compensation patterns to adjust. Over time, other joint movement patterns can become involved in dysfunction. ■

Movements of Joints

Joint movement is named for the plane in which the movement occurs. To define joint and segment motions and to record the location in space of specific points on the body requires a reference point (Figures 8-13 to 8-15). In kinesiology, the three-dimensional rectangular coordinate system is used to describe anatomic relationships of the body. The standard anatomic body position is defined as standing erect with the head, toes, and palms of the hands facing forward and with the fingers extended. Three imaginary planes are arranged perpendicular to each other through the body, with their axes intersecting at the center of gravity of the body (a point slightly anterior to the second sacral vertebra). These planes are called cardinal planes of the body.

The frontal plane divides the body into front and back parts. Motions that occur in this plane are defined as abduction and adduction. *Abduction* is a position or motion of the segment away from the midline, regardless of which segment moves. Abduction of the hip occurs when the thigh segment moves away from the midline or the pelvic segment approaches the thigh, as in tilting to the side while standing on one leg. *Adduction* is a position or motion toward the midline.

The sagittal plane divides the body into right and left sides. Joint motions occurring in the sagittal plane are defined as flexion and extension. *Flexion* indicates that two segments approach each other; for example, flexion of the elbow may be accomplished by flexion of the forearm on the arm or by flexion of the arm on the forearm, as in a pull-up. *Extension* occurs when two segments move away from each other. If extension goes beyond the anatomic reference position, it is called *hyperextension.*

The horizontal plane divides the body into upper and lower parts and is like a view from above. Rotations occur in this plane. Internal rotation, inward or medial rotation, is transverse rotation oriented to the anterior surface of the body. Internal rotation of the hip brings points marked on the anterior surface of the pelvis and femur closer together regardless of which of the segments moves. *Pronation* is the term for internal rotation of the forearm. External rotation, outward or lateral rotation, is in the opposite direction and

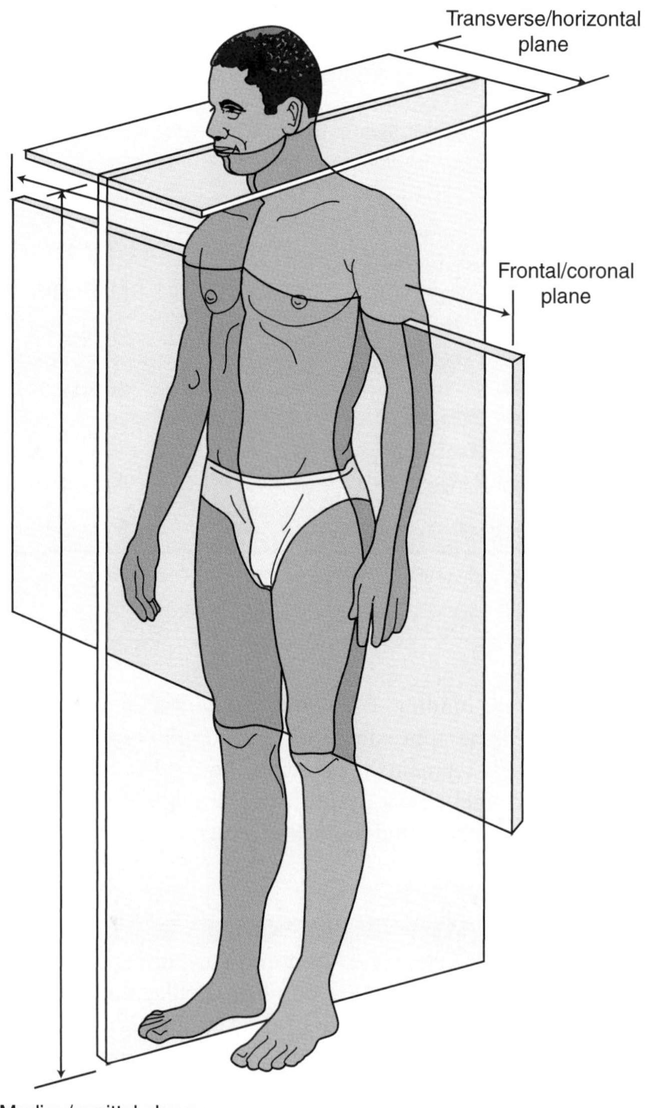

Figure 8-13
Anatomic planes. A person is considered to be in the standard anatomic position when standing with the palms facing forward.

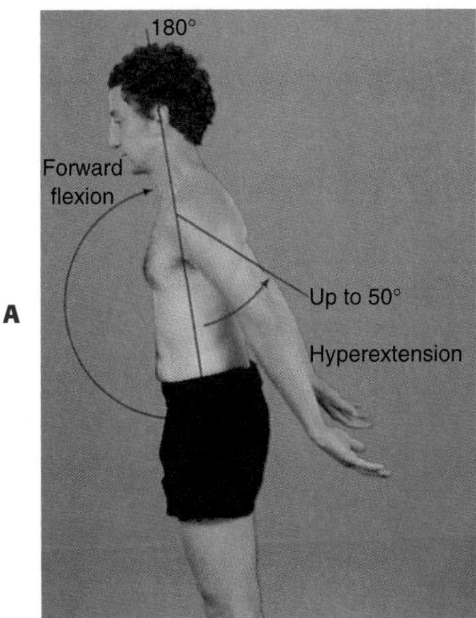

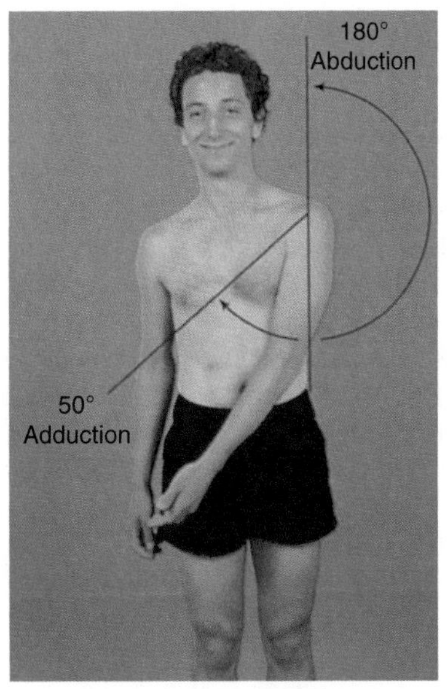

Figure 8-14
Joint movement is measured in degrees. The system presented in this book uses 0 degrees as the reference point for the standard anatomic position (extension, adduction, and neutral rotation). Motions or position of flexion, abduction, and internal and external rotation are recorded as they move toward 180 degrees. Movements and ROM of the shoulder. **A,** Forward flexion, extension (back to anatomical position of 0 degrees), and backward hyperextension up to 50 degrees. **B,** Abduction and adduction. (From Thibodeau GA, Patton KT: *Anatomy and physiology*, ed 5, St Louis, 2003, Mosby.)

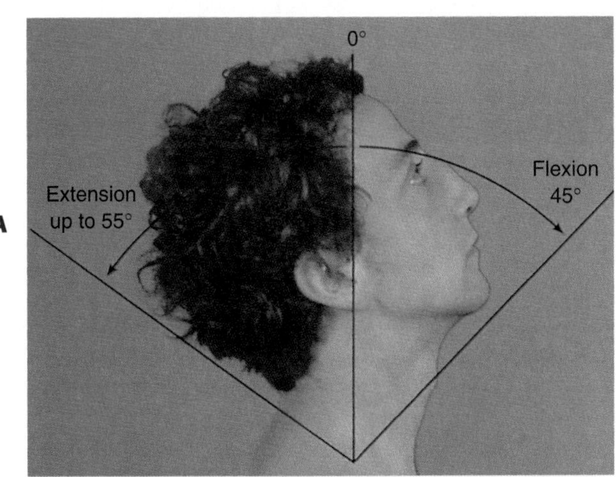

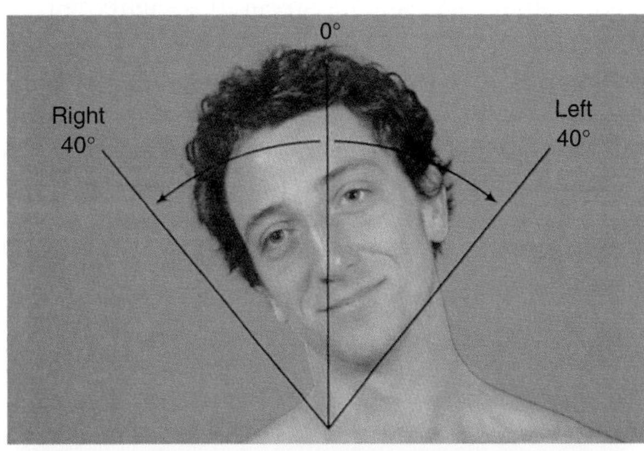

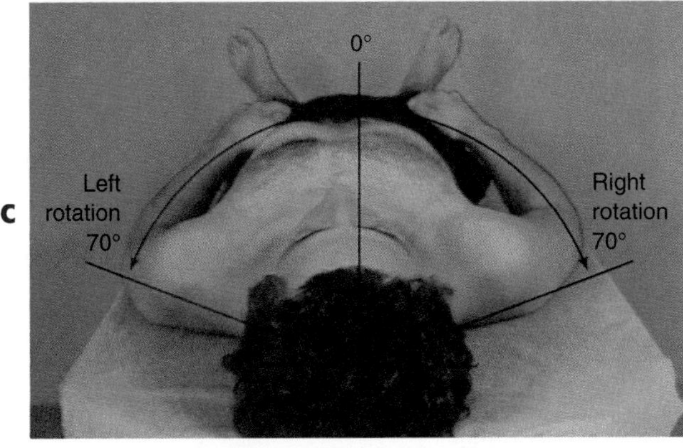

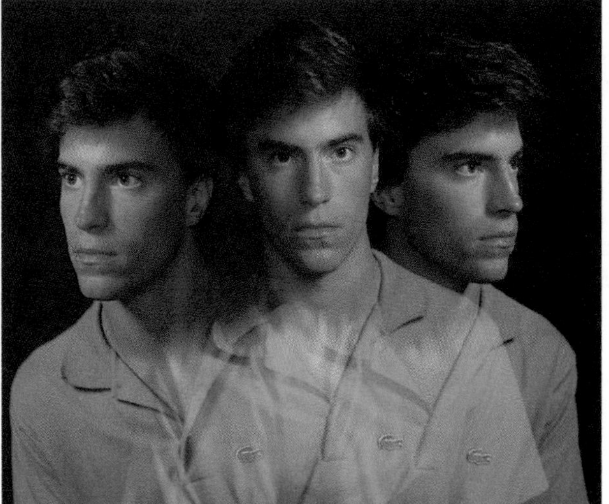

Figure 8-15
Joint movement is measured in degrees. The system presented in this book uses 0 degrees as the reference point for the standard anatomic position (extension, adduction, and neutral rotation). Movements and range of motion (ROM). **A,** Flexion and extension. **B,** Lateral bending. **C,** Rotation (supine position). **D,** Rotation (standing position). (From Thibodeau GA, Patton KT: *Anatomy and physiology*, ed 5, St Louis, 2003, Mosby.)

is oriented to the posterior surface of the body. *Supination* is the term used at the forearm and is the reference point for the anatomic position.

Sagittal, frontal, and horizontal planes may be laid through points other than the center of gravity of the body, but these are secondary planes. For example, laying three planes through the center of a joint, such as the hip joint, may be convenient for determining body points in relation to such a joint.

In the hand the sagittal plane is centered through the third segment; in the foot the sagittal plane is centered through the second segment. Motion or position away from the reference segment is called *abduction,* and motion toward the segment is called *adduction.* At the wrist the motion of abduction frequently is referred to as radial deviation (toward the radius), and adduction is called ulnar deviation. In the anatomic position the foot is at a right angle to the dorsal aspect of the leg in the sagittal plane. Movement of the foot toward the tibia is called *dorsiflexion,* and movement of the sole of the foot away from the tibia is called *plantar flexion.*

The thumb is also a special case because it normally rotates 90 degrees from the plane of the hand. Thus motions of flexion and extension occur in the frontal plane, and abduction and adduction occur in the sagittal plane (Figure 8-16).

Joint design permits many different types of movement. Some joints only permit flexion and extension. Others permit a wide range of movements, depending largely on the joint structure. Some movement terms may be used to describe motion at several joints throughout the body, whereas other terms are specific to a joint or group of joints. Motions or positions of flexion, abduction, and internal and external rotation are recorded as they move toward 180 degrees.

Terms Describing General Joint Movements

The following terms describe joint movements in general:

Flexion: Bending movement that results in a decrease of the angle in a joint by bringing bones together. An example is the elbow joint when the hand is drawn to the shoulder.

Extension: Straightening movement that results in an increase of the angle in a joint by moving bones apart. An example occurs when the hand is on the shoulder and moves away from the shoulder.

Abduction: Lateral movement away from the midline of the trunk. An example is moving the arms or legs away from the side.

Adduction: Movement medially toward the midline of the trunk. An example is moving the arms to the side or the legs back to the anatomic position.

Diagonal abduction: Movement by a limb through a diagonal plane directly across and away from the midline of the body. An example is moving the right arm from in front of the left hip to in front of the right shoulder.

Diagonal adduction: Movement by a limb through a diagonal plane toward and across the midline of the body. An example is the return of the right arm from a flexed position to in front of the left hip.

Horizontal abduction: Movement of the humerus in the horizontal plane away from the midline of the body. The movement also is known as horizontal extension or transverse abduction.

Horizontal adduction: Movement of the humerus in the horizontal plane toward the midline of the body. The movement also is known as horizontal flexion or transverse adduction.

Circumduction: Circular movement of a limb, combining the movements of flexion, extension, abduction, and adduction, to create a cone shape. An example is the shoulder joint moving in a circular fashion around a fixed point, as in doing arm circles.

Rotation: Twisting or turning of a bone on its own axis. An example is turning the head from side to side to indicate "no."

Internal rotation: Rotary movement around the longitudinal axis of a bone toward the midline of the body. The movement also is known as rotation medially, inward rotation, and medial rotation. An example is turning the palms of the hands from the anatomic position to facing backward.

External rotation: Rotary movement around the longitudinal axis of a bone away from the midline of the body. The movement also is known as rotation laterally, outward rotation, and lateral rotation. An example is returning the palms from facing backward to the anatomic position so that they face forward.

Terms Describing Specific Joint Movements of the Forearm, Wrist, Thumb, Ankle, and Foot

The following terms describe movements specific to the forearm, wrist, thumb, ankle, and foot:

Pronation: Internal rotation of the radius where it lies diagonally across the ulna, resulting in the palm-down position of the forearm.

Supination: External rotation of the radius where it lies parallel to the ulna, resulting in the palm-up position of the forearm.

Radial flexion or wrist abduction (deviation): Abduction movement at the wrist of the thumb side of the hand toward the forearm.

Ulnar flexion or wrist adduction (deviation): Adduction movement at the wrist of the little finger side of the hand toward the forearm.

Opposition of the thumb: Diagonal movement of the thumb across the palmar surface of the hand to make contact with the fingers.

Eversion: Turning of the sole of the foot outward or laterally. An example is moving our body weight to the inner edge of the foot.

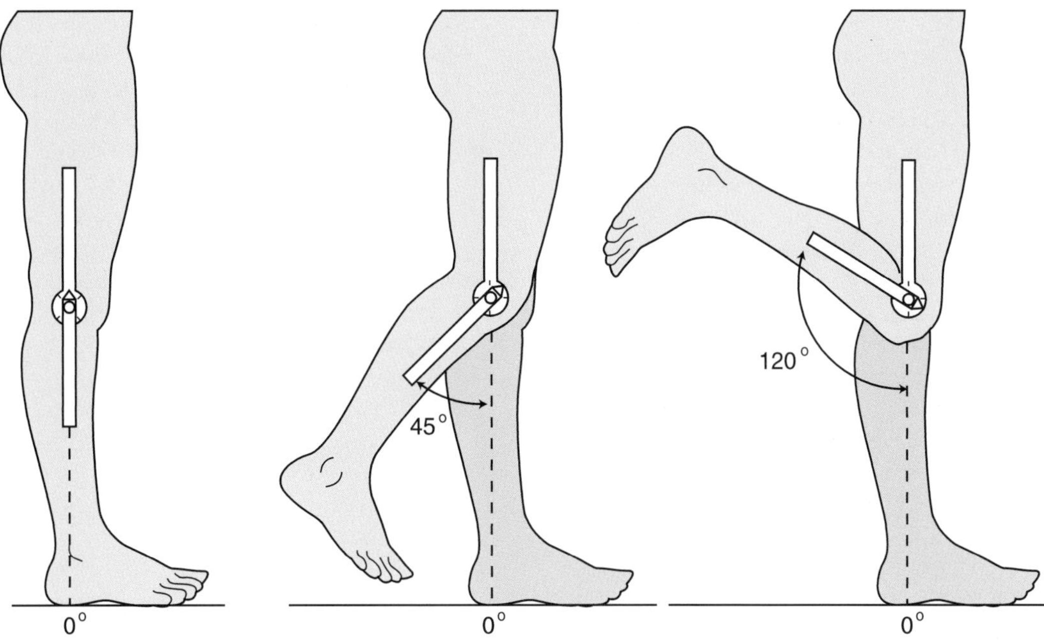

Figure 8-16
Measurement of knee positions in the sagittal plane.

Inversion: Turning of the sole of the foot inward or medially. An example is moving our body weight to the outer edge of the foot.

Dorsal flexion or dorsiflexion: Flexion movement of the ankle that results in the top of the foot moving toward the anterior tibia. An example of this is pointing the toes up.

Plantar flexion: Extension movement of the ankle that results in the foot or toes moving away from the body. An example of this is pointing the toes down.

Terms Describing Specific Joint Movements of the Shoulder Girdle and Shoulder Joint

The following terms describe movements of the shoulder girdle and shoulder joint:

Elevation: Movement of the shoulder girdle to become closer to the ears. Such movement occurs in shrugging of the shoulders.

Depression: Inferior movement of the shoulder girdle. An example is returning to the normal position from a shoulder shrug.

Protraction: Forward movement of the shoulder girdle away from the spine. Such movement occurs in abduction of the scapulae.

Retraction: Backward movement of the shoulder girdle toward the spine. An example is adduction of the scapula.

Rotation downward: Rotary movement of the scapula with the inferior angle of the scapula moving medially and downward. The movement occurs when the acromion process moves down.

Rotation upward: Rotary movement of the scapula with the inferior angle of the scapula moving laterally and upward. The movement occurs when the acromion process moves up.

Terms Describing Specific Joint Movements of the Spine and Pelvis

The following terms describe movements of the spinal joints:

Lateral flexion (side bending): Movement of the head or trunk laterally away from the midline. The movement occurs in abduction of the spine.

Reduction: Return of the spinal column to the anatomic position from lateral flexion. The movement occurs in adduction of the spine (Activity 8-4).

Classification of Synovial Joints by Movements

Traditionally, synovial joints have been divided into three main categories based on the number of axes at which motion occurs. A further subdivision of the joints is made based on the shape and configuration of the ends of the bony components. The three main categories are uniaxial, biaxial, and triaxial.

A *uniaxial joint* is constructed so that visible motion of the bony components is allowed in only one of the planes of the body around a single axis. The two types of joints in this category are **hinge joints** and **pivot joints.**

A *hinge joint* allows flexion and extension in one direction, changing the angle of the bones at the joint, as in a door hinge. Examples include the elbow and interphalangeal joints.

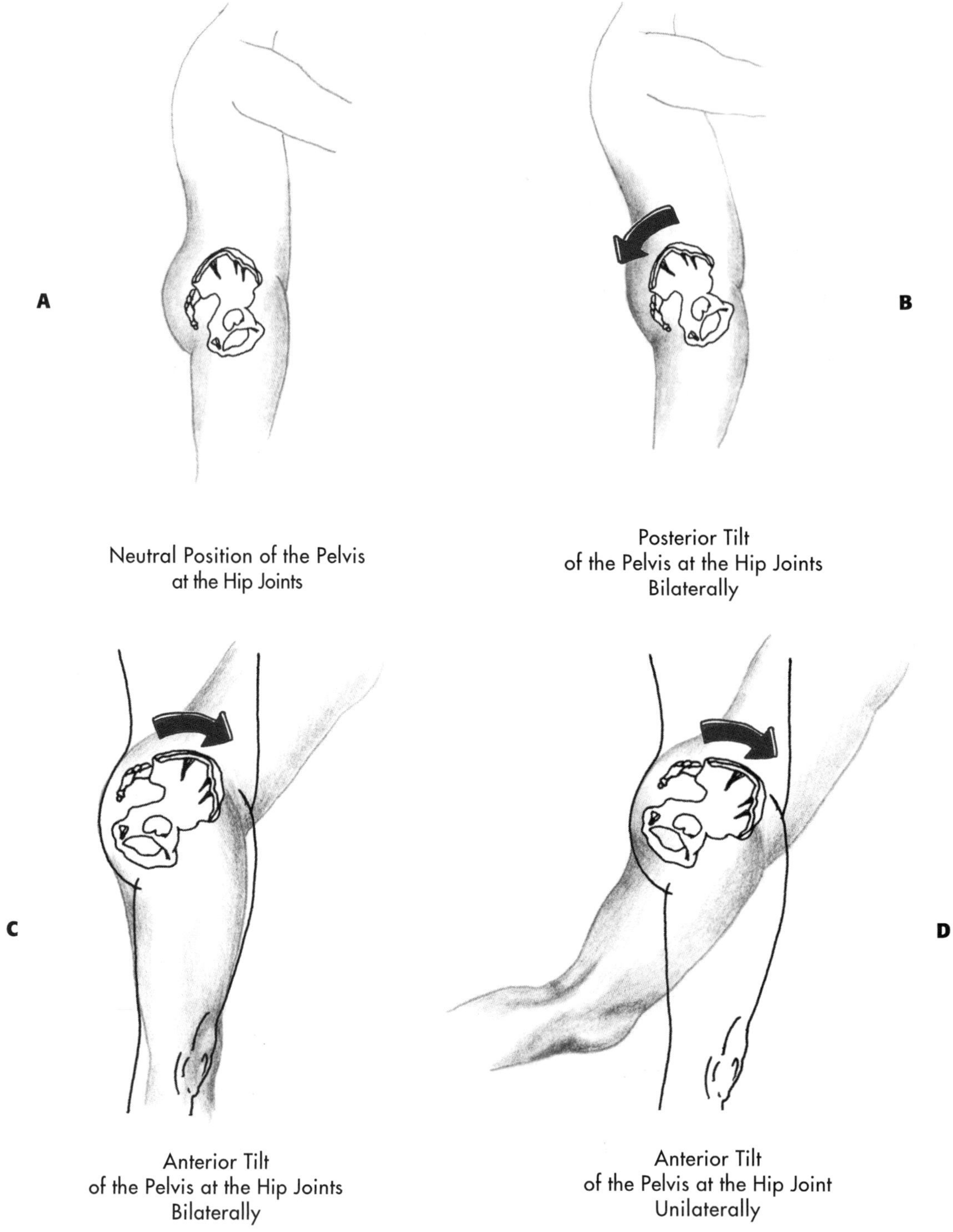

Figure 8-17
Motions or positions of flexion, abduction, and internal and external rotation are recorded as they move toward 180 degrees. (From Muscolino JE: *The muscular system manual: the skeletal muscles of the human body*, St. Louis, 2003, Mosby.)

A *pivot joint* allows rotation around the length of the bone. A pivot (trochoid) joint is a type of joint constructed so that one component is shaped like a ring and the other component is shaped so that it can rotate within the ring. Examples include the joint between the first and second cervical vertebrae and the joint at the proximal ends of the radius and the ulna.

Biaxial joints allow movement in two planes around two axes. The two types of joints in this category are **condyloid joints** and **saddle joints.**

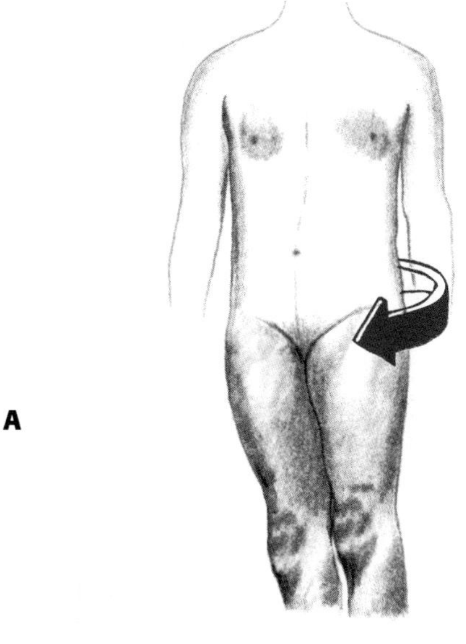

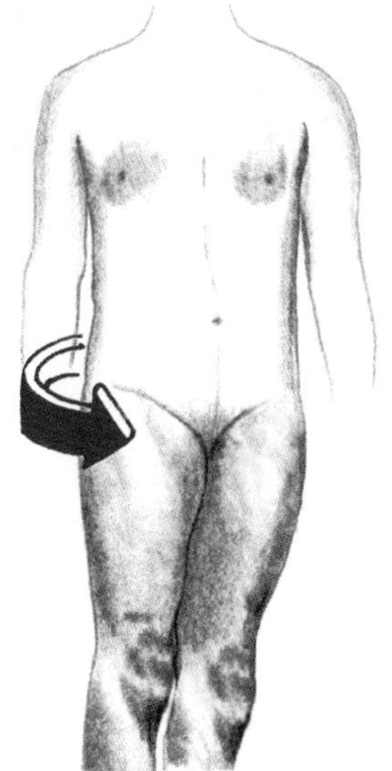

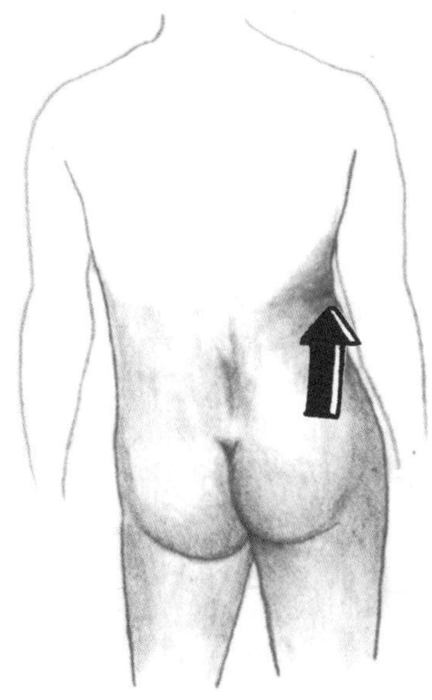

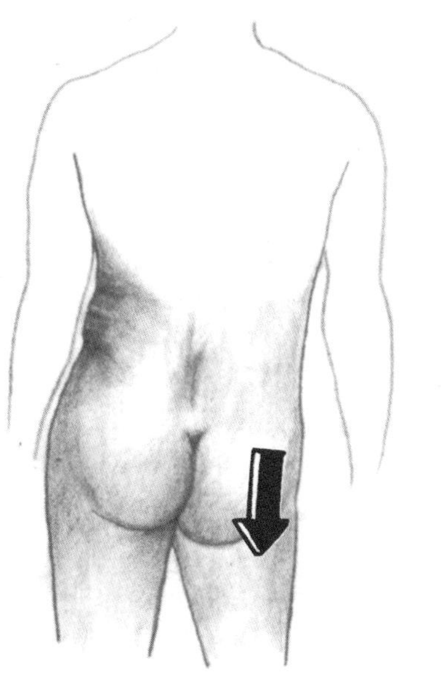

Figure 8-18
Rotation, elevation, and depression of the pelvis. (From Muscolino JE: *The muscular system manual: the skeletal muscles of the human body.* St. Louis, 2003, Mosby.)

A *condyloid joint,* also called a synovial ellipsoid joint, allows movement in two directions, but one motion dominates. The joint surfaces in a condyloid joint are shaped so that the concave surface of one bone slides over the convex surface of another bone in two directions. Movements allowed are flexion, extension, abduction, and adduction. Examples include the wrist joint, metacarpophalangeal joints, metatarsophalangeal joints, and the atlantooccipital joint.

Some condyloid joints allow flexion, extension, and rotation. Examples include the knee and temporomandi-

ACTIVITY 8-4

Find the definitions of the joint movements in Chapter 3 of this text and compare them to the ones you just studied in this chapter. Then, using both definitions, design a joint movement sequence that moves all the synovial joints in your body. An example is provided to get you started.

Example
Flexion
Drop chin to chest, make a fist, bend elbows so that hands touch the shoulders, bring a knee to the chest and then repeat with other knee, bring the heel to the buttocks and then repeat with other heel, curl toes toward the sole of the feet.

Your Turn

Abduction

Adduction

Diagonal abduction

Diagonal adduction

Extension

Horizontal abduction

Horizontal adduction

Circumduction

Rotation

Pronation

Supination

Elevation

Depression

Protraction

Retraction

Rotation downward

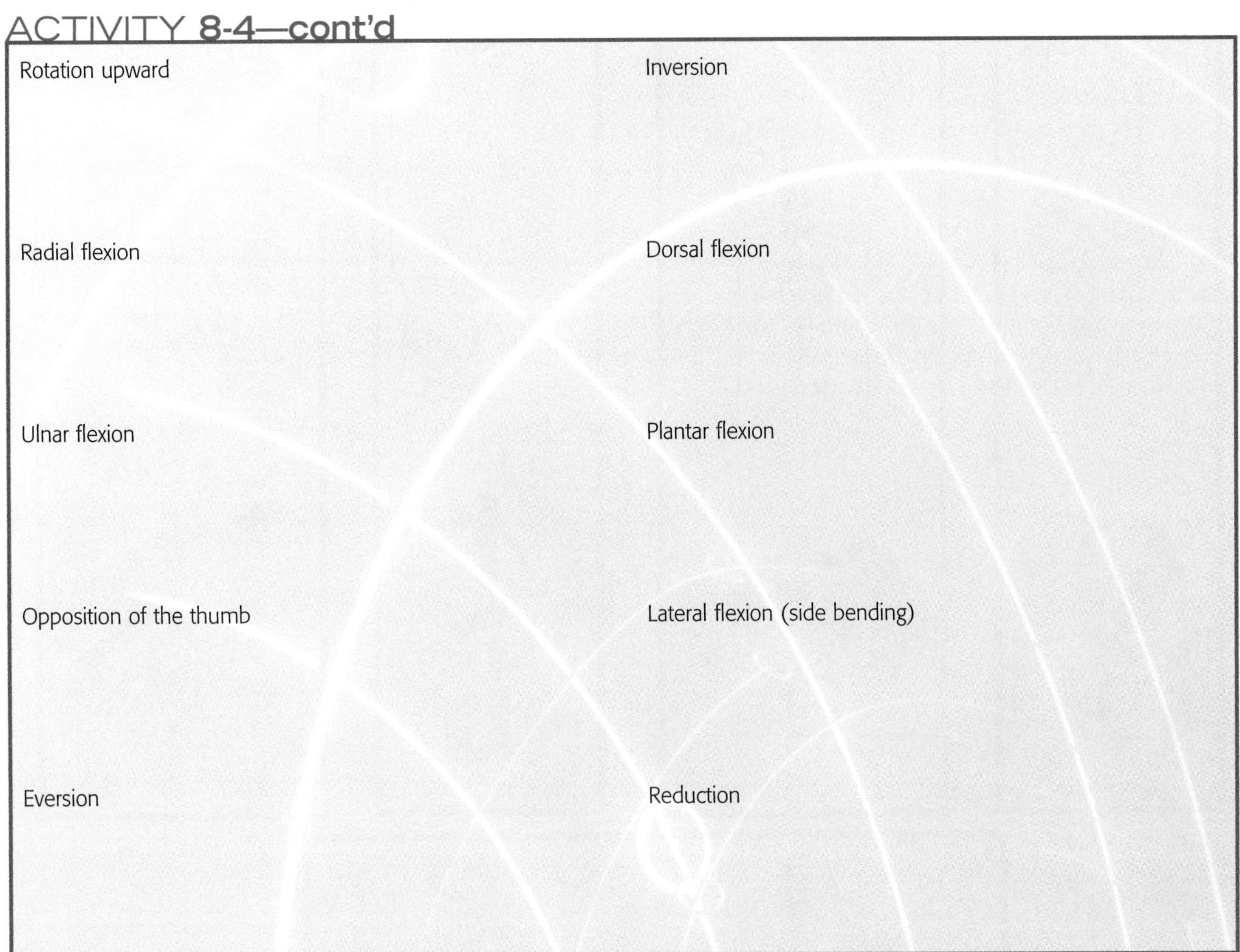

ACTIVITY 8-4—cont'd

Rotation upward

Inversion

Radial flexion

Dorsal flexion

Ulnar flexion

Plantar flexion

Opposition of the thumb

Lateral flexion (side bending)

Eversion

Reduction

bular joint. (The knee often is classified as a hinge joint, but it is more accurately a condyloid joint.)

In a *saddle joint* each joint surface is convex in one plane and concave in the other, and these surfaces fit together similar to a rider on a saddle. Movements allowed are flexion, extension, abduction, adduction, and a small degree of axial rotation.

Examples include the joint between the wrist and the metacarpal bone of the thumb (carpometacarpal joint), sternoclavicular joint, and ankle joint.

Triaxial or *multiaxial joints* are joints in which the bony components are free to move in three planes around the axes. Motion at these joints may also occur in oblique planes. The two types of joints in this category are **ball-and-socket joints** and plane or **gliding joints.**

A *ball-and-socket joint* allows movement in many directions around a central point. Ball-and-socket joints are formed when a ball-shaped convex surface is fitted into a concave socket. Movements allowed are flexion, extension, abduction, adduction, rotation, and circumduction. This type of joint gives the greatest freedom of movement but also is the easiest to dislocate. Examples are the hip and shoulder joints.

Synovial plane joints, most often referred to as *gliding joints,* permit gliding between two or more bones. These joints allow only a gliding motion in various planes. The adjacent surfaces may glide on one another or rotate with respect to one another in any plane. Examples include the sacroiliac joint, superior tibiofibular joint, acromioclavicular joint, costovertebral joints, and zygopophyseal joints between the vertebral arches (Figure 8-19).

Kinematic Chains

Kinematic chains describe the association between joints as they operate in relation to each other. The concept of kinematic chains is useful for analyzing human motion and the effects of injury and disease on the joints of the body. Two types are **closed kinematic chains** and **open kinematic chains.**

Closed Kinematic Chain

Some joints of the human body are linked together into a series in which motion at one of the joints is accompanied by motion at an adjacent joint, which is called a closed kinematic chain. For instance, when a person is standing

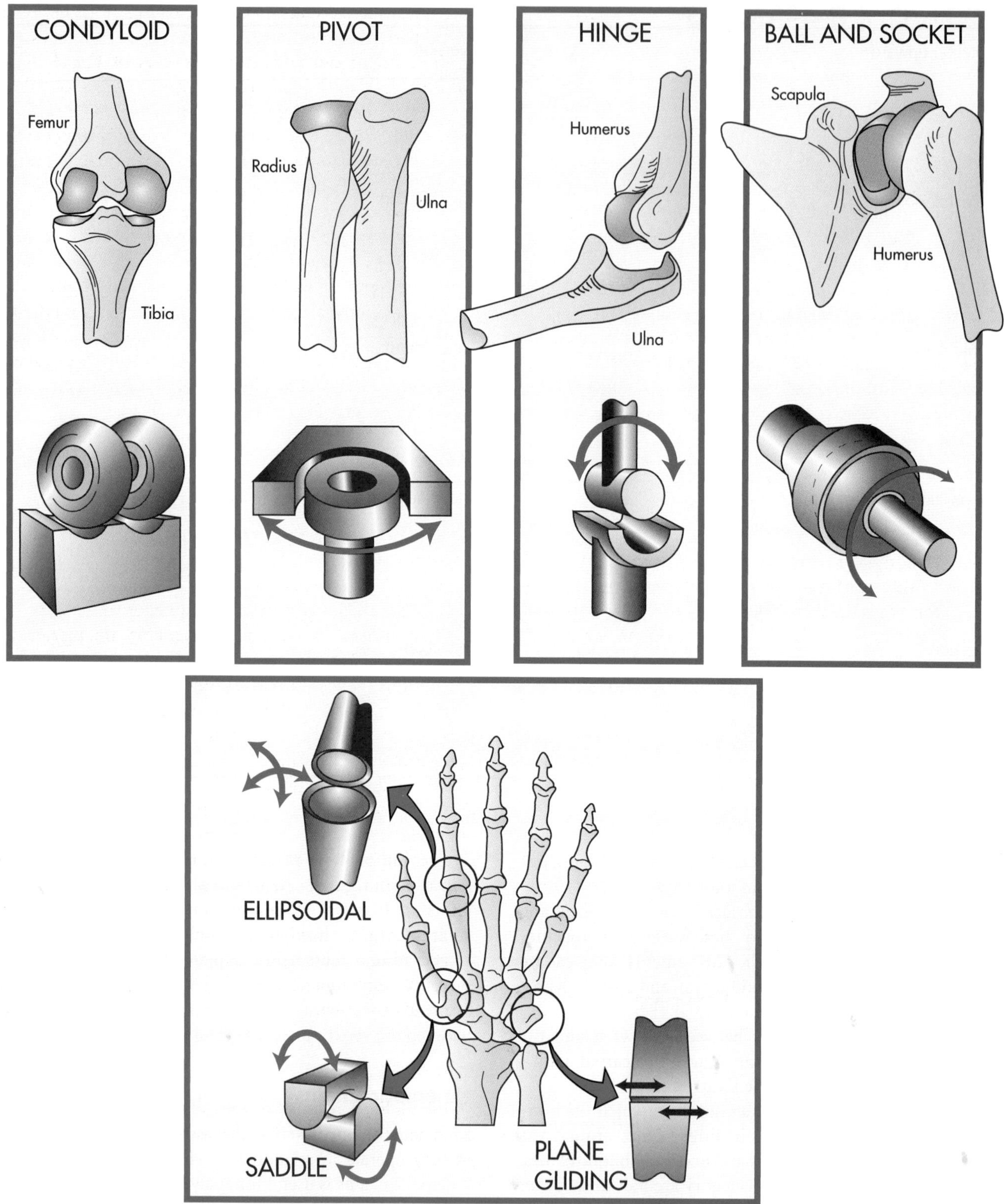

Figure 8-19
Synovial joint types. (Modified from Hamill J, Knutzen K: *Biomechanical basis of human movement,* ed 2, Philadelphia, 2003, Lippincott Williams & Wilkins.)

erect and bends both knees, simultaneous motion must occur at the ankle and hip joints. If the hand applies a compressive force to a fixed object, a closed kinematic chain is created. The interaction between joints in the chain is predictable in terms of linked movement because the joints are interdependent. A change in the structure or function of one joint in the chain usually causes a change in the function of a joint immediately adjacent to the affected joint or at a distal joint. For example, if the ROM at the knee were limited, the hip and ankle joints would have to compensate so that the foot could clear the floor when a person walked to avoid stumbling.

Open Kinematic Chain

When the ends of the limbs or parts of the body are free to move without causing motion at another joint, the system is referred to as an open kinematic chain.

The ends of our limbs often are not fixed but are free to move without necessarily causing motion at another joint. When one lifts the leg from the ground, the knee is free to bend without causing or changing motion at the hip or ankle. The motion of waving the hand may occur at the wrist without causing motion of the elbow or shoulder. In an open kinematic chain, motion does not occur in a predictable fashion because joints may function independently or in unison. For example, you can wave your whole upper limb by moving your arm at the shoulder or by moving only at the wrist.

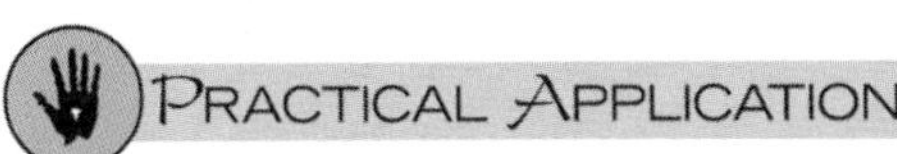

An understanding of joint movement is fundamental to any therapeutic massage system. Many systems, particularly movement modalities, are based on body movement patterns provided by joints. A comparison of these systems, such as yoga, tai chi, or Feldenkrais, reveals the intricate and interactive interplay of the joint moved alone or in a dynamic combination of movement.

All types of athletes depend on proper functioning of their joints, as do dancers and others who purposefully move their bodies. These persons often seek out therapeutic massage to enhance their performance and maintain or restore optimal functioning. Especially when working with closed kinematic chains, the practitioner must address all joints in the pattern for proper function to be restored in any particular area. ■

IDENTIFICATION AND PALPATION OF SPECIFIC JOINTS

Joints of the Skull

The joints of the skull are the cranial sutures and the temporomandibular joint.

Cranial Sutures

The four cranial sutures are these:

- The coronal suture is the articulation of the frontal and the parietal bones.
- The sagittal suture is the articulation of the two parietal bones.
- The squamous suture is the articulation of the parietal and temporal bones.
- The lambdoidal suture is the articulation of the occipital and parietal bones.

The student can palpate the sutures of the skull as follows: Place your fingertips on your eyebrows and slide them firmly up your forehead to the top of your skull to where you feel the first indentation, which is the coronal suture. Pressing your finger firmly into the suture, follow the indentation down on either side to where the suture ends, about midway between the top of the ear and the eye. Move posteriorly along the next indentation that arcs over your ear; this is the squamous suture. Behind the ear, just above the mastoid process, palpate the indentation that moves in an arc superiorly and posteriorly; this is the lambdoidal suture. At the midway point of the lambdoidal suture find the indentation that travels superiorly and anteriorly along the middle of the skull to join with the coronal suture; this is the sagittal suture (Figure 8-20, *A* and *B*).

Temporomandibular Joint

The temporomandibular joint consists of the following structures:

Articulating bones: Temporal bone and mandible

Joint type: Synovial condylar joint

Ligaments: Lateral temporomandibular ligament from the zygomatic arch to the mandible; sphenomandibular ligament from the sphenoid to mandible (not pictured in Figure 8-21); and the stylomandibular ligament from the styloid process to the mandible

The temporomandibular joint allows the following movements: depression, elevation, protrusion, retraction, and lateral movements.

The temporomandibular joint is one of the strongest joints in the body and is the only biarticular joint in the body. This means that the joint has two separate articulating surfaces on one bone joining with two separate bones. This construction requires a balanced action in the joint so that both jointed areas work freely. When this is not the case, the result is temporomandibular joint dysfunction.

The student can palpate the joint just in front of each ear while opening and closing the jaw (Figure 8-21; Activity 8-5).

Joints of the Shoulder

The shoulder joints include the glenohumeral, sternoclavicular, and acromioclavicular joints and the scapulothoracic junction.

ACTIVITY 8-5

Move your temporomandibular joint through each of the movement patterns.

A
Sagittal suture
Parietal bone
Squamous suture
Occipital bone
Lambdoidal suture
Mandible
B
Frontal bone
Coronal suture
Sagittal suture
Parietal bone
Occipital bone

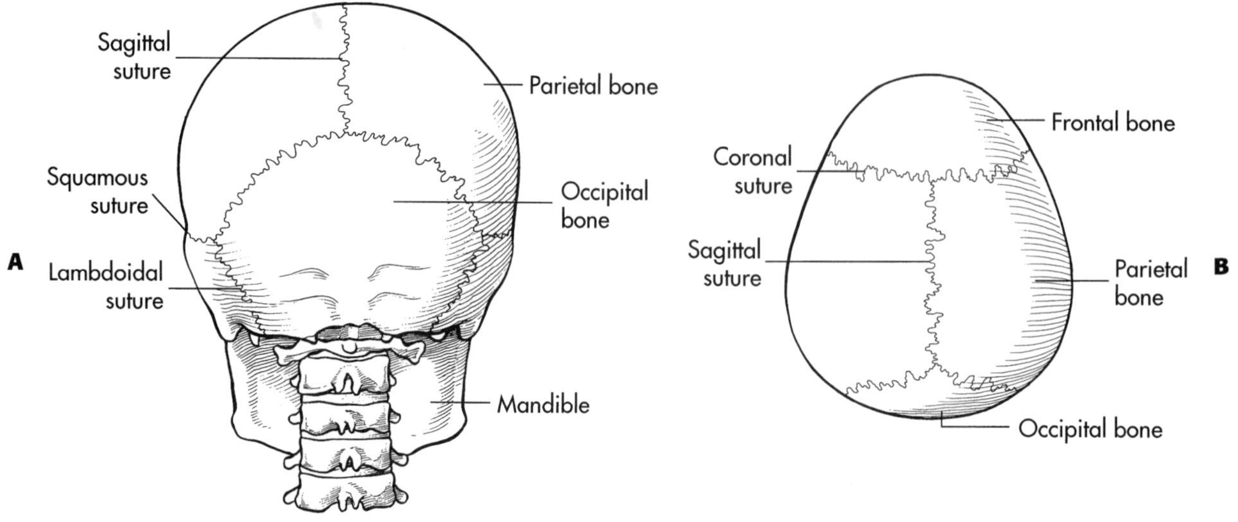

Figure 8-20
A, Posterior skull. **B,** Top view of skull. (Modified from D'Ambrogio KJ, Roth GB: *Positional release therapy: assessment and treatment of musculoskeletal dysfunction*, St Louis, 1997, Mosby.)

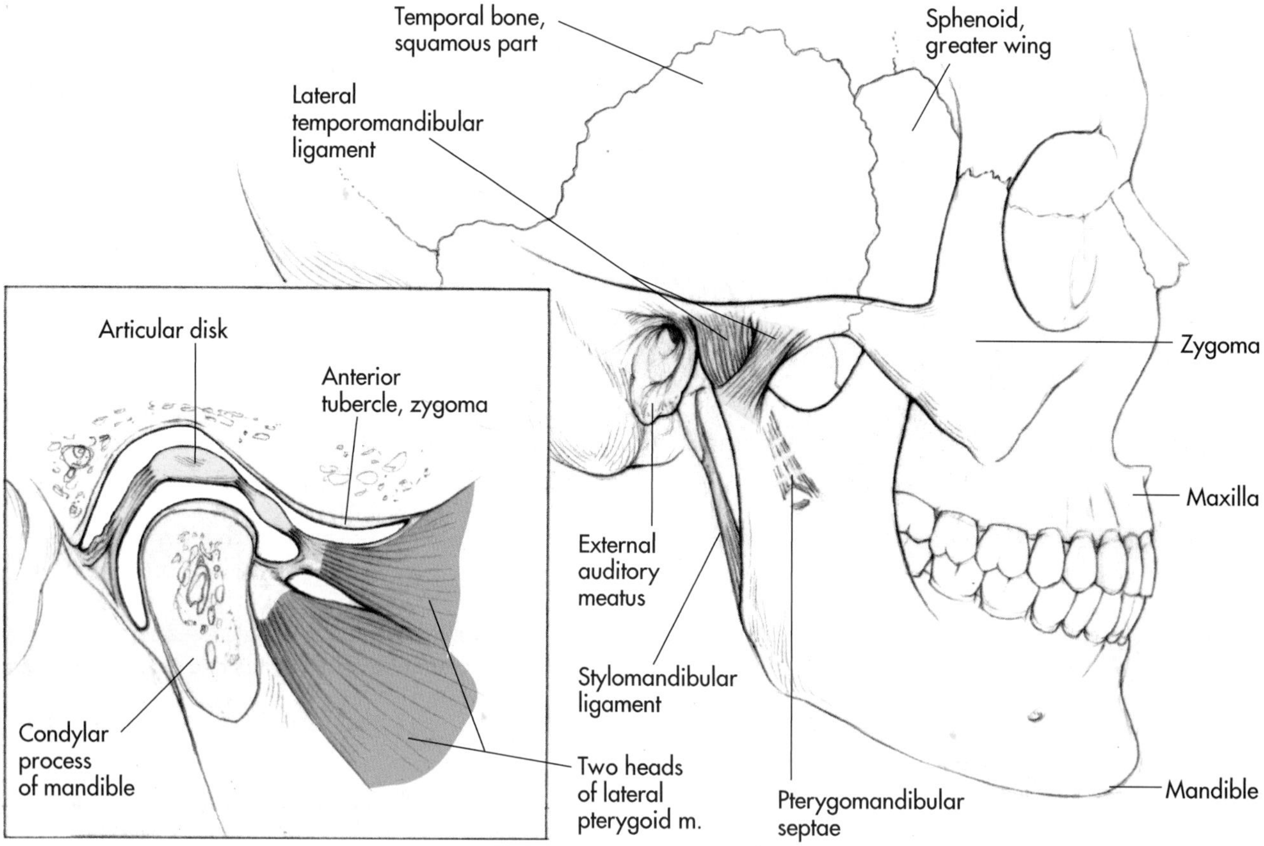

Temporal bone, squamous part
Sphenoid, greater wing
Lateral temporomandibular ligament
Articular disk
Anterior tubercle, zygoma
Zygoma
Maxilla
External auditory meatus
Stylomandibular ligament
Condylar process of mandible
Two heads of lateral pterygoid m.
Pterygomandibular septae
Mandible

Figure 8-21
Temporomandibular joint/inset of articular disk. (From Mathers LH et al: *Clinical anatomy principles*, St Louis, 1996, Mosby.)

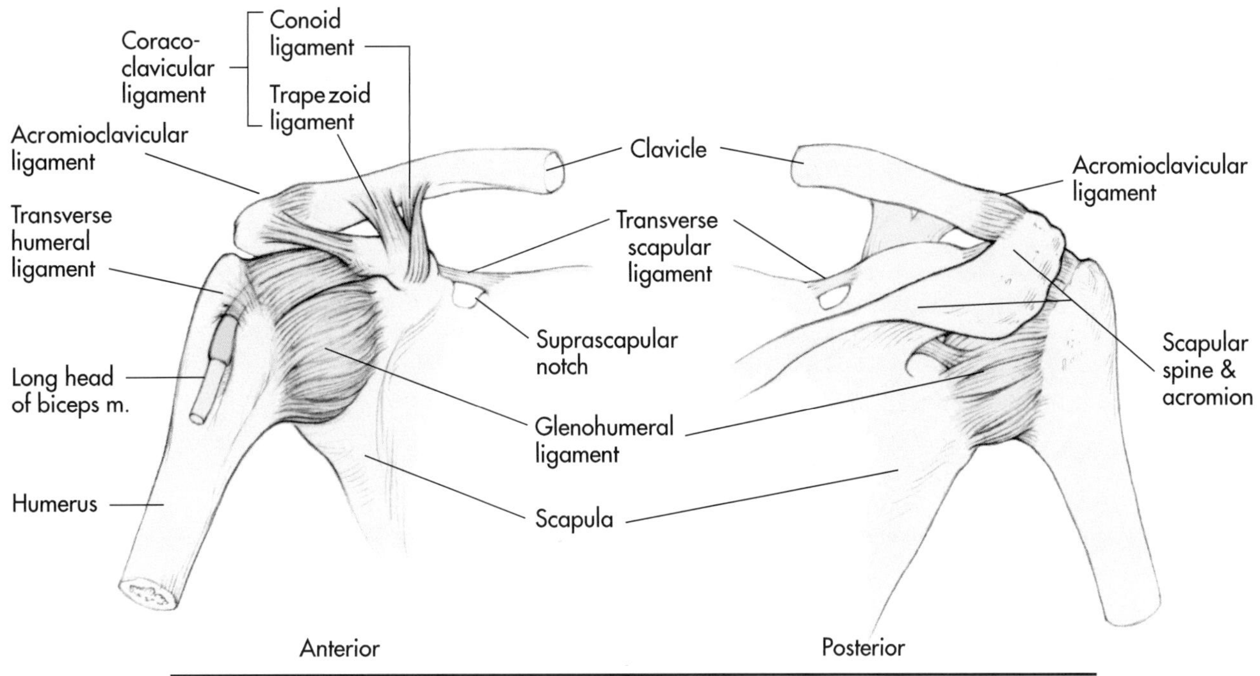

Figure 8-22
Ligaments of the shoulder. Anterior and posterior views. (From Mathers LH et al: *Clinical anatomy principles*, St Louis, 1996, Mosby.)

Glenohumeral Joint

The glenohumeral joint consists of the following structures:

Articulating bones: Humerus and scapula

Joint type: Synovial ball and socket

Ligaments: Glenohumeral: inferior, middle, and superior, from the glenoid cavity of the scapula to head of humerus; coracohumeral ligament from coracoid process to greater and lesser tuberosity of humerus (not pictured in Figure 8-22)

The glenohumeral joint allows the following movements: flexion, extension, abduction, adduction, medial (internal) rotation, lateral (external) rotation, and circumduction.

The glenohumeral joint is the main joint of the shoulder and the most mobile joint in the body. The joint is shallow, which allows for its high degree of mobility, but also accounts for its decreased stability. Most of the support for this joint is provided by the muscles, ligaments, and a loose joint capsule with little support by the bony structures themselves. The tendons of the rotator cuff muscles provide additional stability (Figure 8-22).

Sternoclavicular Joint

The sternoclavicular joint consists of the following structures:

Articulating bones: Clavicle and manubrium

Joint type: Synovial saddle joint

Ligaments: Anterior and posterior sternoclavicular from clavicle to sternum; interclavicular ligament joining both clavicles; costoclavicular ligament from clavicle to first rib; and a fibrocartilaginous (articular) disk located within the joint

The sternoclavicular joint allows the following movements: elevation, depression, anterior and posterior movement, and rotation.

The movements of the sternoclavicular joint follow the movements of the scapula because no muscle works directly on this joint. A decrease or loss of mobility in this joint directly affects shoulder movement. This joint is the only direct connection between the axial skeleton and the shoulder girdle and arm (Figure 8-23).

Acromioclavicular Joint

The acromioclavicular joint consists of the following structures:

Articulating bones: Clavicle and scapula

Joint type: Synovial gliding joint

Ligaments: Acromioclavicular from the acromion process to the clavicle and coracoclavicular ligament from the coracoid process to the clavicle

The acromioclavicular joint may contain a fibrocartilaginous disk. One should note that some persons do not have an acromioclavicular joint because the bones have fused.

The acromioclavicular joint allows the following movements: anterior and posterior gliding, upward and downward rotation, and elevation and depression. Movements that separate the joint are also possible. Although a small joint, the acromioclavicular joint is important in shoulder action (Figure 8-24, *A* and *B*).

Scapulothoracic Junction

Although not a true joint because it does not involve bone-to-bone contact, the scapula moves across the thorax as the

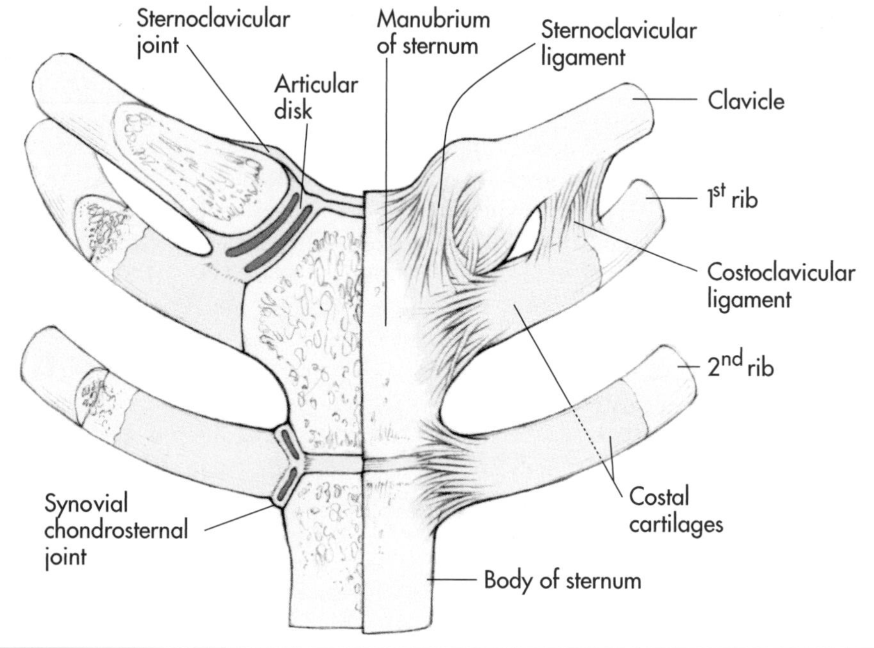

Figure 8-23
Joints of the sternum. The sternoclavicular joint is a double synovial joint, with an articular disk dividing the synovial cavity into two distinct compartments. (From Mathers LH et al: *Clinical anatomy principles*, St Louis, 1996, Mosby.)

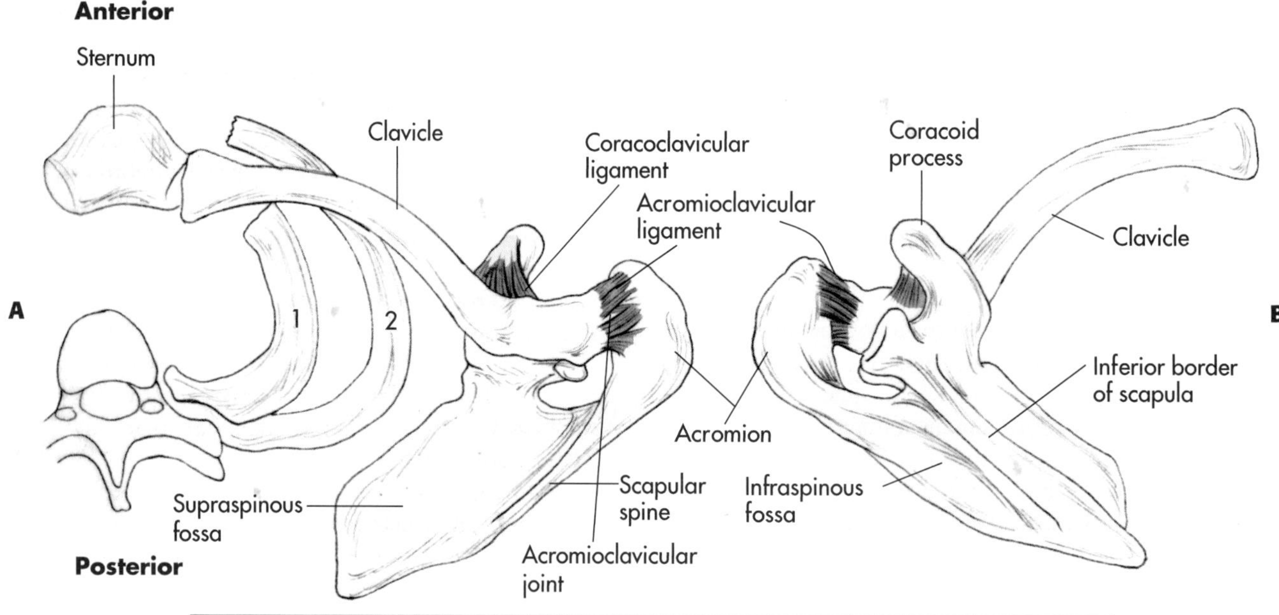

Figure 8-24
Acromial clavicular joint of the shoulder girdle. Superior (**A**) and inferior (**B**) views. The superior view illustrates the attachments of the lateral end of the clavicle, especially to the acromion and coracoid process. (From Mathers LH et al: *Clinical anatomy principles*, St Louis, 1996, Mosby.)

subscapularis and serratus anterior muscles glide over a subscapular bursa and fat pad. Most of the movement results from sternoclavicular action, with the rest of the action provided by movement in the acromioclavicular joint. If the scapula is limited in its movement, all shoulder movement is restricted, although one can compensate for restrictions in adduction most easily. The movements of the scapulothoracic junction include elevation, depression, protraction, retraction, and upward and downward rotation.

The position of three major points—the tip of the acromion, the greater tubercle of the humerus, and the coracoid process—provide clues as to the exact position of the shoulder. **The student can palpate the shoulder as follows:** Beginning at the suprasternal notch, move slightly laterally to locate the sternoclavicular joint. To confirm the location of the joint, hold lightly while moving the same side arm into flexion and extension. Compare this joint movement with the direction of the scapular movements. Continue along the clavicle, following the convex curve of the medial two thirds and the concave curve of the lateral one third. Reach back to the spine of the scapula and follow it laterally; at its end move superiorly and anteriorly, where it becomes the acromion (the high point of the shoulder). This is a large flat area, with a slight concavity. Find the anterior tip of the acromion and move slightly medially; the elevated ridge marks the start of the acromioclavicular joint. Move back to the top of the acromion, then laterally and inferiorly to the outer edge of the greater tubercle of the humerus. Moving anteriorly and medially, locate the lesser tubercle. Continuing medially on to the soft tissues of the anterior chest, press in to locate the coracoid process of the scapula just below the concave portion of the clavicle.

The glenohumeral joint, where the arm connects to the body, is easiest to palpate when the arm is in passive extension or actively moving through circumduction. The fibrous capsule of the rotator cuff (muscles and tendons that surround the joint) often makes feeling the bony structures difficult. Of the four muscles of the rotator cuff, three—the supraspinatus, infraspinatus, and teres minor—insert together on the greater tubercle of the humerus, and their attachments are easiest to palpate. The fourth, the subscapularis, inserts on the lesser tubercle and is not palpated easily (Activity 8-6).

Joints of the Elbow

The joints of the elbow are the ulnarhumeral, radiohumeral, and radioulnar joints.

Ulnarhumeral and Radiohumeral Joints

The ulnarhumeral and radiohumeral joints consist of the following structures:

Articulating bones: Humerus with the ulna and humerus with the radius

Joint type: Synovial hinge

Ligaments: Medial (ulnar) collateral: anterior, posterior, transverse from the medial epicondyle of the humerus and olecranon process of the ulna to the coronoid process; radial collateral from lateral epicondyle of the humerus to the annular ligament; and annular ligament from anterior portion of radial notch around to the posterior margin of radial notch

The ulnarhumeral and radiohumeral joints allow the following movements: flexion and extension.

Because of the bony structure and the support of muscles and ligaments, the elbow is a stable joint. Most elbow action involves the ulnar and humeral portion of the joint, although the radius interacts with the humerus. The radius is on the thumb side of the forearm, and the ulna is on the little finger side. In anatomic position the radius is referred to as lateral and the ulna as medial. During flexion, the trochlear notch of the ulna slides on the humeral trochlea, while the head of the radius slides on the capitulum. In extension the movements are reversed and stop when the olecranon process reaches its anatomic barrier at the olecranon fossa. The elbow is one of the few areas in the body where a hard end feel and anatomic barrier occurs. Hyperextension is possible in those individuals who have a small olecranon process or a large olecranon fossa (Figure 8-25).

Radioulnar Joint

The radioulnar joint consists of the following structures:

Articulating bones: Radius and ulna

Joint type: Synovial pivot

Ligaments: Annular ligament (see the previous joint)

The radioulnar joint allows the following movements: pronation and supination.

The radioulnar joint articulates at the proximal and distal ends (Figure 8-25) and is listed as part of the elbow complex because it has the same soft tissue support as the elbow joint, and most of the actions occur in this area. The head of the radius moves clockwise and counterclockwise around the ulna at the proximal end. During pronation, the radius crosses the ulna and ends diagonal to the ulna, allowing the palm to face down. Supination returns the radius and ulna to parallel positions, with the palm facing up, as in holding a bowl of soup (soup = supination, or *up* as in sUPination—a clue to remembering the position).

The interosseous membrane connects the ulna and radius, and its fibers run in a diagonal pattern perpendicular to one another. This membrane is taut during supination and relaxed in pronation and sometimes is referred to as an articulation, just as the scapulothoracic junction is (Figure 8-26).

The student can locate the medial and lateral epicondyles of the humerus and the olecranon process of the ulna. A bursa lies between the olecranon process and the skin. If the student can palpate the bursa, it will feel like a small bubble. The synovial membrane is most accessible to examination between the olecranon and the epicondyles. One can trace the ulna by following the bony ridge toward the wrist from the olecranon. The area between the medial epicondyle and olecranon may be sensitive because of the proximity of the ulnar nerve.

The student can supinate and pronate the forearm and feel the radius rotate on the ulna (Activity 8-7).

ACTIVITY 8-6

Move your shoulder joints, individually and (if possible) together, through all of the range of motion positions.

ACTIVITY 8-7

Move your elbow through the range of motion positions.

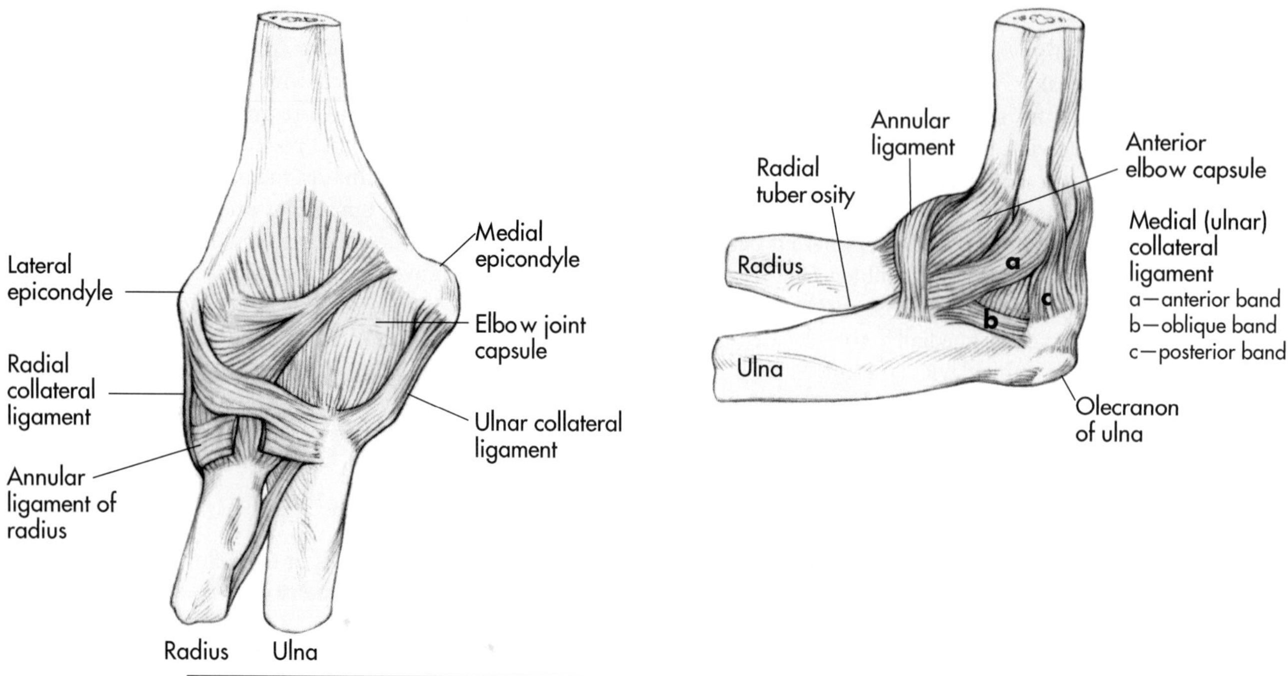

Figure 8-25
Ligaments of the elbow joint. Anterior and lateral views. (From Mathers LH et al: *Clinical anatomy principles*, St Louis, 1996, Mosby.)

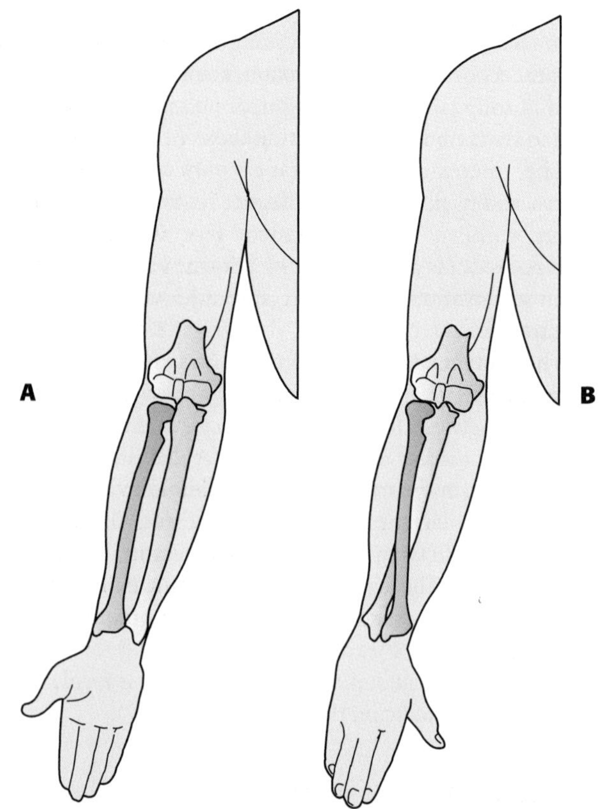

Figure 8-26
A, Supination. **B,** Pronation.

Joints of the Wrist and Hand

The joints of the wrist and hand include the radiocarpal and carpometacarpal joints.

Radiocarpal (Wrist) Joint

The radiocarpal joint consists of the following structures:

Articulating bones: Radius, scaphoid, and lunate with some triquetral bone involvement

Joint type: Synovial condyloid

Ligaments: Palmar radiocarpal ligament from the radius to the scaphoid, lunate, and triquetral bones; palmar ulnocarpal ligament from the ulna to the scaphoid, lunate, and triquetral bones; and dorsal radiocarpal ligament from the radius to the scaphoid, lunate, and triquetral bones. (Figure 8-27 shows the bones that these ligaments connect [ligaments not pictured].)

The radiocarpal joint allows the following movements: flexion, extension, and radial and ulnar flexion.

The wrist is called the radiocarpal joint because the radius alone articulates with the carpal bones. The ulna joins the wrist indirectly by a disk that articulates with the carpal bones. This allows pronation and supination to take place without affecting any wrist movements.

Hand Joints

This intricate pattern of hand joints is where all the movements involving the hand take place. The metacarpals and phalanges, which make up the palm of the hand and the

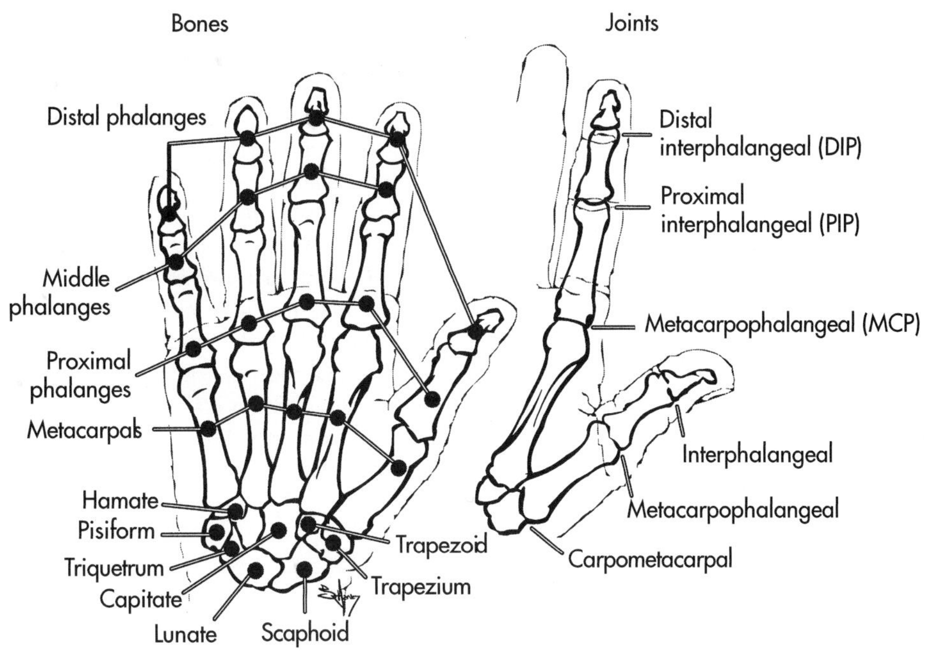

Figure 8-27
Joints of the hand and wrist. (From Brister SJ: *Mosby's comprehensive physical therapist assistant board review,* St Louis, 1996, Mosby.)

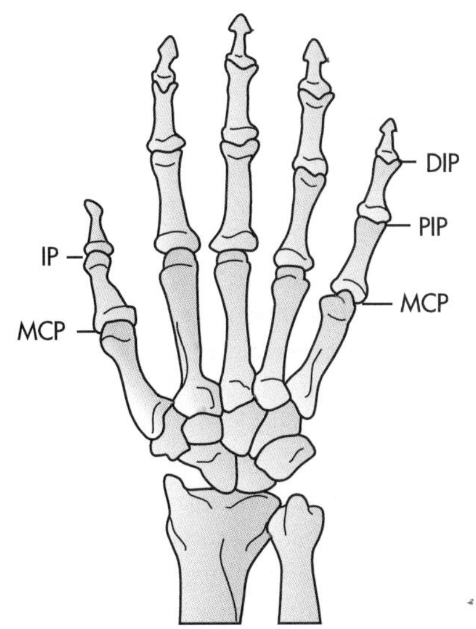

Figure 8-28
Hand joints.

fingers, form hinge joints permitting flexion and extension. These joints are called proximal interphalangeal (PIP) joints, metacarpophalangeal (MCP) joints, and distal interphalangeal (DIP) joints (Figures 8-28 and 8-29).

The first carpometacarpal joint (the thumb) consists of the following structures:

Articulating bones: First metacarpal with trapezium
Joint type: Synovial saddle
Ligaments: Flexor retinaculum from the trapezium to the pisiform, with assistance from the articular capsule

The first carpometacarpal joint allows the following movements: flexion, extension, abduction, adduction, circumduction, and opposition.

The hand is capable of a variety of functions that vary from the precise handling of objects to acts of great strength. The opposable thumb allows us to grasp and manipulate objects. Because the thumb is rotated from the rest of the fingers in the resting position, the thumb faces the rest of the fingers. The joint capsule of the wrist is loose in the superior and inferior directions, allowing easy flexion and extension, but tight laterally and medially, allowing for minimal adduction and abduction. No circumduction occurs at the wrist. Instead, what appears to be a rotation is actually pronation and supination of the forearm combined with wrist flexion.

The student can palpate the wrist as follows: At the wrist, locate the bony tips of the radius (laterally) and the ulna (medially). On the dorsum of the wrist, palpate the groove of the radiocarpal or wrist joint. Each individual carpal bone within the hand cannot be identified readily, so instead palpate the carpal structure while moving the wrist. Palpate each of the five metacarpals and the proximal, middle, and distal phalanges and connecting hinge joints. Remember the thumb lacks a middle phalanx. Partially flex your fingers, and find the groove marking the metacarpophalangeal joint of each finger. The joint is proximal to the first knuckle and is palpated best on either side of the extensor tendon (Activity 8-8).

Joints of the Pelvis and Hip

The joints of the hip and pelvis include the sacroiliac joint, symphysis pubis, and hip joint.

ACTIVITY 8-8

Move your hand and the wrist through each of the range of motion positions.

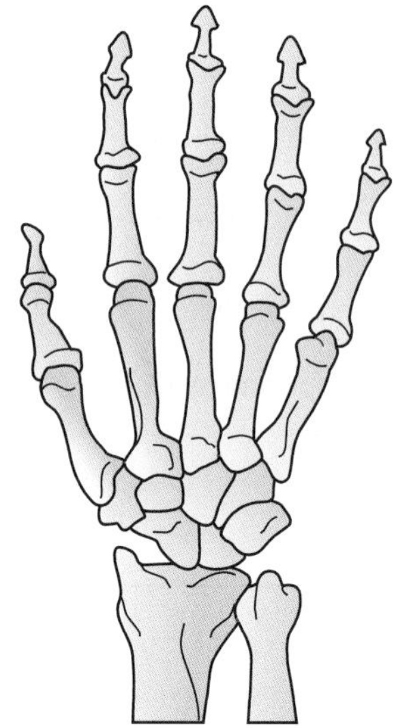

Figure 8-29
Label the hand joints. See Figures 8-27 and 8-28 after you've finished.

Sacroiliac Joint

The sacroiliac joint consists of the following structures:
Articulating bones: Sacrum and the two ilia
Ligaments: The ventral sacroiliac ligament covers the anterior and inferior aspects of the joint; the interosseous sacroiliac ligament links the sacrum and the iliac tuberosity; and the dorsal sacroiliac ligament (on the posterior aspect of the joint to the anterior surface of the sacrum) interfaces with the sacrotuberous ligament. The sacrospinous ligament connects the sacrum to the ischial spine.

This joint connects the pelvis to the trunk, transfers the weight of the body to the hip, and works as a shock absorber during walking and running. The movement allowed is a small but important anterior and posterior and lateral and medial rotation in a side-lying figure-eight pattern. This rotary movement of the hips at the pelvis allows the vertebral column to remain relatively still as we walk. When the sacroiliac joint does not move, the sacral lumbar junction compensates for the lack of rotation, putting strain on the joint. No direct muscle action occurs on this joint. Instead, the sacroiliac joint moves as a result of other joint movements in the area, following the sacral movement.

Ligaments provide much support. They are more relaxed in the female. This laxity increases with hormones released during monthly cycles and especially during pregnancy (Figure 8-30).

Symphysis Pubis

The symphysis pubis consists of the following structures:
Articulating bones: The two pubic bones
Ligaments: The superior pubic ligament supports the anterior, posterior, and superior aspect, and the arcuate pubic ligament supports the inferior aspect (these ligaments are not shown in Figure 8-30).

The symphysis pubis allows the following movement: slight separation, especially during pregnancy and delivery.

The main function of this joint is to provide stability. The joint connects the left and right coxal (hip) bones anteriorly. Should this joint become misaligned, which can happen during childbirth or trauma such as a fall, the stability of the pelvis is compromised and many postural and soft tissue problems can result (see Figure 8-30).

Hip Joint

The hip joint consists of the following structures:
Articulating bones: Ilium, pubis, and ischium, which form the concave surface called the acetabulum; the femur
Ligaments: Iliofemoral ligament from the anterior superior iliac spine to the intertrochanteric line of the femur; ischiofemoral ligament from the ischium to the femur on the posterior side; pubofemoral ligament from the pubis to the intertrochanteric line of the femur on the anterior side; and the ligamentum teres, also known as the ligament of the head of the femur, from the fovea to the acetabulum

A fibrocartilaginous ring called the labrum attaches around the edge of the acetabulum and is reinforced by the transverse acetabular ligament. This ring helps hold the femoral head in place by increasing the depth of the acetabulum (not shown).

The hip joint allows the following movements: flexion, extension, abduction, adduction, medial rotation, lateral rotation, and circumduction.

The hip joint is the most massive of the joints. Although a mobile ball-and-socket joint, the hip joint is less mobile than the shoulder joint because of the round head of the femur fitting into the deep socket of the acetabulum of the pelvis. This structure provides stability. In the anatomic position the femoral head is not fully in the hip socket. A better fit is when the femur is flexed to 90 degrees, slightly abducted, and laterally rotated. The most relaxed position is flexion, abduction, and lateral rotation such as found in relaxed sitting with the leg falling to the side.

The joint capsule is large. All ligaments become tight in lateral rotation and looser in medial rotation. The capsule is looser in flexion than in extension.

Usually the leg moves on the pelvis, but the pelvis can move on the leg if the leg is fixed. With the femur fixed, the pelvis can move forward, which tends to increase the lordosis of the lumbar spine and is called *anteversion. Retroversion* is the opposite movement and decreases lumbar lordosis. The pelvis can flex laterally and medially along with flexion of the lumbar spine (Figure 8-31).

The student can palpate the hip joint as follows: The hip joint lies deep within the body and is not directly palpable.

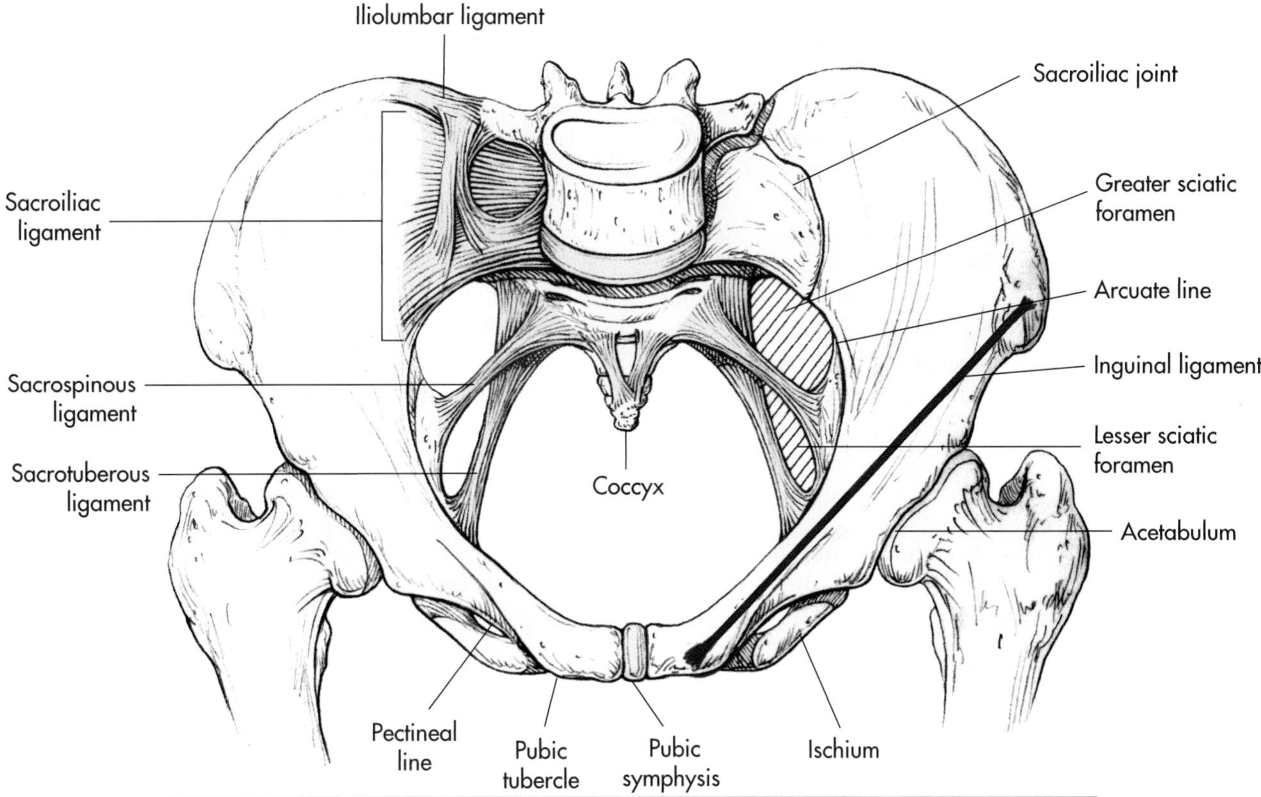

Figure 8-30
Pelvic ligaments, superoanterior view. These important ligaments give the pelvis its strength. (From Mathers LH et al: *Clinical anatomy principles*, St Louis, 1996, Mosby.)

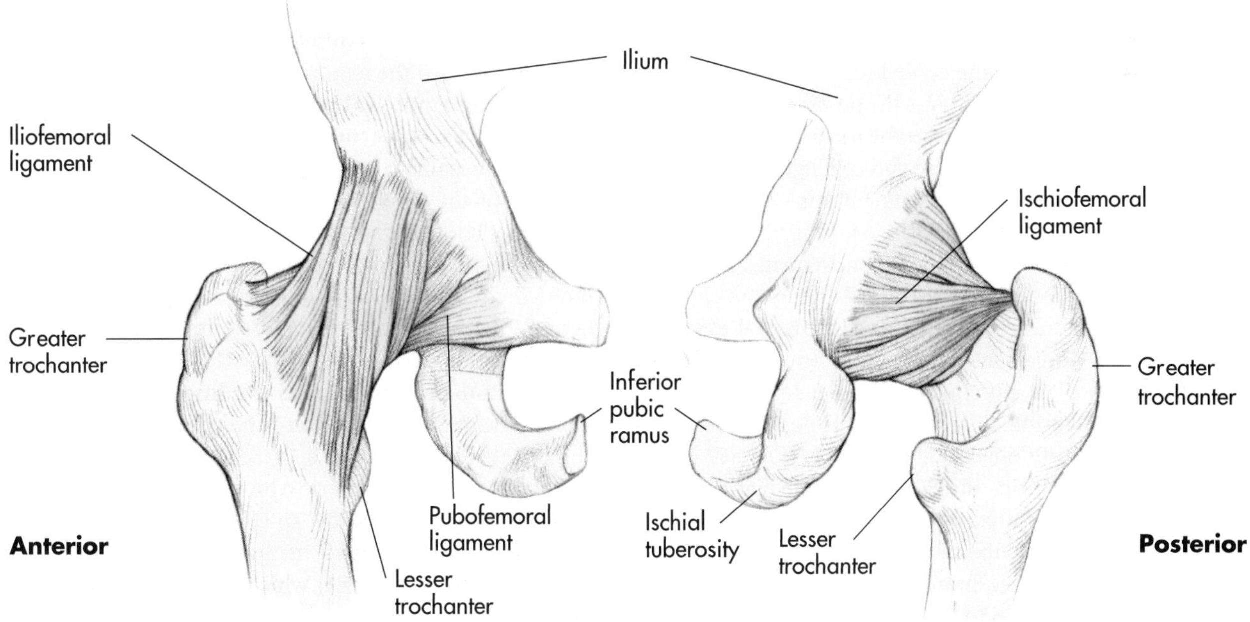

Figure 8-31
Ligaments of the hip joint. The three principal hip joint ligaments are arranged in a continuum that surrounds the joint. The iliofemoral ligament is especially important in limiting the extension of the hip. (From Mathers LH et al: *Clinical anatomy principles*, St Louis, 1996, Mosby.)

The posterior edge of the greater trochanter of the femur is easiest to locate and one can feel it about a palm's width below the iliac crest. The superficial trochanteric bursa lies on the posterolateral surface of the greater trochanter. At the same level as the greater trochanter, locate the pubic tubercles. One can palpate the symphysis pubis at the anterior midline of the body and can palpate the sacroiliac joint just inferior to the posterior superior iliac spine near the dimples of the gluteal area. The sacroiliac joint is not directly palpable because it is covered with ligaments, but one can feel movements there. One can feel a small rotary movement if one holds the finger or thumb in this area while walking, marching in place, or flexing or extending the trunk (Activity 8-9).

Joints of the Knee

The tibiofemoral joint is the two articular areas between the femur and tibia. The patellofemoral joint is found between the patella and the trochlear groove of the femur. These two joints consist of the following structures:

Articulating bones: Femur, tibia, and patella (or knee cap)

Joint type: Synovial condylar

Ligaments: The patellar ligament runs from the patella to the tibial tuberosity (the quadriceps femoris tendon also provides stability to the patella); the oblique popliteal ligament joins the lateral aspect of the fibrous capsule to the lateral condyle of the femur; the tibial (medial) collateral ligament joins the medial epicondyle of the femur to medial condyle of the tibia; the fibular (lateral) collateral ligament joins the lateral epicondyle of the femur to the fibula; the anterior cruciate ligament joins the anterior medial intercondylar area of the tibia to the medial surface of the lateral condyle of the femur; the posterior cruciate ligament joins the posterior intercondylar area of the tibia to the medial condyle of the femur; the posterior meniscofemoral ligament is not described here; the transverse ligament joins the medial meniscus to the lateral meniscus.

The knee joints allow the following movements: flexion, extension, medial rotation, and lateral rotation.

The knee joint is the most complicated joint in the body, is not as stable as other joints, and yet it is one of the most often used joints. The principal movements at the knee are flexion and extension. Some rotation is possible during flexion of the joint. Prolonged standing while the knee is in a slightly flexed position, instead of the normal locked extension position, puts stress on the articular surfaces of the condyles and can damage the cartilage.

The medial condyle is more curved than the lateral condyle, which contributes to the automatic rotation of the knee during flexion and extension. The femoral condyle first rolls off the tibial condyle and then glides, producing a combined rolling-gliding movement. The opposite action occurs in extension of the knee: first a glide and then rolling.

In the male the acetabulum is located almost directly above the knee, which allows for even distribution of weight-bearing forces during movement. In contrast, the wider female pelvis results in the knee being medial to the acetabulum. This arrangement puts strain on the female knee during movement. Female knees are not typically anatomically designed to handle the strain of running and repetitive flexion/extension with impact activities.

The fibrocartilaginous menisci provide more surface contact on the tibia for the femur, which allows for stability between the rounded femoral condyles, which sit on an almost flat tibia. The menisci are attached to muscles and connected by ligaments to each other and to the bones. These shock absorbers protect bone and cartilage and increase the movement of synovial fluid. The menisci move in the joint capsule, depending on the forces imposed on them. If the movement against the menisci is too abrupt or quickly changes direction so that they cannot shift position, the menisci can be crushed or torn.

The joint capsule is slack anteriorly and taut posteriorly in extension and just the opposite in flexion. The posterior knee capsule is thick and consists of two strong bands connecting the femoral and tibial condyles. These ligaments resist hyperextension of the joint and provide stability in the standing position in normal extension. In normal extension all the ligaments are taut, and one can stabilize the joint passively without any muscular action. Extension is the most stable position for the knee.

The patella protects the knee joint from external impact such as falling forward onto the knees. The patella moves in a groove between the femoral condyles by the contraction of the quadriceps muscle. The more flexion, the greater the pull on the patella. The contraction of the quadriceps tends to pull the patella laterally during active extension. The position of the patella becomes somewhat unstable in this position. The patella provides an increased mechanical advantage for the quadriceps muscles when contracting to move the knee into extension. The knee is prone to injury because it relies on soft tissue for much of its support in a flexed position (Figure 8-32).

The student can palpate the knee joint as follows: Landmarks in and around the knee help orient you to this complicated joint. Locate the flat medial surface of the tibia, the shin. Follow its anterior border upward to the tibial tuberosity. Move medially and follow the medial border of the tibia upward until it merges into a bony prominence, the medial tibial condyle, which is higher than the tibial tuberosity. In a comparable location on the other side of the knee, find a similar prominence, the lateral condyle of the knee. Just below the level of the lateral tibial condyle, find the head of the fibula.

Now identify three parts of the distal femur. Bring your fingertips firmly down the medial surface of the thigh along a line where the inner seam of your pant leg would be. Your

ACTIVITY 8-9

Move your hip through each of the range of motion positions.

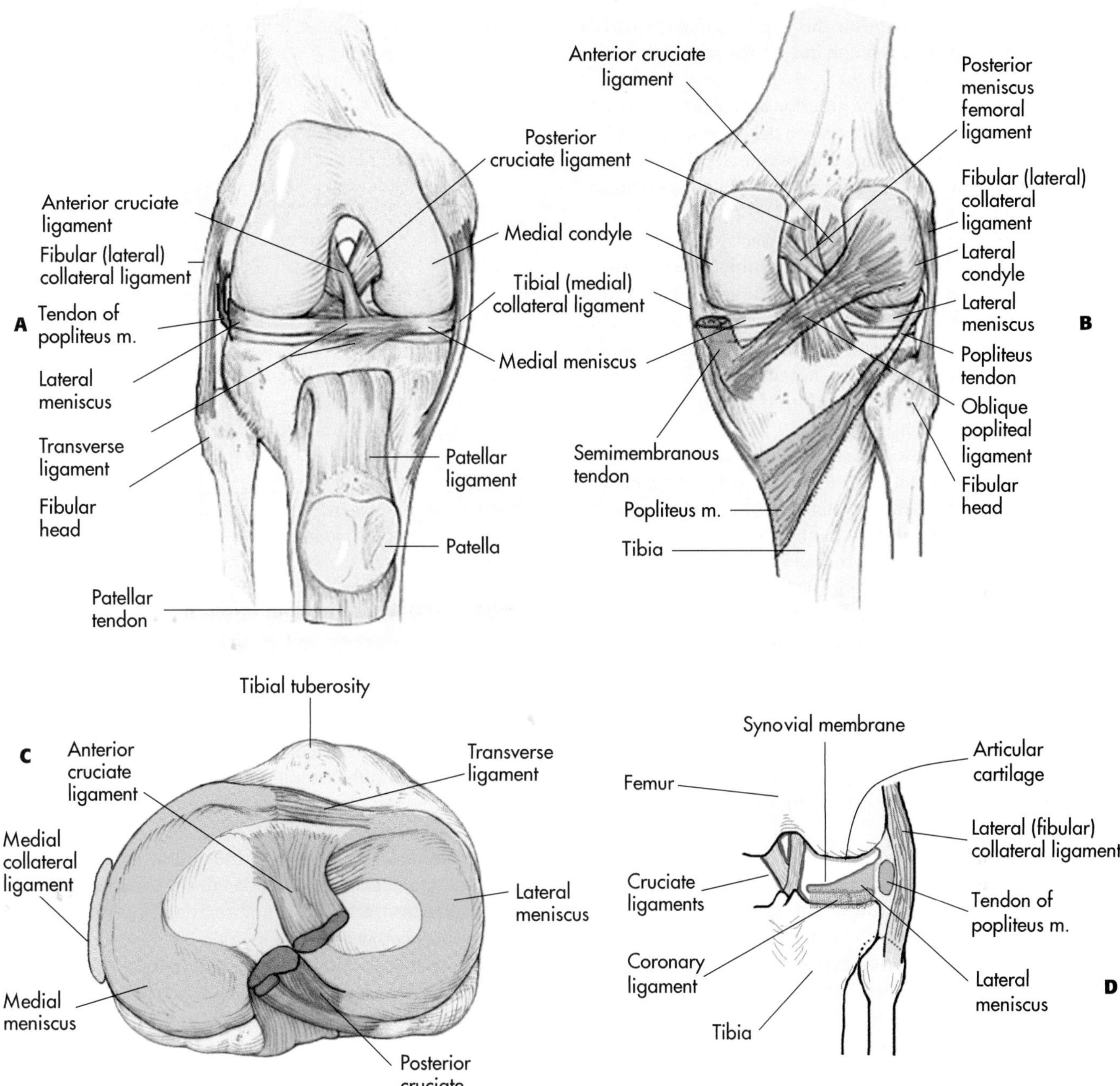

Figure 8-32

Knee joint opened, anterior and posterior view. **A,** Anterior view of the knee joint, opened by folding the patella and patellar ligament inferiorly. On the lateral side is the fibular collateral ligament, separated by the popliteal tendon from the lateral meniscus. On the medial side, the tibial collateral ligament is attached to the medial meniscus. The anterior and posterior cruciate ligaments are seen between the femoral condyles. **B,** Posterior view of the opened knee joint, with a more complete view of the posterior cruciate ligament. **C,** The femur is removed, showing the superior (articular) end of the right tibia. On the medial side is the gently curved medial meniscus and, on the lateral side, the more tightly curved lateral meniscus. The anterior end of the medial meniscus is anchored to the surface of the tibia by the transverse ligament. The cut ends of both the anterior and posterior cruciate ligaments are shown, as well as the meniscofemoral ligament. **D,** This view of the lateral side of the knee illustrates the way the lateral meniscus is attached to the tibial plateau by the coronary ligaments. It is enclosed by synovial membrane, continuous with the general synovial lining of the joint space. (From Mathers LH et al: *Clinical anatomy principles*, St Louis, 1996, Mosby.)

fingers will run up against an abrupt bony prominence, the adductor tubercle. Just below this is the medial epicondyle. The lateral epicondyle is found in a similar area on the other side.

The patella rests on the anterior articulating surface of the femur, roughly midway between the epicondyles, and lies within the tendon of the quadriceps muscles. This structure continues below the knee joint as the patellar ligament and inserts on the tibial tuberosity.

Two collateral ligaments, one on each side of the knee, give medial and lateral stability to the joint. To feel the lateral collateral ligament, cross one leg so that your ankle rests on the opposite knee. Find the firm cord that runs from the lateral epicondyle of the femur to the head of the fibula. The medial collateral ligament is not palpable. Two cruciate ligaments cross obliquely within the knee and give it anteroposterior stability.

With the knee flexed to about 90 degrees, you can press your thumbs—one on each side of the patellar ligament—into the groove of the tibiofemoral joint. Note that the patella lies just above this joint line. As you press your thumbs downward, you can feel the edge of the upper surface of the tibia. Follow it medially, then laterally until you are stopped by the converging femur and tibia.

The medial and lateral menisci, crescent-shaped fibrocartilaginous pads that lie on the tibial plateaus, form cushions between the tibia and femur. By moving your thumbs up and toward the midline to the top of the patella, you can follow the articulating surface of the femur and identify the margins of the joint. The soft tissue in front of the joint space, on either side of the patellar ligament, is the infrapatellar fat pad.

Several bursae lie near the knee. The prepatellar bursa lies between the patella and the overlying skin, whereas the superficial infrapatellar bursa lies anterior to the patellar ligament.

Observe the concavities that are usually evident at each side and above the patella. In these areas is the synovial cavity of the knee joint. Although the synovium is not normally detectable, these areas may become swollen and tender when the joint is inflamed (Activity 8-10).

Joints of the Ankle and Foot

The joints of the ankle and foot include the tibiotalar, inferior tibiofibular, and talocalcaneal joints, interphalangeal, metatarsophalangeal, intertarsal joints, and tarsometatarsal joints (Figure 8-33).

Tibiotalar Joint

The tibiotalar joint consists of the following structures:

> **ACTIVITY 8-10**
>
> Move your knee through each of the range of motion positions.

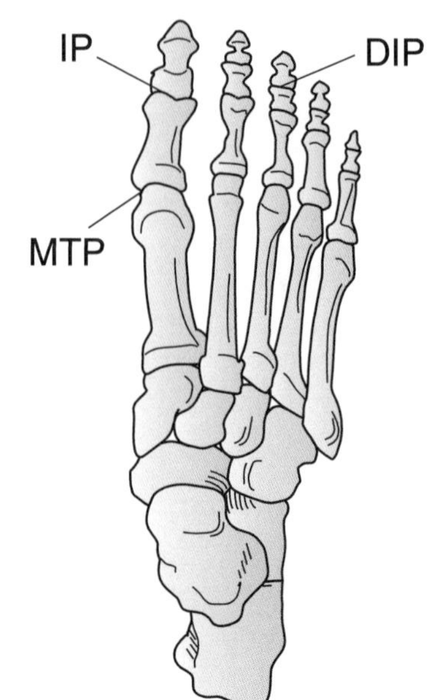

Figure 8-33
Foot joints.

Articulating bones: Tibia, fibula, and talus

Joint type: Synovial saddle joint (Many resources classify as a synovial hinge; the saddle joint classification is based on the accessory movements in plantar flexion.)

Ligaments: Medial collateral or deltoid from the medial malleolus to the navicular, calcaneus, and talus; lateral collateral from the lateral malleolus to the talus and calcaneus; and calcaneofibular from the fibula to the lateral calcaneus

The tibiotalar joint allows the following movements: dorsiflexion (flexion) and plantar flexion (extension) with slight abduction, adduction, and rotation in plantar flexion caused by the other joints.

The metatarsals and phalanges that make up the anterior portion of the foot and the toes form a hinge joint permitting flexion and extension (Figures 8-33 and 8-34).

Inferior Tibiofibular Joint and Talocalcaneal Joint

The inferior tibiofibular joint, a mortise joint, is a fibrous syndesmosis joint that holds the tibia and fibula together as one bone, forming the ankle joint. Immediately distal to the ankle joint is the talocalcaneal joint, or the articulation of the talus with the calcaneus. This joint is reinforced by the joint capsule and interosseous ligaments, which essentially make the talus and calcaneus one bone, just as the tibiofibular joint function makes the tibia and fibula one bone. No muscles insert on the talus, which is moved indirectly by the structures surrounding it. Full dorsiflexion is the more stable position. Most sprained ankles occur in plantar flexion, where less stability is evident. This joint is more stable than mobile because of the structural support, but if these structures are injured, the joint can become unstable.

Motions of the ankle joint itself are limited to dorsiflexion and plantar flexion, as previously stated. Inversion

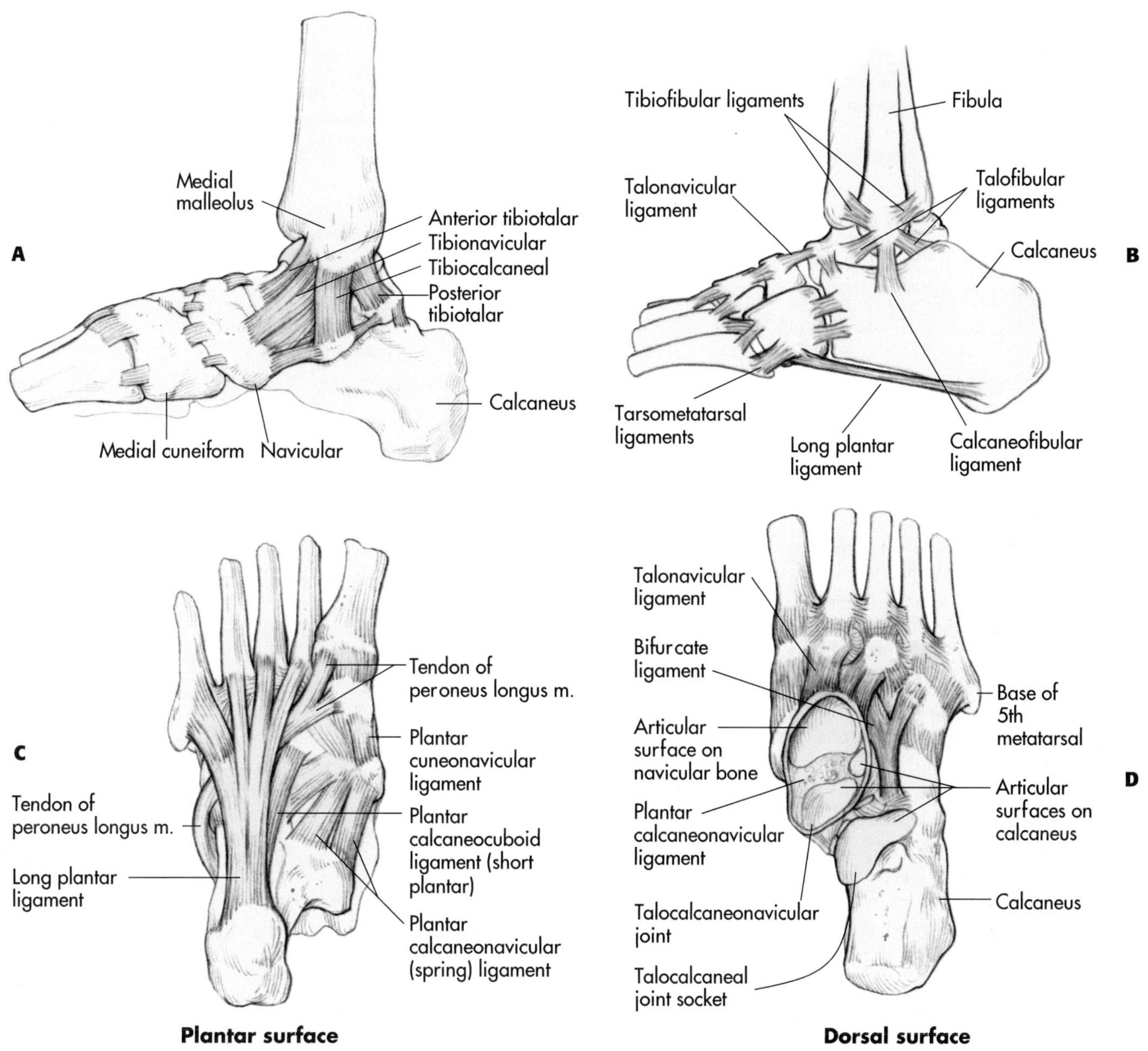

Figure 8-34
A, Deltoid ligament. The deltoid ligament attaches the medial malleolus of the tibia to several underlying bones. It consists of anterior tibiotalar, tibionavicular, tibiocalcaneal, and posterior tibiotalar portions. **B,** Ligaments of the ankle. **C,** Plantar ligaments of the foot, including the long plantar, short plantar, and spring ligaments. **D,** Carpal bones with the talus removed, showing the rounded socket in which it articulates (the talocalcaneonavicular joint). The bifurcate and talonavicular ligaments help stabilize the bones forming this articulation. (From Mathers LH et al: *Clinical anatomy principles*, St Louis, 1996, Mosby.)

and eversion of the foot are functions of the talocalcaneal and transverse tarsal joints (see Figure 8-34).

Foot Joints

The joints between the tarsal bones are called intertarsal joints. The joints between the tarsals and the metatarsals are called tarsometatarsal joints. The joints between the metatarsals and the phalanges are called metatarsophalangeal (MTP) joints. The joints in the toes between the proximal and distal phalanges are called interphalangeal (IP) joints. The great toe has one joint, and the lesser toes each have two joints. The more proximal joint is the proximal interphalangeal (PIP) joint, and the distal joint is the distal interphalangeal joint or the DIP. The interphalangeal joints are hinge joints. The metatarsophalangeal (MTP) joints are condyloid joints. A system of collateral ligaments and the joint capsule secure the joint structure.

The principal landmarks of the ankle are the medial malleolus, the bony prominence at the distal end of the tibia, and the lateral malleolus, at the distal end of the fibula. Ligaments extend from each malleolus into the foot. The heads of the metatarsals are palpable in the ball of the foot.

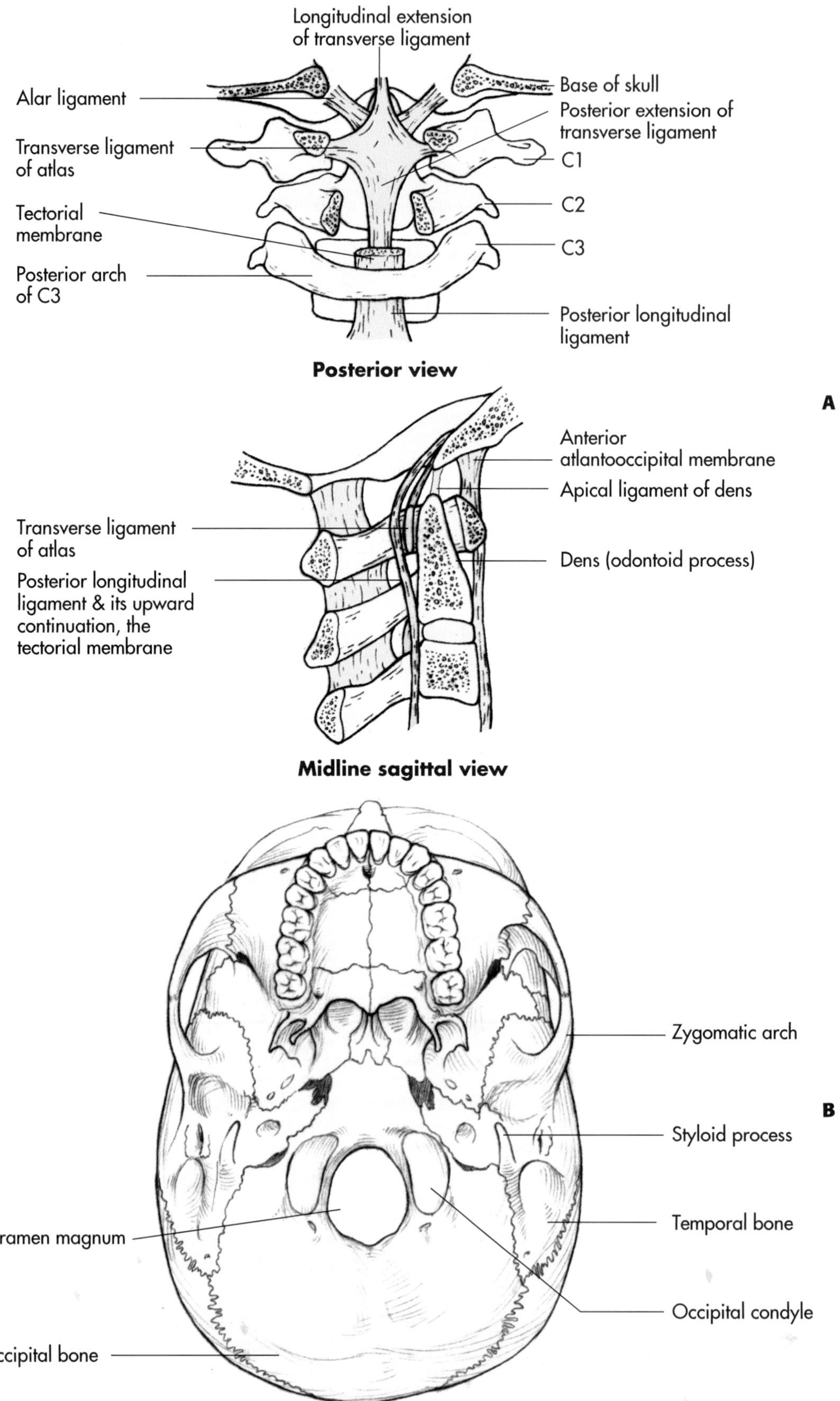

Figure 8-35

A, Ligaments connecting the skull and vertebral column. Both C1 and C2 vertebrae are separately attached to the base of the skull to ensure maximal stability. The transverse ligament of the atlas prevents the dens from moving posteriorly and crushing the spinal cord as it passes through the lumen of the C1 vertebra. With its upward and downward extensions, the transverse ligament forms the cruciform ligament. **B,** Base of the skull. On this view, the large occipital condyles are shown. These are the surfaces at which the skull articulates with the C1 vertebra, the atlas. (From Mathers LH et al: *Clinical anatomy principles*, St Louis, 1996, Mosby.)

ACTIVITY 8-11

Move your ankles and feet through each of the range of motion positions.

These and the associated metatarsophalangeal joints are proximal to the webs of the toes. An imaginary line along the foot bones extending from the heads of the metatarsals to the calcaneus is called the longitudinal arch (Activity 8-11).

Joints of the Spine and Thorax

The spine and thorax joints consist of the atlantooccipital, atlantoaxial, and intervertebral joints, the zygopophyseal joints, and the costovertebral, costotransverse, costochondral, and chondrosternal joints.

Atlantooccipital Joint

The atlantooccipital joint consists of the following structures (Figure 8-35):

Articulating bones: Atlas C1 and occipital bone at the occipital condyles

Joint type: Synovial condyloid (ellipsoid) joint

The atlantooccipital joint allows the following movements: flexion, extension, and lateral flexion.

Atlantoaxial Joint (Atlantoepistropheal Joint)

The atlantoaxial joint consists of the following structures:

Articulating bones: Atlas C1 and axis C2

Joint type: Synovial pivot

The atlantoaxial joint allows rotation.

Intervertebral Joints

The intervertebral joints consist of the following structures (Figure 8-36):

Articulating bones: Adjacent vertebrae

Joint type: Cartilaginous symphysis

Individual intervertebral joints allow minimal movement; movement of spine as a whole unit is much larger.

Zygopophyseal Joints

The zygopophyseal joints consist of the following structures:

Articulating bones: Superior and inferior articulating facets of adjacent vertebrae

Joint type: Synovial gliding joints

Ligaments: The supraspinous ligament and interspinous ligaments run along the ends of the spinous processes of each vertebra; the supraspinous ligament enlarges in the cervical region and becomes the ligamentum nuchae in the cervical area; intertransverse ligaments connect the transverse processes; ligamenta flava connect adjacent laminae in the trunk; the anterior longitudinal ligament,

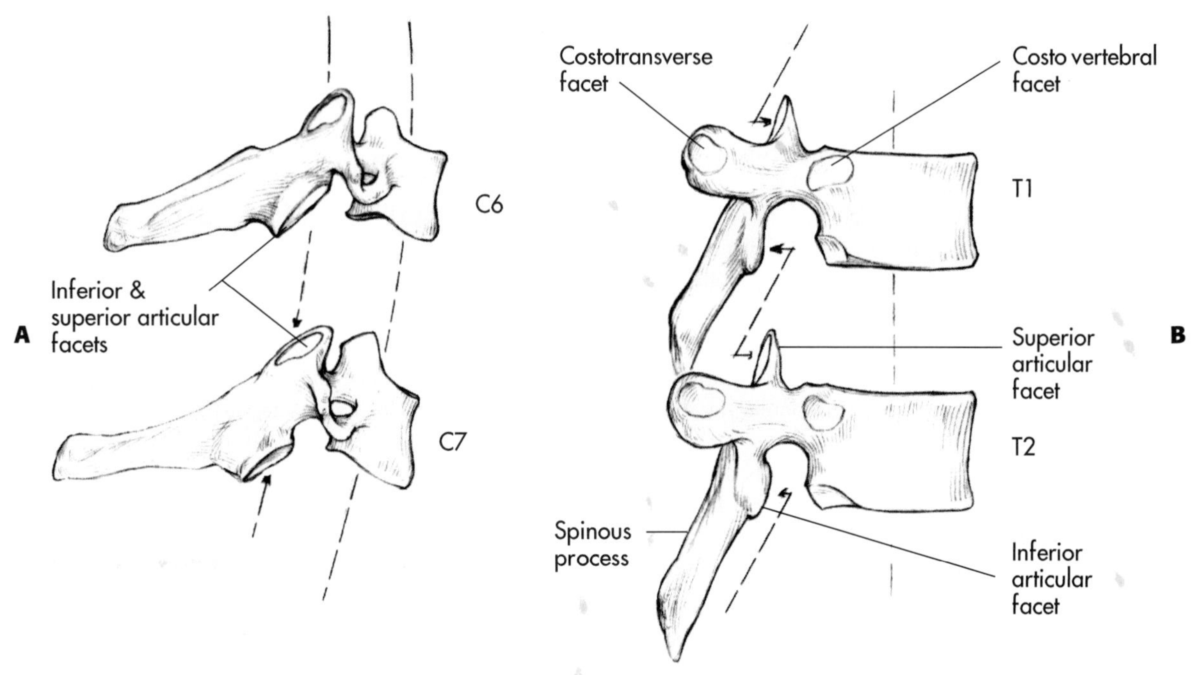

Figure 8-36
Vertebral articulations. In these two examples, pairs of articulated cervical and thoracic vertebrae are separated to show their points of attachment. In cervical vertebrae (**A**) the superior and inferior articular facets are nearly in the horizontal plane, whereas for thoracic vertebrae (**B**), they are in the frontal plane. (In lumbar vertebrae [not shown] the articular facets are in the sagittal plane.) In **A,** the dashed lines indicate the position of the anterior and posterior borders of the spinal cord. In **B,** the vertical dashed line indicates the articulation of adjacent vertebral bodies. The jagged dashed lines indicate the way articular facets align with one another. (From Mathers LH et al: *Clinical anatomy principles*, St Louis, 1996, Mosby.)

which connects the anterior vertebral body and disk to the anterior vertebral body and disk located directly above, runs the entire length of the spine; and the posterior longitudinal ligament, which connects the posterior vertebral body and disk to the above posterior vertebral body and disk, runs the entire length of the spine.

The zygopophyseal joints allow the following movements: flexion, extension, lateral flexion, rotation, and gliding.

Movements of individual vertebrae are slight, but the cumulative effect of main movements occurs at C7 to T1, the cervical thoracic junction; T12 to L1, the thoracolumbar junction; and L5 to S1, the sacral lumbar junction. These areas, where one curve ends and another begins, are more flexible and more prone to injury. In flexion the body of the vertebra moves forward, compressing the disk anteriorly and expanding it posteriorly. The fluid nucleus moves toward the back. The posterior ligaments stabilize. In extension the opposite occurs.

Lateral flexion creates a similar pattern. Compression on the side of the flexion increases pressure in the disk on the opposite side. The action of the disks and the ligaments is more involved in movement than the actual bony components of the spine (Figures 8-37 and 8-38).

Costovertebral Joints and Costotransverse Joints

The costovertebral joints consist of the following structures:

Articulating bones: Rib with facets on adjoining vertebrae

Joint type: Synovial plane joints

Ligaments: Intraarticular ligament from the disk to the head of the rib and radiate ligaments from the head of the rib to the vertebral body

The costovertebral joints allow gliding (Figure 8-39).

Costochondral and Chondrosternal Joints

The costochondral and chondrosternal joints consist of the following structures:

Articulating bones: Costochondral joints: The first through the seventh ribs articulate with the costal cartilage. Chondrosternal joints: The cartilage articulates with the sternum.

Ligaments: Costochondral joints are synchondroses and have no ligaments for support; chondrosternal joints are synovial and are supported by an intraarticular ligament and a thin capsule.

The costochondral and chondrosternal joints allow the following movement: similar to the movement of a handle on a bucket, movement of the thoracic cage occurs during respiration. Small movement of the ribs at the costovertebral joints produces large movements anteriorly of the sternum and laterally of the rib shafts. The result is a change in diameter of the thoracic cage that shifts intrathoracic pressure and enables inspiration to occur (Figure 8-40).

The student can palpate the spine and thorax joints as follows: Beginning just below the skull, palpate the spinous processes of the cervical vertebrae. The spinous processes of C7 and often T1 are larger and more prominent. Continue along the thoracic spine, noticing the bony prominences of each vertebra. A line drawn between the iliac crests runs between the spinous processes of L4 and L5. This point is used most often as a reference to locate the other vertebrae.

Viewed laterally, the spine has cervical and lumbar concavities and a thoracic convexity. The sacral curve forms a second convexity.

The most mobile portion of the spine is the neck. Flexion and extension occur chiefly between the head and the first cervical vertebrae, rotation occurs primarily between the first and second vertebrae, and lateral bending involves the cervical spine from the second to the seventh vertebra.

Movements of the rest of the spine (i.e., from the sacrum to the base of the neck) are more difficult to measure than those in the neck and are subject to considerable individual variation. The most mobile areas are at the thoracolumbar junction of T11 to T12, L1, L4 to L5, and the lumbosacral joint. The angle at the lumbosacral joint is tipped anteriorly so that when the lumbar vertebra wants to slide forward, contact between the articular facets of S1 and the inferior articular process of L5 prevent the movement.

In the thoracic region, follow each rib from its costovertebral joint to the costal cartilage. Feel for the bucket-handle motion of the ribs during breathing. Palpate each of the vertebrae, locating each spinous process. Then palpate again during rotation of the spine and identify the thoracolumbar junction of T11 to T12, L1, L4 to L5, and the lumbosacral joint.

What looks like spinal flexion takes place partly at the hips. For this reason, and because persons differ in the length of their limbs, flexion cannot be estimated accurately by noting the distance of our fingertips from the floor when we bend over. On forward flexion, watch the lumbar area; its normal concavity should flatten (Activity 8-12).

PATHOLOGY OF JOINTS

Generalized Joint Disorders

Any process or event that disturbs the normal function of a specific joint usually sets up a chain of events that eventually affects every part of a joint and its surrounding structures. Most pathologic joint conditions fall into the following categories: injury, immobilization, and repetitive overuse.

Injury

Joint injuries usually are classified as dislocations and sprains. A dislocation is a dislodging of the joint parts. A sprain is the wrenching of a joint with rupture or tearing of the ligaments.

ACTIVITY 8-12

Move your spine and thorax through each of the range of motion positions.

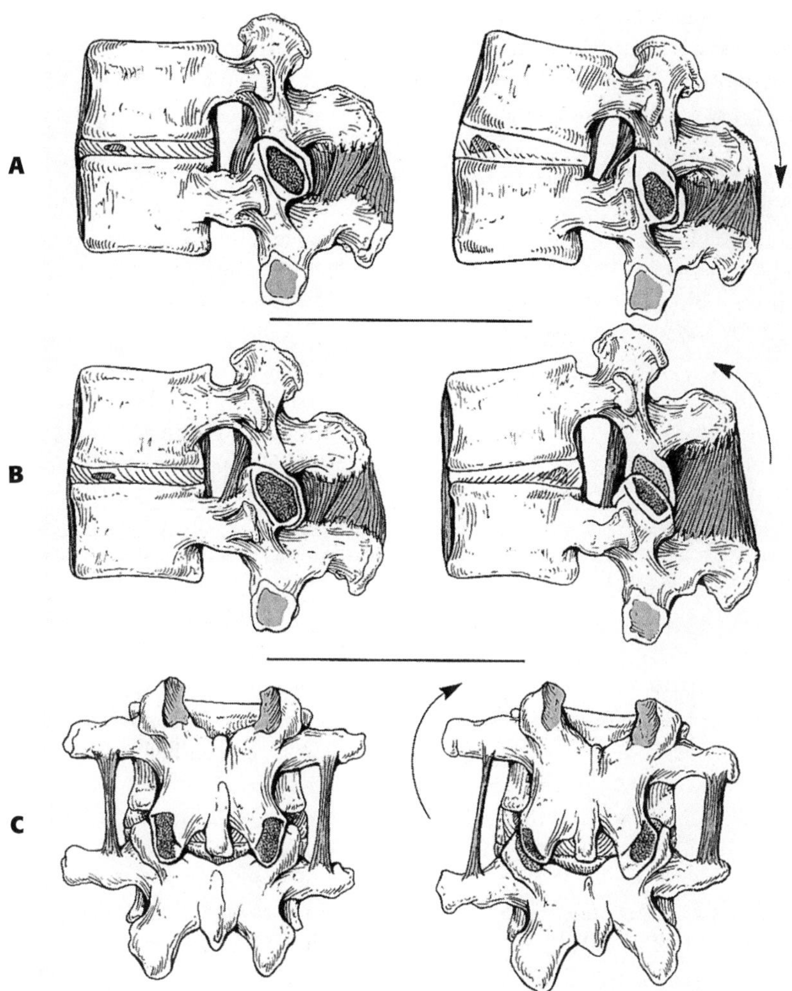

Figure 8-37
Motion between adjacent vertebrae. **A** through **C,** *Left,* Vertebrae in their neutral positions. **A,** *Right,* Vertebra in extension. The anterior longitudinal ligament is becoming taut. **B,** *Right,* Vertebra in flexion. Notice that the interspinous and supraspinous ligaments, as well as the ligamentum flavum, are being stretched. **C,** *Right,* Vertebra in lateral flexion. The left intertransverse ligament is becoming taut, and the right superior articular process is making contact with the right lamina. (From Cramer GD, Darby SA: *Basic and clinical anatomy of the spine, spinal cord and ANS,* St Louis, 1995, Mosby.)

Injury such as the tearing of a ligament results in a lack of support for the joint. Instability causes the separation of the articulating bones with wobbling or deviation from the normal alignment of the bones of the joint. These changes in alignment create an abnormal joint distraction on the side where a ligament is torn. As a result, the other ligaments, tendons, and the joint capsule may become excessively stretched in the area of the injury.

Injury on one side of the joint also can affect the other side by subjecting it to abnormal compression during weight bearing or movement. Compensation in movement patterns, from instability and pain, can result in uneven pressure on the joint. Protective muscle spasms develop called guarding, which limits movement. In the short-term acute phase of injury, this action provides effective splinting of the area, but if the restriction in ROM continues, immobilization can result. Joint injury usually is measured as follows:

First degree: a partial tear (5%) with pain and swelling but with the ability to bear weight and move through the normal range of motion

Second degree: larger tearing of structures with pain and swelling and inability to bear weight without pain and weakness that compromises range of motion

Third degree: extensive injury to joint structures including full ligament tears and the inability to bear weight and loss of normal range of motion.

Immobilization

Immobilization is detrimental to joint structure and function and can be caused by a cast or other form of external restraining mechanism such as a reaction to pain and inflammation or by paralysis. Immobilization affects the surrounding soft tissues, the articular surfaces of the joint, and the underlying bone. The detrimental effects of immo-

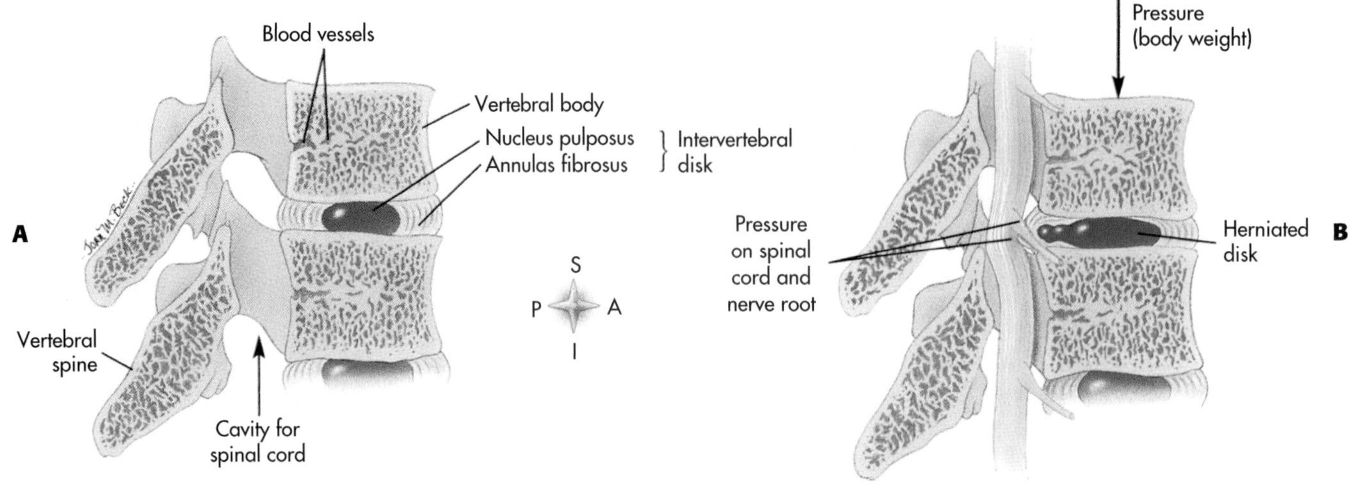

Figure 8-38
Vertebrae. Sagittal section of vertebrae showing (**A**) normal and (**B**) herniated disks. (From Thibodeau GA, Patton KT: *Anatomy and physiology*, ed 5, St Louis, 2003, Mosby.)

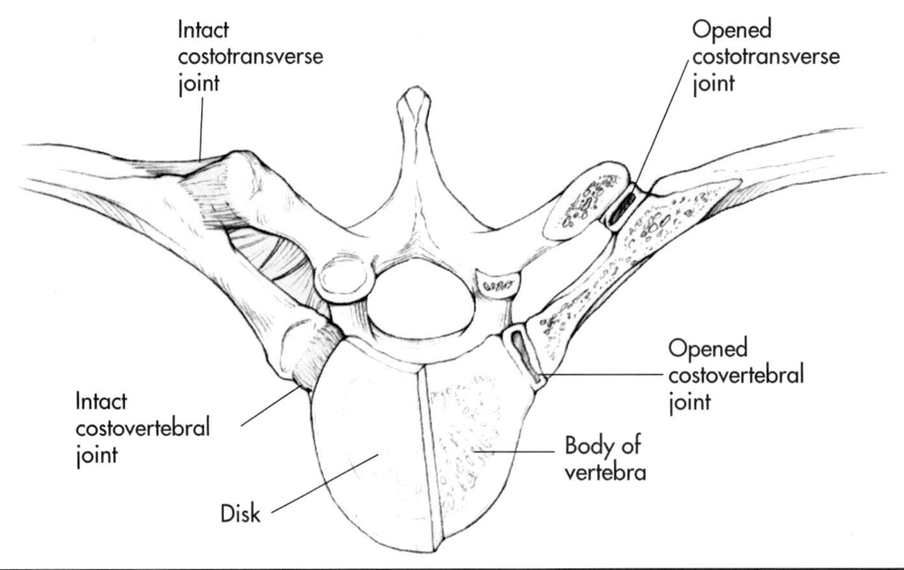

Figure 8-39
Joints between the ribs and vertebrae. On the left are shown the intact costovertebral and costotransverse joints, reinforced by ligaments. On the right the joints have been opened, revealing the synovial spaces within. (From Mathers LH et al: *Clinical anatomy principles*, St Louis, 1996, Mosby.)

bilization include development of fibrofatty connective tissue within the joint space, adhesions between the folds of the synovium, atrophy of cartilage, regional osteoporosis, weakening of ligaments at insertion sites, and a decrease in the water content of articular cartilage, tendons, ligaments, and the joint capsule. Swelling or immobilization of a joint also inhibits and weakens the muscles surrounding the joint; therefore the joint is unable to function normally and is at high risk for additional injury.

An injured joint subjected to inflammation and swelling assumes a least-packed position of comfort to minimize the pressure within the joint space. Pain decreases in this position. If the joint movement is restricted for a few weeks in the position of comfort, contractures can develop in the surrounding soft tissues and the joint capsule. As a result, normal range of joint motion is compromised.

INDICATIONS CONTRAINDICATIONS

For Therapeutic Massage

One can overcome pain and swelling of joint injury with the judicious and short-term use of pain medication, ice, and appropriate rehabilitative exercise. Soft tissue methods such as massage, myofascial release, and trigger point work are often effective after the acute phase (2 to 3 days). The application of ice along with rehabilitative exercise is beneficial. The practitioner

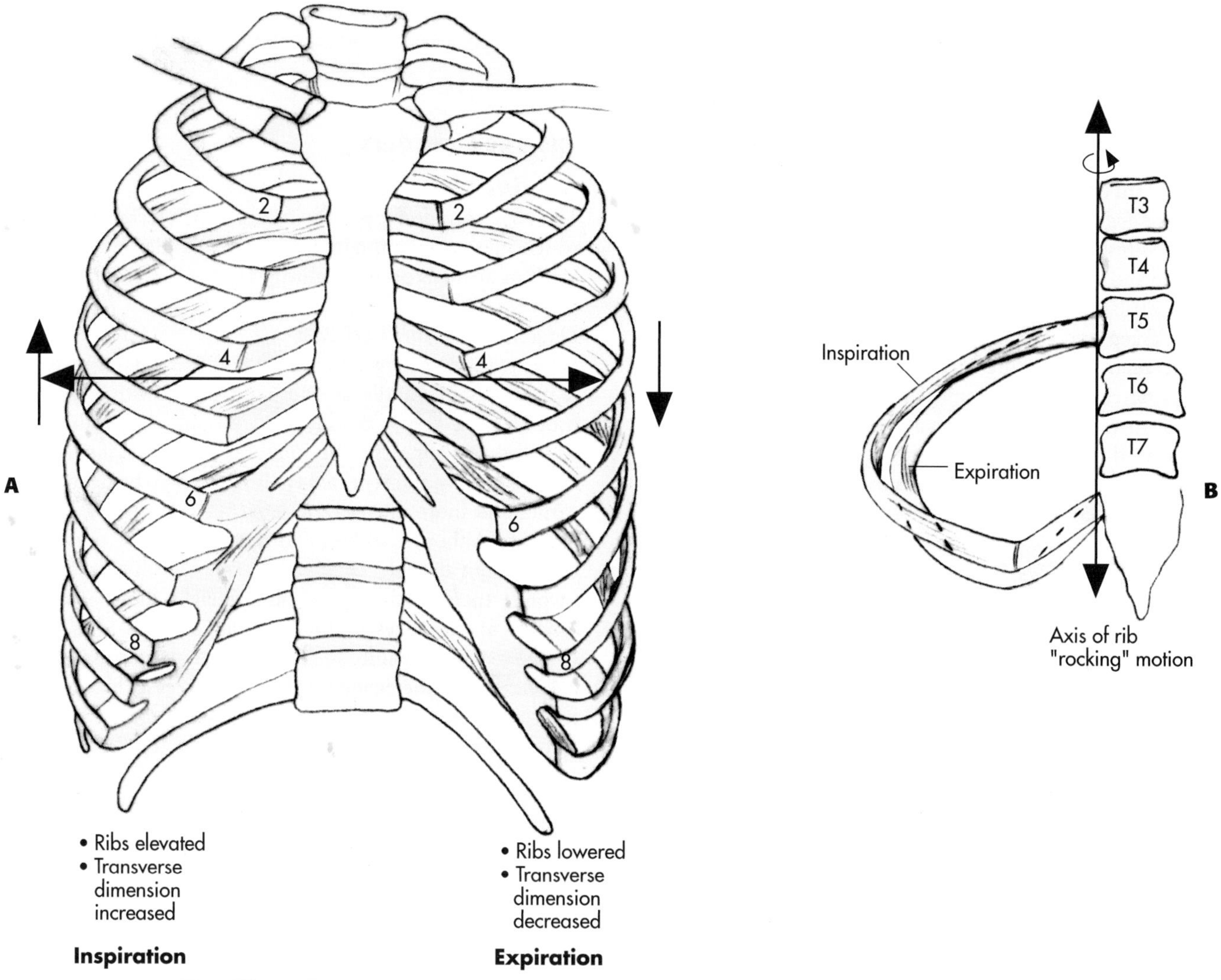

Figure 8-40
Rib cage and respirations. **A,** The rib cage in inspiration and expiration, illustrating the upward and lateral excursion that takes place at inspiration. This results in an increase in intrathoracic volume and the movement of air into the tracheobronchial tree. **B,** The "bucket handle" motion of a sample single rib during inspiration and expiration. (From Mathers LH et al: *Clinical anatomy principles*, St Louis, 1996, Mosby.)

needs to give attention to the scope of practice and appropriate training to deal with rehabilitation programs. Management and rehabilitation of joint problems is a long-term process often requiring a multidisciplinary approach. Ice, massage, and rehabilitative exercise are often methods of choice because they are drugless therapies. Ice is contraindicated in some conditions and thus should be used with caution. All three methods require active participation by the client, and the methods are not always pleasant. Compliance can be a problem, and the client needs to be motivated toward healing for the best results.

Immobilization from casts, splints, and so on is more difficult to handle. Physicians recognize that prolonged immobilization is undesirable and have developed forms of external stabilization that allow mobility. Dynamic movable splinting devices such as air casts and continuous passive motion devices that are capable of moving joints passively and repeatedly through a specified position of the physiologic ROM have been beneficial in reducing immobilization in joints. Therapeutic massage can be used to maintain pliability in accessible connective tissue structures. Therapeutic massage methods and movement approaches are beneficial in assisting a return to normal function after removal of the splinting.

Massage therapy also can aid management of compensatory patterns that develop because of casting and other forms of immobilization. Although direct work over an area that is actively healing is contraindicated unless supervised, massage and other forms of soft tissue work, coupled with movement therapies, can manage the tension and possible pain that the rest of the body may develop from the changes in movement, sleeping positions, and so forth caused from the casting, immobilization process, gait changes, and other compensation patterns.

In paralysis conditions, therapeutic massage helps to maintain and in some instances restore pliability of connective tissues. Joint movement applications can passively replace lost joint movement and mimic compressive forces on the bones and jointed areas, helping to prevent contracture and any other detrimental effects of immobilization. Massage intervention for those with paralysis must be supervised as part of a total treatment program. The practitioner must take care with pressure and intensity because normal feedback mechanisms are disrupted. ■

Repetitive Overuse

Constant static stress on the joints such as occurs in prolonged standing, sitting, or squatting can damage joint structures. Ligaments subjected to constant tensile loads creep and can undergo excessive lengthening.

Cartilage subjected to constant compressive loading also can creep and may undergo excessive deformation. Joints and their supporting structures subjected to repetitive loading can be injured and fail because they do not have time to recover their original dimensions before they are subjected to another loading cycle. These types of injuries are common in athletes, dancers, musicians, and factory and office workers.

INDICATIONS CONTRAINDICATIONS

For Therapeutic Massage

Rest, rehabilitative exercise, ergonomically correct equipment, education, and other similar methods often are used to treat and manage overuse syndromes. Massage can restore and manage some types of connective tissue dysfunctions. Movement modalities, such as active and passive joint movement, can be used to balance movement function and reduce tension patterns. ■

Specific Disorders

Arthritis

The most common type of joint disorder is termed *arthritis,* which means "inflammation of the joint." Several different kinds of arthritis occur (Figure 8-41).

Degenerative Joint Disease

Osteoarthritis, or degenerative joint disease (DJD), usually first occurs in middle age and progresses with the aging process as a result of normal wear and tear. Although osteoarthritis appears to be a natural result of aging, factors such as obesity and repeated trauma can help bring it about earlier and more intensely. Osteoarthritis may be a genetic disorder. Although some inflammation may be present, it results from the degenerative process. The disease process involves the growth of new bone (called spurs or osteophytes) at the edges of the articular surfaces, thickening of the synovial membrane, atrophy of the cartilage, and calcification of the ligaments. Friction increases between the joint surfaces, further increasing the degenerative process. Osteoarthritis occurs mostly in joints used in weight

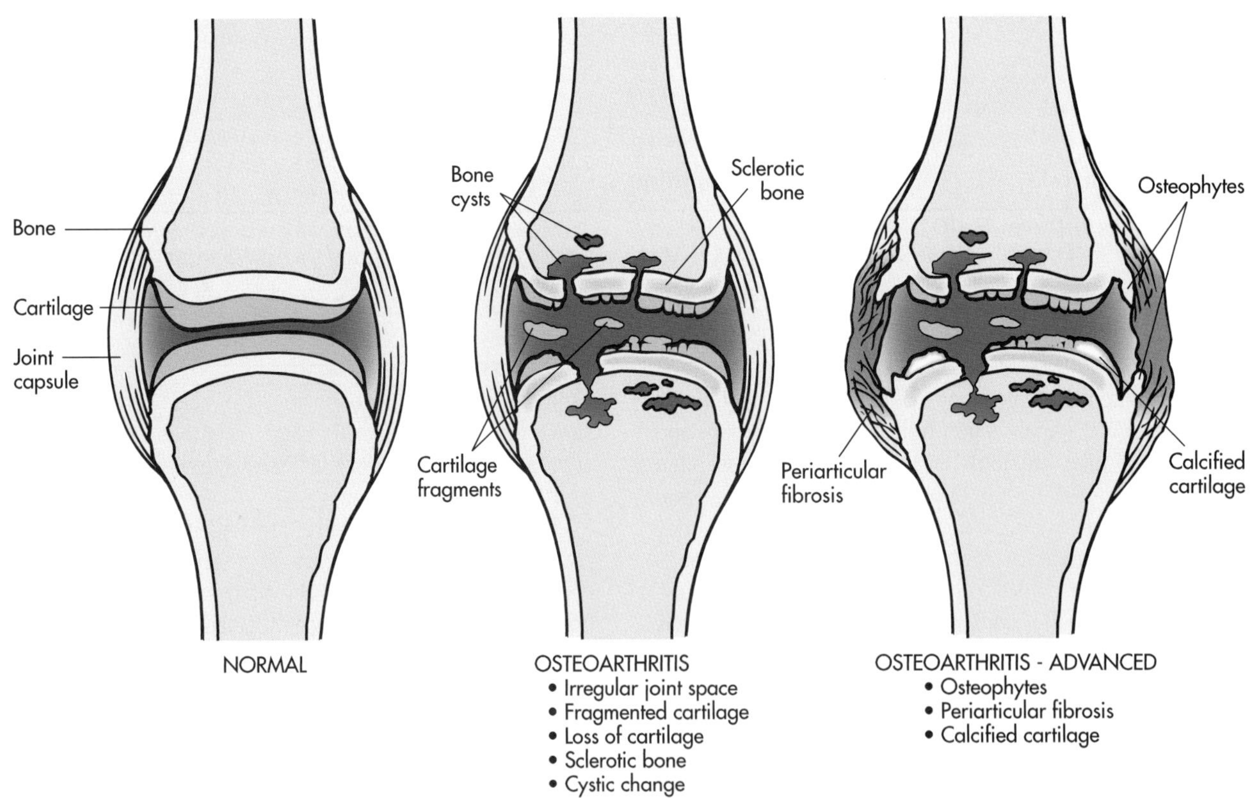

Figure 8-41
Schematic presentation of the pathologic changes in osteoarthritis. Fragmentation and loss of cartilage denude the subchondral bone, which undergoes sclerosis and cystic change. Osteophytes form on the lateral sides and protrude into the adjacent soft tissues, causing irritation, inflammation, and fibrosis. (From Damjanov I: *Pathology for the health-related professions*, ed 2, Philadelphia, 2000, Saunders.)

bearing, such as the hips, knees, and spinal column, but it can occur in most joints. For joints that have been previously injured to develop some arthritis later is not uncommon. Pain is usually less intense in the morning and steadily worsens throughout the day.

In the hands, nodules on the dorsal lateral aspects of the distal interphalangeal joints, called Heberden's nodes, result from the bony overgrowth of osteoarthritis. Flexion and deviation deformities may develop. Usually hard and painless, they affect the middle-aged or elderly and often are associated with arthritic changes in other joints.

Methods of treatment include the use of nonsteroidal antiinflammatory and pain medications. Nonpharmaceutical interventions include moderate exercise that does not cause pain, the use of ice, and topical counterirritant ointments such as capsicum-based preparations. Therapeutic massage can manage excessive protective muscle spasms that may develop. Gentle traction or distraction methods can provide temporary relief. General systemic changes in the neurotransmitters and hormones that accompany exercise and many forms of massage therapy can elevate mood and thus reduce pain perception.

Inflammatory Joint Disease

The three types of inflammatory joint disease are immune-related, crystal-induced, and infectious.

Immune-related disease. *Rheumatoid arthritis* is the most common immune-related form of inflammatory joint disease. Lupus erythematosus can cause immune-related arthritis. Rheumatoid arthritis has many characteristics similar to other autoimmune disorders in which antibodies attack normal body tissues. The disease is a crippling condition characterized by swelling of the joints in the hands, feet, and other parts of the body as a result of inflammation and overgrowth of the synovial membranes and other joint tissues. The disease process changes the composition and quantity of the synovial fluid, altering the lubrication of the joint. The articular cartilage gradually is destroyed, the joint cavity develops adhesions, and the surfaces become stuck together. The joints stiffen and may eventually become useless. The cause of rheumatoid arthritis is uncertain, and the interaction of multiple agents is probable. Genetic factors may influence susceptibility.

Treatment includes the use of various nonsteroidal antiinflammatory drugs. The administration of steroids and gold salts may provide some relief in severe conditions. Localized injection of steroids can reduce severe acute localized symptoms. The use of steroids is controversial, and benefits do not always outweigh the risks of long-term use.

INDICATIONS CONTRAINDICATIONS

For Therapeutic Massage

Because the progression and flare-ups of the disease are often stress related, the generalized gentle stress reduction methods provided by massage therapy may be beneficial in long-term management of the condition, if supervised as part of a total care program. The practitioner should avoid frictioning techniques or any other forms of massage therapy that cause inflammation. General systemic changes in the neurotransmitters and hormones that accompany exercise and many forms of massage therapy can elevate mood and thus reduce pain perception.

Crystal-induced disease. *Gout* is a form of arthritis caused by a disturbance of metabolism. One of the by-products of metabolism is uric acid, which normally is excreted in the urine. If an overproduction of uric acid occurs or for some reason not enough is excreted, the accumulated uric acid forms crystals, which are deposited as masses around the joints and other parts of the body. Gout is characterized by a painful and tender, hot, dusky red swelling that extends beyond the margin of the joint. Gout is easily mistaken for cellulitis. Any joint can be involved, but the one most commonly affected is the metatarsophalangeal joint of the great toe. Most victims of gout are men past middle age. Treatment includes dietary modifications.

Massage therapy is regionally contraindicated.

Infectious arthritis. Infectious arthritis can be brought on by infections such as rheumatic fever, gonorrhea, and tuberculosis. Gonorrheal arthritis is becoming widespread because of the tremendous increase in the number of cases of gonorrhea.

The joints and bones themselves are subject to attack by the tuberculosis organism, and the result may be gradual destruction of parts of the bone near the joint. The organism is carried by the bloodstream, usually from the lungs or lymph nodes, and may cause considerable damage before being discovered. Several vertebrae sometimes are affected, or one hip or other single joint may be diseased. The client may complain only of difficulty in walking, and diagnosis is difficult unless an accompanying lung tuberculosis has been found. This disorder is most common in children. Referral for proper diagnosis is important.

INDICATIONS CONTRAINDICATIONS

For Therapeutic Massage

Infectious disease is a contraindication for massage unless directly supervised by appropriate health care professionals.

Ganglion

Ganglia are cystic, round, usually nontender swellings located along tendon sheaths or joint capsules. The dorsum of the hand and wrist is a frequent site of involvement. Flexion of the wrist makes ganglia more prominent, whereas extension tends to obscure them. Ganglia also may develop elsewhere on the hands, wrists, ankles, and feet.

INDICATIONS CONTRAINDICATIONS

For Therapeutic Massage

Massage methods are regionally contraindicated.

Bursitis

Bursitis is one of the most common causes of joint pain. Inflammation of the bursae, especially those located between the bony prominences and a muscle or tendon such as in the shoulder, elbow, hip, or knee, usually results from trauma. Repetitive overuse, or rheumatoid or gouty arthritis, also may cause bursitis. A common treatment includes the use of rest during the acute phase but only for a short time to avoid pathologic immobilization. Analgesics and local injections of antiinflammatory medications also can be helpful. Ice can reduce inflammation and pain. Massage that reduces any muscle tension contributing to the development of inflammation and a readjustment of activities to reduce strain on the bursa are beneficial. Often a postural deviation changes the angle of function at a joint, resulting in irritation at an area of a bursa. Restoring normal postural alignment alleviates the irritation, and the bursitis may resolve itself.

Lateral Epicondylitis

Lateral epicondylitis (tennis elbow) follows repetitive extension of the wrist or pronation-supination of the forearm. Pain and tenderness develop at the lateral epicondyle and possibly in the proximal extensor muscles. When the wrist is extended against resistance, pain increases. Treatment is as for bursitis.

Medial Epicondylitis

Medial epicondylitis (golfer's or pitcher's elbow) follows repetitive wrist flexion, as in throwing. Tenderness is maximal at the medial epicondyle. Wrist flexion against resistance increases the pain. Again, treatment is as for bursitis.

Adhesive Capsulitis (Frozen Shoulder)

Adhesive capsulitis refers to a mysterious fibrosis of the glenohumeral joint capsule, manifested by diffuse, dull, aching pain in the shoulder and progressive restriction of motion but usually no localized tenderness. The condition is usually unilateral and most often occurs in persons 50 to 70 years of age. Onset often is preceded by some sort of pathologic condition, resulting in the joint being immobilized. Pathologic immobilization sets in. The course is chronic, lasting months to years, but the disorder often resolves itself spontaneously, at least partially. Treatment is with physical therapy, including ROM exercises.

INDICATIONS CONTRAINDICATIONS

For Therapeutic Massage

Therapeutic massage can be a beneficial adjunct treatment, especially with the symptomatic management of pain in supporting increase in range of motion. ■

Backache

Backache is a common complaint. Although persons most often complain of lower back pain, neck or cervical pain is also common. The usual cause is muscular and is discussed later. A list of some joint causes of backache follows.

In disorders of the intervertebral disks, pain may be severe, with muscle spasms and the resulting nerve impingement extending symptoms along the course of the nerve to the legs and groin. The condition can degenerate to a ruptured disk, which is most commonly a posterior or posterolateral protrusion of the nucleus pulposus through a tear in the annulus fibrosus, placing pressure on nerves.

Abnormalities of the vertebrae or ligaments and other supporting structures include the following:

- Strains on the lumbosacral joint (where the lumbar region joins the sacrum) or strains on the sacroiliac joint (where the sacrum joins the ilium)
- Spondylolisthesis, or the moving forward of part of one vertebra on another, which usually occurs at the L5/S1 junction
- Spondylitis, or inflammation of more than one vertebra
- Ankylosing spondylitis, or rheumatoid inflammatory disorder, in which the articular hyaline cartilage is destroyed, the bones fuse, and the spinal ligaments ossify. The disease tends to begin in the sacroiliac joints and progress up the spine.
- Spondylosis, or the formation of bony spurs at the disk margin of the vertebral bodies. The disease causes degenerative changes in the intervertebral disks.

Abnormal Spinal Curvatures

Abnormal spine curvatures result from postural deviation, especially the forward head position. Several types occur.

Flattening of the lumbar curve results in muscle spasm in the lumbar area and decreased spinal mobility. This combination of signs suggests the possibility of a herniated lumbar disk or, especially in men, ankylosing spondylitis.

Lordosis is an accentuation of the normal lumbar curve that develops to compensate for the protuberant abdomen of pregnancy or obesity. Lordosis also may compensate for kyphosis and flexion deformities of the hips.

Kyphosis—a rounded thoracic convexity—is common in aging and occurs especially in women.

Gibbus is an angular deformity of a collapsed vertebra. Causes include metastatic cancer and tuberculosis of the spine.

List is a lateral tilt of the spine. When a plumb line dropped from the spinous process of T1 falls to one side of the gluteal cleft, a list is present. Causes include a herniated disk and painful spasms of the paravertebral muscles.

Scoliosis is a lateral S curvature of the spine and may be structural or functional. Structural scoliosis typically is associated with rotation of the vertebrae on one another, and the rib cage is deformed accordingly. This deformity is seen best when the client bends forward. On the side of the thoracic convexity, the ribs bulge posteriorly and are separated widely. On the opposite side, they are displaced anteriorly and are close together.

Functional scoliosis compensates for other abnormalities such as unequal leg lengths and involves neither vertebral rotation nor thoracic deformity. The scoliosis disappears with forward flexion.

Indications/Contraindications

For Therapeutic Massage

Most backaches are preventable. One should not use the back muscles for lifting. One should bring weight close to the body, above the hips if possible, and allow the legs to do the actual lifting. An adequate exercise program is also important.

Massage therapy modalities are effective in managing backache. The benefits derived are from reduction in protective muscle spasm compensation (guarding) and generalized pain-modulating effects. The practitioner should be aware that protective spasm provides stabilization. The goal is not to eliminate protective spasm but to support the body in managing dysfunctional patterns. Complex backache involving the joint structures requires that therapeutic massage be incorporated into a total treatment program with supervision by the appropriate health care professional. ■

SUMMARY

A comprehensive understanding of joint structure and function is necessary for the effective practice of therapeutic massage for the joints. One can use massage methods to support joint health and provide benefits in managing joint dysfunction.

The health and strength of joint structures depend on a certain amount of stress and strain. Cartilage and bone nutrition and growth depend on joint movement and muscle contraction. Cartilage nutrition depends on joint movement through a full ROM to ensure that all of the articular cartilage receives the nutrients necessary for health. Ligaments and tendons depend on a normal amount of stress and strain to maintain and increase strength. Bone density and strength increase after the stress and strain created by muscle and joint activity. In contrast, bone density and strength decrease when stress and strain are absent.

Without stress and strain the joints do not function well, but with too much stress and strain a pathologic condition may develop. Persons are similar. We need to be exposed to challenges in life, but attempting to deal with too much can be overwhelming. The concept of balance is illustrated again—in joint health and personal well-being.

evolve

View the image bank on the EVOLVE site accompanying this book under Course Materials Chapter 8 for more explanation of range of motion.

Workbook Section

Workbook Section • Workbook Section • Workbook Section • Workbook Section • Workbo

Short Answer

1. Describe the elementary principles of joint design.

2. Define the two main types of joints.

3. Define arthrokinematics and osteokinematics and the three categories of range of motion.

4. Describe joint play.

5. List the structures that contribute to joint stability.

6. Identify the generalized joint disorders and describe a treatment protocol used for each.

WORKBOOK SECTION

FILL IN THE BLANK

(1) ________________ refers to the amount of motion available to a joint within the anatomic limits of the joint structure. An articulation, or (2) ________________, is where two or more bones meet to connect parts and allow for movement in the body.

(3) ________________ are flat sacs of synovial membrane in which the inner sides of the sacs are separated by a fluid film. Bursae are located where moving structures are apt to (4) ________________.

A (5) ________________ occurs when joints of the human body are linked together into a series in such a way that motion at one of the joints is accompanied by motion at an adjacent joint.

The (6) ________________ is the only position in a synovial joint in which the surfaces fit precisely together and maximal contact occurs between the opposing surfaces. Because the joint surfaces are (7) ________________, they permit no movement, and the joint possesses its greatest stability.

Collagen is a fibrous tissue that provides stability to (8) ____________ tissue structures. (9) ____________ is a fibrous tissue that has elastic properties and allows flexibility of connective tissue structures.

A diarthrosis is a freely movable (10) ______________ joint.

(11) ________________ is a connective tissue that permits little motion in joints and structures. It is found in places such as the intervertebral disks and forms our ears.

Hyaline cartilage is the thin covering of (12) __________ connective tissue on the ends of the bones in freely movable joints in the adult skeleton.

Hypermobility occurs when the range of motion of a joint is (13) ________________ than normally would be permitted by the structure. It results in (14) __________.

(15) ________________ occurs when the ROM of a joint is less than what normally would be permitted by the structure. It results in (16) ________________ ROM.

The joint (17) ________________ is a connective tissue structure that indirectly connects the bony components of a joint.

Joint play is the (18) ________________ movement that occurs between articular surfaces, which has nothing to do with the ROM of a joint produced by (19) ________________. It is an essential component of joint motion and must occur for normal functioning of the joint.

The least-packed position is the position of a synovial joint where the joint capsule is at its most (20) ______________. Joints tend to assume this position when (21) __________ occurs to accommodate the increased volume of synovial fluid.

Open kinematic chain occurs when the ends of the limbs or parts of the body are free to move without causing (22) ________________ at another joint.

(23) ________________ ROM is the amount of motion at a joint that fails to reach the normal physiologic range or exceeds normal anatomic limits of motion of that joint.

Physiologic ROM is the amount of motion available to a joint determined by the nervous system from information provided by joint (24) ________________ receptors. This information usually prevents a joint from being positioned where (25) ________________ could occur.

(26) A ________________ is a limited movement, nonsynovial joint.

A suture is a (27) ________________ joint in which two bony components are united by a thin layer of dense fibrous tissue.

A symphysis is a (28) ________________ joint in which the two bony components are joined directly by fibrocartilage in the form of a disk or plate.

WORKBOOK SECTION

A synchondrosis is a joint in which the material used for connecting the two components is (29) ______________ growth cartilage.

A syndesmosis is a (30) ______________ joint in which two bony components are joined directly by a ligament, cord, or aponeurotic membrane.

(31) ______________ fluid is a thick, colorless, lubricating fluid secreted by the membrane of the joint cavity.

Types of (32) ______________ joints include the following:

Hinge joints allow flexion and extension movements in (33) ______________ direction, changing the angle of the bones at the joint, similar to a door hinge.

(34) ______________ joints allow rotation around the length of the bone.

Condyloid (condylar) joints allow movement in (35) ______________ directions, but one motion predominates.

A saddle joint is (36) ______________ in one plane and concave in the other, and these surfaces fit together like a rider on a saddle.

A (37) ______________ joint allows movement in many directions around a central point.

Gliding joints, also known as synovial (38) __________ joints, allow only a gliding motion in various planes.

(39) ______________ is the combination of resistance offered by a fluid to a change of form and the ability of material to return to its original state after deformation. This term is used to describe (40) ______________ tissue.

PROBLEM SOLVING

Read the problem presented. There is no correct answer; rather the exercise is intended to assist the student in developing the analytic and decision-making skills necessary in a professional practice. After reading the problem, follow the next six steps.

1. Identify the facts presented in the information.
2. Identify the possibilities ("what if" statements) presented or develop your own possibilities that relate to the facts.
3. Evaluate each possibility in terms of the logical cause and effect and pros and cons.
4. Consider the effect on the persons involved.
5. Write each answer in the space provided.
6. Develop your solution by answering the question posed.

Problem

All movement involves joints. Individuals who move for a living such as professional athletes or dancers are particularly susceptible to joint dysfunction. Injury is more than an inconvenience; it can put an end to a career. Many of these persons continue to work in pain. They do not allow proper healing time, and additional damage may result.

Young children who begin to train for competition before puberty develop a more pliable joint structure. Hypermobility may result. As these persons age, joint structure is compromised by laxity in the joints, and pain and various degrees of disability can result.

Question

In what ways can a massage therapist use the information presented in this chapter to educate the vulnerable client about the need for support of the joints so that accumulating damage does not continue?

Facts

1. Persons who move professionally are susceptible to joint injury.
2. ____
3. ____

Possibilities

1. Persons may work with joint injury.
2. ____
3. ____

Logical Cause and Effect

1. Performance would not be as good.
2. ____
3. ____

Effect

1. The massage professional may feel frustrated working with someone who will not or cannot take time off for appropriate healing.
2. ______
3. ______

In what ways can a massage therapist use the information presented in this chapter to educate the vulnerable client about the need for support of the joints so that accumulating damage does not continue?

Professional Application

Connective tissue plays an important role in joint health. What are the specific massage applications to affect connective tissue function? What other knowledge would you require to work more effectively with connective tissues? What referral base would be necessary to support best a client with connective tissue dysfunction affecting the joints?

FURTHER STUDY

Using additional resource material (see the Works Consulted list at the back of this book), elaborate on the following topics:

Connective tissue

Cartilage

WORKBOOK SECTION

Kinematic chains

Immobilization pathology

Repetitive overuse syndrome

Ergonomics

Answer Key

SHORT ANSWER

1. Some joints provide stability. Some joints provide mobility. The structure of the joint determines the function of the joint. A breakdown or change of any joint structure affects the entire joint function. Joints connect two or more bones. The design of a joint depends on its function. Each part of the joint has a specific function that is essential to the whole function of the joint. Complex joints are more likely to malfunction than simple joints. Effective functioning of the whole body depends on the integrated action of many joints. Generally, stability must be achieved before mobility. Most joints serve a dual function of mobility and stability. Simple joints provide more stability. Complex joints provide more mobility.
2. The two main types of joints are synarthroses, which are nonsynovial, limited-movement joints and consist of fibrous joints, and cartilaginous joints. Diarthroses, which are synovial, freely movable joints, consist of the following:

- A joint capsule formed of fibrous tissue
- Hyaline cartilage covering the joint surfaces
- A joint cavity enclosed by the joint capsule
- Synovial fluid forming a film over the joint surfaces
- A synovial membrane lining the inner surface of the capsule

3. *Arthrokinematics* refers to movements of joint surfaces. A *roll* refers to the rolling of one joint surface on another. *Sliding* refers to the gliding of one component over another. *Spin* refers to a rotation of the movable component. *Osteokinematics* refers to the movement of the bones rather than the movement of the articular surfaces. Three categories of range of motion exist: anatomic, physiologic, and pathologic. The *anatomic range of motion* refers to the amount of motion available to a joint within the anatomic limits of the joint structure. The anatomic range of motion may extend the limits of available range of motion to where joint injury can occur. Therefore many joints have established a physiologic range of motion set by the nervous system from information provided by joint sensory receptors. Usually this physiologic range of motion is somewhat less than the anatomic range of motion, preventing a joint from being positioned where injury could occur. Pathologic range of motion occurs when motion at a joint fails to reach the normal physiologic range or exceeds normal anatomic limits of motion. Two main pathologic conditions exist: hypomobility and hypermobility.
4. The involuntary movement that occurs between articular surfaces, which has nothing to do with the range of motion of a joint produced by muscles, is an essential component of joint motion and must occur for the joint to function normally. In an optimal situation a joint has a sufficient amount of play to allow normal motion of the joint. If the supporting joint structures are lax, the joint may have too much play and become unstable. If the joint structures are tight, the joint has too little movement between the articular surfaces, and the amount of motion is restricted.
5. Structures contributing to bone stability include bone shape, ligaments, joint capsule, fibrocartilaginous rings, tendons, fasciae, and muscles.
6. Most joint disorders fall into the following categories: injury, immobilization, and repetitive overuse. Joint injuries usually are classified as dislocations and sprains. A dislocation is a dislodging of the joint parts. A sprain is the wrenching of a joint with rupture or tearing of the ligaments.

   Immobilization can be caused by a cast or other form of external restraining mechanism, as a reaction to pain and inflammation, or from paralysis. The detrimental effects of immobilization include development of fibrofatty connective tissue within the joint space; adhesions between the folds of the synovium; atrophy of cartilage; regional osteoporosis; weakening of ligaments at insertion sites; and a decrease in the water content of articular cartilage, tendons, ligaments, and the joint capsule. Swelling or immobilization of a joint also inhibits and weakens the muscles surrounding the joint; therefore the joint is unable to function normally and is at high risk for additional injury.

   Repetitive overuse results from constant static stress on the joints such as occurs in prolonged standing, sitting, or squatting; it can damage joint structures. Ligaments subjected to constant tensile loads creep and can undergo excessive lengthening.

   Cartilage subjected to constant compressive loading also can creep and may undergo excessive deformation. Joints and their supporting structures subjected to repetitive loading can be injured and fail because they do not have time to recover their original dimensions before they are subjected to another loading cycle.

   Therapeutic massage also helps manage compensatory patterns that develop because of casting and other forms of immobilization. Although direct work over an area in an active healing process is contraindicated, massage and other forms of soft tissue work, coupled with movement therapies, can manage the tension and possible pain that the rest of the body may develop from the changes in movement, sleeping positions, and so on.

   Rest, rehabilitative exercise, ergonomically correct equipment, and education are used to treat and manage overuse syndromes. Therapeutic massage can both restore and manage some types of connective tissue dysfunctions. One can use movement modalities to balance movement function and reduce tension patterns.

Fill in the Blank

1. Anatomic range of motion
2. joint
3. Bursae
4. rub
5. closed kinematic chain
6. close-packed position
7. compressed
8. connective
9. Elastin
10. synovial
11. Fibrocartilage
12. articular
13. more
14. instability
15. Hypomobility
16. restricted
17. capsule
18. involuntary
19. muscles
20. lax
21. inflammation
22. motion
23. Pathologic
24. sensory
25. injury
26. Synarthrosis
27. synarthrotic
28. cartilaginous
29. hyaline
30. fibrous
31. Synovial
32. synovial
33. one
34. Pivot
35. two
36. convex
37. ball-and-socket
38. plane
39. Viscoelasticity
40. connective

Muscles

▼ CHAPTER OBJECTIVES

After completing this chapter, the student will be able to perform the following:

- Describe the functions of muscles.
- List the three types of muscles.
- Describe the types of skeletal muscle fiber.
- List the components of myotatic units.
- Identify the attachments, function, synergist, antagonist, and common trigger points of individual muscles.
- Apply knowledge of the muscular system to therapeutic massage application.

▼ CHAPTER OUTLINE

MUSCLE STRUCTURE AND FUNCTION
- Muscle Tissue and the Whole Body
- Types of Muscle Contraction
- Anatomy and Physiology of Muscle Fibers
- Pathologic Connective Tissue Changes
- Myotatic Units (Functional Muscle Groups)
- Proprioceptors and Reflexes
- Muscle Firing Patterns
- Function of Cardiac and Smooth Muscle Tissue

INDIVIDUAL MUSCLES
- How Muscles Are Named
- How to Palpate Muscles
- Activity Explanation
- Muscles of the Face and Head
- Muscles of the Neck
- Deep Muscles of the Back and Posterior Neck
- Muscles of the Torso
- Muscles of the Gluteal Region
- Muscles of the Anterior and Lateral Leg
- Muscles of the Posterior Leg
- Intrinsic Muscles of the Foot
- Muscles of Scapular Stabilization
- Muscles of the Musculotendinous (Rotator) Cuff
- Muscles of the Shoulder Joint
- Muscles of the Elbow and Radioulnar Joints
- Muscles of the Wrist and Hand Joints
- Intrinsic Muscles of the Hand

PATHOLOGIC CONDITIONS
- Mechanisms of Disease
- Specific Disorders

SUMMARY

▼ KEY TERMS

Agonist (ag-on-ist) A muscle that causes or controls joint motion through a specified plane of motion; also known as a mover.

All-or-none response The property of a muscle fiber (cell) contraction by which, when contraction is initiated, the fiber contracts to its full ability or does not contract at all.

Antagonist (an-TAG-a-nist) A muscle usually located on the opposite side of a joint from the mover (agonist) and having the opposite action. The antagonist must lengthen when the mover contracts and shortens.

Aponeurosis (ap-O-nu-RO-sis) A broad, flat sheet of fibrous connective tissue.

Concentric contraction (kon-sen-trik) A contraction in which the muscle shortens with tone because its contractile force is greater than the opposing force at the attachments of the muscle. Concentric contractions are contractions of a mover (i.e., an agonist) wherein it creates the movement of a body part.

Contractility (kon-trak-TIL-i-tee) The ability of a muscle to shorten forcibly with adequate stimulation. This property sets muscle apart from all other types of tissue.

Deep fascia A coarse sheet of fibrous connective tissue that binds muscles into functional groups and forms partitions, called intermuscular septa, between muscle groups.

Dynamic force Force applied to an object that produces movement in or of the object.

Eccentric contraction (EK-sen-trik) A contraction in which the muscle lengthens with tone because its contractile force is less

Continued

than the opposing force at the attachments of the muscle. Eccentric contractions are contractions of an antagonist that usually restrain or control the action of the prime mover. Eccentric contractions sometimes are described as negative contractions.

Elasticity The ability of a muscle to recoil and resume its original resting length after being stretched.

Excitability The ability of a muscle to receive and respond to a stimulus.

Extensibility (eks-tensi-BIL-i-tee) The ability of a muscle to be stretched or extended.

Fascia (fash-ea) A fibrous or loose type of connective tissue; a fibrous membrane covering, supporting, and separating muscles; the subcutaneous tissue that connects the skin to the muscles.

Fixator (fik-SAY-tor) A stabilizing muscle located at a joint or body part that contracts to fix, or stabilize, the area, enabling another limb or body segment to exert force and move. The fixator also may be described as a muscle (or other force) that stops one attachment of a muscle from moving so that the other attachment of the muscle must move.

Insertion The attachment of a muscle that moves (or usually moves) when the muscle contracts. The insertion of a muscle is usually the distal attachment of the muscle. For muscles located on the axial body, the insertion is usually the superior attachment of the muscle or the part of the muscle that attaches farthest from the midline, or center, of the body.

Isometric contraction (I-SO-me-trik) A contraction in which the muscle stays the same length with tone because its contractile force equals that of the opposing force at the attachments of the muscle. The muscle tenses but does not produce movement. Isometric contractions are usually contractions of a fixator/stabilizer muscle (or neutralizer muscle) that acts to hold (i.e., stabilize or fix) a body part in position while another joint action is occurring.

Isotonic contraction (I-SO-ton-ik) The action of the muscle that occurs when tension develops in the muscle while it shortens or lengthens.

Maximal stimulus The point at which all motor units of a muscle have been recruited and the muscle is unable to increase in strength.

Motor unit A motor neuron and all of the muscle fibers it controls.

Origin The attachment of a muscle that does not move (or usually does not move) when the muscle contracts. The origin of a muscle is usually the proximal attachment of the muscle. For muscles located on the axial body, the origin is usually the inferior attachment of the muscle or the part of the muscle that attaches closest to the midline, or center, of the body.

Oxygen debt The extra amount of oxygen that must be taken in to remove the buildup of lactic acid from anaerobic respiration of glucose (to convert lactic acid to glucose or glycogen).

Reverse action When a muscle contracts and the attachment that normally stays fixed (the origin) moves, and the attachment that usually moves (the insertion) stays fixed.

Static force Force applied to an object in such a way that it does not produce movement.

Synergist (SIN-er-jist) Synergists may be defined narrowly as movers of a joint other than the prime mover(s), that is, assistant, secondary, or emergency movers. Synergists may be more broadly defined as any muscle that helps the action occur (i.e., also may be fixator, neutralizer, or support muscles, as well as other movers).

Threshold stimulus The stimulus at which the first observable muscle contraction occurs.

Tone The state of tension in resting muscles.

Trigger points A hyperirritable locus within a taut band of skeletal muscle, located in the muscular tissue or its associated fascia. The spot is painful on compression and can evoke characteristic referred pain and autonomic phenomena.

MUSCLE STRUCTURE AND FUNCTION

Volumes have been written about the intricacies of soft tissue structure and function. This text, by necessity, limits itself to the most functionally practical information as it relates to the methods used by massage therapists. Also, because this chapter is by no means an exhaustive study, the student is encouraged to make use of the list of Works Consulted at the back of this text. The wise student also should commit to continual formal study and self-study of this material.

When studying anatomy and physiology, we must continue to see the body as a whole, in structure and function, and this is especially true in the study of the muscles. Unfortunately, the nature of the study of muscles is to look at the isolating anatomy of an individual muscle instead of the magnificent, interrelated complex of the neurochemical myofascial unit. Physiologically, one muscle does not operate independently of others. Structural design knits together the muscles, bones, and connective tissue structures into intertwining spans that are necessary for stability and mobility. By necessity, this chapter breaks the anatomy into isolated segments. Fortunately, Chapter 10 puts all these pieces back together.

Muscles and their associated connective tissue make up the soft tissues of our bodies. In artistic terms, you could say that muscles and connective tissue are the medium of massage practitioners. Just as a sculptor needs to understand clay, the massage therapist needs to understand muscles. Because soft tissue accounts for about half the tissue mass of the body and most pain patterns find themselves connected to soft tissue dysfunctions of various types, the careful study of this area of anatomy and physiology is obviously important.

The body has three types of muscle tissue: skeletal muscle, cardiac muscle, and smooth muscle. This chapter focuses on skeletal muscle tissue and provides a brief overview of cardiac and smooth muscle.

A prominent functional characteristic of muscle is its ability to transform chemical energy from adenosine triphosphate (ATP) into mechanical energy. When this happens, muscle can exert force. Force is energy applied in such a way that it initiates motion, changes the speed or direction of a motion, or alters the size and shape of an object.

Energy is defined technically as the capacity to do work. Many cultures use the words *force* and *energy* in referring to esoteric concepts. We find it in Eastern philosophy as Qi or Prana and in the Star Wars movies as "The Force"—all these words translate to energy, vital force, life force. One does not have to stretch the imagination too far to see the metaphor of muscles in these more expansive concepts.

When a muscle contracts, muscle tissue transforms one form of energy into another and is able to produce force. ***Dynamic force*** creates movement and change; ***static force*** produces no movement or noticeable change, yet still expends energy. If therapeutic interaction can help transform static force into dynamic force, the energy to achieve therapeutic goals can be released; this often is the objective that massage professionals are seeking to achieve with their clients.

The author would like to thank Joseph E. Muscolino, DC, for his diligent review of this chapter. His expertise is much appreciated.

Muscle Tissue and the Whole Body

The functions of the three muscle types are integral to the maintenance of homeostasis of the whole body. The four major functions of muscle are these:

1. To produce movement
2. To stabilize joints
3. To maintain posture
4. To generate heat

All three types of muscle tissue produce the movement necessary for survival. Skeletal muscle moves the skeleton at the joints so that we can seek shelter, gather food, and protect ourselves. Skeletal, cardiac, and smooth muscles produce movement, such as that involved in breathing, the heartbeat, digestion, and elimination.

Stabilization of joint structures is an often overlooked function of muscle. Especially in the more mobile joints, which by nature have a loose structural design, the dynamic and static contraction of muscles surrounding the joint provides external stability, supporting the structures of the joint.

Maintenance of a stable body posture is primarily a function of the musculoskeletal system. The dynamic tension of muscle contraction opposes the force of gravity.

The relative constancy of the internal temperature of the body could not be maintained in a cool external environment if not for the "waste" heat generated by muscle tissue during contraction.

Muscles have the following four functional characteristics:

1. **Excitability:** Excitability is the ability to receive and respond to a stimulus. A stimulus is a change in the internal or external environment. One of the major reasons massage applications are beneficial is that they provide specific forms of stimulus to the muscles, which in turn stimulate maintenance of homeostasis.
2. **Contractility:** Contractility is the ability to shorten forcibly with adequate stimulation. This property sets muscle apart from all other types of tissue. As mentioned earlier, muscle tissue interacts with all body systems, but it makes a unique contribution: the ability to contract allows the entire organism to move.
3. **Extensibility:** Extensibility is the ability to be stretched or extended. In a typical movement pattern, one group of muscles contracts (concentrically shortens) while the other group on the other side allows this action to occur by lengthening. Together, these two groups achieve an integrated function of stability, balance, and the ability to return to the neutral position. This interaction is the

foundation of homeostasis, the ability to respond to demands and return to balance.

4. **Elasticity:** Elasticity is the ability to recoil and resume the original resting length after being stretched. Elasticity also includes the ability to remember where the process began and return to the previous position (Activity 9-1).

A number of systems support the function of muscle tissues. The nervous system directly controls the contraction of skeletal muscle and smooth muscle and also influences the rate of rhythmic contraction in cardiac muscle and visceral smooth muscle. The endocrine system produces hormones that promote repair of muscle tissue and assist the nervous system in regulating muscle contraction throughout the body. The blood delivers nutrients and carries away waste products. Nutrients for the muscles ultimately are procured by the digestive system. Work done by the body requires ATP, and glucose is the fuel for the manufacture of ATP. Potassium and insulin are required for glucose to enter the muscle cell. The digestive, respiratory, and urinary systems eliminate the waste products of muscle metabolism. Lactic acid can be an end product of muscle work and can be broken down within the muscle cell by the Krebs cycle or can be transported by the bloodstream to the liver to be converted back to glucose (these processes use oxygen). The immune system helps defend muscle tissue against infection and cancer, as it does for all body tissues. Because the systems of the body function interdependently, muscle tissue gives to and receives from the entire body.

ACTIVITY 9-1

Using the functional characteristics of muscle as a metaphor, provide examples of the ways in which your learning thus far has functioned like a muscle. Examples are provided to get you started.

Example

Excitability: The ability to receive and respond to a stimulus. Learning the names of the muscles is a new stimulus.

Contractility: The ability to shorten forcibly and produce movement when adequately stimulated. Using the information about the endocrine system has helped me better understand mood so that I can move more deliberately from one mood to another.

Extensibility: The ability to be stretched or extended. Seeking to understand the Eastern concepts in this text has stretched my belief system.

Elasticity: The ability to recoil and resume the original resting length after being stretched. My self-awareness has been reinforced by acquiring knowledge about my body.

Your Turn

Excitability: The ability to receive and respond to a stimulus.

Contractility: The ability to shorten forcibly and produce movement when adequately stimulated.

Extensibility: The ability to be stretched or extended.

Elasticity: The ability to recoil and resume the original resting length after being stretched.

Types of Muscle Contraction

Muscles can contract in different ways depending on the demand. Muscle contractions are classified as isometric or isotonic.

Isometric Contraction

An ***isometric contraction*** occurs when tension develops within a muscle but no appreciable change occurs in the joint angle or the length of the muscle. In other words, no movement occurs. Isometric contractions are static contractions because large amounts of tension develop in the muscle to maintain the joint angle in a static or stable position. Fixing or stabilizing a proximal joint so that a distal joint can move is an example of the way the body uses isometric contractions. Isometric contractions function to maintain joint stability and upright posture (Figure 9-1, *A*).

Isotonic Contraction

An ***isotonic contraction*** occurs when tension develops in the muscle while it shortens or lengthens. Isotonic contractions are dynamic contractions because the varying degrees of tension in the muscle cause the joint angles to change. Isotonic contractions produce movement. Isotonic muscle contractions can be classified as *concentric* or *eccentric* based on whether shortening or lengthening occurs.

In a ***concentric contraction*** the muscle develops tension as it shortens, and the contraction develops enough force to overcome any applied resistance. Concentric contractions cause movement against gravity or resistance and are described as being positive contractions. Concentric contractions occur as the angle of the joint decreases. An example is the biceps brachii curl, in which one lifts a weight toward the shoulder by moving the forearm toward the arm by bending the elbow (Figure 9-1, *C*).

Eccentric contractions take place when the muscle lengthens while under tension and changes in tension to control the descent of the resistance. Eccentric contractions control movement with gravity or resistance and are described as negative contractions. Typically, eccentric contractions happen as an antagonist pattern lengthens in a controlled fashion in response to a force (usually a force

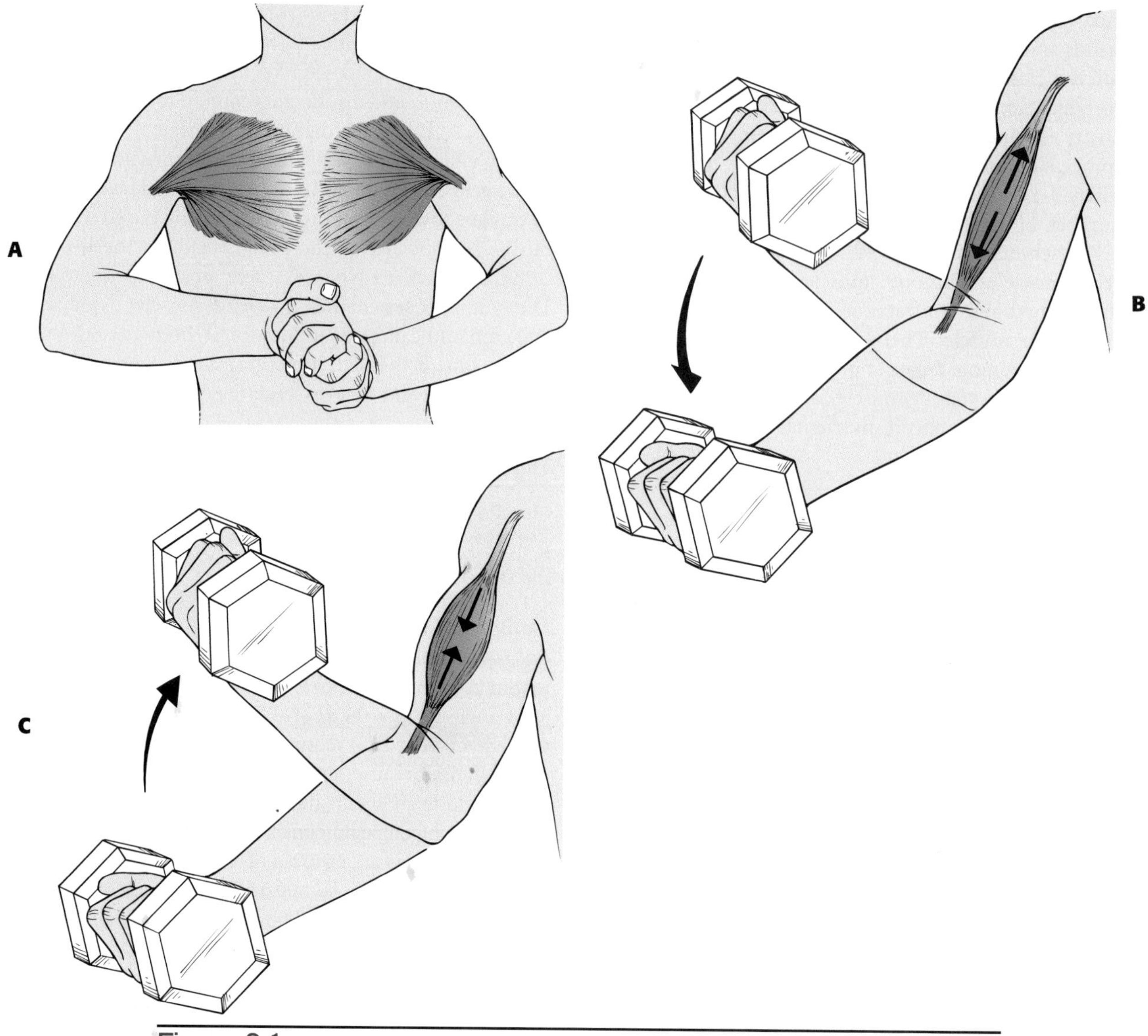

Figure 9-1
A, Isometric exercise is muscle activity with no change in length. No work is performed. **B,** Eccentric muscle activity. Muscle lengthens during tension production. **C,** Concentric muscle activity. Muscle shortens during tension production. (From Greenstein GM: *Clinical assessment of neuromusculoskeletal disorders,* St Louis, 1997, Mosby.)

external to the body) that is moving a body part at the joint in the opposite direction. The muscle slowly yields to resistance, allowing itself to be lengthened. Eccentric contractions occur as the angle of a joint increases. An example is the reverse of the biceps curl such as when one lowers a weight from the shoulder by extending the forearm at the elbow joint (Figure 9-1, *C*). Gravity, which is the prime mover, creates the action while the eccentric contraction of the biceps brachii keeps the movement under control. The amount of tension in the muscle may increase or decrease, depending on the weight of the object providing the resistance to gravity. Using the previous example, if the object is light, the biceps brachii decreases in tension as it lengthens. If the weight is substantial, the contraction of the biceps brachii increases in tension (Figure 9-1, *B*).

Anatomy and Physiology of Muscle Fibers

Each skeletal muscle is an individual organ made of hundreds or thousands of muscle fibers (or cells), large amounts of connective tissue and nerve fibers, and many blood vessels (Figure 9-2).

Skeletal muscle fibers are long, cylindric, tapered cells that have cross-striations created by the contractile structure inside. The *sarcolemma* is the plasma membrane that covers muscle cells. Numerous nuclei lie beneath the sarcolemma. The *sarcoplasm* of a muscle fiber is similar to the cytoplasm of other cells but contains large amounts of stored glycogen and a unique oxygen-binding protein called myoglobin. *Myoglobin* is a red pigment similar to hemoglobin that stores oxygen within the muscle cells.

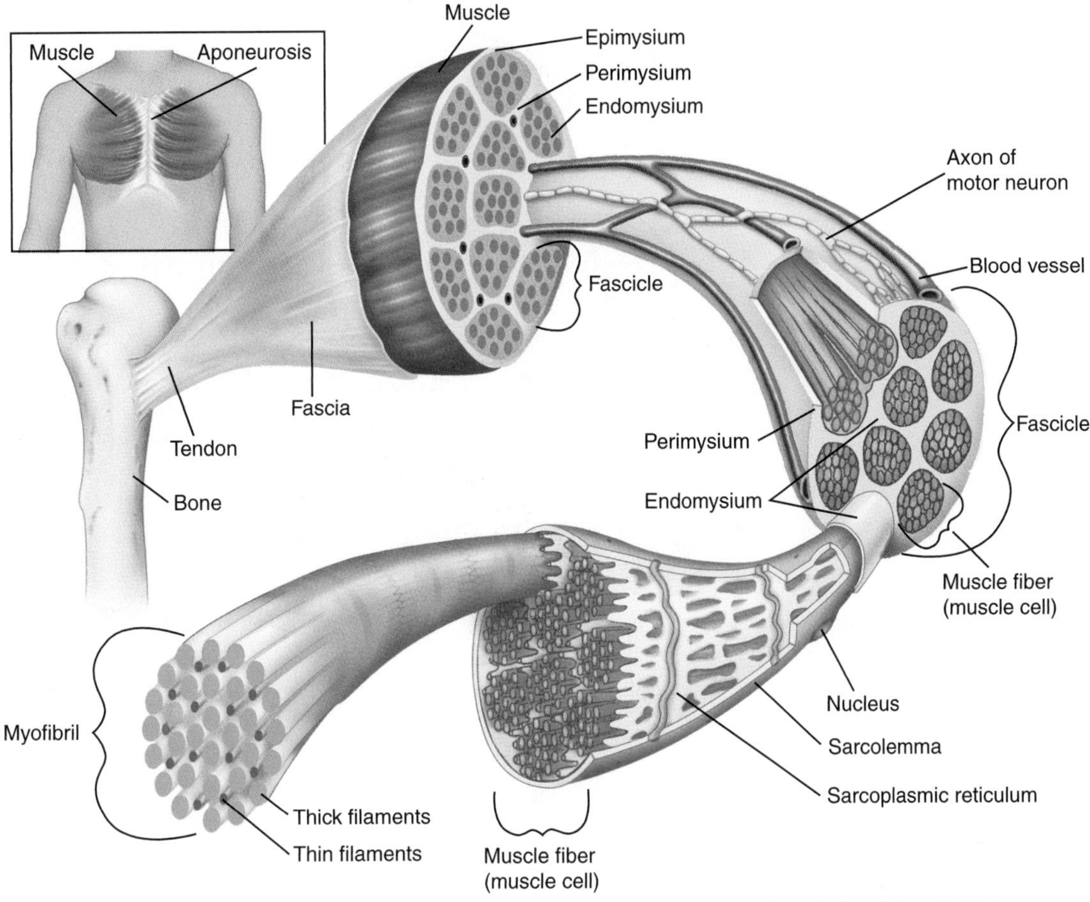

Figure 9-2
Structure of a muscle organ. The connective tissue coverings—the epimysium, perimysium, and endomysium—are continuous with each other and with the tendon. Muscle fibers are held together by the perimysium in groups called fascicles. (From Thibodeau GA, Patton KT: *Anatomy and physiology,* ed 5, St Louis, 2003, Mosby.)

Sarcomeres are the structural units of contraction in skeletal muscle fibers. *Myofibrils,* which are chains of sarcomeres, are packed side by side within the sarcoplasm. Thus the functional units of skeletal muscles are small portions of the myofibrils, and each myofibril is a chain of sarcomere units laid end to end. These structures are held together by various layers of connective tissue (Figure 9-3).

When a muscle cell contracts, its individual sarcomeres shorten. Within a neuromuscular unit, once a contraction has been initiated, it cannot be stopped, and the muscle fibers contract to their full ability or do not contract at all. This is called the ***all-or-none response.***

Shortening of a sarcomere (causing muscle contraction) occurs because of the two types of filaments found within the myofibril. The thick filaments are *myosin,* and the thin filaments are *actin.* The actin and myosin filaments slide over one another, shortening (contracting) the myofibrils.

When the nervous system activates muscle fibers by stimulating the motor neuron, the neurotransmitter acetylcholine crosses the synapses between the motor neuron and the muscle cell. Then cross-bridges from the myosin attach to active sites on the actin subunits of the filaments, and the sliding begins. Each cross-bridge attaches and detaches several times during a contraction, working like a tiny ratchet to generate tension and pull the thin actin filaments toward the center of the sarcomere. As this event occurs simultaneously in the sarcomeres throughout the cell, the muscle cell shortens. The attachment of myosin cross-bridges to actin requires *calcium,* and the nerve impulse leading to contraction causes an increase in calcium ions within the muscle cell (Figure 9-4). Sliding of these filaments continues as long as the calcium signal and ATP are present. Relaxation occurs when the nerve impulse no longer stimulates calcium release and the myosin can no longer grip the actin, and the sliding reverses.

Length-Tension Relationship

A direct relationship exists between tension development in a muscle and the length of the muscle. An optimum length exists at which the muscle is capable of developing maximal tension. Muscles can develop maximal tension because the actin and myosin filaments are positioned to form the maximum number of cross-bridges. If the muscles are shortened or lengthened beyond the optimum length, the amount of tension that the muscle is able to generate decreases.

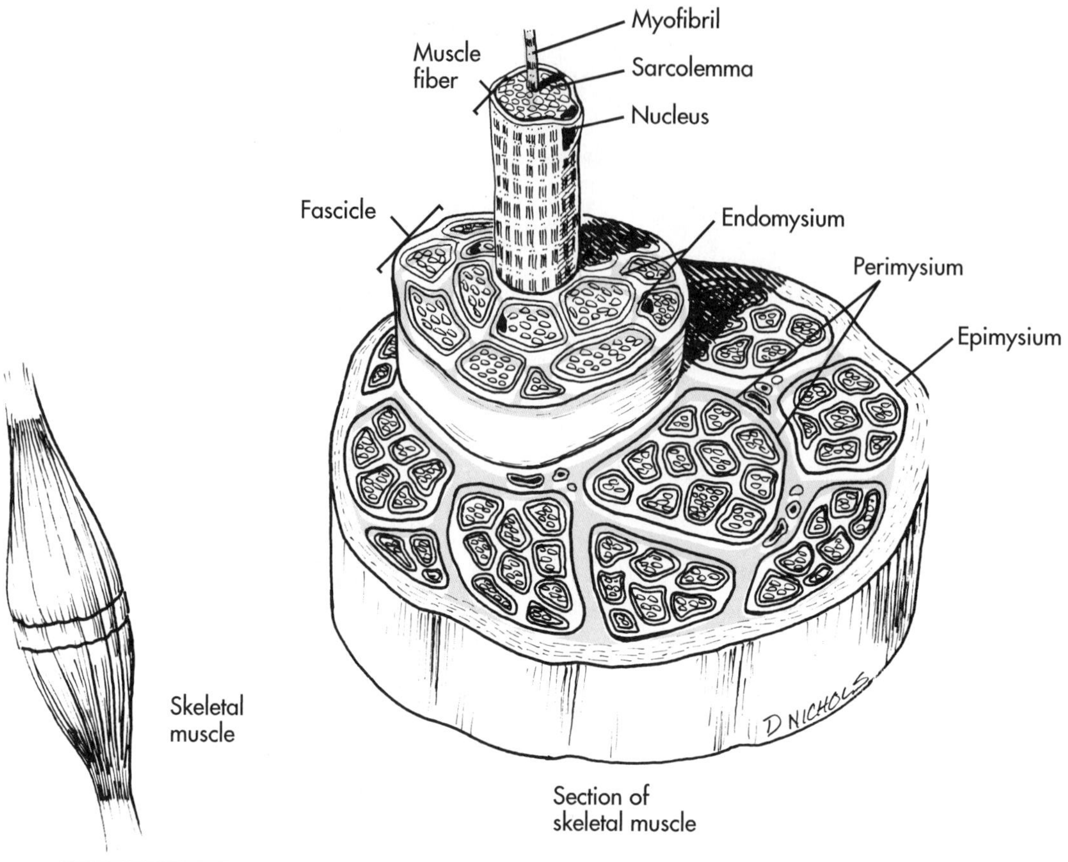

Figure 9-3

Section of skeletal muscle with contractile and noncontractile connective tissue. (From Shankman GA: *Fundamental orthopedic management for the physical therapist assistant,* St Louis, 1997, Mosby.)

Innervation

The autonomic division of the peripheral nervous system innervates the cardiac and smooth muscles. The somatic division of the peripheral nervous system innervates the skeletal muscles. Motor nerves stimulate the skeletal muscles to contract. The area of contact between the motor nerve and the muscle is the *motor end plate,* or myoneural (neuromuscular) junction. The motor end plate is a modified synapse consisting of a terminal bud of a nerve cell axon and a muscle fiber. When the nerve is stimulated, the terminal bud releases acetylcholine, and contraction follows (Figure 9-5).

A *motor point* is the location where the motor neuron enters the muscle and a visible contraction can be elicited with a minimal amount of stimulation. Motor points most often are located in the belly of the muscle. Muscles with a large belly may have more than one motor point. The motor point works in the same way a pilot light does in a gas furnace. Even though all the burners in the furnace are not on (much as with a muscle at rest), because of the pilot light, the furnace can respond quickly to the signal of the thermostat for more heat. The same holds true for the motor point area. Because the motor point is always "on the alert," it quickly can trigger the rest of the muscle to respond if needed. The increased activity in these areas logically could lead to localized hyperstates in the muscle called **trigger points.** The classic definition of a trigger point, from the master of trigger point knowledge, Janet Travell, is this: "A myofascial trigger point is a hyperirritable locus within a taut band of skeletal muscle, located in the muscular tissue and/or its associated fascia. The spot is painful on compression and can evoke characteristic referred pain and autonomic phenomena." Trigger points occur for many reasons including motor end plate dysfunction, ATP and calcium imbalance, and ischemia (lack of oxygen because of decreased blood flow).

A single motor neuron innervates many muscle fibers, delivering stimuli to each one and making them all contract as a group; such a group is called a **motor unit.** The muscle fibers in a single motor unit are not clustered together but are spread throughout the muscle; thus the stimulation of a single motor unit causes a weak contraction of the entire muscle. The more strength that is needed, the more motor units are recruited. The size of the motor units determines whether a muscle contracts forcefully or delicately. Large motor units with 700 fibers are found in the quadriceps femoris and other large, strong muscles that participate in running and walking. At the other extreme, 5 to 10 fibers per motor unit provide the extrinsic muscles of the eyeball with the ability to produce delicate eye motions.

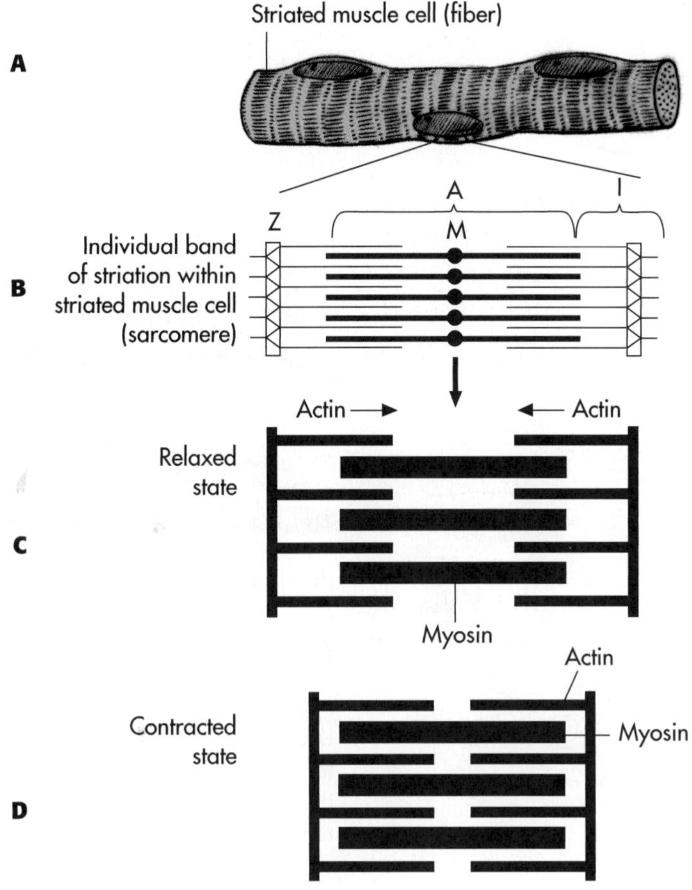

Figure 9-4
Striated muscle. Part of a single muscle cell, or fiber, with peripherally located nuclei. Vertical striations are evident within the cell. The repeating unit of this striation is the sarcomere (*B*); its major constituents are the proteins actin (*B*) and myosin (*M*), which slide in relation to each other to effect relaxation and elongation (*C*) or contraction (*D*). Neural signals stimulate the movement of calcium ions in the muscle fiber, and these ions stimulate the sliding movement of actin and myosin. (From Mathers LH et al: *Clinical anatomy principles,* St Louis, 1996, Mosby.)

PRACTICAL APPLICATION

Most massage applications manage trigger points effectively. First, the practitioner introduces some sort of sensory stimulation to the trigger point area that interrupts the existing neurologic signal and calcium flow so the myosin can release from the actin. Then the practitioner lengthens the muscle to restore the normal resting length. The traditional approach, called ischemic compression, involves compressing the trigger point with direct pressure or by pinching the point. One holds the pressure for up to 30 seconds. After the application of pressure, the practitioner lengthens the area of the trigger point in a muscle to reestablish an optimal tension length relationship. More recently, the recommended approach has been to use a series of deep strokes across the trigger point. Muscle energy methods that use various types of muscle contraction, directed to the muscle or its antagonist, assist in the lengthening process.

This theme has many variations; for example, applying ice over the trigger point instead of compression, followed by lengthening, is often successful. Methods that position the muscle fiber, holding the trigger point in an eased, nonpainful position and then gently lengthening it, are effective for tender trigger points. If fibrotic tissue changes have occurred around the trigger point, connective tissue stretching is necessary to elongate the connective tissue structures in the area. Realizing that lengthening is different than stretching is important. Lengthening involves neurochemical responses of the muscle fiber. Stretching is a mechanical force directed to altering connective tissue structure.

A strong correlation exists between the locations of motor points, acupuncture points, and trigger points. However, assuming that these are the same anatomic structure is simplistic. Researchers disagree about the differences and similarities of these areas. Acupuncture points correspond to motor point locations and the locations of the Golgi tendon organs; this explains why trigger and acupuncture points can be found in the belly and near the attachment ends of a muscle. Some agreement has been reached that these points correspond to

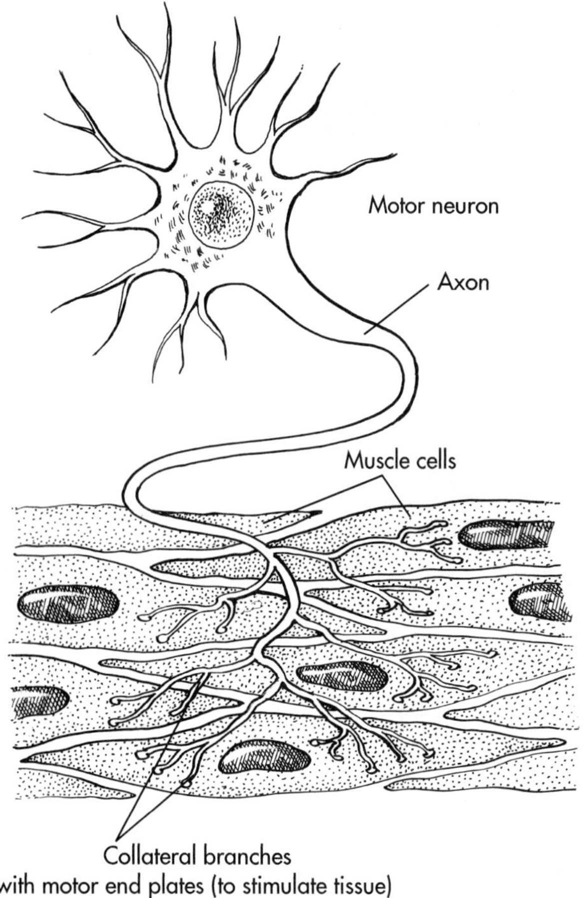

Figure 9-5
Motor unit. (From Scuderi GR, McCann PD, Bruno PJ: *Sports medicine: principles of primary care,* St Louis, 1997, Mosby.)

neurovascular bundles in the muscles; this supports the idea of a neurologic and a vascular component of pathologic conditions of these points and the benefits of acupuncture and trigger point methods. Acupuncture points may be the nervous system aspect of the point phenomenon, and the trigger point may be the myofascial aspect of the same phenomenon. In this chicken-and-egg situation, the logical step is to follow the teaching of an old, wise, and experienced Russian physician, who said, "Where is pain, I rub" (Activity 9-2). ■

Resting Muscle Tone

When the synapses in normal muscles stop firing, the muscles relax. Even so, they maintain a certain amount of contraction that keeps them ready to respond; this minimal amount of tautness is known as resting **tone.** Resting tone maintains the natural firmness of our muscles and their state of ready responsiveness. Appropriate amounts of resting tone help stabilize our joints and maintain our posture. Resting muscle tone is controlled by small signals from the spinal cord, brain, and spindles of the individual muscles. Because the stimulation occurs alternately to different sets of motor units within the muscle itself, some parts of the muscle contract while others relax. This keeps the muscle, especially postural muscle, from fatiguing.

This changeover in the signaling, which maintains resting muscle tone, can be demonstrated. Hold a heavy book in your hand as you slowly start to flex your forearm at the elbow joint. The small twitch in the muscle occurs with a changeover in motor units. Sometimes it feels like a small loss of strength that quickly returns.

Threshold Stimulus

The stimulus at which the first noticeable muscle contraction occurs is called the ***threshold stimulus.*** Beyond this point the muscle contracts more vigorously as the intensity of the stimulus increases. The stimulus intensity beyond which the muscle fails to increase in strength is called the ***maximal stimulus,*** or the point at which all the motor units of the muscle have been recruited. Thus the same muscle can apply a gentle stroke and a firm slap depending on the intensity of the stimulus.

Treppe

The first contraction of a muscle unit may be as little as one half the strength of those that occur in succession after it; this is called treppe. Many factors cause this stair step effect; for example, as the muscle begins work and produces heat, the muscle enzyme systems become more efficient, releasing more calcium ions, and this produces a stronger contraction with each successive twitch during the beginning phase of muscle activity. Treppe is one reason why warming up before exercise is important.

Energy Sources for Muscle Contraction

The energy required for muscular contraction comes from ATP.

Efficient contraction of muscle fibers requires glucose and oxygen. Glucose is a nutrient molecule that contains many chemical bonds. The potential energy stored in these chemical bonds is released during catabolic reactions (breaking apart) in the sarcoplasm and mitochondria. Some muscle fibers store glucose in the form of glycogen. Oxygen is needed for a catabolic process known as *aerobic respiration* and also is stored by muscle cells in myoglobin. *Myoglobin* contains iron groups that attract oxygen molecules and hold them temporarily. When the oxygen concentration inside a muscle fiber decreases rapidly, such as occurs during exercise, myoglobin can resupply it quickly. Muscle fibers that contain large amounts of myoglobin are deep red and are called red fibers (slow twitch). Muscle fibers with little myoglobin in them are light pink and are called white fibers (fast twitch). Most muscle tissues contain a mixture of red and white fibers.

When the oxygen concentration is low, muscle fibers can shift use to another catabolic process called *anaerobic respiration,* which does not require the immediate use of oxygen. Muscle fibers having difficulty getting oxygen or fibers that generate a great deal of force quickly may rely on anaerobic respiration.

ACTIVITY 9-2

Do you think the statement "Where is pain, I rub" is a valid therapeutic approach? Use the clinical reasoning model to formulate your position.

What are the facts?
What is considered normal or balanced function?
What has happened?
What caused the imbalance?
What was done or is being done?
What has worked or not worked?

What are the possibilities?
What does my intuition suggest?
What are the possible patterns of dysfunction?
What are the possible contributing factors?
What are possible interventions?
What might work?
What are other ways to look at the situation?
What do the data suggest?

What is the logical progression of the symptom pattern, contributing factors, and current behaviors?
What are the logical consequences of each intervention identified as a possibility?

What are the pros and cons of each intervention suggested?
What are the consequences of not acting?
What are the consequences of acting?

In terms of each intervention considered, what would be the impact on the persons involved: client, practitioner, and other professionals working with the client?
How does each person involved feel about the possible interventions?
Does the practitioner feel qualified to work with such situations?
Does a feeling of cooperation and agreement exist among all parties involved?

Summarize your reasons for determining the validity or invalidity of the statement "Where is pain, I rub."

Anaerobic respiration results in the formation of lactic acid, which may accumulate in muscle tissue during activity in which insufficient oxygen is available. The lactic acid then can be broken down via aerobic respiration if oxygen becomes present or can diffuse into the blood and be taken to the liver where it is converted to glucose. These processes require oxygen. After heavy exercise, the lack of oxygen in some tissues is called **oxygen debt.** *Oxygen debt* is defined as the extra amount of oxygen that must be taken in to break down or convert the lactic acid. A person may continue to breathe heavily to repay the oxygen debt. The extra oxygen gained by heavy breathing is used to process the lactic acid via aerobic respiration in the muscle cell or in the liver.

Types of Muscle Fiber

Muscles contain fast-, slow-, and intermediate-twitch fibers, which contract at different rates and with different characteristics, allowing muscles a wide range of action.

Fast-twitch (white) fibers contract more rapidly and forcefully, are larger than red fibers, and belong to larger motor units that activate when the nervous system demands rapid, powerful motion. They fatigue quickly and are considered *anaerobic* because they do not require much oxygen to contract. Muscles that need to respond quickly for short range-of-motion movements predominantly have fast twitch fibers.

Slow-twitch (red) fibers are smaller, contract more slowly and with less intensity, and belong to smaller motor units that respond during slower, more delicate movements. Red fibers do not fatigue quickly and can hold a contraction for a long period, making them highly efficient in muscles that maintain posture. They contain much larger quantities of myoglobin and are classified as aerobic because they require oxygen for contraction. Some texts divide red fibers into fast and slow types.

Intermediate fibers combine the qualities of red and white fibers to provide a rapid, moderately forceful contraction with moderate fatigue resistance. Muscles of the limbs are an example.

Although the fiber composition varies from muscle to muscle, on the average 50% of the fibers in a muscle are red, 35% are intermediate, and 15% are white. Up to 90% of the fibers in postural muscles are red, whereas leg muscles contain a higher proportion of white and intermediate fibers.

Genetics greatly determines the fiber configuration, but this can change as a result of demands made on the muscles. For example, the most successful sprinters are born with more white fibers in their leg muscles. To a certain extent, some others can be trained to be sprinters because the fiber configuration adjusts to demand.

White fibers, which are anaerobic, obtain ATP by converting glucose to lactic acid in the absence of oxygen. As a result, they fatigue more easily because the lactic acid accumulates and interferes with contractions. As previously mentioned, the liver needs oxygen to convert the lactic acid to glucose or glycogen. Heavy breathing is triggered primarily by a high level of lactic acid in the blood, which stimulates the respiratory center of the brain. When the oxygen debt has been paid and lactic acid has been converted, breathing returns to normal.

Because of their aerobic quality, red fibers do not produce lactic acid. For this reason, postural muscles, which are composed mainly of red fibers, can sustain a contraction longer without fatiguing.

Muscle Fatigue

Muscle fatigue is a state of exhaustion (a loss of strength or endurance) produced by strenuous muscular activity. Two types of muscle fatigue are *physiologic* and *psychologic.* Low levels of ATP cause *physiologic muscle fatigue,* and the myosin cross-bridges become incapable of producing the force required for further muscle contractions. The lack of ATP that produces fatigue may result from a depletion of oxygen or glucose in muscle fibers or from the inability to regenerate ATP quickly enough. High levels of lactic acid or other metabolic waste products also contribute to physiologic fatigue. Complete physiologic fatigue seldom occurs. Usually *psychologic fatigue* is what produces the exhausted feeling that stops us from continuing a muscular activity. We feel tired and do not want to continue an activity. The mechanism is protective and keeps the body from continually functioning at maximal levels and producing physiologic fatigue that is stressful and draining on the whole body.

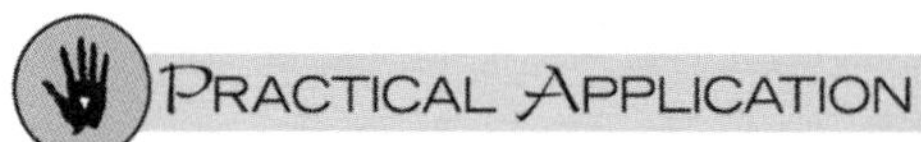

The primary type of fiber in a muscle can affect the length of application of pressure methods (e.g., compression, direct pressure, and acupressure) and tension methods (e.g., tensing and relaxing) that are used in progressive relaxation and muscle energy approaches. Red fibers often take longer to respond to these methods than white fibers. ■

Heat

Heat is a by-product of muscle activity. Several homeostatic mechanisms such as radiation of heat from the skin surface and sweating prevent heat buildup from reaching dangerous levels. Shivering causes muscle contraction, which produces more heat.

Blood Supply

Contracting muscle fibers use tremendous amounts of oxygen and nutrients while giving off large amounts of metabolic waste. The blood delivers oxygen and nutrients and takes away waste products. Muscle tissue is highly vascularized, and the structure of capillaries in muscle has been modified so that they are long and winding. Thus when a muscle stretches, the capillaries can easily accommodate the change in shape.

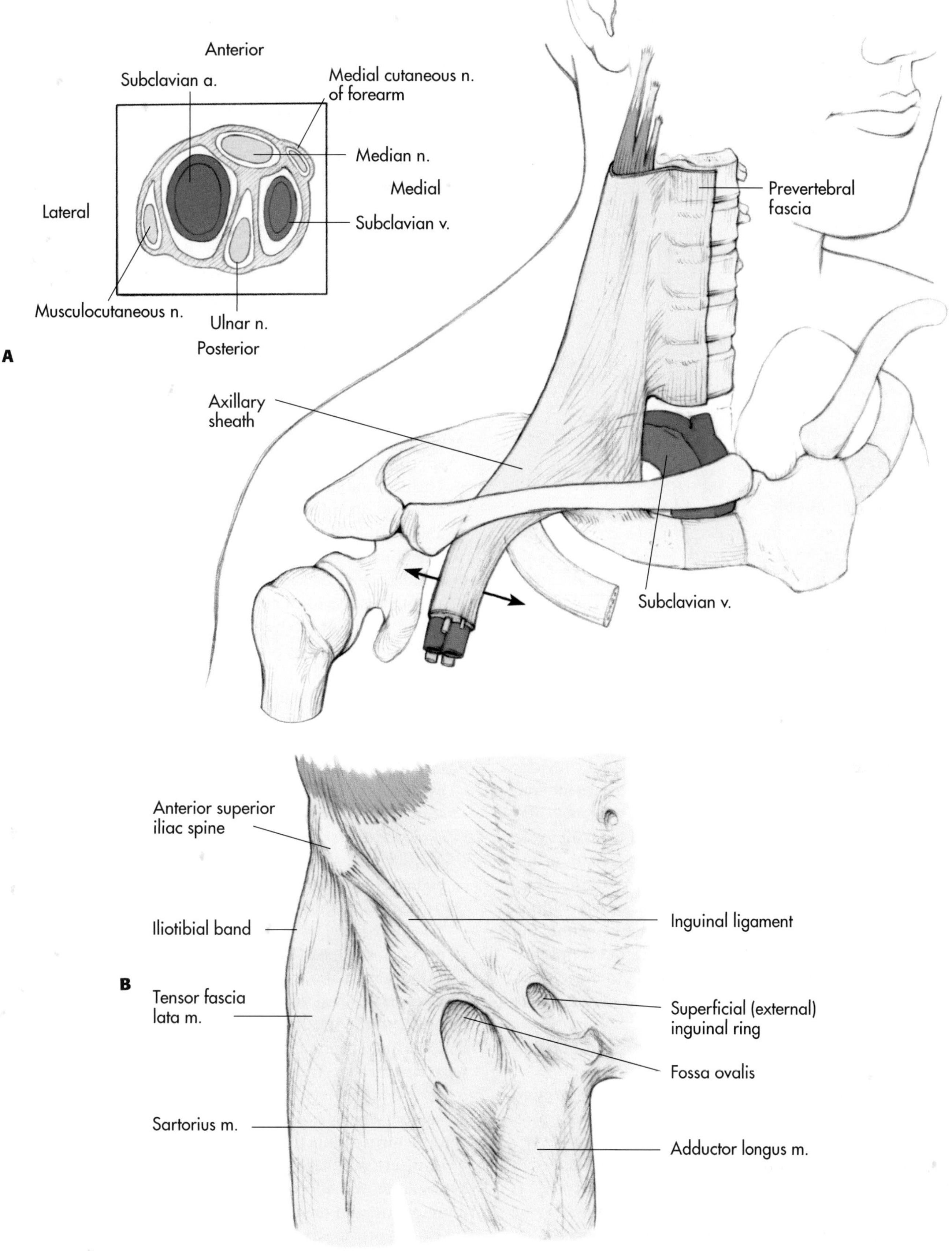

Figure 9-6

A, Cervical fascia and the axillary sheath. Inset in the upper left shows the relationships of structures within the axillary sheath, cut in cross-section where marked by the arrows. **B,** Fascia of the upper anterior thigh.

Continued

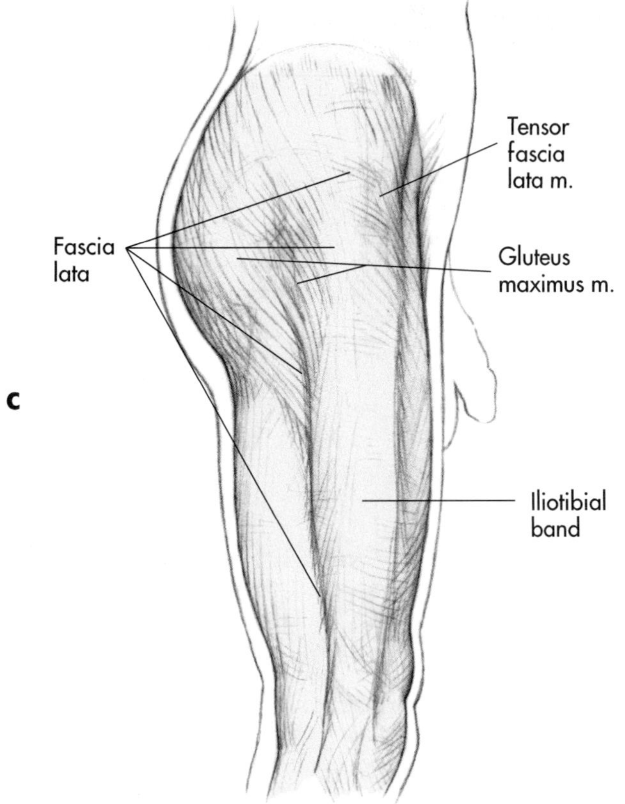

Figure 9-6, cont'd.
C, Deep fascia of the lateral thigh. On the lateral side of the thigh, the fascia lata thickens to form the elongated iliotibial band. (From Mathers LH et al: *Clinical anatomy principles,* St Louis, 1995, Mosby.)

Connective Tissue Component of Muscle

The fascial network surrounds and permeates muscles (Figure 9-6). **Fascia** is one form of connective tissue and comprises one integrated and totally connected network, from the attachments on the inner aspects of the skull to the fascia in the soles of the feet and from the skin to the innermost center of the body. If any part of a fascial structure becomes deformed or distorted, adverse affects can occur on any of the interconnected structures within the network. Chapters 1 and 8 previously discussed connective tissue structure and function in relationship to tissue types and joint structure and function. Now we discuss fascia again in relationship to muscles.

Fascia is involved in numerous complex biochemical activities:

- Connective tissue provides a supporting matrix for more highly organized structures and attaches extensively to and invests into muscles.
- Connective tissue sheaths cover muscle structures.
- Because connective tissue contains mesenchymal cells of an embryonic type, it provides a generalized tissue capable of developing into more specialized elements.
- Connective tissue provides (by its fascial planes) pathways for nerves and blood and lymphatic vessels and structures.
- Many of the neural structures in fascia are sensory.
- Fascia supplies restraining mechanisms in the form of retention bands and fibrous pulleys, therefore assisting in the coordination of movement.
- Where connective tissue has a loose texture, it allows movement between adjacent structures and by the formation of bursal sacs reduces the effects of pressure and friction.
- **Deep fascia** ensheaths and preserves the characteristic contour of the limbs and promotes circulation in the veins and lymphatic vessels.
- The superficial fascia, which forms the adipose tissue, allows for the storage of fat and also provides a surface covering that aids in the conservation of body heat.
- Because of its fibroblastic activity, connective tissue aids in the repair of injuries by generating collagenous fibers, creating scar tissue.
- The ensheathing layer of deep fascia, as well as intermuscular septa and interosseous membranes, provides vast surface areas used for muscular attachment.
- The mesh of loose connective tissue contains the tissue fluid and provides an essential medium through which to bring the cellular elements of other tissues into functional contact with blood and lymph.
- Connective tissue has a nutritive function and contains about a quarter of all body fluids.
- Fascia is a major location of inflammatory processes.
- Fluids and infectious processes often travel along fascial planes.
- Chemical (nutritional) factors influence the strength of connective tissue coverings of muscles and bones.
- The histiocytes of connective tissue comprise part of an important defense mechanism against bacterial invasion by their phagocytic activity. They also play a part as scavengers in removing cell debris and foreign material.
- Connective tissue represents an important neutralizer or detoxifier to endogenous toxins (those produced in the body from physiologic processes) and exogenous toxins (from outside the body).
- The mechanical barrier presented by fascia has important defensive functions in cases of infectious pathogen invasion.

Fascia is involved deeply in almost all of the fundamental processes of the structure, function, and metabolism of the body. In therapeutic terms, trying to consider muscle as a separate structure from fascia is illogical because they are related so intimately. Remove connective tissue from the scene, and any muscle left would be a jellylike structure without form or functional ability (Boxes 9-1 and 9-2).

Muscle tissue has elasticity that allows it to withstand deformation when force or pressure is applied, but fascia is more plastic, and therefore these forces can be detrimental. When one uses massage to introduce various forces, one can reverse the detrimental changes. Applying force is called *loading,* and releasing force is called *unloading.* When one gradually applies either undesirable forces or desirable

BOX 9-1

Biomechanical Laws: The Influence on the Fascia and Muscle Unit

Basic laws govern the mechanical principles influencing the body neurologically and anatomically.

Wolff's law states that biologic systems (including soft and hard tissues) deform in relation to the lines of force imposed on them.

Hooke's law states that deformation (resulting from strain) imposed on an elastic body is in proportion to the stress (force load) placed on it.

Newton's third law states that when two bodies interact, the force exerted by the first on the second is equal in magnitude and opposite in direction to the force exerted by the second on the first.

Ardnt-Schultz's law states that weak stimuli excite physiologic activity, moderately strong ones favor it, strong ones retard it, and very strong ones arrest it.

Hilton's law states that the nerve supplying a joint also supplies the muscles that move the joint and the skin covering the articular insertion of those muscles.

These biomechanical laws influence the behavior of the fascia/muscle fiber unit: the myofascial complex. Application of massage must respect these laws for massage to be effective. Appropriate application of force introduced into the tissue by massage is the key. Depth of pressure and direction coupled with drag and duration are qualities of massage application that determine the type of force introduced. Wolff's law, Hooke's law, and Newton's law in particular describe how forces interact. For example, if a client shows a connective tissue shortening in a diagonal pattern from the top of the shoulder at the acromioclavicular joint to the lumbar dorsal fascia, the forces imposed by the massage have to interact with that same directional line.

Muscle and fascia are anatomically inseparable. Therefore fascia moves during muscular activities acting on bone, joints, ligaments, and tendons. Sensory receptors of the nervous system exist in fascia and relate to proprioception and pain reception.

Fascia is colloidal, as is most of the soft tissue of the body. A colloid consists of particles of solid material suspended in fluid like wallpaper paste; the colloid conforms to the shape of the container it is in and responds to pressure in predictable ways. The amount of resistance colloids offer to pressure applied to the tissues increases proportionally to the velocity (how fast) of force applied to them. This response makes a slow touch a fundamental requirement of massage application; one is to avoid resistance when attempting to produce a change in, or release of, restricted fascial structures.

(Adapted from Chaitow L, DeLany J: *Clinical applications of neuromuscular technique*, vol 1, New York, 2002, Churchill Livingstone.)

BOX 9-2

Biomechanical Terms Relating to Fascia

Creep Continued deformation (increasing strain) of a viscoelastic material under constant load (traction, compression, twist)

Hysteresis Process of energy loss caused by friction when tissues are loaded and unloaded

Load The degree of force (stress) applied to an area

Strain Change in shape as a result of stress

Stress Force (load) normalized over the area on which it acts (all tissues exhibit stress-strain responses)

Thixotropy A quality of colloids in which the more rapidly force is applied (load), the more rigid the tissue response is

Viscoelastic The potential to deform elastically when load is applied and to return to the original nondeformed state when load is removed

Viscoplastic A permanent deformation resulting from the elastic potential having been exceeded or pressure forces sustained

(Adapted from Chaitow L, DeLany J: *Clinical applications of neuromuscular technique*, vol 1, New York, 2002, Churchill Livingstone.)

therapeutic forces to fascia, at first an elastic reaction occurs in which a degree of slack is allowed to be taken up, and then the tissue begins to creep because of the *viscoelastic nature. Creep* describes the slow, delayed, and continuous deformation that occurs in response to a sustained, slowly applied load. Creep can be caused from inappropriate forces imposed on the soft tissues. Therapeutically, the goal is to produce creep to elongate shortened and binding tissue to a more normal position. The forces created by massage application produce creep and must be applied with slow and appropriate pressure with a sustained drag quality without causing injury.

Thixotropy relates to the quality of colloids in which the more rapidly the force is applied (load), the more rigid and the less pliable the tissue response will be. Muscle tissue that is rigid or feels dense may have undergone thixotropic changes. If one gradually applies force, as described earlier, the tissues absorb and store energy. To increase connective tissue pliability, massage application must not be abrupt or the tissue will become more rigid. *Hysteresis* describes the process of energy loss because of friction and to minute structural damage that occurs when tissues are loaded and unloaded repetitively. The tissues produce heat as they are loaded and unloaded. During massage application, the loading and unloading occurs with on-and-off pressure application. Creating hysteresis reduces stiffness and improves the way the tissue responds to subsequent demands. The properties of hysteresis and creep provide much of the rationale for myofascial release techniques of therapeutic massage.

If the elastic potential of fascia has been exceeded or pressure forces are sustained for an extended period of time, a *viscoplastic* response develops and deformation can become permanent. This response results in either a dysfunctional change or a therapeutic change to reverse dysfunction. Elastic recoil occurs when the application of force ceases to prevent recoil, especially if released quickly. One should release force introduced during massage gradually. A viscoplastic permanent deformation change depends on the uptake of water by the tissues. Subclinical dehydration contributes to dysfunctional changes. Therefore drinking water for proper hydration is essential to support therapeutic change.

A muscle cannot be separated from its extensive connective tissue network. Each individual muscle fiber is wrapped by several different layers of connective tissue. Each muscle fiber is surrounded by a fine sheath of collagenic connective tissue called the *endomysium.* Several muscle fibers are wrapped together in side-by-side bundles, called *fascicles,* which in turn are wrapped in a collagenic sheath, the *perimysium.* The fascicles are bound together with more dense, fibrous connective tissue called the *epimysium,* which surrounds the entire muscle. External to the epimysium is the deep fascia, an even coarser sheet of fibrous connective tissue that binds muscles into functional groups. The deep fascia forms partitions between muscle groups called *intermuscular septa.* All these connective tissue sheaths are continuous with one another. Near the ends of muscles the actual muscle fiber ends, but the connective tissue continues and converges to become the tendons and aponeuroses that join muscles to bones or other connective tissue structures. Tendons and aponeuroses are the continuation of the endomysium, perimysium, and epimysium minus the muscle fibers. The connective tissue in tendons is arranged in a parallel fashion. Tendons and aponeuroses make the transition of the attachment from the muscle to bone. The difference between a tendon and an **aponeurosis** is one of shape. A tendon by definition is round and cordlike; an aponeurosis is a broad, flat sheet. The point where the muscle fiber ends and the tendon begins is called the *musculotendinous junction.* When muscle fibers contract, they pull on the connective tissue sheaths, which transmit the force to the bone to be moved. Because the individual skeletal muscle fibers are fragile, the connective tissue supports each cell, reinforces the muscle as a whole, and gives muscle tissue its natural elasticity. These sheaths also provide entry and exit routes for the blood vessels and nerve fibers that serve the muscles, as well as a vast surface area for muscular attachment (Figure 9-7).

The entire connective tissue network is one structure. Muscles do not just stick on bones; the connective tissue structure of the muscle and the bone blend into one tissue. Nerve and blood vessels do not just pass though holes in the connective tissue; rather they are contained and supported in wrappings of connective tissue that intertwine into the entire fascial network. Movement of any one body part creates a force that can be transmitted along fascial planes far and away in your body. Pulling on your big toe could transmit a force all the way to your head and every other structure in your body. No dysfunction is isolated; everything is connected (Figure 9-8).

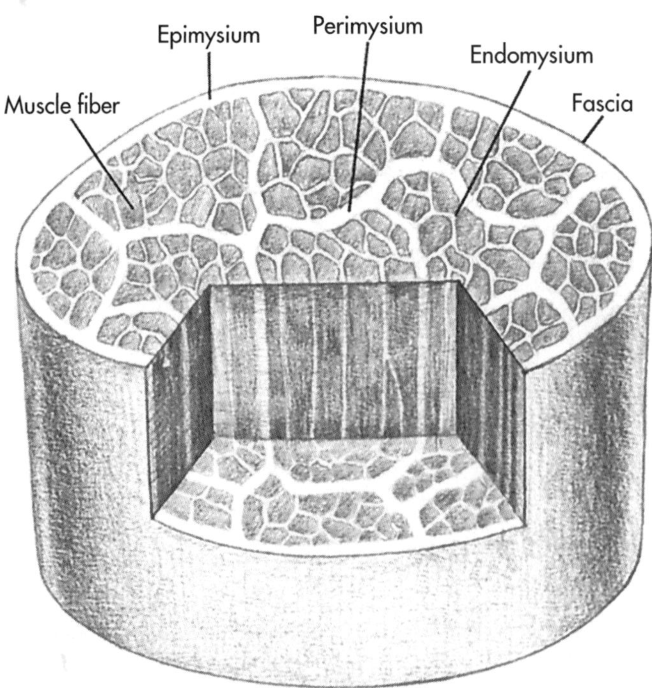

Figure 9-7
Structure of muscle fibers and their coverings. (From Thompson JM et al: *Mosby's clinical nursing,* ed 4, St Louis, 1997, Mosby.)

A

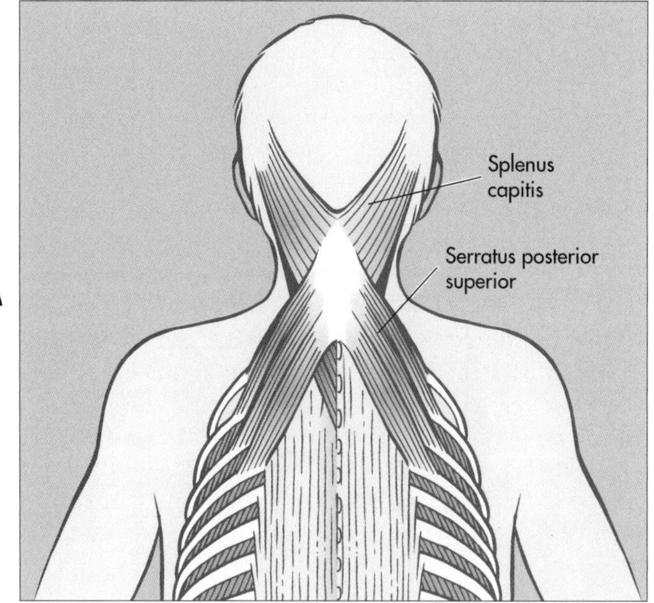

B

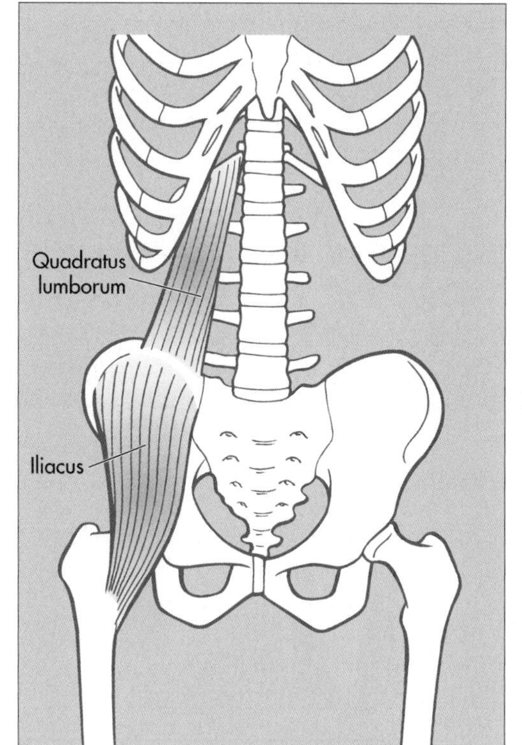

C

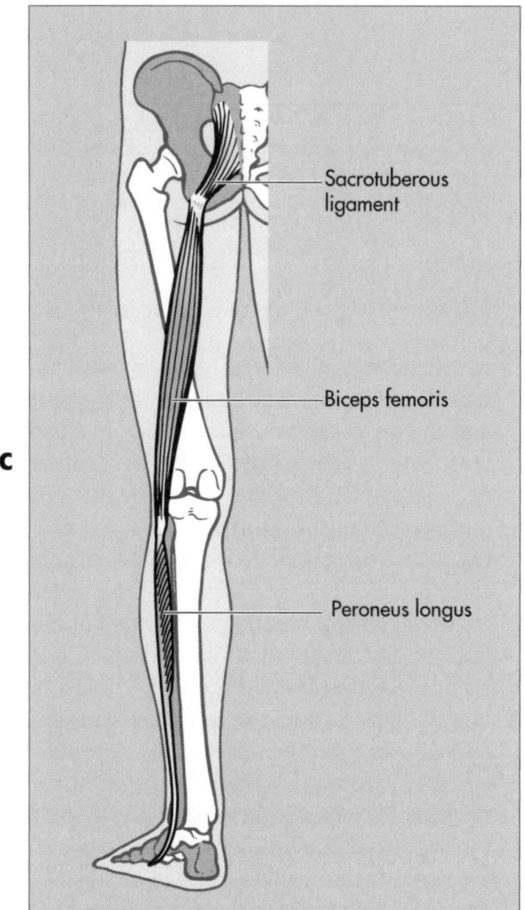

Figure 9-8

A, The opening myofascial continuity of the Spiral Line is a mechanical connection through the spinous processes. A branch line connection could also be made to the serratus posterior superior muscle, which goes underneath the rhomboids but over the erector fascia to attach to the ribs.. **B,** The outer line of the hip-spine locals comprises the iliacus, linking into the quadratus lumborum. **C,** The lower back part of the Spiral Line connects the lateral arch to the sacrum and the sacroiliac joint. One should consider the lateral arch and fibular placement when dealing with chronic sacroiliac dysfunction.

Continued

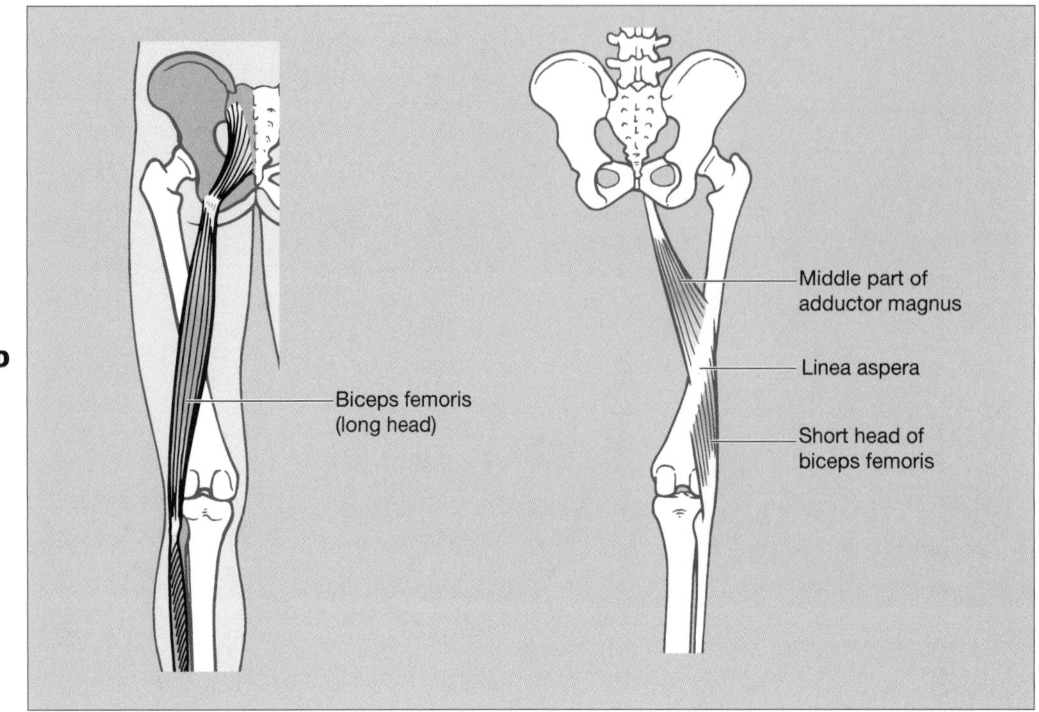

Figure 9-8, cont'd.
D, The long head of the biceps femoris is a two-joint 'express.' Below it lie the one-joint 'locals' of the short head of the biceps connecting across the linea aspera to the middle of the adductor magnus muscle. The two locals closely mirror individually the collective action of the express. (From Myers T: *Anatomy trains: myofascial meridians for manual and movement therapists,* London, 2002, Churchill Livingstone.)

Myofascial Integration

As explained by Tom Myers in his text *Anatomy Trains: Myofascial Meridians for Manual and Movement Therapists,* muscles operate across functionally integrated bodywide continuities within the fascial network. These sheets and lines follow the network of the connective tissue system, weaving a pattern of interconnected myofascial structures (Figure 9-9). Strain, tension, fixation, compensations, and most movement are distributed along these lines.

The term *myofascial continuity* describes the connection between two adjacent and aligned structures within the structural webbing. They create lines of pull, which transmit strain and movement through the myofascia around the skeleton.

According to Myers, *tensegrity* was coined from the phrase "tension integrity" by the designer R. Buckminster Fuller (working from original structures developed by artist Kenneth Snelson). The term refers to structures that maintain their integrity primarily because of a balance of continuous tensile forces through the structure (Figure 9-10). Although every structure ultimately is held together by a balance between tension and compression, tensegrity structures, according to Fuller, are characterized by continuous tension and local compression. Tension forces naturally transmit the shortest distance between two points, so the components of tensegrity structures are positioned to withstand stress best. The bones, muscle, and fascia create a tensegric structure. The bones are the compression members and the myofascia is the surrounding tension member of a tensegrity system of the body. That soft tissue balance is necessary to hold the skeleton upright is evident. The bones are "spacers" pushing out into the soft tissue, and the tone of the tensile myofascia becomes the determinant of balanced structure.

The geometry of tensegrity is not confined to the human body by any means. Many natural systems, including carbon atoms, water molecules, proteins, viruses, cells, tissues, and other living creatures are constructed using tensegrity.

We often view the skeleton as a continuous compression structure, like a brick wall: the weight of the head and neck rests on the seventh cervical vertebra, the head, neck, and thorax rest on the fifth lumbar vertebra, and so on down to the feet, which must bear the whole weight of the body and transmit that weight to the earth. According to this concept, the muscles hang from this skeleton and move it around, the way the cables move a crane around. This mechanical model lends itself to the traditional picture of the actions of individual muscles on the bones and the forces are localized. For example, if a tree falls on one corner of a rectangular building, that corner will collapse, perhaps without damaging the rest of the structure. Most modern manipulative therapy works off this idea: if a part is injured, the

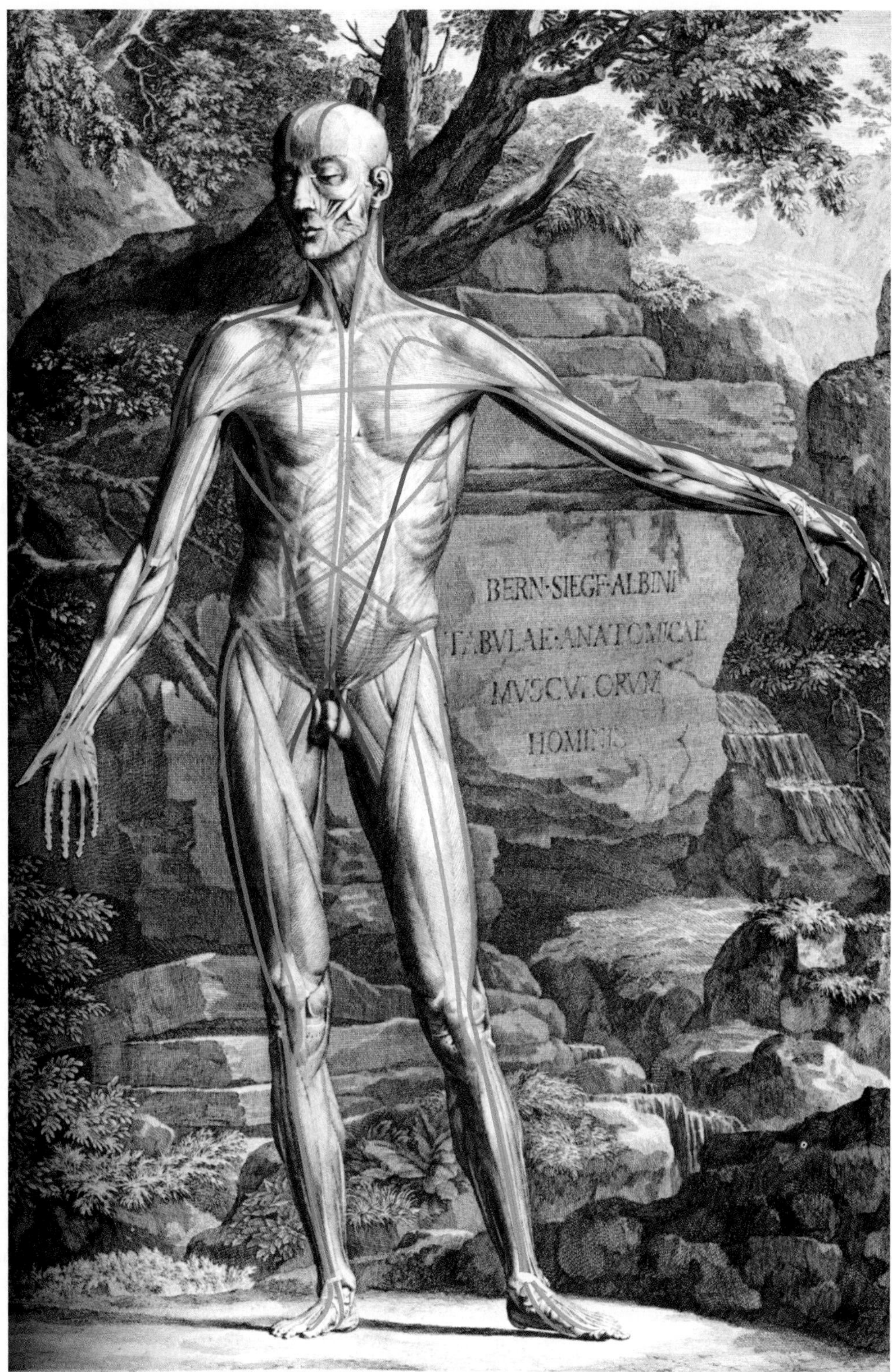

Figure 9-9
Pattern of interconnected myofascial structures. (Reprinted with permission of Dover Publications.)

injury is caused by localized forces that have overcome local tissues, and local relief and repair are necessary. This, however, is a limited view and seldom addresses the cause of the problem. Because of this spot work is seldom effective.

A tensegrity model of the body presents a different picture. A tensegrity model is difficult to describe, but the principles are simple. A tensegrity structure combines tension and compression components, but the compression members are islands, floating in a sea of continuous tension.

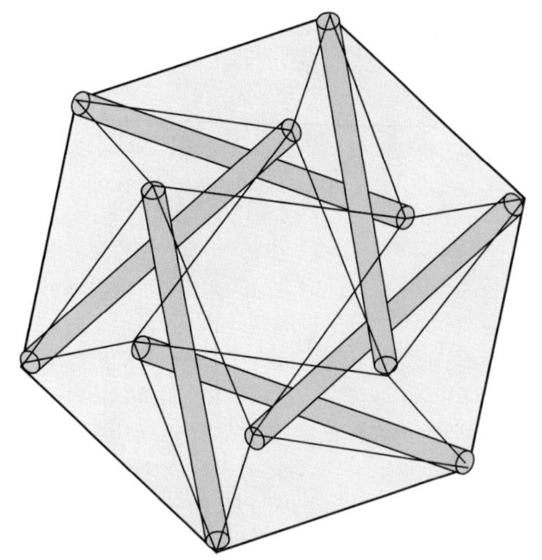

Figure 9-10
An abstract image of a cell that is kept together by tensegrity.

The compression members push outward against the tension members that pull inward. As long as the two sets of forces are balanced, the structure is stable. A tent made of canvas, poles, and tension supplied by ropes is a good example.

The stability of a tensegrity structure is less stiff and more resilient than the continuous compression structure. Load one "corner" of a tensegrity structure, and the whole structure gives a little to accommodate. Load the structure too much and the structure ultimately breaks, but not necessarily anywhere near the load. Because the structure distributes strain throughout the structure along the lines of tension, the tensegrity structure may give at some weak point away from the area of applied strain. A principle of massage application that supports this process is to identify the symptoms (the weak part), look elsewhere for the cause (origin of the strain).

In fact, all the interconnected structural elements of a tensegrity model rearrange themselves in response to a local stress. And as the applied stress increases, more of the components come to lie in the direction of the applied stress, resulting in a linear stiffening of the material.

In other words, tensegrity structures show resiliency, becoming more stable the greater the load is. Through response to piezoelectric charges, as well as to simple pull (take a wad of loose cotton batten and gently pull on the ends to see the multidirectional fibers suddenly line up in a similar way), the fibrous body reacts as a tensegrity structure when confronted with extra strain.

Myers further indicates that tensegrity concepts create a system or interconnected view of body structure and function, viewing the body as an integrated system. An injury at any given site often can be caused by long-term strain in other parts. Discovering these pathways and easing chronic strain at some point removes the painful portion and then becomes a natural part of restoring systemic ease and preventing future injuries. Full-body massage applications best address the tensegric nature of the body. Full-body massage that addresses these areas of strain creates ease in the tensegrity system. Spot work often is directed at the symptom and not the cause and therefore is less effective.

Pathologic Connective Tissue Changes

Pathologic changes in connective tissue result in alterations such as thickening, shortening, calcification, and erosion. These changes may result from sudden or sustained torsion, tension, compression, and bind and shear forces. Sustained inappropriate forces cause the fascia to adapt and result in reduced pliability and may lead to varying degrees of fascial entrapment of nerve structures and consequently a wide range of symptoms and dysfunctions. Nerve receptors within the fascia report to the central nervous system as part of any adaptation process. The pacinian corpuscles are particularly important because they inform the central nervous system about the rate of acceleration of movement taking place in the area. This involvement can affect reflex responses. Other sensing input in response to biomechanical stress involves fascial structures, such as tendons and ligaments, which contain highly specialized and sensitive mechanoreceptor and proprioceptor reporting stations. Fascial changes adversely influence many of these sensing receptors, which are implicated in pain syndromes.

Apparently the fascial tonus might be influenced and regulated by the state of the autonomic nervous system. Intervention in the fascial system might have an effect on the autonomic nervous system in general and on the organs that are affected directly by it.

In ground substance, collagen molecules bind together and orient along the lines of tension and piezoelectric charge. This adaptive process can be beneficial or dysfunctional. If dysfunction occurs, the muscles become overworked and undernourished and may develop trigger point pain, weakness, increased density in the surrounding ground substance, and increased metabolite toxicity. As previously mentioned, counterforces introduced by methods such as massage, exercise, and stretching can reduce strain. The fascia remodels, and the muscles can be restored to full function. Two elements, however, are necessary for successful resolution of these situations, whether achieved through movement or soft tissue manipulation:

1. A restoring of normal structure of the tissue to help restore fluid content, muscle function, and connection with the sensory-motor system
2. An easing of the force that caused the increased stress on that tissue in the first place

Either of these alone produces temporary or unsatisfactory results. One must address the cause and the effect in a therapeutic intervention.

Pathologic and therapeutic viscoplastic changes are not absolutely permanent because collagen has a limited half-life (300 to 500 days) and then is replaced by new tissue formation. One can modify negative stresses (such as poor posture and use) for the better, impose positive (therapeutic) forces by means of appropriate massage methods, or exercise the system for positive results. Dysfunctional connective tissue changes usually improve in about a year with ongoing therapeutic intervention. However, the client often requires long-term maintenance to support the therapeutic changes.

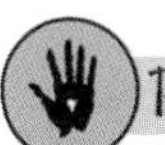

PRACTICAL APPLICATION

The massage application influences the muscle fibers most if it affects the nervous system and responds to approaches that introduce stimulation to restore or support homeostasis.

The connective tissue network is influenced more by a mechanical approach that affects the viscous (colloid) and plastic components of this tissue. As described in Chapter 8 and again in this chapter, sustained, slow elongation of connective tissue at an intensity sufficient to cause a change in the plastic properties is necessary to affect these structures therapeutically. If one applies too much force too fast to the tissue, the colloid gel responds with increased resistance. If one does not apply enough force, the intensity will not be sufficient to effect change. As one stretches the fascia and applies manipulative mechanical force, the viscous component becomes softer and more pliable.

Most researchers agree that connective tissue changes are part of a degenerative process. Restoration of function helps reverse degenerative processes, supporting a return to homeostasis and an increase in well-being. Myofascial shortening in one area affects alignment of the tensegrity structure. The myofascial tracts, or meridians as Myers calls them, are integral in myofascial performance. Appropriate massage intervention helps restore the balance of the myofascial spans interconnected with the bone and joint structure (Figure 9-11). ■

Repair of Muscle

Most of an adult's muscle cells are already in place at birth. As we grow, existing muscle fibers enlarge (hypertrophy) by as much as 30% of their original size. An injured muscle often is repaired with connective tissue. The body has a specific repair process for regenerating muscle cells. Within hours of an injury, enzymes in the body begin to digest the damaged cell portion. Satellite cells, which are inactive during normal muscle activity, begin to form the new fibers by creating myotubes, which combine to form myofibrils. These new cells take on the characteristics of muscle fibers. Exercise influences the growth of satellite cells and aids in maintaining plasticity of connective tissue. Cardiac muscle has no satellite cells, and its damaged cells are replaced with fibrous connective tissue. Smooth muscle is able to regenerate itself throughout life.

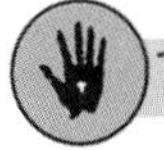

PRACTICAL APPLICATION

The goals for supporting healing of the skeletal muscle injury are to promote satellite cell repair processes and manage the development of scar tissue. This process allows the connective tissue structures that develop to be as normal as possible and to stay pliable so that they do not interfere with the function of the muscles. Stimulation of muscle function seems to encourage the satellite cells and support muscle regeneration. Movement therapies can support these functions. Massage methods can encourage appropriate mobile connective tissue development so that adhesions do not develop. Because connective tissue originates along the direction of tension, scar tissue can be encouraged to form along lines of external pressure provided by methods that orient by stroking and pulling the tissue in the direction of the desired connective tissue formation.

Areas of muscle healing formed primarily from connective tissue with adhesion and random directional formation can be encouraged to reheal through the use of massage methods that introduce therapeutic inflammation. These methods must be followed with appropriate rehabilitation processes, including broadening contractions to encourage mobility in the scar and decrease adhesion formation. One applies the techniques to small areas. Friction, which is a massage method that moves muscle tissue against the muscle fiber configuration pattern, is the approach most commonly used. Stretching methods that exceed the elastic range of connective tissue to alter the plastic range can pull apart adhesions and can be used to create the controlled area of inflammation. ■

Muscle Attachments

Most of our individual skeletal muscles span joints and are attached to bones or other structures in at least two places. In most cases a muscle starts on one bone and ends on another.

The terms most commonly used in the past to describe these attachments are ***origin*** and ***insertion.*** Classically, the origin of a muscle has been defined as the attachment that does not move when the muscle contracts; the origin is usually the proximal attachment or the attachment closer to the midline or center of the body. The insertion has been defined as the attachment that does move when the muscle contracts; the insertion is usually the distal attachment or the attachment farther from the midline or center of the body. However, this terminology can lead to confusion and a lack of proper understanding of how muscles function. Persons learning origins and insertions of a muscle often do not realize that the origin and insertion of a muscle can switch, that is, the insertion could stay fixed while the origin moves. When this situation happens, the movement that occurs often is called a **reverse action.** Simple examples of reverse actions are when the biceps brachii contracts and causes the arm to move toward the forearm (instead of the forearm moving toward the arm) when doing a chin-up or when the quadriceps femoris group contracts and causes the thigh to move toward the leg (instead of the leg moving toward the thigh) when standing up from a seated position.

In an effort to simplify the learning and understanding of muscles and their attachments and actions, a simpler terminology is becoming more widespread and accepted; that is simply to name the attachments of a muscle by the locations of the attachments. For example, the attachments of the biceps brachii onto the scapula would be called the proximal attachments and the attachment onto the forearm would be called the distal attachment. This system is used in this text.

Muscles also may be said to have two types of attachments, direct and indirect. In *direct attachments,* which are uncommon, the epimysium of the muscle blends into the periosteum of the bone or the perichondrium of cartilage. The more common form of muscle attachments is the *indirect attachment,* in which the muscle fascia extends beyond the muscles in a ropelike tendon or flat, broad aponeurosis. The tendon or aponeurosis blends and wraps into the connective tissue coverings and structures, including ligaments and other tendons, or into a seam of fibrous connective tissue, called a raphe, at the attachment site. One must realize that muscle attachments do not stick on bone but wrap around the bone so the muscles can lift the bone when they contract (Figure 9-12, *A*). The middle of the muscle or the area with the largest and broadest concentration of muscle fibers is the belly of the muscle (Figure 9-12, *B*).

Muscle Shapes

The bundles of muscle fibers known as fascicles form different patterns in muscles, resulting in the different shapes of muscles (Figure 9-13). These fascicle forms affect function, primarily the strength and direction of movement. The following are the more common patterns of fascicle arrangement:

Parallel: The fascicles are long and oriented parallel with the longitudinal axis of the muscle. Some of these muscles are straplike (e.g., the sartorius), and others are fusiform with an expanded belly (e.g., the biceps brachii).

Convergent: The fascicle pattern begins with a broad origin and converges to blend with a much smaller tendon. The result is a triangular muscle (e.g., the pectoralis major).

Pennate: The fascicles are short, lie at an angle to the muscle, and attach to one or more tendons running the length of the muscle. A *unipennate muscle* (e.g., the extensor digitorum longus) has fascicles that insert on only one side of the tendon. A *bipennate muscle* (e.g., the rectus femoris) has fascicles that insert into the tendon from both sides; the result looks like a feather. A muscle resembling many feathers, all inserted into one large tendon, is called a *multipennate muscle.*

Circular: The fascicles are arranged in concentric rings around external body openings. These muscles, which contract to close the openings, are called sphincters.

The various patterns of fascicle arrangement determine the strength and amount of movement a muscle provides. Skeletal muscles can shorten to about 50% of their resting length when contracted. The longer and more parallel the muscle fibers to the long axis of the muscle, the greater the muscle shortening. Parallel muscles shorten as a direct result of the shortening of their fibers; these muscles produce the greatest amount of shortening. They do this at the expense of strength; parallel muscles are not powerful. The fibers of pennate muscles rotate around their tendon attachments. Pennate muscles can pack more fibers into the same amount of space as parallel fibers and so can produce the stronger contraction, albeit over a shorter range of motion (Activity 9-3).

Myotatic Units (Functional Muscle Groups)

Myotatic units neurologically interconnect muscle function. Only rarely does any muscle act independently. Most muscles play a part in a movement pattern, just as actors do in a play. Roles can change, depending on the response required. A muscle can be the star, or prime mover, and in the next instant become one of the supporting cast. A moment later the same muscle can assume the opposite role. As previously described, three types of contractions exist:

ACTIVITY 9-3

Draw the following muscle shapes:

Parallel

Pennate

Convergent

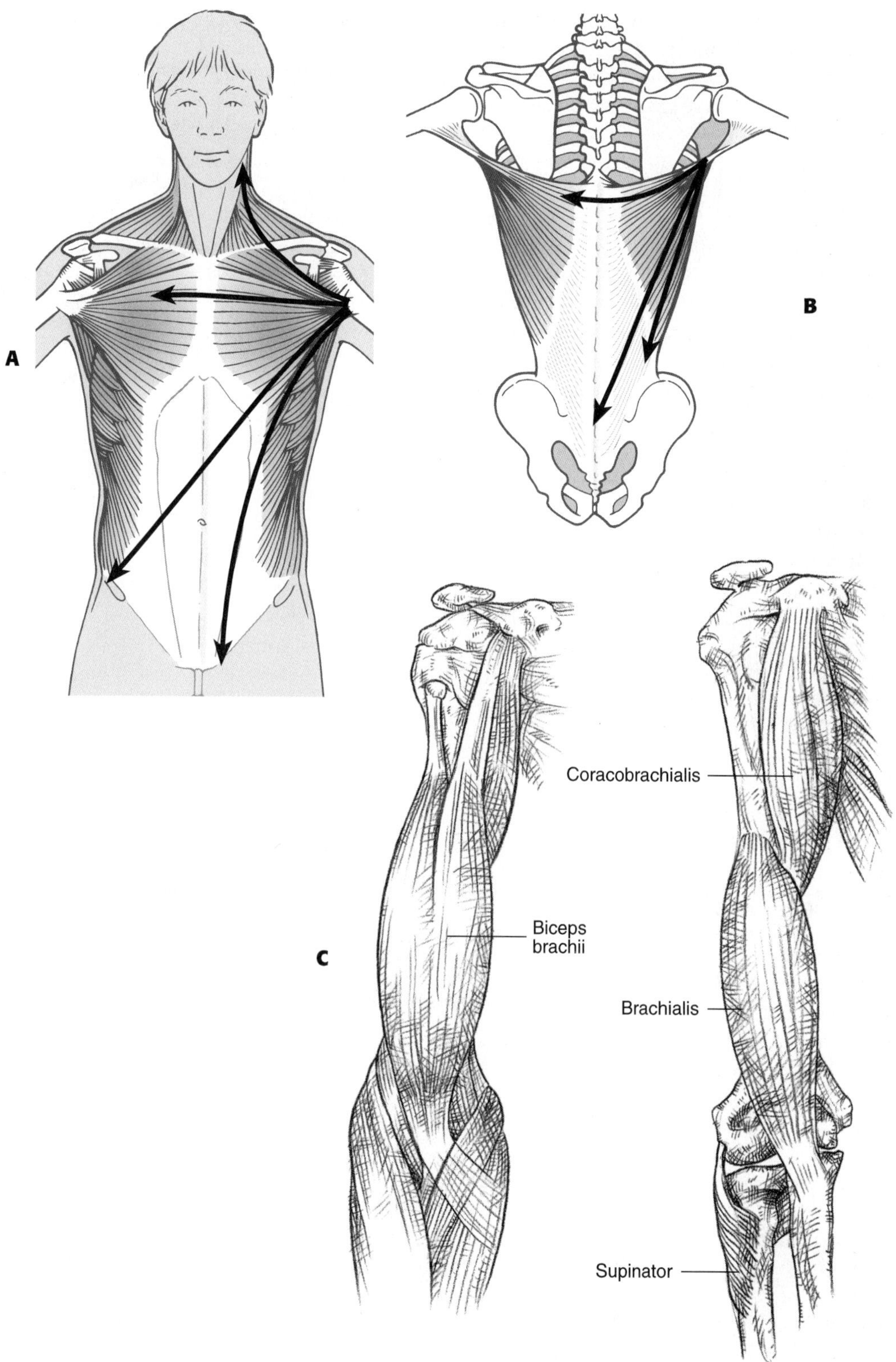

Figure 9-11
A, A tennis forehand connects the Superficial Front Arm Line to its partner on the opposite side. **B,** A backhand shot could similarly join the Superficial Back Arm Line to its opposite partner. **C,** The biceps brachii function at three joints. Deep to the biceps lie three local (functions at one joint) muscles, each of which duplicates the biceps action on the individual joints. (From Myers T: *Anatomy trains: myofascial meridians for manual and movement therapists,* London, 2002, Churchill Livingstone.)

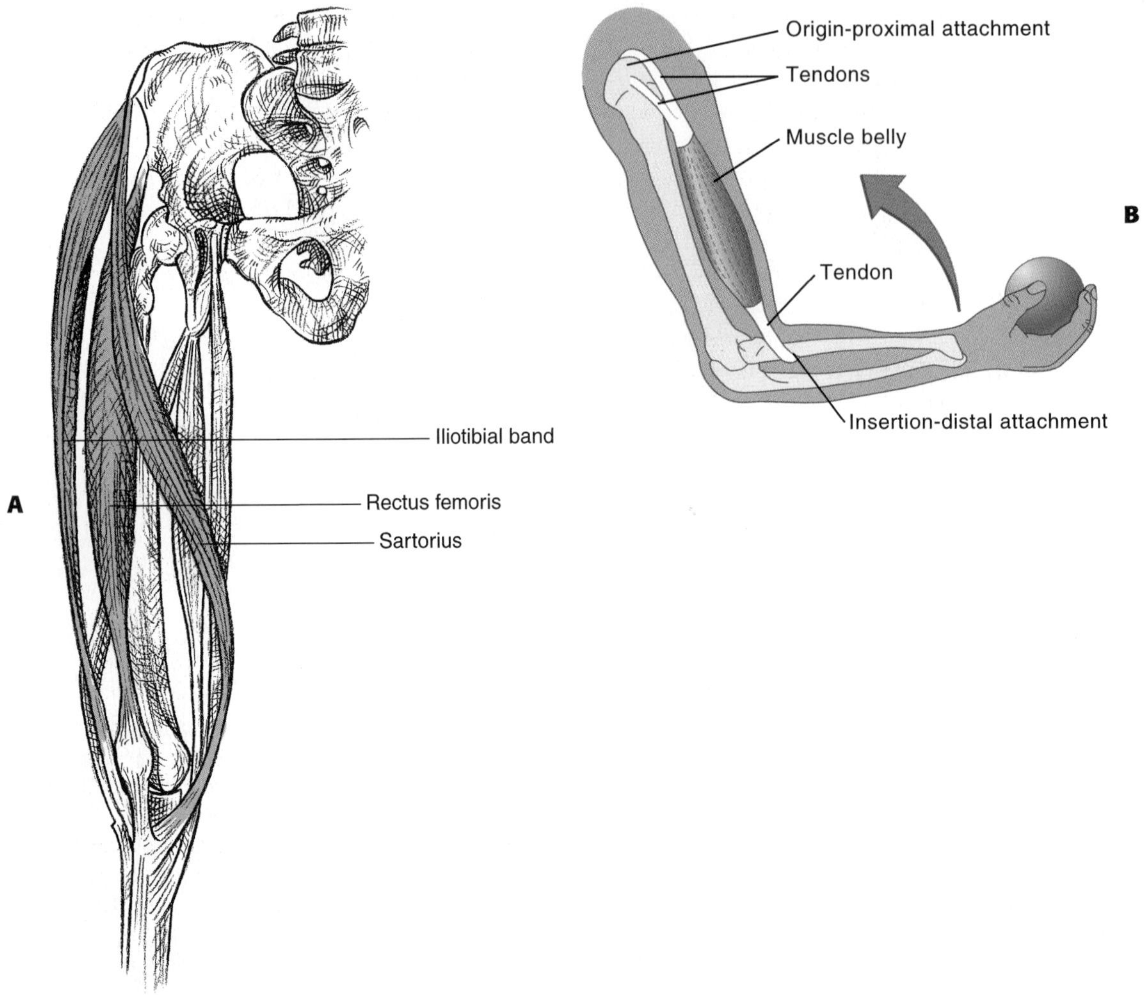

Figure 9-12
A, Example of how muscles wrap around bones and weave into each other. **B,** Attachments of a skeletal muscle. A muscle originates at a relatively stable part of the skeleton (origin) and inserts at the skeletal part that is moved when the muscle contracts (insertion). (**A** from Myers T: *Anatomy trains: myofascial meridians for manual and movement therapists,* London, 2002, Churchill Livingstone. **B** from Thibodeau GA, Patton KT: *Anatomy and physiology,* ed 5, St Louis, 2003, Mosby.)

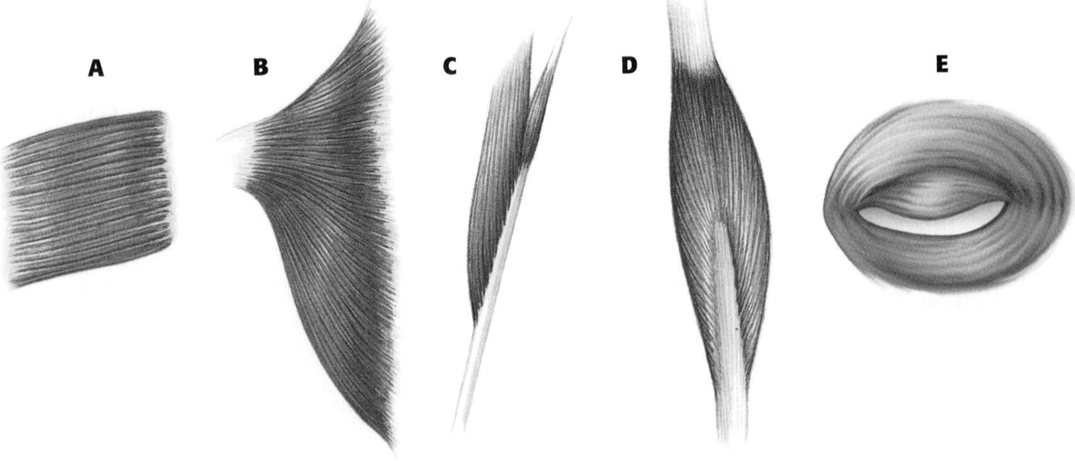

Figure 9-13
Muscle shape and fiber arrangement. **A,** Parallel. **B,** Convergent. **C,** Pennate. **D,** Bipennate. **E,** Circular. (From Thibodeau GA, Patton KT: *Anatomy and physiology,* ed 5, St Louis, 2003, Mosby.)

concentric contraction, in which the muscle shortens (acceleration) and the joint angle decreases; eccentric contraction, in which the muscle maintains a controlled lengthening (deceleration) response as the joint angle increases; and isometric contraction, in which the muscle shortens but produces no movement. The terms **mover** ***(agonist),*** **prime mover,** ***antagonist, fixator*** *(stabilizer),* **neutralizer, support** and ***synergist*** describe the function of muscles in a complete movement pattern. Because the central nervous system processes movement patterns, understanding the interaction of muscles in functional units is important. This integrated function often is called the kinetic chain and is explained in depth in Chapter 10 (Box 9-3).

The mover/antagonist interaction is easy to visualize in muscles such as the biceps brachii/triceps brachii unit but becomes more complex when we consider that the deltoid and quadriceps femoris and the adductors and hamstrings form a functional unit because of our gait, or walking pattern. The various functional units that require muscles to cooperate in producing bodywide movements (e.g., walking or maintaining balance) need sophisticated reflex control by the nervous system. The student would benefit from reviewing the section on reflex arcs in Chapter 4. When the role of stabilization is factored into a movement pattern, the functional (or myotatic) muscle group interaction becomes complex. Whenever maintaining posture is part of the pattern, a bodywide process is involved. Chapter 10 presents more on biomechanics.

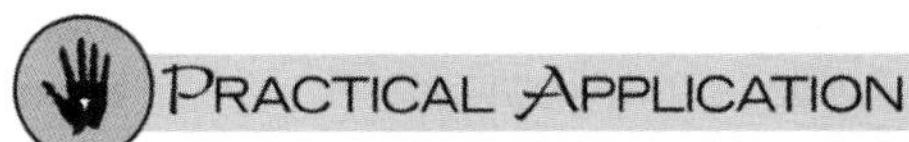

Often, effective applications of massage depend on unraveling complex functional groups of muscles. In many cases, addressing the entire body during each session in what is called a general constitutional approach is just as

BOX 9-3

Names of Muscles by Function

Mover (agonist) A muscle or muscles using concentric contractions that are the main force causing a joint motion through a specified plane of motion; the mover or movers most responsible for the action can be called the prime mover(s).

Antagonist A muscle that has the opposite action to the mover and usually is located on the opposite side of the joint and eccentrically contracts and lengthens, restraining and controlling an opposite force (usually a force external to the body such as gravity).

Fixator (stabilizer) A muscle that surrounds the joint or body segment and isometrically contracts to support or stabilize one attachment of the mover (or antagonist), enabling the other attachment of the mover (or antagonist) to work effectively. Usually the fixator establishes a firm base for the more distal attachment to carry out movements.

Neutralizer A muscle that stops an unwanted action of the mover (or antagonist) at the attachment of the mover (or antagonist) that is moving. Like fixators, neutralizers work via isometric contractions.

Support muscle A support muscle acts at a joint other than where the action in question is occurring to hold a body part in position while the action in question is occurring. Support muscles generally work via isometric contractions.

Synergist Defined as a helper mover (assistant mover or emergency mover) of the action that is occurring or more broadly defined as any muscle that helps an action occur. Synergists are sometimes known as guiding muscles.

Mover and antagonist muscles can contract at the same time in what is called a co-contraction. The result is no movement because the forces generated resist each other. Isometric contraction occurs, providing stability.

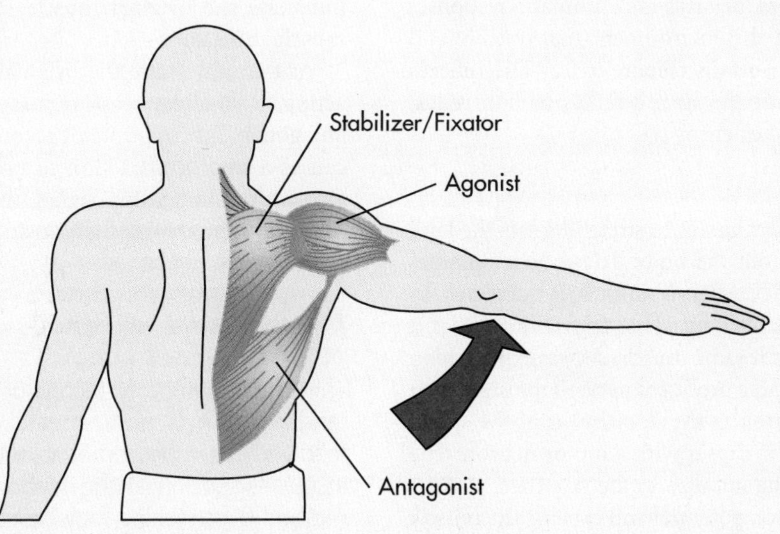

effective. Interventions that bring more general demand on the body to respond naturally address these complex patterns. Spot work or addressing an isolated area and excluding the rest of the body is less effective. When considering myotatic units and the development of patterns of compensation to any change in the body, one may assume logically that any alteration in musculoskeletal function has a bodywide effect. For example, the arm and thigh muscles are connected in agonist/antagonist patterns through the gait reflex and the neck and trunk muscles interact together through the ocular/pelvic and righting reflexes that keep us upright and eyes forward. Because the components of the body are interdependent, everything affects everything else. Methods and treatment plans developed around generalized whole-body responses honor the innate body wisdom. ■

Proprioceptors and Reflexes

If the central nervous system is to coordinate motion, it must be aware constantly of any muscle action. Proprioceptors are sensory receptors that provide the central nervous system with information about position, movement, muscle tension, joint activity, and equilibrium. Methods that move, stretch, and apply tension to the muscles and joints stimulate the following receptors:

1. Muscle spindles: Respond to sudden and prolonged stretch.
2. Tendon organs: Respond to tension in the muscle that is relayed to the tendon; ligaments contain receptors that respond to strain at the joint and feed back information to adjust the tension patterns of associated muscles.
3. Joint kinesthetic receptors in the joint capsule: Respond to pressure, acceleration, and deceleration of joint movement. The two main types of joint kinesthetic receptors are type II cutaneous mechanoreceptors and pacinian (lamellated) corpuscles.

Somatic reflex arcs interpret and process stimulation of nervous system receptors. Reflexes are automatic responses triggered by changes in the environment that quickly and predictably restore homeostasis (Figure 9-14). The reflexes most often stimulated are the stretch reflex, tendon reflex, flexor reflex, and crossed extensor reflex.

Stretch Reflex

The sensitivity of muscle spindles to stretching sets the level of muscle tone throughout the body. The muscle spindles activate the stretch reflex when a muscle is subjected to sudden or prolonged stretching. This activation causes a reflexive contraction of the same muscle. As was explained in Chapter 5, a muscle spindle produces nerve impulses that it sends via a sensory neuron to the dorsal root of the spinal cord, where an impulse synapses with a motor neuron. The motor neuron carries the impulse to the stretched muscle, generating a muscle action potential and causing the muscle and its synergists to contract. Muscle contraction stops spindle cell discharge unless the muscle is held in a lengthened state, and a small amount of stretch reflex continues to be generated. The effect of the muscle fiber length stimulates the stretch reflex, resulting in facilitation and concentric shortening of the muscle.

The principle of *reciprocal inhibition* comes into play during the stretch reflex. At the same time the original muscle is stimulated to contract, sensory signals synapse with association neurons to its antagonist(s), inhibiting any signal through the motor neurons to the antagonists; this results in relaxation of the antagonist. To simplify, when one muscle contracts, its antagonist or opposing muscle group must relax. One can initiate the pathway of this inhibition circuitry (reciprocal innervation) therapeutically to assist in muscle relaxation.

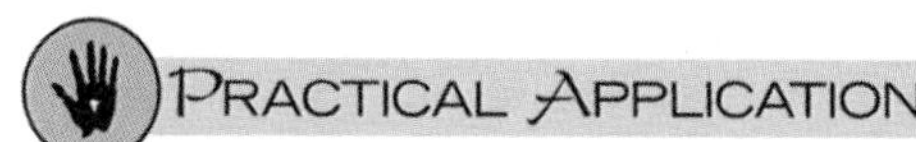

Therapeutic methods can activate or strengthen weakened muscle patterns by lengthening the muscles and initiating the stretch reflex. An awareness of this reflex response is important in all methods intended to lengthen and relax the muscles. In these instances, one must avoid the stretch reflex. This system of reflexes frequently becomes hyperactive, resulting in an increase of muscle tension. Techniques using isometric and isotonic muscle contractions to relax and lengthen muscles are helpful in resetting muscle tension patterns. ■

Tendon Reflex

The tendon reflex operates as a feedback mechanism that monitors and controls muscle tension by inducing muscle relaxation. This reflex is mediated by the tendon organs that detect and respond to changes in muscle tension caused by a sudden or intense muscle contraction. When the tendon organ is stimulated, it sends a signal along a sensory neuron to the spinal cord, where it synapses with an inhibitory association neuron, which inhibits the motor neurons that innervate the original muscle. This inhibition causes the muscle to relax.

At the same time the original muscle is inhibited from acting, a small increase occurs in the signal sent to the antagonist. The opposite of reciprocal inhibition, this signal causes a small contraction to take place in the antagonist. One can initiate this signal therapeutically to assist in relaxing a tense muscle and in stimulating its antagonist.

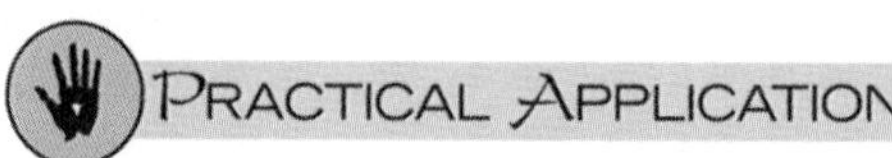

The most common technique used to stimulate the tendon reflex is an isometric (or isotonic) contraction, followed by postisometric relaxation. This technique increases tension at the tendon to elicit relaxation. This method of stretching may be called PNF (proprio-neuro-facilitation) stretching. ■

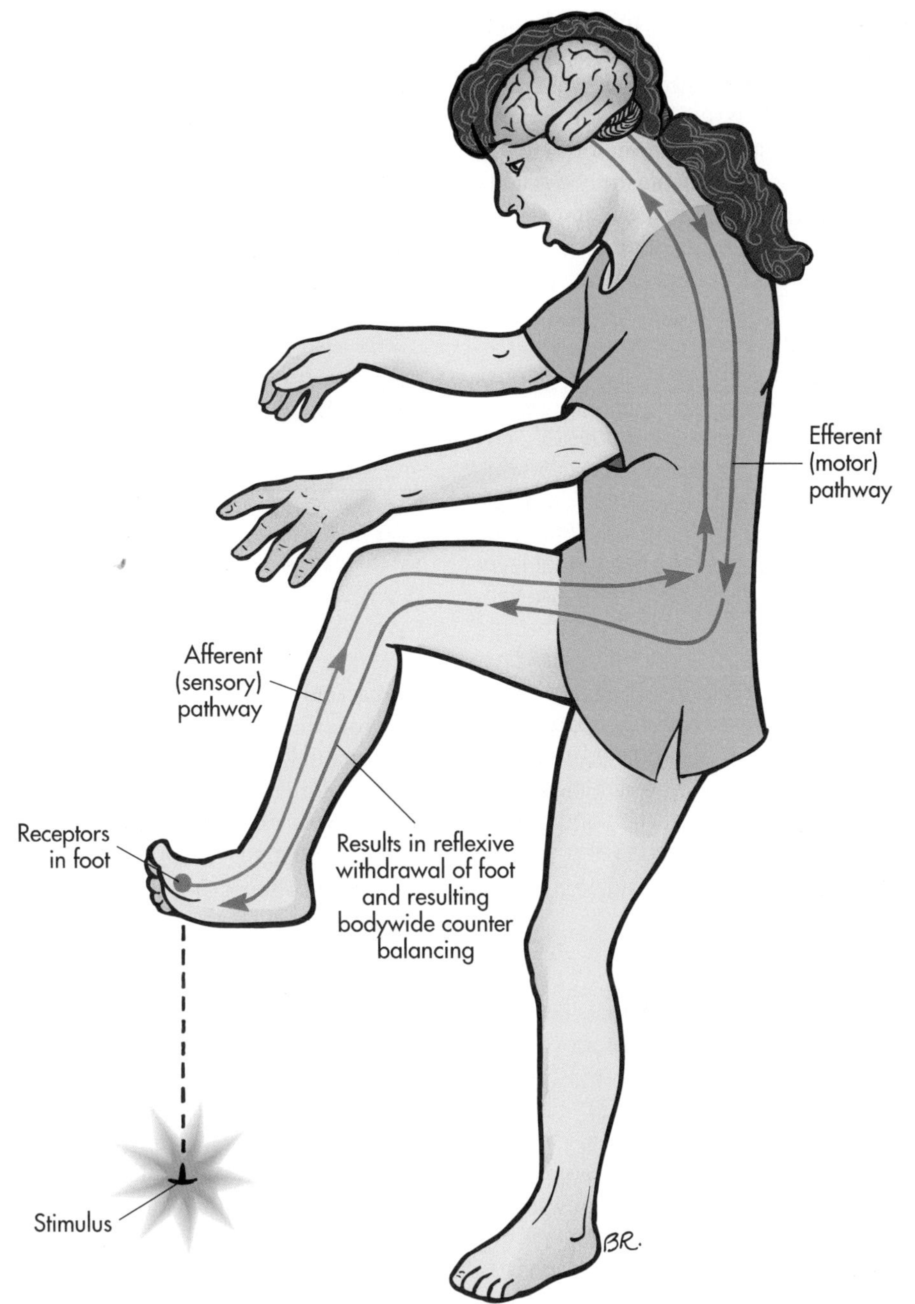

Figure 9-14
Reflex response. Local stimulation of a few specific receptors leads to a large number of outgoing impulses, which affect many muscles. (From Fritz S: *Mosby's fundamentals of therapeutic massage,* ed 3, St Louis, 2004, Mosby.)

Flexor Reflex and Crossed Extensor Reflex

The flexor (withdrawal) and crossed extensor reflexes are polysynaptic reflex arcs. A single sensory neuron, most likely located in the skin, can activate several motor neurons. Stimulation of these reflexes affects both sides of the body through intersegmental reflex arcs. The flexor reflex withdraws the limb from an unpleasant or painful stimulus, while the crossed extensor reflex extends the limb on the opposite side of the spinal cord to maintain balance. The circuitry of contralateral reflex arcs synchronizes control over the contracting and inhibited muscles. These reflexes also explain why one seldom finds tension patterns only on one side of the body. As with the stretch reflex, the principle of reciprocal inhibition is active in flexor and extensor reflexes.

Postural Reflexes

In addition, a series of reflexes maintain posture and the position of the head so that the eyes remain in the horizontal plane and oriented forward. These righting and tonic neck reflexes together with oculopelvic reflexes coordinate position and function of the neck, trunk, and pelvic muscles.

Looking back over the head or tipping the head back activates the extensors and inhibits the flexors. Looking down toward the navel or tipping the head down activates the flexors and inhibits the extensors. Looking left or turning the head to the left activates muscles that would rotate the body left and inhibits those that would rotate the body right. Losing postural balance during eye and head movement causes the opposite reaction, returning the body to an upright position in gravity.

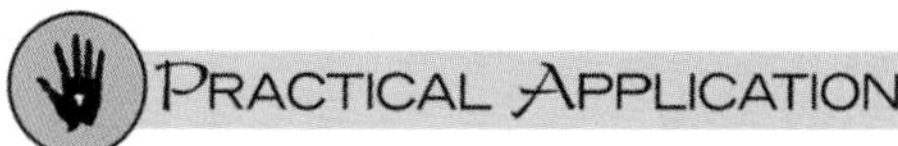

The withdrawal response can stimulate opposite side patterns of tension or weakness. The response is powerful because flexor or withdrawal reflexes take priority over all other reflex activity taking place simultaneously. Massage can reset reflex patterns that are unproductive or that lead to discomfort and postural distortion from uneven contraction and relaxation muscle patterns. The effectiveness of the techniques depends on how efficiently one stimulates the receptors for these reflexes. The practitioner must stimulate the targeted receptor with the appropriate technique and intensity to allow the stimulated reflex to function appropriately. One can use the positioning of the eyes and head to influence muscle interaction and during muscle energy methods to initiate facilitation (contraction) or inhibition of muscle. ■

Muscle Firing Patterns

Reflex patterns also regulate in what order muscles contract to produce movement. The prime movers contract first. Then stabilization occurs so that fixators or co-contraction patterns (mover and antagonist) contract next. Fixators often are located in the deep layers of muscles. Muscles that are shorter and cross only one joint have the best mechanical advantage to start or initiate and guide a joint movement contract third in the sequence. These muscles are often the middle layer of muscles and may be classified as synergists. This pattern is general and exceptions occur, but the pattern provides a framework for understanding muscle interaction. Disruption of the firing pattern causes labored movement, and muscle fatigue often occurs. Chapter 10 provides more discussion on muscle firing patterns, but considering the firing sequence when learning about reflex patterns and the coordination of muscle movement is helpful.

Function of Cardiac and Smooth Muscle Tissue

Cardiac and smooth muscle tissues operate by mechanisms similar to those in skeletal muscle tissues.

Cardiac Muscle

Cardiac muscle (Figure 9-15), also known as striated involuntary muscle, is found in only one organ of the body, the heart. Forming the bulk of the wall of each heart chamber,

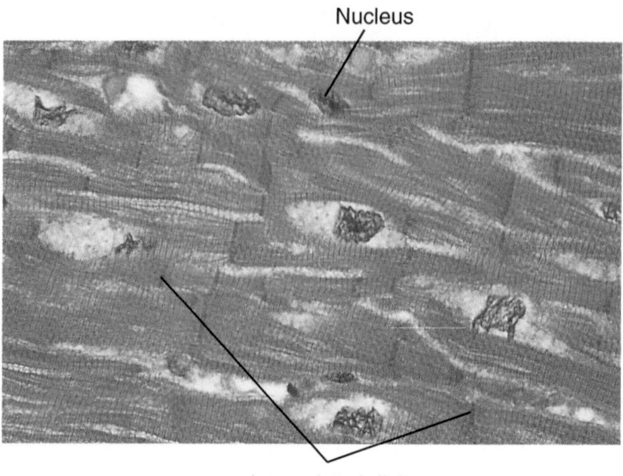

Figure 9-15
Cardiac muscle. The dark bands, called intercalated disks, are characteristic of cardiac muscle and are clearly visible in this tissue section. (From Thibodeau GA, Patton KT: *Anatomy and physiology,* ed 5, St Louis, 2003, Mosby.)

cardiac muscle contracts rhythmically and continuously to provide the pumping action necessary to maintain a consistent blood flow through our internal environment.

The functional anatomy of cardiac muscle tissue resembles that of skeletal muscle but has specialized features related to the role of pumping blood continuously. Each cardiac muscle fiber contains parallel myofibrils composed of sarcomeres that give the whole fiber a striated appearance. However, the cardiac muscle fiber does not taper like a skeletal muscle fiber; rather, it forms strong, electrically coupled junctions (intercalated disks) with other fibers. Cardiac muscle forms a continuous contractile band around the heart that conducts a single impulse across a continuous sarcolemma, allowing for an efficient, coordinated pumping action. This means that even though many adjacent cardiac muscle cells contract simultaneously, they have a prolonged contraction rather than a rapid twitch. Cardiac muscle does not normally run low on ATP and thus does not experience fatigue. Obviously, this characteristic of cardiac muscle is vital for keeping the heart pumping continuously.

Unlike skeletal muscle, in which a nervous impulse is necessary to excite the sarcolemma to produce its own impulse, cardiac muscle can be self-exciting. Cardiac muscle cells can have a continuing rhythm of excitation and contraction on their own, although the rate of self-induced impulses is usually too slow to allow for strenuous activity. Central nervous system control of the heart is usual, is considered healthy, and is necessary for strenuous activity as well as generally altering the rate of the heart contractions to meet the demands placed on the heart.

Smooth Muscle

Smooth muscle comprises small, tapered cells with single nuclei (Figure 9-16). Smooth muscle fibers lack striations because the thick and thin myofilaments are arranged differently than in skeletal or cardiac muscle fibers. These

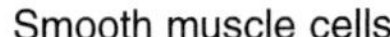

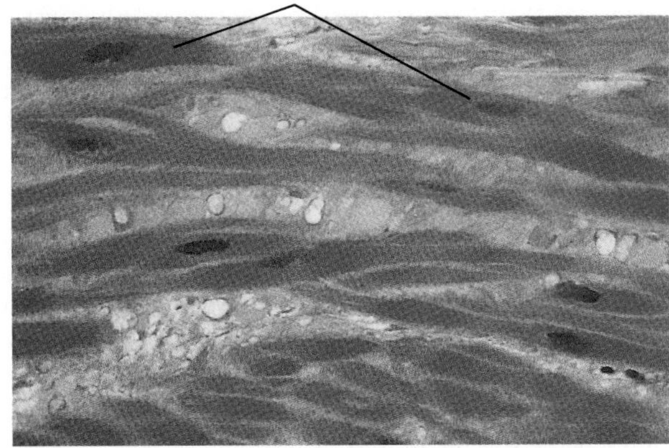

Figure 9-16
Smooth muscle. The central placement of nuclei in the spindle-shaped smooth muscle fibers is notable. (From Thibodeau GA, Patton KT: *Anatomy and physiology,* ed 5, St Louis, 2003, Mosby.)

arrangements of myofilaments crisscross the cell and attach at their ends to the plasma membrane of the cell.

When cross-bridges pull the thin filaments together, the muscle balls up and thus contracts the cell. Because the myofilaments are not organized into sarcomeres, they have more freedom of movement and can contract a smooth muscle fiber to shorter lengths than in skeletal and cardiac muscle.

The two types of smooth muscle tissue are visceral muscle and multiunit muscle. In visceral or single-unit muscles, gap junctions join individual smooth muscles into large, continuous sheets, much like the fibers observed in cardiac muscle. Visceral muscle is the most common type of smooth muscle and forms the muscular layer in the walls of many hollow structures such as in the digestive, urinary, and reproductive tracts.

Similar to cardiac muscle, visceral smooth muscle commonly has a rhythmic self-excitation, or autorhythmicity (meaning self-rhythm), that spreads across the entire tissue. When these rhythmic, spreading waves of contraction become strong enough, they can push the contents of a hollow organ progressively along its lumen (the interior of a tubular structure). This type of contraction, called peristalsis, moves food along the digestive tract, assists the flow of urine to the bladder, and pushes a baby out of the womb during labor. Such contractions also can be coordinated to produce mixing movements in the stomach and other organs.

Multiunit smooth muscle tissue does not act as a single unit, as does visceral muscle; instead, it comprises many independent, single-cell units. Each independent fiber does not generate its own impulse but rather responds only to nervous input. Although this type of smooth muscle can form thin sheets, as in the walls of large blood vessels, it more often is found in bundles (e.g., the erector pili muscles of the skin) or as single fibers, such as those surrounding small blood and lymph vessels.

INDIVIDUAL MUSCLES

Although we understand that the body operates as a unit, the massage practitioner must know the pieces making up that unit. The following section describes the individual muscles most often discussed by massage professionals. We discuss their primary function or functions, attachments (origin and insertion), innervation, synergists, antagonists, and if applicable, common trigger point areas and referred pain patterns. The primary function of muscles occurs during concentric contraction. Almost all muscles have eccentric function wherein they restrain and control movement during lengthening, and isometric function when acting as stabilizers (fixators) and neutralizers. When these functions of muscles are specifically important to the massage profession, we discuss them as well. Activities such as palpation, movement, coloring, drawing and labeling the attachment points, and locating common trigger points reinforce your knowledge of the structure and function of individual muscles or groups of muscles.

Ideally, we would remember every single detail of each muscle, but most of us are not able to do so because the amount of information is so great. A more realistic expectation in this study is for you to get to know the muscles as you would a new friend. Knowing where to find them, what they do, who their friends are, and what bothers them is helpful. To appreciate them as individuals, you do not need to know every single detail of the friend's life. If you need to know more about a muscle, you can always ask questions and look up additional material in reference texts as needed (one such reference is Joseph Muscolino's *The Muscular System Manual: The Skeletal Muscles of the Human Body,* Mosby, 2003). Not all references agree about specific details, and different books list slightly different attachment sites, functions, and so forth. Do not let this confuse you; as with most differing opinions, the answer is not black or white but somewhere in between in a range of gray.

This book uses the terminology of naming attachments simply as *From* and *To.* To translate to the origin/insertion terminology, one should note that the commonly accepted origin of a muscle is stated first and the commonly accepted insertion is stated second. As previously mentioned, for muscles that attach onto the extremities, the proximal attachment of the muscle is usually the origin, and the distal attachment is usually the insertion; for muscles of the axial body, the inferior attachment is usually the origin and the superior attachment is usually the insertion.

Muscles are arranged in layers, and most body areas have three to five layers of muscles. Those muscles considered deep lie closest to the bone, and those considered superficial lie closest to the skin.

When studying the individual muscles, the student should pay attention to all elements provided for each muscle and to referred pain patterns, because these are the symptoms persons will complain about if dysfunction with the muscle occurs (see Appendix B).

How Muscles Are Named

Muscle names seem more logical and therefore easier to learn when one understands the reasons for the names. Many of the muscles of the body are named using one or more of the following features:

- Location: Many muscles are named as a result of their location using medical terminology. The brachialis (arm muscle) and gluteus (buttock) muscles are examples.
- Function: The function of a muscle is frequently a part of its name. The adductor muscles of the thigh adduct or move the thigh at the hip joint toward the midline of the body.
- Shape: Shape is a descriptive feature used for naming many muscles. The deltoid (triangular) muscle covering the shoulder is shaped like a delta or triangle.
- Direction of fibers: Muscles may be named according to the orientation of their fibers. The term *rectus* means straight. The fibers of the rectus abdominis muscle run straight up and down (vertically) and are parallel to each other.
- Number of heads or divisions: The number of divisions or heads (points of attachment) may be used to name a muscle. The word part *–cep* means head. The bicep (two), triceps (three), and quadriceps (four) refer to multiple heads or points of attachment. The biceps brachii is a muscle having two heads located in the arm.
- Points of attachment: A muscle attaches from one site to another site. These attachment sites may be used to name a muscle. For example, the sternocleidomastoid has an attachment on the sternum and clavicle and another attachment on the mastoid process of the temporal bone.
- Size of muscle: The size of a muscle can be used to name a muscle, especially if it is compared to the size of nearby muscles. For example, the gluteus maximus is the largest muscle of the gluteal (Greek *glautos,* meaning buttock) region. Nearby is a small gluteal muscle, gluteus minimus, and midsize gluteal muscle, gluteus medius.

How to Palpate Muscles

One can palpate muscles that are relaxed or contracted as follows: With relaxed muscles, locating the muscle depends on anatomic knowledge and the ability to identify bony landmarks. Distinguishing whether you are touching the correct muscle is difficult at times because many structures such as tendons, fascia, and ligaments can attach in the same place. To palpate muscles when they are relaxed, read the attachment descriptions carefully and place your hand on the location described. Then trace the path of the muscle between the attachments. Notice the fiber direction, which determines the angle of pull when the muscle shortens. The largest area of the muscle is usually near the middle of the muscle and is called the belly. Remember that three or more layers of muscles cover each area. The more superficial muscles are easier to palpate than the deeper muscles. Palpation of deeper muscles requires more pressure but should not feel painful or pokey to the massage client.

To identify a specific muscle, first identify the attachments and belly of the muscle while the muscle is relaxed and then have the client actively contract the muscle. One can do this by placing the muscle in the concentric function position and then having the person hold that position or move the muscle a bit between concentric and eccentric patterns. While the person holds the position or slightly contracts the specific muscle, you should be able to feel the muscle tensing, bunching up, or pushing out. Again, identifying the deeper muscle layers is more difficult. The deeper muscles usually have smaller movement patterns, so a slight contraction to initiate a tiny movement to differentiate the smaller deeper layers is helpful. Then one initiates a larger or stronger contraction to identify the more superficial layers of the muscle.

Activity Explanation

This section provides a color illustration of each muscle along with composite pictures. Composite illustrations are presented in black and white format to be used as a color activity if desired.* Skeletal pictures are provided for you on which to draw individual muscles or muscle groups. If the activity requires more than one muscle to be drawn on the same picture, you should color each muscle a different color. Label the attachment sites with different colors, and use those colors consistently throughout all the activities. Mark the trigger point or points in yet a third color, again being consistent throughout the activities. Fine-point colored pencils work best for these activities.

Muscles of the Face and Head

The superficial muscles of the head, including those of the scalp and face, produce movement for facial expressions, which are vital to nonverbal communication (Figures 9-17 and 9-18). The muscles vary in shape and strength. Many adjacent muscles tend to be fused together. Unlike most skeletal muscles, which attach onto bones of the skeleton, many muscles of facial expression attach into skin or other muscles. Muscles of the head and face lift our eyebrows, flare our nostrils, and open and close our eyes and mouth. Many of these muscles are implicated in headaches and tend to tense when a person is stressed, especially if they are in pain. Careful massage to the area can be soothing and effective in managing tension headaches.

---

*Composite art is taken from Muscolino JE: *The muscular system manual: the skeletal muscles of the human body,* St Louis, 2003, Mosby. More complete musculoskeletal activities can be found in Muscolino JE: *Musculoskeletal anatomy coloring book,* St Louis, 2004, Mosby.

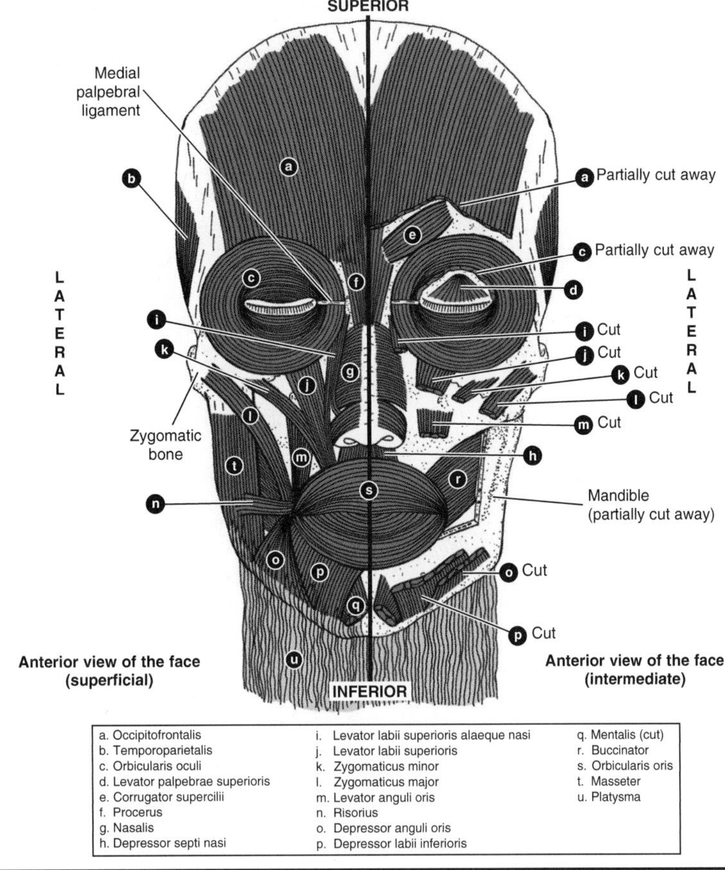

Figure 9-17
Anterior view of the head. (Modified from Muscolino JE: *The muscular system manual: the skeletal muscles of the human body*, ed 2, St Louis, 2005, Mosby.)

Muscles of Facial Expression

Occipitofrontalis (ok-SIP-ih-toe-fron-TAL-iss)

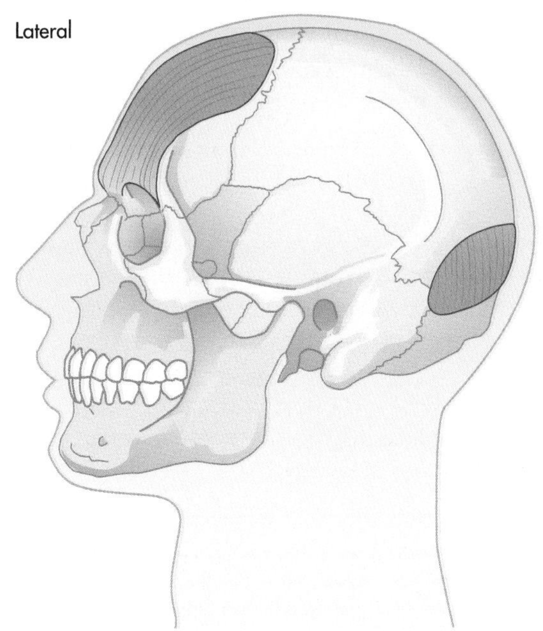

Also called the epicranius, occipitofrontalis means back of the head and related to the forehead. The muscle sometimes is described as separate muscles, the occipitalis and the frontalis.

Concentric function:

Draws the scalp anteriorly and posteriorly, elevates the eyebrows, and wrinkles the forehead.

From:

Occipital belly—Lateral two thirds of the highest nuchal line of the occipital bone and the mastoid area of the temporal bone

Frontal belly—Galea aponeurotica near the coronal suture

To:

Occipital belly—Galea aponeurotica

Frontal belly—Fascia and skin superior to the eye and nose

Innervation:

Occipitalis—Posterior auricular branch of the facial nerve (cranial nerve VII)

Frontalis—Temporal branches of the facial nerve (cranial nerve VII)

Major synergists:

Occipitalis—No major synergists

Frontalis—No major synergists

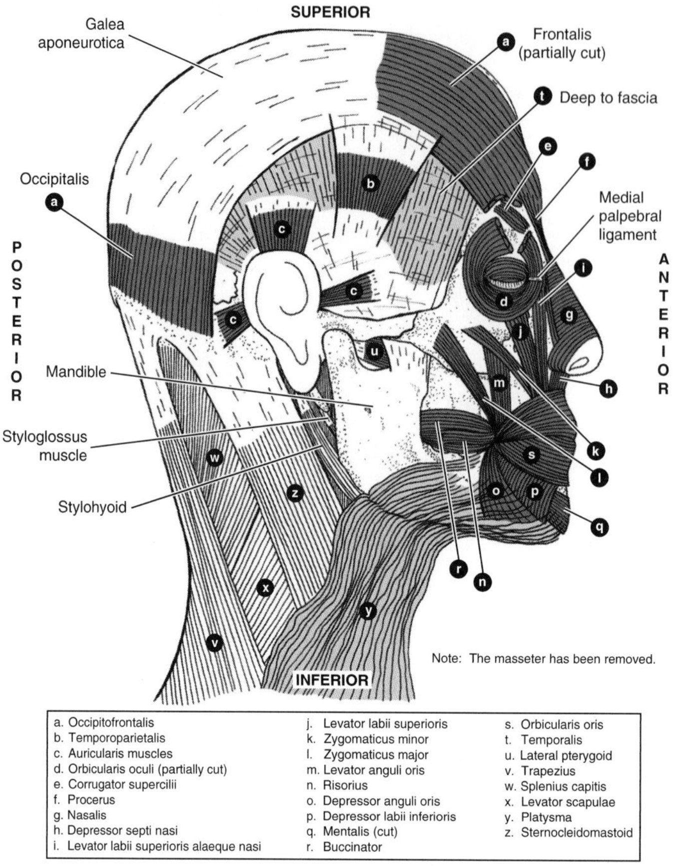

Figure 9-18
Lateral view of the head. (Modified from Muscolino JE: *The muscular system manual: the skeletal muscles of the human body,* ed 2, St Louis, 2005, Mosby.)

Major antagonists:
Occipitalis—Frontalis
Frontalis—Occipitalis, corrugator supercilii, and procerus

Trigger points:
Occipitalis—Near attachment at the galea aponeurotica
Frontalis—Belly of the muscle superior to the eyebrow

Referred pain patterns:
Eye, ear, and the scalp superior to the ear and deep occipital pain

See Activity 9-4.

ACTIVITY 9-4

1. Draw and color the occipitofrontalis in the space provided.
2. Label the proximal and distal attachment points: *P* for proximal; *D* for distal.
3. Place an X on the trigger points.
4. Palpate this muscle; identify the attachment points and the belly of the muscle.
5. Move this muscle on yourself.

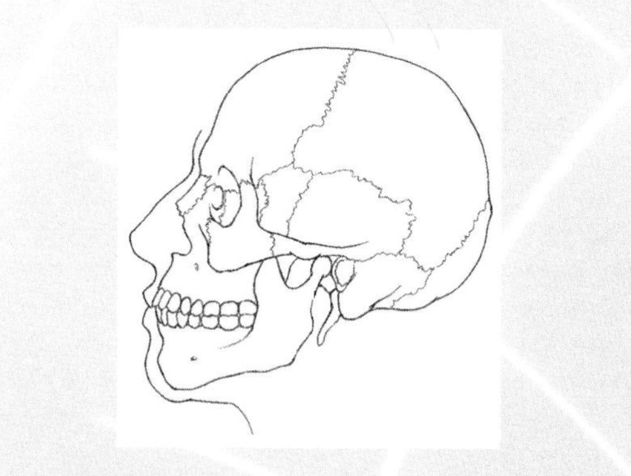

Much of the material in this section is modified from Edwards D: *Mosby's anatomy flashcards: the musculature, bones, and joints,* St Louis, 1998, Mosby.

Procerus (pro-SEHR-us)

Procerus means tall.

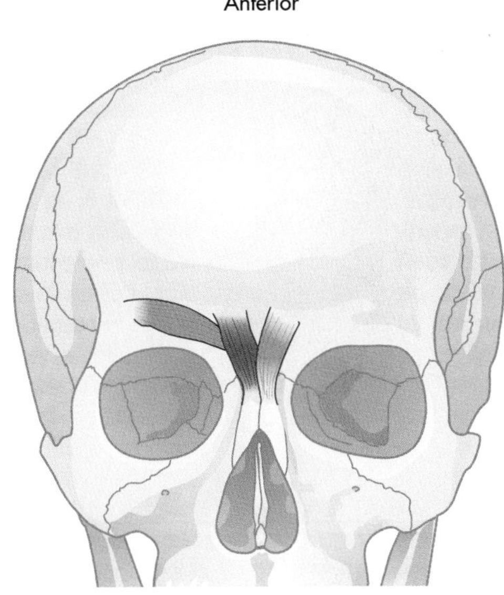

Concentric function:
Draws medial angle of the eyebrow downward and produces transverse wrinkles over the bridge of the nose.
From:
Fascia covering the inferior part of the nasal bone and the superior part of the lateral nasal cartilage
To:
Skin over the lower forehead between the eyebrows
Innervation:
Superior buccal branch of the facial nerve (cranial nerve VII)
Major synergist:
Corrugator supercilii
Major antagonist:
Occipitofrontalis
Trigger point:
No common trigger point identified

See Activity 9-5.

ACTIVITY 9-5

1. Draw and color the procerus in the space provided.
2. Label the proximal and distal attachment points: *P* for proximal; *D* for distal.
3. Palpate this muscle; identify the attachment points and the belly of the muscle.
4. Move this muscle on yourself.

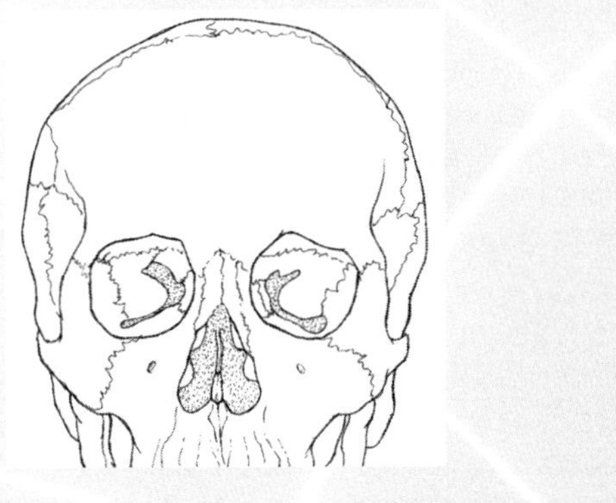

Corrugator supercilii (kor-U-GA-tor su-per-SIL-ee-eye)

Corrugator supercilii means to wrinkle the eyebrows.

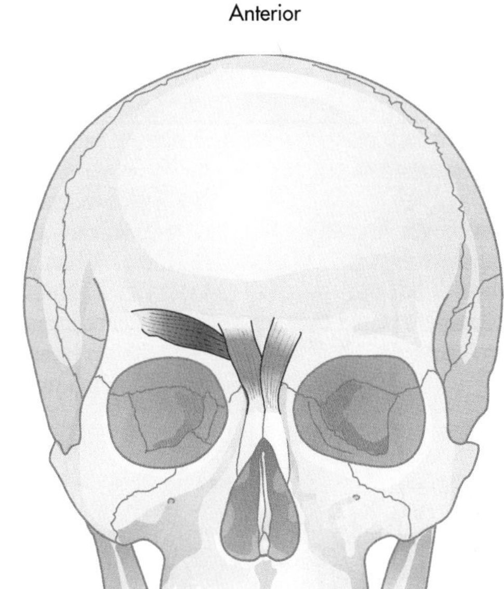

Concentric function:
Draws the eyebrow inferiorly and medially.
From:
Medial end of the superciliary arch of the frontal bone
To:
Skin deep to the medial portion of the eyebrow
Innervation:
Temporal branch of the facial nerve (cranial nerve VII)
Major synergist:
Procerus
Major antagonist:
Occipitofrontalis
Trigger point:
No common trigger point identified

See Activity 9-6.

ACTIVITY 9-6

1. Draw and color the corrugator supercilii in the space provided.
2. Label the proximal and distal attachment points: *P* for proximal; *D* for distal.
3. Palpate this muscle; identify the attachment points and the belly of the muscle.
4. Move this muscle on yourself.

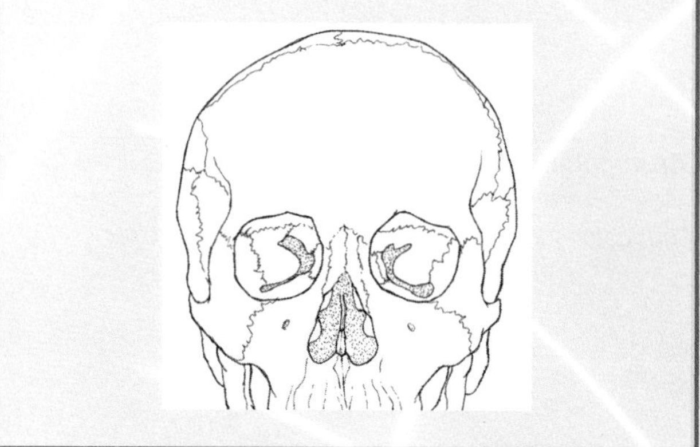

ACTIVITY 9-7

1. Draw and color the transverse and alar nasalis in the space provided.
2. Label the proximal and distal attachment points: *P* for proximal; *D* for distal.
3. Palpate this muscle; identify the attachment points and the belly of the muscle.
4. Move this muscle on yourself.

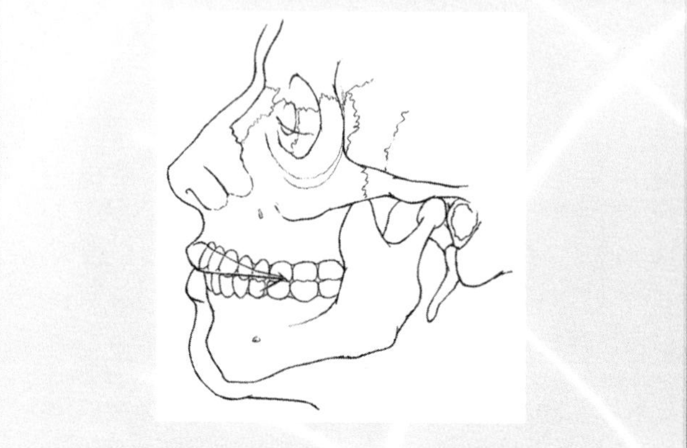

Nasalis (nay-SAL-iss)

Nasalis means related to the nose.

Lateral

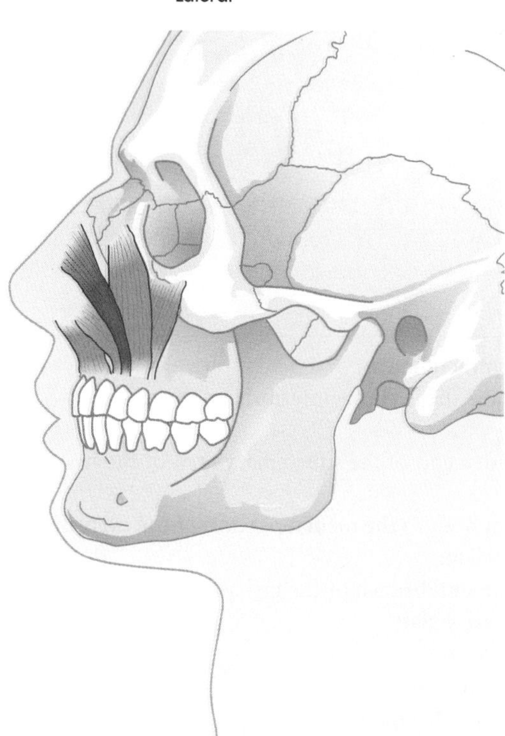

Concentric function:
Flares the nasal aperture.

From:
Transverse part—Maxilla, lateral to the nose
Alar part—Nasal notch of the maxilla and lesser alar cartilage

To:
Aponeurosis of the procerus and the same muscle on the opposite side and cartilage of the nose

Innervation:
Superior buccal branch of the facial nerve (cranial nerve VII)

Major synergist:
Levator labii superioris alaeque nasi

Major antagonist:
Depressor septi nasi

Trigger point:
No common trigger point identified

See Activity 9-7.

All subsequent activity figures in this chapter are taken from or modified from Edwards D: *Mosby's anatomy flashcards: musculature, bones, and joints,* St Louis, 1998, Mosby.

Ear Muscles

Auricularis (aw-RIK-u-lar-iss) muscles

Auricularis means belonging to the ear. As a group, these muscles move the ear.

Auricularis anterior

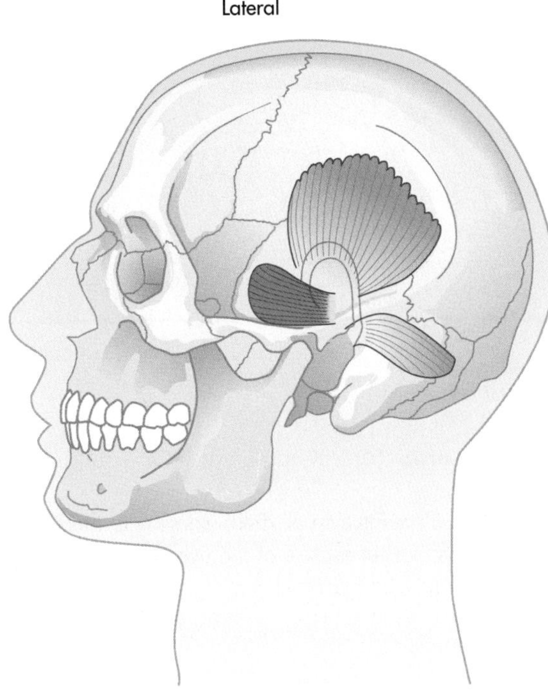

Concentric function:
Draws the ear anteriorly and tightens and moves the scalp.

From:
Lateral edge of the galea aponeurotica

To:
Spine of the helix of the ear

Innervation:
Temporal branches of the facial nerve (cranial nerve VII)

Auricularis posterior

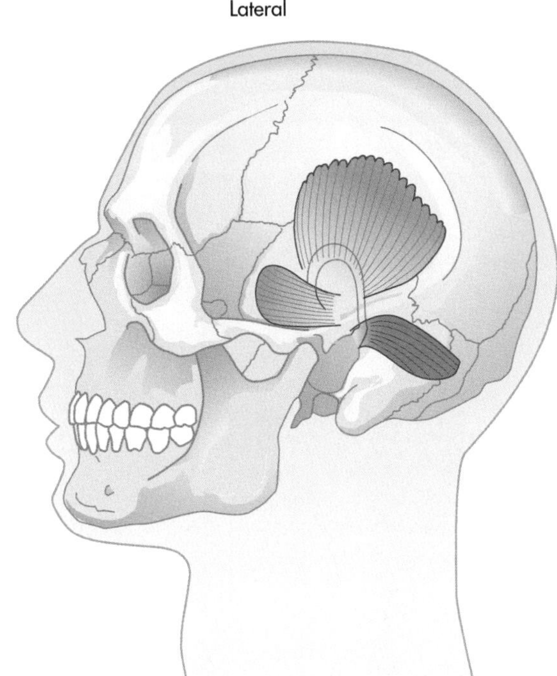

Concentric function:
Draws ear posteriorly.

From:
Mastoid area of the temporal bone

To:
Inferior part of the cranial part of the conchae of the ear

Innervation:
Posterior auricular branches of the facial nerve (cranial nerve VII)

Auricularis superior

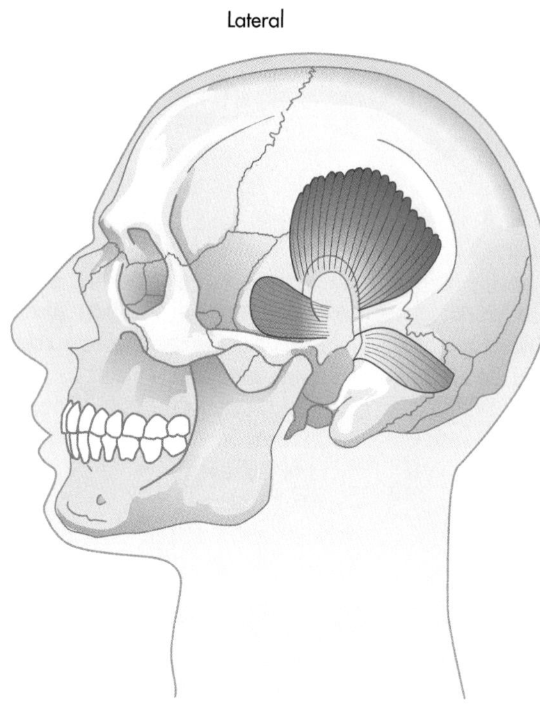

Concentric function:
Elevates the ear and tightens and moves the scalp.

From:
Galea aponeurotica

To:
Superior part of the cranial surface of the ear

Innervation:
Temporal branches of the facial nerve (cranial nerve VII)

Major synergist:
Temporoparietalis

Major antagonists:
Auricularis anterior and auricularis posterior are antagonistic

Trigger point:
No common trigger point identified

See Activity 9-8.

ACTIVITY 9-8

1. Draw and color the anterior, posterior, and superior auricular muscles in the space provided.
2. Label the proximal and distal attachment points: *P* for proximal; *D* for distal.
3. Palpate these muscles; identify the attachment points and the bellies of the muscles.
4. Move these muscles on yourself.

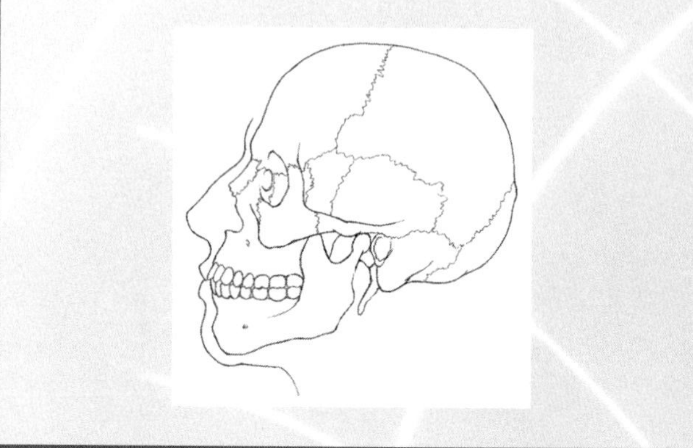

Eye Muscles

Orbicularis oculi (or-BIK-you-LAR-iss OK-you-li)

Orbicularis oculi means a small disk belonging to the eye. This muscle is a sphincter muscle of the eye and has three parts: orbital, palpebral, and lacrimal.

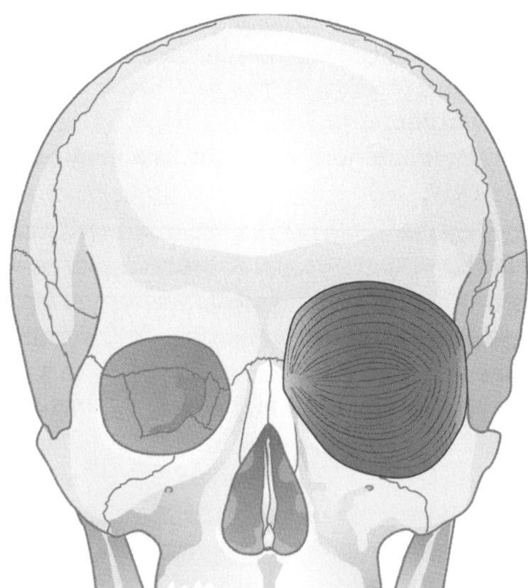

Concentric function:
Closes and squints the eye, depresses the upper eyelid, and elevates the lower eyelid.

From:
Orbital portion—Medial orbital margin
Palpebral (eyelid) portion—Medial palpebral ligament
Lacrimal portion—Lacrimal bone

ACTIVITY 9-9

1. Draw and color the orbicularis oculi in the space provided.
2. Label the proximal and distal attachment points: *P* for proximal; *D* for distal.
3. Place an X on the trigger point.
4. Palpate this muscle; identify the attachment points and the belly of the muscle.
5. Move this muscle on yourself.

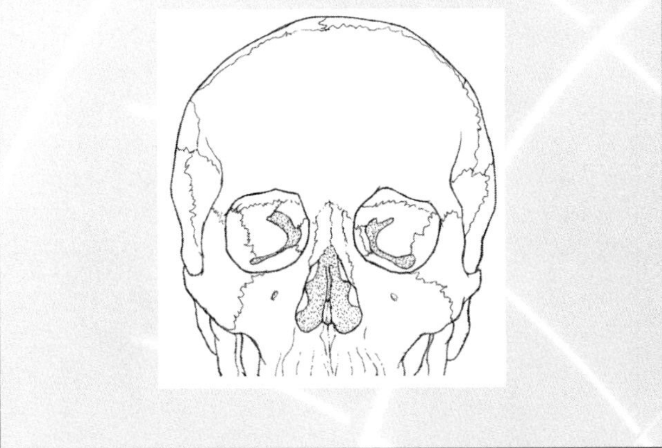

To:

Orbital portion—Medial orbital margin (this muscle returns to attach to the same place from which it originated)

Palpebral portion—Lateral palpebral ligament

Lacrimal portion—Medial palpebral raphe

Innervation:

Temporal and zygomatic branches of the facial nerve (cranial nerve VII)

Major synergists:

No major synergists

Major antagonist:

Levator palpebrae superioris

Trigger point:

Orbital area superior to the eyelid

Referred pain pattern:

To the nose

See Activity 9-9.

Muscles That Move the Mouth

Orbicularis oris (or-BIK-you-LAR-iss OR-iss)

Orbicularis oris means a small disk belonging to the mouth.

Anterior

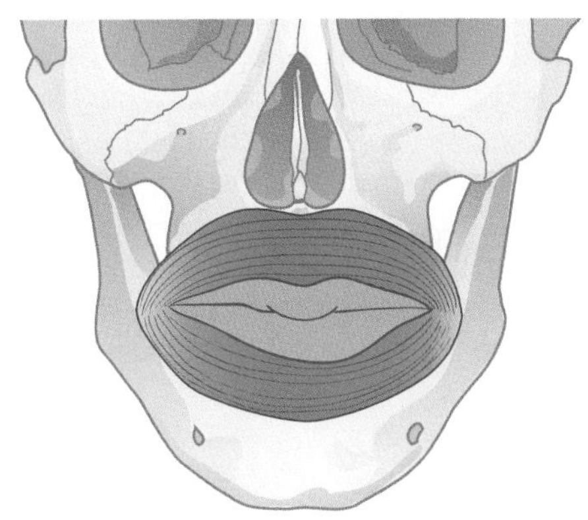

Concentric function:

Closes the mouth, protracts the lips (causes the lips to protrude anteriorly), and draws the angle of the mouth medially.

From and To:

Skin and fascia of the lips and tissue surrounding the lips

Innervation:

Lower buccal and mandibular branches of the facial nerve (cranial nerve VII)

Major synergist:

Mentalis

Major antagonists:

Depressor labii inferioris, platysma, and levators of the upper lip

Trigger points:

No common trigger points identified

Depressor anguli oris (de-PRESS-or ANG-you-li OR-iss)

Depressor anguli oris means to press down the corner belonging to the mouth.

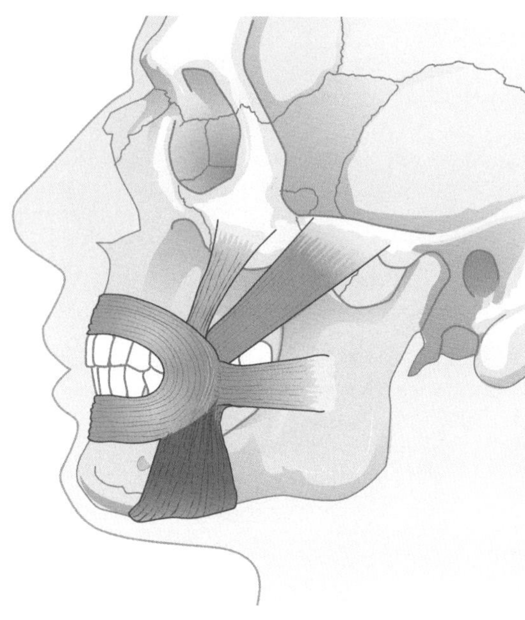

Concentric function:
Draws the angle of the mouth downward and laterally. (This muscle is involved in opening the mouth and in expressions of sadness.)

From:
Oblique line of the mandible, inferior and lateral to the depressor labii inferioris

To:
Angle of the mouth

Innervation:
Mandibular branch of the facial nerve (cranial nerve VII)

Major synergists:
Risorius and zygomaticus major

Major antagonists:
Levator anguli oris and zygomaticus major

Trigger points:
No common trigger points identified. Trigger points that form likely are located in the belly of the muscle.

Risorius (rih-ZOR-ee-us)

Risorius means to cause one to laugh.

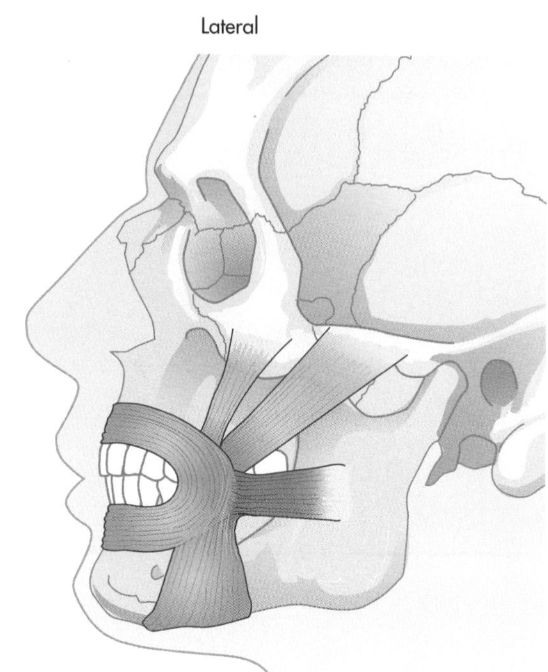

Concentric function:
Draws the angle of the mouth laterally.

From:
Parotid fascia superficial to the masseter muscle

To:
Fascia at the lateral angle of the mouth

Innervation:
Mandibular branches of the facial nerve (cranial nerve VII)

Major synergists:
Zygomaticus major and depressor anguli oris

Major antagonist:
Orbicularis oris

Trigger points:
No common trigger points identified. Trigger points that form likely are located in the belly of the muscle.

Zygomaticus major (ZYE-go-MAT-ik-us)

Zygomaticus means connected to the yoke or connector; *major* means larger.

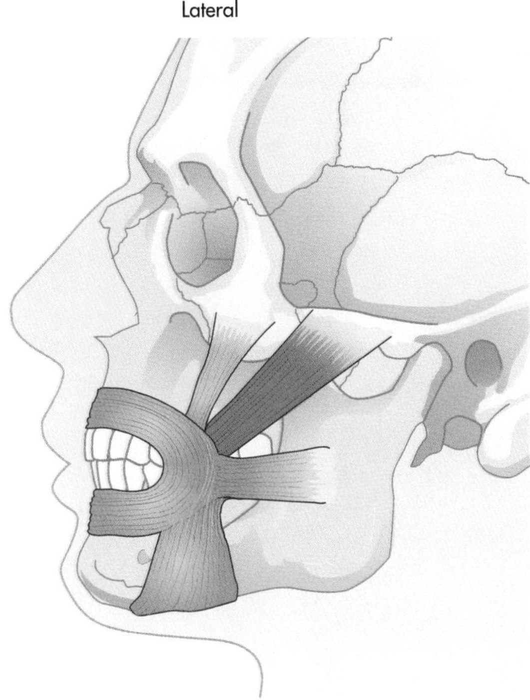

Concentric function:
Elevates and draws the angle of the mouth laterally (as in laughing).

From:
Zygomatic bone anterior to the zygomaticotemporal suture

To:
Angle of the mouth, blending with the levator anguli oris and the orbicularis oris

Innervation:
Buccal branches of the facial nerve (cranial nerve VII)

Major synergist:
Levator anguli oris

Major antagonist:
Depressor anguli oris

Trigger points:
No common trigger points identified. Trigger points that form likely are located in the belly of the muscle.

Zygomaticus minor (ZYE-go-MAT-ik-us)

Zygomaticus means connected to the yoke or connector; *minor* means smaller.

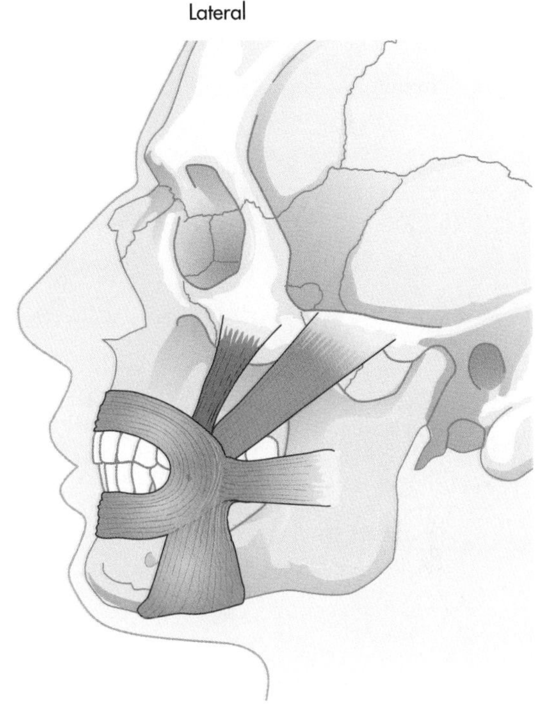

Concentric function:
Elevates and everts the upper lip and produces the nasolabial sulcus.

From:
Lateral surface of the zygomatic bone, immediately posterior to the zygomaticomaxillary suture

To:
Angle of the mouth, blending with the levator labii superioris

Innervation:
Buccal branches of the facial nerve (cranial nerve VII)

Major synergists:
Levator labii superioris and levator labii superioris alaeque nasi

Major antagonist:
Orbicularis oris

Trigger points:
No common trigger points identified. Trigger points that form likely are located in the belly of the muscle.

Levator labii superioris (le-VAY-tor LAY-bee-eye su-PEER-ee-OR-iss)

Levator labii means one that raises the lip; *superioris* means above or upper.

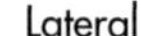

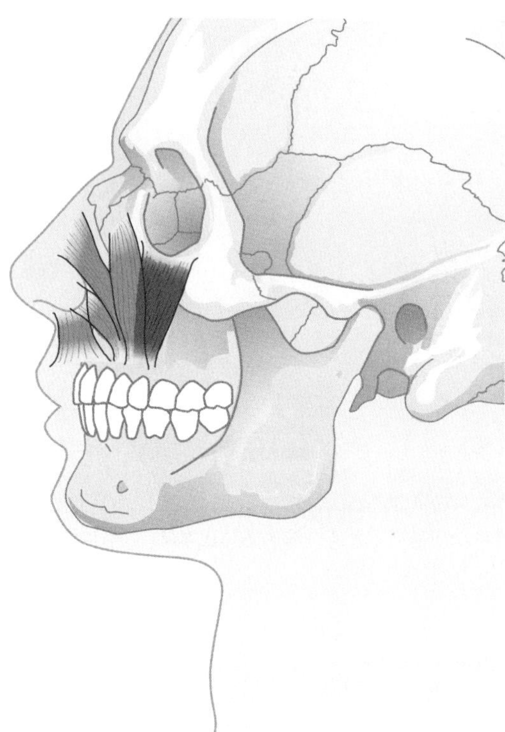

Concentric function:
Elevates and everts the upper lip.

From:
Maxilla and zygomatic bone, from the lower margin of the orbital opening immediately superior to the infraorbital foramen

To:
Muscular substance of the lateral part of the upper lip

Innervation:
Buccal branches of the facial nerve (cranial nerve VII)

Major synergists:
Levator labii superioris alaeque nasi and zygomaticus minor

Major antagonist:
Orbicularis oris

Trigger points:
No common trigger points identified. Trigger points that form likely are located in the belly of the muscle.

Levator labii superioris alaeque nasi (le-VAY-tor LAY-bee-eye su-PEER-ee-OR-iss AL-ek-wee NAY-see)

Levator labii and *alaeque nasi* mean one that raises the lip and belonging to the wing of the nose, respectively; *superioris* means above or upper.

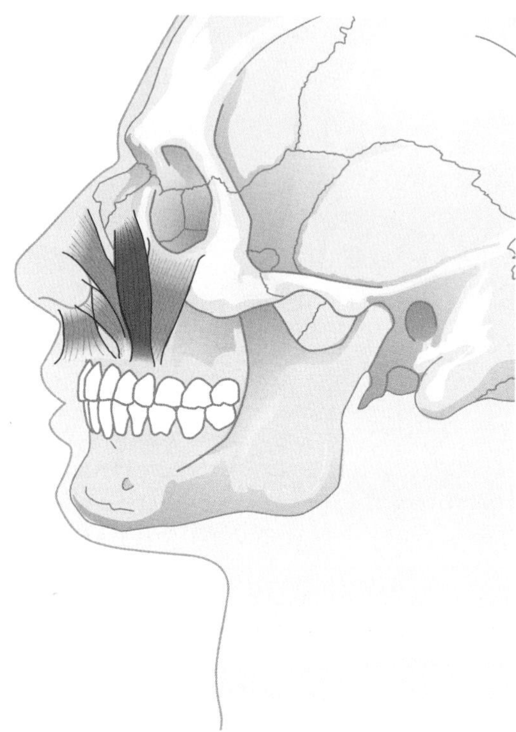

Concentric function:
Elevates and everts the upper lip and flares the nostril.

From:
Frontal process of the maxilla

To:
The muscle divides into the lateral slip, which inserts into the lateral part of the upper lip, and the medial slip, which inserts into the greater alar cartilage and the skin of the nose.

Innervation:
Buccal branches of the facial nerve (cranial nerve VII)

Major synergists:
Levator labii superioris and zygomaticus minor

Major antagonists:
Orbicularis oris and depressor septi nasi

Trigger points:
No common trigger points identified. Trigger points that form likely are located in the belly of the muscle.

Depressor labii inferioris (de-PRESS-or LAY-bee-eye in-FEAR-ee-or-iss)

Depressor labii means to press down the lip; *inferioris* means lower or beneath.

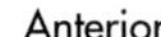

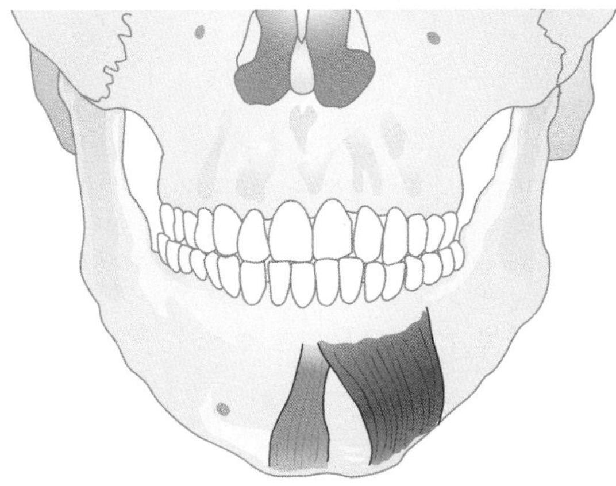

Concentric function:
Depresses, everts, and draws the lower lip laterally.

From:
Oblique line of the mandible, between the symphysis menti and the mental foramen

To:
Skin of the lower lip, blending with the orbicularis oris

Innervation:
Buccal branches of the facial nerve (cranial nerve VII)

Major synergist:
Platysma

Major antagonists:
Mentalis and orbicularis oris

Trigger points:
No common trigger points identified. Trigger points that form likely are located in the belly of the muscle.

Levator anguli oris (le-VAY-tor ANG-you-li OR-iss)

Levator anguli oris means one that raises the corner of the mouth.

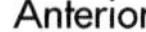

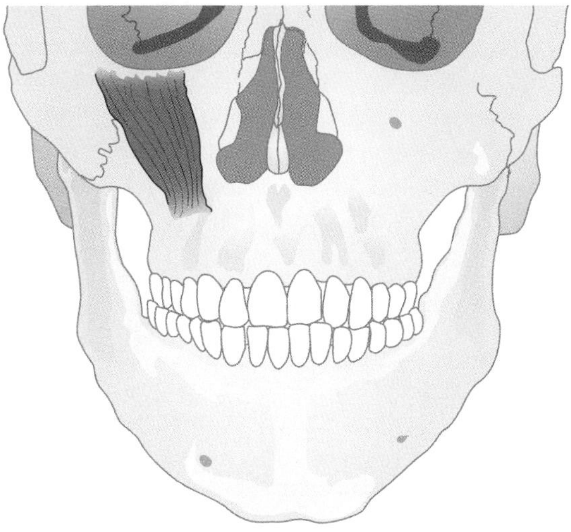

Concentric function:
Elevates the angle of the mouth and produces the nasolabial sulcus.

From:
Canine fossa of the maxilla, just inferior to the infraorbital foramen

To:
Angle of the mouth, blending with the zygomaticus major, depressor anguli oris, and orbicularis oris

Innervation:
Buccal branches of the facial nerve (cranial nerve VII)

Major synergist:
Zygomaticus major

Major antagonist:
Depressor anguli oris

Trigger points:
No common trigger points identified. Trigger points that form likely are located in the belly of the muscle.

Buccinator (BUK-sin-ate-or)

Buccinator means trumpeter.

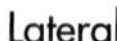

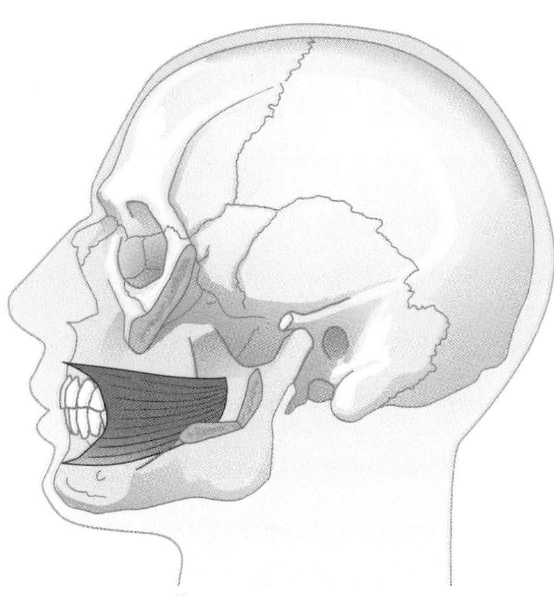

Concentric function:
Compresses the cheek against the teeth. (This muscle aids in mastication and forcing air out between the lips.)

From:
Alveolar processes of the maxilla and mandible and the pterygomandibular raphe

To:
Angle of the mouth

Innervation:
Lower buccal branches of the facial nerve (cranial nerve VII)

Major synergists:
No major synergist

Major antagonists:
No major antagonist

Trigger points:
No common trigger points identified. Trigger points that form likely are located in the belly of the muscle.

Platysma (PLAH-tiz-ma)

Platysma means a flat plate.

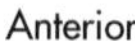

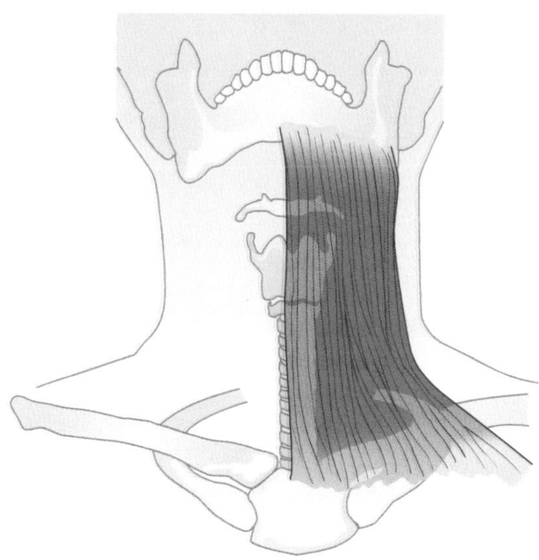

Concentric function:
Draws up the skin of the superior chest and neck, creating ridges of skin in the neck; depresses and draws the lower lip laterally; and depresses the mandible at the temporomandibular joint.

From:
Fascia covering the superior parts of the pectoralis major and deltoid

To:
Mandible and the fascia of the lower face (blending with the contralateral platysma and many other muscles of facial expression)

Innervation:
Cervical branch of the facial nerve (cranial nerve VII)

Major synergists:
Depressor labii inferioris and depressors of the mandible

Major antagonists:
Mentalis, orbicularis oris, and elevators of the mandible

Trigger points:
No common trigger points identified. Trigger points that form likely are located in the belly of the muscle.

Mentalis (men-TAL-iss)

Mentalis means related to the chin.

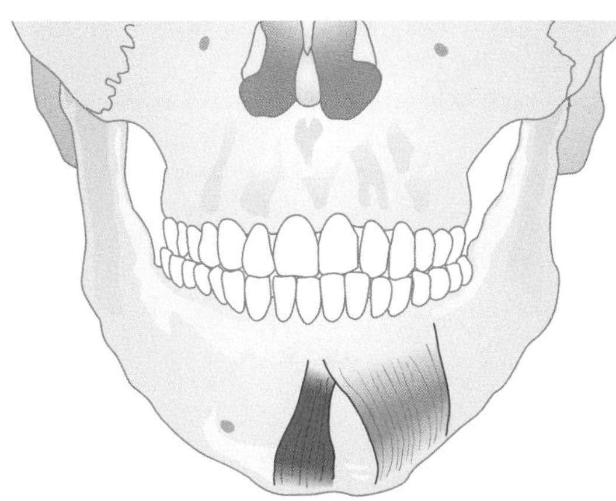

Concentric function:
Elevates, everts, and protracts the lower lip and wrinkles the skin of the chin.

From:
Incisive fossa of the mandible

To:
Skin of the chin

Innervation:
Mandibular marginal branch of the facial nerve (cranial nerve VII)

Major synergists:
Orbicularis oris and depressor labii inferioris

Major antagonists:
Platysma and depressor labii inferioris

Trigger points:
No common trigger points identified. Trigger points that form likely are located in the belly of the muscle.

See Activity 9-10.

Muscles of Mastication (Chewing)

Four main pairs of muscles are involved in mastication (chewing) because they move the temporomandibular joint (TMJ). These muscles are powerful. The masseter and temporalis muscles are the prime movers of jaw closure (elevation of the mandible at the TMJ). The medial and lateral pterygoid muscles provide side-to-side grinding movements. Tension and tone imbalance in these groups of muscles are common causes of TMJ dysfunction. The buccinator muscles keep the cheeks close to the teeth to help us chew. The tongue is composed of specialized muscle fibers that curl, squeeze, and fold the tongue.

ACTIVITY 9-10

1. Draw and color the following muscles in the space provided: orbicularis oris, depressor anguli oris, risorius, zygomaticus major and zygomaticus minor, levator labii superioris, levator labii superioris alaeque nasi, depressor labii inferioris, levator anguli oris, buccinator, platysma, and mentalis.
2. Label the proximal and distal attachment points: *P* for proximal; *D* for distal.
3. Palpate these muscles; identify the attachment points and the bellies of the muscles.
4. Move these muscles on yourself.

Note: Levators help us smile.
Depressors help us frown.

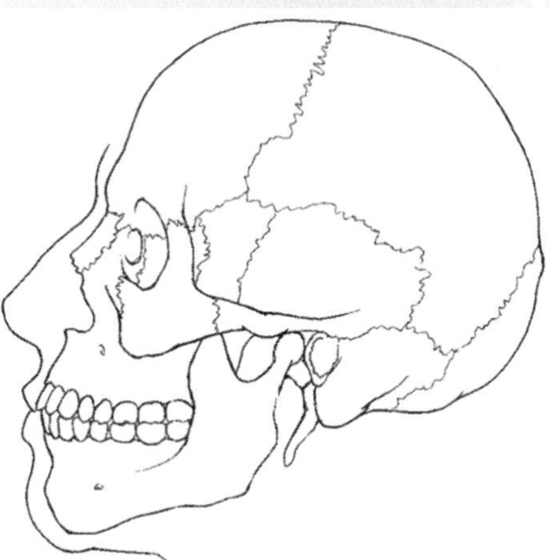

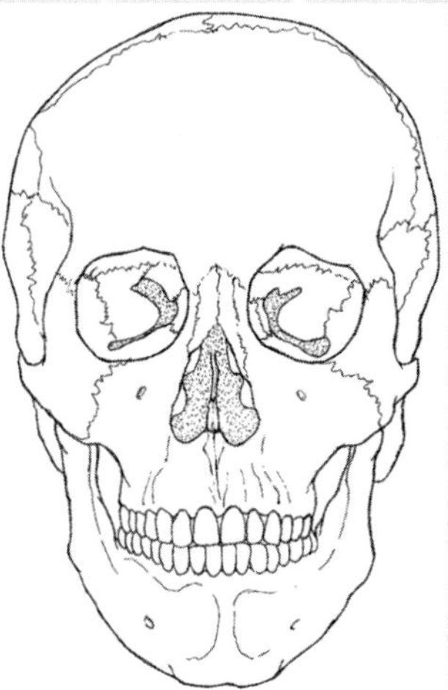

Masseter (MAS-sit-er)

Masseter means one who chews.

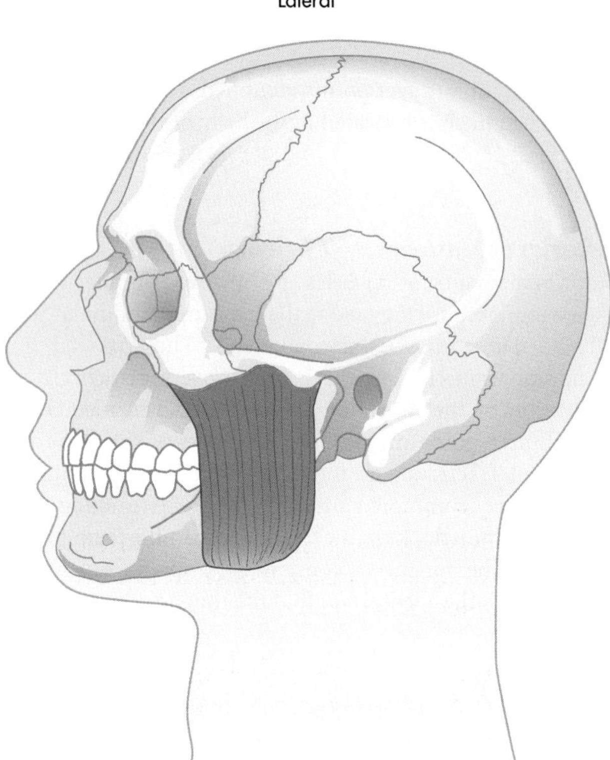

Concentric function:
Elevates the mandible at the TMJ.

Eccentric function:
Restrains depression of the mandible.

From:
Superficial portion—Anterior two thirds of the inferior border of the zygomatic arch
Deep portion—Medial surface of the zygomatic arch

To:
Coronoid process, ramus, and angle of the mandible

Innervation:
Mandibular division of the trigeminal nerve (cranial nerve V)

Major synergists:
Temporalis and medial pterygoid

Major antagonists:
Suprahyoid muscles

Trigger points:
Superior at the tendinous junction near the zygomatic arch and in the belly of the muscle

Referred pain patterns:
Upper jaw (maxillary region) and lower jaw (mandibular region), the ear, and the eyebrow

See Activity 9-11.

ACTIVITY 9-11

1. Draw and color the masseter in the space provided.
2. Label the proximal and distal attachment points: *P* for proximal; *D* for distal.
3. Place an X on the trigger points.
4. Palpate this muscle; identify the attachment points and the belly of the muscle.
5. Move this muscle on yourself.

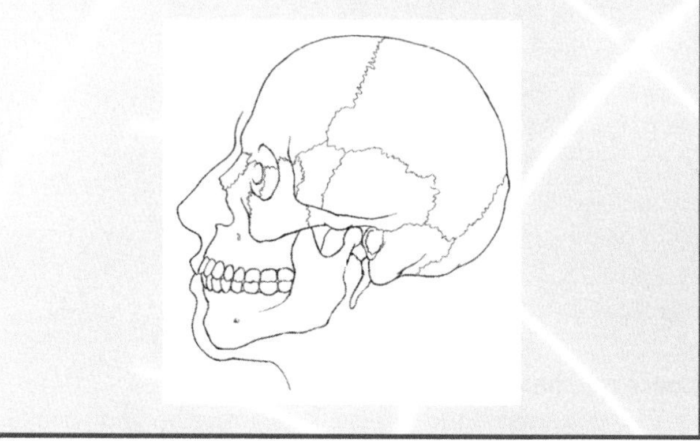

Temporalis (temp-or-AL-iss)

Temporalis means related to the temple of the head.

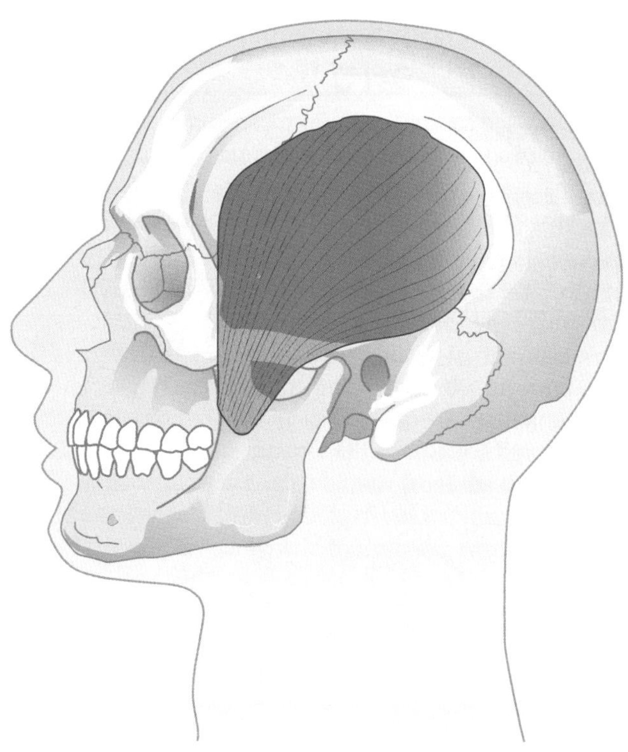

Concentric function:
Elevates the mandible at the TMJ.

Eccentric function:
Restrains depression of the mandible.

ACTIVITY 9-12

1. Draw and color the temporalis in the space provided.
2. Label the proximal and distal attachment points: *P* for proximal; *D* for distal.
3. Place an X on the trigger points.
4. Palpate this muscle; identify the attachment points and the belly of the muscle.
5. Move this muscle on yourself.

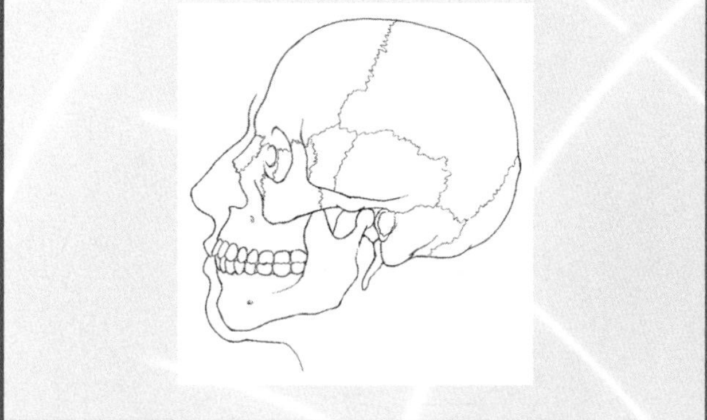

From:
Temporal fossa and deep surface of the temporal fascia

To:
Ramus of the mandible and medial surface and anterior border of the coronoid process

Innervation:
Anterior and posterior deep temporal nerve from the mandibular portion of the trigeminal nerve (cranial nerve V)

Major synergists:
Masseter and medial pterygoid

Major antagonists:
Suprahyoid muscles

Trigger points:
Anterior, medial, and posterior along the inferior aspect of the muscle near the tendinous junction at the coronoid process of the mandible

Referred pain patterns:
Temporal region, eyebrow, and upper teeth

See Activity 9-12.

Lateral (external) pterygoid (TER-ih-goyd)

Pterygoid means wing shaped; *lateral* means to the side.

Lateral

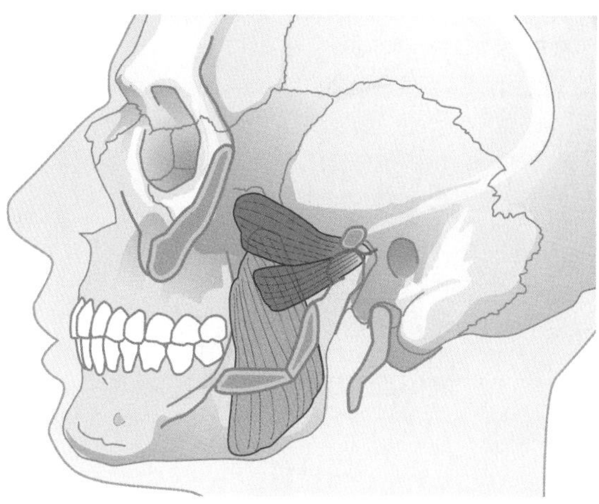

Concentric functions:
Protraction and contralateral deviation (movement to the opposite side) of the mandible at the temporomandibular joint

From:
Superior head—Greater wing of the sphenoid bone
Inferior head—Lateral surface of the lateral pterygoid plate of the sphenoid bone

To:
Anterior surface of the neck of the mandible and articular capsule and disk of the TMJ

Innervation:
Mandibular division of the trigeminal nerve (cranial nerve V)

Major synergist:
Medial pterygoid

Major antagonists:
Opposite-sided lateral and medial pterygoids

Trigger points:
Belly of both divisions of the muscle

Referred pain pattern:
Cheek and TMJ

The student should note that one palpates the lateral pterygoid from inside the mouth. See Activity 9-13.

ACTIVITY 9-13

1. Draw and color the lateral pterygoid in the space provided.
2. Label the proximal and distal attachment points: *P* for proximal; *D* for distal.
3. Place an X on the trigger points.
4. Palpate this muscle; identify the attachment points and the belly of the muscle.
5. Move this muscle on yourself.

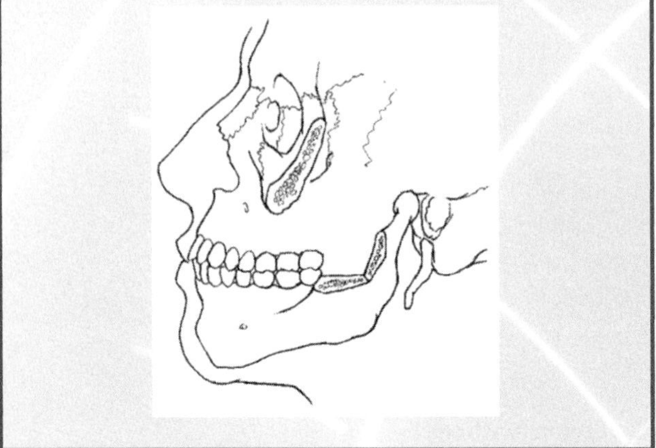

ACTIVITY 9-14

1. Draw and color the medial pterygoid in the space provided.
2. Label the proximal and distal attachment points: *P* for proximal; *D* for distal.
3. Place an X on the trigger points.
4. Palpate this muscle; identify the attachment points and the belly of the muscle.
5. Move this muscle on yourself.

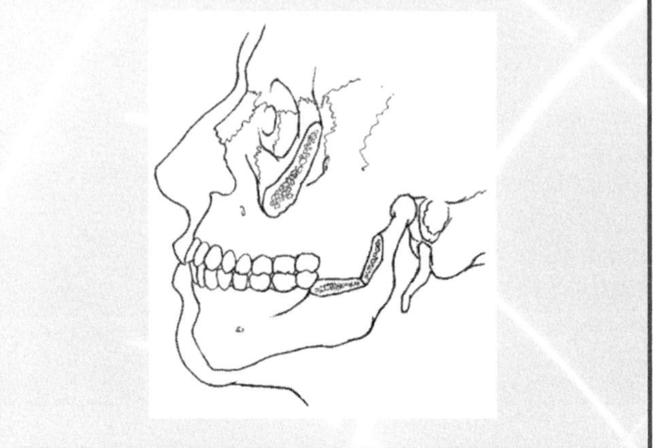

Medial (internal) pterygoid (TER-ih-goyd)

Pterygoid means wing shaped; *medial* means related to the middle.

Lateral

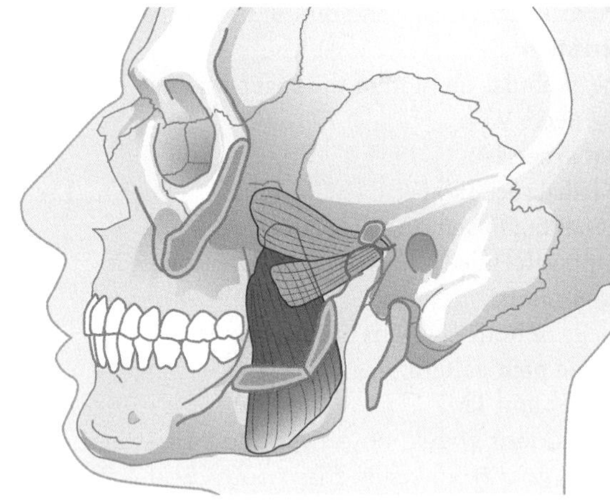

Concentric function:
Elevation, protraction, and contralateral deviation (movement to the opposite side) of the mandible at the TMJ

From:
Medial surface of the lateral pterygoid plate of the sphenoid bone, pyramidal surface of the palatine bone, and tuberosity of the maxilla

To:
Internal surface of the angle and inferior ramus of the mandible

Innervation:
Mandibular division of the trigeminal nerve (cranial nerve V)

Major synergists:
Lateral pterygoid, temporalis, and masseter

Major antagonists:
Suprahyoid muscles and opposite-sided lateral and medial pterygoids

Trigger points:
Belly of the muscle, with best access from inside the mouth

Referred pain pattern:
Back of the throat and into the ear

See Activity 9-14.

Muscles of the Neck

The sternocleidomastoid muscles divide the neck into the anterior and posterior triangles. Muscles of the neck move the neck at the cervical spinal joints. Most of the muscles of the anterior neck also assist in swallowing. Muscles of the neck that attach to the head provide movements of the head on the neck at the atlanto-occipital joint. The sternocleidomastoid muscles are the major neck flexors. The sternocleidomastoid and deeper neck muscles, including the scalenes, and several straplike muscles of the vertebral column at the back of the neck provide lateral flexion of the neck. The posterior muscles of the neck, including the upper trapezius and other deeper musculature, provide extension of the neck. The sternocleidomastoid assists in head extension if the neck is stabilized. Tension and muscle imbalances of the neck muscles are a major cause of headaches and arm and shoulder pain and dysfunction because of impingement of the cervical and brachial plexuses of nerves. These muscles do more than just provide head movement. They isometrically act to stabilize and balance the head in an upright, eyes-forward position and therefore are involved in righting and postural reflexes. These muscles often act in sequence with trunk flexors and extensors. Therefore neck muscle problems are a common finding with low back pain and with hamstring and quadriceps dysfunction. Because the head is so heavy, these muscles often become short and increase in tension especially with a postural imbalance. Because many of these muscles attach to the upper ribs, they function as accessory breathing muscles and can become dysfunctional if these muscles are used excessively during breathing. In massage that targets this area, one must address muscles of the region effectively while being cautious of underlying nerves and vessels (Figures 9-19 and 9-20).

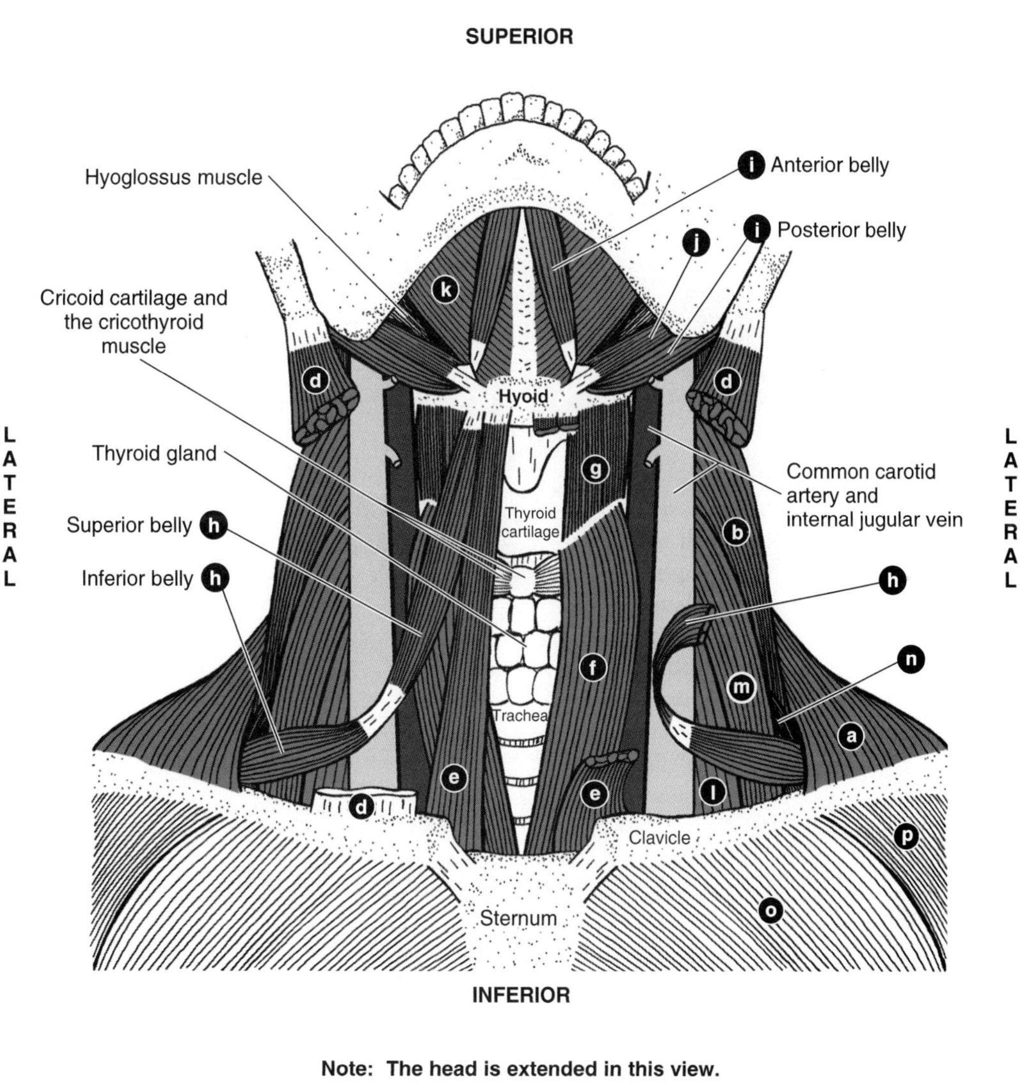

Note: The head is extended in this view.

a. Trapezius	i. Digastric
b. Levator scapulae	j. Stylohyoid
c. Platysma (removed)	k. Mylohyoid
d. Sternocleidomastoid (cut)	l. Anterior scalene
e. Sternohyoid (cut on our right)	m. Middle scalene
f. Sternothyroid	n. Posterior scalene
g. Thyrohyoid	o. Pectoralis major
h. Omohyoid (cut and reflected on our right)	p. Deltoid

Figure 9-19
Anterior view of the neck (intermediate). (Modified from Muscolino JE: *The muscular system manual: the skeletal muscles of the human body,* ed 2, St Louis, 2005, Mosby.)

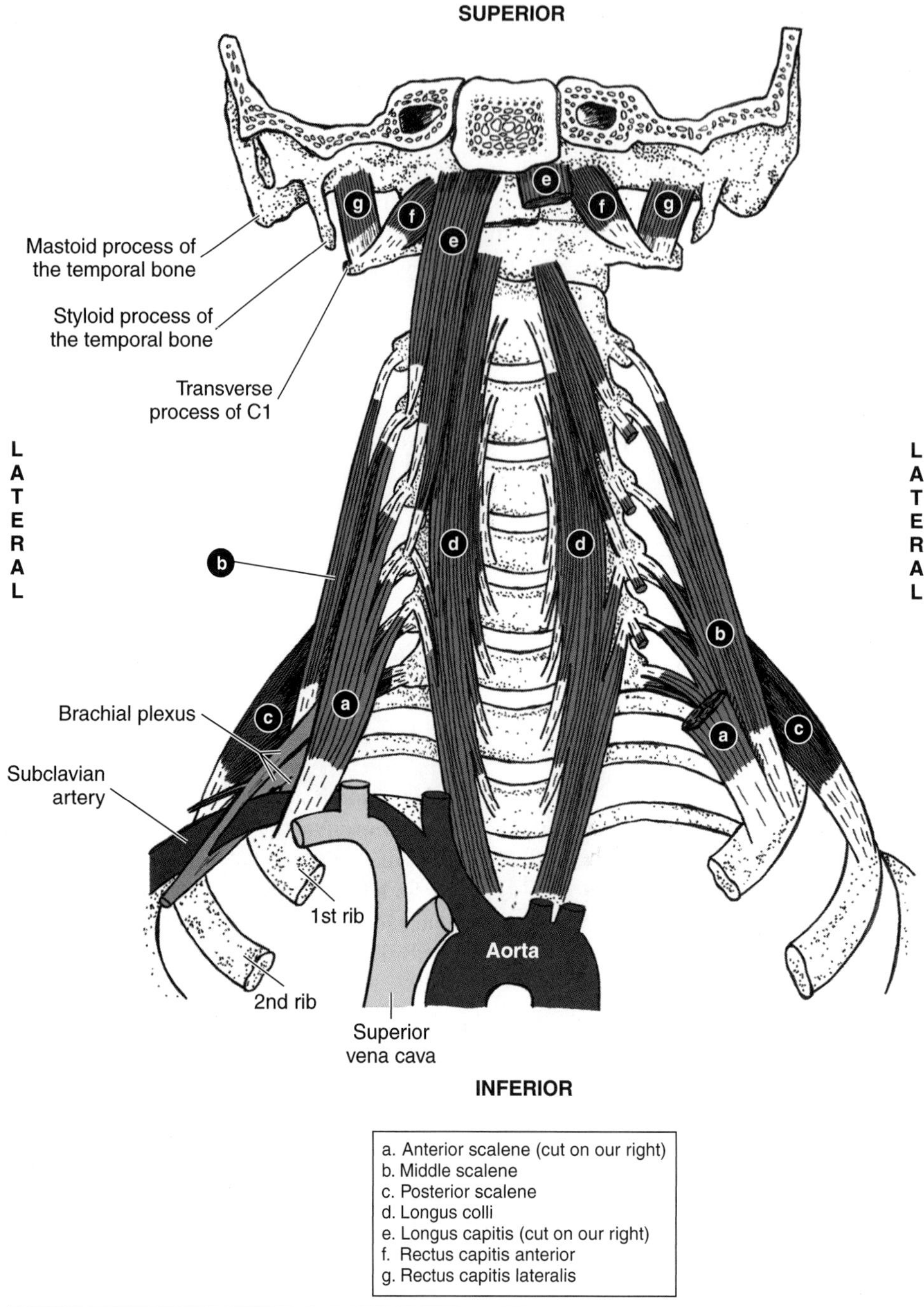

a. Anterior scalene (cut on our right)
b. Middle scalene
c. Posterior scalene
d. Longus colli
e. Longus capitis (cut on our right)
f. Rectus capitis anterior
g. Rectus capitis lateralis

Figure 9-20
Anterior view of the neck (deep). (Modified from Muscolino JE: *The muscular system manual: the skeletal muscles of the human body,* ed 2, St Louis, 2005, Mosby.)

Sternocleidomastoid (STER-no-CLY-do-mas-toyd)

Sternocleidomastoid means connecting to the sternum, clavicle, and mastoid process of the skull.

Anterior

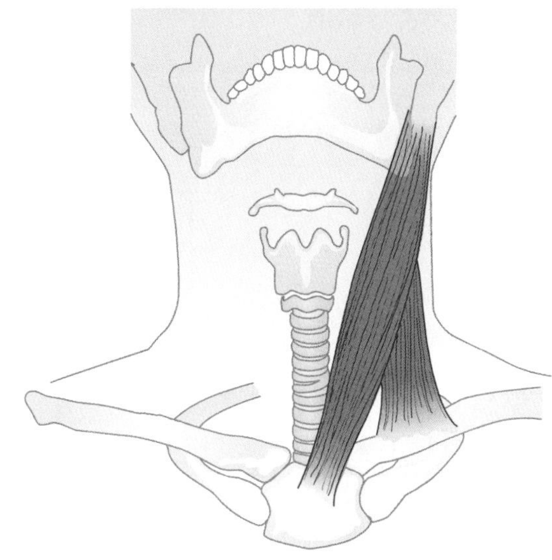

ACTIVITY 9-15

1. Draw and color the sternocleidomastoid in the space provided.
2. Label the proximal and distal attachment points: *P* for proximal; *D* for distal.
3. Place an X on the trigger points.
4. Palpate this muscle; identify the attachment points and the belly of the muscle.
5. Move this muscle on yourself.

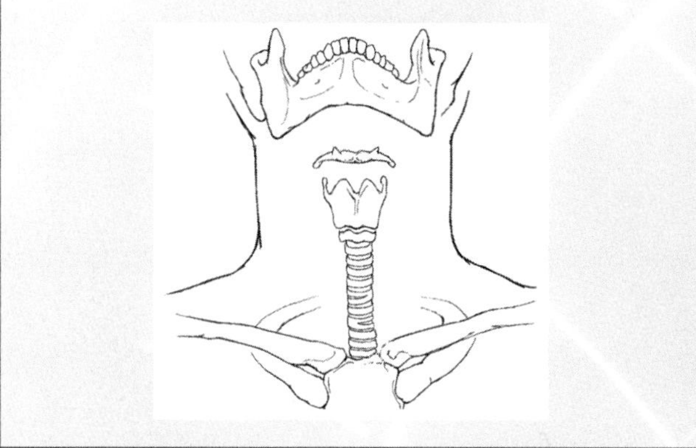

Concentric function:

Flexion of the neck at the spinal joints, lateral flexion and contralateral rotation of the neck and the head at the spinal joints, and extension of the head at the atlanto-occipital joint

Eccentric function:

Restrains extension of the neck, contralateral lateral flexion of the neck and head, ipsilateral rotation of the neck and head, and flexion of the head.

Isometric function:

Assists in stabilizing the head in space when the mandible moves.

From:

Sternal head—Superior aspect of anterior surface of manubrium of the sternum

Clavicular head—Superior border of the anterior surface of the medial third of the clavicle

To:

Superior surface of the mastoid process and lateral half of the superior nuchal line of occiput

Innervation:

Spinal accessory nerve (cranial nerve XI) and ventral rami of second and third cervical spinal nerves

Major synergists:

Scalenes, opposite-sided splenius capitis, and suboccipital muscles

Major antagonists:

Upper trapezius and semispinalis capitis (opposite-sided sternocleidomastoid)

Trigger points:

Several points along the entire length of both divisions of the muscle

Referred pain pattern:

Head and face, particularly the occipital region, ear, and forehead. Autonomic nervous system phenomena and proprioceptive disturbances are common.

See Activity 9-15.

Anterior Triangle of the Neck

Suprahyoid muscles. As a group these muscles are located superior to the hyoid bone. These muscles can elevate the hyoid bone, which affects the movement of the tongue and other movements necessary for swallowing. If the mandible and hyoid bone are stabilized, this group of muscles can act as weak accessory flexors of the neck at the spinal joints.

Digastric (dye-GAS-trik)

Digastric means two bellies.

Anterior

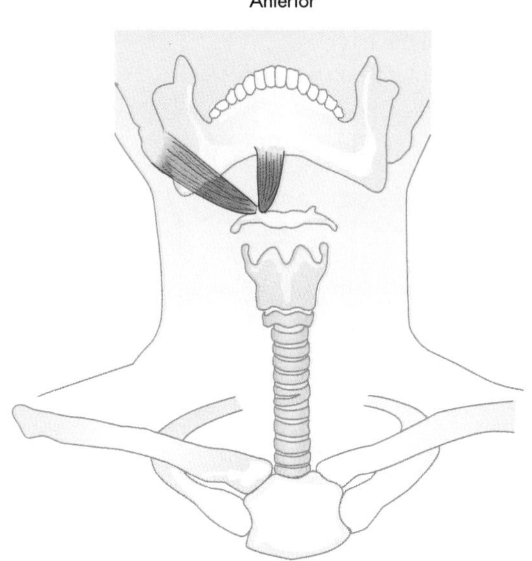

Concentric function:
Elevates the hyoid and depresses the mandible at the TMJ. (The posterior belly of this muscle is especially active in swallowing and chewing.)

Eccentric function:
Restrains depression of the hyoid and elevation of the mandible.

Isometric function:
Stabilizes the hyoid bone.

From:
Posterior belly—Mastoid notch of the temporal bone
Anterior belly—Digastric fossa on the base of the mandible

To:
Body of the greater cornu of the hyoid bone via a fibrous sling of tissue

Innervation:
Trigeminal (cranial nerve V) and facial (cranial nerve VII) nerves

Major synergists:
Other suprahyoids

Major antagonists:
Infrahyoids, temporalis, and masseter

Trigger points:
Belly of each division of the muscle

Referred pain pattern:
Sternocleidomastoid area and bottom front teeth

See Activity 9-16.

ACTIVITY 9-16

1. Draw and color the digastric in the space provided.
2. Label the proximal and distal attachment points: *P* for proximal; *D* for distal.
3. Place an X on the trigger points.
4. Palpate this muscle; identify the attachment points and the bellies of the muscle.
5. Move this muscle on yourself.

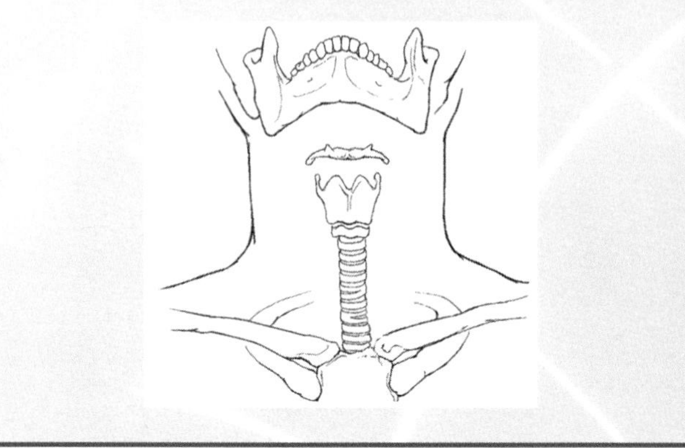

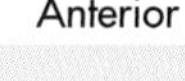

Stylohyoid (STY-low-HY-oyd)

Stylohyoid means pen and U-shaped.

Anterior

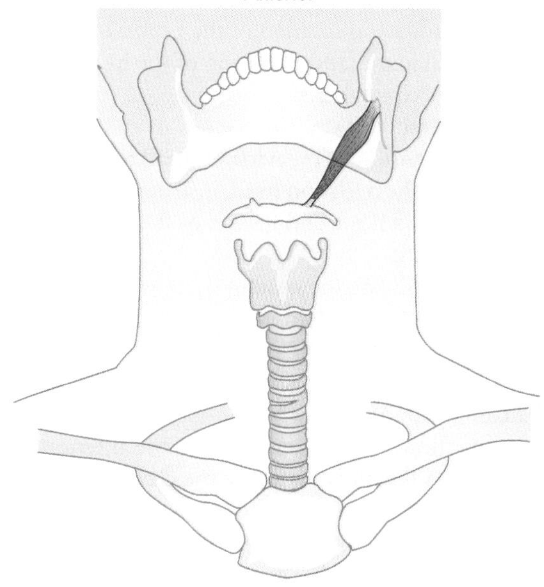

Concentric function:
Elevates the hyoid. (This muscle is effective at elevating the tongue.)

Eccentric function:
Restrains depression of the hyoid.

Isometric function:
Stabilizes the hyoid bone.

From:
Posterior surface of the styloid process

To:
Body of the hyoid bone, at the junction with the greater cornu

Innervation:
Facial nerve (cranial nerve VII, stylohyoid branch)
Major synergists:
Other suprahyoids
Major antagonists:
Infrahyoids, temporalis, and masseter
Trigger points:
Likely to form in the belly

Mylohyoid (MY-lo-HY-oyd)

Mylohyoid means molar and U-shaped.

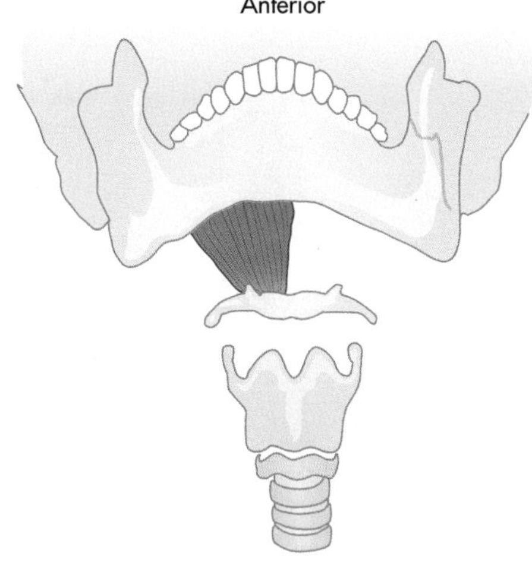

Concentric function:
Elevates the hyoid and depresses the mandible at the TMJ. (This muscle is important in elevating the floor of the mouth during the first stage of swallowing.)
Eccentric function:
Restrains depression of the hyoid and elevation of the mandible.
Isometric function:
Stabilizes the hyoid bone.
From:
Mylohyoid line of the mandible
To:
Posterior fibers—Anterior surface of the body of the hyoid bone near the inferior border
Middle and anterior fibers—Median fibrous raphe stretching from the symphysis menti to the hyoid bone
Innervation:
Mylohyoid branch of the inferior alveolar nerve of the trigeminal nerve (cranial nerve V)
Major synergists:
Other suprahyoids
Major antagonists:
Infrahyoids, temporalis, and masseter
Trigger points:
Likely to form in the belly

Geniohyoid (JEEN-ee-oh-HY-oyd)

Geniohyoid means chin and U-shaped.

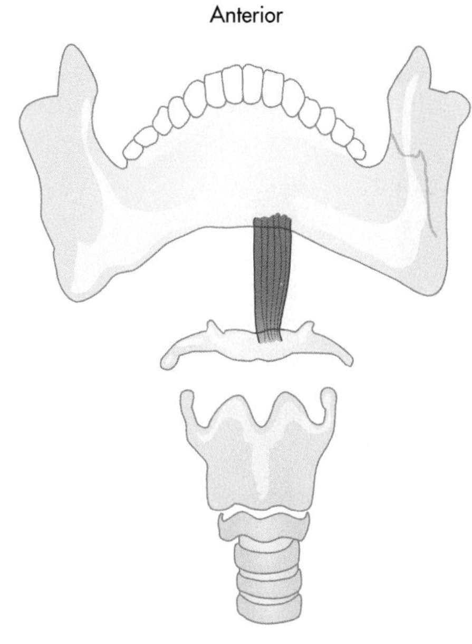

Concentric function:
Elevates the hyoid (this muscle elevates the tongue and draws it forward) and depresses the mandible at the TMJ.
Eccentric function:
Restrains depression of the hyoid and elevation of the mandible.
Isometric function:
Stabilizes the hyoid bone.
From:
Inferior mental spine on the posterior surface of the symphysis of the mandible
To:
Anterior surface of the body of the hyoid bone
Innervation:
Hypoglossal nerve (cranial nerve XII)
Major synergists:
Other suprahyoids
Major antagonists:
Infrahyoids, temporalis, and masseter
Trigger points:
Likely to form in the belly

Infrahyoid muscles

These muscles are located inferior to the hyoid bone. As a group they depress the hyoid bone and influence swallowing and the production of sound.

Sternohyoid (STERN-oh-HY-oyd)

Sternohyoid means chest and U-shaped.

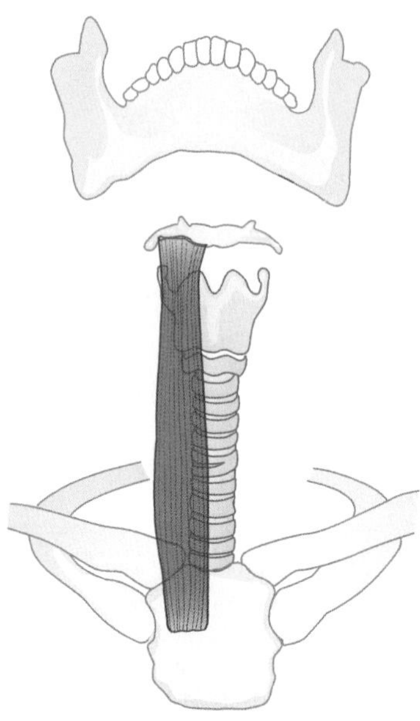

Concentric function:
Depresses the hyoid. (This muscle plays a part in speech and mastication.)

Eccentric function:
Restrains elevation of the hyoid.

Isometric function:
Stabilizes the hyoid bone.

From:
Posterior surface of the medial end of the clavicle, posterior sternoclavicular ligament, and superior and posterior parts of the manubrium

To:
Inferior border of the body of the hyoid bone

Innervation:
Branches from the ansa cervicalis of the cervical plexus

Major synergists:
Thyrohyoid and omohyoid

Major antagonists:
Suprahyoids

Trigger points:
Likely to form in the belly

Sternothyroid (STERN-oh-THY-royd)

Sternothyroid means chest and shaped like a shield.

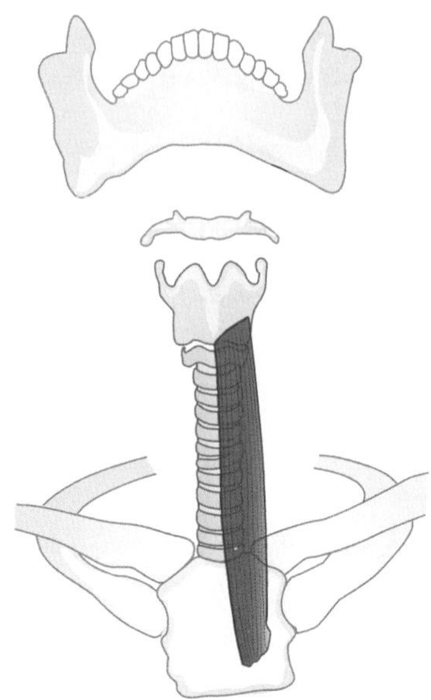

Concentric function:
Depresses the thyroid cartilage.

Eccentric function:
Restrains elevation of the thyroid cartilage.

Isometric function:
Assists stabilization of the hyoid bone through its pull on the thyroid cartilage.

From:
Posterior surface of the manubrium and cartilage of the first rib

To:
Oblique line on the lamina of the thyroid cartilage

Innervation:
Branches from the ansa cervicalis of the cervical plexus

Major synergists:
Sternohyoid and omohyoid (if the thyroid cartilage is fixed to the hyoid bone)

Major antagonist:
Thyrohyoid

Trigger points:
Likely to form in the belly

Omohyoid (OH-mo-HY-oyd)

Omohyoid means shoulder and U-shaped.

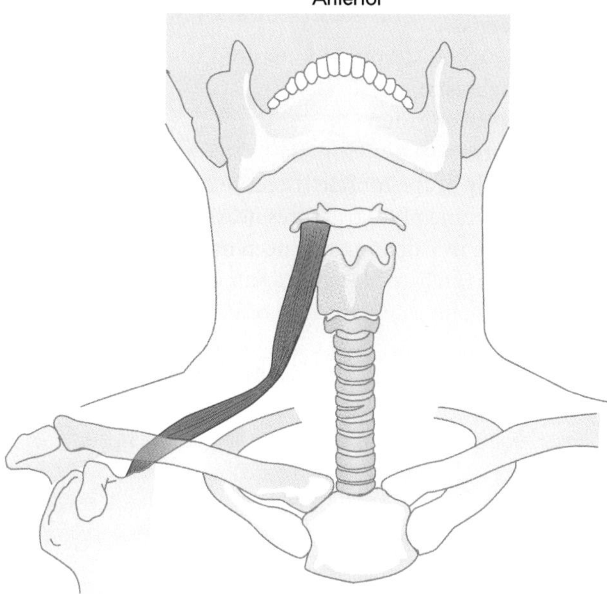

Concentric function:
Depresses the hyoid.
Eccentric function:
Restrains elevation of the hyoid.
Isometric function:
Stabilizes the hyoid bone.
From:
Inferior belly—Superior border of the scapula near the scapular notch and suprascapular ligament (ends at its central tendon attaching to the clavicle by a fibrous sling of tissue deep to the sternocleidomastoid)
Superior belly—From its central tendon at the clavicle
To:
Inferior border of the body of the hyoid bone
Innervation:
Branches from the ansa cervicalis of the cervical plexus
Major synergists:
Sternohyoid and thyrohyoid
Major antagonists:
Suprahyoids
Trigger points:
Likely to form in the belly

Thyrohyoid (THY-ro-HY-oyd)

Thyrohyoid means shaped like a shield and U-shaped.

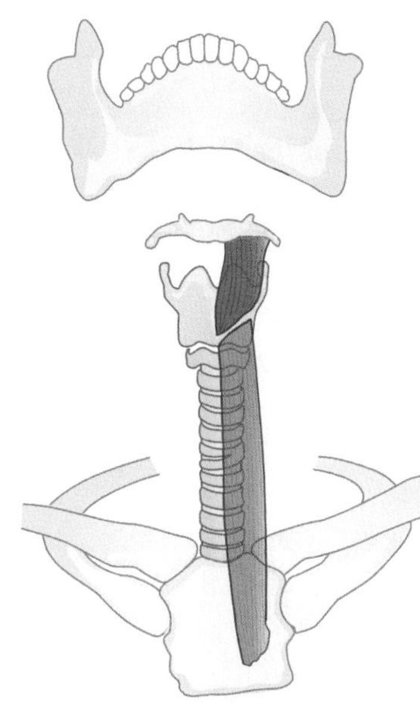

Concentric function:
Depresses the hyoid and elevates the thyroid cartilage.
Eccentric function:
Restrains elevation of the hyoid and depression of the thyroid cartilage.
Isometric function:
Stabilizes the hyoid bone and the thyroid cartilage.
From:
Lamina of the thyroid cartilage at the oblique line
To:
Inferior border of the greater cornu and the body of the hyoid bone
Innervation:
First cervical spinal nerve via the hypoglossal nerve (cranial nerve XII)
Major synergists:
Infrahyoids for depression of the hyoid and suprahyoids for elevation of the thyroid cartilage (if the thyroid cartilage is fixed to the hyoid bone)
Major antagonists:
Suprahyoids for elevation of the hyoid and sternothyroid for depression of the thyroid cartilage
Trigger points:
Likely to form in the belly

See Activity 9-17.

ACTIVITY 9-17

1. Palpate the suprahyoid and infrahyoid muscles as groups.
2. Swallow to identify the hyoid bone and the action of these muscles.
3. Identify the attachment points and the bellies of the muscles.

Posterior Triangle of the Neck

Longus colli (LONG-us KOAL-ee)

Longus colli means long and belonging to the neck.

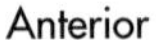

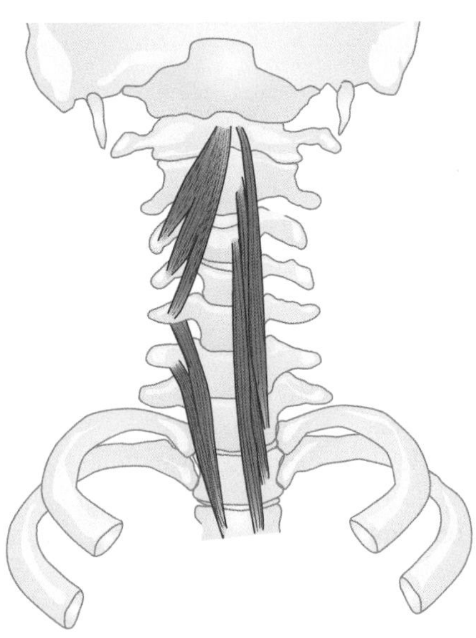

Concentric function:
Flexion, lateral flexion, and contralateral rotation of the neck at the spinal joints

Eccentric function:
Restrains extension, contralateral lateral flexion, and ipsilateral rotation of the neck.

Isometric function:
Stabilizes the cervical spine and can be compared with the psoas major and psoas minor in the lumbar region.

From:
Superior oblique portion—Anterior tubercles of the transverse processes of the third, fourth, and fifth cervical vertebrae
Inferior oblique portion—Anterior bodies of the first three thoracic vertebrae
Vertical portion—Anterior bodies of the lower three cervical vertebrae and the upper three thoracic vertebrae

To:
Superior—Anterior arch of the atlas
Inferior—Anterior tubercles of the transverse processes of the fifth and sixth cervical vertebrae
Vertical—Anterior bodies of the second, third, and fourth cervical vertebrae

Innervation:
Ventral rami of the second through sixth cervical spinal nerves

Major synergists:
Longus capitis, sternocleidomastoid, and scalenes

Major antagonists:
Neck extensor group

Trigger points:
In the belly of the muscle (Because of the presence of many vulnerable structures nearby, one must use caution in palpating this deep muscle.)

The longus colli and longus capitis are important muscles to consider in any whiplash type of neck injury.

Longus capitis (LONG-us KAP-ih-tiss)

Longus capitis means long and belonging to the head.

Anterior

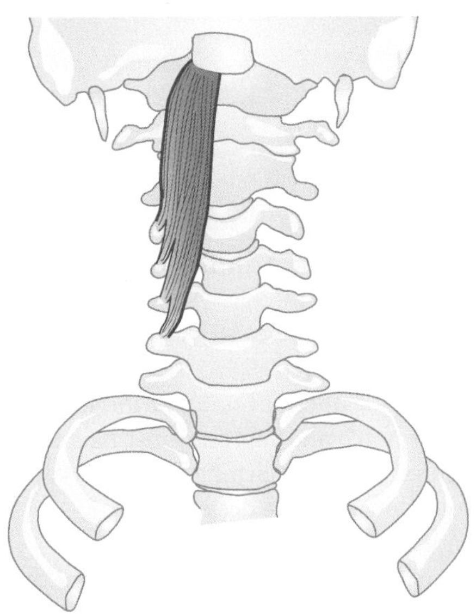

Concentric function:
Flexion and lateral flexion of the head and the neck at the spinal joints

Eccentric function:
Restrains extension and contralateral lateral flexion of the head and neck.

Isometric function:
Stabilizes the cervical spine.

From:
Anterior tubercles of the transverse processes of the third through sixth cervical vertebrae

To:
Inferior surface of the basilar part of the occipital bone just anterior to the foramen magnum

Innervation:
Ventral rami of the first through third cervical spinal nerves

ACTIVITY 9-18

1. Draw and color the longus colli and longus capitis in the space provided.
2. Label the proximal and distal attachment points: *P* for proximal; *D* for distal.
3. Move these muscles on yourself.

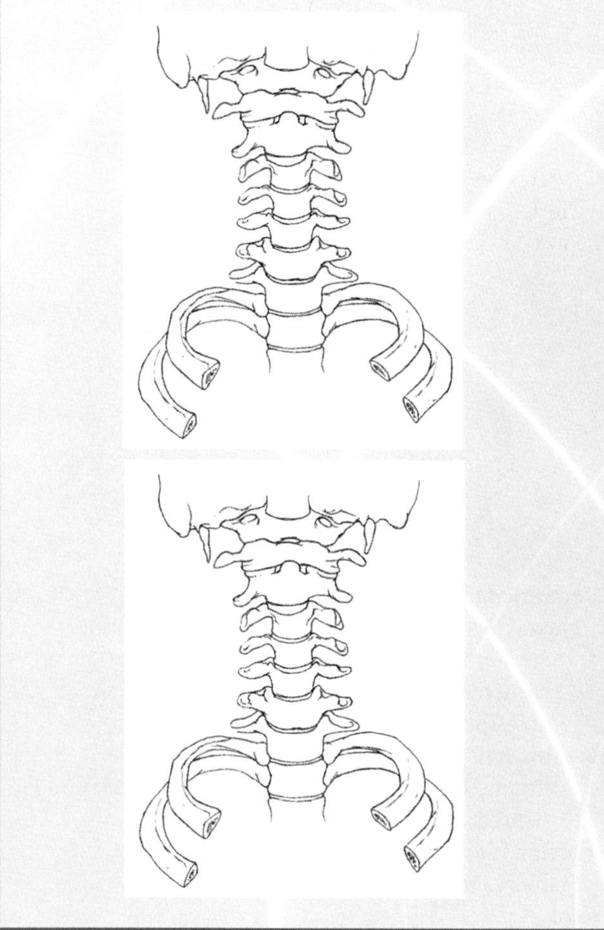

Major synergists:
Longus colli, sternocleidomastoid, and scalenes

Major antagonists:
Neck extensor group

Trigger points:
In the belly of the muscle (Because of the presence of many vulnerable structures nearby, one must use caution in palpating this deep muscle.)

The longus colli and longus capitis are important muscles to consider in any whiplash type of neck injury.

See Activity 9-18.

Scalene Group

Scalenus anterior (skay-LEE-nus)

Scalenus means triangular with unequal sides; *anterior* means before or in front.

Anterior

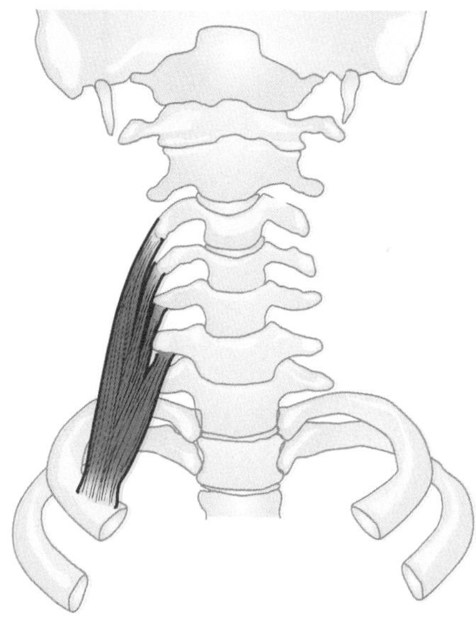

Concentric function:
Flexion and lateral flexion of the neck at the spinal joints; elevation of the first rib at the sternocostal and costovertebral joints (thus functioning as an accessory muscle of respiration)

Eccentric function:
Restrains extension and contralateral lateral flexion of the neck and depression of the first rib.

Isometric function:
Stabilizes the cervical spine.

From:
Anterior tubercles of the transverse processes of the third through sixth cervical vertebrae

To:
Scalene tubercle on the inner border of the first rib and superior surface of the first rib

Innervation:
Ventral rami of the fourth through sixth cervical spinal nerves

Major synergists:
Middle and posterior scalenes and sternocleidomastoid

Major antagonists:
Neck extensors and lateral flexors on the opposite side of the neck

Trigger points:
Belly of the muscle near the rib attachment

Referred pain pattern:
Pectoral region, rhomboid region, and the entire length of the arm into the hand

Scalenus medius (skay-LEE-nus)

Scalenus means triangular with unequal sides; *medius* means middle.

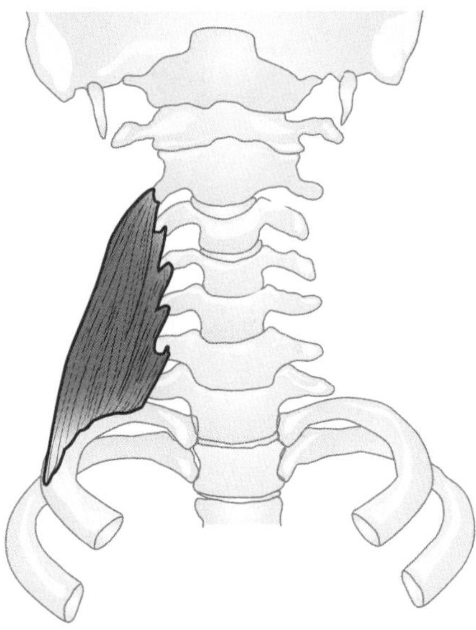

Concentric function:
Flexion and lateral flexion of the neck at the spinal joints and elevation of the first rib at the sternocostal and costovertebral joints (thus functioning as an accessory muscle of respiration)

Eccentric function:
Restrains extension and contralateral lateral flexion of the neck and depression of the first rib.

Isometric function:
Stabilizes the cervical spine.

From:
Posterior tubercles of the transverse processes of the second through seventh cervical vertebrae

To:
Superior surface of the first rib

Innervation:
Ventral rami of the third through eighth cervical spinal nerves

Major synergists:
Anterior and posterior scalenes and sternocleidomastoid

Major antagonists:
Neck extensors and lateral flexors on the opposite side of the neck

Trigger points:
Belly of the muscle near the rib attachment

Referred pain pattern:
Pectoral region, rhomboid region, and the entire length of the arm into the hand

Scalenus posterior (skay-LEE-nus)

Scalenus means triangular with unequal sides; *posterior* means behind.

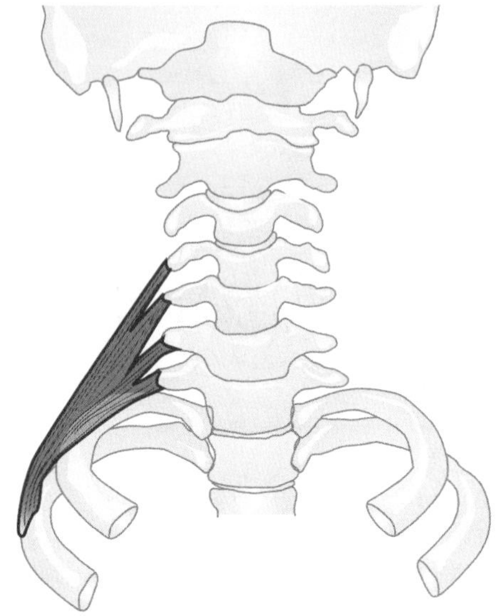

Concentric function:
Lateral flexion of the neck at the spinal joints and elevation of the second rib at the sternocostal and costovertebral joints (thus functioning as an accessory muscle of respiration)

Eccentric function:
Restrains contralateral lateral flexion of the neck and depression of the second rib.

Isometric function:
Stabilizes the cervical spine.

From:
Posterior tubercles of the transverse processes of the fifth through seventh cervical vertebrae

To:
Outer surface of the second rib

Innervation:
Ventral rami of the sixth through eighth cervical spinal nerves

Major synergists:
Anterior and middle scalenes and sternocleidomastoid

Major antagonists:
Lateral flexors on the opposite side of the neck

Trigger points:
Belly of the muscle near the rib attachment

Referred pain pattern:
Pectoral region, rhomboid region, and the entire length of the arm into the hand

See Activity 9-19.

ACTIVITY 9-19

1. Draw and color the scalenus anterior, scalenus medius, and scalenus posterior in the space provided.
2. Label the proximal and distal attachment points: *P* for proximal; *D* for distal.
3. Place an X on the trigger points.
4. Palpate these muscles; identify the attachment points and the bellies of the muscles.
5. Move these muscles on yourself.

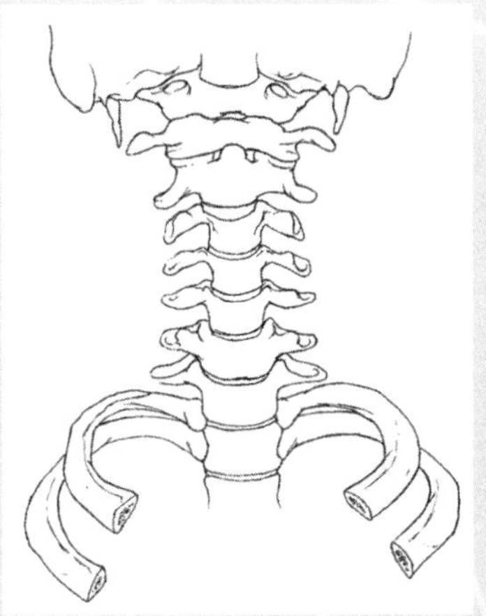

Deep Muscles of the Back and Posterior Neck

When concentrically contracted, the splenius muscles are responsible for neck and head extension, lateral flexion, and rotation. The deep or intrinsic back muscles associated with the vertebral column affect trunk movements. Isometrically, these muscles also play an important role in maintaining the normal curvature of the spine. The deep muscles of the back form a complex column that extends from the sacrum to the skull. Thinking of each of the individual deep back muscles as a string that when pulled causes one or more vertebrae to move on the vertebrae below is helpful. Because the attachments of the different muscle groups overlap extensively, entire regions of the vertebral column can move simultaneously and smoothly. Concentrically acting together, the deep back muscles can extend the trunk, neck, or head. Contraction of muscles on only one side causes extension, lateral flexion, and rotation of the trunk, neck, or head. Eccentric contraction restrains the opposite actions, primarily flexion, lateral flexion to the opposite side, and perhaps rotation.

The largest deep back muscle group is the erector spinae group. Assisting the long muscles of the back are a number of short muscles that extend from one vertebra to the next; these small intrinsic muscles act primarily as stabilizers for the spine. Postural deviation of any type—including forward head position or scoliosis, excessive kyphosis, and excessive lordosis or any rotational adaptation of the shoulder girdle and pelvic girdle—strains the deep postural muscles. These muscles are more involved in stabilizing than mobility; therefore when dysfunctional patterns exist, these muscles tend to shorten because of sustained isometric contraction. Massage affecting these muscles must be deep enough to access them while not causing protective tensing (guarding) of the more superficial muscles. Massage is most effective when applied with a slow, sustained, broad-based compressive force that penetrates through the superficial layers to affect the deep muscles.

Deep Posterior Cervical Muscles

Splenius capitis and splenius cervicis (SPLEEN-ee-us KAP-ih-tiss, SIR-vih-siss)

Splenius means bandage; *capitis* means head; and *cervicis* means belonging to the neck.

Posterior

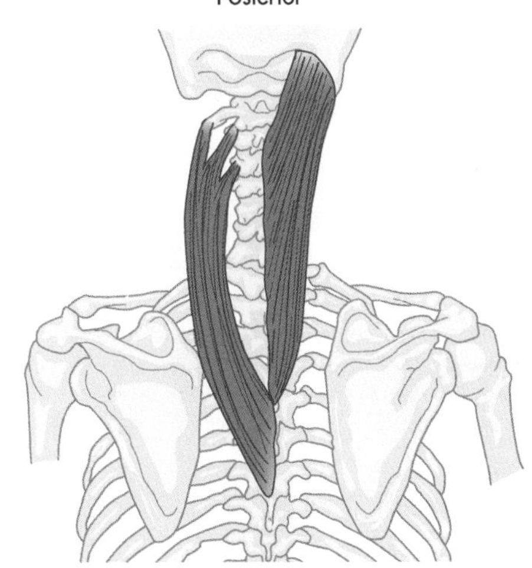

Concentric function:

Extension, lateral flexion, and ipsilateral rotation of the head and the neck at the spinal joints

Eccentric function:

Restrains flexion, contralateral lateral flexion, and contralateral rotation of the neck and the head.

Isometric function:
Stabilizes the cervical spine.

From:
Capitis—Nuchal ligament and the spinous processes of the seventh cervical and first four thoracic vertebrae
Cervicis—Spinous processes of the third through sixth thoracic vertebrae

To:
Capitis—Lateral one third of the superior nuchal line of the occipital bone deep to the attachment of the sternocleidomastoid and the mastoid process of the temporal bone
Cervicis—Posterior tubercles of the transverse processes of the upper three cervical vertebrae

Innervation:
Capitis—Dorsal rami of the middle cervical spinal nerves
Cervicis—Dorsal rami of the lower cervical spinal nerves

Major synergists:
Posterior cervical extensors, opposite-sided upper trapezius, and opposite-sided sternocleidomastoid

Major antagonists:
Anterior cervical flexors, same-sided upper trapezius, and same-sided sternocleidomastoid

Trigger points:
Belly of the muscles closer to the head

Referred pain patterns:
To the top of the skull (the pain often feels as if it is inside the head), to the eye, and into the shoulder

See Activity 9-20.

Vertical Muscles, Erector Spinae Group

Also called the sacrospinalis muscles, the muscles in the erector spinae (ee-REK-tor SPIN-aye) group are the principal extensors of the spinal joints.

ACTIVITY 9-20

1. Draw and color the splenius capitis and splenius cervicis in the space provided.
2. Label the proximal and distal attachment points: *P* for proximal; *D* for distal.
3. Place an X on the trigger points.
4. Palpate these muscles; identify the attachment points and the bellies of the muscles.
5. Move these muscles on yourself.

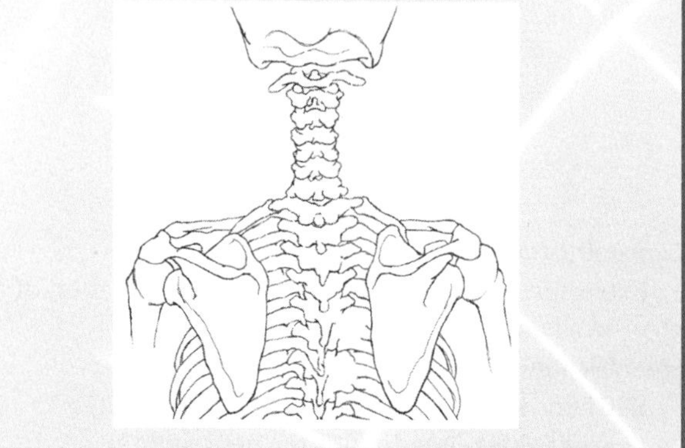

Iliocostalis lumborum, iliocostalis thoracis, and iliocostalis cervicis (ILL-ee-oh-kos-TAL-iss lum-BOR-um, thor-AH-siss, SIR-vih-siss)

Iliocostalis means connecting the ilium to the loins (lumborum), ribs (costa), chest (thoracis) and neck (cervicis).

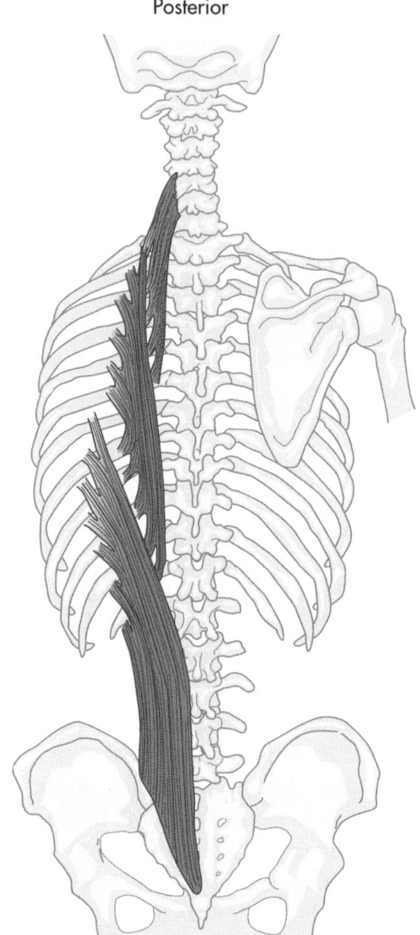

Concentric function:
Extension, lateral flexion, and ipsilateral rotation of the trunk and neck at the spinal joints and anterior tilt of the pelvis at the lumbosacral joint

Eccentric function:
Restrains flexion, contralateral lateral flexion, and contralateral rotation of the trunk and neck and allows posterior tilt of the pelvis.

Isometric function:
Stabilizes the spine and pelvis.

From:
Lumborum—Medial iliac crest and medial and lateral sacral crests
Thoracis—Lower six ribs medial to the tendons of the iliocostalis lumborum
Cervicis—Angles of the third through sixth ribs

To:
Lumborum—Inferior border at the angles of the ribs 7 to 12

Thoracis—Superior border at the angles of ribs 1 to 6 and transverse process of seventh cervical vertebra
Cervicis—Posterior tubercles of the transverse processes of the fourth through sixth cervical vertebrae

Innervation:
Dorsal rami of the lower cervical, thoracic, and lumbar spinal nerves

See Activity 9-21.

Longissimus thoracis, longissimus cervicis, and longissimus capitis (lon-GISS-ih-mus thor-AH-siss, SIR-vih-siss, KAP-ih-tiss)

Longissimus means the longest; these muscles relate to the thorax, neck, and head, respectively.

Posterior

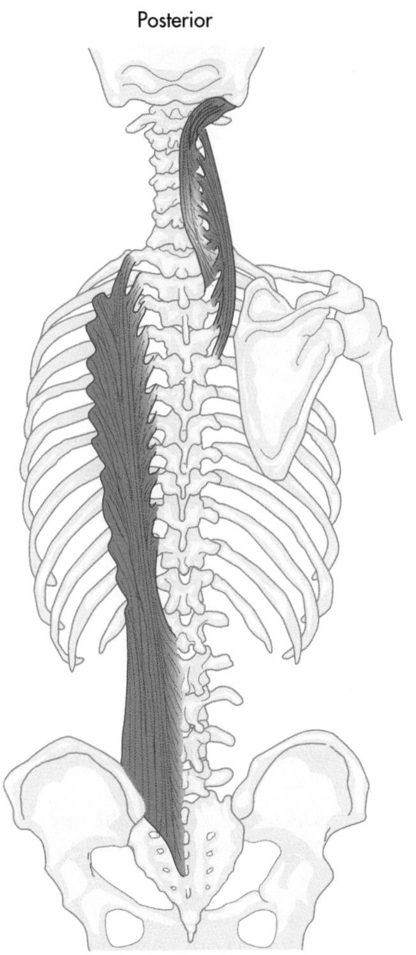

Concentric function:
Extension, lateral flexion, and ipsilateral rotation of the trunk, neck, and head at the spinal joints and anterior tilt of the pelvis at the lumbosacral joint

Eccentric function:
Restrains flexion, contralateral lateral flexion, and contralateral rotation of the trunk, neck, and head and allows posterior tilt of the pelvis.

Isometric function:
Stabilizes the spine and pelvis.

From:
Thoracis—Transverse processes of the lumbar vertebrae, lumbocostal aponeurosis, and medial iliac crest and posterior sacrum
Cervicis—Transverse processes of the upper five thoracic vertebrae
Capitis—Transverse processes of the upper four or five thoracic vertebrae and articular processes of the lower three or four cervical vertebrae

To:
Thoracis—Transverse processes of all thoracic vertebrae and lower 9 or 10 ribs
Cervicis—Posterior tubercles of the transverse processes of the second through sixth cervical vertebrae
Capitis—Mastoid process of the temporal bone

Innervation:
Dorsal rami of the lower cervical, thoracic, and lumbar spinal nerves

Spinalis thoracis, spinalis cervicis, and spinalis capitis (spy-NAL-iss thor-AH-ciss, SIR-vih-ciss, KAP-ih-tiss)

Spinalis means related to the spine; these muscles relate to the chest, neck, and head, respectively.

Posterior

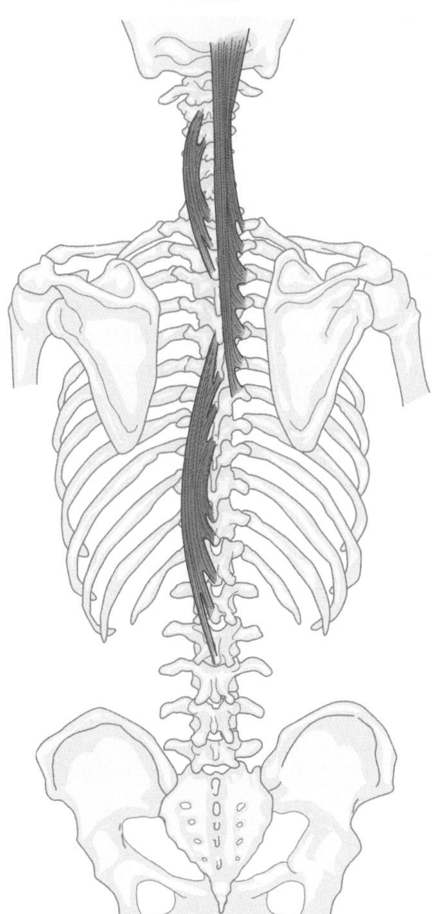

Concentric function:
Extension, lateral flexion, and ipsilateral rotation of the trunk, neck, and head at the spinal joints

Eccentric function:
Restrains flexion, contralateral lateral flexion, and contralateral rotation of the trunk, neck, and head.
Isometric function:
Stabilizes the spine.
From:
Thoracis—Spinous processes of the first two lumbar and the last two thoracic vertebrae
Cervicis—Spinous processes of the first and second thoracic and the seventh cervical vertebrae
Capitis—Transverse processes of the upper seven thoracic and the seventh cervical vertebrae and articular processes of the fourth through sixth cervical vertebrae
To:
Thoracis—Spinous processes of the fourth through eighth thoracic vertebrae
Cervicis—Spinous processes of the second and third cervical vertebrae
Capitis—Between the superior and inferior nuchal lines of the occipital bone
Innervation:
Dorsal rami of the lower cervical, thoracic, and lumbar spinal nerves
Elements common to the erector spinae and transversospinalis group
Major antagonists:
Flexors of the trunk (abdominals)
Major synergists:
Extension is assisted by the serratus posterior inferior and the quadrutus lumborum; rotation is assisted by the abdominal obliques
Trigger points:
The most common site for trigger points is the superficial long-fibered, longitudinal muscles in the erector spinae group; trigger points usually are found in the midscapular and lumbar regions
Referred pain patterns:
Scapular, lumbar, abdominal, and gluteal areas. Also local area and adjacent spinal segment.

See Activity 9-21.

Oblique Muscles, Transversospinales Group

This group of muscles extends, laterally flexes, and contralaterally rotates the spinal joints and also functions to move and stabilize the pelvis.

Semispinalis thoracis, semispinalis cervicis, and semispinalis capitis (sem-ee-spy-NAL-us thor-AH-siss, SIR-vih-siss, KAP-ih-tiss)

Semispinalis means half and the spine; these muscles relate to the chest, neck, and head, respectively.

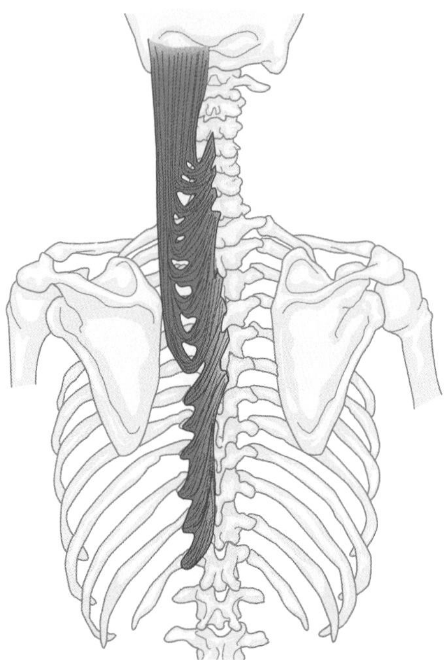

Concentric function:
Extension and lateral flexion of the trunk, neck, and head at the spinal joints and contralateral rotation of the trunk and neck at the spinal joints
Eccentric function:
Allows flexion and contralateral lateral flexion of the trunk, neck, and head and allows ipsilateral rotation of the trunk and neck.
Isometric function:
Stabilizes the spine.
From:
Thoracis—Transverse processes of the last six thoracic vertebrae
Cervicis—Transverse processes of the upper six thoracic and articular processes of the lower four cervical vertebrae
Capitis—Transverse processes of the upper six thoracic vertebrae and the seventh cervical vertebrae; articular processes of the fourth through sixth cervical vertebrae
To:
Thoracis—Spinous processes of the first four thoracic and the last two cervical vertebrae
Cervicis—Spinous processes of the second through fifth cervical vertebrae
Capitis—Between the superior and inferior nuchal lines of the occipital bone
Innervation:
Thoracis—Dorsal rami of the upper six thoracic spinal nerves

Cervicis—Dorsal rami of the lower three cervical spinal nerves
Capitis—Dorsal rami of the first six cervical spinal nerves

Major synergists:
Multifidus and rotatores and extensors of the neck and head

Major antagonists:
Flexors of the trunk (abdominals)

Trigger points:
Belly of the muscles

Referred pain patterns:
Local area

See Activity 9-21.

Multifidus (mul-tih-FYE-dus)

Multifidus means many split parts.

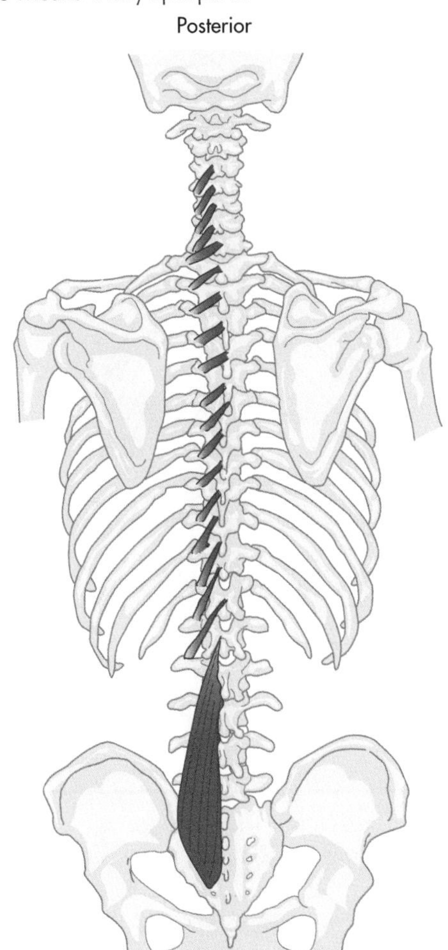

Concentric function:
Contralateral rotation, lateral flexion, and extension of the trunk and neck at the spinal joints and anterior tilt and elevation of the pelvis at the lumbosacral joint

Eccentric function:
Allows ipsilateral rotation, contralateral lateral flexion, and flexion of the trunk and neck and allows posterior tilt and depression of the pelvis.

Isometric function:
Stabilizes the spine and pelvis.

This muscle group provides proprioceptive input about posture and movement.

From:
Articular processes of the last four cervical vertebrae, transverse processes of all thoracic vertebrae, mammillary processes of the lumbar vertebrae, posterior superior iliac spine, posterior sacroiliac ligaments, and posterior surface of the sacrum

To:
Spinous processes of the vertebrae two to four levels superior to the vertebrae of origin

Innervation:
Dorsal rami of the spinal nerves

Major synergists:
Semispinalis and rotatores

Major antagonists:
Flexors of the trunk (abdominals)

Trigger points:
Belly of the muscles

Referred pain patterns:
Local area and sacroiliac joint

See Activity 9-21.

Rotatores (ro-TA-to-reez)

Rotatores means one that rotates.

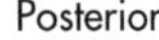

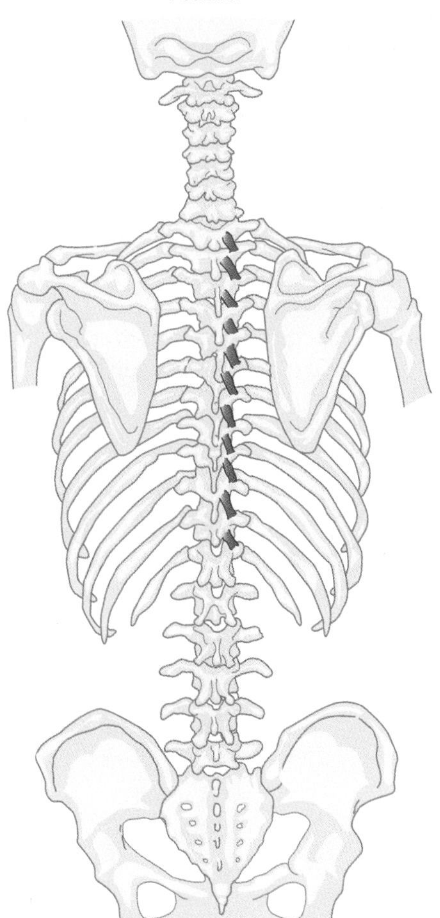

Concentric function:
Contralateral rotation and extension of the trunk and neck at the spinal joints

Eccentric function:
Restrains ipsilateral rotation and flexion of the trunk and neck.

Isometric function:
Stabilizes the vertebral column particularly on the transverse plane between each vertebra.
The rotatores are an important muscle group (with the multifidi) in providing proprioceptive posture information to the central nervous system.

From:
Transverse process of one thoracic vertebra (11 pairs total)

To:
Laminae of the vertebrae one to two levels superior

Innervation:
Dorsal rami of spinal nerves

Major synergists:
Same-sided contralateral rotators of the trunk and neck and opposite-sided ipsilateral rotators of the trunk and neck.

Major antagonists:
Opposite-sided contralateral rotators of the trunk and neck and same-sided ipsilateral rotators of the trunk and neck.

Trigger points:
Belly of the muscles

Referred pain patterns:
Local area

See Activity 9-21.

ACTIVITY 9-21

1. Draw and color the erector spinae and transversospinalis in the space provided.
2. Label the proximal and distal attachment points: *P* for proximal; *D* for distal.
3. Place an X on the trigger points.
4. Palpate these muscles; identify the attachment points and the bellies of the muscles.
5. Move these muscles on yourself.

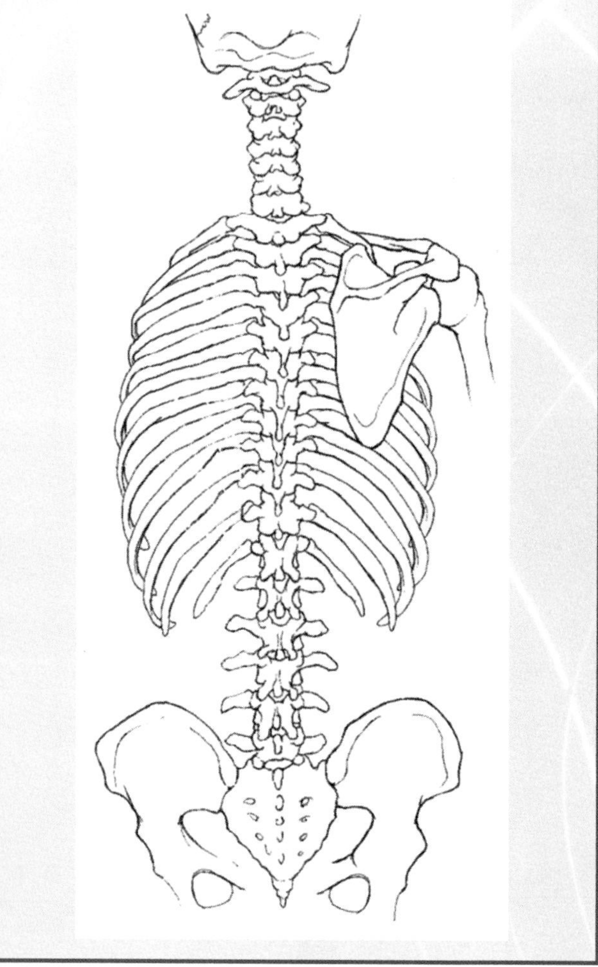

Intertransversarii lumborum, intertransversarii thoracis, and intertransversarii cervicis (INTER-TRANS-ver-SAIR-ee-ee lum-BOR-um, thor-AH-siss, SIR-vih-siss)

Intertransversarii means between or among the transverse processes of the vertebrae; these muscles relate to the loins, thorax, and neck, respectively.

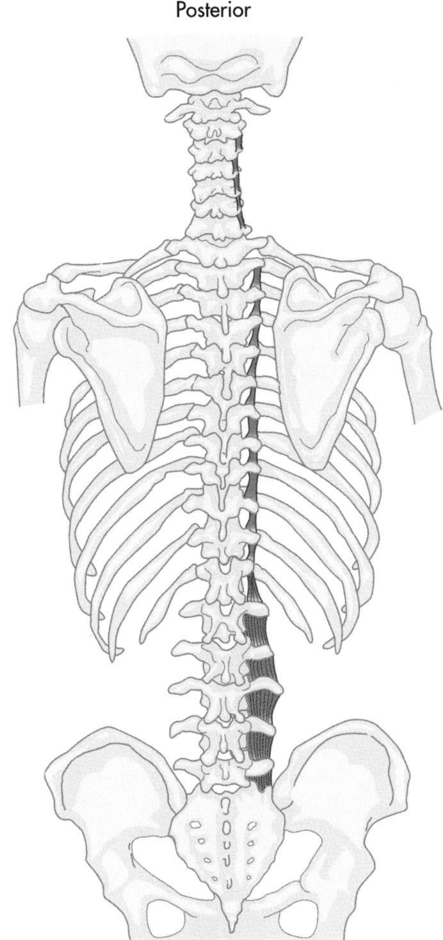

Concentric function:
Lateral flexion of the trunk and neck at the spinal joints

Eccentric function:
Restrains contralateral lateral flexion of the trunk and neck.

Isometric function:
Provides intersegmental stability of the spine in the frontal plane.
The intertransversarii muscles are active in proprioceptive input to the central nervous system.

From and To:
Between transverse processes of the cervical, thoracic, and lumbar vertebrae (best developed in the cervical and lumbar regions)

Innervation:
Ventral and dorsal rami of the spinal nerves

Major synergists:
Ipsilateral lateral flexors of the trunk and neck

Major antagonists:
Contralateral lateral flexors of the trunk and neck

Trigger points:
Belly of the muscles

Referred pain patterns:
Local area

See Activity 9-21.

Interspinalis lumborum, interspinalis thoracis, and interspinalis cervicis (inter-spy-NAL-eez lum-BOR-um, thor-AH-siss, SIR-vih-siss)

Interspinalis means between or among the parts of the spine; these muscles relate to the loins, chest, and neck, respectively.

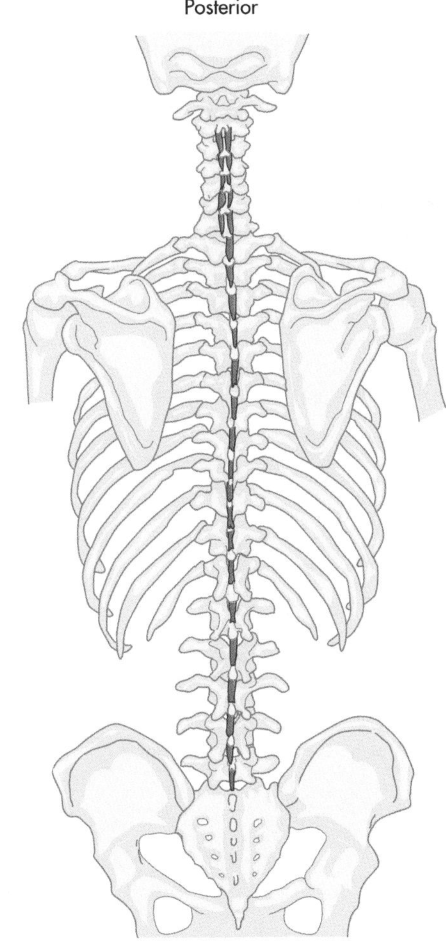

Concentric function:
Extension of the trunk and neck at the spinal joints

Eccentric function:
Restrains vertebral flexion.

Isometric function:
Provides intersegmental stability of the spine in the sagittal plane.
Interspinalis muscles provide proprioceptive input concerning spinal stabilization and neuromuscular control.

From and To:
Between the spinous processes of the vertebrae
Innervation:
Dorsal rami of the spinal nerves
Major synergists:
Extensors of the trunk and neck
Major antagonists:
Flexors of the trunk and neck
Trigger points:
Belly of the muscle
Referred pain patterns:
Local area

See Activity 9-21.

Suboccipital Muscles

As a group, these muscles extend and rotate the head at the atlanto-occipital joint in small and precise movements. More often, these muscles isometrically function as stabilizers of the head. These muscles are also important postural muscles and are neurologic reporting stations on balance and proprioceptive monitors of cervical spine and head position.

Rectus capitis posterior major (REK-tus KAP-ih-tiss)

Rectus means straight, *capitis* means belonging to the head, *posterior* means behind, and *major* means larger.

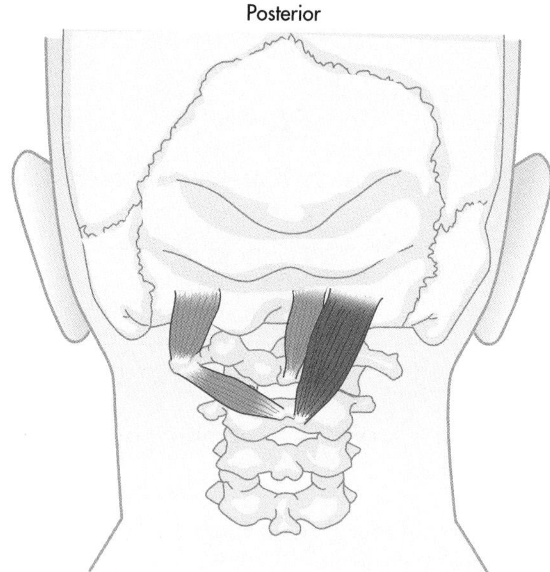

Concentric function:
Extension, lateral flexion, and ipsilateral rotation of the head at the atlanto-occipital joint
Eccentric function:
Restrains flexion, contralateral lateral flexion, and contralateral rotation of the head.
Isometric function:
Stabilizes the upper cervical spine and head.
From:
Spinous process of the axis
To:
Lateral aspect of the inferior nuchal line of the occipital bone lateral to the rectus capitis posterior minor
Innervation:
Dorsal ramus of the first cervical spinal nerve (the suboccipital nerve)
Major synergists:
Semispinalis capitis, rectus capitis posterior minor, and the splenius capitis on the same side
Major antagonists:
Rectus capitis anterior and the sternocleidomastoid on the same side
Trigger points:
Belly of the muscle, located with deep palpation at the base of the skull
Referred pain pattern:
Around the ear on the same-side, sensation of compressed junction of skull and neck, and bandlike headache

Rectus capitis posterior minor (REK-tus KAP-ih-tiss)

Rectus means straight, *capitis* means belonging to the head, *posterior* means behind, and *minor* means smaller.

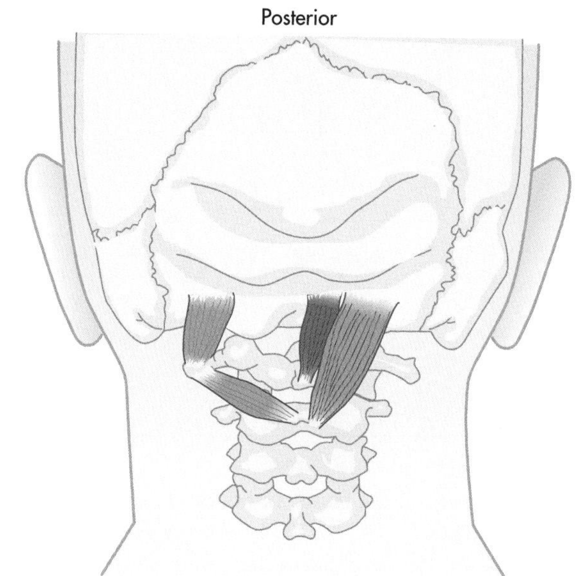

Concentric function:
Extension of the head at the atlanto-occipital joint (See under Isometric function.)
Eccentric function:
Restrains flexion of the head.
Isometric function:
Stabilizes the upper cervical spine and head.
Recent myographic studies indicate that this muscle does not act in extension beyond neutral position but rather functions more importantly as a restraint to flexion and forward movement of the head; its proximal attachment weaves into the dura through the foramen magnum (Greenman, 1996). This

muscle actively provides proprioceptive input on positioning and posture to the central nervous system.

From:
Posterior tubercle of the atlas

To:
Medial aspect of the inferior nuchal line of the occipital bone just superior to the foramen magnum

Innervation:
Dorsal ramus of the first cervical spinal nerve (the suboccipital nerve)

Major synergists:
Semispinalis capitis and rectus capitis posterior major

Major antagonists:
Rectus capitis anterior and longus capitis on the opposite side

Trigger points:
Belly of the muscle, located with deep palpation at the base of the skull

Referred pain pattern:
Around the ear on the same-side, sensation of compressed junction of skull and neck, and bandlike headache

Obliquus capitis superior (oh-BLI-kwus KAP-ih-tiss)

Obliquus means slanting, *capitis* means head, and *superior* means above or higher.

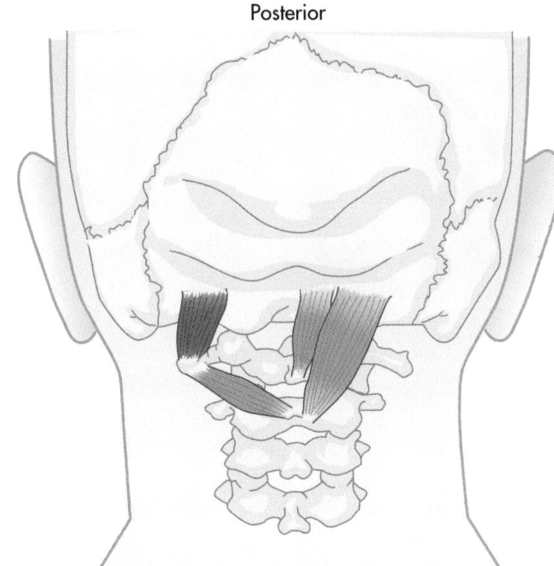

Concentric function:
Extension and lateral flexion of the head at the atlanto-occipital joint

Eccentric function:
Restrains flexion and contralateral lateral flexion of the head.

Isometric function:
Stabilizes the upper cervical spine and head.

From:
Superior surface of the transverse process of the atlas

To:
Between the superior and inferior nuchal lines of the occipital bone and lateral to the semispinalis capitis

Innervation:
Dorsal ramus of the first cervical spinal nerve (the suboccipital nerve)

Obliquus capitis inferior (oh-BLI-kwus KAP-ih-tiss)

Obliquus means slanting, *capitis* means head, and *inferior* means lower or beneath.

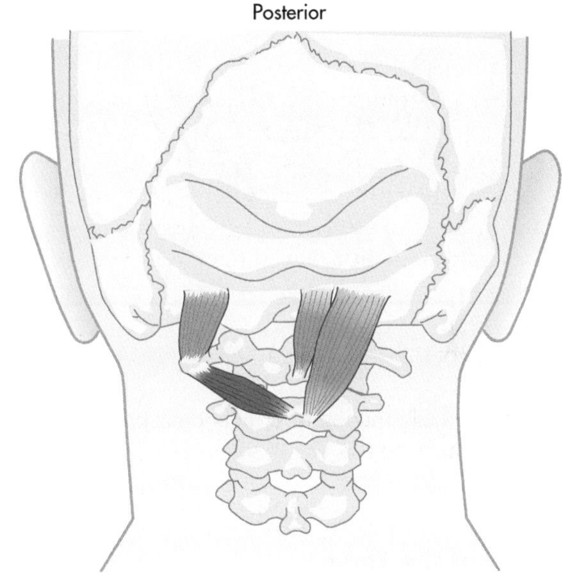

Concentric function:
Ipsilateral rotation of the atlas at the atlantoaxial joint

Eccentric function:
Restrains contralateral rotation of the atlas.

Isometric function:
Stabilizes the upper cervical spine.

From:
Superior part of the spinous process of the axis

To:
Inferior and posterior aspect of the transverse process of the atlas

Innervation:
Dorsal ramus of the first cervical spinal nerve (the suboccipital nerve)

Major synergists:
Semispinalis capitis and the rectus capitis posterior major and rectus capitis posterior minor

Major antagonists:
Rectus capitis anterior and rectus capitis lateralis on the opposite side

Trigger points:
Belly of the muscle, located with deep palpation at the base of the skull

Referred pain pattern:
Around the ear on the same-side, sensation of

ACTIVITY 9-22

1. Draw and color the suboccipital muscles in the space provided.
2. Label the proximal and distal attachment points: *P* for proximal; *D* for distal.
3. Place an X on the trigger points.
4. Palpate these muscles; identify the attachment points and the bellies of the muscles.
5. Move these muscles on yourself.

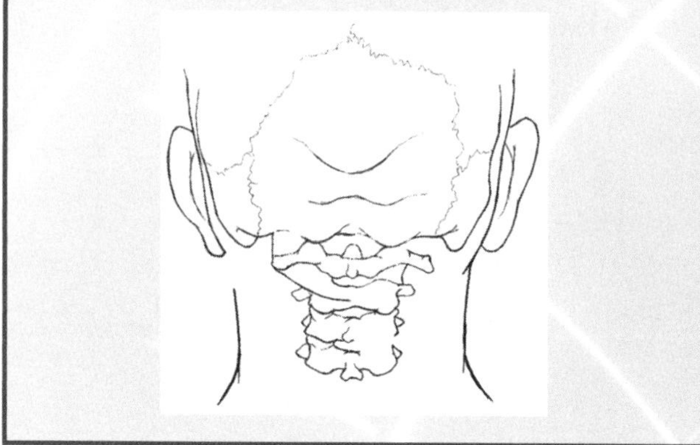

compressed junction of skull and neck, and bandlike headache

See Activity 9-22.

Muscles of the Torso

Figures 9-21 to 9-24 illustrate the muscles of the torso.

Muscles of the Thorax and Posterior Abdominal Wall

The primary function of the deep muscles of the thorax is to create movements necessary for breathing. Contraction of the diaphragm creates relaxed, quiet inspiration. Relaxed, quiet expiration requires no muscular contractions at all; rather expiration is caused by the elastic recoil of the soft tissues (the lungs themselves and the abdominal viscera) that were stretched during inspiration. Forced inspiration and forced expiration result from the contraction of accessory muscles of respiration in addition to the diaphragm.

Some anatomists have considered the abdominal and thorax muscle groups as one group. However, unlike the abdominal muscles, the thoracic muscles are short, extending between the ribs. When they contract, they may elevate or depress the ribs. The external intercostals (most superficial layer) generally are accepted as elevating the ribs for inspiration, whereas the internal intercostals (from the intermediate layer) depress the ribs for expiration. The transversus thoracis (the deepest layer) is involved in depression of ribs.

The diaphragm is the most important muscle of inspiration and forms a muscular partition between the thoracic and abdominopelvic cavities. When relaxed, the diaphragm is dome shaped, but when contracted, its central dome moves inferiorly and flattens, increasing the volume of the thoracic cavity. The alternating contraction and relaxation of the diaphragm causes pressure changes in the abdominopelvic cavity that assist the return of lymph fluid to the venous blood and to the heart. One can contract the diaphragm to increase the intraabdominal pressure voluntarily to help evacuate urine or feces or to deliver a baby. An increase in intraabdominal pressure also aids in lifting weight. When we take a deep breath to fixate our diaphragm, we can increase the abdominal pressure enough to support the spine while lifting a heavy weight. Fibers from the quadratus lumborum and psoas muscles weave into the diaphragm. With this direct relationship, we can see how low back function and breathing function are interrelated.

Forced breathing involves a number of other muscles that insert into the ribs. During forced inspiration the scalenes and sternocleidomastoid muscles may assist in lifting the ribs. Contraction of the abdominal wall muscles assists respiration. Massage in this area can influence effective breathing positively.

Diaphragm (DYE-ah-fram)

Diaphragm means a partition or wall (between the thoracic and abdominal cavities).

Anterior-Inferior

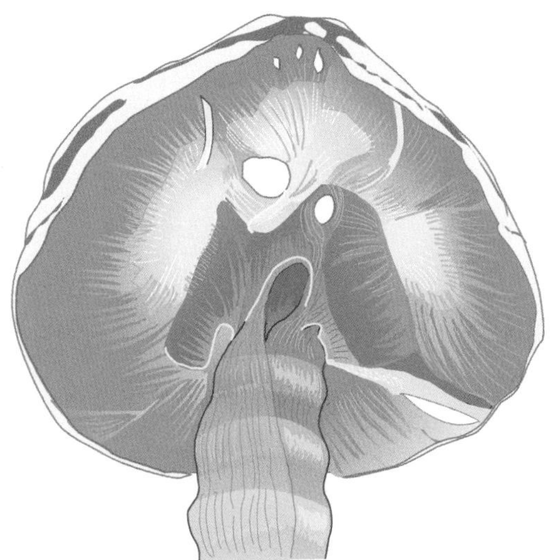

Concentric function:
Inspiration (breathing in); diaphragmatic contractions increase the volume of the thoracic cavity.

Eccentric function:
Restrains expiration as the diaphragm relaxes (eccentrically contracts).

Isometric function:
Stabilizes the thoracic and abdominopelvic cavities during breath holding and stabilizes the thoracic and lumbar spine.

From:
First three lumbar vertebrae, the lower six costal

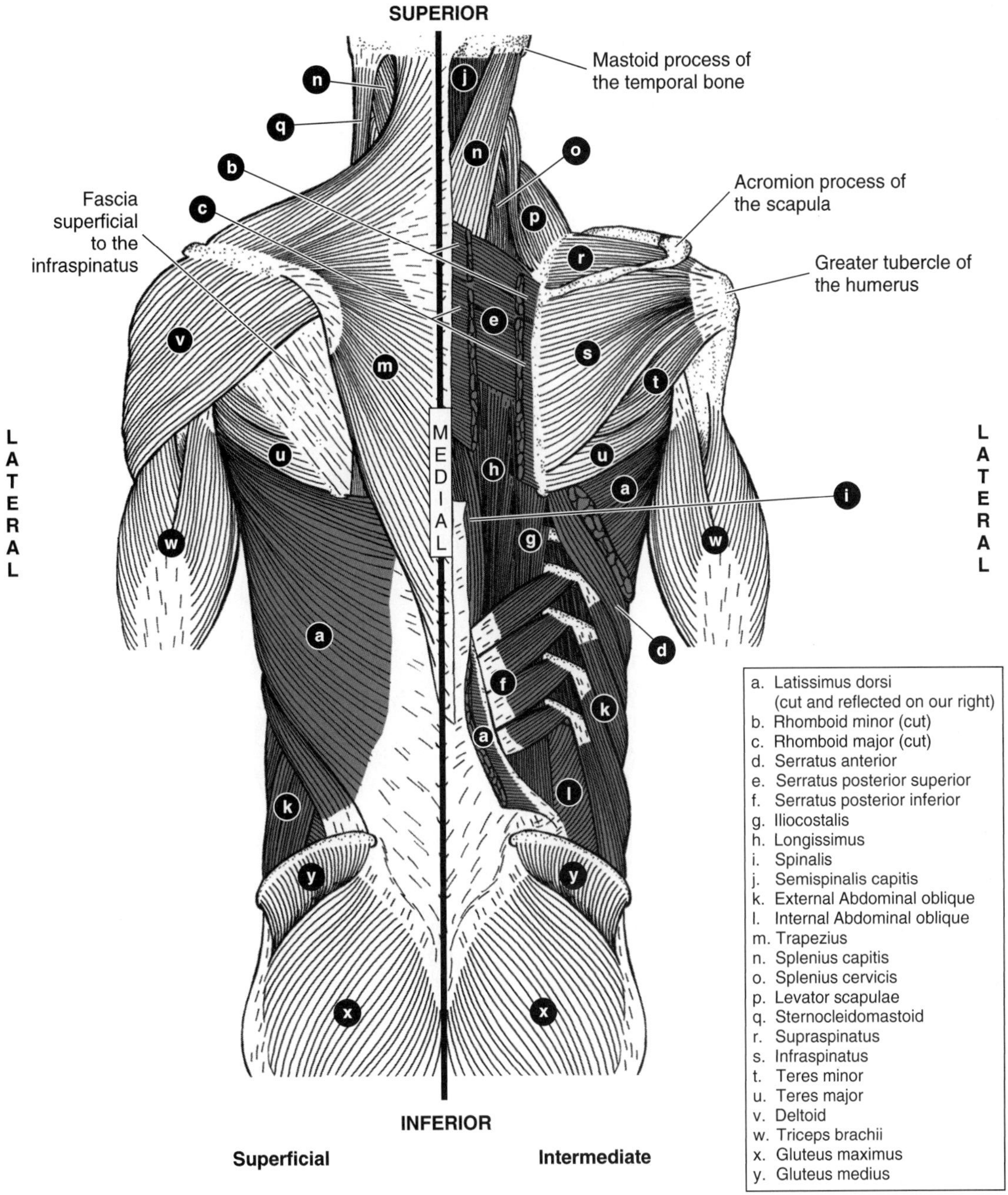

Figure 9-21
Posterior view of the trunk (superficial and intermediate). (Modified from Muscolino JE: *The muscular system manual: the skeletal muscles of the human body,* ed 2, St Louis, 2005, Mosby.)

cartilages, and the inner surface of the xiphoid process

To:

Muscle fibers arch superiorly and inward to end in tendinous fibers, which form the central tendon; the central tendon is a large aponeurosis.

The diaphragm is a broad, thin muscle that spans the thoracoabdominal cavity, separating the thorax from the abdomen. One can visualize it as plastic wrap around the edges of a bowl. The central tendon (the insertion) is not attached to any solid structure; rather the middle of the plastic wrap becomes a thickened fascial structure. When the muscle component of the diaphragm contracts, it pulls and flattens the central tendon, which increases the volume of the thoracic cavity.

Innervation:

Phrenic nerve (C3 to C5)

Major synergists:

Accessory muscles of inspiration: external intercostals, scalenes, and sternocleidomastoids

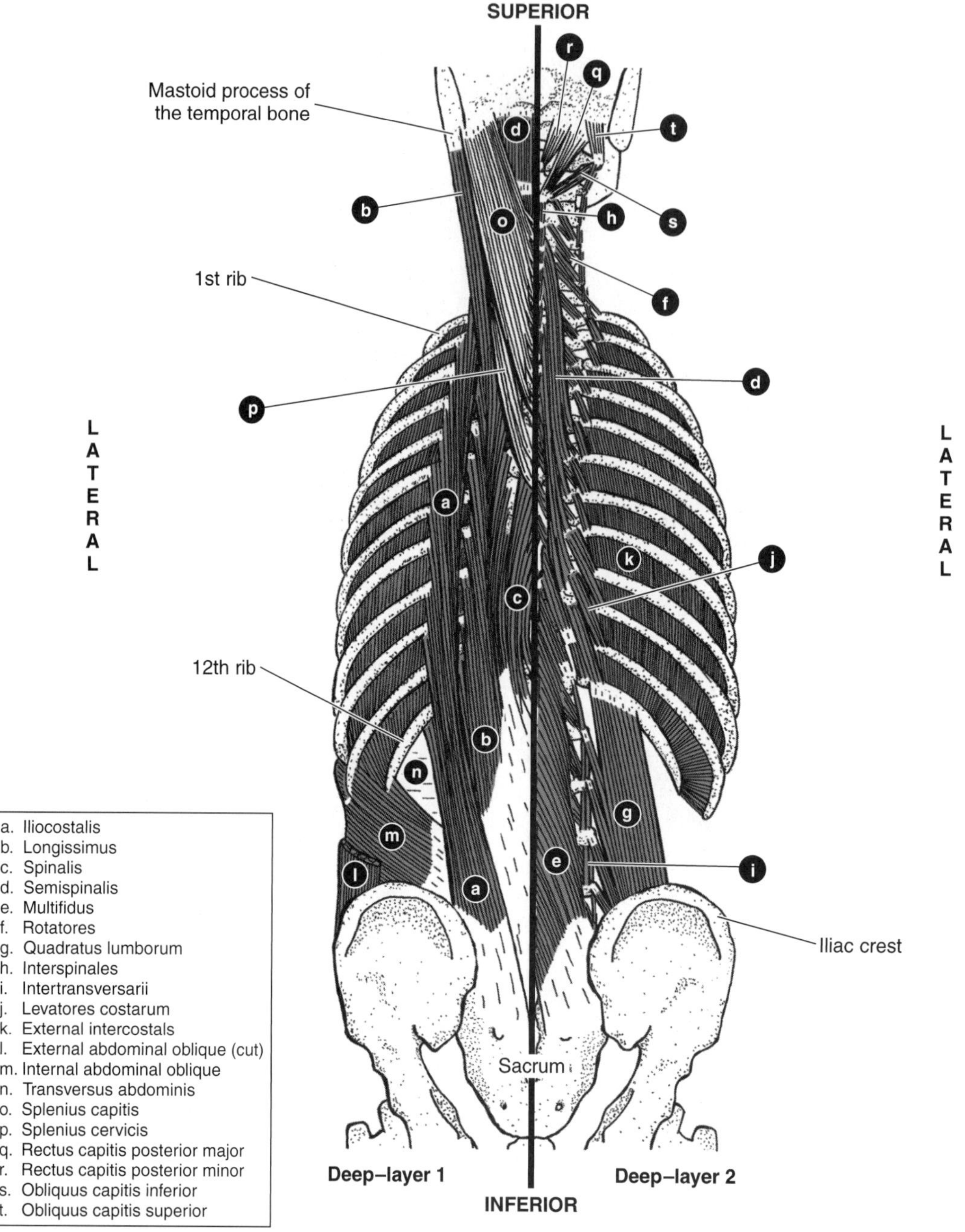

Figure 9-22

Posterior view of the trunk (deep layers). (Modified from Muscolino JE: *The muscular system manual: the skeletal muscles of the human body,* ed 2, St Louis, 2005, Mosby.)

Major antagonists:

Accessory muscles of expiration: internal intercostals and anterior and anterolateral muscles of the abdominal wall. The elastic recoil of the soft tissues of the thoracic and abdominal cavities also provides an opposing force. The pelvic floor muscles may act as antagonists as well.

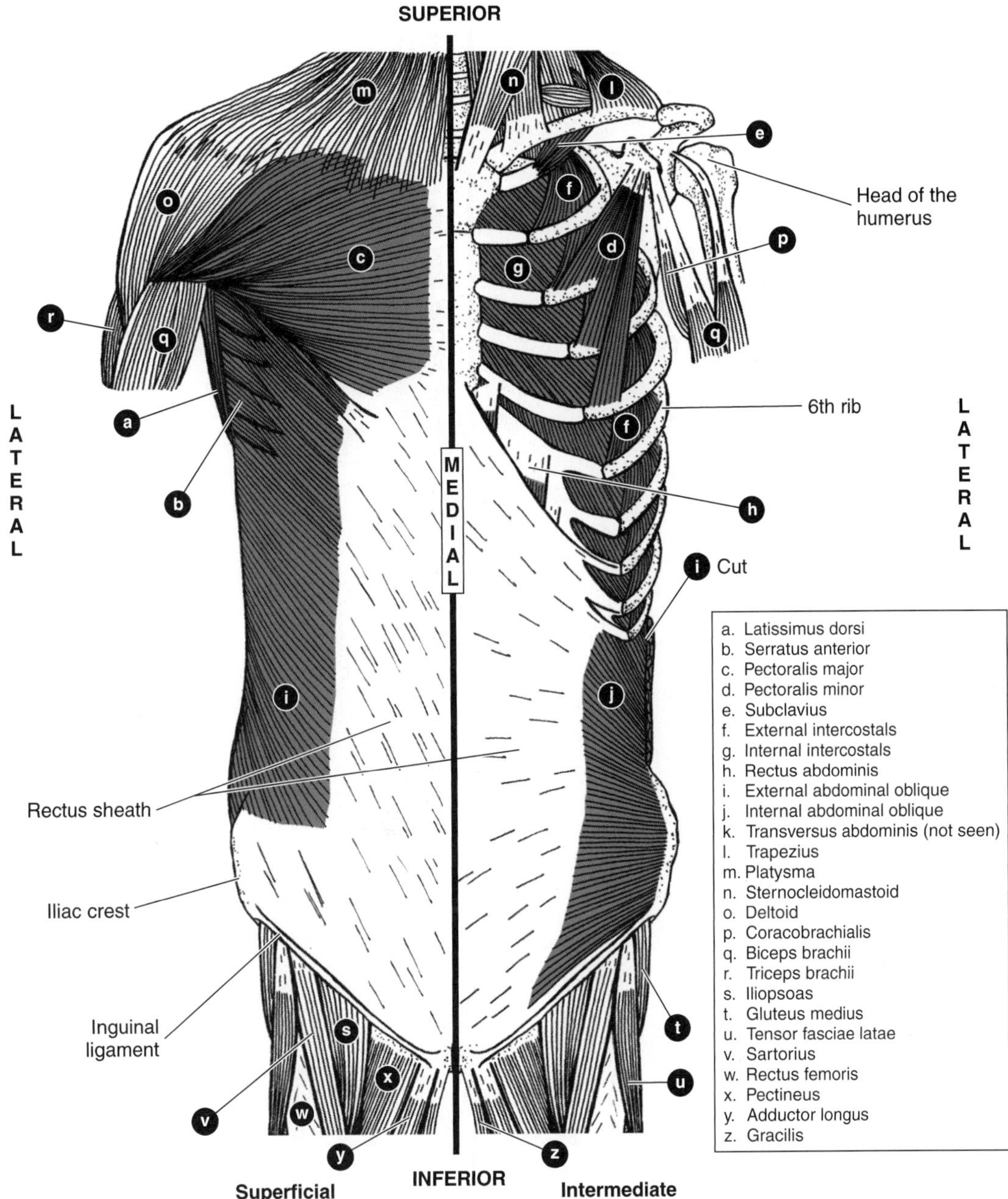

Figure 9-23
Anterior view of the trunk (superficial and intermediate). (Modified from Muscolino JE: *The muscular system manual: the skeletal muscles of the human body,* ed 2, St Louis, 2005, Mosby.)

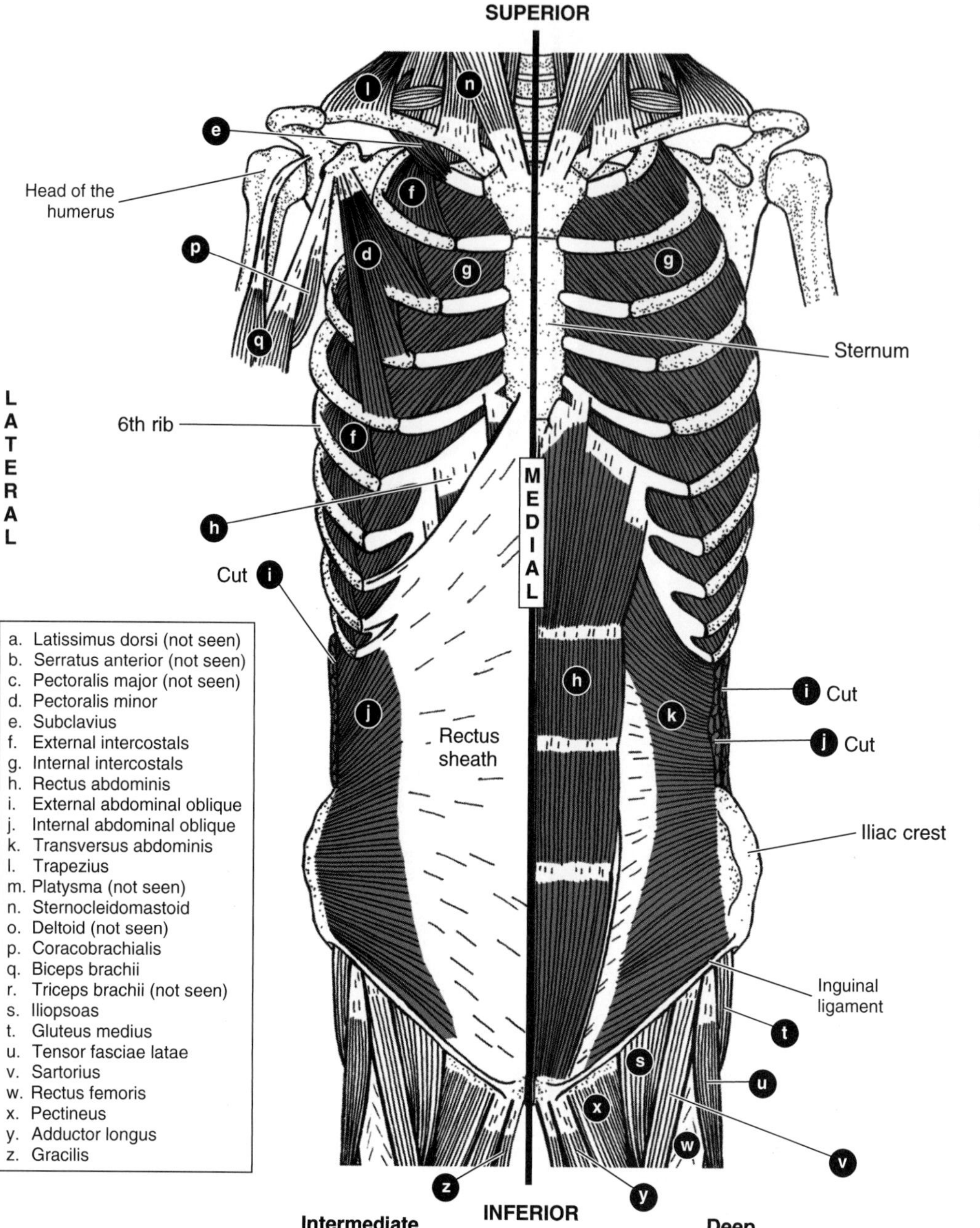

Figure 9-24

Anterior view of the trunk (intermediate and deep). (Modified from Muscolino JE: *The muscular system manual: the skeletal muscles of the human body,* ed 2, St Louis, 2005, Mosby.)

Serratus posterior superior (suhr-RATE-us)

Serratus means saw-shaped, *posterior* means behind, and *superior* means above.

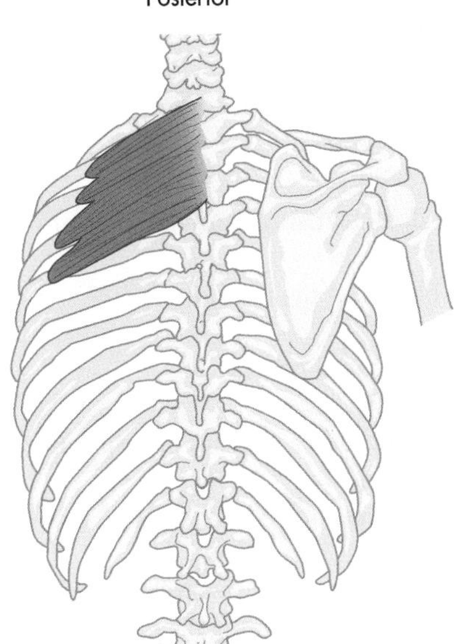

Concentric function:
Elevates ribs 2 to 5 at the sternocostal and costovertebral joints during inspiration.

Eccentric function:
Restrains depression of ribs 2 to 5.

Isometric function:
Stabilizes the ribcage.

From:
Lower portion of the nuchal ligament and spinous processes of vertebrae C7 to T3

To:
Superior borders and external surfaces of the second through fifth ribs, just lateral to their angles

This muscle lies deep to the rhomboids.

Innervation:
Second through fifth intercostal nerves

Major synergists:
Diaphragm and other muscles of inspiration

Major antagonists:
Muscles of expiration including the serratus posterior inferior

Trigger points:
Deep to the scapula near the insertion of the muscle on the ribs

Referred pain pattern:
Deep to the superior portion of the scapula into the posterior deltoid, elbow, wrist, and ulnar portion of the hand

Serratus posterior inferior (suhr-RATE-us)

Serratus means saw-shaped, *posterior* means behind, and *inferior* means below.

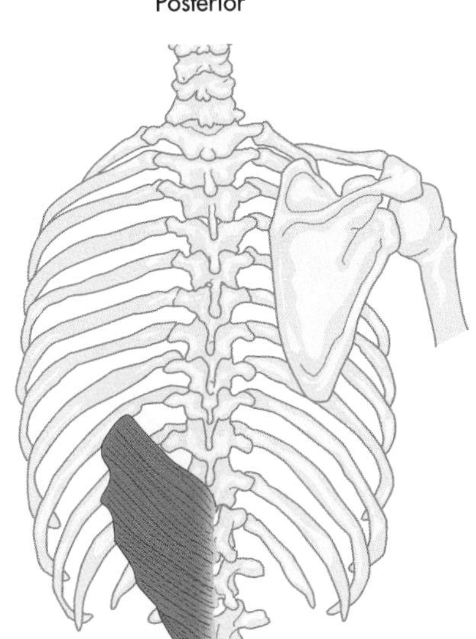

Concentric function:
Depresses ribs 9 to 12 at the sternocostal and costovertebral joints during expiration.

Eccentric function:
Restrains elevation of ribs 9 to 12.

Isometric function:
Stabilizes the ribcage.

Some studies disagree that depression of ribs 9 to 12 for expiration is the function, finding no electromyographic activity of this muscle during respiration. Perhaps the serratus posterior inferior acts as a stabilizer during forced expirations such as coughing, which would be a concentric function.

From:
Spines of T11, T12, and L1 to L3; supraspinous ligament; and thoracolumbar fascia

To:
Inferior borders and outer surfaces of the lower four ribs (9 to 12) just lateral to the angles

Innervation:
Subcostal nerve and intercostal nerves 9 to 11

Major synergists:
Other muscles of expiration

Major antagonists:
Diaphragm and serratus posterior superior

Trigger points:
Belly of the muscle near the eleventh rib

Referred pain pattern:
Nagging ache in the area of the muscle

See Activity 9-23.

ACTIVITY 9-23

1. Draw and color the serratus posterior superior and serratus posterior inferior in the space provided.
2. Label the proximal and distal attachment points: *P* for proximal; *D* for distal.
3. Place an X on the trigger points.
4. Palpate these muscles; identify the attachment points and the bellies of the muscles.
5. Move these muscles on yourself.

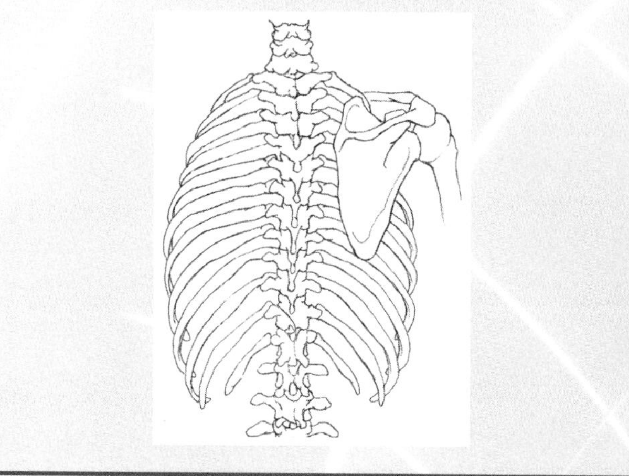

External intercostals (inter-KOS-talz)

Intercostal means between or among the ribs; *external* means on the outside.

Lateral

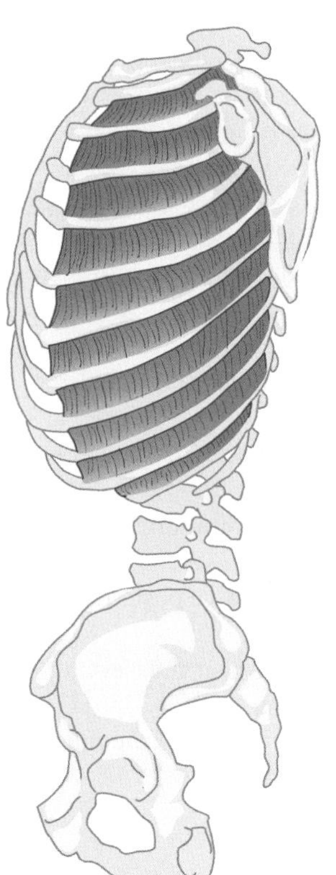

Concentric function:

Elevates the ribs at the sternocostal and costovertebral joints, increasing the volume of the thoracic cavity for inspiration

The external intercostals also may contribute to contralateral rotation of the trunk.

Eccentric function:

Restrains depression of ribs.

Isometric function:

Stabilizes the ribcage.

From:

Eleven total, each arising from the inferior border of a rib

To:

Superior border of the inferior rib

Innervation:

Adjacent intercostal nerves

Major synergists:

Diaphragm and other muscles of inspiration

Major antagonists:

Muscles of expiration

Trigger points:

The external intercostals can develop trigger points, which one can locate by palpating the muscles between the ribs.

Referred pain pattern:

Spans the intercostal segment, especially noticed with deep breathing or rotational movement.

Internal intercostals (inter-KOS-talz)

Intercostal means between or among the ribs; *internal* means on the inside.

Lateral

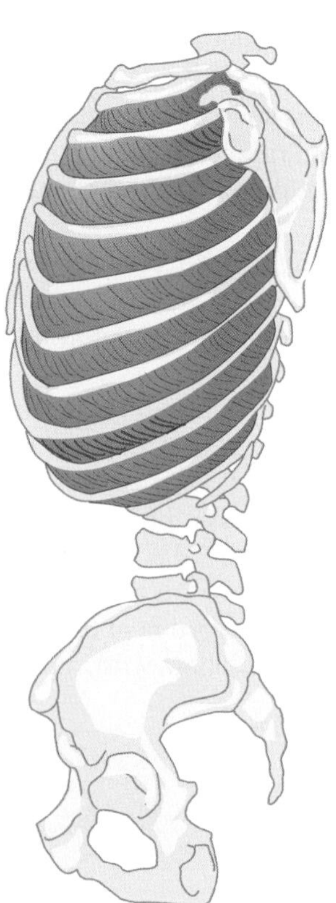

Concentric function:
Depresses the ribs at the sternocostal and costovertebral joints, decreasing the volume of the thoracic cavity for expiration.
The internal intercostals also may contribute to ipsilateral rotation of the trunk.

Eccentric function:
Restrains elevation of ribs.

Isometric function:
Stabilizes the ribcage.

From:
Eleven total, each arising from the ridge of the inner surface of a rib and corresponding costal cartilage

To:
Inferior border of the superior rib

Innervation:
Adjacent intercostal nerves

Major synergists:
Muscles of expiration

Major antagonists:
Diaphragm and other muscles of inspiration

Trigger points:
The internal intercostals can develop trigger points, which one can locate by palpating the muscles between the ribs.

Referred pain pattern:
Spans the intercostal segment, especially noticeable with deep breathing or rotational movement.

Innermost intercostals (inter-KOS-talz)

Intercostal means between or among the ribs.

The muscles of this small group attach to the internal aspects of two adjoining ribs. They are believed to act with the internal intercostals.

Transversus thoracis (trans-VER-sus thor-AH-siss)

Transversus means lying crosswise, and *thoracis* means related to the chest.

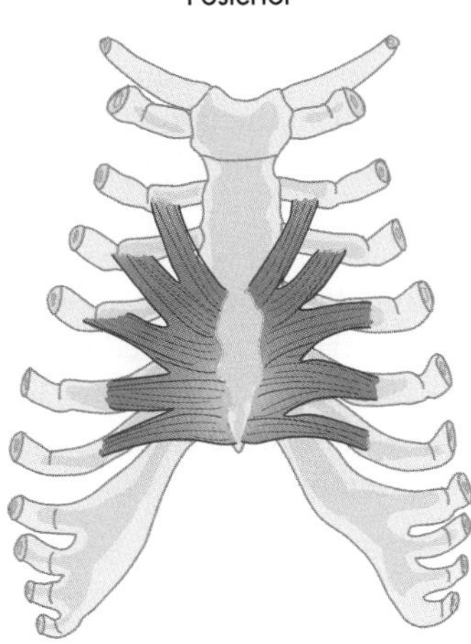

Concentric function:
Depresses ribs 2 to 6 at the sternocostal and costovertebral joints.

Eccentric function:
Restrains elevation of ribs 2 to 6.

Isometric function:
Stabilizes the ribcage.

From:
Inner surface of the body of the sternum (caudal one third), xiphoid process, and sternal ends of the costal cartilages of ribs 4 to 7

To:
Costal cartilages of the second through sixth ribs

Innervation:
Adjacent intercostal nerves
This muscle is on the inside of the ribcage.

Major synergists:
Muscles of expiration

Major antagonists:
Diaphragm and other muscles of inspiration

Trigger points:
Because of its location, this muscle is difficult to palpate for trigger points.

Referred pain pattern:
Spans the intercostal segment, especially noticeable with deep breathing or rotational movement.

See Activity 9-24.

ACTIVITY 9-24

1. Draw and color the external and internal intercostals in the space provided.
2. Label the proximal and distal attachment points: *P* for proximal; *D* for distal.
3. Place an X on the trigger points.
4. Palpate these muscles; identify the attachment points and the bellies of the muscles.
5. Move these muscles on yourself.

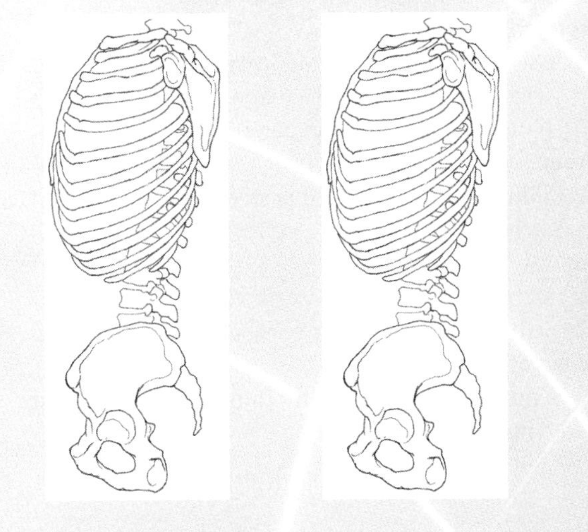

Quadratus lumborum (kwad-RATE-us lum-BOR-um)

Quadratus means square shaped, and *lumborum* means of the loins.

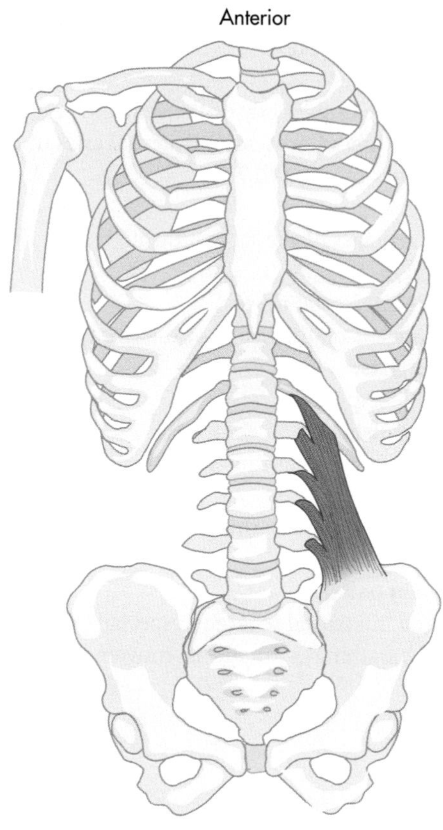

Concentric function:
Elevation and anterior tilt of the pelvis at the lumbosacral joint, lateral flexion and extension of the trunk at the spinal joints, and depression of the twelfth rib at the costovertebral joints

Eccentric function:
Allows depression and posterior tilt of the pelvis, allows contralateral lateral flexion and flexion of the trunk, and elevation of the twelfth rib.

Isometric function:
Assists normal inspiration by stabilizing the twelfth rib against the pull of the diaphragm and also stabilizes the lumbar spine and pelvis.

From:
Iliolumbar ligament and posterior portion of the iliac crest

To:
Inferior border of the last rib and transverse processes of the first four lumbar vertebrae

Innervation:
Ventral rami of the twelfth thoracic and upper three lumbar spinal nerves

ACTIVITY 9-25

1. Draw and color the quadratus lumborum in the space provided.
2. Label the proximal and distal attachment points: *P* for proximal; *D* for distal.
3. Place an X on the trigger points.
4. Palpate this muscle; identify the attachment points and the belly of the muscle.
5. Move this muscle on yourself.

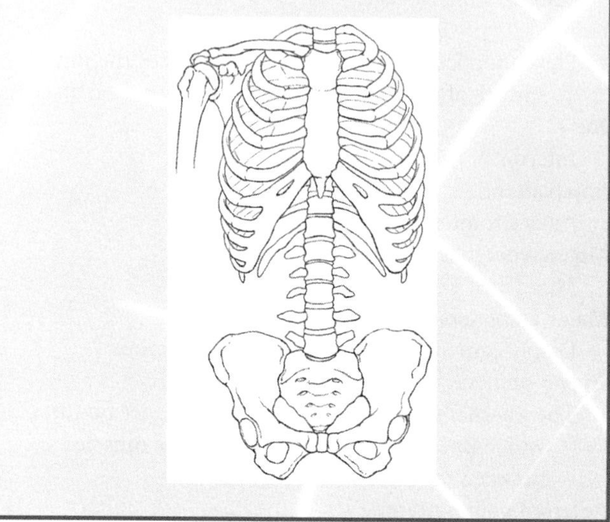

Major synergists:
Erector spinae group
The quadratus lumborum also functions with the gluteus medius, fascia lata, and adductors to stabilize the body in the frontal plane.

Major antagonists:
Posterior fibers of gluteus medius and the anterior and contralateral anterolateral abdominal wall muscles

Trigger points:
Laterally near the rib or iliac attachment and medially near the iliac attachment at the transverse processes of the lumbar vertebra

Referred pain pattern:
Gluteal and groin area, sacroiliac joint and greater trochanter; these points are implicated in most low back pain. The dual function of lumbar stabilization (isometric function) and respiration (concentric function) can cause severe pain in the low back with a cough or sneeze if these trigger points are active. Low back pain often is related more to maintenance of posture than trigger point activity; therefore finding corresponding pain patterns in the muscles that laterally flex the head and neck, such as the scalenes, is common.

See Activity 9-25.

Psoas major (SO-as)

Psoas means of the loins; *major* means larger.

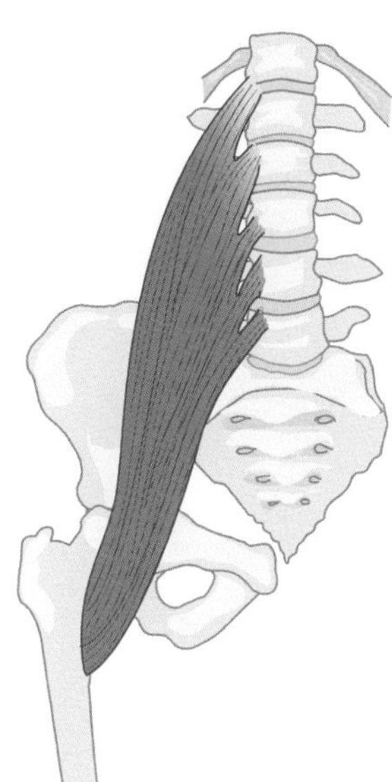

Concentric function:
Flexion and lateral rotation of the thigh at the hip joint, flexion and lateral flexion of the trunk at the spinal joints, and anterior tilt of the pelvis at the hip joint

Eccentric function:
Allows extension and medial rotation of the thigh and allows extension and contralateral lateral flexion of the trunk and posterior tilt of the pelvis.

Isometric function:
Stabilizes the lumbar spine and the lumbosacral and hip joints.

From:
Bodies and corresponding intervertebral disks of last thoracic and all lumbar vertebrae, anterior surface of transverse processes of all lumbar vertebrae, and tendinous arches extending across the sides of the bodies of the lumbar vertebrae

To:
Lesser trochanter of the femur

Innervation:
Ventral rami of lumbar plexus nerves (L1 to L3)

Major synergists:
Iliacus, sartorius, rectus femoris, and anterior and anterolateral abdominal wall muscles

Major antagonists:
Extensors of the thigh, extensors of the trunk, and posterior tilters of the pelvis

Trigger points:
Near both attachment points

Referred pain pattern:
Entire lumbar area into the superior gluteal region, as well as the anterior thigh; may be associated with menstrual aching and can mimic appendicitis. Shortening of this muscle is a major cause of low back pain and often occurs during the isometric stabilization function. If tension or trigger point activity is located at the distal attachment, pain can mimic a groin pull. Because of postural reflexes, muscles that flex the head and neck are facilitated with psoas major activation. A common correlation exists between neck pain and stiffness to psoas major pain and low back stiffness. The massage therapist often must address both areas in sequence to be effective.

Psoas major and psoas minor are located on the anterior spine posterior to the abdominal muscles and viscera.

Psoas minor (SO-as)

Psoas means of the loins; *minor* means smaller.

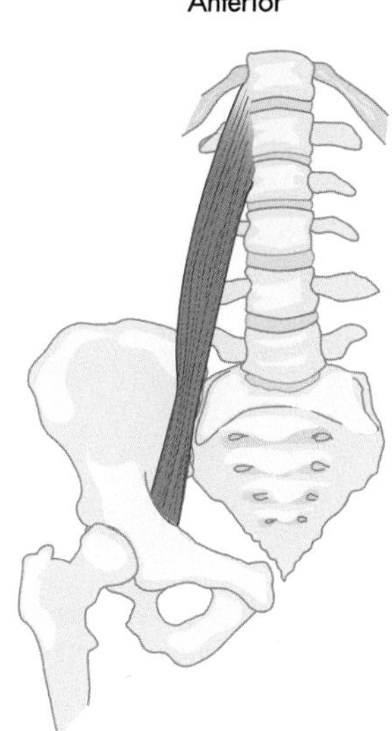

Concentric function:
Flexion of the trunk at the spinal joints and posterior tilt of the pelvis at the lumbosacral joint

Eccentric function:
Restrains extension of the trunk and anterior tilt of the pelvis.

This muscle is absent in approximately half of all human beings.

From:
Sides of the bodies of the twelfth thoracic and first lumbar vertebrae and from the intervertebral disk between them

To:
Pectineal line of the pubis and the iliopectineal eminence of the ilium and pubis

Innervation:
Branch from L1 spinal nerve

Psoas major and psoas minor are located on the anterior spine posterior to the abdominal muscles and viscera.

Major synergists:
Anterior and anterolateral abdominal wall muscles

Major antagonists:
Erector spinae group
Trigger points:
Belly of the muscle
Referred pain pattern:
Lumbar

Iliacus (ILL-ee-AK-us)

Iliacus means of the hip.

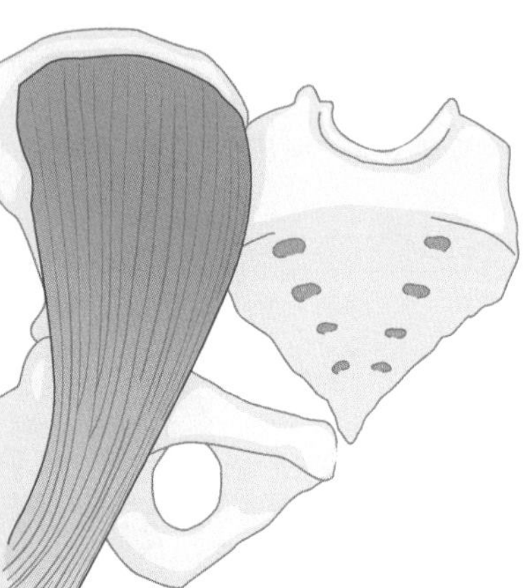

Concentric function:
Flexion and lateral rotation of the thigh at the hip joint and anterior tilt of the pelvis at the lumbosacral joint
Eccentric function:
Allows extension and medial rotation of the thigh and allows posterior tilt of the pelvis.
Isometric function:
Stabilizes the pelvis and the hip joint.
From:
Internal lip of the iliac crest; anterior sacroiliac, lumbosacral, and iliolumbar ligaments; superior two thirds of the iliac fossa; and ala of the sacrum
To:
Lesser trochanter of the femur, into the posterior side of the psoas major tendon
Innervation:
Femoral nerve (L2 to L3)
Major synergist:
Psoas major
Major antagonists:
Gluteus maximus and hamstrings
Trigger points:
Inner border of the ilium posterior to the anterior superior iliac spine

ACTIVITY 9-26

1. Draw and color the psoas major and psoas minor and the iliacus in the space provided.
2. Label the proximal and distal attachment points: *P* for proximal; *D* for distal.
3. Place an X on the trigger points.
4. Palpate these muscles; identify the attachment points and the bellies of the muscles.
5. Move these muscles on yourself.

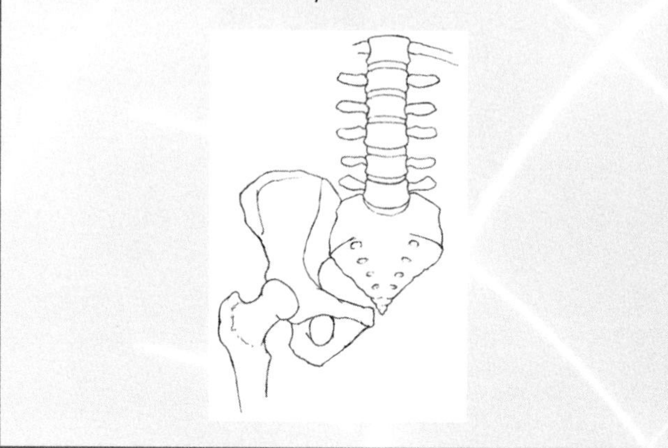

Referred pain pattern:
Hip and groin

See Activity 9-26.

Muscles of the Anterior and Anterolateral Abdominal Wall

The abdominal muscles and extensive fascia form the anterior and anterolateral abdominal wall. The muscle fiber arrangement produces a crisscross fiber pattern similar to plywood, with vertical support provided by the rectus abdominis and the pyramidalis. These muscles attach directly or indirectly to a strong, fibrous cord in the midline of the abdomen called the linea alba, which is formed from the fusion of the two anterior abdominal aponeuroses (each abdominal aponeurosis is formed from the fusion of the aponeuroses of the external abdominal oblique, and the transversus abdominis). The linea alba extends from the xiphoid process to the symphysis pubis and contains the umbilicus.

As a group these muscles act to compress the abdominal contents during expiration, urination, and defecation. They help maintain pressure on the curve of the low back, resisting excessive lumbar lordosis. Isometric stabilization is an important function of this group. Along with the deep muscles of the back, the abdominal muscles provide stability for the entire trunk of the body. The muscles also work with the adductors of the thighs at the hip joint to maintain upright posture. Massage application to this area is important because the muscles are involved in posture and breathing. The fascial aponeuroses may shorten, and the muscles are frequently weak and long. Methods to encourage normal muscle tone are effective. These exercises are usually called core training.

Transversus abdominis (trans-VER-sus ab-DAHM-in-iss)

Transversus means lying crosswise, and *abdominis* means of the abdomen.

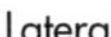

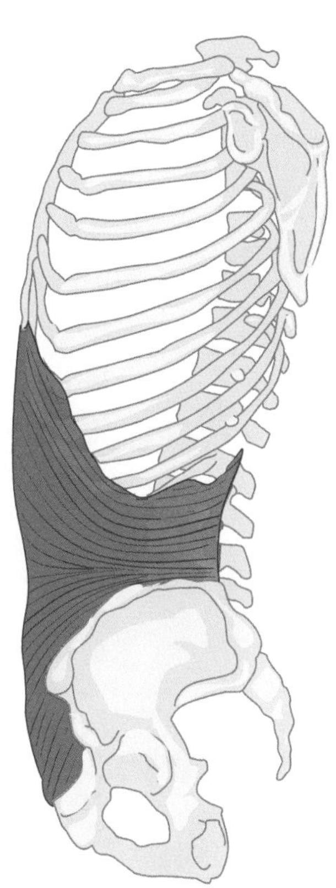

The transversus abdominis is the innermost layer of the abdominal wall just superficial to the peritoneum.

Concentric/isometric function:

Compresses the contents of the abdomen, increasing intraabdominal pressure and thereby supporting the abdominal viscera and assisting in forced expiration.

From:

Inner surfaces of the cartilages of the last six ribs, anterior three fourths of the iliac crest, lateral one third of the inguinal ligament, and thoracolumbar fascia

To:

Linea alba, abdominal aponeurosis, and pubis

Innervation:

Ventral rami of the lower six thoracic and first lumbar spinal nerves

Major synergists:

Rectus abdominis and external and internal abdominal obliques

Major antagonists:

Not clearly defined

Internal abdominal oblique (ab-DAHM-in-al oh-BLEEK)

This muscle is located within the anterolateral abdominal wall, deep to the external abdominal oblique and superficial to the transversus abdominis. It is positioned at a slant.

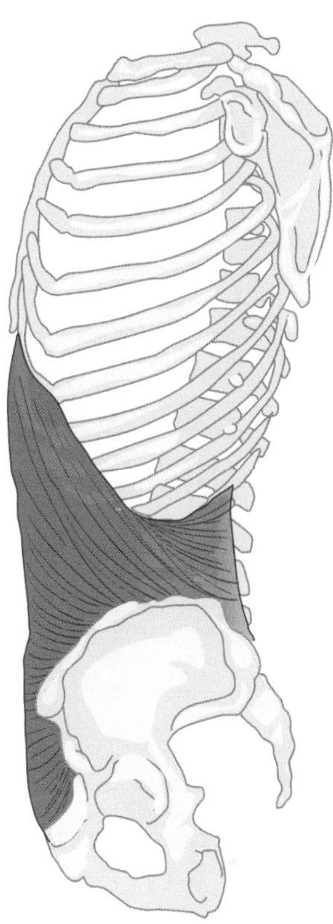

Concentric function:

Flexion, lateral flexion, and ipsilateral rotation of the trunk at the spinal joints; posterior tilt of the pelvis at the lumbosacral joint; and compression of the contents of the abdominal cavity (thereby supporting the abdominal viscera and assisting in forced expiration)

Eccentric function:

Allows extension, contralateral lateral flexion, and contralateral rotation of the trunk and allows anterior tilt of the pelvis.

From:

Inguinal ligament, iliac fascia, anterior two thirds of the middle lip of the iliac crest, and lumbar fascia

To:

Upper fibers into cartilages of last three ribs; the remainder into the aponeurosis extending from the tenth costal cartilage to the pubic bone into the linea alba

Innervation:

Ventral rami of the lower six thoracic and first lumbar spinal nerves

Major synergists:
Opposite-sided external abdominal oblique and the rectus abdominis

Major antagonists:
Extensors of the spine and opposite-sided internal abdominal oblique

External abdominal oblique (ab-DAHM-in-al oh-BLEEK)

This muscle is located within the abdominal wall, superficial to the internal abdominal oblique; its fibers are slanted like pockets of a coat.

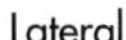

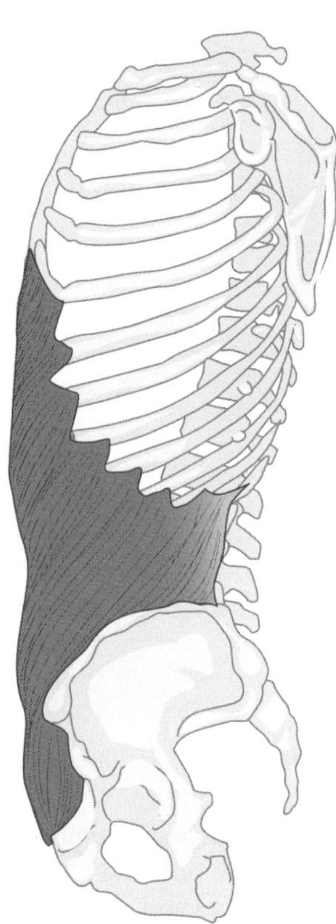

Concentric function:
Flexion, lateral flexion, and contralateral rotation of the trunk at the spinal joints; posterior tilt of the pelvis at the lumbosacral joint; and compression of the contents of the abdominal cavity (thereby supporting the abdominal viscera and assisting in forced expiration)

Eccentric function:
Allows extension, contralateral lateral flexion, and ipsilateral rotation of the trunk and allows anterior tilt of the pelvis.

From:
Outer lip of the iliac crest, pubic bone, and the linea alba

To:
External surface of the lower eight ribs by interdigital slips

Innervation:
Ventral rami of the lower six thoracic spinal nerves

Major synergists:
Opposite-sided internal abdominal oblique and the rectus abdominis

Major antagonists:
Extensors of the spine and opposite-sided external abdominal oblique

Rectus abdominis (REK-tus ab-DAHM-in-iss)

Rectus means straight, and *abdominis* means of the abdomen.

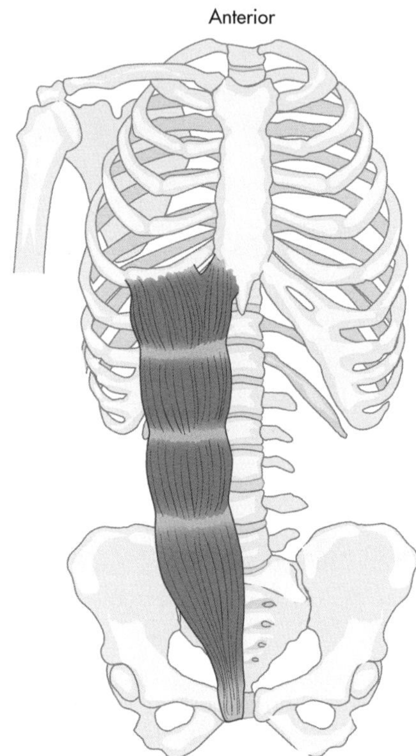

Concentric function:
Flexion and lateral flexion of the trunk at the spinal joints, posterior tilt of the pelvis at the lumbosacral joint, and compression of the contents of the abdominal cavity (thereby supporting the abdominal viscera and assisting in forced expiration)

Eccentric function:
Allows extension and contralateral lateral flexion of the trunk and allows anterior tilt of the pelvis.

From:
Pubis and the pubic symphysis

To:
Cartilages of the fifth, sixth, and seventh ribs and the xiphoid process of the sternum

Major synergists:
External and internal abdominal obliques

Major antagonists:
Extensors of the spine

Innervation:
Anterior primary rami of the lower six intercostal nerves

Pyramidalis (peer-AM-id-al-iss)

Pyramidalis means pyramid shaped.

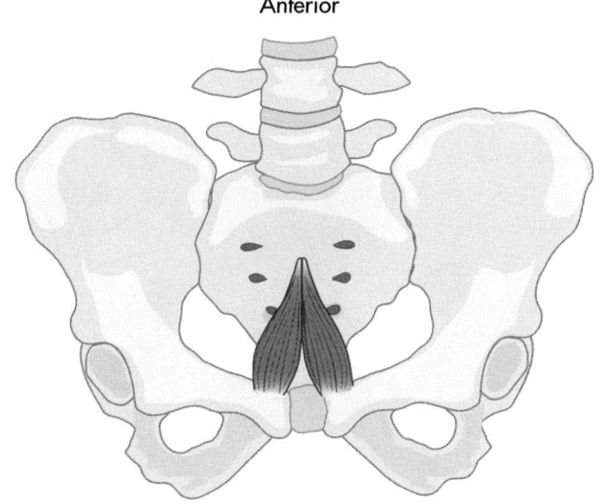

Function:

Tenses the linea alba to compress the contents of the abdominal cavity (thereby supporting the abdominal viscera and assisting in forced expiration).

Although the pyramidalis is a striated muscle, it usually is not under voluntary control.

From:

Ventral surface of the pubis and the pubic ligament

To:

Linea alba (between the pubis and the umbilicus)

Innervation:

Subcostal nerve (ventral ramus of T12)

Cremaster (KREE-mast-er)

Cremaster means a suspender.

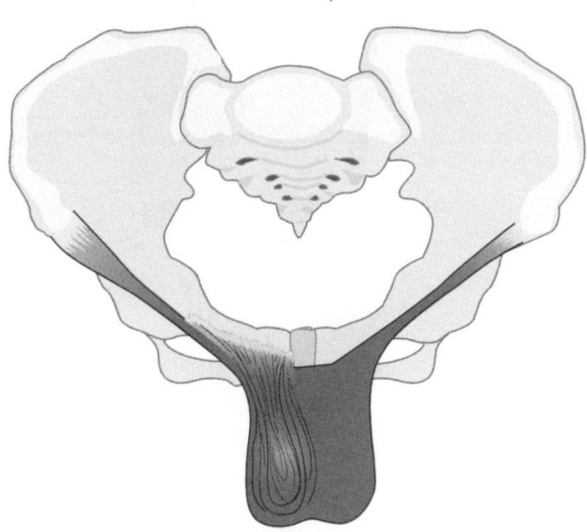

Function:

Pulls the testes superiorly (to help regulate their temperature).

From:

Lower edge of the internal oblique muscle and the middle aspect of the inguinal ligament

To:

Pubic tubercle and the crest of the pubis

Innervation:

Genital branch of the genitofemoral nerve (L1 to L2)

{Elements common to muscles of the anterior abdominal}

Elements common to the anterior abdominal wall muscles

Synergists:

Quadratus lumborum and diaphragm; rotation – lower

ACTIVITY 9-27

1. Draw and color the anterior abdominal wall muscles in the space provided.
2. Label the proximal and distal attachment points: *P* for proximal; *D* for distal.
3. Place an X on the trigger points.
4. Palpate these muscles; identify the attachment points and the bellies of the muscles.
5. Move these muscles on yourself.

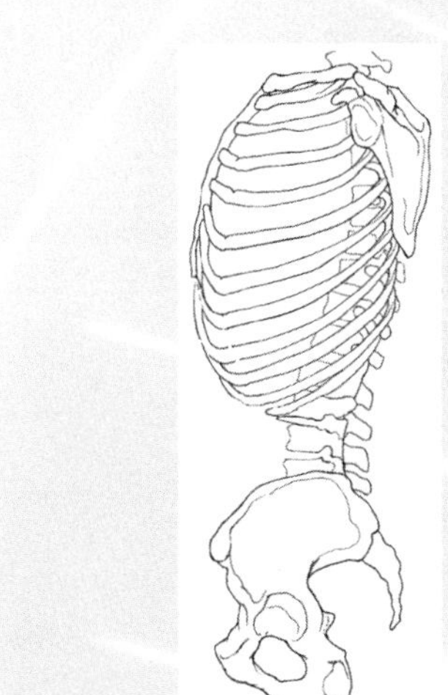

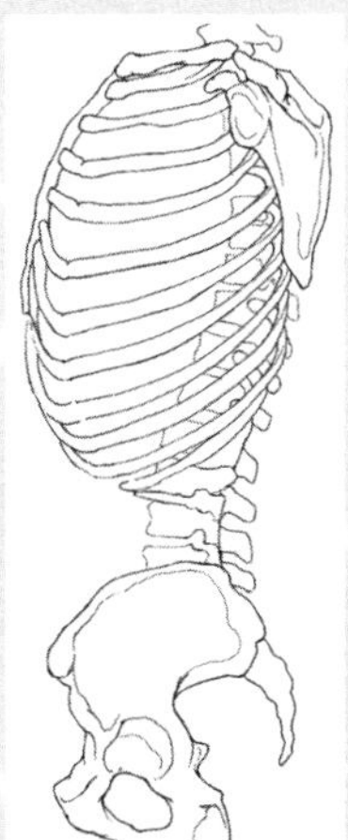

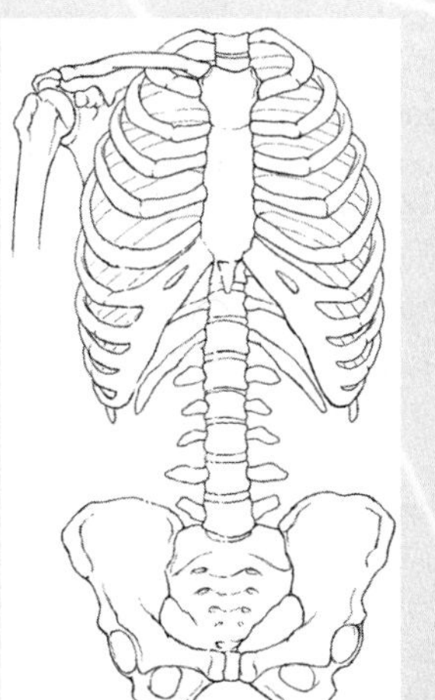

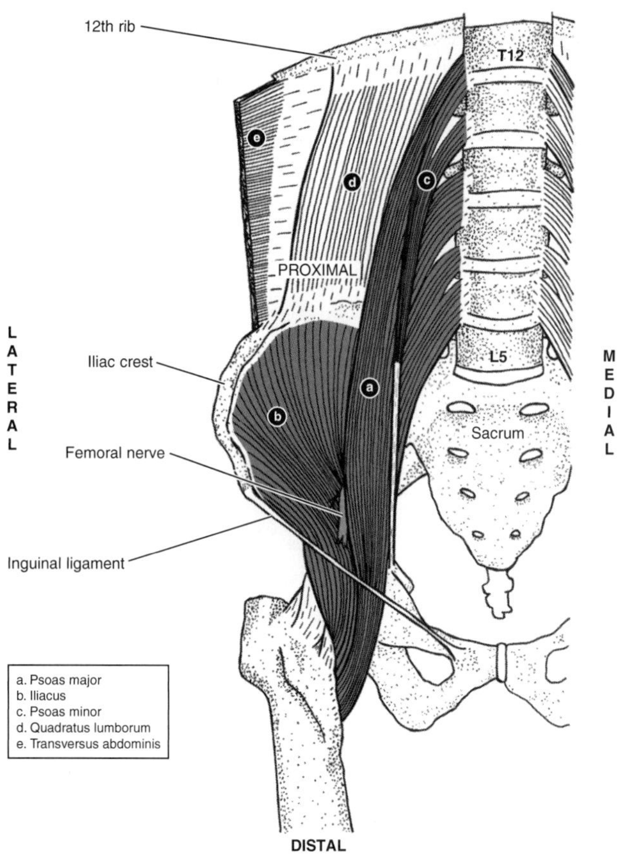

Figure 9-25
Anterior view of the right pelvis. (Modified from Muscolino JE: *The muscular system manual: the skeletal muscles of the human body,* ed 2, St Louis, 2005, Mosby.)

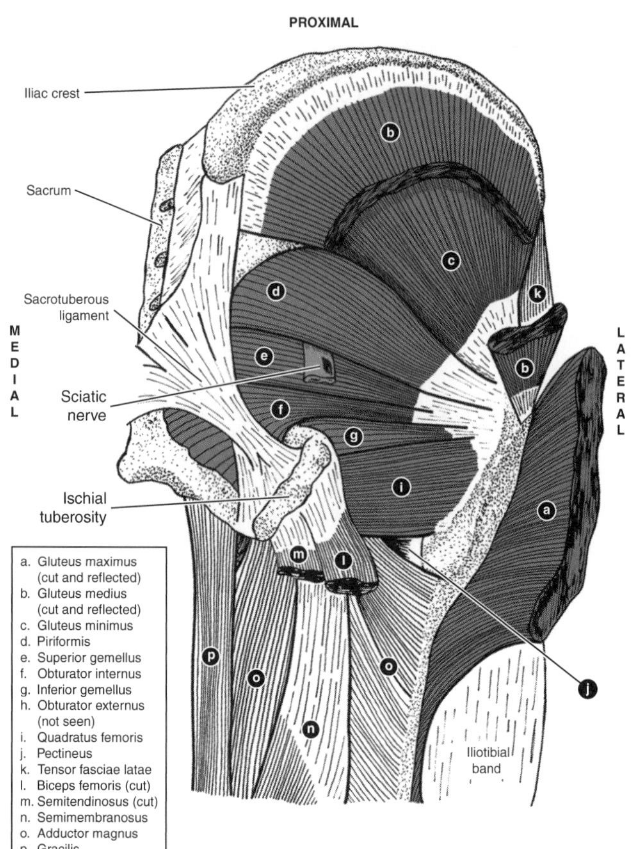

Figure 9-26
Posterior view of the right pelvis (deep). (Modified from Muscolino JE: *The muscular system manual: the skeletal muscles of the human body,* ed 2, St Louis, 2005, Mosby.)

serratus anterior and posterior, latissimus doris, iliocostalis

Antagonists:
Flexion – paraspinal extensor group; rotation – contralateral muscles

Trigger points:
Located throughout the area but concentrated more in the external circle of the abdominal wall rather than toward the middle near the umbilicus; the exceptions are points often found in the rectus abdominis just below the umbilicus on either side of the linea alba

Referred pain pattern:
Pain likely to appear in the same quadrant and in the back; these trigger points are capable of causing somatovisceral responses (e.g., vomiting, nausea, intestinal problems, diarrhea, bladder symptoms, and pain).

See Activity 9-27.

Pelvic and Perineal Muscles

The levator ani and the coccygeus muscles form the pelvic floor (also called the pelvic diaphragm) (Figures 9-25 and 9-26). These muscles close the inferior outlet of the pelvis, support and elevate the pelvic floor, and counterbalance increased intraabdominal pressure, which would expel the contents of the bladder, rectum, and uterus. The pelvic diaphragm has openings for the rectum, urethra, and vagina. One usually does not massage this area with direct methods; however, attention to antagonistic and synergistic muscles that are accessed more easily is indicated. Isometric stabilization is a major function of these muscles.

Levator ani (le-VAY-tor AIN-eye)

Levator means one that raises; *ani* means belonging to the anus or rectum.

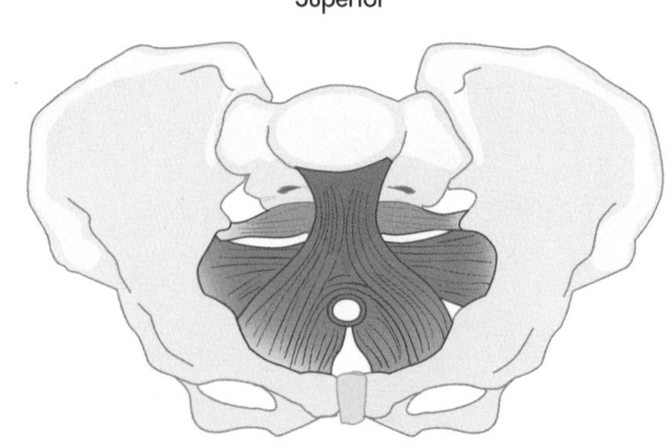

Function:

Forms the floor of the pelvic cavity, constricts the lower end of the rectum and vagina, and supports and slightly raises the pelvic floor.

From:

Pelvic surfaces of the pubis, inner surface of the ischial spine, and the obturator fascia

To:

Last two segments of the coccyx, anococcygeal raphe uniting with fibers from the opposite side, and the sides of the rectum anterior into the perineal body

Innervation:

Muscular branches of the perineal division of the pudendal nerve

Coccygeus (kok-SIH-jee-us)

Coccygeus means related to the coccyx or tailbone.

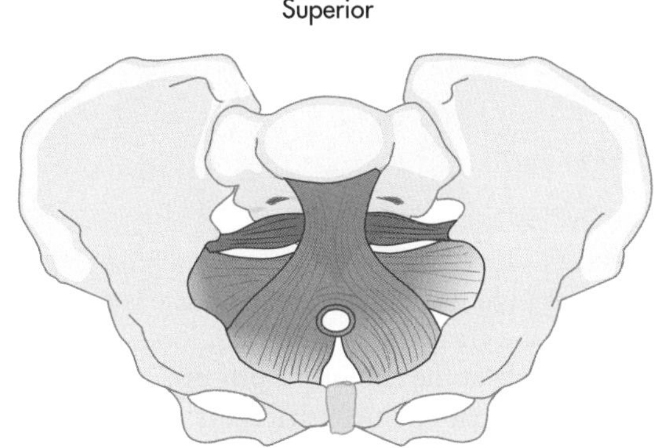

Function:

Pulls forward and supports the coccyx; exerts rotary tension on the sacroiliac joint; and, with the levator ani and piriformis muscles, assists in closing the posterior part of the pelvic outlet and forms the supporting muscular diaphragm for the pelvic viscera.

From:

Pelvic surface of the spine of the ischium and the sacrospinous ligament

To:

Margin of the coccyx and the side of the fifth segment of the sacrum

Innervation:

Branch of the fourth and fifth sacral nerves

External sphincter ani (SFINK-tur AIN-eye)

External means on the outside, *sphincter* means band, and *ani* means related to the anus or rectum.

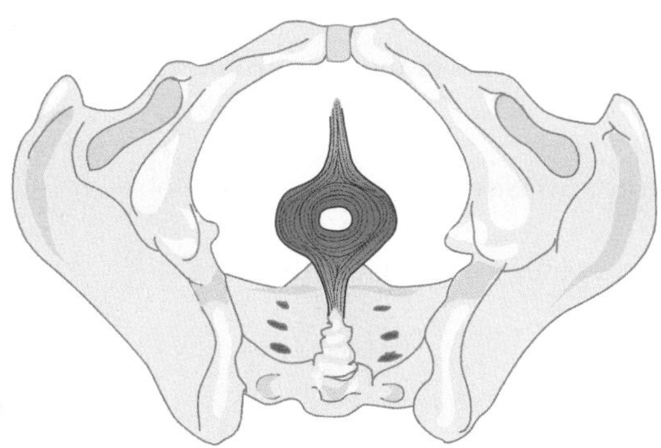

Function:

Closes the anal orifice.

From:

Superficial fibers from the anococcygeal raphe; deeper fibers surround the anal canal.

To:

Superficial fibers surround the anus, meeting posteriorly at the coccyx and anteriorly at the central point of the perineum.

Innervation:

Perineal branch of the fourth sacral nerve and the inferior rectal branch of the pudendal nerve

Deep transverse perineals (pair-i-NEE-als)

Transverse means crossing or around; *perineal* means to empty or defecate.

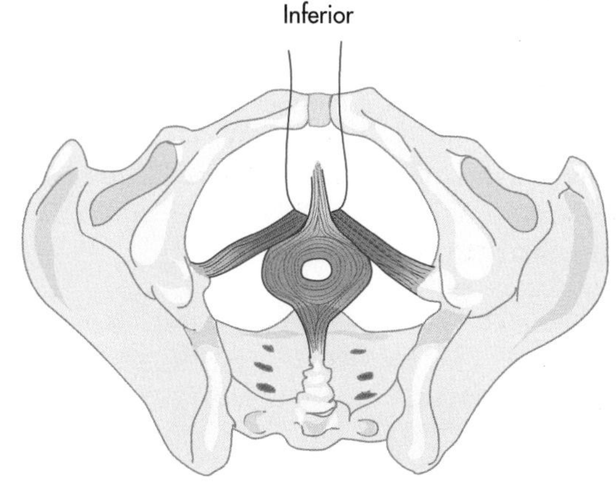

Function:
Simultaneous contraction of both muscles helps to fix the perineal body.
From:
Medial and anterior part of the ischial tuberosity
To:
Central tendinous point of the perineum
Innervation:
Perineal branches of the pudendal nerve

Ischiocavernosus (ISS-she-oh-KAV-ern-oh-sus)

Ischiocavernosus means hip and cavernlike.

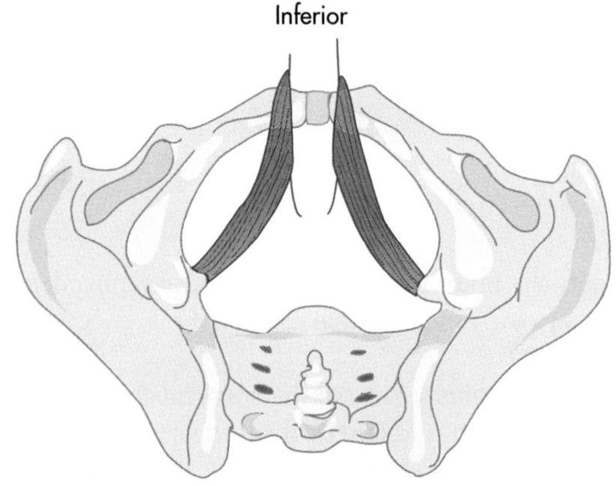

Function:
Compresses the crus penis, which obstructs venous return and therefore is believed to play a part in maintaining erection of the penis or clitoris.
From:
Inner surface of the ischial tuberosity behind the crus penis or clitoris and the ramus of the ischium on both sides of the crus
To:
Aponeuroses on the sides and undersurface of the crus penis or clitoris
Innervation:
Perineal branch of the pudendal nerve (S2 to S4)

Bulbospongiosus (BUL-bo-SPON-jee-oh-sus)

Bulbospongiosus means bulb and spongy.

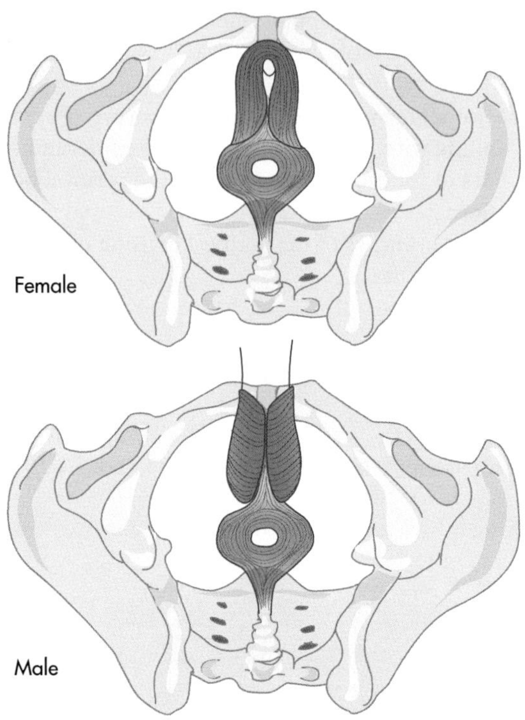

Function:
Aids in emptying the urethra; the muscle is relaxed during the greater part of micturition, coming into action only at the end of the process, and can be used to assist urination; it constricts the orifice of the vagina and contributes to erection of the penis and clitoris.
From:
Central tendinous point of the perineum, with fibers surrounding the vaginal orifice and vestibular bulbs (female)
To:
Lower surface of the perineal membrane, dorsal surface of the corpus spongiosum, deep fascia on the dorsum of the penis, and corpora cavernosa clitoris (female)
Innervation:
Perineal branch of the pudendal nerve (S2 to S4)

The following elements are common to the pelvic and perineal muscles:

Synergists: All muscles are synergistic; the gluteus maximus supports the closure of the anus.

Antagonists: No direct antagonist pattern to the pelvic floor has been identified in the literature; however, because the gluteus maximus is powerfully synergistic with these muscles, one could assume that antagonist patterns to the gluteus maximus, such as the psoas, would have an antagonistic influence on the pelvic floor muscles. The diaphragm muscle also may act as an antagonist to this muscle group.

ACTIVITY 9-28

Move your pelvic floor muscles.

Trigger points: Trigger points do develop in these muscles; one can usually palpate these trigger points internally, rectally or vaginally.

Referred pain patterns: To the pelvic floor itself and to the coccyx region

See Activity 9-28.

Muscles of the Gluteal Region

The muscles of the gluteal region are some of the most powerful muscles of the body (see Figure 9-26). The more superficial muscles, especially the large gluteus maximus, extend the thigh during forceful extension. The gluteus maximus also stabilizes the iliotibial band and thoracolumbar fascia. The gluteus medius and gluteus minimus are especially strong at abduction and medial (internal) rotation of the thigh. The deep lateral (external) rotators of the thigh at the hip joint are six small, deep muscles of the gluteal region that oppose medial rotation. As a group, the gluteal muscles are related to shoulder extensors and flexors and arm medial and lateral rotators because of gait (walking) reflex patterns to promote the appropriate counterbalancing arm swing. Facilitation between muscles of the arms that flex and extend along with thigh muscles in contralateral patterns occurs. One usually needs to consider the muscles of the shoulder joint with muscles of the hip joint and apply massage in a correlated pattern. Although not listed with synergists and antagonists, the flexors of the thigh at the hip joint work with flexors of the arm at the shoulder joint on the opposite side (i.e., right with left and left with right). These muscles also display inhibitory patterns with each other. For example, right extensors of the thigh at the hip joint are inhibitory to left flexors of the arm at the shoulder joint. On the same side (right arm with right thigh, left arm with left thigh), flexors and extensors work with each other. Adductors and medial rotators of the shoulder joint work with adductors and medial rotators of the hip joint on the opposite side. This same concept is true for abductors and lateral rotators. Conversely, same-side adductors of the shoulder and hip are inhibitory to each other, as are same-side abductors and lateral rotators. Although these patterns seem confusing, the connection becomes apparent if one takes a step and analyzes the patterns of what muscles are working together.

Gluteus maximus (GLUE-tee-us MAX-uh-mus)

Gluteus means buttocks; *maximus* means greatest or largest.

Posterior

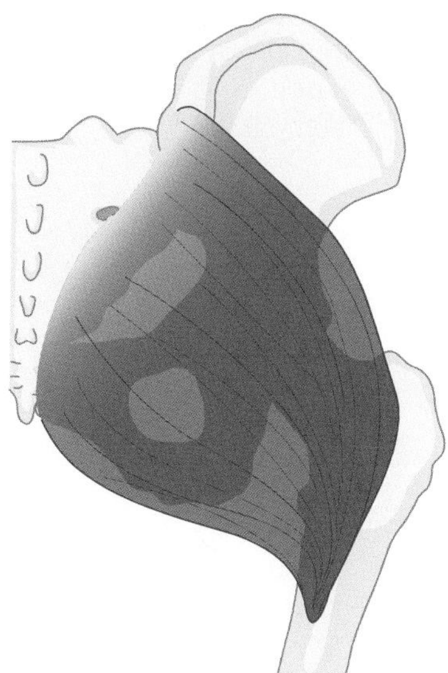

Concentric function:
Extends and laterally rotates the thigh at the hip joint; the upper fibers abduct the thigh at the hip joint, and the lower fibers adduct the thigh at the hip joint; and provides posterior tilt of the pelvis at the hip joint. (The gluteus maximus is active primarily during strenuous activity, such as running, jumping, and climbing stairs.)

Eccentric function:
Restrains flexion and medial rotation of the thigh and anterior tilt of the pelvis; the upper fibers restrain adduction of the thigh, and lower fibers restrain abduction of the thigh.

Isometric function:
These muscles are important postural muscles that help maintain the upright posture, stabilize the pelvis, and provide tension to the iliotibial band to keep the fascial band taut.

From:
Posterior gluteal line of the ilium, dorsal surface of the lower aspect of the sacrum and the side of the coccyx, sacrotuberous ligament and gluteal aponeurosis, and aponeurosis of the erector spinae

To:
Iliotibial band of the fascia lata and gluteal tuberosity of the femur

Innervation:
Inferior gluteal nerve (L5 to S2)

Major synergists:
Hamstring muscles and piriformis

Major antagonists:
Iliopsoas, tensor fasciae latae, and gluteus medius (anterior fibers)

ACTIVITY 9-29

1. Draw and color the gluteus maximus in the space provided.
2. Label the proximal and distal attachment points: *P* for proximal; *D* for distal.
3. Place an X on the trigger points.
4. Palpate this muscle; identify the attachment points and the belly of the muscle.
5. Move this muscle on yourself.

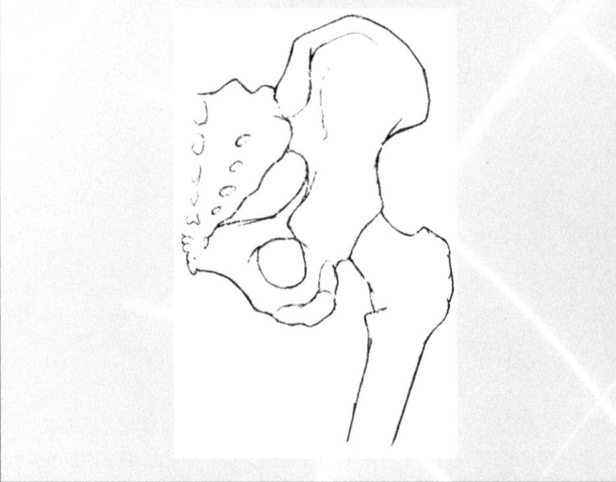

Trigger points:
Three main areas—near the sacrum at the musculotendinous junction midway down from the iliac crest, near the ischial tuberosity, and in the belly of the muscle closer to the lower fibers

Referred pain pattern:
Regionally into the gluteal area, especially to the ischial tuberosity, the tip of the greater trochanter, and the sacrum. A shortened and tight gluteus maximus can be responsible for tightness of the iliotibial band and thoracolumbar fascia. These superficial muscles are thick and require firm massage application to be effective. The smaller deeper muscle layers have to be accessed by pressure that penetrates through the gluteus maximus. Positioning the client so that this muscle is in a passive contraction by propping the client so the attachments of the muscle are closer together is helpful. If no active contraction is taking place, the area becomes softer and is easier for compressive forces of massage to reach the underlying muscle layers.

See Activity 9-29.

Gluteus medius (GLUE-tee-us MEED-ee-us)

Gluteus means buttocks; *medius* means middle.

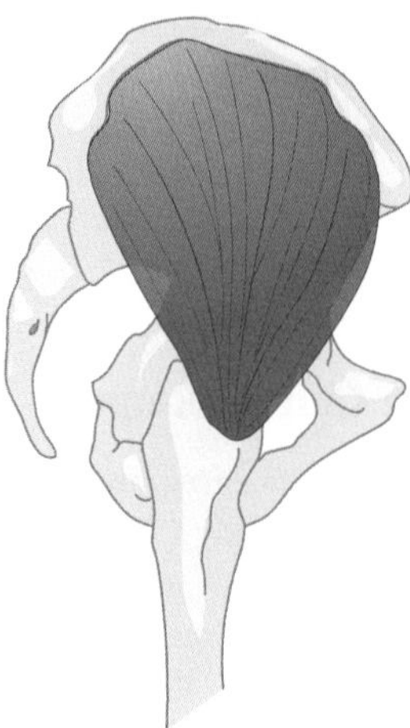

Concentric function:
Abducts the thigh at the hip joint; anterior fibers medially rotate and flex the thigh at the hip joint and allow anterior tilt of the pelvis at the hip joint; posterior fibers laterally rotate and extend the thigh at the hip joint and allow posterior tilt of the pelvis at the hip joint.

Eccentric function:
Restrains adduction of the thigh; the anterior fibers restrain extension and lateral rotation of the thigh and posterior tilt of the pelvis; the posterior fibers restrain flexion and medial rotation of the thigh and anterior tilt of the pelvis.

Isometric function:
Stabilizes the pelvis (especially when a person is standing on one foot).

From:
External surface of the ilium inferior to the iliac crest, between the anterior and posterior gluteal lines, and the gluteal aponeurosis

To:
Lateral surface of the greater trochanter of the femur

Innervation:
Superior gluteal nerve (L4 to S1)

Major synergists:
Gluteus minimus, tensor fasciae latae, and piriformis

Major antagonists:
The adductors of the thigh

Trigger points:
Along the musculotendinous junction at the iliac crest

Referred pain pattern:
Low back, posterior crest of the ilium to the sacrum, and to the posterior and lateral areas of the buttock into the upper thigh

See Activity 9-30.

ACTIVITY 9-30

1. Draw and color the gluteus medius in the space provided.
2. Label the proximal and distal attachment points: *P* for proximal; *D* for distal.
3. Place an X on the trigger points.
4. Palpate this muscle; identify the attachment points and the belly of the muscle.
5. Move this muscle on yourself.

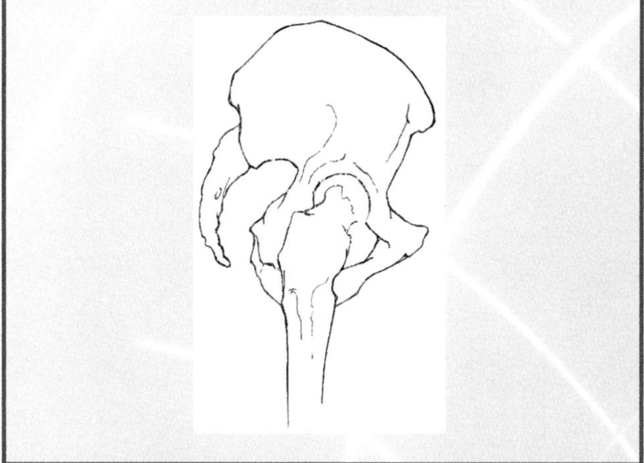

ACTIVITY 9-31

1. Draw and color the gluteus minimus in the space provided.
2. Label the proximal and distal attachment points: *P* for proximal; *D* for distal.
3. Place an X on the trigger points.
4. Palpate this muscle; identify the attachment points and the belly of the muscle.
5. Move this muscle on yourself.

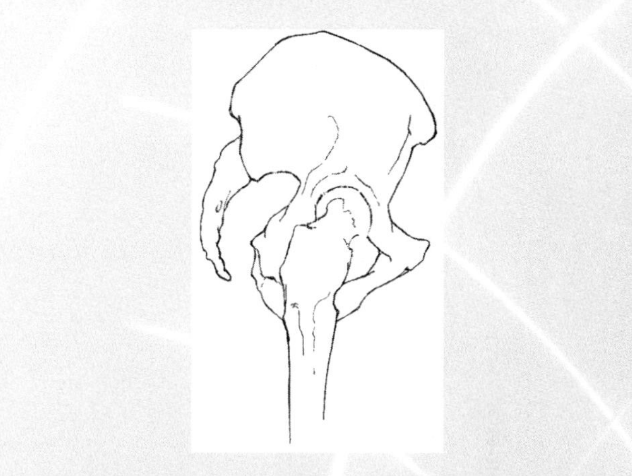

Gluteus minimus (GLUE-tee-us MIN-ih-mus)

Gluteus means buttocks; *minimus* means smallest.

Lateral

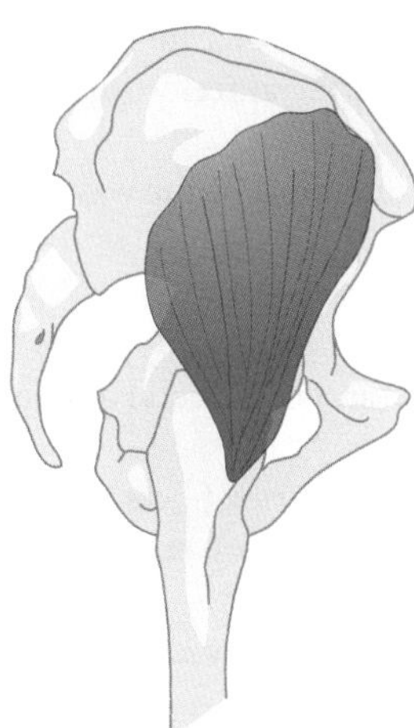

Concentric function:
Abducts the thigh at the hip joint, medially rotates and flexes the thigh at the hip joint, and allows anterior tilt of the pelvis at the hip joint.

Eccentric function:
Restrains adduction of the thigh; the anterior fibers restrain extension and lateral rotation of the thigh and posterior tilt of the pelvis.

Isometric function:
Stabilizes the pelvis (especially when a person is standing on one foot).

From:
External surface of the ilium inferior to the iliac crest, between the anterior and inferior gluteal lines

To:
Anterior border of the greater trochanter of the femur

Innervation:
Superior gluteal nerve (L4 to S1)

Major synergist:
Gluteus medius

Major antagonists:
Adductors of the thigh

Trigger points:
Belly of the muscle

Referred pain pattern:
Lower lateral buttock and down the lateral to posterior aspect of the thigh, knee, and leg to the ankle

See Activity 9-31.

Tensor fasciae latae (TEN-sore FAH-she-a LAT-uh)

Tensor means one that stretches, *fasciae* means bands or bandages, and *latae* means wide.

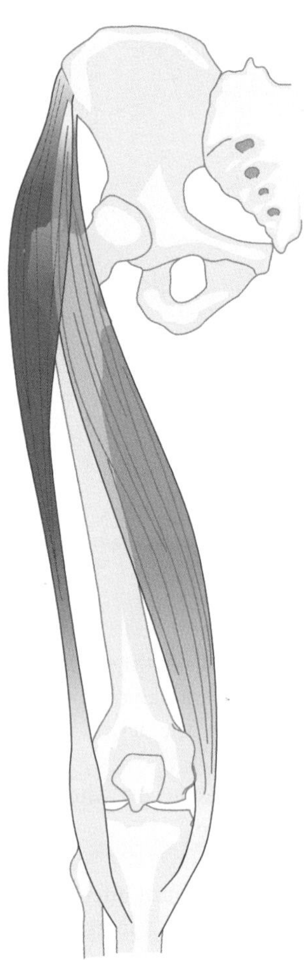

Concentric function:
Flexion, medial rotation, and abduction of the thigh at the hip joint; anterior tilt of the pelvis at the hip joint; and extension of the leg at the knee joint

Eccentric function:
Restrains extension, lateral rotation, and adduction of the thigh and allows posterior tilt of the pelvis and flexion of the leg.

Isometric function:
Tenses the iliotibial band, counterbalancing the backward pull of the gluteus maximus on the iliotibial band, and stabilizes the pelvis and the knee.

ACTIVITY 9-32

1. Draw and color the tensor fasciae latae in the space provided.
2. Label the proximal and distal attachment points: *P* for proximal; *D* for distal.
3. Place an X on the trigger points.
4. Palpate this muscle; identify the attachment points and the belly of the muscle.
5. Move this muscle on yourself.

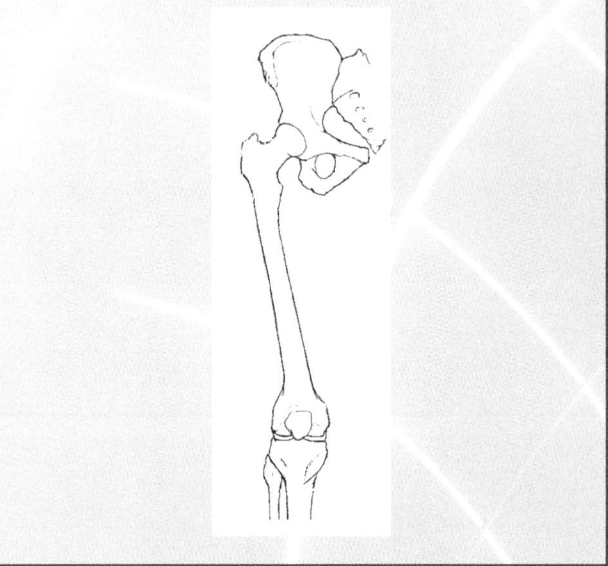

From:
Anterior aspect of the outer lip of the iliac crest and outer surface of the anterior superior iliac spine

To:
Iliotibial band, one third of the way down the thigh

Innervation:
Superior gluteal nerve (L4 to S1)

Major synergists:
Gluteus medius (anterior fibers) and iliopsoas

Major antagonists:
Gluteus medius (posterior fibers), adductors of the thigh group, gluteus maximus, and hamstrings

Trigger points:
In the belly of the muscle and near the distal attachment

Referred pain pattern:
Localized in the hip and down the lateral side of the thigh to the knee

See Activity 9-32.

Deep Lateral Rotators of the Thigh at the Hip Joint

Piriformis (PEER-ih-FOR-miss)

Piriformis means pear shaped.

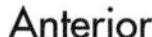

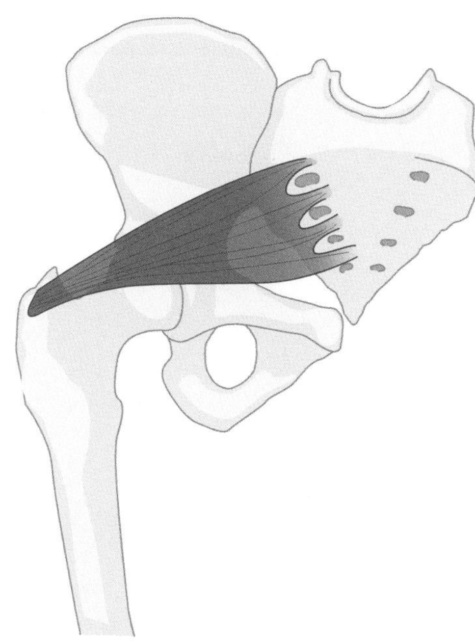

Concentric function:
Lateral rotation of the thigh at the hip joint and abduction and medial rotation of the thigh at the hip joint if the thigh is first in a position of flexion at the hip joint

Eccentric function:
Restrains medial rotation of the thigh and also may restrain adduction and lateral rotation of the thigh (if the thigh is in a position of flexion).

Isometric function:
Stabilizes the hip joint.

From:
Anterior surface of the sacrum between the first through fourth sacral foramina and the pelvic surface of the sacrotuberous ligament

To:
Superior border of the greater trochanter of the femur

Innervation:
Lumbosacral plexus (L5 to S2)

Major synergists:
All deep lateral rotators of the thigh at the hip joint are synergistic with one another; posterior fibers of the gluteus medius.

Major antagonists:
Anterior fibers of the gluteus medius, gluteus minimus, and the tensor fasciae latae

Trigger points:
The main trigger points in the piriformis muscle are near the attachments. The belly may have trigger points as well. Tension in this muscle can cause entrapment of the sciatic nerve, which normally passes inferior to the piriformis but in some individuals passes through the muscle, predisposing the person to symptoms of sciatica.

Referred pain pattern:
Sacroiliac region, entire buttock, and down the posterior thigh to just proximal to the knee

Obturator internus OB-tur-ATE-or in-TER-nus)

Obturator means one that covers an opening; *internus* means interior.

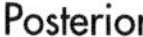

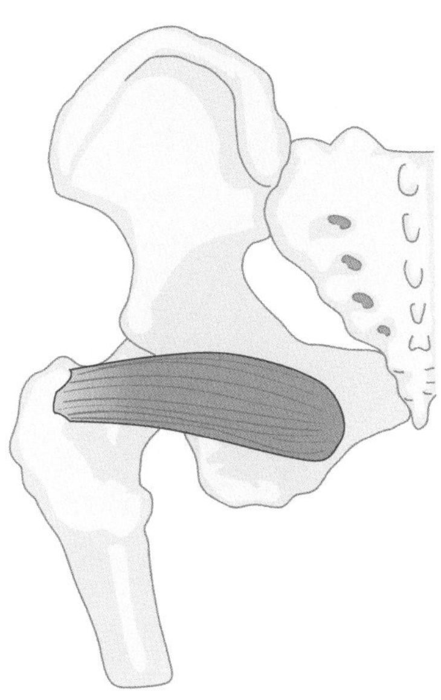

Concentric function:
Lateral rotation of the thigh at the hip joint and abduction of the thigh at the hip joint if the thigh is first in a position of flexion at the hip joint

Eccentric function:
Restrains medial rotation of the thigh and also may restrain adduction of the thigh (if the thigh is in a position of flexion).

Isometric function:
Stabilizes the hip joint.

From:
Internal surface of the obturator membrane and the margins of the obturator foramen (on the ilium, ischium, and pubis)

To:
Medial surface of the greater trochanter of the femur

Innervation:
Nerve to obturator internus from the lumbosacral plexus (L5 to S1)

Major synergists:
All deep lateral rotators of the thigh at the hip joint are synergistic with one another; posterior fibers of the gluteus medius.

Major antagonists:
Anterior fibers of the gluteus medius, gluteus minimus, and the tensor fasciae latae

Trigger points:
The belly of the muscle

Referred pain pattern:
Sacroiliac region, entire buttock, and down the posterior thigh to just proximal to the knee joint

Obturator externus (OB-tur-ATE-or ex-STIR-nus)

Obturator means one that covers an opening; *externus* means exterior.

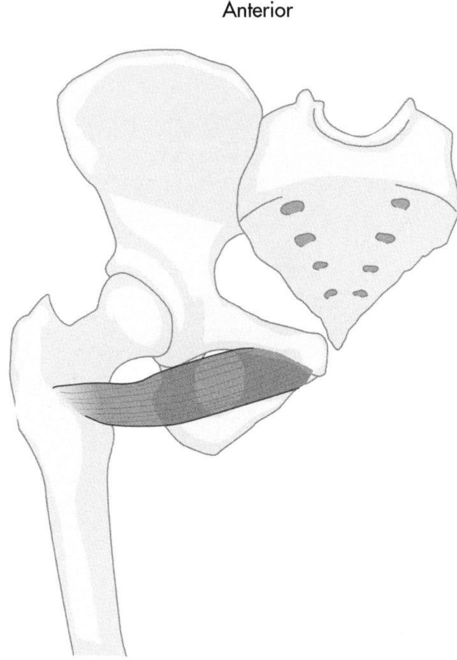

Concentric function:
Lateral rotation of the thigh at the hip joint

Eccentric function:
Restrains medial rotation of the thigh.

Isometric function:
Stabilizes the hip joint.

From:
External surface of the obturator membrane and the margins of the obturator foramen (on the ischium and pubis)

To:
Trochanteric fossa of the femur

Innervation:
Obturator nerve (L3 to L4)

Major synergists:
All deep lateral rotators of the thigh at the hip joint are synergistic with one another; posterior fibers of the gluteus medius.

Major antagonists:
Anterior fibers of the gluteus medius, gluteus minimus, and the tensor fasciae latae

Trigger points:
The belly of the muscle

Referred pain pattern:
Sacroiliac region, entire buttock, and down the posterior thigh to just proximal to the knee joint

Quadratus femoris (kwad-RATE-us FEM-or-iss)

Quadratus means square shaped; *femoris* means related to the thigh.

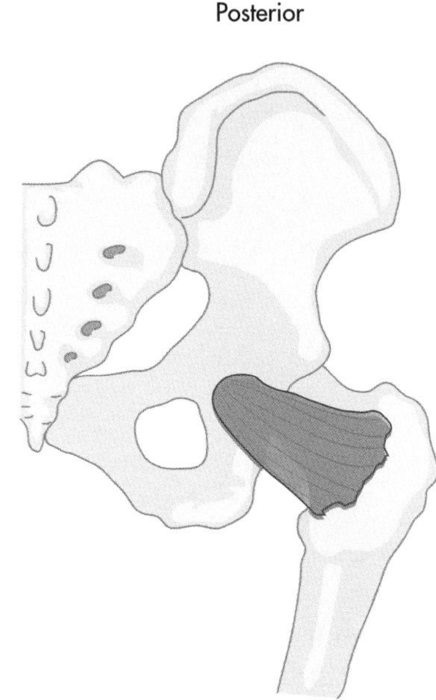

Concentric function:
Lateral rotation and adduction of the thigh at the hip joint (if the thigh is in a position of flexion).

Eccentric function:
Restrains medial rotation of the thigh and also may restrain abduction of the thigh

Isometric function:
Stabilizes the hip joint.

From:
Lateral border of the ischial tuberosity

To:
Small tubercle on the upper part of the intertrochanteric crest of the femur

Innervation:
Nerve to quadratus femoris from the lumbosacral plexus (L5 and S1)

Major synergists:
All deep lateral rotators of the thigh at the hip joint are synergistic with one another; posterior fibers of the gluteus medius.

Major antagonists:
Anterior fibers of the gluteus medius, gluteus minimus, and the tensor fasciae latae

Trigger points:
The belly of the muscle

Referred pain pattern:
Sacroiliac region, entire buttock, and down the posterior thigh to just proximal to the knee joint

Gemellus superior (JEM-ell-us)

Gemellus means twin; *superior* means above.

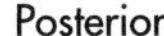

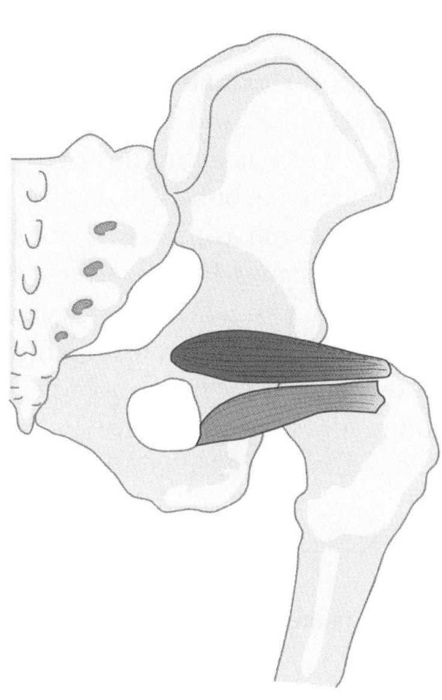

Concentric function:
Lateral rotation of the thigh at the hip joint and abduction of the thigh at the hip joint if the thigh is first in a position of flexion at the hip joint

Eccentric function:
Restrains medial rotation of the thigh and also may restrain adduction of the thigh (if the thigh is in a position of flexion).

Isometric function:
Stabilizes the hip joint.

From:
Dorsal surface of the ischial spine

To:
Medial surface of the greater trochanter of the femur

Innervation:
Nerve to obturator internus (L5 to S1)

Major synergists:
All deep lateral rotators of the thigh at the hip joint are synergistic with one another; posterior fibers of the gluteus medius.

Major antagonists:
Anterior fibers of the gluteus medius, gluteus minimus, and the tensor fasciae latae

Trigger points:
The belly of the muscle

Referred pain pattern:
Sacroiliac region, entire buttock, and down the posterior thigh to just proximal to the knee joint

Gemellus inferior (JEM-ell-us)

Gemellus means twin; *inferior* means below.

Posterior

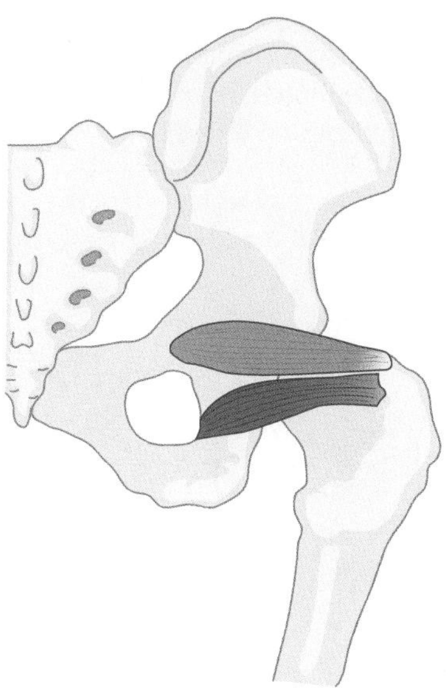

Concentric function:
Lateral rotation of the thigh at the hip joint and abduction of the thigh at the hip joint if the thigh is first in a position of flexion at the hip joint

Eccentric function:
Restrains medial rotation of the thigh and also may restrain adduction of the thigh (if the thigh is in a position of flexion).

Isometric function:
Stabilizes the hip joint.

From:
Upper part of the ischial tuberosity

To:
Medial surface of the greater trochanter

Innervation:
Lumbosacral plexus

Major synergists:
All deep lateral rotators of the thigh at the hip joint are synergistic with one another; posterior fibers of the gluteus medius.

Major antagonists:
Anterior fibers of the gluteus medius, gluteus minimus, and the tensor fasciae latae

Trigger points:
The belly of the muscle

Referred pain pattern:
Sacroiliac region, entire buttock, and down the posterior thigh to just proximal to the knee joint

See Activity 9-33.

ACTIVITY 9-33

1. Draw and color the deep lateral rotators in the space provided.
2. Label the proximal and distal attachment points: *P* for proximal; *D* for distal.
3. Place an X on the trigger points.
4. Palpate these muscles; identify the attachment points and the bellies of the muscles.
5. Move these muscles on yourself.

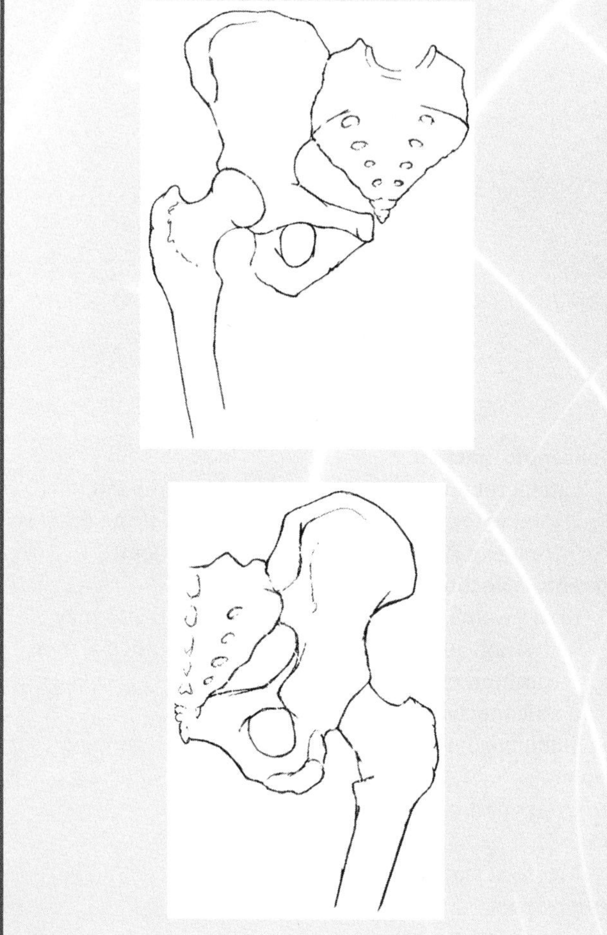

Muscles of the Posterior Thigh

Figure 9-27 illustrates the muscles of the posterior thigh.

The hamstring muscle group crosses two joints, the hip and the knee. These muscles posteriorly tilt the pelvis at the hip joint, extend the thigh at the hip joint, and flex the leg at the knee joint. The muscles of the massive hamstring group are the main extensors of the thigh. Because these muscles are active during walking, all gait reflexes are involved with the shoulder muscles to promote the appropriate counter-balancing arm swing. Facilitation between muscles of the arms that flex and extend occur along with thigh muscles in contralateral patterns. One usually needs to consider the muscles of the shoulder joint with muscles of the hip and so massage in a correlated pattern. Although not listed with synergists and antagonists, the flexors of the arm at the shoulder joint work with the flexors of the thigh at the hip joint on the opposite side (i.e., right with left and left with right). This concept is also true for the extensors of the arm and thigh. These muscles show patterns of inhibition as well (for example, right-side extensors of the thigh at the hip joint inhibit right-side extensors of the arm at the shoulder joint.) Adductors and medial rotators of the arm at the shoulder joint work with adductors and medial rotators of the thigh at the hip joint on the opposite side. This concept holds true for abductors and lateral rotators as well. Of course, these muscles also exhibit inhibitory patterns.

These muscles are thick, and massage application must address the muscles adequately but not painfully compress them against the underlying bone. The side-lying position is most suitable for applying compressive force during the massage and moving the muscles away from the bone. These muscles have a tendency to adhere together, and although this may be a compensation pattern for repetitive movement in extension of the thigh at the hip joint or flexion of the leg at the knee joint, adhesion can reduce and interfere with range of motion of the associated joints.

Semimembranosus (SEM-ee-MEM-bran-oh-sus)

Semimembranosus means half membrane.

Posterior

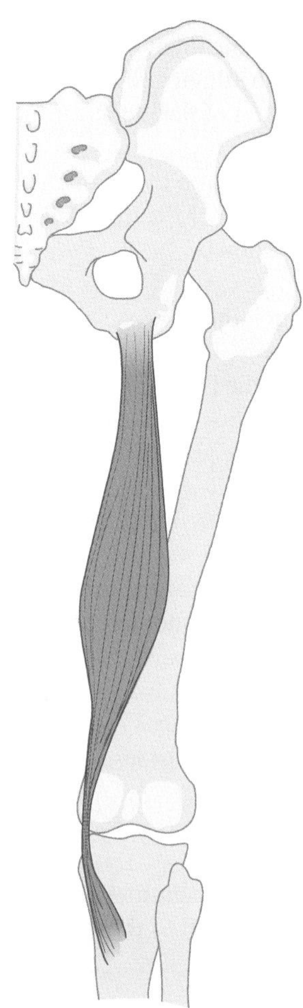

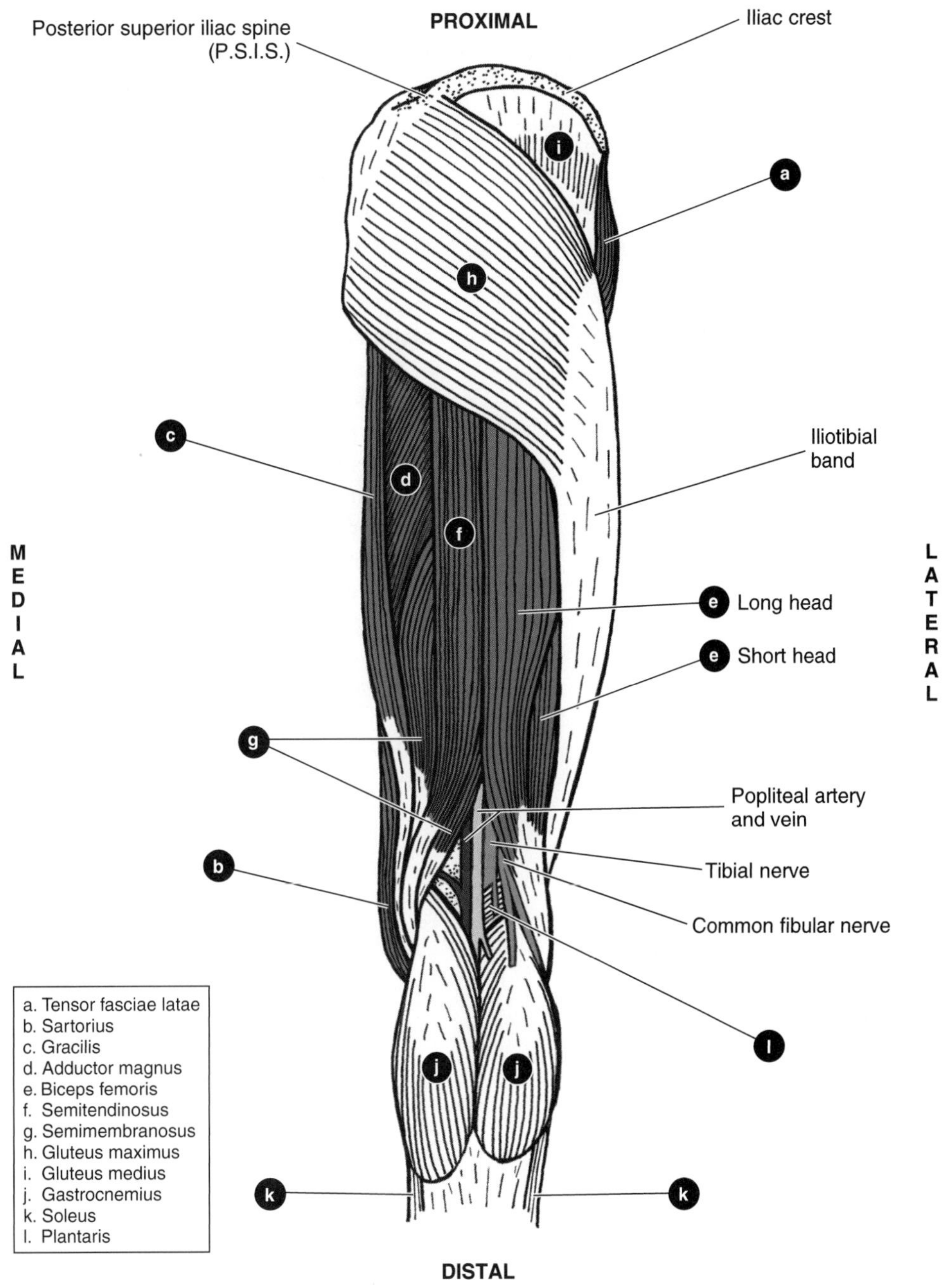

Figure 9-27
Posterior view of the right thigh (superficial). (Modified from Muscolino JE: *The muscular system manual: the skeletal muscles of the human body,* ed 2, St Louis, 2005, Mosby.)

Concentric function:
Flexion and medial rotation of the leg at the knee joint (the knee joint must be semiflexed for medial rotation to occur), extension of the thigh at the hip joint, and posterior tilt of the pelvis at the hip joint; the semimembranosus also serves to move the medial meniscus posteriorly during knee flexion.

Eccentric function:
Restrains extension and lateral rotation of the leg and allows flexion of the thigh and anterior tilt of the pelvis.

Isometric function:
Stabilizes the knee and hip joints.

From:
Upper lateral aspect of the ischial tuberosity

To:
Posteromedial surface of the medial condyle of the tibia; attaches to the medial meniscus.

Innervation:
Tibial portion of the sciatic nerve (L5 to S2)

Major synergists:
Semitendinosus, biceps femoris, and gluteus maximus

Major antagonists:
Quadriceps femoris group, iliopsoas, and tensor fasciae latae

Trigger points:
Several areas in the belly of the muscle and at the musculotendinous junction near the knee joint

Referred pain pattern:
Ischial tuberosity, back of the knee, and the entire posterior thigh and leg to midcalf

Semitendinosus (SEM-ee-TEN-din-oh-sus)

Semitendinosus means half tendon.

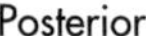

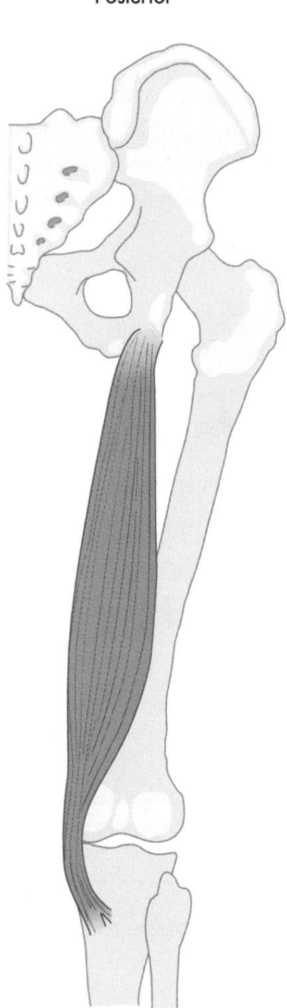

Concentric function:
Flexion and medial rotation of the leg at the knee joint (the knee joint must be semiflexed for medial rotation to occur), extension of the thigh at the hip joint, and posterior tilt of the pelvis at the hip joint

Eccentric function:
Restrains extension and lateral rotation of the leg and allows flexion of the thigh and anterior tilt of the pelvis.

Isometric function:
Stabilizes the knee and hip joints.

From:
Distal part of the medial aspect of the ischial tuberosity

To:
Proximal anteromedial tibia at the pes anserinus tendon and deep fascia of the leg

Innervation:
Tibial portion of the sciatic nerve (L5 to S2)

Major synergists:
Semimembranosus, biceps femoris, and gluteus maximus

Major antagonists:
Quadriceps femoris group, iliopsoas, and tensor fasciae latae

Trigger points:
Several areas in the belly of the muscle and at the musculotendinous junction near the knee joint

Referred pain pattern:
Ischial tuberosity, back of the knee, and the entire posterior thigh and leg to midcalf

Biceps femoris (BI-seps FEM-or-iss)

Biceps means two headed; *femoris* means related to the thigh.

Posterior

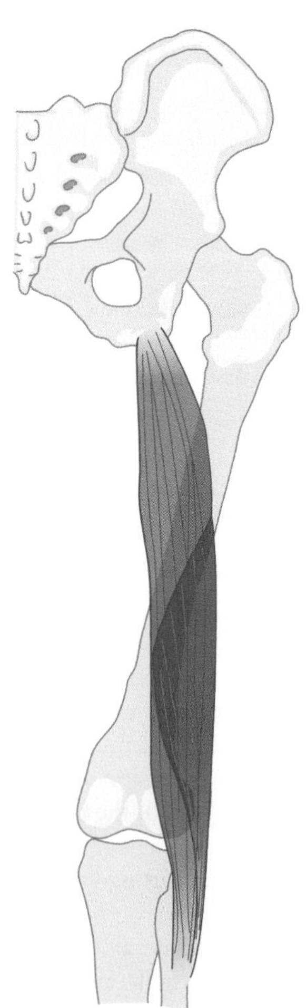

Concentric function:

Entire muscle—Flexion and lateral rotation of the leg at the knee joint (The knee joint must be semiflexed for lateral rotation to occur.)

Long head—Extension of the thigh at the hip joint and posterior tilt of the pelvis at the hip joint

Eccentric function:

Restrains extension and medial rotation of the leg and restrains flexion of the thigh and anterior tilt of the pelvis.

Isometric function:

Stabilizes the hip and knee joints.

From:

Long head—Posterior part of the ischial tuberosity and the sacrotuberous ligament

Short head—Lateral lip of the linea aspera, lateral intermuscular septum, and proximal two thirds of the supracondylar line

To:

Lateral side of the fibular head, lateral condyle of the tibia, and deep fascia on the lateral aspect of the leg

Innervation:

Tibial and common fibular portions of the sciatic nerve (L5 to S2)

Major synergists:

Semitendinosus, semimembranosus, and gluteus maximus

Major antagonists:

Quadriceps femoris group, iliopsoas, and tensor fasciae latae

Trigger points:

Several areas in the belly of the muscle and at the musculotendinous junction near the knee joint

Referred pain pattern:

Ischial tuberosity, back of the knee, and the entire posterior thigh and leg to midcalf

See Activity 9-34.

Muscles of the Medial Thigh

The medial thigh muscles, called the adductor group of the thigh, adduct the thigh at the hip joint (Figure 9-28). Interaction between abduction and adduction of the thighs (co-contraction) keeps the weight of the body balanced over

ACTIVITY 9-34

1. Draw and color the muscles of the hamstring group (the semimembranosus, semitendinosus, and biceps femoris) in the space provided.
2. Label the proximal and distal attachment points: *P* for proximal; *D* for distal.
3. Place an X on the trigger points.
4. Palpate these muscles; identify the attachment points and the bellies of the muscles.
5. Move these muscles on yourself.

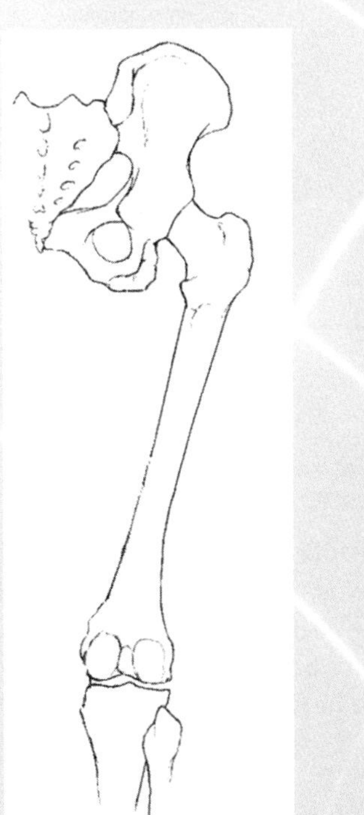

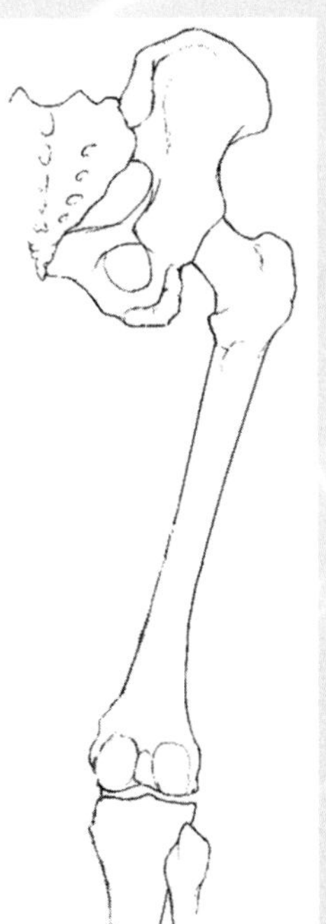

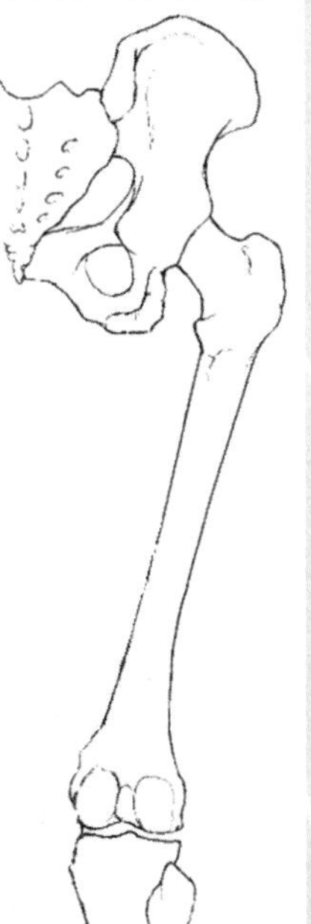

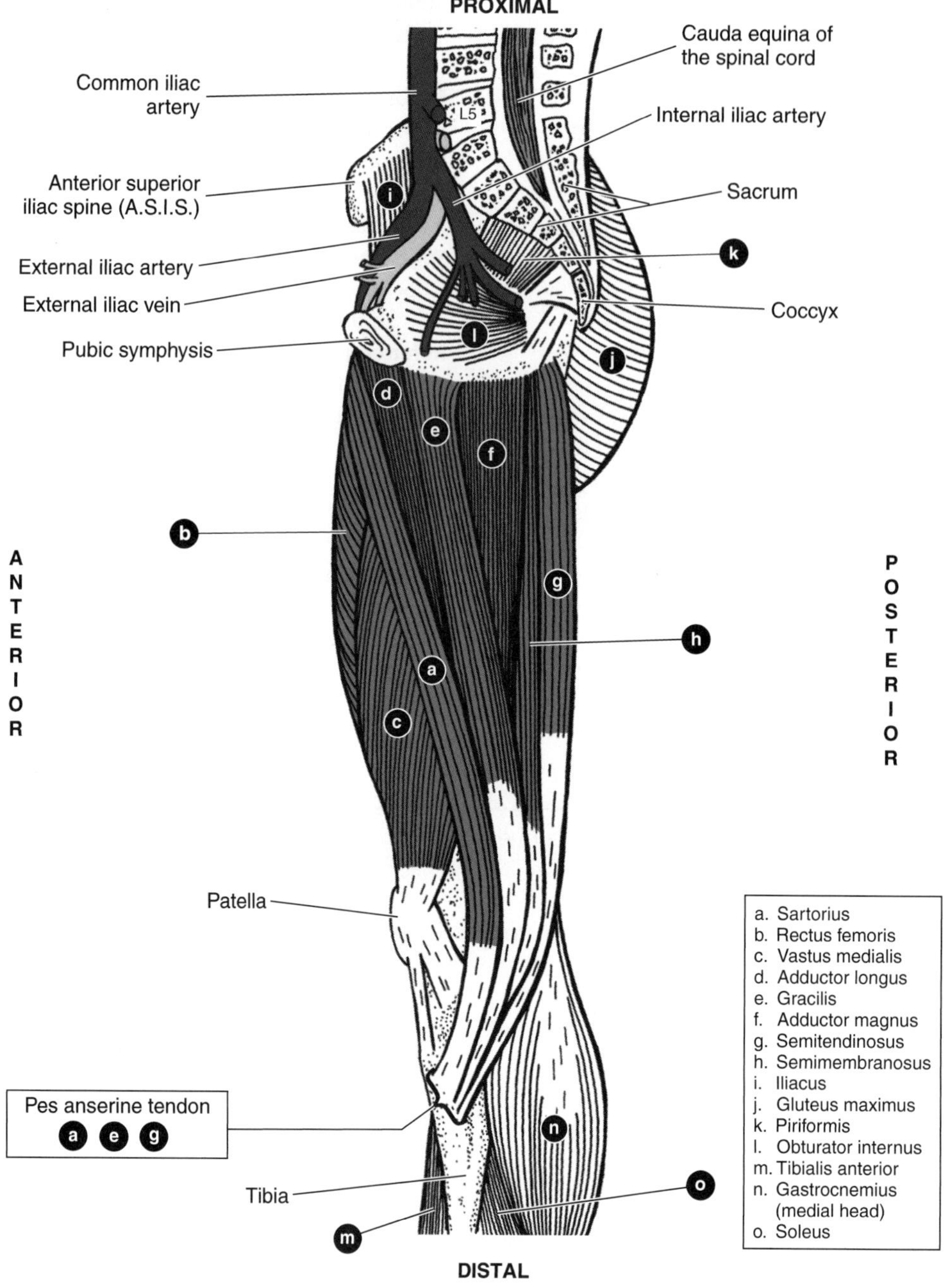

Figure 9-28
Medial view of the right thigh. (Modified from Muscolino JE: *The muscular system manual: the skeletal muscles of the human body,* ed 2, St Louis, 2005, Mosby.)

the weight-bearing lower extremity when a person is walking. Because of gait reflexes, these muscles work with adductors of the arm at the shoulder joint and inhibit abductors of the arm at the shoulder joint on the opposite side. These muscles also work with the abdominals to support the trunk and pelvis in an upright position. This muscle group is massive, and one can manage it most easily with the client in the side-lying position with the top lower extremity bent and forward to expose the adductor muscles of the bottom thigh.

Pectineus (PEK-tih-NEE-us)

Pectineus means related to the pubic bone.

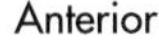

Anterior

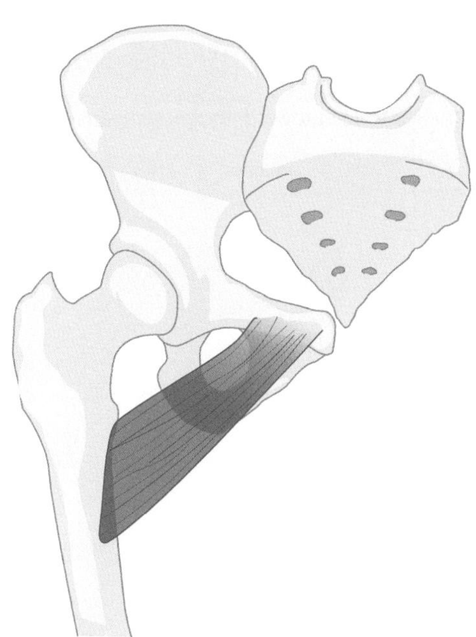

Concentric function:
Adduction and flexion of the thigh at the hip joint and anterior tilt of the pelvis at the hip joint

Eccentric function:
Restrains abduction and extension of the thigh and posterior tilt of the pelvis.

Isometric function:
Stabilizes the pelvis at the hip joint.

From:
Pectineal line of the pubis (on the superior ramus of the pubis)

To:
Pectineal line of the femur (line extending from the lesser trochanter of the femur to the linea aspera)

Innervation:
Femoral nerve (L2 to L3)

Major synergists:
The adductor group of the thigh is synergistic; iliopsoas.

Major antagonists:
Gluteus medius and gluteus minimus, tensor fasciae latae, and hamstrings

Trigger points:
Within the belly of each muscle and near the ischial tuberosity attachment

Referred pain pattern:
Deep in the groin, into the medial thigh and downward to the knee and leg; may mimic hamstring tension.

Adductor brevis (ad-DUCK-tur BREV-us)

Adductor means to lead toward; *brevis* means short.

Anterior

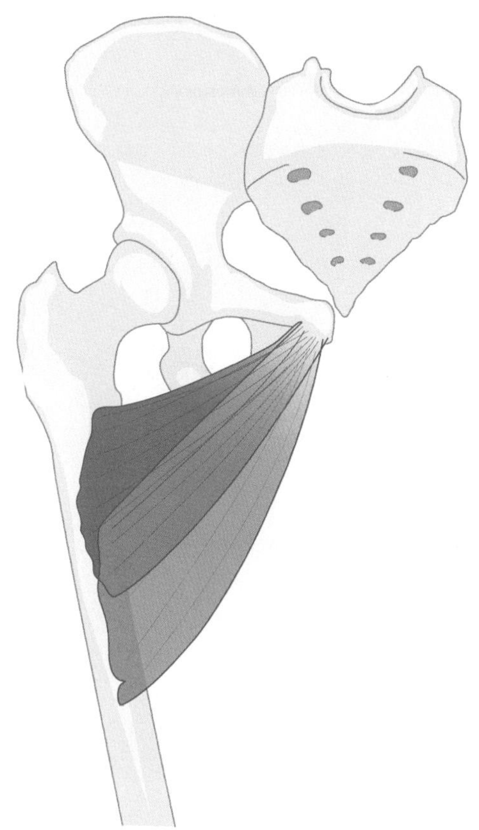

Concentric function:
Adduction and flexion of the thigh at the hip joint and anterior tilt of the pelvis at the hip joint

Eccentric function:
Restrains abduction and extension of the thigh and posterior tilt of the pelvis.

Isometric function:
Stabilizes the pelvis at the hip joint.

From:
Outer surface of the inferior ramus of the pubis between the gracilis and the obturator externus

To:
Linea aspera of the femur

Innervation:
Obturator nerve (L2 to L3)

Major synergists:
The adductor group of the thigh group is synergistic; iliopsoas.

Major antagonists:
Gluteus medius and gluteus minimus, tensor fasciae latae, and hamstrings

Trigger points:
Within the belly of each muscle and near the ischial tuberosity attachment

Referred pain pattern:
Deep in the groin, into the medial thigh and downward to the knee and leg; may mimic hamstring tension.

Adductor longus (ad-DUCK-tur LONG-us)

Adductor means to lead toward; *longus* means long.

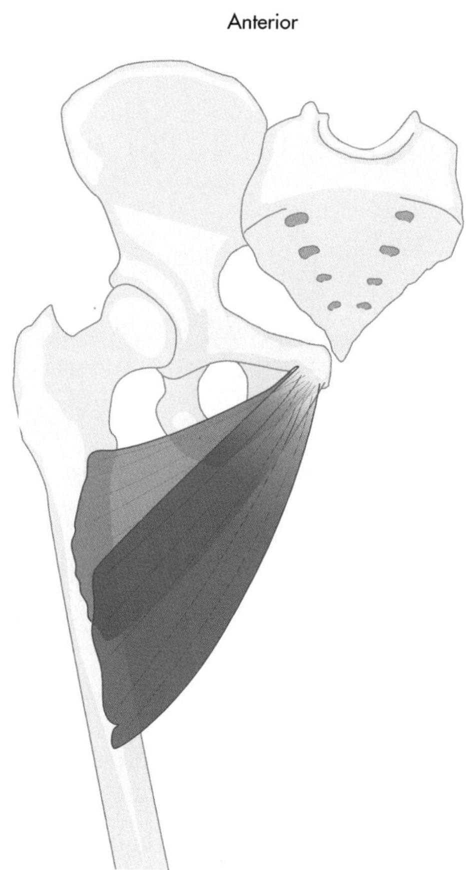

Concentric function:
Adduction and flexion of the thigh at the hip joint and anterior tilt of the pelvis at the hip joint

Eccentric function:
Restrains abduction and extension of the thigh and posterior tilt of the pelvis.

Isometric function:
Stabilizes the pelvis at the hip joint.

From:
Anterior pubis between the crest and symphysis

To:
Middle one third of the medial lip of the linea aspera of the femur

Innervation:
Obturator nerve (L2 to L4)

Major synergists:
The adductor group of the thigh is synergistic; iliopsoas.

Major antagonists:
Gluteus medius and gluteus minimus, tensor fasciae latae, and hamstrings

Trigger points:
Within the belly of each muscle and near the ischial tuberosity attachment

Referred pain pattern:
Deep in the groin, into the medial thigh and downward to the knee and leg; may mimic hamstring tension.

Adductor magnus (ad-DUCK-tur MAG-nus)

Adductor means to lead toward; *magnus* means great.

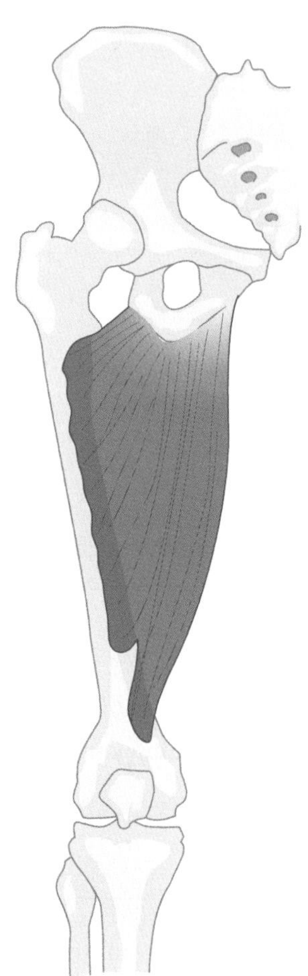

Concentric function:
Adduction and extension of the thigh at the hip joint and posterior tilt of the pelvis at the hip joint

Eccentric function:
Restrains abduction and flexion of the thigh and anterior tilt of the pelvis.

Isometric function:
Stabilizes the pelvis at the hip joint.

From:
Inferior ramus of the pubis and the ramus of the ischium (anterior fibers) and posterior fibers attach to the ischial tuberosity

To:
Gluteal tuberosity, linea aspera, medial supracondylar line, and adductor tubercle of the femur

Innervation:
Obturator and tibial division of sciatic nerves (L2 to L4)

Major synergists:
The adductor group of the thigh is synergistic; hamstrings.

Major antagonists:
Gluteus medius and gluteus minimus, tensor fasciae latae, and iliopsoas

Trigger points:
Within the belly of each muscle and near the ischial tuberosity attachment

Referred pain pattern:
Deep in the groin, into the medial thigh and downward to the knee and leg; may mimic hamstring tension.

Gracilis (gra-SIL-iss)

Gracilis means slender.

Anterior

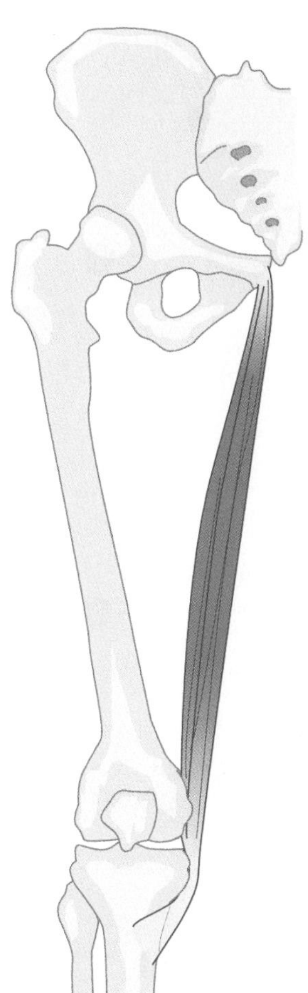

Concentric function:
Adduction and flexion of the thigh at the hip joint, anterior tilt of the pelvis at the hip joint, and flexion and medial rotation of the leg at the knee joint (The knee joint must be semiflexed for medial rotation to occur.)

Eccentric function:
Restrains abduction and extension of the thigh and allows posterior tilt of the pelvis and extension and lateral rotation of the leg.

Isometric function:
Stabilizes the pelvis at the hip joint and assists in controlling and stabilizing the valgus angulation of the knee joint.

From:
Inferior one half of the symphysis pubis and inferior ramus of the pubic bone

To:
Proximal anteromedial tibia at the pes anserinus tendon

Innervation:
Obturator nerve (L2 to L3)

Major synergists:
The adductor group of the thigh is synergistic; iliopsoas and sartorius.

Major antagonists:
Gluteus medius and gluteus minimus, tensor fasciae latae, and hamstrings

Trigger points:
Within the belly of each muscle and near the ischial tuberosity attachment

Referred pain pattern:
Deep in the groin, into the medial thigh and downward to the knee and leg; may mimic hamstring tension.

See Activity 9-35.

ACTIVITY 9-35

1. Draw and color the muscles of the medial thigh (the pectineus, adductor brevis, adductor longus, adductor magnus, and gracilis) in the space provided.
2. Label the origin and insertion points: *O* for the origin; *I* for the insertion.
3. Place an X on the trigger points.
4. Palpate these muscles; identify the attachment points and the bellies of the muscles.
5. Move these muscles on yourself.

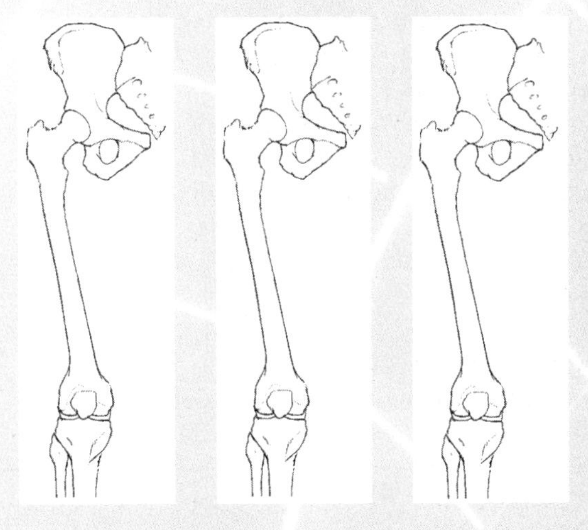

Muscles of the Anterior Thigh

The majority of the musculature of the anterior thigh is composed of the muscles of the quadriceps femoris group; the main action of this group is to extend the leg at the knee joint (Figure 9-29). The quadriceps femoris and hamstring muscle groups obviously are antagonistic, yet together they ensure the stability of the knee joint. The vastus lateralis and vastus medialis of the quadriceps femoris group also function together for proper tracking of the patella. The rectus femoris of the quadriceps femoris group is the only one that also crosses the hip joint. Because rectus femoris crosses the hip joint anteriorly, it can flex the thigh at the hip joint. Another muscle of the anterior thigh is the sartorius, which also flexes the thigh at the hip joint and flexes the leg at the knee joint. The rectus femoris and sartorius fall into gait patterns and reflexes with flexors and extensors of the arm at the shoulder joint. The remaining quadriceps femoris muscles work with muscles that flex and extend the forearm at the elbow joint, these patterns being synergistic on opposite sides and antagonistic on the same side. Muscles of

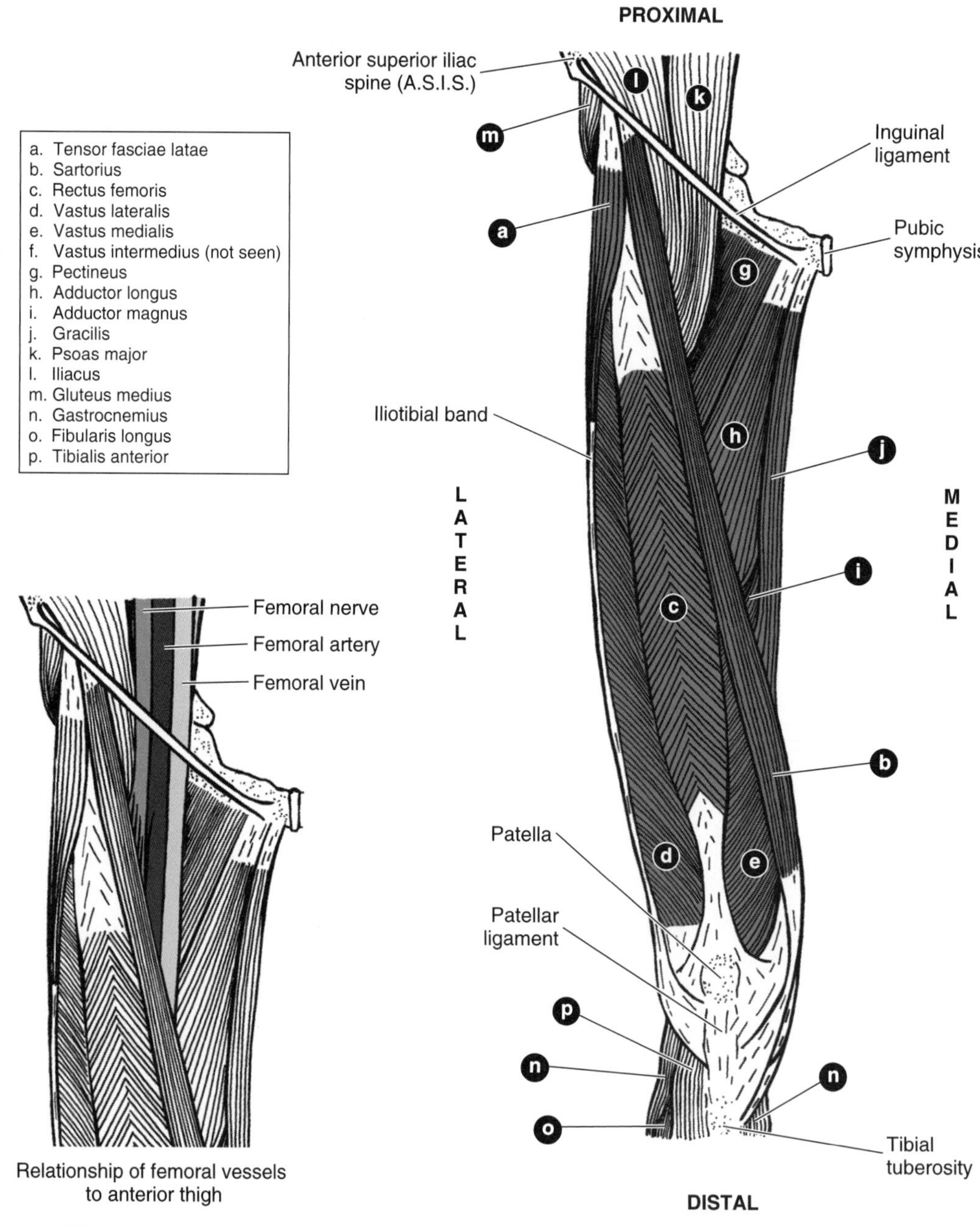

Figure 9-29
Anterior view of the right thigh (superficial). (Modified from Muscolino JE: *The muscular system manual: the skeletal muscles of the human body,* ed 2, St Louis, 2005, Mosby.)

the anterior thigh can adhere to each other, particularly the rectus femoris to the underlying vastus intermedius. Should this happen, the rectus femoris will not have the necessary functional range during flexion of the thigh at the hip joint and extension of the leg at the knee joint. Adhesion compromises range of motion and pain occurs, usually in the knee.

A major function of the quadriceps femoris group is to move the thigh into extension at the knee; this is sometimes called a reverse action because the proximal attachment moves in this situation and the distal attachment stays fixed. Examples would be standing up from a seated position or coming up into a straight leg position from a squat. This action requires moving the upper body and the thigh. Therefore the quadriceps femoris group is large and strong.

Sartorius (sar-TOR-ee-us)

Sartorius means tailor.

Anterior

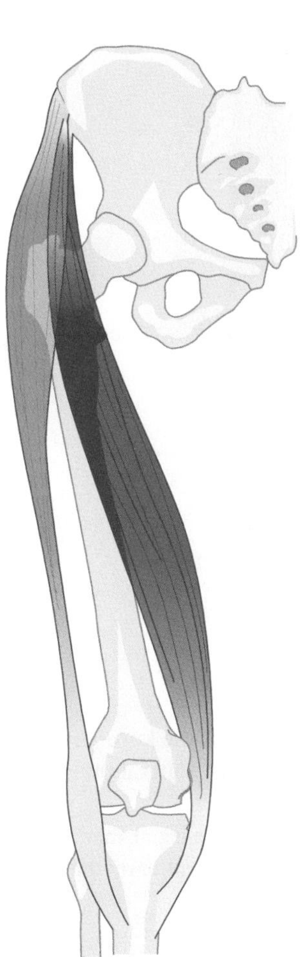

Concentric function:
Flexion, lateral rotation, and abduction of the thigh at the hip joint; flexion and medial rotation of the leg at the knee joint (the knee joint must be semiflexed for medial rotation to occur); and anterior tilt of the pelvis at the hip joint

Eccentric function:
Restrains extension, medial rotation, and adduction of the thigh and allows extension and lateral rotation of the leg and posterior tilt of the pelvis.

Isometric function:
Stabilizes the knee and hip joints.

From:
Anterior superior iliac spine

To:
Proximal anteromedial tibia at the pes anserinus tendon

Innervation:
Femoral nerve (L2 to L3)

Major synergists:
Iliopsoas, rectus femoris, lateral rotator group of the thigh, gluteus medius

Major antagonists:
Hamstrings, tensor fasciae latae, adductor group of the thigh, quadriceps femoris group

Trigger points:
Three or four areas along the belly of the muscle

Referred pain pattern:
Entire anterior thigh, with concentration at the knee

Quadriceps femoris group (KWAD-rih-seps FEM-or-iss)

Quadriceps means four headed; *femoris* means related to the thigh.

Rectus femoris (REK-tus FEM-or-iss)

Rectus means straight or upright; *femoris* means related to the thigh.

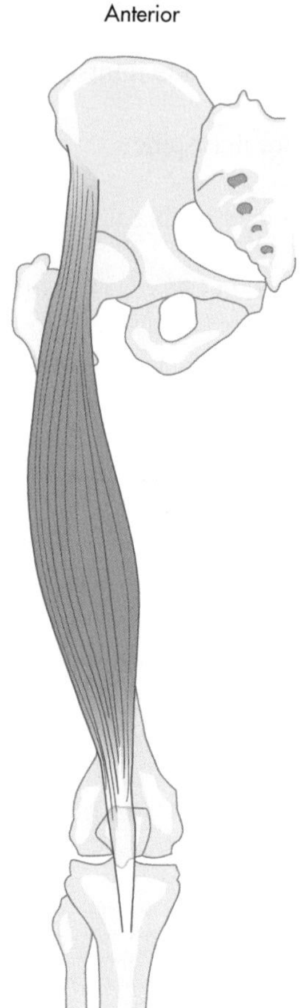

Concentric function:
Extension of the leg at the knee joint, flexion of the thigh at the hip joint, and anterior tilt of the pelvis at the hip joint

Eccentric function:
Restrains flexion of the leg and allows extension of the thigh and posterior tilt of the pelvis.

Isometric function:
Stabilizes the knee and hip joints.

From:
Anterior inferior iliac spine; groove above the rim of the acetabulum

To:
Tibial tuberosity, via the patella and patellar ligament

Innervation:
Femoral nerve (L2 to L4)

Major synergists:
All quadriceps femoris muscles are synergistic; iliopsoas and sartorius.

Major antagonists:
Hamstrings and gluteus maximus

Trigger points:
Near the attachment at the pelvis

Referred pain pattern:
Entire anterior thigh, with concentration at the knee

Vastus lateralis (VAS-tus LAT-ter-al-us)

Vastus means vast or large; *lateralis* means related to the side.

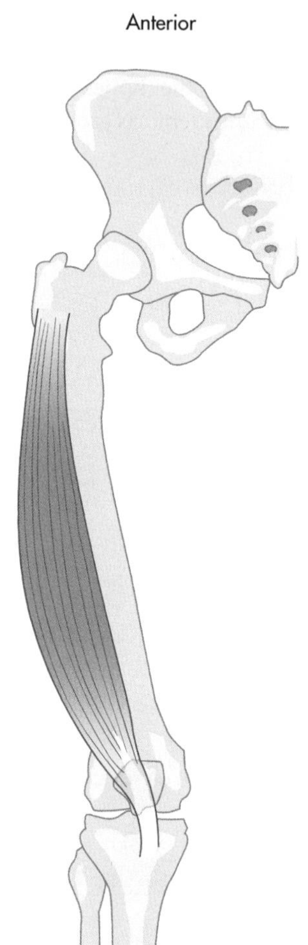

Concentric function:
Extension of the leg at the knee joint (The vastus lateralis also exerts a lateral pull on the patella.)

Eccentric function:
Restrains flexion of the leg at the knee joint (the vastus lateralis also restrains the medial pull on the patella by the vastus medialis).

Isometric function:
Stabilizes the patella and the knee joint (and the iliotibial band).

From:
Linea aspera, anterior aspect of the greater trochanter, gluteal tuberosity, and lateral intermuscular septum

To:
Tibial tuberosity, via the patella and patellar ligament

Innervation:
Femoral nerve (L2 to L4)

Major synergists:
All quadriceps femoris muscles are synergistic.

Major antagonists:
Hamstrings.

Trigger points:
Several locations at each attachment and in the belly of the muscle

Referred pain pattern:
Entire anterior thigh, with concentration at the knee
A tight vastus lateralis, not the iliotibial band, is usually responsible for shortening and pain in the lateral thigh

Vastus medialis (VAS-tus MEE-dee-al-us)

Vastus means vast or large; *medialis* means related to the middle.

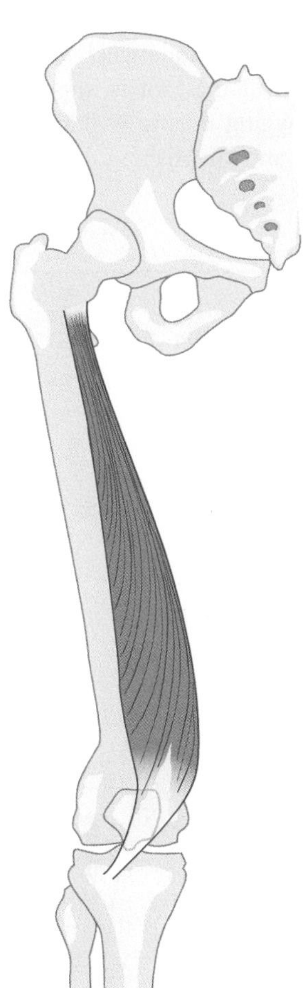

Concentric function:
Extension of the leg at the knee joint (The vastus medialis also exerts a medial pull on the patella.)

Eccentric function:
Restrains flexion of the leg at the knee joint (the vastus medialis also restrains the lateral pull on the patella by the vastus lateralis).

Isometric function:
Stabilizes the patella and the knee joint.

From:
Linea aspera, intertrochanteric line, medial supracondylar line, and medial intermuscular septum

To:
Tibial tuberosity, via the patella and patellar ligament
The lower fibers of the vastus medialis often are called the VMO (vastus medialis oblique); the upper fibers often are called the VML (vastus medialis longus).

Innervation:
Femoral nerve (L2 to L4)

Major synergists:
All quadriceps femoris muscles are synergistic.

Major antagonists:
Hamstrings

Trigger points:
In the belly of the muscle, near the attachment just above the knee, and in the oblique portion (VMO)

Referred pain pattern:
Entire anterior thigh, with concentration at the knee

Vastus intermedius (VAS-tus inter-MEE-dee-us)

Vastus means vast or large; *intermedius* means among the middle.

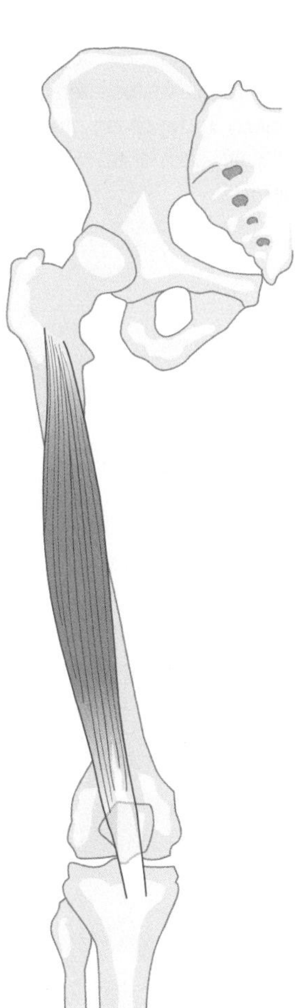

Concentric function:
Extension of the leg at the knee joint
Eccentric function:
Restrains flexion of the leg.
Isometric function:
Stabilizes the patella and the knee joint.
From:
Linea aspera, anterior and lateral surfaces of the proximal two thirds of the shaft of the femur, and intermuscular septum
To:
Tibial tuberosity, via the patella and patellar ligament

A portion of vastus intermedius can be considered a separate muscle called articularis genus, which is responsible for lifting the joint capsule of the knee during extension so it is not pinched between the patella and femur.

Innervation:
Femoral nerve (L2 to L4)
Major synergists:
All quadriceps femoris muscles are synergistic.
Major antagonists:
Hamstrings
Trigger points:
Near the proximal attachment at the musculotendinous junction
Referred pain pattern:
Entire anterior thigh, with concentration at the knee

See Activity 9-36.

Muscles of the Anterior and Lateral Leg

The muscles of the leg are primarily important for their actions at the foot (Figure 9-30, *A*, *B*). These muscles produce dorsiflexion and plantar flexion movements of the foot at the ankle joint and inversion and eversion movements of the foot at the tarsal (subtalar) joints. (The terms *pronation* and *supination* often are used for movements of the foot at the tarsal joints. Pronation of the foot primarily consists of eversion; supination of the foot primarily consists of inversion.) Many of these muscles also flex and extend the toes at the metatarsophalangeal and interphalangeal joints. The muscles of the anterior leg primarily provide dorsiflexion of the foot at the ankle joint and extension of the toes at the metatarsophalangeal and interphalangeal joints. The muscles of the posterior leg primarily provide plantar flexion of the foot at the ankle joint and flexion of the toes at the metatarsophalangeal and interphalangeal joints. Dorsiflexion of the foot is important in preventing the toes from dragging during walking; plantar flexion of the foot is important for pushing off during walking. The

ACTIVITY 9-36

1. Draw and color the muscles of the anterior thigh (the sartorius, rectus femoris, vastus lateralis, vastus medialis, and vastus intermedius) in the space provided.
2. Label the proximal and distal attachment points: *P* for proximal; *D* for distal.
3. Place an X on the trigger points.
4. Palpate these muscles; identify the attachment points and the bellies of the muscles..
5. Move these muscles on yourself.

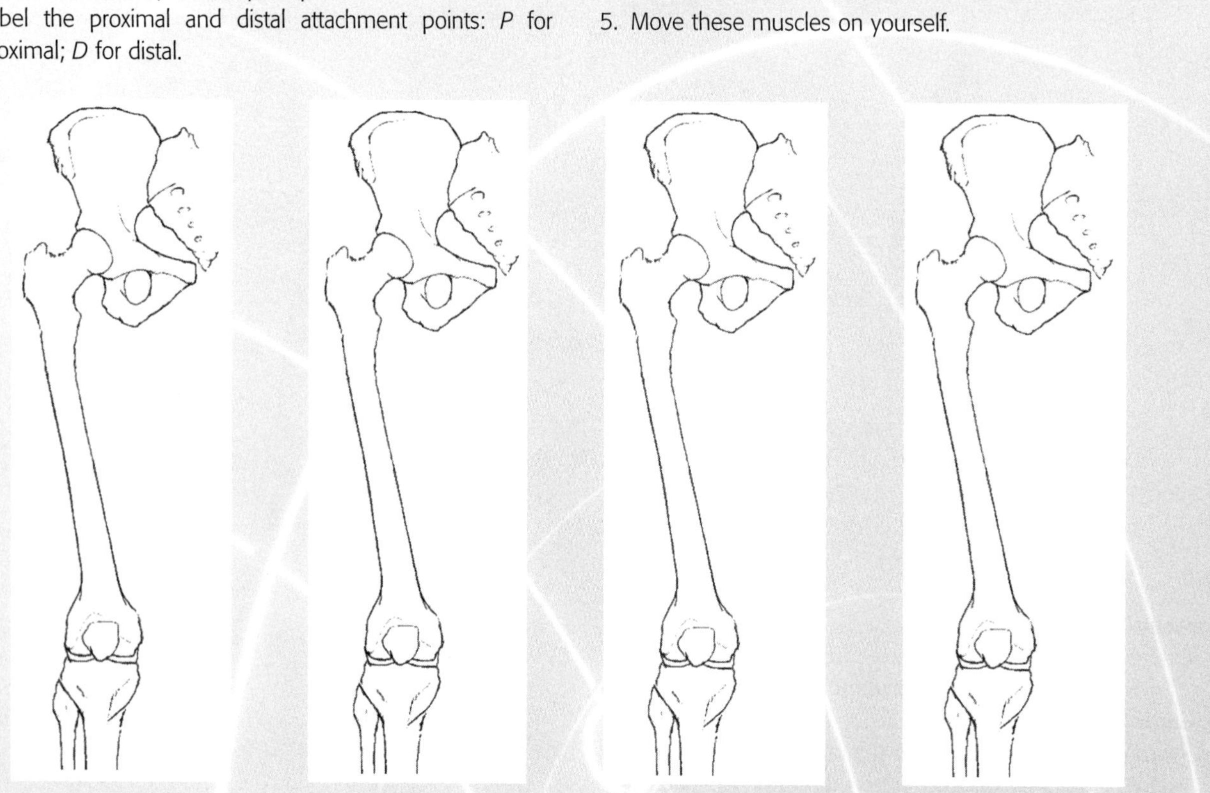

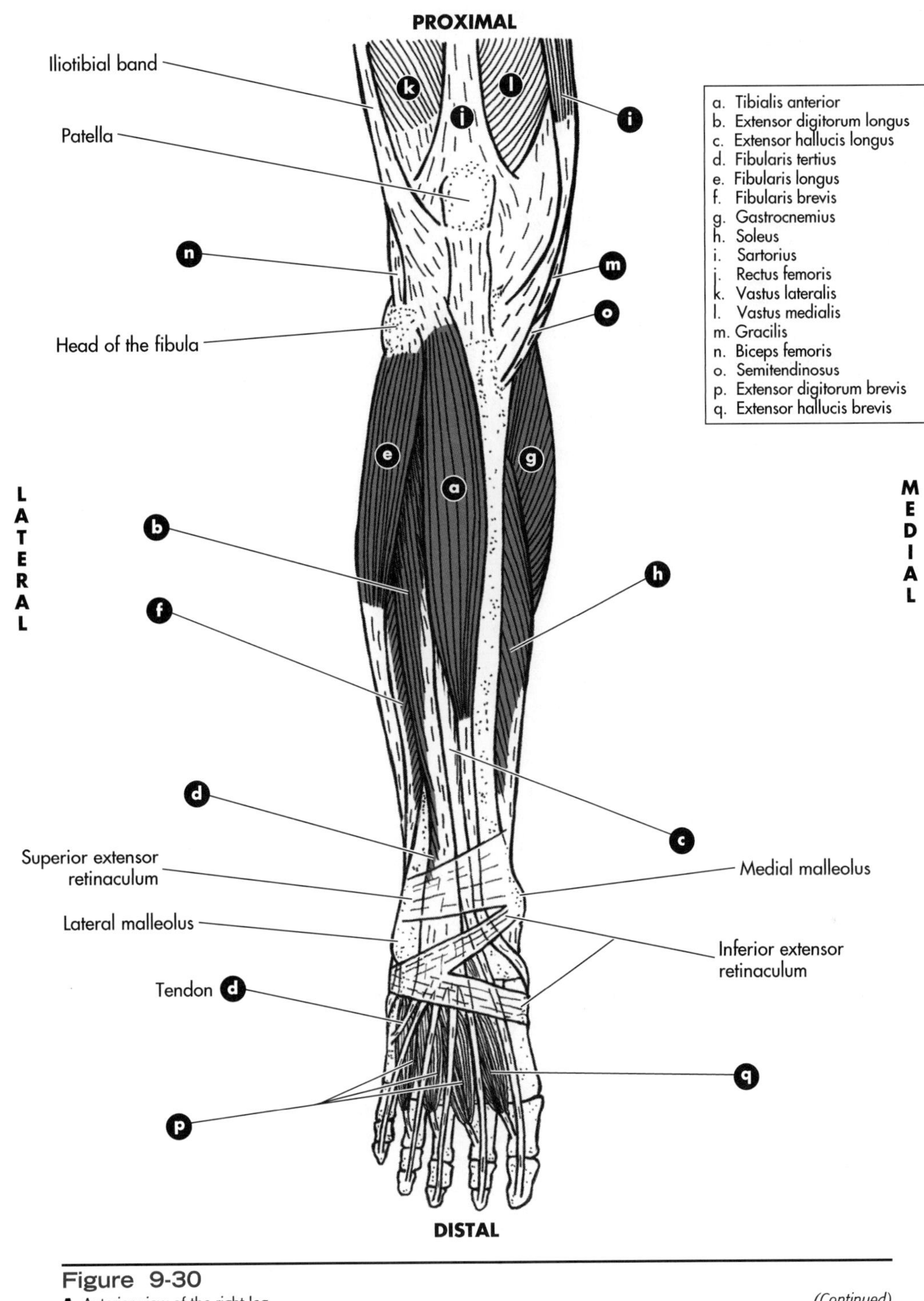

Figure 9-30
A, Anterior view of the right leg.

(Continued)

lateral leg muscles evert the foot at the tarsal (subtalar) joints and provide plantar flexion of the foot at the ankle joint.

The deep fascia of the leg is continuous with the iliotibial band, which expands and ensheathes the thigh and binds the leg muscles together. This construction helps prevent excessive swelling of the muscles during exercise. This same fascial sheath supports a pumping action that aids the circulation of blood and lymph, particularly venous return flow. The fascia divides the leg muscles into the anterior, lateral, and posterior compartments, each with its own nerve and blood supply. The leg fascia thickens at the ankles to form the retinaculae, which secure the muscle tendons in place as they cross the ankles into the feet. Because of this

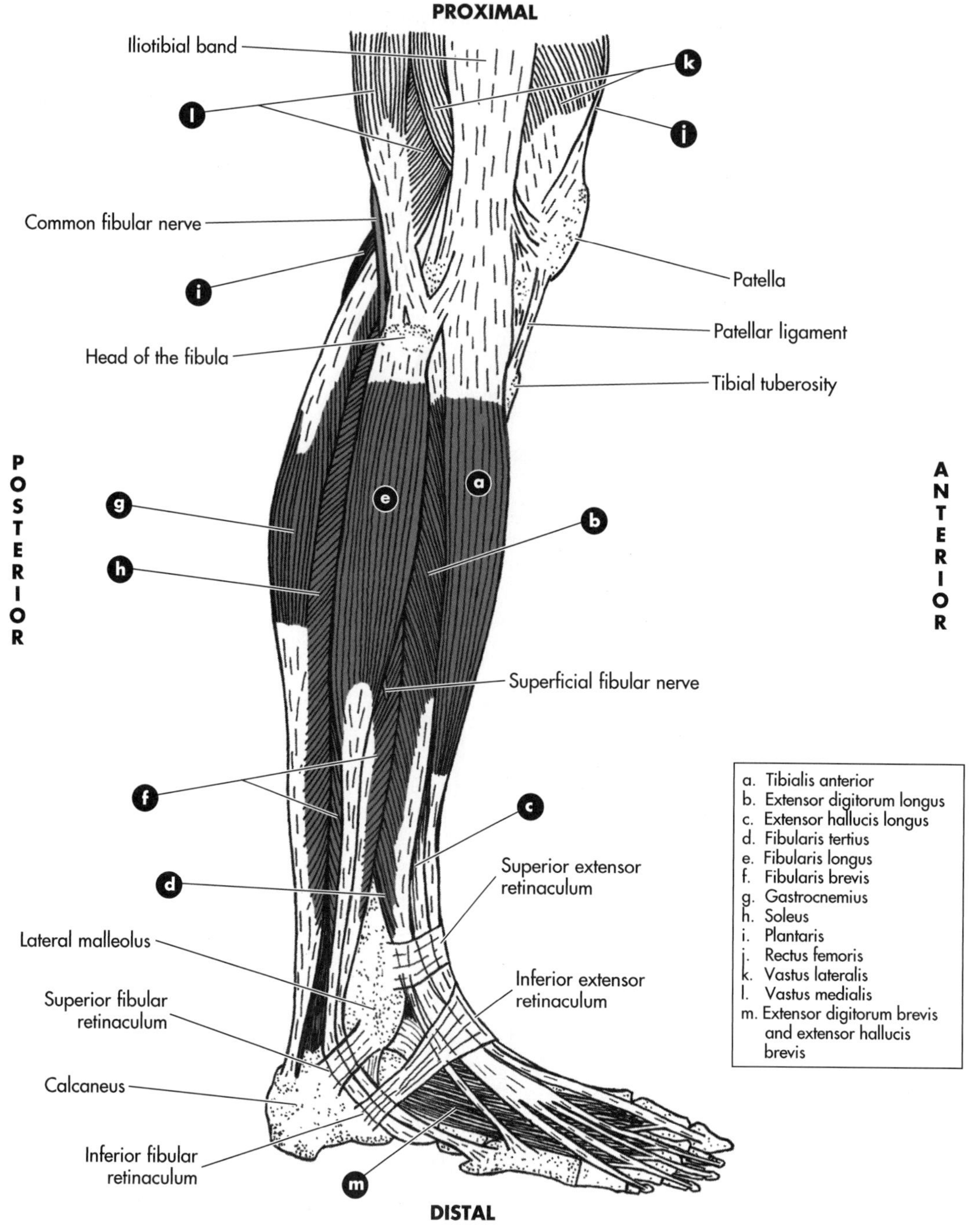

Figure 9-30—cont'd.
B, Lateral view of the right leg. (Modified from Muscolino JE: *The muscular system manual: the skeletal muscles of the human body,* ed 2, St Louis, 2005, Mosby.)

extensive fascial structure, the practitioner applies effective massage in a slow, sustained manner with a drag that addresses the viscous quality of the tissue. Although most of these muscles primarily produce movements of the foot, any muscle that crosses the knee joint is involved in the function and dysfunction of the knee joint. Because the hip, knee, and ankle joints function as a complex unit and closed kinematic chain when standing, all muscles affecting these joints interact with each other.

Anterior Muscles

See Figure 9-30, *A* for the anterior muscles of the leg.

Tibialis anterior (TIB-ee-AL-iss)

Tibialis means related to the shinbone; *anterior* means before or in front.

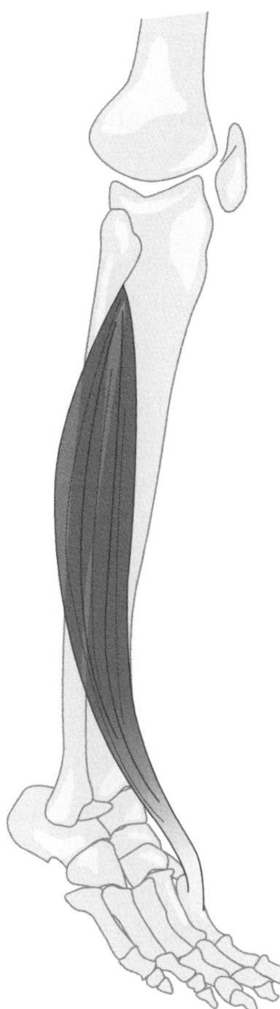

Concentric function:
Dorsiflexion of the foot at the ankle joint and inversion of the foot at the tarsal joints

Eccentric function:
Restrains plantar flexion and eversion of the foot.

Isometric function:
Stabilizes the ankle joint.

From:
Lateral condyle and proximal two thirds of the anterior surface of the tibia, interosseous membrane, deep fascia, and lateral intermuscular septum

To:
At the foot on the medial plantar surface of the medial cuneiform bone and base of the first metatarsal bone

Innervation:
Deep fibular nerve (L4 to L5)

Major synergists:
Extensor digitorum longus, extensor hallucis longus, and tibialis posterior

Major antagonists:
Gastrocnemius, soleus, and fibularis muscles

Trigger points:
In the belly of the muscle

Referred pain pattern:
Down the leg to the ankle and into the toes

Extensor digitorum longus (ex-STEN-sur DIH-jih-TOR-um LONG-us)

Extensor means one that stretches, *digitorum* means of the fingers and toes, and *longus* means long.

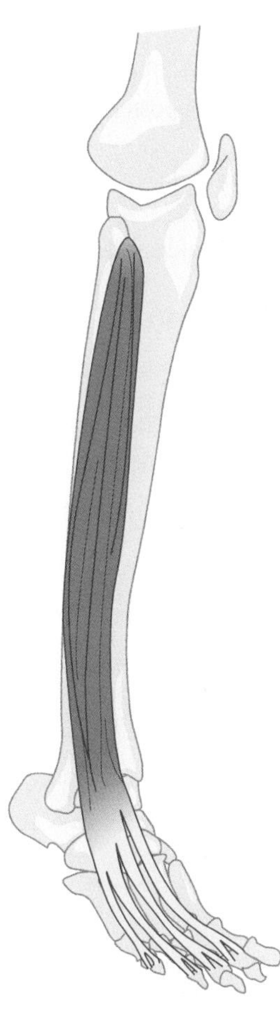

Concentric function:
Extension of toes 2 to 5 at the metatarsophalangeal and interphalangeal joints, dorsiflexion of the foot at the ankle joint, and eversion of the foot at the tarsal joints

Eccentric function:
Restrains flexion of the toes and allows plantar flexion and inversion of the foot.

Isometric function:
Stabilizes joints of the ankle and foot.

From:
Lateral condyle of the tibia, proximal two thirds of the anterior surface of the shaft of the fibula, interosseous membrane, deep fascia, and intermuscular septa

To:

By four tendons to the second through fifth digits; each tendon divides into an intermediate slip, which attaches to the base of the middle phalanx, and two lateral slips, which attach to the base of the distal phalanx.

The distal tendons of the extensor digitorum longus create the dorsal digital expansion of toes 2 to 5.

Innervation:

Deep fibular nerve (L5 to S1)

Major synergists:

Extensor digitorum brevis, tibialis anterior, and fibularis muscles

Major antagonists:

Flexor digitorum longus, flexor digitorum brevis, tibialis anterior, and tibialis posterior

Trigger points:

In the belly of the muscle

Referred pain pattern:

Down the leg to the ankle and into the toes

Extensor hallucis longus (ex-STEN-sur HAL-uh-siss LONG-us)

Extensor means one that stretches, *hallucis* means related to the big toe, and *longus* means long.

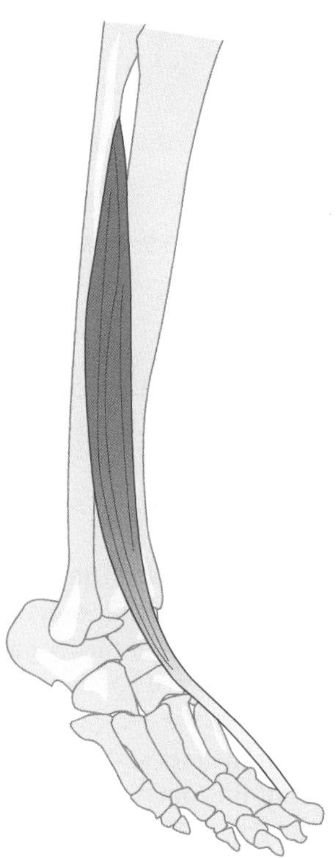

Concentric function:

Extension of the big toe at the metatarsophalangeal and interphalangeal joints, dorsiflexion of the foot at the ankle joint, and inversion of the foot at the tarsal joints

Eccentric function:

Restrains flexion of the great toe and allows plantar flexion and eversion of the foot.

Isometric function:

Stabilizes the great toe and assists in stabilizing the ankle.

From:

Middle third of the anterior surface of the fibula and adjacent interosseous membrane

To:

Base of the distal phalanx of the great toe

Innervation:

Deep fibular nerve (L5 to S1)

Major synergists:

Tibialis anterior, digitorum longus, peroneus tertius and extensor hallucis longus are synergistic for dorsiflexion

Major antagonists:

Eversion and inversion—Tibialis anterior, digitorum longus

Dorsiflexion—Gastrocnemius, soleus, peroneus longus and brevis, flexors of the toes, tibialis posterior

Trigger points:

In the belly of each muscle

Referred pain pattern:

Down the leg to the ankle and into the toes

Fibularis (peroneus) tertius (fib-you-LAR-iss TER-she-us)

Fibularis means related to the pin or fibula; *tertius* means the third.

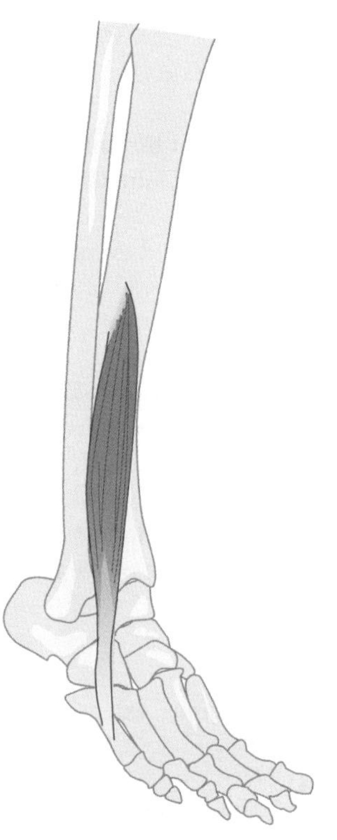

ACTIVITY 9-37

1. Draw and color the anterior leg muscles (the tibialis anterior, extensor digitorum longus, extensor hallucis longus, and peroneus [fibularis] tertius) in the space provided.
2. Label the proximal and distal attachment points: *P* for proximal; *D* for distal.
3. Place an X on the trigger points.
4. Palpate these muscles; identify the attachment points and the bellies of the muscles.
5. Move these muscles on yourself.

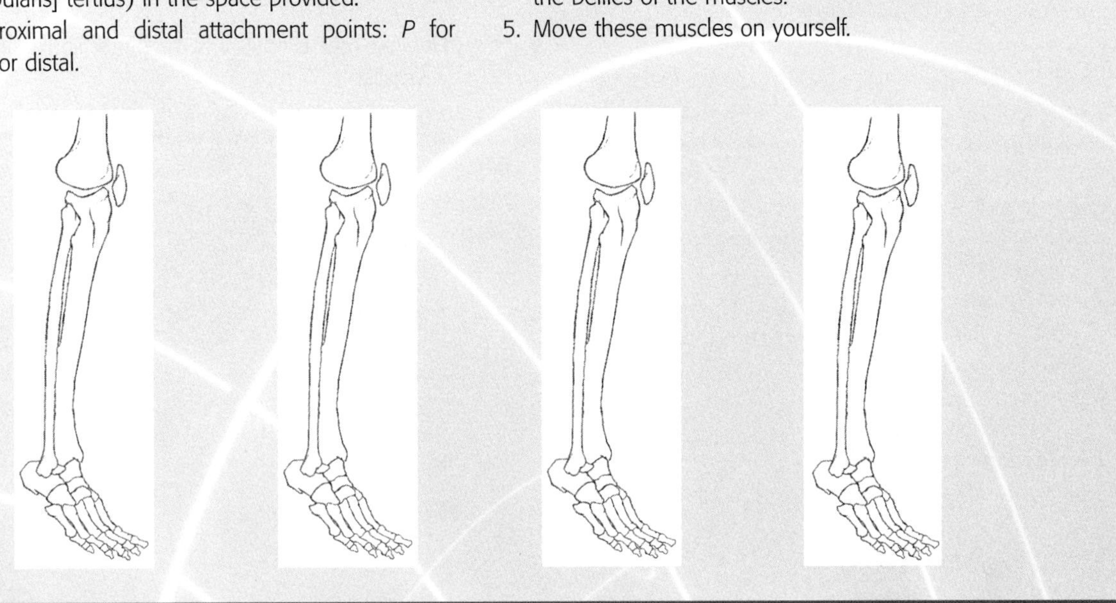

Concentric function:

Dorsiflexion of the foot at the ankle joint and eversion of the foot at the tarsal joints

Eccentric function:

Restrains plantar flexion and inversion of the foot.

Isometric function:

Assists in stabilizing the ankle joint.

From:

Distal one third of the anterior surface of the fibula, interosseous membrane, and intermuscular septum

To:

Dorsal surface of the base of the fifth metatarsal bone

Innervation:

Deep fibular nerve (L5 to S1)

Major synergists:

Extensor hallucis brevis and tibialis anterior

Major antagonists:

Flexor hallucis longus, flexor hallucis brevis, and fibularis muscles

Trigger points:

In the belly of the muscle

Referred pain pattern:

Down the leg to the ankle and into the toes

See Activity 9-37.

Lateral Muscles

See Figure 9-30, *B* for the lateral muscles of the leg.

Fibularis (peroneus) longus (fib-you-LAR-iss LONG-us)

Fibularis means related to the pin or fibula; *longus* means long.

Lateral

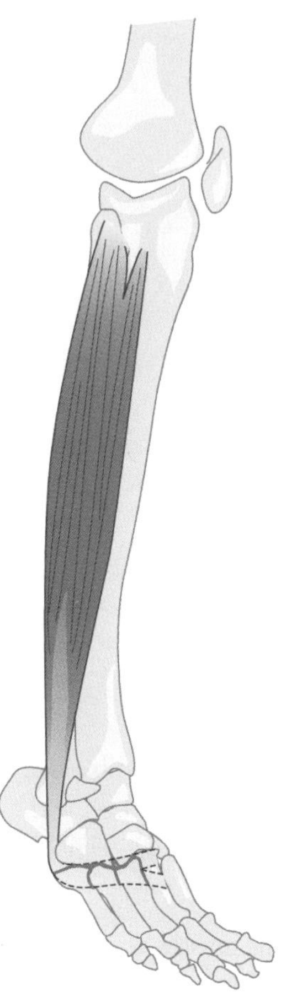

Concentric function:
Eversion of the foot at the tarsal joints and plantar flexion of the foot at the ankle joint

Eccentric function:
Restrains inversion and dorsiflexion of the foot.

Isometric function:
Stabilizes the ankle joint.

From:
Lateral condyle of the tibia, head and proximal one half of the lateral surface of the fibula, intermuscular septa, and adjacent deep fascia

To:
Lateral side of the base of the first metatarsal bone and the medial cuneiform bone

Innervation:
Superficial fibular nerve (L5 to S1)

Major synergist:
Fibularis brevis

Major antagonist:
Tibialis anterior

Trigger points:
Located at the origin and insertion near the musculotendinous junction

Referred pain pattern:
To the lateral malleolus and the heel

Fibularis (peroneus) brevis (fib-you-LAR-iss BREV-us)

Fibularis means related to the pin or fibula; *brevis* means smaller.

Lateral

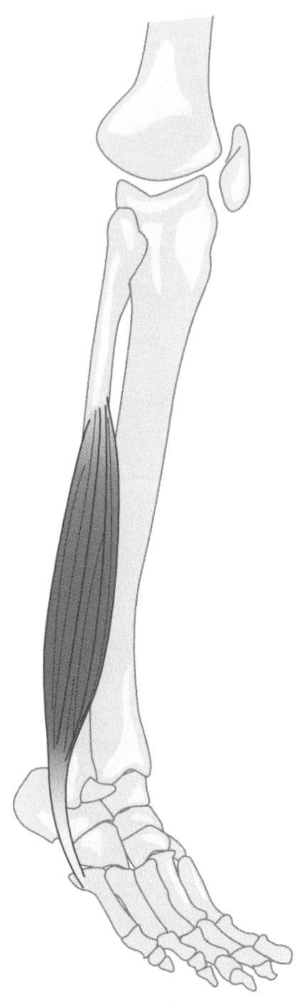

Concentric function:
Eversion of the foot at the tarsal joints and plantar flexion of the foot at the ankle joint

Eccentric function:
Restrains inversion and dorsiflexion of the foot.

Isometric function:
Stabilizes the ankle joint.

From:
Distal one half of the lateral surface of the fibula and adjacent intermuscular septum

To:
Tuberosity at the base of the fifth metatarsal bone on the lateral side

Innervation:
Superficial fibular nerve (L5 to S1)

Major synergist:
Fibularis longus

Major antagonist:
Tibialis anterior

ACTIVITY 9-38

1. Draw and color the lateral leg muscles (the peroneus [fibularis] longus and peroneus [fibularis] brevis) in the space provided.
2. Label the proximal and distal attachment points: *P* for proximal; *D* for distal.
3. Place an X on the trigger points.
4. Palpate these muscles; identify the attachment points and the bellies of the muscles.
5. Move these muscles on yourself.

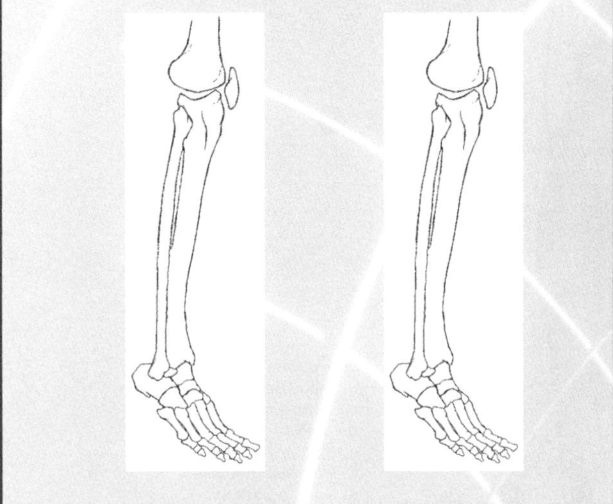

Trigger points:

Located at the origin and insertion near the musculotendinous junction

Referred pain pattern:

To the lateral malleolus and the heel

See Activity 9-38.

Muscles of the Posterior Leg

The majority of the posterior leg muscles provide plantar flexion of the foot at the ankle joint and invert the foot at the tarsal joints; many of them also flex the toes at the metatarsophalangeal and interphalangeal joints (Figure 9-31). Plantar flexion lifts the entire weight of the body to allow a person to stand on tiptoe and provides the necessary forward thrust for walking and running. Plantar flexion is a powerful movement. The popliteus muscle, which crosses the knee, is important in unlocking the extended knee (by medial rotation of the leg at the knee joint) in preparation for flexion of the leg at the knee joint. Because they cross the knee joint posteriorly, the gastrocnemius and plantaris muscles assist with flexion of the leg at the knee joint. The gastrocnemius and soleus can become adhered together, which interferes with the function of the gastrocnemius, often causing knee pain, stiffness, and ankle restriction.

Popliteus (pop-LIT-ee-us)

Popliteus means hollow of the knee.

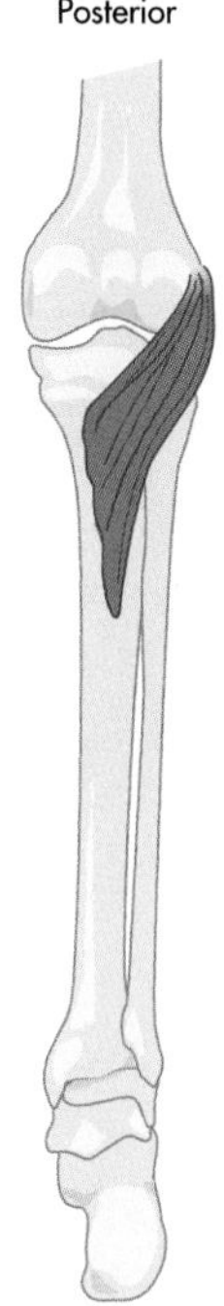

Concentric function:

With the proximal attachment (origin) fixed, medial rotation and flexion of the leg at the knee joint

The medial rotation of the knee joint is considered to be important for flexing the fully extended knee. The reverse action of lateral rotation of the thigh at the knee joint is also important for beginning flexion of the thigh at the knee joint in a weight-bearing lower extremity. The popliteus also moves the lateral meniscus posteriorly during knee flexion.

Eccentric function:

Restrains lateral rotation and extension of the leg.

Isometric function:

Stabilizes the knee joint.

From:

Lateral surface of the lateral condyle of the femur, oblique popliteal ligament, and lateral meniscus of the knee.

To:

Triangular area above the soleal line on the posterior and medial surfaces of the tibia, as well as the fascia covering its surface

Innervation:

Tibial nerve (L4 to S1)

Major synergists:

Semitendinosus, semimembranosus, sartorius, and gracilis

Major antagonists:

Biceps femoris and the quadriceps femoris group

Trigger points:

Belly of the muscle

Referred pain pattern:

To the back of the knee

See Activity 9-39.

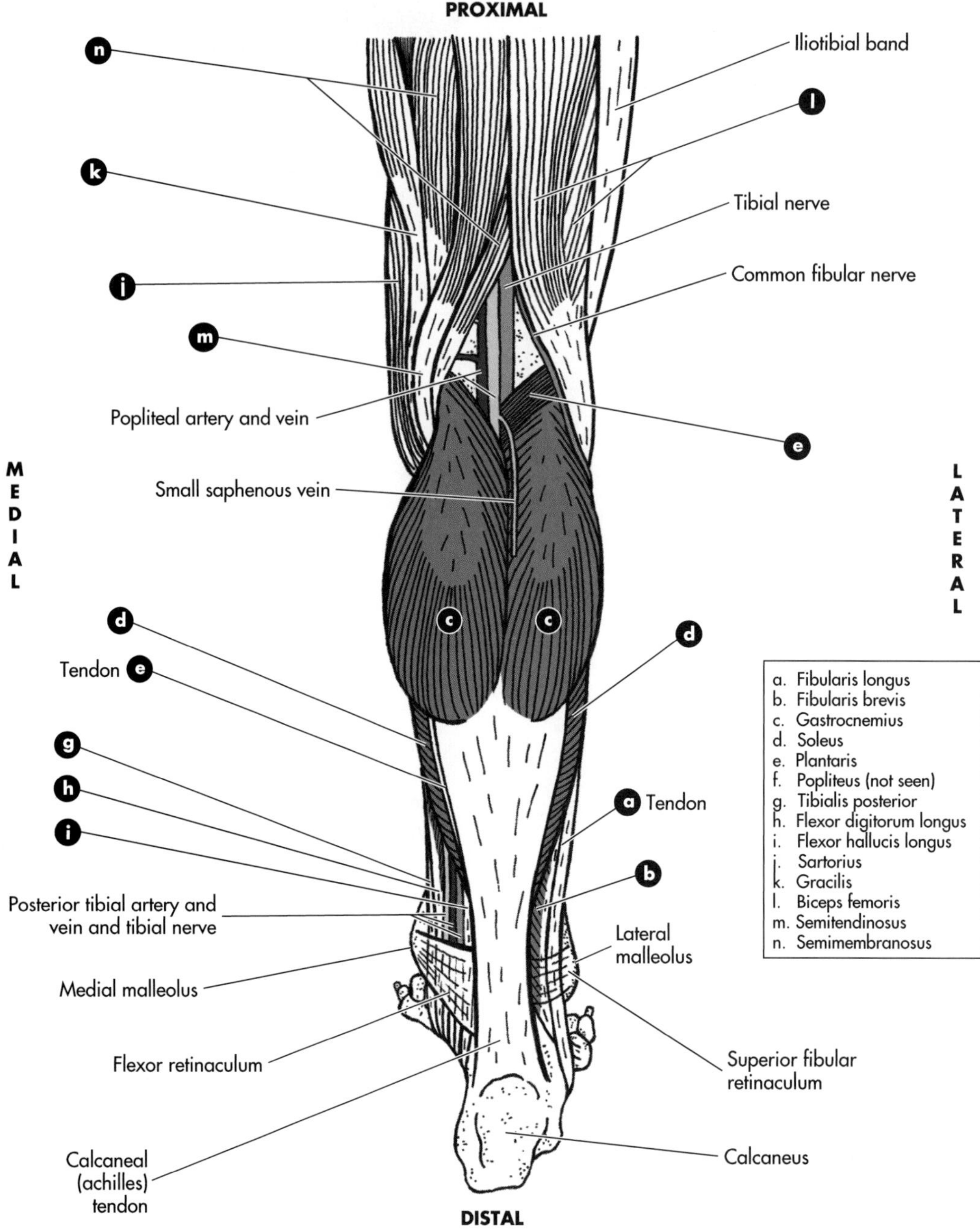

Figure 9-31
Posterior view of the right leg (superficial). (Modified from Muscolino JE: *The muscular system manual: the skeletal muscles of the human body,* ed 2, St Louis, 2005, Mosby.)

ACTIVITY 9-39

1. Draw and color the popliteus in the space provided.
2. Label the proximal and distal attachment points: *P* for proximal; *D* for distal.
3. Place an X on the trigger points.
4. Palpate this muscle; identify the attachment points and the belly of the muscle.
5. Move this muscle on yourself.

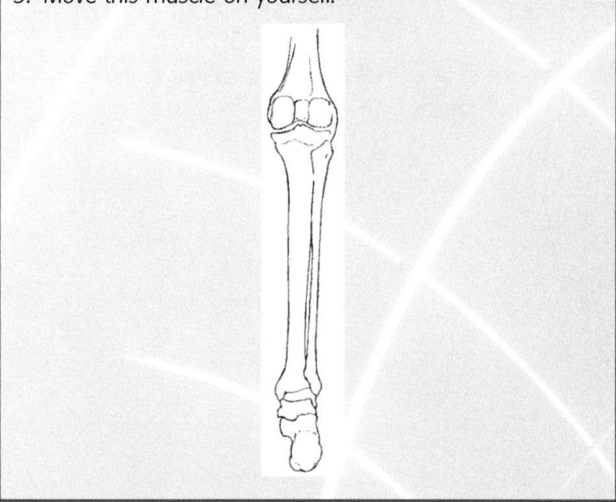

Tibialis posterior (TIB-ee-AL-iss)

Tibialis means related to the shinbone; *posterior* means coming after or behind.

Posterior/Inferior

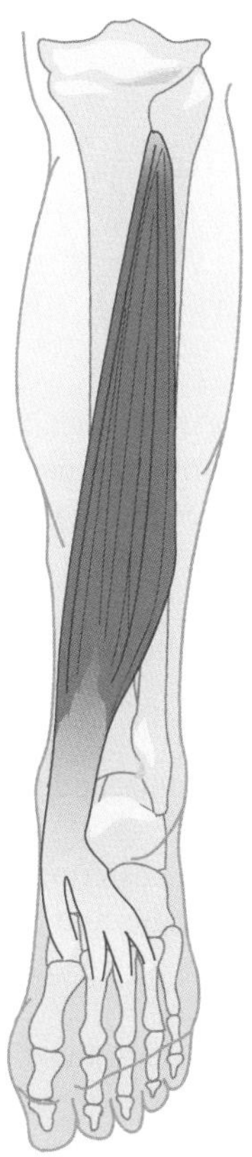

Concentric function:
Plantar flexion of the foot at the ankle joint and inversion of the foot at the tarsal joints

Eccentric function:
Restrains dorsiflexion and eversion of the foot.

Isometric function:
Stabilizes the ankle joint.

From:
Proximal two thirds of the posterior surface of the tibia, fibula, and the interosseous membrane and intermuscular septa

To:
Tuberosity of the navicular bone, calcaneus, three cuneiforms and the cuboid, and bases of the second through fourth metatarsal bones (sole of foot)

Innervation:
Tibial nerve (L4 to L5)

Major synergists:
Tibialis anterior, flexor digitorum longus, and flexor hallucis longus

Major antagonists:
Fibularis longus, fibularis brevis, and tibialis anterior

Trigger points:
Belly of the muscle near the knee joint

Referred pain pattern:
Down the posterior leg to the heel and the sole of the foot into the plantar surface of the toes; can be a factor in knee pain and restricted mobility of the knee and ankle.

Flexor digitorum longus (FLEKS-or DIH-jih-TOR-um LONG-us)

Flexor means to bend, *digitorum* means related to the fingers or toes, and *longus* means long.

Posterior/Inferior

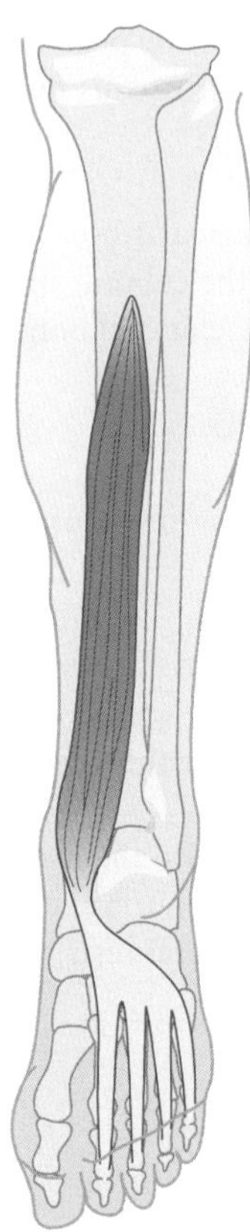

Concentric function:
Flexion of toes 2 to 5 at the metatarsophalangeal and interphalangeal joints, plantar flexion of the foot at the ankle joint, and inversion of the foot at the tarsal joints

Eccentric function:
Allows extension of the toes and allows dorsiflexion and eversion of the foot.

Isometric function:
Stabilizes the ankle joint and the toes.

From:
Middle one third of the posterior surface of the shaft of the tibia and the fascia covering the tibialis posterior

To:
Bases of the distal phalanges of the second through fifth digits (sole of foot)

Innervation:
Tibial nerve (L5 to S2)

Major synergist:
Flexor digitorum brevis

Major antagonists:
Extensor digitorum longus and extensor digitorum brevis

Trigger points:
In the belly of the muscle

Referred pain pattern:
Down the posterior leg to the heel and the sole of the foot into the plantar surface of the toes; can be a factor in knee pain and restricted mobility of the knee and ankle.

Flexor hallucis longus (FLEKS-or HAL-uh-siss LONG-us)

Flexor means to bend, *hallucis* means related to the big toe, and *longus* means long.

Posterior/Inferior

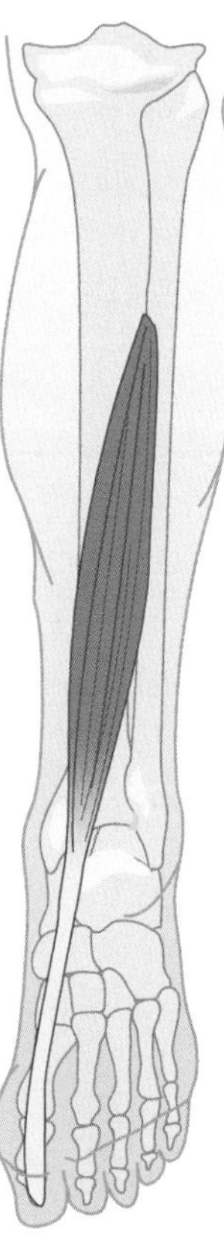

Concentric function:
Flexion of the big toe at the metatarsophalangeal and interphalangeal joints, plantar flexion of the foot at the ankle joint, inversion of the foot at the tarsal joints

Eccentric function:
Restrains extension of the big toe and dorsiflexion and eversion of the foot.

Isometric function:
Stabilizes the big toe, ankle, and foot.

From:
Distal two thirds of the posterior surface of the fibula, interosseous membrane, and adjacent intermuscular septum and fascia

To:
Plantar aspect of the base of the distal phalanx of the big toe (sole of foot)

Innervation:
Tibial nerve (L5 to S2)
Major synergist:
Flexor hallucis brevis
Major antagonists:
Extensor hallucis longus and extensor hallucis brevis
Trigger points:
In the belly of the muscle
Referred pain pattern:
Down the posterior leg to the heel and the sole of the foot into the plantar surface of the toes; can be a factor in knee pain and restricted mobility of the knee and ankle.

Plantaris (plan-TAR-iss)

Plantaris means the sole of the foot.

Posterior

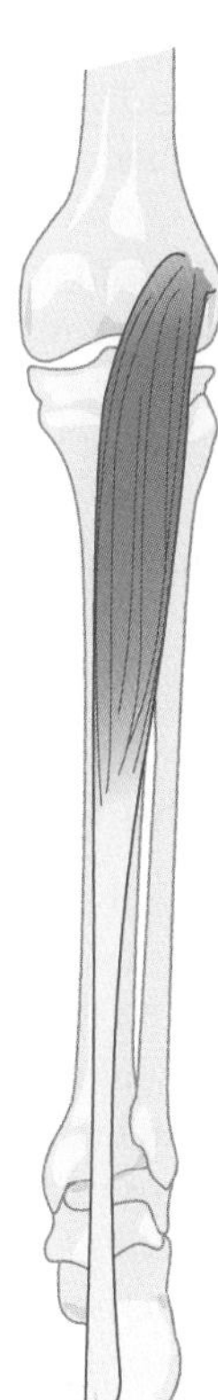

Concentric function:
Plantar flexion of the foot at the ankle joint and flexion of the leg at the knee joint
Eccentric function:
Restrains dorsiflexion of the foot and extension of the leg.
Isometric function:
Stabilizes the ankle and knee joints.
From:
Distal part of the lateral supracondylar line of the femur and oblique popliteal ligament
To:
Posterior medial part of the calcaneus with the calcaneal tendon

Innervation:
Tibial nerve (S1 to S2)
Major synergists:
Gastrocnemius and soleus
Major antagonists:
Tibialis anterior and quadriceps femoris group
Trigger points:
In the belly of the muscle at the back of the knee joint
Referred pain pattern:
Down the posterior leg to the heel and the sole of the foot into the plantar surface of the toes; can be a factor in knee pain and restricted mobility of the knee and ankle.

Soleus (SOL-ee-us)

Soleus means sandal or sole of the foot.

Posterior

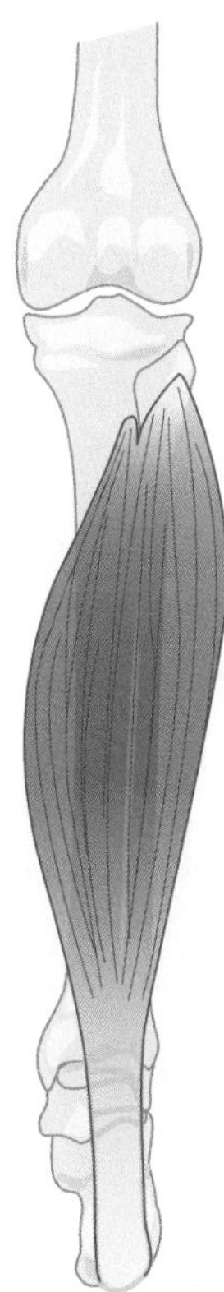

Concentric function:
Plantar flexion of the foot at the ankle joint and inversion of the foot at the tarsal joints.
Eccentric function:
Restrains dorsiflexion and eversion of the foot.
Isometric function:
Stabilizes the ankle joint.

Because of its thick, large venous sinuses, tough fascial covering, and vein structure, the soleus is an effective musculovenous pump that functions as a "second heart," especially during strenuous running and jumping activities.
From:
Posterior surface of the head and proximal one third of

the posterior surface of the fibula, soleal line of the tibia, and fibrous band between the tibia and the fibula

To:

Calcaneus (with the gastrocnemius) via the calcaneal (Achilles) tendon

Innervation:

Tibial nerve (S1 to S2)

Major synergist:

Gastrocnemius

Major antagonists:

Tibialis anterior, extensor digitorum longus, and extensor hallucis longus

Trigger points:

Near the proximal and distal attachments

Referred pain pattern:

Down the posterior leg to the heel and the sole of the foot into the plantar surface of the toes; can be a factor in knee pain and restricted mobility of the knee and ankle.

Gastrocnemius (GAS-trok-NEEM-ee-us)

Gastrocnemius means belly and shin or leg.

Posterior

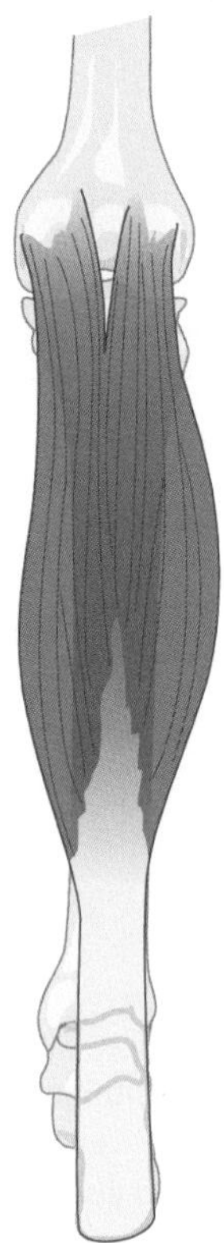

Concentric function:

Plantar flexion of the foot at the ankle joint, inversion of the foot at the tarsal joints, and flexion of the leg at the knee joint

Eccentric function:

Allows dorsiflexion and eversion of the foot and allows extension of the leg.

Isometric function:

Stabilizes the knee and ankle joints and is involved in maintaining balance in static standing.

From:

Medial head—Proximal posterior part of the medial condyle of the femur and capsule of the knee joint

Lateral head—Distal part of the lateral supracondylar line and lateral condyle of the femur and capsule of the knee joint

To:

Calcaneus (with the soleus) via the calcaneal (Achilles) tendon

Innervation:

Tibial nerve (S1 to S2)

Major synergists:

Soleus and hamstring muscles

Major antagonists:

Tibialis anterior, extensor digitorum longus, extensor hallucis longus, and quadriceps femoris muscles

Trigger points:

In the belly of the muscle and at the attachment near the knee in each head of this muscle

Referred pain pattern:

Down the posterior leg to the heel and the sole of the foot into the plantar surface of the toes; can be a factor in knee pain and restricted mobility of the knee and ankle.

See Activity 9-40.

Intrinsic Muscles of the Foot

Intrinsic muscles of the foot are small muscles located wholly within the foot (i.e., they originate and insert within the foot) (Figures 9-32 and 9-33). The muscles of the sole of the foot work concentrically and eccentrically to help flex, extend, abduct, and adduct the toes; they also work isometrically with the tendons of the leg muscles to support the arches of the foot. These muscles are numerous, their arrangement is complex, and their actions are interdependent. Although only the classic concentric mover functions of these muscles are listed, one should note that the primary function of these muscles is stabilization and proprioceptive feedback on foot position.

ACTIVITY 9-40

1. Draw and color the tibialis posterior, flexor digitorum longus, flexor hallucis longus, plantaris, soleus, and gastrocnemius in the space provided.
2. Label the proximal and distal attachment points: *P* for proximal; *D* for distal.
3. Place an X on the trigger points.
4. Palpate these muscles; identify the attachment points and the bellies of the muscles.
5. Move these muscles on yourself.

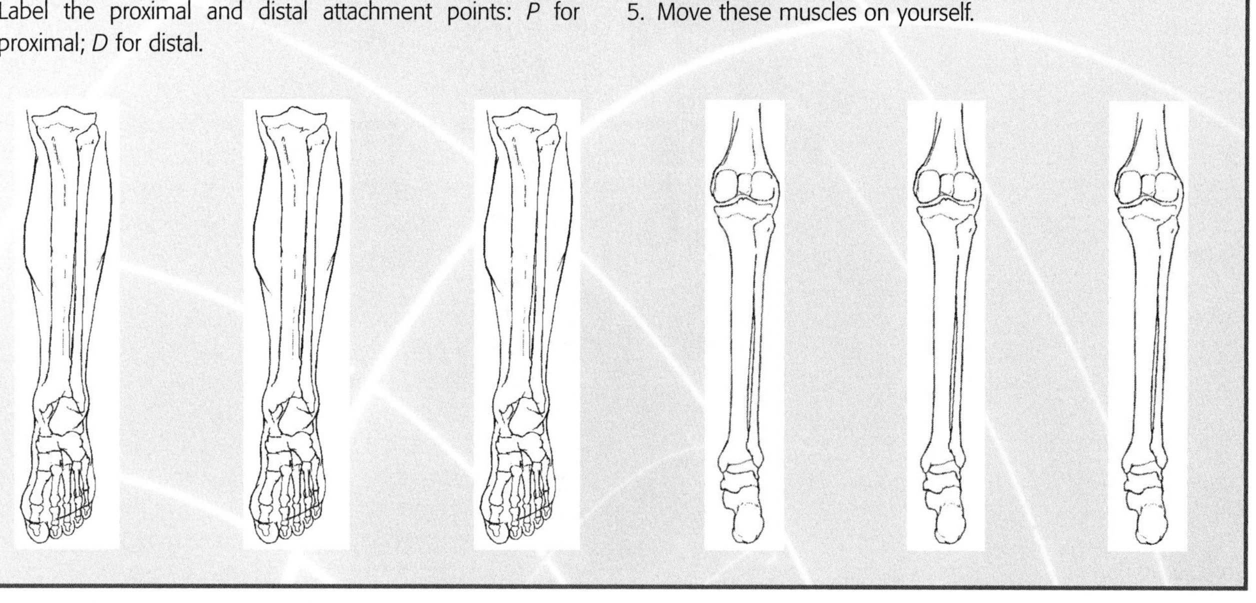

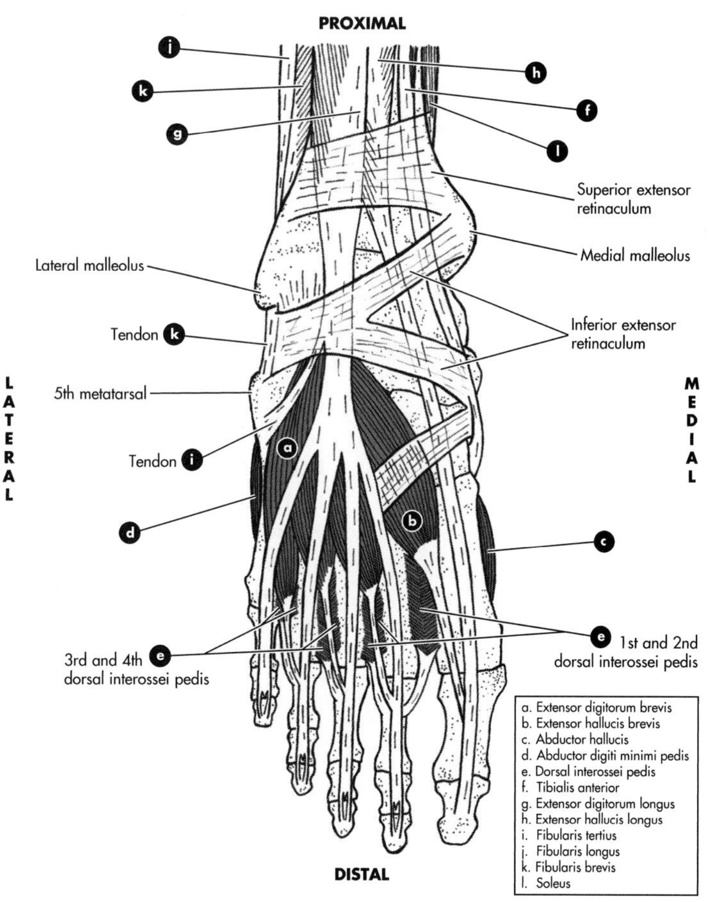

Figure 9-32
Dorsal view of the right foot. (Modified from Muscolino JE: *The muscular system manual: the skeletal muscles of the human body,* ed 2, St Louis, 2005, Mosby.)

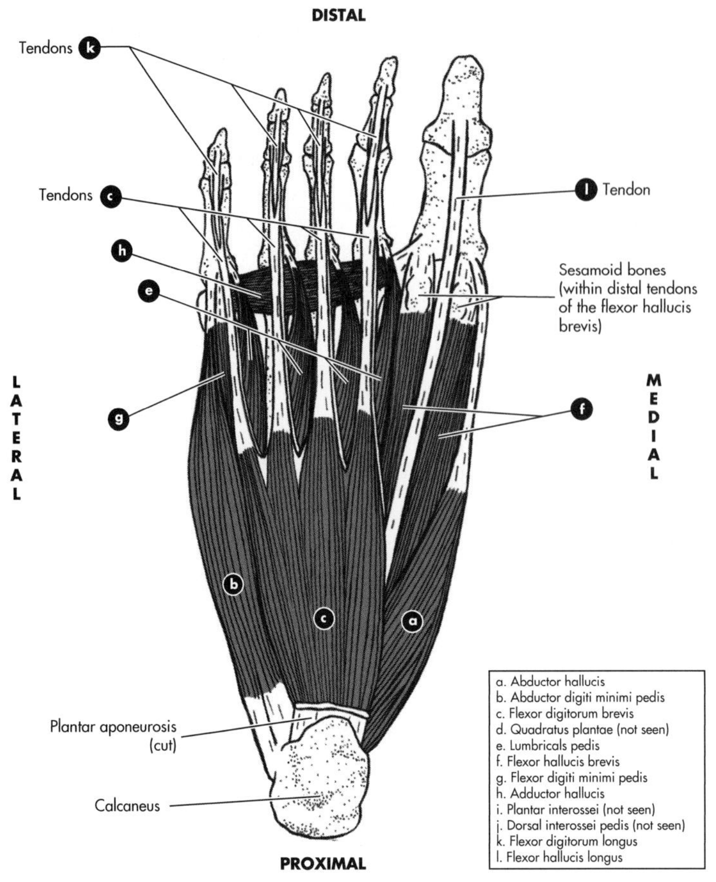

Figure 9-33
Plantar view of the right foot (superficial muscular layer). (Modified from Muscolino JE: *The muscular system manual: the skeletal muscles of the human body,* ed 2, St Louis, 2005, Mosby.)

Dorsal Aspect

Extensor digitorum brevis (ex-STEN-sur DIH-jih-TOR-um BREV-us)

Extensor means to stretch, *digitorum* means related to the fingers or toes, and *brevis* means short.

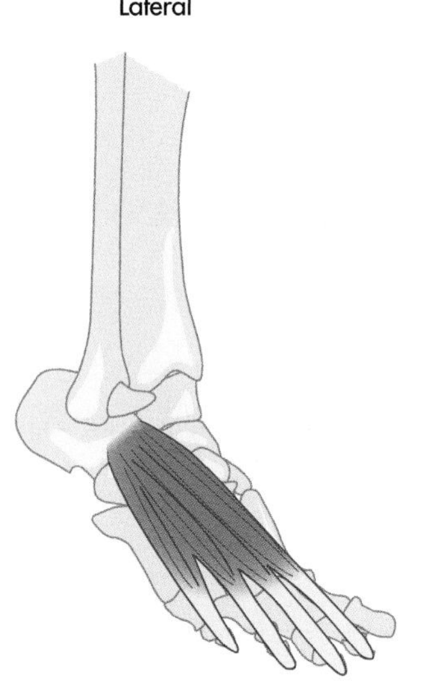

The most medial portion of the extensor digitorum brevis inserts into the dorsal surface of the base of the proximal phalanx of the big toe and sometimes is called the extensor hallucis brevis muscle.

Concentric function:
Extension of the big toe at the metatarsophalangeal joint and extension of toes 2 to 4 at the metatarsophalangeal and interphalangeal joints

Eccentric function:
Restrains flexion of the big toe and flexion of toes 2 to 4.

From:
Dorsal surface of the calcaneus, lateral talocalcaneal ligament, and inferior extensor retinaculum

To:
First tendon into the dorsal surface of the base of the proximal phalanx of the great toe and lateral sides of the tendons of the extensor digitorum longus (dorsal digital expansion) to the second, third, and fourth toes

Innervation:
Deep fibular nerve (L5 to S1)

Major synergists:
Extensor digitorum longus and extensor hallucis longus

Major antagonists:
Flexor digitorum longus, flexor hallucis longus, and flexor digitorum brevis

Trigger points:
The belly of the muscle
Referred pain pattern:
The entire foot with areas concentrated at the large toe, the ball of the foot, and the heel

Plantar Aspect: Superficial Layer

Abductor hallucis (ab-DUCK-tur HAL-uh-siss)

Abductor means to lead away from; *hallucis* means big toe.

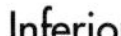

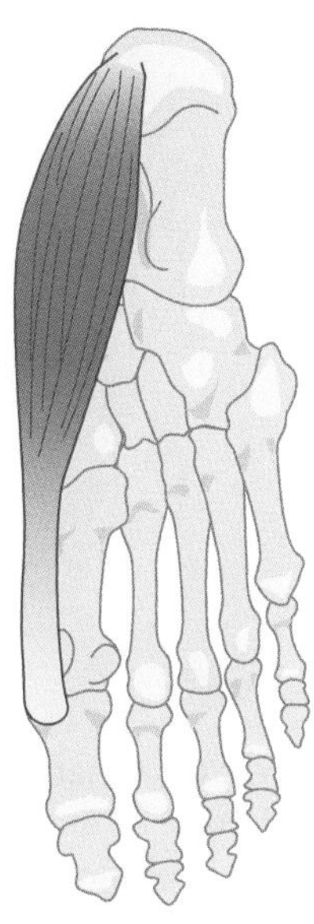

Concentric function:
Abduction and flexion of the big toe at the metatarsophalangeal joint
Eccentric function:
Restrains adduction and extension of the big toe.
From:
Medial process of the calcaneal tuberosity, flexor retinaculum, plantar aponeurosis, and adjacent intermuscular septum
To:
Medial side of the base of the proximal phalanx of the great toe
Innervation:
Medial plantar nerve (S1 to S2)
Major synergist:
Flexor hallucis brevis
Major antagonist:
Adductor hallucis
Trigger points:
The belly of the muscle
Referred pain pattern:
The entire foot with areas concentrated at the large toe, the ball of the foot, and the heel

Flexor digitorum brevis (FLEKS-or DIH-jih-TOR-um BREV-us)

Flexor means to bend, *digitorum* means related to fingers or toes, and *brevis* means short.

Inferior

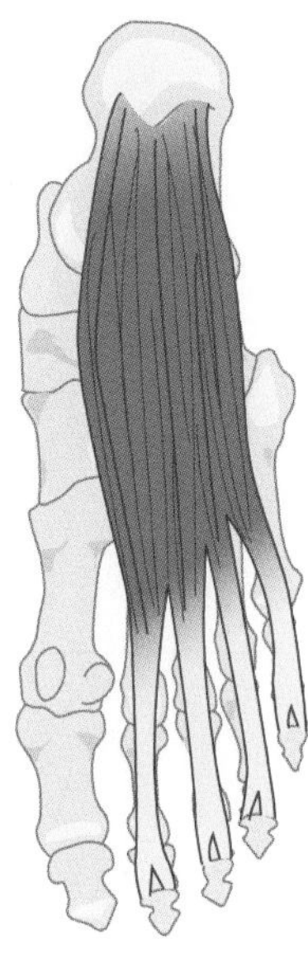

Concentric function:
Flexion of toes 2 to 5 at the metatarsophalangeal and proximal interphalangeal joints
Eccentric function:
Restrains extension of toes 2 to 5.
From:
Medial process of the calcaneal tuberosity, plantar aponeurosis, and adjacent intermuscular septa
To:
Medial and lateral sides of the middle phalanges of the second through fifth toes
Innervation:
Medial plantar nerve (S1 and S2)
Major synergists:
Flexor digitorum longus and quadratus plantae
Major antagonists:
Extensor digitorum longus and extensor digitorum brevis
Trigger points:
The belly of the muscle
Referred pain pattern:
The entire foot with areas concentrated at the large toe, the ball of the foot, and the heel

Abductor digiti minimi pedis (ab-DUCK-tur DIH-jih-tee MIN-ih-mee PEE-dis)

Abductor means to lead away from, *digiti* means related to the fingers or toes, *minimi* means smallest, and *pedis* means of the foot.

Inferior

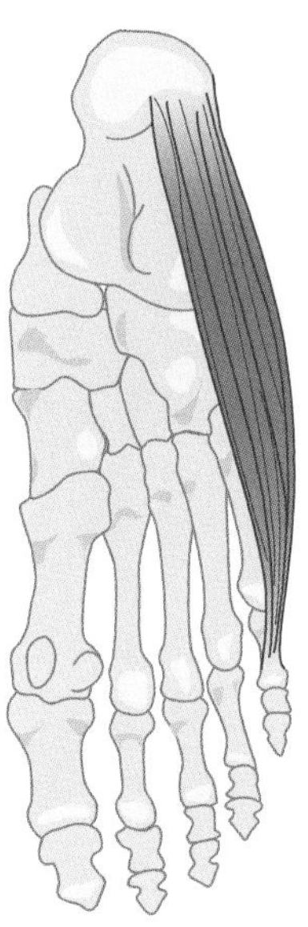

Concentric function:
Abduction and flexion of the little toe at the metatarsophalangeal joint

Eccentric function:
Restrains adduction and extension of the little toe.

From:
Lateral process of the calcaneal tuberosity, plantar aponeurosis, and intermuscular septum

To:
Lateral side of the base of the proximal phalanx of the fifth toe

Innervation:
Lateral plantar nerve (S2 to S3)

Major synergists:
Flexor digitorum brevis

Major antagonist:
Plantar interosseous (No. 3)

Trigger points:
The belly of the muscle

Referred pain pattern:
The entire foot with areas concentrated at the large toe, the ball of the foot, and the heel

Plantar Aspect: Second Layer

Quadratus plantae (kwad-RATE-us PLAN-tie)

Quadratus means square shaped; *plantae* means for the sole of the foot.

Inferior

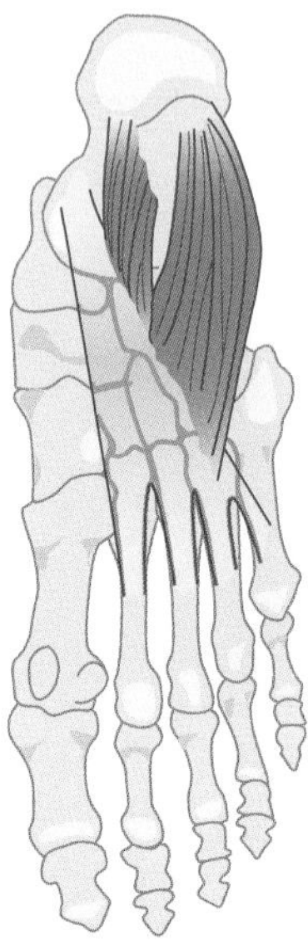

Concentric function:
Flexion of toes 2 to 5 at the metatarsophalangeal and interphalangeal joints (The quadratus plantae acts to modify the line of pull of the flexor digitorum longus.)

Eccentric function:
Restrains extension of toes 2 to 5.

From:
Medial head—Medial surface of the calcaneus and medial border of the long plantar ligament

Lateral head—Lateral inferior surface of the calcaneus, lateral border of the plantar surface of the calcaneus, and lateral border of the long plantar ligament

To:
Lateral margin of the flexor digitorum longus tendon

Innervation:
Lateral plantar nerve (S2 to S3)

Major synergists:
Flexor digitorum longus and flexor digitorum brevis

Major antagonists:
Extensor digitorum longus and extensor digitorum brevis

Trigger points:
The belly of the muscle

Referred pain pattern:
The entire foot with areas concentrated at the large toe, the ball of the foot, and the heel

Lumbricales pedis (LUM-brih-kal-es PEE-dis)

Lumbricales means earthworms; *pedis* means of the foot.

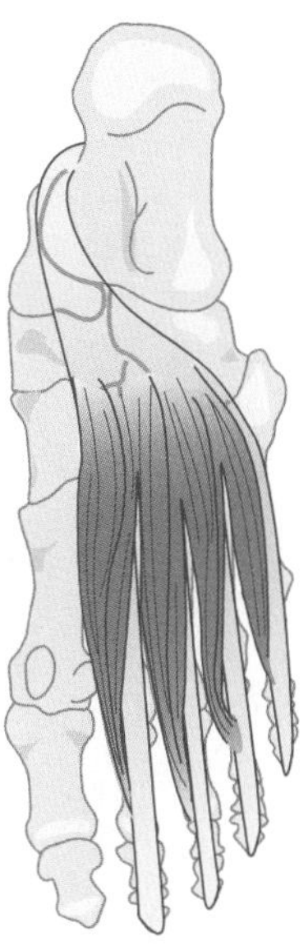

Concentric function:
Flexion of toes 2 to 5 at the metatarsophalangeal joints and extension of toes 2 to 5 at the proximal and distal interphalangeal joints

Eccentric function:
Restrains extension and flexion of toes 2 to 5.

From:
First—From the medial side of the first flexor digitorum longus tendon
Second—From adjacent sides of the first and second flexor digitorum longus tendons
Third—From adjacent sides of the second and third flexor digitorum longus tendons
Fourth—From adjacent sides of the third and fourth flexor digitorum longus tendons

To:
Distal tendons of the extensor digitorum longus (dorsal digital expansion) into the base of the middle and distal phalanges of the second through fifth toes

Innervation:
Medial and lateral plantar nerves (S1 to S3)

Major synergists:
Flexor digitorum longus and extensor digitorum longus

Major antagonists:
Flexor digitorum longus and extensor digitorum longus

Trigger points:
The belly of the muscle

Referred pain pattern:
The entire foot with areas concentrated at the large toe, the ball of the foot, and the heel

Plantar Aspect: Third Layer

Flexor hallucis brevis (FLEKS-or HAL-uh-siss BREV-us)

Flexor means to bend, *hallucis* means big toe, and *brevis* means short.

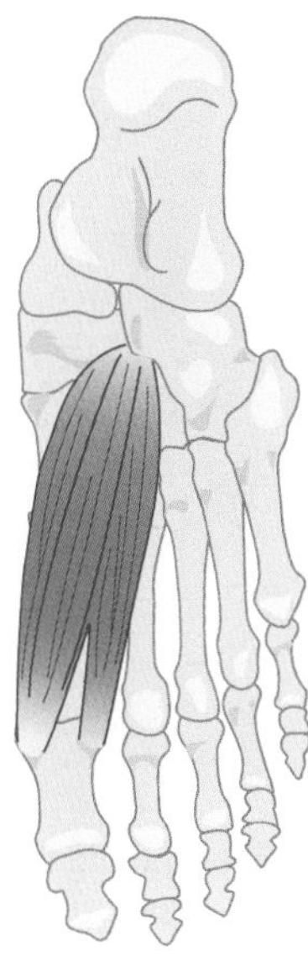

Concentric function:
Flexion of the big toe at the metatarsophalangeal joint

Eccentric function:
Restrains extension of the big toe.

From:
Medial aspect of the plantar surface of the cuboid bone, lateral cuneiform bone, and from the tendon of the tibialis posterior

To:
Medial and lateral sides of the base of the proximal phalanx of the great toe

Innervation:
Medial plantar nerve (S1 to S2)

Major synergist:
Flexor hallucis longus

Major antagonists:
Extensor hallucis longus and extensor digitorum brevis (medial part)

Trigger points:
The belly of the muscle

Referred pain pattern:
The entire foot with areas concentrated at the large toe, the ball of the foot, and the heel

Adductor hallucis (ad-DUCK-tur HAL-uh-siss)

Adductor means to lead toward; *hallucis* means big toe.

Inferior

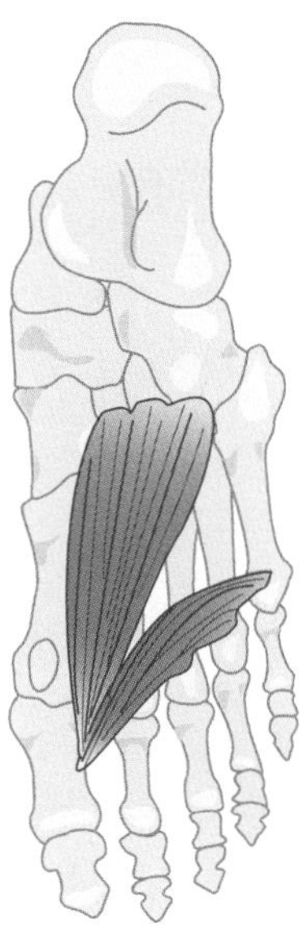

Concentric function:
Adduction and flexion of the big toe at the metatarsophalangeal joint

Eccentric function:
Restrains abduction and extension of the big toe.

From:
Oblique head—Bases of the second, third, and fourth metatarsal bones and sheath of the tendon of the fibularis longus
Transverse head—Plantar metatarsophalangeal ligaments of the third, fourth, and fifth digits and deep transverse metatarsal ligament of the sole

To:
Lateral side of the base of the proximal phalanx of the big toe

Innervation:
Lateral plantar nerve (S2 to S3)

Major synergists:
Flexor hallucis longus and flexor hallucis brevis

Major antagonist:
Abductor hallucis

Trigger points:
The belly of the muscle

Referred pain pattern:
The entire foot with areas concentrated at the large toe, the ball of the foot, and the heel

Flexor digiti minimi pedis (FLEKS-or DIH-jih-tee MIN-ih-mee PEE-dis)

Flexor means to bend, *digiti* means related to the fingers and toes, *minimi* means smallest, and *pedis* means of the foot.

Inferior

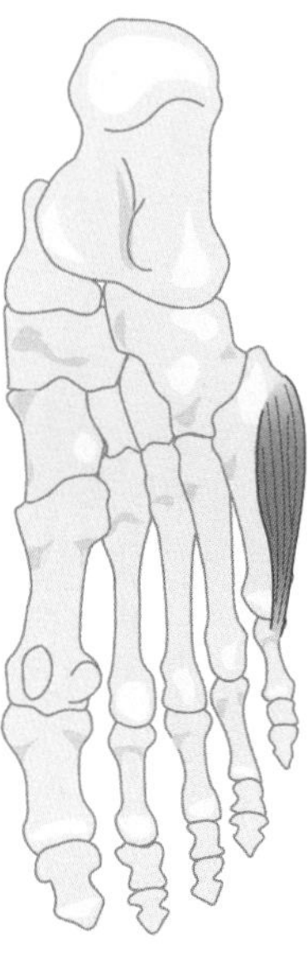

Occasionally, some of the deeper fibers of the flexor digiti minimi pedis reach the lateral part of the distal half of the fifth metatarsal bone; this sometimes is described as a distinct muscle, the opponens digiti minimi pedis

Concentric function:
Flexion of the little toe at the metatarsophalangeal joint

Eccentric function:
Restrains extension of the little toe.

From:
Medial part of the plantar surface of the base of the fifth metatarsal bone and sheath of the fibularis longus

To:
Plantar surface of the base of the proximal phalanx of the little toe

Innervation:
Lateral plantar nerve (S2 to S3)

Major synergists:
Flexor digitorum longus and flexor digitorum brevis

Major antagonist:
Extensor digitorum longus

Trigger points:
The belly of the muscle

Referred pain pattern:
The entire foot with areas concentrated at the large toe, the ball of the foot, and the heel

Plantar Aspect: Fourth Layer

Interossei plantares (INT-er-OSS-ee-eye plan-TAR-es)

Interossei means between the bones; *plantares* means sole of the foot.

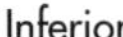

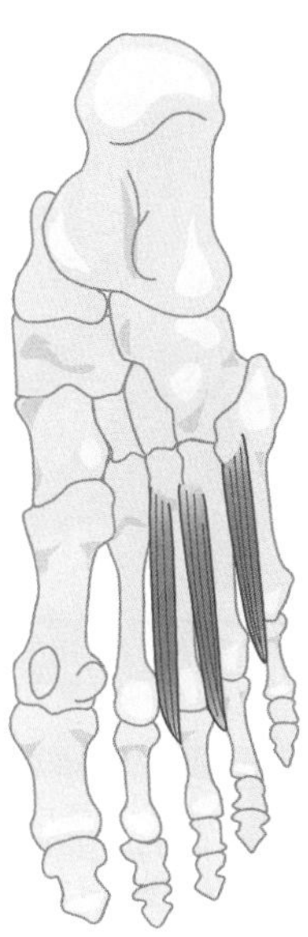

Concentric function:

Adduction of toes 3 to 5 at the metatarsophalangeal joints (adduction of a toe is a movement toward an imaginary line drawn through the middle of the second toe), flexion of toes 3 to 5 at the metatarsophalangeal joints, and extension of toes 3 to 5 at the proximal and distal interphalangeal joints

Eccentric function:

Restrains abduction, extension, and flexion of toes 3 to 5.

From:

Three interossei plantares arise from the base and medial sides of the shafts of the third, fourth, and fifth metatarsals.

To:

Medial sides of the bases of the proximal phalanges of the same toes and the dorsal digital expansion

Innervation:

Lateral plantar nerve (S2 to S3)

Major synergists:

Lumbricales pedis

Major antagonists:

Interossei dorsales pedis

Trigger points:

The belly of the muscle

Referred pain pattern:

The entire foot with areas concentrated at the large toe, the ball of the foot, and the heel

Interossei dorsales pedis (INT-er-OSS-ee-eye door-SAL-es PEE-dis)

Interossei means between the bones, *dorsales* means on or near the back, and *pedis* means of the foot.

Inferior

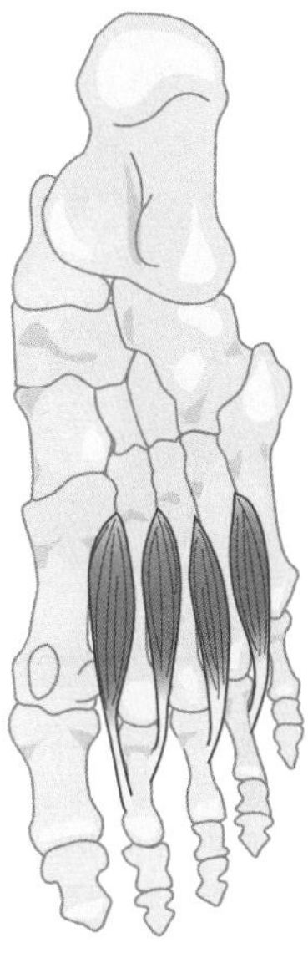

Concentric function:

Abduction of toes 2 to 4 at the metatarsophalangeal joints (abduction of a toe is a movement away from an imaginary line drawn through the middle of the second toe), flexion of toes 2 to 4 at the metatarsophalangeal joints, and extension of toes 2 to 4 at the proximal and distal interphalangeal joints

Eccentric function:

Restrains adduction, extension, and flexion of toes 2 to 4.

From:

Each arises via two heads from adjacent sides of the metatarsal bones between which they are placed.

To:

Bases of the proximal phalanges of toes 2 to 4 and distal tendons of the extensor digitorum longus (dorsal digital expansion)

Innervation:

Lateral plantar nerve (S2 to S3)

Major synergists:

Lumbricales pedis

Major antagonists:

Interossei plantares

Trigger points:

The belly of the muscle

Referred pain pattern:

The entire foot with areas concentrated at the large toe, the ball of the foot, and the heel

See Activity 9-41.

ACTIVITY 9-41

1. Draw and color the muscles of the foot in the space provided.
2. Label the proximal and distal attachment points: *P* for proximal; *D* for distal.
3. Place an X on the trigger points.
4. Palpate these muscles; identify the attachment points and the bellies of the muscles.
5. Move these muscles on yourself.

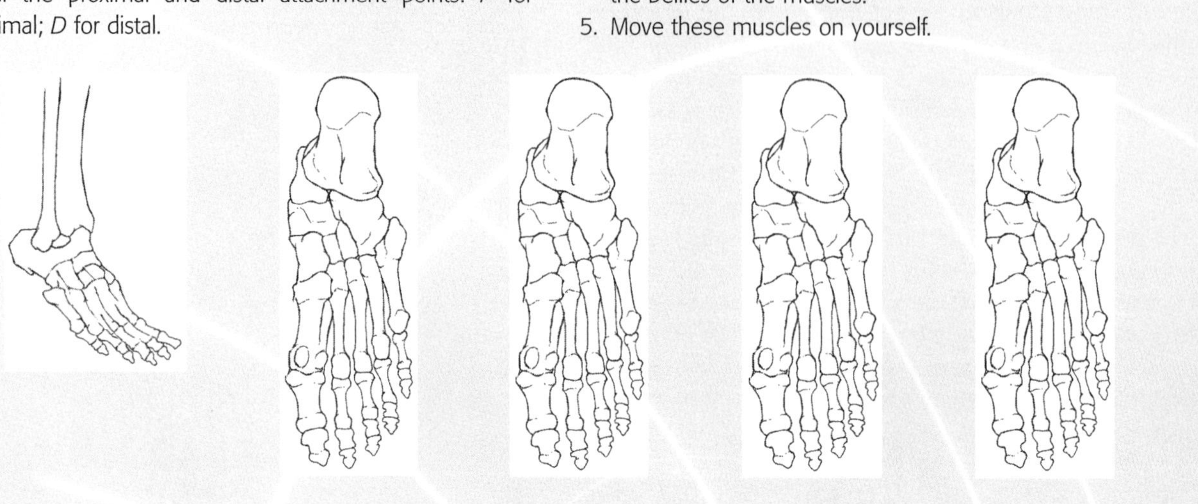

Muscles of Scapular Stabilization

The muscles of scapular stabilization hold the scapula to the ribcage (wall of the thorax) during isometric function and move the scapula during concentric and eccentric function (Figure 9-34, *A*, *B*). The arrangement of the muscle attachments to the scapula requires cooperative concentric, eccentric, and isometric interaction to produce movement. Several muscles must act together to elevate or depress the scapula or to effect other scapular movements at the scapulocostal joint.

The prime movers of scapular elevation at the scapulocostal joint (shrugging the shoulder) are the upper trapezius and the levator scapulae. The opposite rotational effects of the trapezius and levator scapulae on the scapula counterbalance each other.

Scapular depression at the scapulocostal joint results largely from gravitational pull, but when the scapula is depressed against resistance, the lower trapezius and serratus anterior are active. Serratus anterior activity creates the forward (pushing) movements of protraction (abduction) of the scapula at the scapulocostal joint on the chest wall. The trapezius and the rhomboids provide retraction (adduction) of the scapula at the scapulocostal joint.

Although the serratus anterior and trapezius muscles are antagonists in the anterior/posterior movements of the scapula, they act together to create upward rotation of the scapula at the scapulocostal joint.

Clavicular movements accompany scapular movements. The clavicles rotate around their own axes as they move with scapular movements, giving these movements stability and precision. Therapeutic massage methods easily address these more superficial muscles.

Trapezius (TRA-PEE-zee-us)

Trapezius means a figure with four unequal sides (a trapezoid).

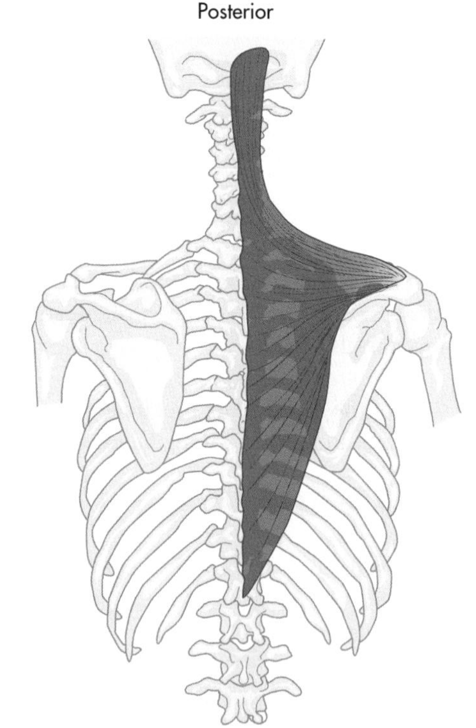

The trapezius usually is considered to consist of three functional parts: the upper trapezius, middle trapezius, and lower trapezius. Concentric, eccentric, and isometric contraction can occur simultaneously in different aspects of the muscle.

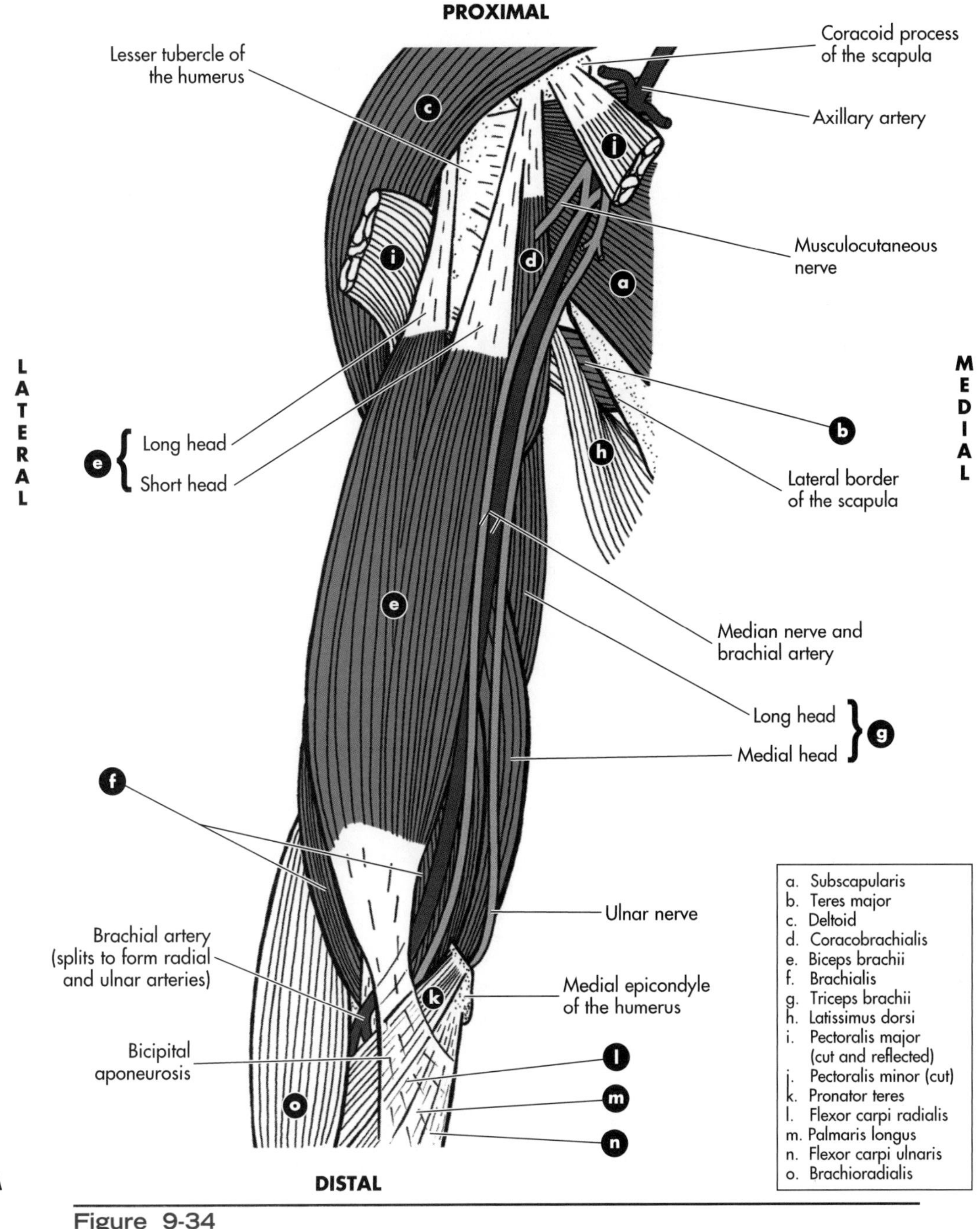

Figure 9-34
A, Anterior view of the right arm (superficial). *(Continued)*

Concentric function:

Extension, lateral flexion, and contralateral rotation of the neck and head at the spinal joints (upper trapezius); elevation of the scapula at the scapulocostal joint (upper trapezius); retraction of the scapula at the scapulocostal joint (entire trapezius); depression of the scapula at the scapulocostal joint (lower trapezius); upward rotation of the scapula at the scapulocostal joint (upper and lower trapezius); and extension of the trunk at the spinal joints (middle and lower trapezius)

Many books divide the actions of the trapezius (and other muscles of the neck and trunk) into the actions created when the muscle contracts on one side (unilaterally) and when the right and left muscles contract (bilaterally). In this division they often describe these actions in a manner that may be misleading. For example, they might state that the unilateral contraction of the upper trapezius causes lateral flexion and contralateral rotation of the neck at the spinal joints and that bilateral contraction of the upper trapezius muscles causes extension of the neck at the spinal joints. Although the bilateral trapezius contraction causes

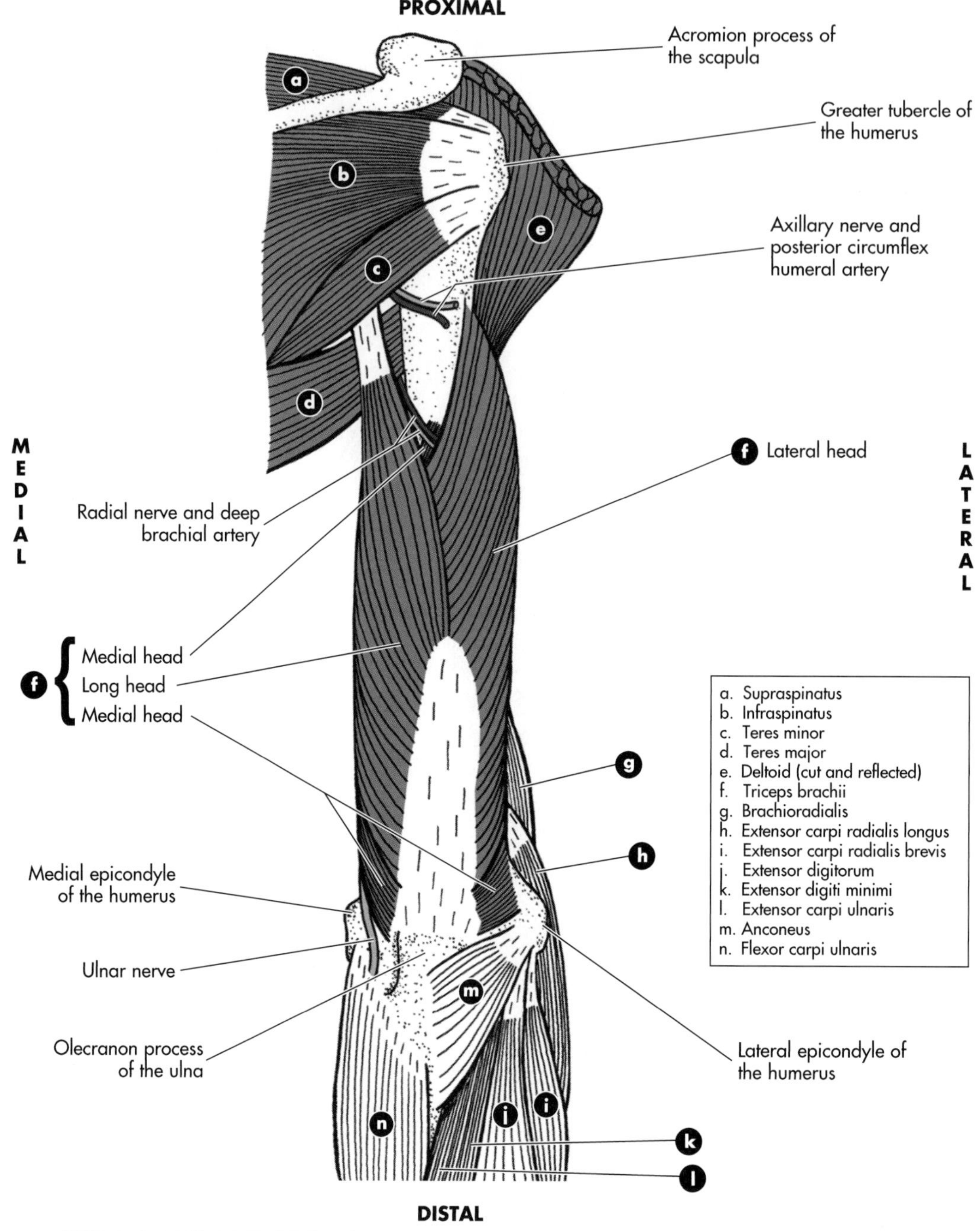

Figure 9-34—cont'd.
B, Posterior view of the right arm. (Modified from Muscolino JE: *The muscular system manual: the skeletal muscles of the human body,* ed 2, St Louis, 2005, Mosby.)

extension of the neck (and in fact is pure extension because the opposite lateral flexions and opposite rotations cancel each other out), unilateral trapezius contraction also causes extension of the neck. One may not realize this when actions are worded this way. No muscle can cause extension bilaterally if it cannot cause extension unilaterally.

What is valuable to take from this type of description is that when any muscle of the neck and trunk contracts bilaterally, its lateral flexion and rotation components always cancel each other out and the resulting joint action is a pure sagittal plane movement, that is, flexion or extension. The other important thing to realize with all muscles of the neck and trunk is that the muscle on one side of the body always can be an antagonist to the same muscle on the other side of the body; for example, the right upper trapezius causes right lateral flexion of the neck and the left upper trapezius causes left lateral flexion of the neck, hence they are antagonistic; also, the right upper trapezius causes left rotation of the neck and the left upper trapezius causes right rotation of the neck, hence they are antagonistic. Of course, regarding extension of the neck, because both sides can cause extension of the neck, they are synergistic. These principles are true and should be kept in mind for all muscles of the neck and trunk. As a rule, this text does not usually list the same muscle on the opposite side of the body in the synergist and antagonist sections.

Eccentric function:
Restrains flexion, contralateral lateral flexion, and ipsilateral rotation of the neck and head; depression, protraction (abduction), elevation, and downward rotation of the scapula; and flexion of the trunk

Isometric function:
Stabilizes the scapula and cervical spine.

From:
Upper trapezius—External occipital protuberance; superior nuchal line, nuchal ligament; and spinous process of the seventh cervical vertebrae
Middle trapezius—Spinous processes of the first through fifth thoracic vertebrae
Lower trapezius—Spinous processes of the sixth through twelfth thoracic vertebrae

To:
Upper trapezius—Lateral one third of the clavicle and acromion process of the scapula
Middle trapezius—Acromion process and spine of the scapula
Lower trapezius—Root of the spine of the scapula

Innervation:
Spinal accessory nerve (cranial nerve XI) and ventral rami of third and fourth cervical spinal nerves

Major synergists:
Upper trapezius—Semispinalis capitis, levator scapulae, serratus anterior, and sternocleidomastoid
Middle trapezius—Rhomboids and spinal extensors
Lower trapezius—Serratus anterior, pectoralis minor, and spinal extensors

Major antagonists:
Upper trapezius—Lower trapezius, rhomboids, and flexors of the neck
Middle trapezius—Pectoralis minor and serratus anterior
Lower trapezius—Upper trapezius and levator scapulae

Trigger points:
Upper trapezius near the acromion and clavicular attachments, middle trapezius near the spine of the scapula, and lower trapezius in the belly of the muscle

Referred pain patterns:
Neck posterior to the ear and to the temple, subscapular area, and acromial pain

See Activity 9-42.

ACTIVITY 9-42

1. Draw and color the trapezius in the space provided.
2. Label the proximal and distal attachment points: *P* for proximal; *D* for distal.
3. Place an X on the trigger points.
4. Palpate this muscle; identify the attachment points and the belly of the muscle.
5. Move this muscle on yourself.

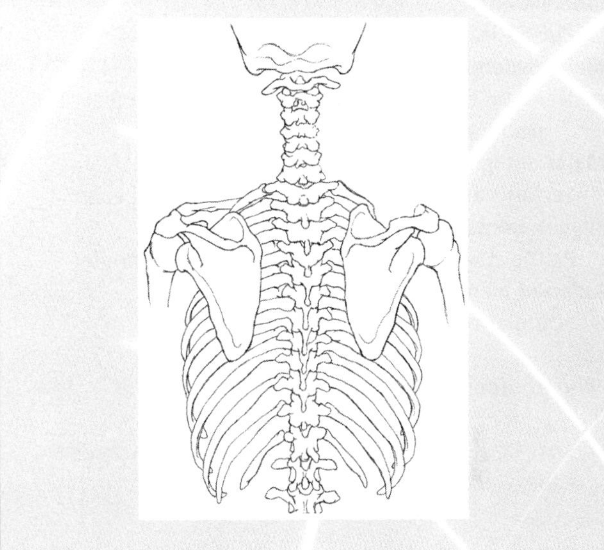

Rhomboideus major (rom-BOYD-ee-us)

Rhomboideus means shaped like a rhombus (a diamond shape); *major* means larger.

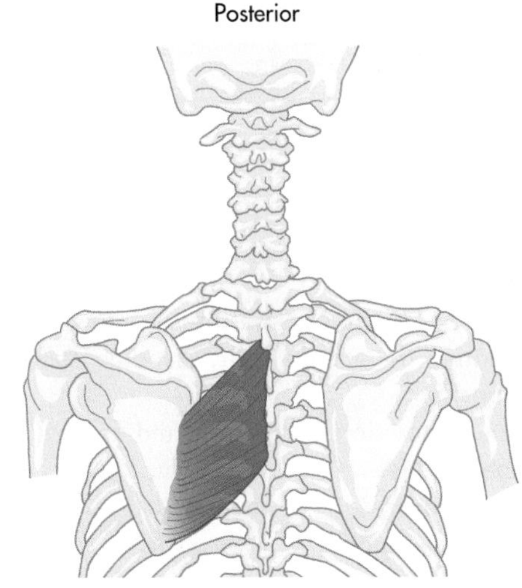

Concentric function:
Retraction (adduction), elevation, and downward rotation of the scapula at the scapulocostal joint

Eccentric function:
Restrains protraction (abduction), depression, and upward rotation of the scapula.

Isometric function:
Stabilizes the scapula.

From:
Spinous processes of the second through fifth thoracic vertebrae

To:
Medial border of the scapula, between the spine and the inferior angle

Innervation:
Dorsal scapular nerve (C4 to C5)

Major synergists:
Rhomboideus minor, trapezius, levator scapulae, and pectoralis minor

Major antagonists:
Serratus anterior, pectoralis minor, and trapezius

Trigger points:
At the attachment point near the scapular border

Referred pain pattern:
Scapular region

ACTIVITY 9-43

1. Draw and color the rhomboideus major and rhomboideus minor in the space provided.
2. Label the proximal and distal attachment points: *P* for proximal; *D* for distal.
3. Place an X on the trigger points.
4. Palpate these muscles; identify the attachment points and the bellies of the muscles.
5. Move these muscles on yourself.

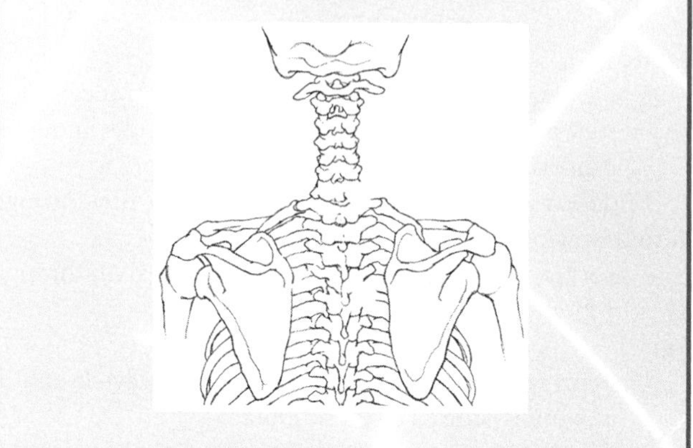

Rhomboideus minor (rom-BOYD-ee-us)

Rhomboideus means shaped like a rhombus (a diamond shape); *minor* means smaller.

Posterior

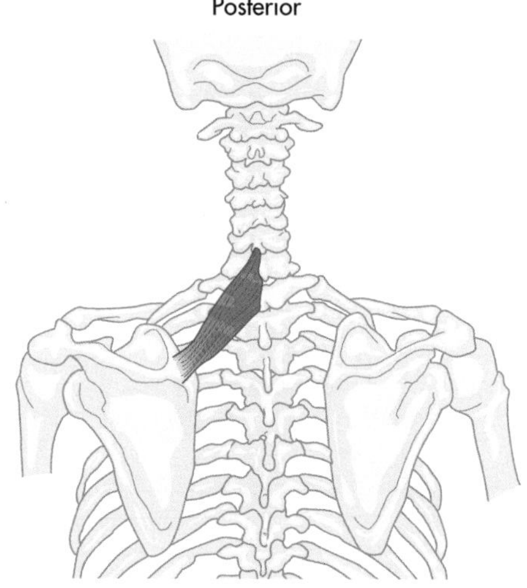

Concentric function:
Retraction (adduction), elevation, and downward rotation of the scapula at the scapulocostal joint

Eccentric function:
Restrains protraction, depression, and upward rotation of the scapula.

Isometric function:
Stabilizes the scapula.

From:
Ligamentum nuchae and spinous processes of the seventh cervical and first thoracic vertebrae

To:
Medial border of the scapula at the root of the spine of the scapula

Innervation:
Dorsal scapular nerve (C4 to C5)

Major synergists:
Rhomboideus major, trapezius, levator scapulae, and pectoralis minor

Major antagonists:
Serratus anterior, pectoralis minor, and trapezius

Trigger points:
At the attachment point near the scapular border

Referred pain pattern:
Scapular region

See Activity 9-43.

Levator scapulae (le-VAY-tor SKAP-you-lee)

Levator scapulae means to elevate the scapula.

Posterior

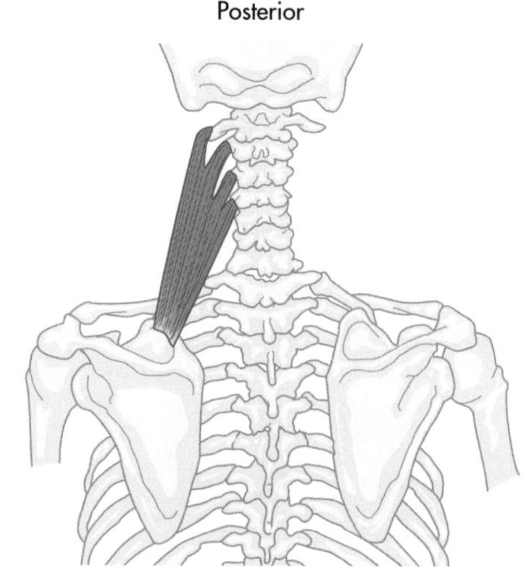

Concentric function:
Elevation and retraction (adduction) of the scapula at the scapulocostal joint, and extension, lateral flexion, and ipsilateral rotation of the neck at the spinal joints

Eccentric function:
Allows depression and protraction (abduction) of the scapula and restrains flexion, contralateral lateral flexion, and contralateral rotation of the neck.

Isometric function:
Stabilizes cervical/scapular function.

From:
Transverse processes of the atlas and axis and the third and fourth cervical vertebrae

To:
Medial border of the scapula between the superior angle and the root of the spine

The levator scapulae is a large muscle and has a rotation, or twist, that occurs in its design so that the attachments at the atlas and axis are from muscle fibers that attach to the inferior portion of the medial border of the scapula and the attachments at C4 are from fibers at the superior portion of the medial border.

Innervation:
Dorsal scapular nerve (C3 to C5)

Major synergists:
Splenius cervicis and the upper trapezius

Major antagonists:
Serratus anterior and the sternocleidomastoid

Trigger points:
Belly of the muscle just as it begins the twist in its fibers and at the attachment near the scapula

Referred pain patterns:
Angle of the neck at the trigger point and along the vertebral border of the scapula and stiff neck in rotation

See Activity 9-44.

ACTIVITY 9-44

1. Draw and color the levator scapulae in the space provided.
2. Label the proximal and distal attachment points: *P* for proximal; *D* for distal.
3. Place an X on the trigger points.
4. Palpate this muscle; identify the attachment points and the belly of the muscle.
5. Move this muscle on yourself.

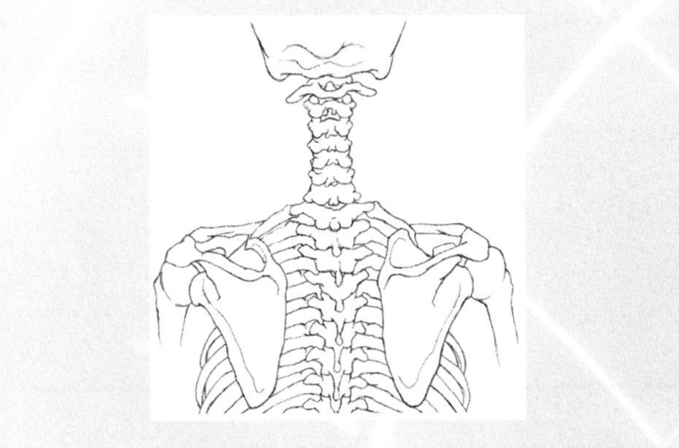

Pectoralis minor (PEK-tor-al-iss)

Pectoralis means related to the chest; *minor* means smaller.

Anterior

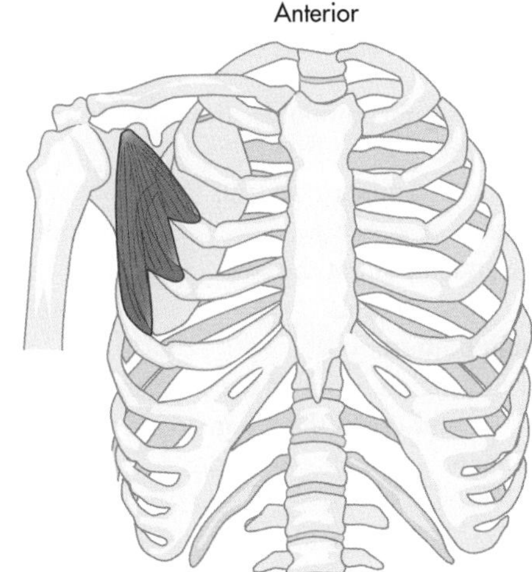

Concentric function:
Protraction (abduction), depression, and downward rotation of the scapula at the scapulocostal joint and elevation of ribs 3 to 5 at the sternocostal and costovertebral joints (This action assists in forced inspiration; therefore the pectoralis minor is an accessory respiratory muscle.)

Eccentric function:
Allows retraction (adduction), elevation, and upward rotation of the scapula and allows depression of ribs 3 to 5.

Isometric function:
Stabilizes the scapula.

ACTIVITY 9-45

1. Draw and color the pectoralis minor in the space provided.
2. Label the proximal and distal attachment points: *P* for proximal; *D* for distal.
3. Place an X on the trigger points.
4. Palpate this muscle; identify the attachment points and the belly of the muscle.
5. Move this muscle on yourself.

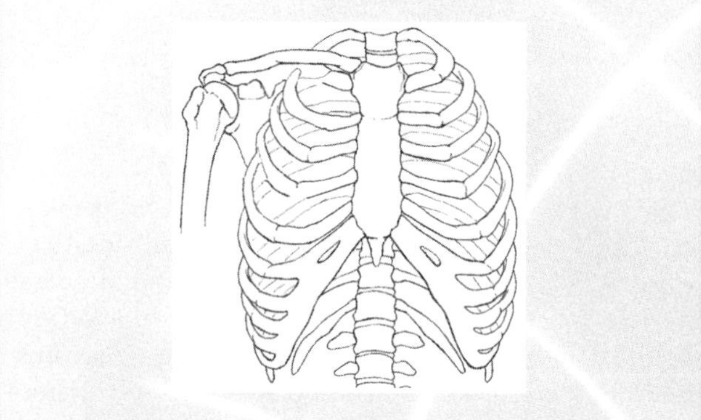

From:
Third, fourth, and fifth ribs near the cartilage and the aponeurosis covering the intercostals

To:
Coracoid process of the scapula

Innervation:
Medial and lateral pectoral nerves (C5 to T1)

Major synergists:
Serratus anterior, rhomboids, and lower trapezius

Major antagonists:
Rhomboids and upper trapezius

Trigger points:
Near the attachment at the coracoid process and at the belly of the muscle

Referred pain pattern:
May mimic angina; front of the chest from the shoulder and down the ulnar side of the arm into the fingers.

See Activity 9-45.

Serratus anterior (suhr-RATE-us)

Serratus means sawlike; *anterior* means toward the front.

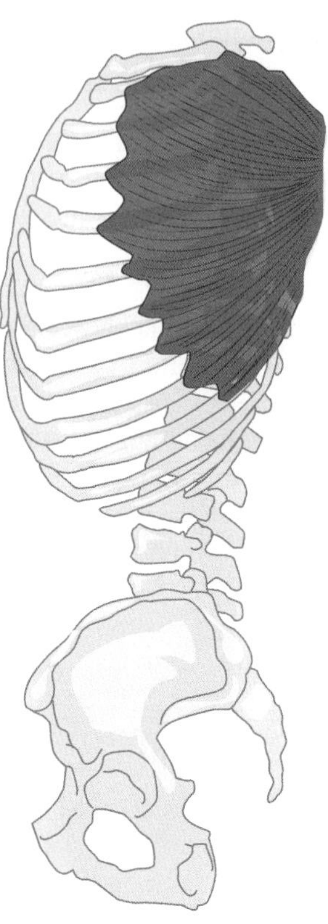

Concentric function:
Protraction (abduction) and upward rotation of the scapula at the scapulocostal joint and elevation of ribs 7 to 9 (assisting forced inspiration; therefore the serratus anterior is an accessory muscle of respiration)

Eccentric function:
Restrains retraction and downward rotation of the scapula.

Isometric function:
Holds the medial border of the scapula firmly against the thorax, thereby preventing winging of the scapula.

From:
External surfaces and superior borders of the upper eight or nine ribs

To:
Costal surface of the medial border of the scapula
This muscle lies along the ribcage and is deep to the scapula.

Innervation:
Long thoracic nerve (C5 to C7)

Major synergists:
Pectoralis minor and upper trapezius

Major antagonists:
Rhomboids and middle trapezius

ACTIVITY 9-46

1. Draw and color the serratus anterior in the space provided.
2. Label the proximal and distal attachment points: *P* for proximal; *D* for distal.
3. Place an X on the trigger points.
4. Palpate this muscle; identify the attachment points and the belly of the muscle.
5. Move this muscle on yourself.

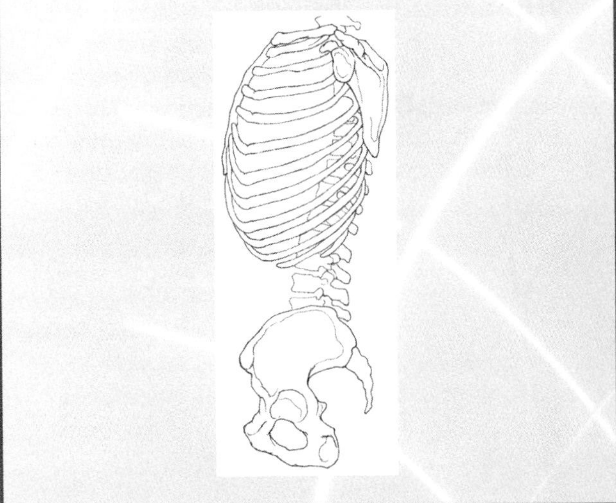

Trigger points:
Along the midaxillary line near the ribs

Referred pain patterns:
Side and back of the chest and down the ulnar aspect of the arm into the hand

Injury may result in shortness of breath and pain during inhalation.

See Activity 9-46.

Muscles of the Musculotendinous (Rotator) Cuff

Nine muscles cross over the ball-and-socket joint of the shoulder to stabilize and move this joint (Figures 9-35 and 9-36). Of these nine, the four "SITS" muscles are known as the rotator cuff muscles: the supraspinatus, infraspinatus, teres minor, and subscapularis. These muscles originate on the scapula, and their distal tendons blend into each other (and with the fibrous capsule of the shoulder joint). The main functions of these muscles are to hold the head of the humerus in the glenoid cavity and to reinforce the joint capsule; therefore they often sustain isometric contraction. Except for the subscapularis, one can access these muscles easily during massage. Because the subscapularis is located deep to the scapula, the best access position is supine with pressure applied through the axilla and toward the scapula. One must take care not to press on the nerves and vessels in the area.

Supraspinatus (SOO-prah-spy-NAH-tus)

Supraspinatus means above the spine (of the scapula).

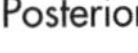

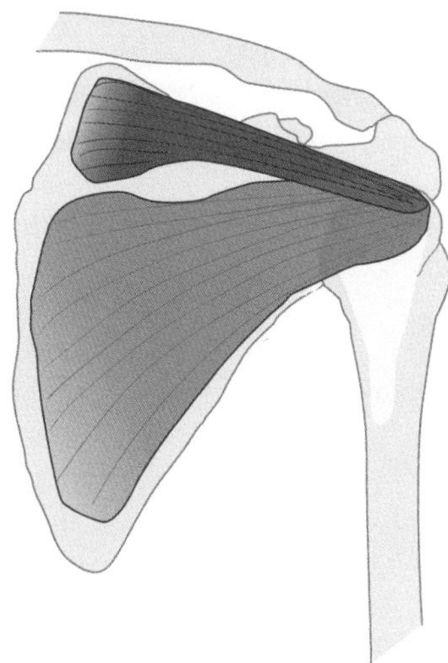

Concentric function:
Abduction of the arm at the shoulder joint

Eccentric function:
Restrains adduction of the arm.

Isometric function:
Acts to stabilize the humeral head in the glenoid cavity during movements of the arm.

From:
Medial two thirds of the supraspinous fossa of the scapula

To:
Superior facet of the greater tubercle of the humerus and the capsule of the shoulder joint

Innervation:
Suprascapular nerve (C5 to C6)

Major synergist:
Deltoid (The rotator cuff muscles assist one another in stabilizing the head of the humerus in the glenoid fossa.)

Major antagonists:
Latissimus dorsi, teres major, and pectoralis major

Trigger points:
In the belly of the muscle and near the tendon at the humerus

Referred pain pattern:
Shoulder, deltoid, and down the arm to the elbow, often experienced as a dull ache

See Activity 9-47.

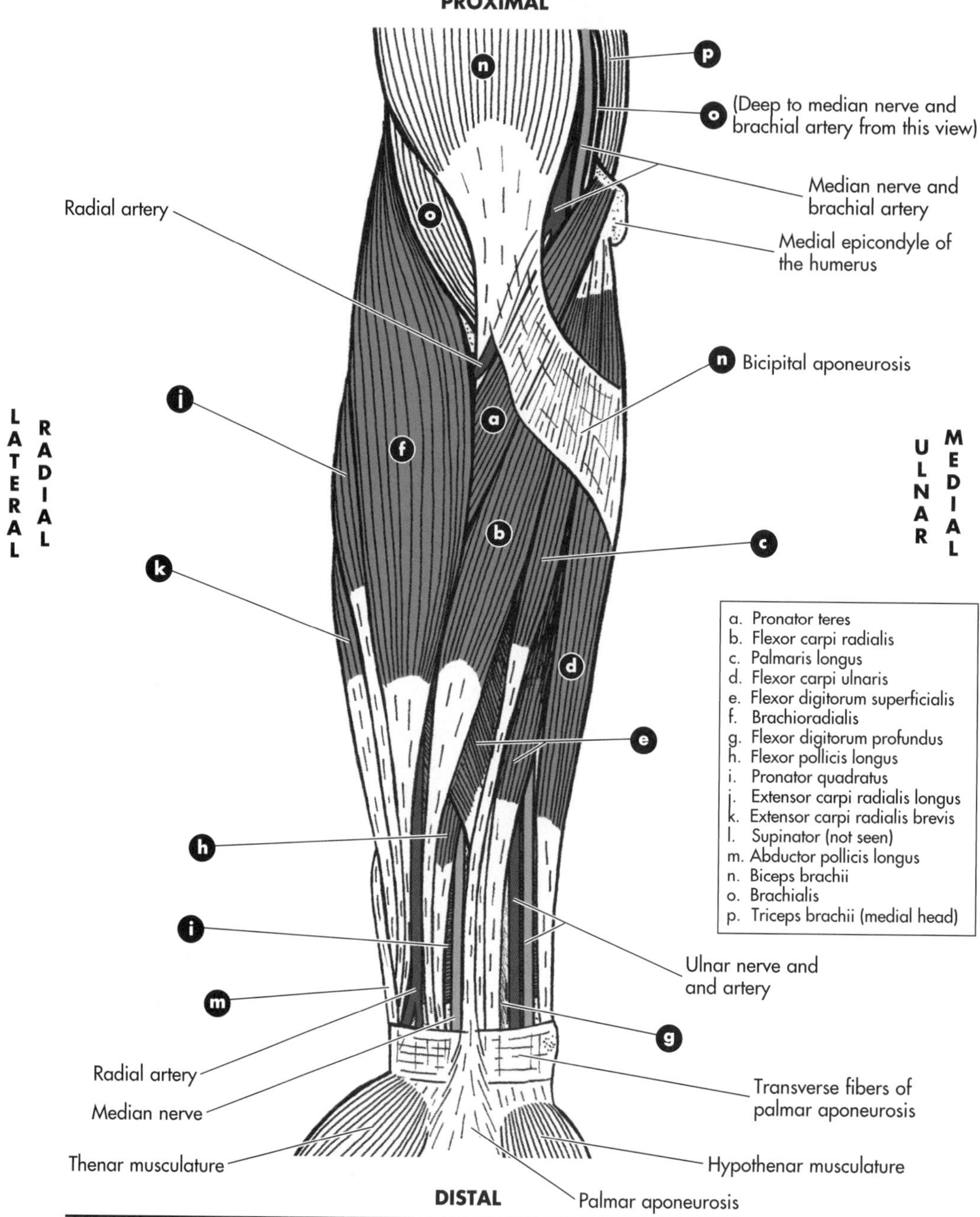

Figure 9-35

Anterior view of the right forearm (superficial). (Modified from Muscolino JE: *The muscular system manual: the skeletal muscles of the human body,* ed 2, St Louis, 2005, Mosby.)

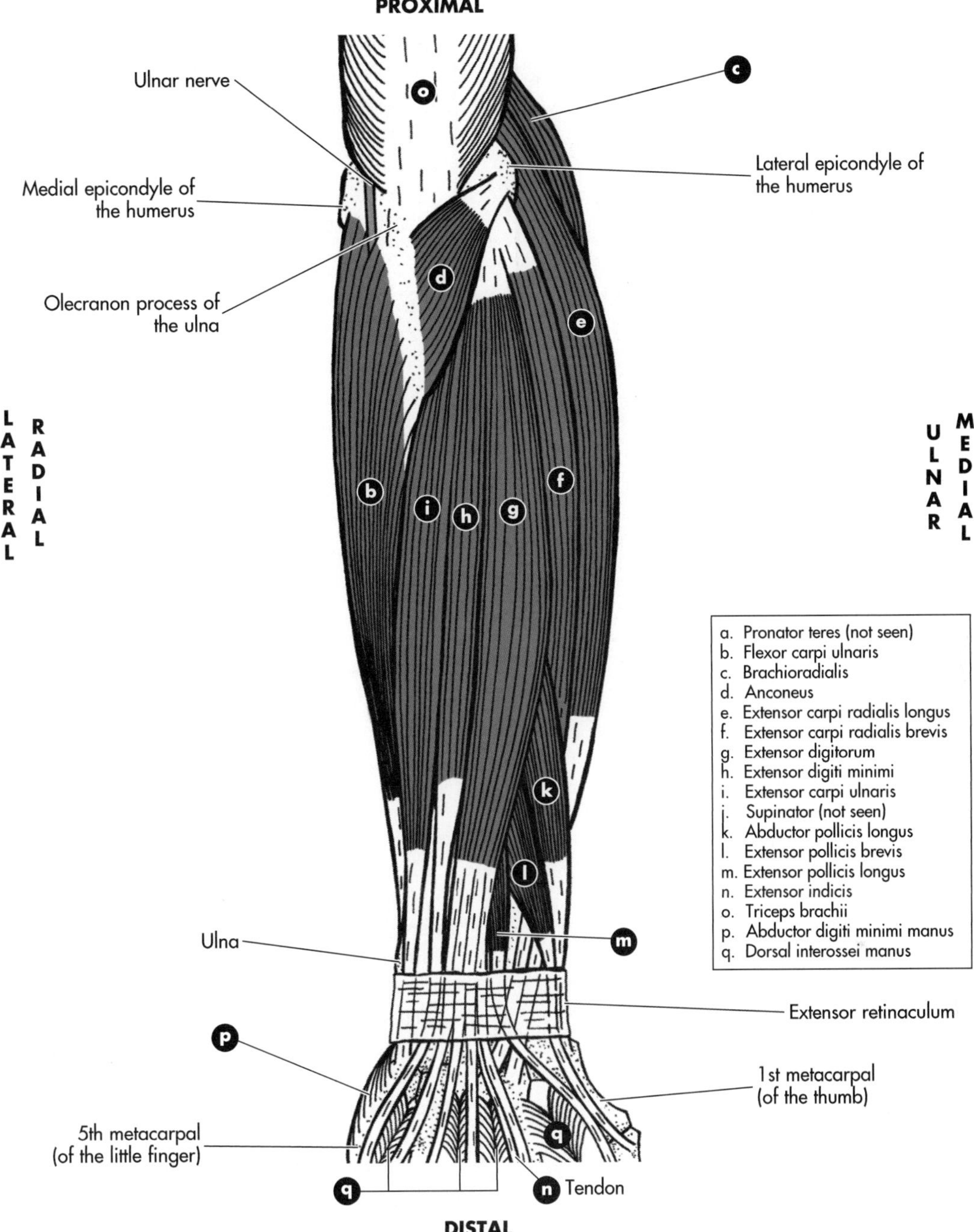

Figure 9-36

Posterior view of the right forearm (superficial). (Modified from Muscolino JE: *The muscular system manual: the skeletal muscles of the human body,* ed 2, St Louis, 2005, Mosby.)

ACTIVITY 9-47

1. Draw and color the supraspinatus in the space provided.
2. Label the proximal and distal attachment points: *P* for proximal; *D* for distal.
3. Place an X on the trigger points.
4. Palpate this muscle; identify the attachment points and the belly of the muscle.
5. Move this muscle on yourself.

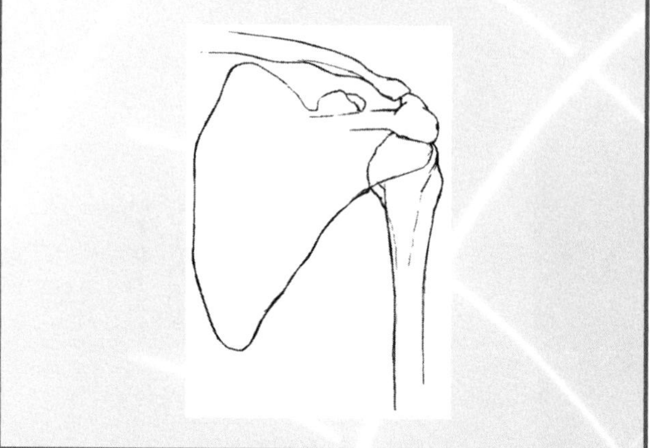

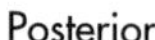

ACTIVITY 9-48

1. Draw and color the infraspinatus in the space provided.
2. Label the proximal and distal attachment points: *P* for proximal; *D* for distal.
3. Place an X on the trigger points.
4. Palpate this muscle; identify the attachment points and the belly of the muscle.
5. Move this muscle on yourself.

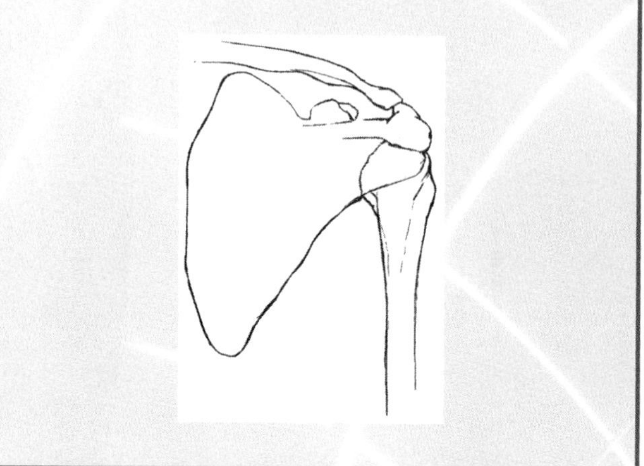

Infraspinatus (in-fra-spy-NAH-tus)

Infraspinatus means below the spine (of the scapula).

Posterior

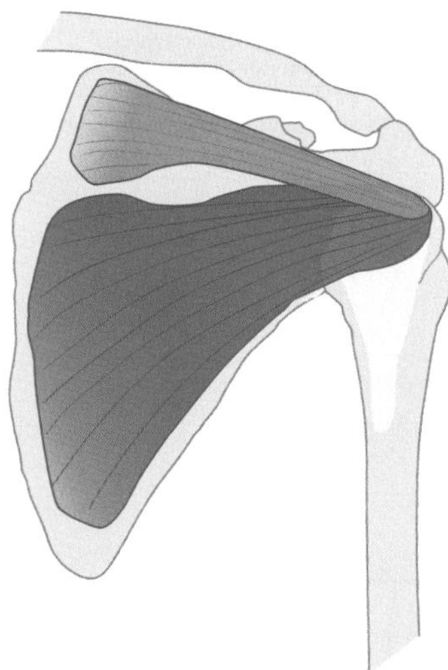

Concentric function:
Lateral rotation of the arm at the shoulder joint

Eccentric function:
Restrains medial rotation of the arm.

Isometric function:
Acts to stabilize the humeral head in the glenoid cavity during movements of the arm.

From:
Medial two thirds of the infraspinous fossa

To:
Middle facet of the greater tubercle of the humerus and the capsule of the shoulder joint

Innervation:
Suprascapular nerve (C5 to C6)

Major synergists:
Teres minor and posterior deltoid (The rotator cuff muscles assist one another in stabilizing the head of the humerus in the glenoid fossa.)

Major antagonists:
Subscapularis, pectoralis major, anterior deltoid, latissimus dorsi, and teres major

Trigger points:
Belly of the muscle below the spine of the scapula and near the medial border of the scapula

Referred pain patterns:
Deep into the shoulder and deltoid area, down the arm, suboccipital area, and medial border of the scapula, which limits the ability to reach behind the back

See Activity 9-48.

Teres minor (TER-eze)

Teres means smooth and round; *minor* means smaller.

Posterior

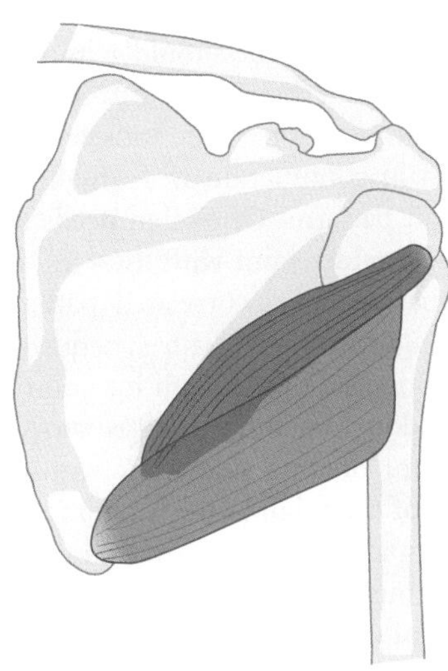

Concentric function:
Lateral rotation and adduction of the arm at the shoulder joint

Eccentric function:
Restrains medial rotation and abduction of the arm.

Isometric function:
Acts to stabilize the humeral head in the glenoid cavity during movements of the arm.

From:
Superior two thirds, dorsal surface of the lateral border of the scapula

To:
Inferior facet of the greater tubercle of the humerus and the capsule of the shoulder joint

Innervation:
Axillary nerve (C5 to C6)

Major synergists:
Infraspinatus, posterior deltoid, and latissimus dorsi (The rotator cuff muscles assist one another in stabilizing the head of the humerus in the glenoid fossa.)

Major antagonists:
Subscapularis, pectoralis major, anterior deltoid, and supraspinatus

Trigger points:
Belly of the muscle closer to the attachment on the humerus

Referred pain pattern:
Posterior deltoid region often has limited range of motion for reaching behind the back, such as putting hands in back pocket of pants.

See Activity 9-49.

ACTIVITY 9-49

1. Draw and color the teres minor in the space provided.
2. Label the proximal and distal attachment points: *P* for proximal; *D* for distal.
3. Place an X on the trigger points.
4. Palpate this muscle; identify the attachment points and the belly of the muscle.
5. Move this muscle on yourself.

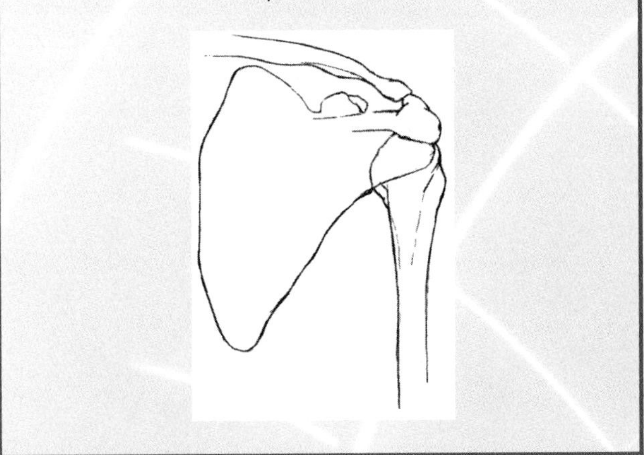

Subscapularis (sub-SKAP-you-LAR-iss)

Subscapularis means under (deep to) the shoulder blade.

Anterior

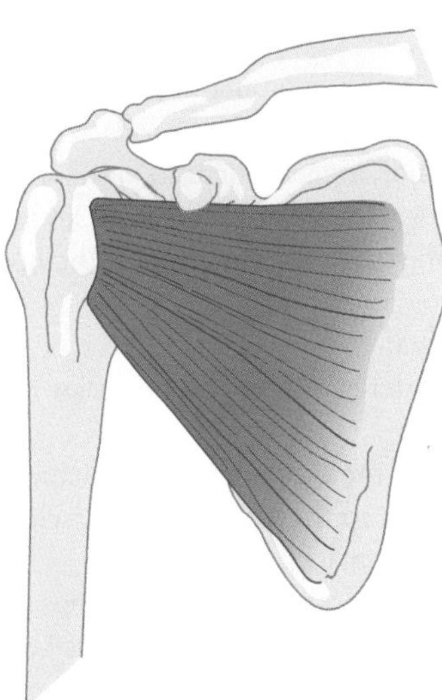

This muscle often is implicated in "frozen shoulder" syndromes.

Concentric function:
Medial rotation of the arm at the shoulder joint

Eccentric function:
Restrains lateral rotation of the arm.

Isometric function:
Acts to stabilize the humeral head in the glenoid cavity during movements of the arm.

From:
Subscapular fossa of the scapula

ACTIVITY 9-50

1. Draw and color the subscapularis in the space provided.
2. Label the proximal and distal attachment points: *P* for proximal; *D* for distal.
3. Place an X on the trigger points.
4. Palpate this muscle; identify the attachment points and the belly of the muscle.
5. Move this muscle on yourself.

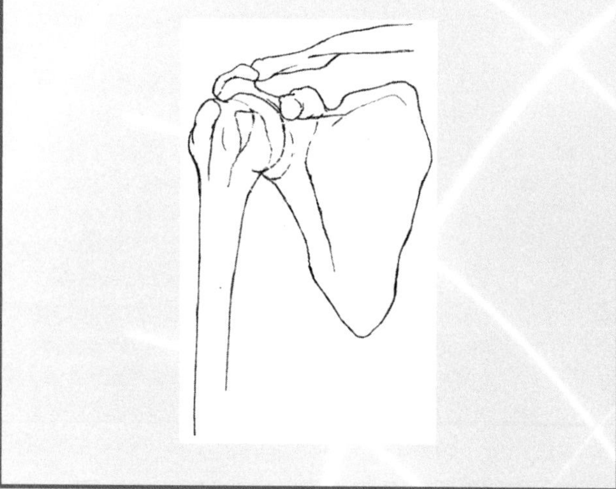

To:

Lesser tubercle of the humerus and the capsule of the shoulder joint

Innervation:

Upper and lower subscapular nerves (C5 to C6)

Major synergists:

Pectoralis major, anterior deltoid, latissimus dorsi, and teres major (The rotator cuff muscles assist one another in stabilizing the head of the humerus in the glenoid fossa.)

Major antagonists:

Infraspinatus, teres minor, and posterior deltoid

Trigger points:

Access through the axilla near the attachment at the humerus and in the belly of the muscle.

Referred pain pattern:

Posterior deltoid, scapular region, triceps area and into the wrist, often mistaken for bursitis because the pain often refers to insertion at the shoulder

See Activity 9-50.

Muscles of the Shoulder Joint

In general, any muscle that crosses the shoulder joint anteriorly can flex the arm at the shoulder joint, and any muscle that crosses the shoulder joint posteriorly can extend the arm at the shoulder joint (see Figure 9-34). The deltoid is the prime mover of arm abduction at the shoulder joint but also is involved in flexion and extension of the arm at the shoulder joint. The main antagonists to abduction of the arm at the shoulder joint are the pectoralis major anteriorly and the latissimus dorsi posteriorly. Depending on the location and insertion points, the various muscles acting on the arm also provide lateral (external) and medial (internal) rotation of the arm at the shoulder joint. The interaction of these muscles is complex, and each muscle contributes to more than one movement.

Because these muscles are active during walking, all gait reflexes are involved with the shoulder muscles to promote the appropriate counterbalancing arm swing to the thigh swing. Facilitation occurs between muscles of the arms that flex and extend in conjunction with thigh muscles during contralateral gait patterns. One often needs to consider the muscles of the shoulder joint with muscles of the hip joint and provide massage in a correlated pattern to be most effective. Although not listed with synergists, the shoulder joint flexors on one side work with hip joint flexors on the opposite side. Adductors and medial rotators of the arm at the shoulder joint on one side work with adductors and medial rotators of the thigh at the hip joint on the opposite side. The same pattern applies to lateral rotation. These muscles inhibit muscles on the same side of the body, that is, medial rotation of the arm at the shoulder joint and thigh at the hip joint on the right inhibit each other, as do the lateral rotators. Obviously, the same patterns occur on the left. Also, during normal gait, flexors and extensors of the arm at the shoulder joints interact. The flexors on the right work with extensors on the left and inhibit flexors on the left and vice versa. The extensors on the right work with flexors on the left and inhibit the extensors on the left and vice versa. Although this seems confusing, the patterns become apparent when one observes gait. To understand this, the student should take a step and freeze and then notice what muscles are interacting.

Deltoid (DEL-toyd)

Deltoid means triangular.

Posterior

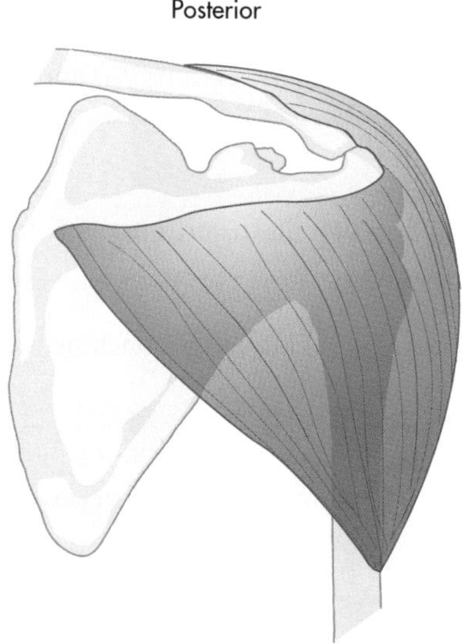

This muscle functions in three distinct patterns and can be thought of as three different muscles.

Concentric Function:

Anterior deltoid—Flexion, medial rotation, and abduction of the arm at the shoulder joint

Middle deltoid—Abduction of the arm at the shoulder joint

Posterior deltoid—Extension, lateral rotation, and abduction of the arm at the shoulder joint

Eccentric function:

The anterior deltoid restrains extension, lateral rotation, and adduction of the arm. The middle deltoid restrains adduction of the arm. The posterior deltoid restrains flexion, medial rotation, and adduction of the arm.

Isometric function:

Stabilizes glenohumeral joint during arm movement.

From:

Anterior deltoid—Superior surface, lateral third of the clavicle

Middle deltoid—Lateral margin of the spine of the scapula and superior surface of the acromion

Posterior deltoid—Posterior border of the spine of the scapula

To:

Deltoid tuberosity of the humerus

Innervation:

Axillary nerve (C5 to C6)

Major synergists:

Anterior deltoid—Coracobrachialis, clavicular head of the pectoralis major, and biceps brachii

Middle deltoid—Supraspinatus

Posterior deltoid—Latissimus dorsi, teres major, and infraspinatus

Major antagonists:

Pectoralis major and latissimus dorsi; the anterior and posterior deltoids are antagonistic to each other.

Trigger points:

Anterior deltoid—Near the clavicular attachment

Posterior and middle deltoid—In the belly of the muscles

Referred pain pattern:

Deltoid region and down the lateral side of the arm

See Activity 9-51.

ACTIVITY 9-51

1. Draw and color the deltoid in the space provided.
2. Label the proximal and distal attachment points: *P* for proximal; *D* for distal.
3. Place an X on the trigger points.
4. Palpate this muscle; identify the attachment points and the belly of the muscle.
5. Move this muscle on yourself.

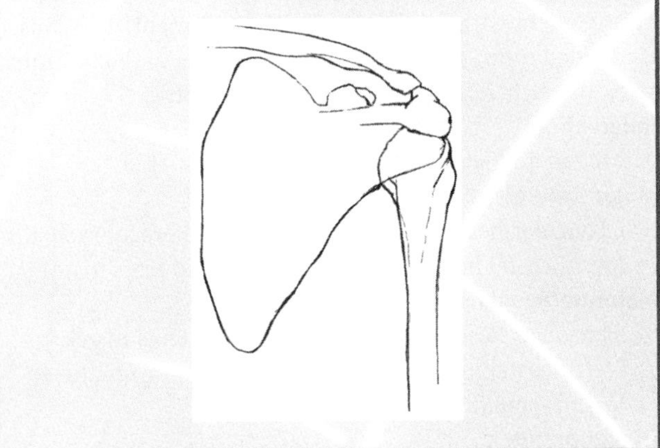

Pectoralis major (PEK-tor-al-iss)

Pectoralis means of the chest; *major* means larger.

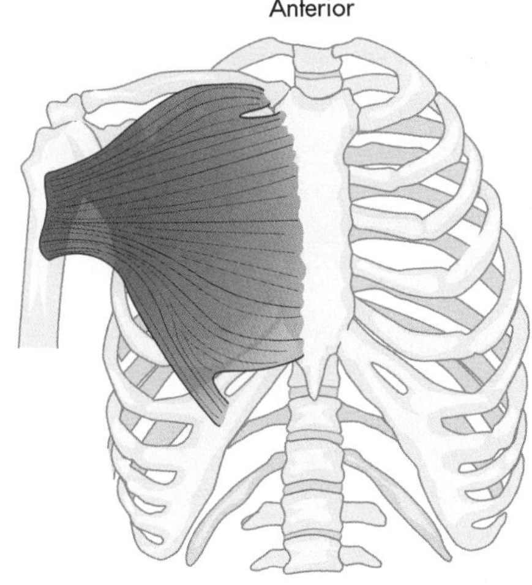

Concentric function:

Entire muscle—Adduction and medial rotation of the arm at the shoulder joint

Clavicular head—Flexion of the arm at the shoulder joint

Sternocostal head—Extension of the arm at the shoulder joint

Eccentric function:

Restrains abduction and lateral rotation of the arm and also can restrain extension and flexion of the arm.

Isometric function:

Stabilizes the shoulder during overhead activity.

From:

Ventral surface of the sternum down to the seventh rib, medial half of the clavicle, cartilage of ribs 1 to 7, and aponeurosis of the external abdominal oblique muscle

To:

Lateral lip of the bicipital groove of the humerus

The attachment pattern for this muscle is complex and consists of several overlapping sheets of muscles in a fan arrangement with a spiraling distal attachment. The muscle is divided into clavicular, sternal, costal, and abdominal sections, each able to function independently.

Innervation:

Medial and lateral pectoral nerves (C5 to T1)

Major synergists:

Clavicular head—Anterior deltoid and coracobrachialis

Sternocostal head—Latissimus dorsi and teres major

Major antagonists:

Clavicular head—Latissimus dorsi and teres major

Sternocostal head—Anterior deltoid, supraspinatus, infraspinatus, and teres minor

Trigger points:

Belly of the muscle

Referred pain pattern:

Chest and breast and down the ulnar aspect of the arm and forearm to the fourth and fifth fingers

Subclavius (sub-KLAVE-ee-us)

Subclavius means below and little key (referring to the clavicle).

Anterior

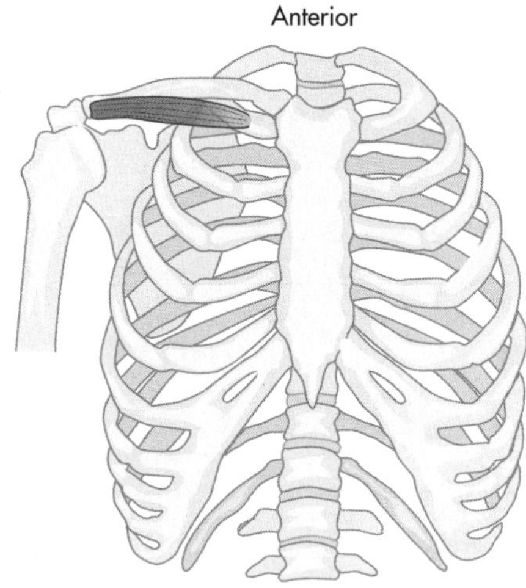

This muscle often is considered with the clavicular portion of the pectoralis major.

Concentric function:

Protraction and depression of the clavicle at the sternoclavicular joint

Eccentric function:

Restrains retraction and elevation of the clavicle at the sternoclavicular joint.

Isometric function:

Stabilizes the clavicle.

ACTIVITY 9-52

1. Draw and color the pectoralis major and the subclavius in the space provided.
2. Label the proximal and distal attachment points: *P* for proximal; *D* for distal.
3. Place an X on the trigger points.
4. Palpate these muscles; identify the attachment points and the bellies of the muscles.
5. Move these muscles on yourself.

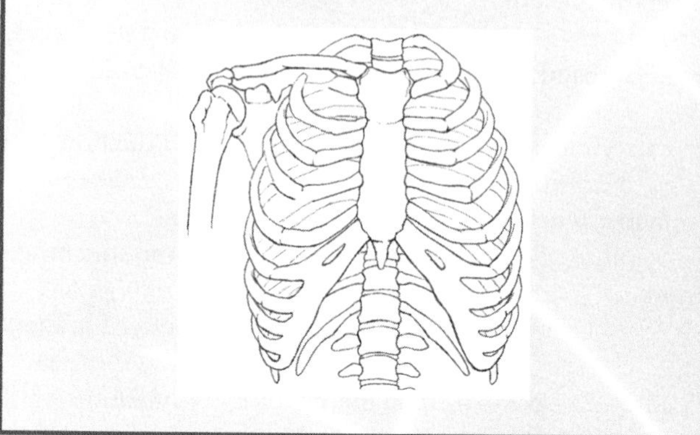

From:

Junction of the first rib and its costal cartilage

To:

Inferior surface of the clavicle

Innervation:

Fifth and sixth cervical nerves (C5 to C6)

Major synergists:

Deltoid and pectoralis major

Major antagonists:

Sternocleidomastoid and upper trapezius

Trigger points:

Belly of the muscle

Referred pain pattern:

Chest and breast region

See Activity 9-52.

Latissimus dorsi (la-TISS-ih-mus DOR-see)

Latissimus means widest; *dorsi* means belonging to the back.

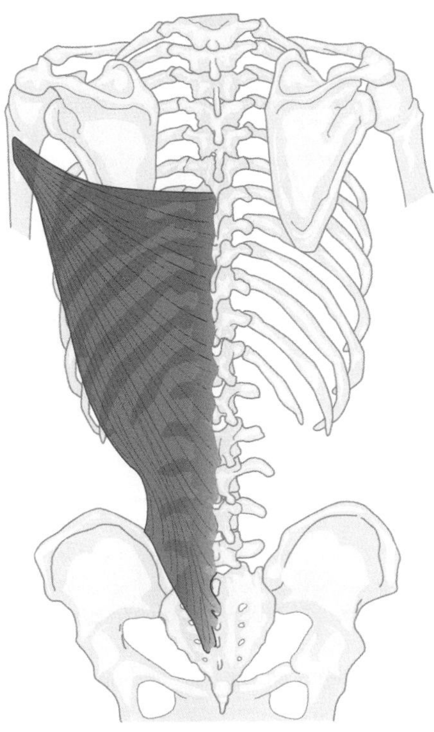

ACTIVITY 9-53

1. Draw and color the latissimus dorsi in the space provided.
2. Label the proximal and distal attachment points: *P* for proximal; *D* for distal.
3. Place an X on the trigger points.
4. Palpate this muscle; identify the attachment points and the belly of the muscle.
5. Move this muscle on yourself.

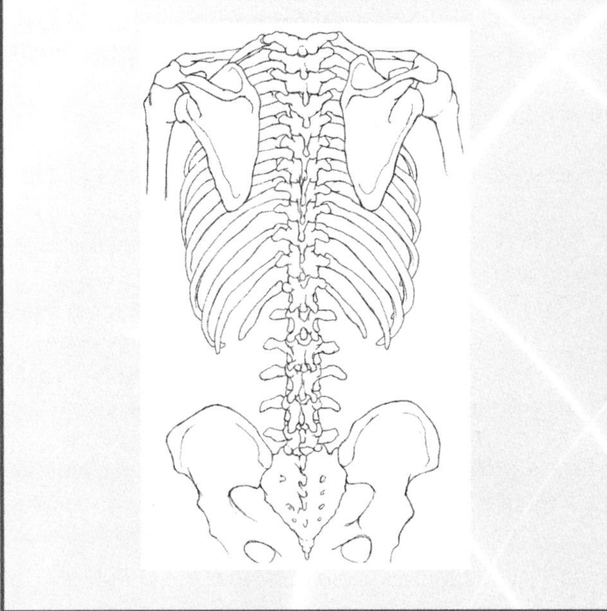

Concentric function:
Medial rotation, adduction, and extension of the arm at the shoulder joint; depression of the scapula at the scapulocostal joint; extension of the trunk at the spinal joints; and anterior tilt and elevation of the pelvis at the lumbosacral joint

Eccentric function:
Restrains lateral rotation, abduction, and flexion of the arm, elevation of the scapula, flexion of the trunk, and posterior tilt and depression of the pelvis.

Isometric function:
Stabilizes the lumbar and pelvic area by maintaining tension on the thoracolumbar fascia.

From:
Spinous processes of T7 through L5, posterior one third of the external lip of the iliac crest, posterior layer of the thoracolumbar fascia, and lower three or four ribs

To:
Medial lip of the bicipital groove of the humerus just as the muscle begins to twist around the teres major

The latissimus dorsi is fan shaped and has a twist in its fibers such that the superior fibers attach more distally on the humerus and the inferior fibers attach more proximally on the humerus. Shortening in this muscle limits arm movement over the head and can cause the back of the lumbar area to feel tight.

Innervation:
Thoracodorsal nerve (C6 to C8)

Major synergists:
Teres major, the long head of the triceps brachii, sternocostal head of the pectoralis major, subscapularis, and anterior deltoid

Major antagonists:
Clavicular head of the pectoralis major, teres minor, infraspinatus, deltoid, supraspinatus, levator scapulae, and rectus abdominis

Trigger points:
Posterior axillary area and belly of the muscle near the rib attachments

Referred pain pattern:
Just below the scapula and into the ulnar side of the arm and anterior deltoid region and abdominal oblique area

See Activity 9-53.

Teres major (TER-eze)

Teres means smooth and round; *major* means larger. This muscle may be fused with the latissimus dorsi.

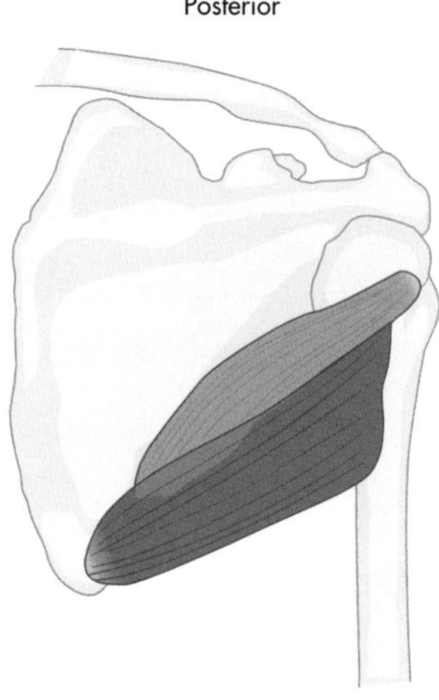

Concentric function:
Medial rotation, adduction, and extension of the arm at the shoulder joint and upward rotation of the scapula at the scapulocostal joint

Eccentric function:
Restrains lateral rotation, abduction, and flexion of the arm and restrains downward rotation of the scapula.

Isometric function:
Stabilizes the glenohumeral joint.

From:
Dorsal surfaces of inferior angle and lower third of lateral border of scapula

To:
Medial lip of bicipital groove of the humerus

Innervation:
Lower subscapular nerve (C5 to C7)

Major synergists:
Latissimus dorsi, subscapularis, and trapezius

Major antagonists:
Teres minor, infraspinatus, supraspinatus, anterior deltoid, and pectoralis minor

Trigger points:
Near the musculotendinous junction at both attachments and points at the attachments at the humerus; one can reach these best through the axilla.

Referred pain pattern:
Posterior deltoid region and down the dorsal portion of the arm

See Activity 9-54.

ACTIVITY 9-54

1. Draw and color the teres major in the space provided.
2. Label the proximal and distal attachment points: *P* for proximal; *D* for distal.
3. Place an X on the trigger points.
4. Palpate this muscle; identify the attachment points and the belly of the muscle.
5. Move this muscle on yourself.

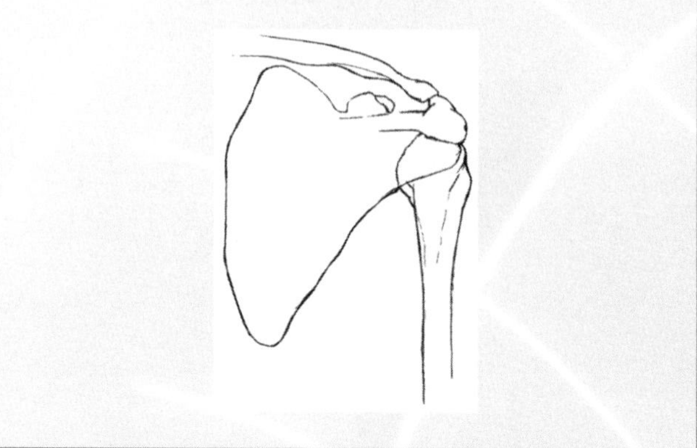

Coracobrachialis (KORE-a-koe-BRAY-kee-AL-iss)

Coracobrachialis means crow's beak and of the arm.

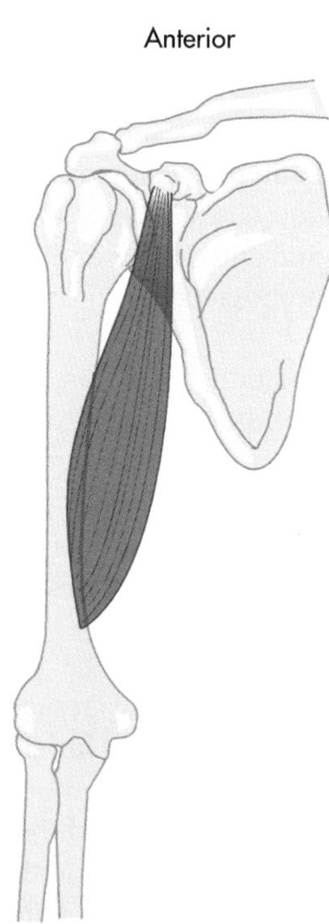

Concentric function:
Flexion and adduction of the arm at the shoulder joint

Eccentric function:
Restrains extension and abduction of the arm.

Isometric function:
Stabilizes the shoulder and scapula.

ACTIVITY 9-55

1. Draw and color the coracobrachialis in the space provided.
2. Label the proximal and distal attachment points: *P* for proximal; *D* for distal.
3. Place an X on the trigger points.
4. Palpate this muscle; identify the attachment points and the belly of the muscle.
5. Move this muscle on yourself.

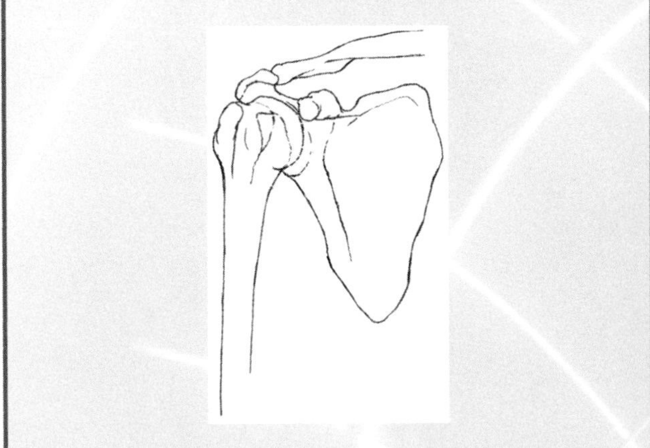

From:
Tip of the coracoid process of the scapula

To:
Anteromedial surface of the middle of the shaft of the humerus, opposite the deltoid tuberosity

Innervation:
Musculocutaneous nerve (C5 to C7)

Major synergists:
Pectoralis major and short head of biceps brachii

Major antagonist:
Posterior deltoid

Trigger points:
Near the musculotendinous junction and the coracoid attachment

Referred pain pattern:
Front of shoulder and posterior aspect of the arm down the triceps and posterior forearm into the posterior hand

See Activity 9-55.

Muscles of the Elbow and Radioulnar Joints

The elbow is a hinge joint, and movements produced by the muscles at the elbow joint are limited entirely to flexion and extension of the forearm. Posterior arm muscles produce extension of the forearm at the elbow joint; anterior arm muscles produce flexion of the forearm at the elbow joint. The strongest elbow flexor is the brachialis. Reverse actions of flexion and extension of the arm at the elbow joint are also common. Pronation and supination take place at the radioulnar joints. Because of contralateral joint reflexes involved with gait, flexors of the forearm at the elbow joint work with flexors of the leg at the knee joint on the opposite side of the body, and extensors of the forearm at the elbow joint work with extensors of the leg at the knee joint on the opposite side of the body. Massage application is more effective when one observes these interactions and considers the bodywide patterns. Dysfunction is common with static posture. Static position requires these muscles to hold contraction for prolonged periods of time. Examples are driving a car, holding a phone, computer work, and using hand tools. Repetitive use activities such as using a hammer or wrench also strain this group of muscles.

Biceps brachii (BI-seps BRAY-kee-eye)

Biceps means two heads; *brachii* means of the arm.

Anterior

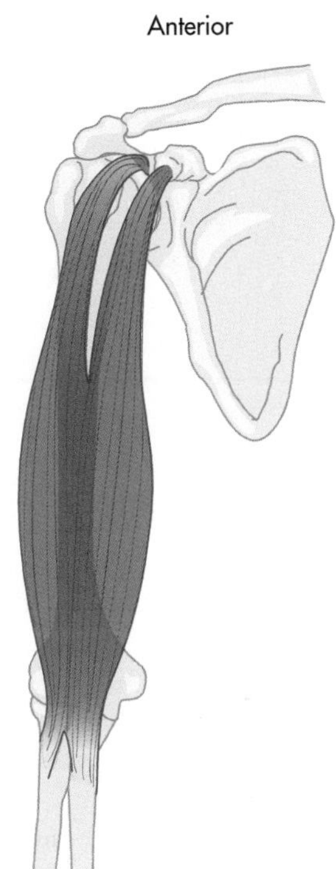

Concentric function:
Flexion of the forearm at the elbow joint, supination of the forearm at the radioulnar joints, and flexion of the arm at the shoulder joint (A common reverse action is flexion of the arm at the elbow joint such as when doing a pull-up or chin-up.)

Eccentric function:
Restrains extension and pronation of the forearm and extension of the arm.

Isometric function:
Stabilizes the humerus at the shoulder and elbow joints during full extension and stabilizes the elbow joint when flexed and holding a weight.

From:
Long head—Supraglenoid tubercle of the scapula
Short head—Tip of the coracoid process of the scapula

To:
Tuberosity of the radius and aponeurosis of the proximal attachment (origin) of the wrist flexor muscles in the forearm

ACTIVITY 9-56

1. Draw and color the biceps brachii in the space provided.
2. Label the proximal and distal attachment points: *P* for proximal; *D* for distal.
3. Place an X on the trigger points.
4. Palpate this muscle; identify the attachment points and the belly of the muscle.
5. Move this muscle on yourself.

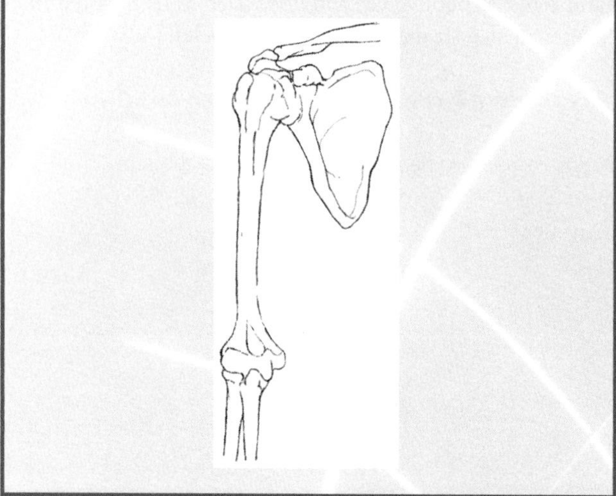

Innervation:
Musculocutaneous nerve (C5 to C6)

Major synergists:
Brachialis, brachioradialis, supinator, and anterior deltoid

Major antagonists:
Triceps brachii, pronator teres, pronator quadratus, and posterior deltoid

Trigger points:
In the belly of the long and short heads, closer to the elbow

Referred pain pattern:
Front of the shoulder at the anterior deltoid region and into the scapular region and also into the antecubital space (front of the elbow)

See Activity 9-56.

Brachialis (BRAY-kee-AL-iss)

Brachialis means of the arm.

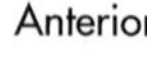

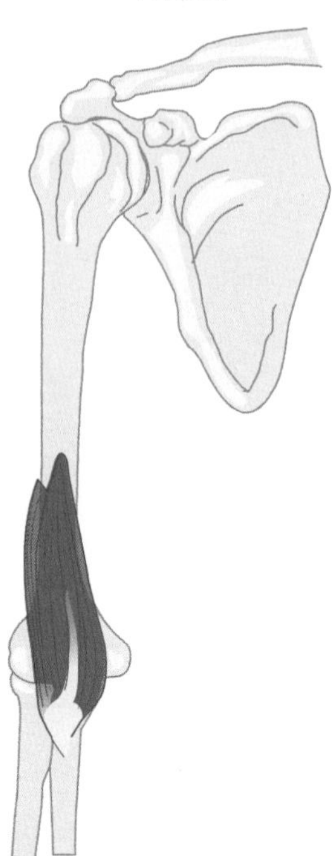

Concentric function:
Flexion of the forearm at the elbow joint

Eccentric function:
Restrains extension of the forearm.

Isometric function:
Stabilizes the elbow joint.

From:
Distal one half of the anterior surface of the humerus and the medial and lateral intermuscular septae

To:
Coronoid process and tuberosity of the ulna

Innervation:
Musculocutaneous nerve (C5 to C7)

Major synergists:
Biceps brachii and brachioradialis

Major antagonist:
Triceps brachii

Trigger points:
Several locations in the belly of the muscle

Referred pain pattern:
Primarily to the thumb, with some pain in the anterior deltoid area and at the elbow

See Activity 9-57.

ACTIVITY 9-57

1. Draw and color the brachialis in the space provided.
2. Label the proximal and distal attachment points: *P* for proximal; *D* for distal.
3. Place an X on the trigger points.
4. Palpate this muscle; identify the attachment points and the belly of the muscle.
5. Move this muscle on yourself.

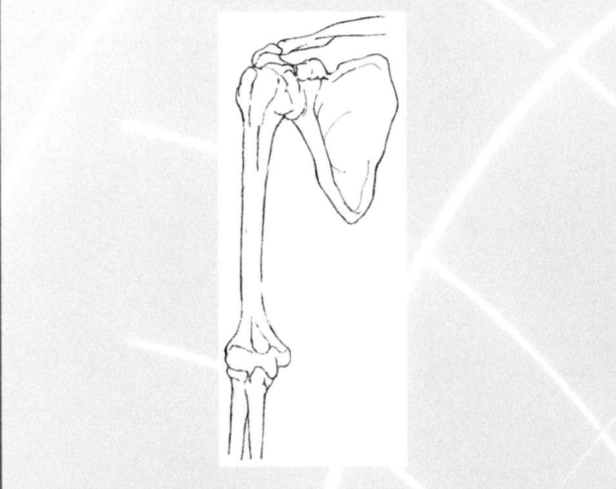

Brachioradialis (BRAY-kee-oh-RAY-dee-AL-iss)

Brachioradialis means related to the arm and radius.

Anterior

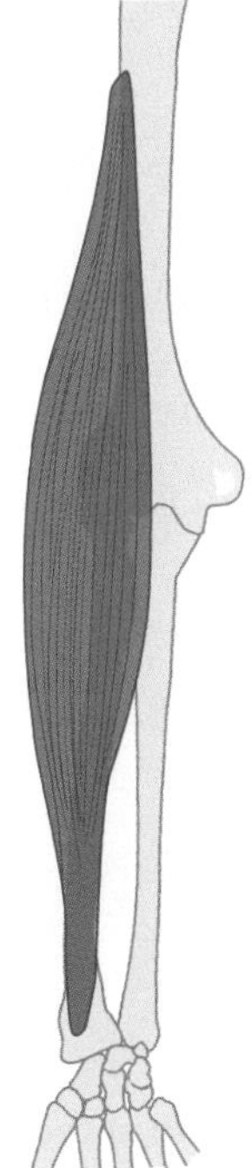

Concentric function:

Flexion of the forearm at the elbow joint; the brachioradialis also can assist in pronation and supination of the forearm at the radioulnar joints to midposition (halfway between full pronation and full supination).

Eccentric function:

Restrains extension of the forearm and can restrain pronation and supination of the forearm (beyond midposition).

Isometric function:

Stabilizes the elbow joint.

From:

Proximal two thirds of the lateral supracondylar ridge of the humerus and lateral intermuscular septum

To:

Lateral side of the base of the styloid process of the radius

Innervation:

Radial nerve (C5 to C6)

Major synergists:

Biceps brachii, brachialis, supinator, pronator teres, and pronator quadratus

Major antagonists:

Triceps brachii, supinator, pronator teres, and pronator quadratus

Trigger points:

Belly of the muscle

Referred pain pattern:

Wrist and base of the thumb in the web space between the thumb and index finger and to the lateral epicondyle at the elbow

See Activity 9-58.

ACTIVITY 9-58

1. Draw and color the brachioradialis in the space provided.
2. Label the proximal and distal attachment points: *P* for proximal; *D* for distal.
3. Place an X on the trigger points.
4. Palpate this muscle; identify the attachment points and the belly of the muscle.
5. Move this muscle on yourself.

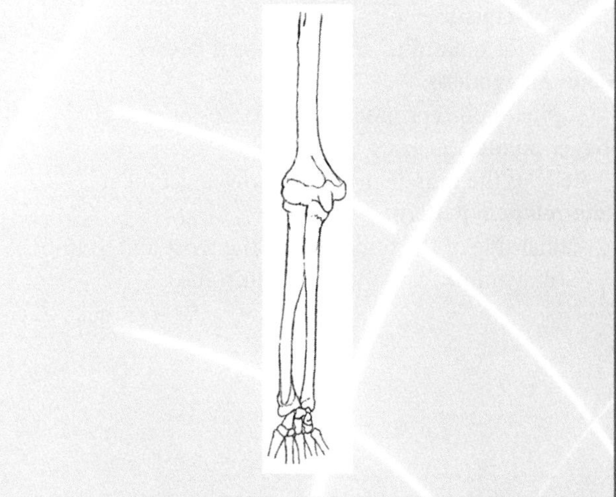

Pronator teres (PRO-nay-tor TER-eez)

Pronator means one that causes pronation; *teres* means round and smooth.

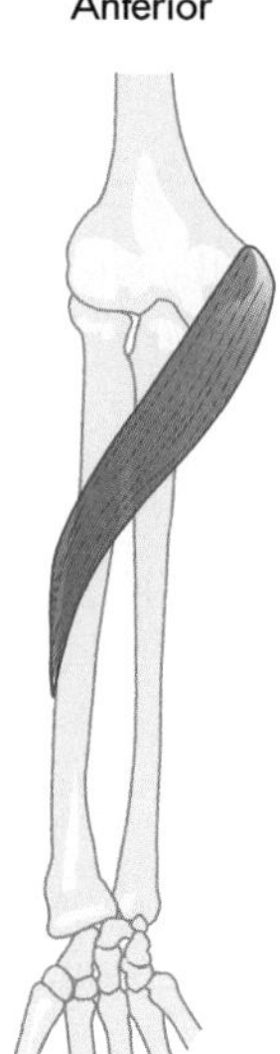

Concentric function:
Pronation of the forearm at the radioulnar joints and flexion of the forearm at the elbow joint

Eccentric function:
Restrains supination and extension of the forearm.

Isometric function:
Stabilizes the elbow joint and the radioulnar joints.

From:
Humeral head—Medial epicondyle of the humerus, common flexor tendon, and deep antebrachial fascia
Ulnar head—Medial side of the coronoid process of the ulna

To:
Middle of lateral surface of radius

Innervation:
Median nerve (C6 to C7)

Major synergists:
Pronator quadratus and all forearm flexors

Major antagonists:
Supinator, biceps brachii, and triceps brachii

Trigger points:
Belly of the muscle near the elbow attachment

Referred pain pattern:
Radial side of the forearm into the wrist and thumb; may mimic carpal tunnel syndrome.

See Activity 9-59.

ACTIVITY 9-59

1. Draw and color the pronator teres in the space provided.
2. Label the proximal and distal attachment points: *P* for proximal; *D* for distal.
3. Place an X on the trigger points.
4. Palpate this muscle; identify the attachment points and the belly of the muscle.
5. Move this muscle on yourself.

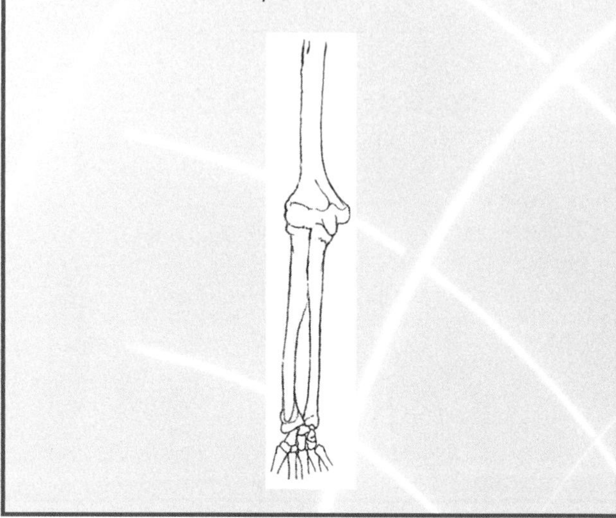

Supinator (SOOP-in-ATE-or)

Supinator means one that causes supination.

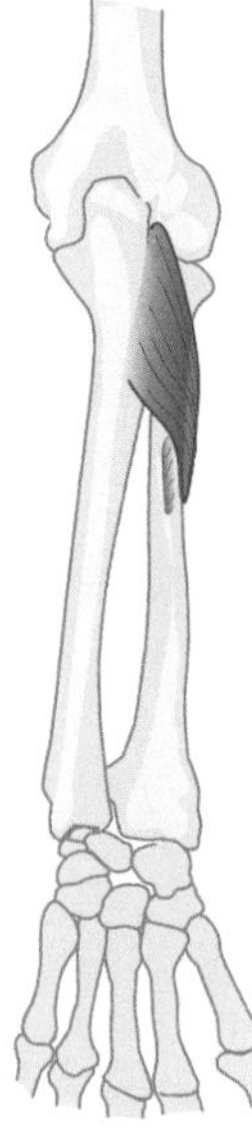

Concentric function:
Supination of the forearm at the radioulnar joints

Eccentric function:
Restrains pronation of the forearm.

Isometric function:
Stabilizes the elbow and radioulnar joints.

From:

Lateral epicondyle of the humerus, radial collateral ligament of the elbow joint, annular ligament of the radius, and supinator crest of the ulna

To:

Lateral surface of the proximal one third of the shaft of the radius, covering part of the anterior, medial, and posterior surfaces

The supinator is a large muscle that wraps around the bones of the forearm.

Innervation:

Deep branch of the radial nerve (C6 to C7)

Major synergist:

Biceps brachii

Major antagonists:

Pronator teres and pronator quadratus

Trigger points:

Near the radius in the antecubital space

Referred pain pattern:

Local area

Pronator quadratus (PRO-nay-tor kwad-RATE-us)

Pronator means one that causes pronation; *quadratus* means square shaped.

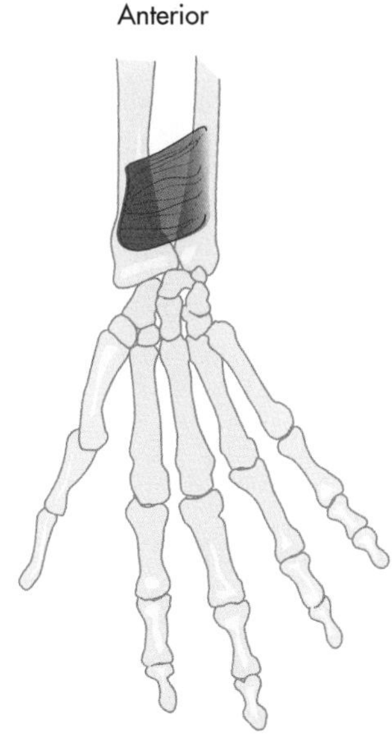

Concentric function:

Pronation of the forearm at the radioulnar joints

Eccentric function:

Restrains supination of the forearm.

The pronator quadratus is the prime mover of pronation of the forearm.

From:

Medial side and anterior surface of the distal one fourth of the ulna

To:

Lateral side and anterior surface of the distal one fourth of the radius

ACTIVITY 9-60

1. Draw and color the supinator quadratus and the pronator quadratus in the space provided.
2. Label the proximal and distal attachment points: *P* for proximal; *D* for distal.
3. Place an X on the trigger points.
4. Palpate these muscles; identify the attachment points and the bellies of the muscles.
5. Move the muscles on yourself.

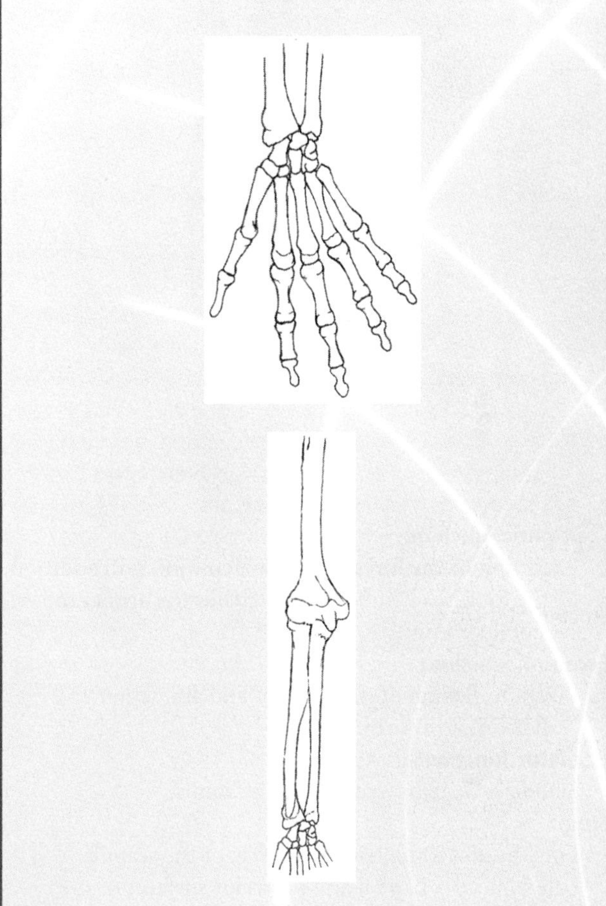

Innervation:

Anterior interosseous branch of the median nerve (C7 to C8)

Major synergist:

Pronator teres

Major antagonists:

Supinator and biceps brachii

Trigger points:

Belly of muscle

Referred pain pattern:

Local area

See Activity 9-60.

Triceps brachii (TRY-seps BRAY-kee-eye)

Triceps means three heads; *brachii* means of the arm.

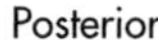

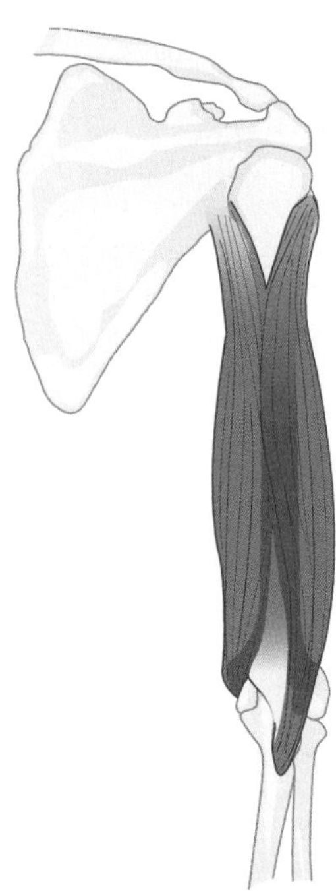

Concentric function:
Extension of the forearm at the elbow joint; in addition, the long head adducts and extends the arm at the shoulder joint.

Eccentric function:
Restrains flexion of the forearm and abduction and flexion of the arm.

Isometric function:
Stabilizes the elbow and shoulder joints.

From:
Long head—Infraglenoid tubercle of the scapula
Lateral head—Lateral and posterior surfaces of the proximal one half of the shaft of the humerus and the lateral intermuscular septum
Medial (deep) head—Distal one half of the medial and posterior surfaces of the shaft of the humerus distal to the radial groove and the medial intermuscular septum

To:
Posterior surface of the olecranon process of the ulna and antebrachial fascia

Innervation:
Radial nerve (C6 to C8)

Major synergist:
Anconeus

Major antagonists:
Brachialis and biceps brachii

Trigger points:
Belly of each head

Referred pain pattern:
Length of the posterior arm

Anconeus (an-Ko-nee-us)

Anconeus means elbow.

Posterior

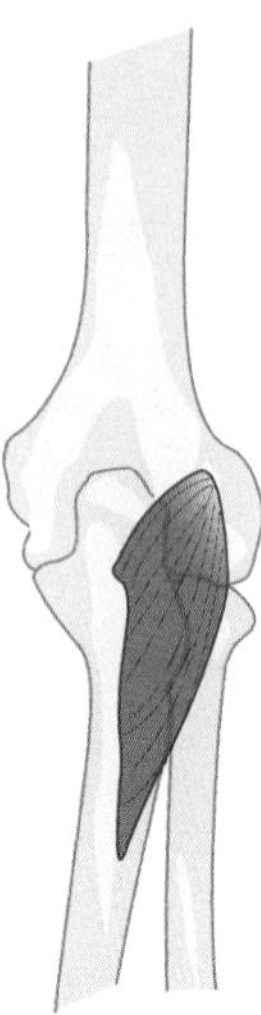

Concentric function:
Extension of the forearm at the elbow joint

Eccentric function:
Restrains flexion of the forearm.

Isometric function:
Stabilizes the elbow joint.

From:
Posterior surface of the lateral epicondyle of the humerus

To:
Lateral side of the olecranon process and proximal one fourth of the posterior surface of the shaft of the ulna

Innervation:
Radial nerve (C6 to C8)

Major synergist:
Triceps brachii

Major antagonists:
Biceps brachii and brachialis

Trigger points:
In the belly

Referred pain pattern:
Elbow at the lateral epicondyle

See Activity 9-61.

Muscles of the Wrist and Hand Joints

If all the muscles that move the hand actually were located in the hand, the hand would be too bulky to be functional. Instead, the bellies of these muscles are located closer to the elbow, tapering to long insertion tendons in the wrist and hand (Figure 9-37, *A, B*). Strong ligaments, called the flexor and extensor retinacula, secure the long, tendinous insertions much like a bracelet at the wrist. Synovial tendon sheaths surround the tendons to assist their movements and reduce friction. Many of the forearm muscles attach on the

ACTIVITY 9-61

1. Draw and color the triceps brachii and the anconeus in the space provided.
2. Label the proximal and distal attachment points: *P* for proximal; *D* for distal.
3. Place an X on the trigger points.
4. Palpate these muscles; identify the attachment points and the bellies of the muscles.
5. Move these muscles on yourself.

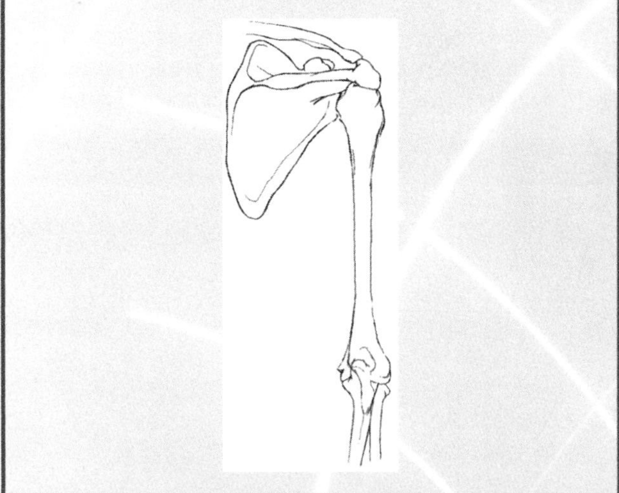

humerus and cross the elbow and the wrist joints; however, their action on the elbow is usually insignificant. The forearm muscles are subdivided by fascial sheets into the anterior and posterior compartments, each having a superficial and a deep layer of muscles. Most muscles of the anterior compartment are wrist and finger flexors; the muscles of the posterior compartment are mainly wrist and finger extensors. These muscles have distinct layers, and massage application requires careful and gradual access to the deeper layers by penetrating through the superficial layers using a broad-base compressive force. A narrow-pointed contact with the tissue usually results in tensing and guarding by the superficial muscles.

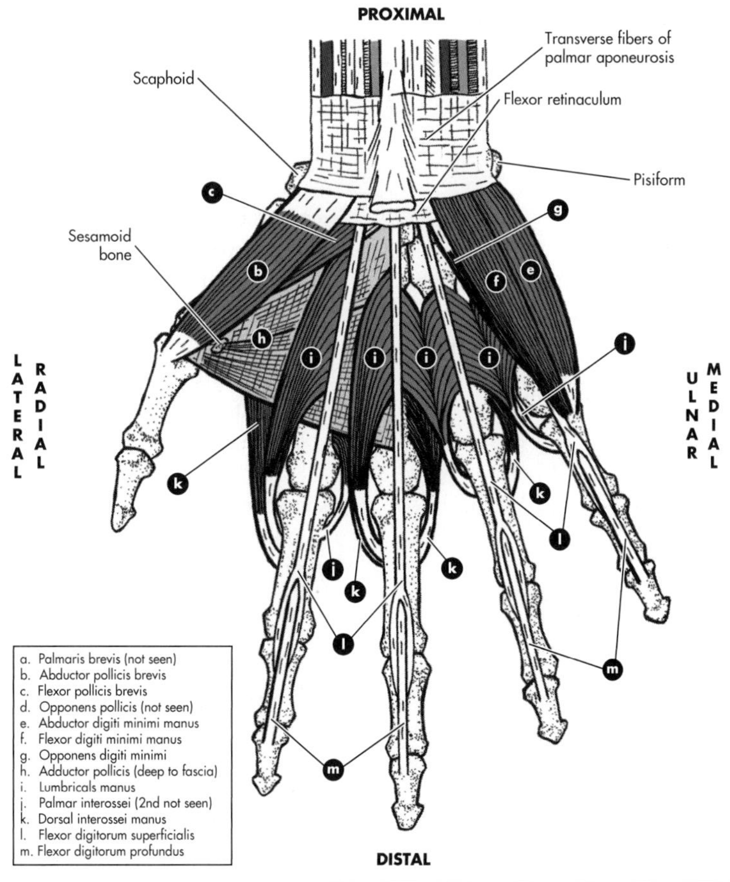

Figure 9-37
A, Palmar view of the right hand (superficial muscular layer).

(Continued)

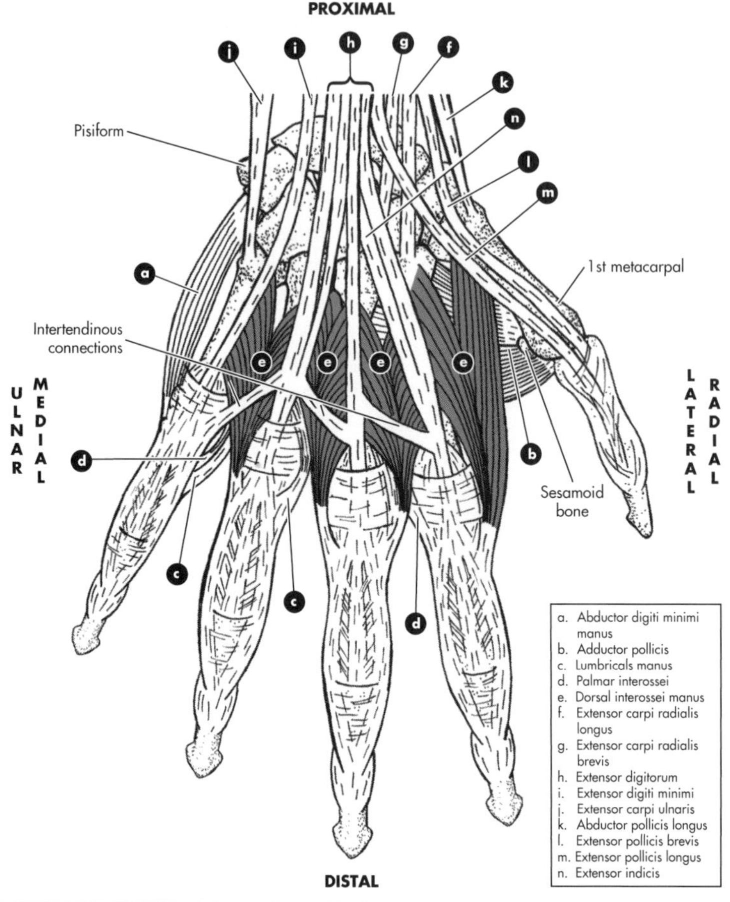

Figure 9-37—cont'd.
B, Dorsal view of the right hand. (Modified from Muscolino JE: *The muscular system manual: the skeletal muscles of the human body,* ed 2, St Louis, 2005, Mosby.)

Anterior Flexor Group: Superficial Layer

Flexor carpi radialis (FLEKS-or KAR-pee RAY-dee-AL-iss)

Flexor means to bend, *carpi* means of the wrist, and *radialis* means related to the radius.

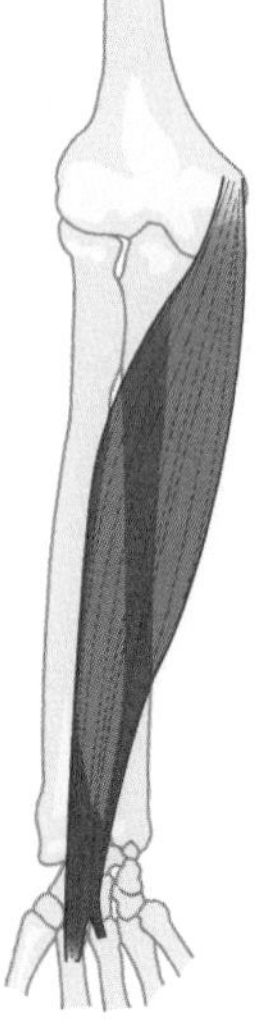

Concentric function:
Flexion and radial deviation (abduction) of the hand at the wrist joint, flexion of the forearm at the elbow joint, and pronation of the forearm at the radioulnar joints

Eccentric function:
Restrains extension and ulnar deviation (adduction) of the hand and extension and supination of the forearm.

Isometric function:
Stabilizes the wrist.

From:
Common flexor tendon from the medial epicondyle of the humerus and deep antebrachial fascia

To:
Base of the second and third metacarpal bones

Innervation:
Median nerve (C6 to C7)

Major synergists:
All flexors of the hand and the extensor carpi radialis longus and extensor carpi radialis brevis

Major antagonists:
All extensors of the hand and the flexor carpi ulnaris

Palmaris longus (pal-MAR-iss LONG-us)

Palmaris means related to the palm; *longus* means long.

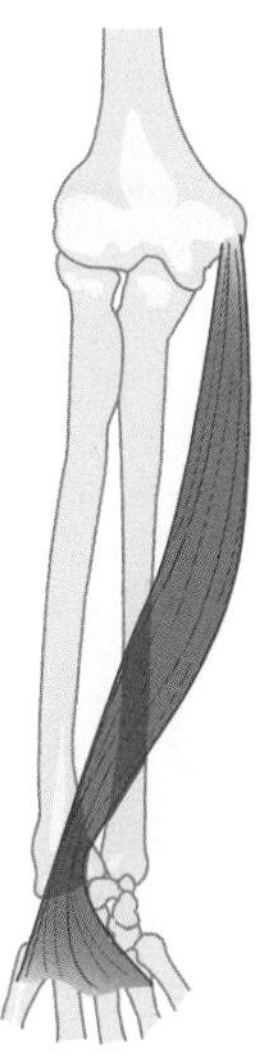

Concentric function:
Flexion of the hand at the wrist joint, flexion of the forearm at the elbow joint, and pronation of the forearm at the radioulnar joints

Eccentric function:
Restrains extension of the hand and extension and supination of the forearm.

Isometric function:
Tenses the palmar fascia.

From:
Common flexor tendon from the medial epicondyle of the humerus and deep antebrachial fascia

To:
Flexor retinaculum and palmar aponeurosis

Innervation:
Median nerve (C7 to C8)

Major synergists:
All flexors of the hand and the palmaris brevis

Major antagonists:
All extensors of the hand

The tendon of the palmaris longus is superficial to the antebrachial fascia of the wrist and is visible if one cups the hand and slightly flexes the wrist. This muscle is absent in about one fourth of the population.

Flexor carpi ulnaris (FLEKS-or KAR-pee ul-NAR-iss)

Flexor means to bend, *carpi* means of the wrist, and *ulnaris* means related to the ulna.

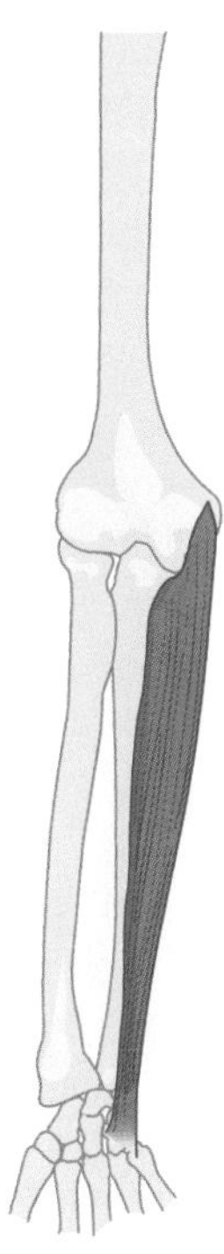

Concentric function:
Flexion and ulnar deviation (adduction) of the hand at the wrist joint and flexion of the forearm at the elbow joint

Eccentric function:
Restrains extension and radial deviation (abduction) of the hand and extension of the forearm.

Isometric function:
Stabilizes the wrist.

From:
Humeral head—Common flexor tendon from the medial epicondyle of the humerus
Ulnar head—Olecranon, proximal two thirds of the posterior border of the ulna, and deep antebrachial fascia

To:
Pisiform bone and, indirectly, by ligaments to the hamate and fifth metacarpal bones

Innervation:
Ulnar nerve (C7 to C8)

Major synergists:
All flexors of the hand and the extensor carpi ulnaris

Major antagonists:
All extensors of the hand and the flexor carpi radialis

Anterior Flexor Group: Intermediate Layer

Flexor digitorum superficialis (FLEKS-or DIH-jih-TOR-um SOO-per-fish-ee-AL-us)

Flexor means to bend, *digitorum* means of the fingers or toes, and *superficialis* means related to the top or surface.

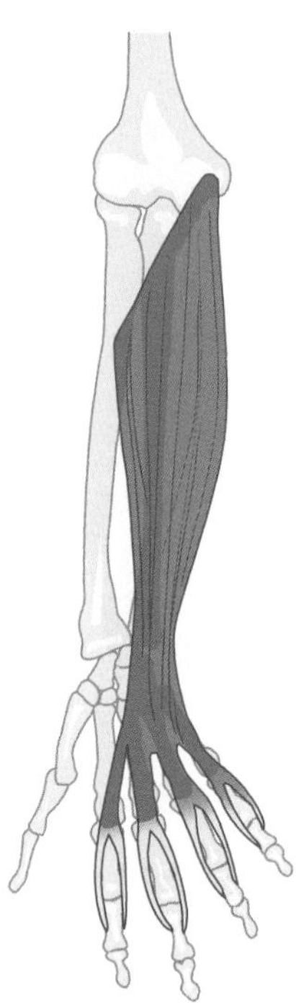

Concentric function:
Flexion of fingers 2 to 5 at the metacarpophalangeal and proximal interphalangeal joints and flexion of the hand at the wrist joint

Eccentric function:
Restrains finger extension and hand extension.

Isometric function:
Stabilizes wrist and finger joints.

From:
Humeral head—Common flexor tendon from the medial epicondyle of the humerus, ulnar collateral ligament of the elbow joint, and deep antebrachial fascia
Ulnar head—Medial side of the coronoid process of the ulna
Radial head—Oblique line of the radius

To:
Sides of the palmar surface of the middle phalanges of the second through fifth fingers

Innervation:
Median nerve (C7 to T1)

Major synergist:
Flexor digitorum profundus

Major antagonist:
Extensor digitorum

Anterior Flexor Group: Deep Layer

Flexor digitorum profundus (FLEKS-or DIH-jih-TOR-um pro-FUND-us)

Flexor means to bend, *digitorum* means related to the fingers or toes, and *profundus* means deep.

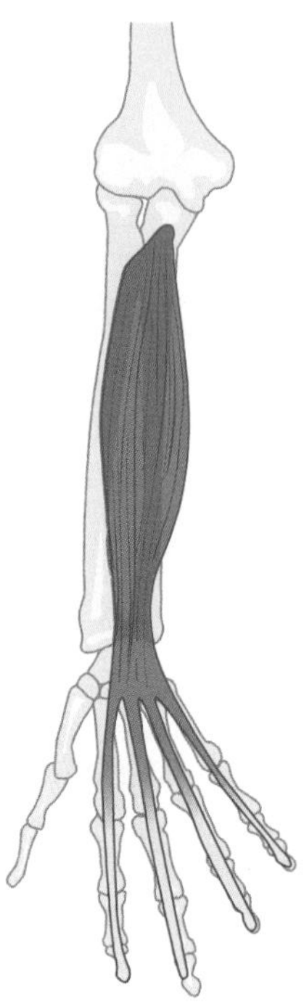

Concentric function:
Flexion of fingers 2 to 5 at the metacarpophalangeal, proximal, and distal interphalangeal joints and flexion of the hand at the wrist joint

Eccentric function:
Restrains extension of the fingers and extension of the hand.

Isometric function:
Stabilizes wrist and finger joints.

From:
Medial and anterior surfaces of the proximal one half of the ulna, interosseous membrane, and deep antebrachial fascia

To:
By four tendons into the distal phalanges of fingers 2 to 5 on the anterior surface

Innervation:
Ulnar nerve and interosseous branch of the median nerve (C7 to T1)

Major synergist:
Flexor digitorum superficialis

Major antagonist:
Extensor digitorum

Flexor pollicis longus (FLEKS-or POLL-is-iss LONG-us)

Flexor means to bend, *pollicis* means of the thumb, and *longus* means long.

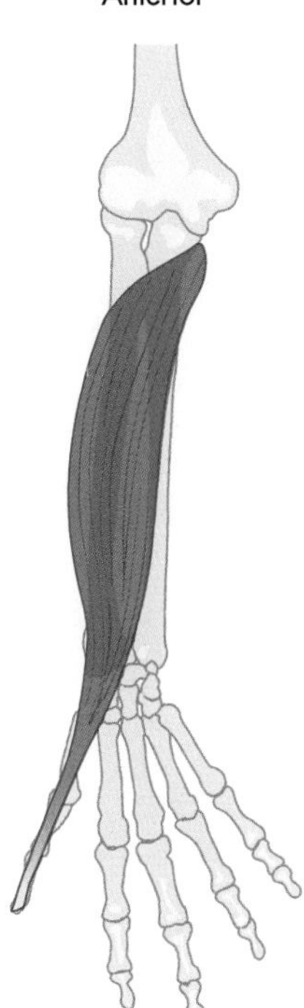

Concentric function:
Flexion of the thumb at the carpometacarpal, metacarpophalangeal, and interphalangeal joints

Eccentric function:
Restrains extension of the thumb.

Isometric function:
Stabilizes the thumb.

From:
Anterior surface of the radius distal to the tuberosity, medial border of the coronoid process of the ulna, and interosseous membrane

To:
Palmar surface of the base of the distal phalanx of the thumb

Innervation:
Anterior interosseous branch of the median nerve (C7 to C8)

Major synergist:
Flexor pollicis brevis

Major antagonists:
Extensor pollicis longus and extensor pollicis brevis
Elements common to the anterior flexion group:

Trigger points:
In the belly

Referred pain pattern:
Into the wrist, associated fingers, or thumb and occasionally into the elbow

See Activity 9-62.

ACTIVITY 9-62

1. Draw and color the anterior flexor group in the space provided.
2. Label the proximal and distal attachment points: *P* for proximal; *D* for distal.
3. Place an X on the trigger points.
4. Palpate these muscles; identify the attachment points and the bellies of the muscles.
5. Move these muscles on yourself.

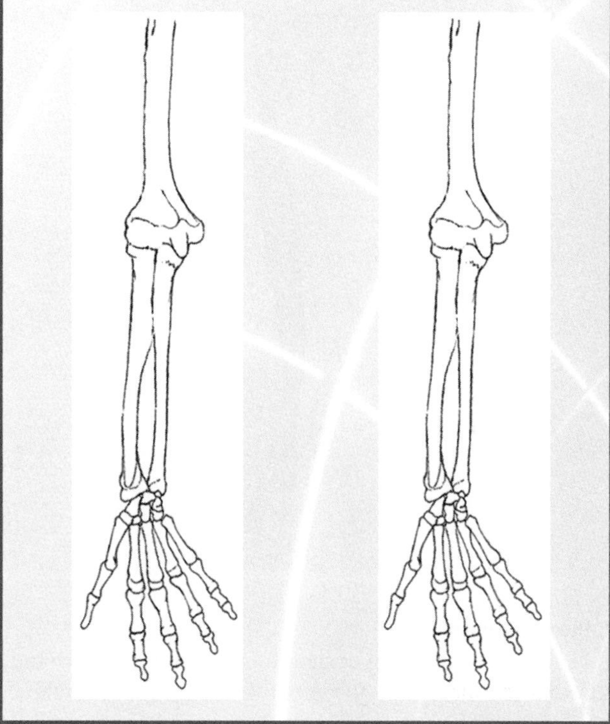

Posterior Extensor Group: Superficial Layer

Extensor carpi radialis longus (ex-STEN-sur KAR-pee RAY-dee-AL-iss LONG-us)

Extensor means one that stretches, *carpi* means related to the wrist, *radialis* means related to the radius, and *longus* means long.

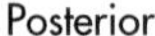

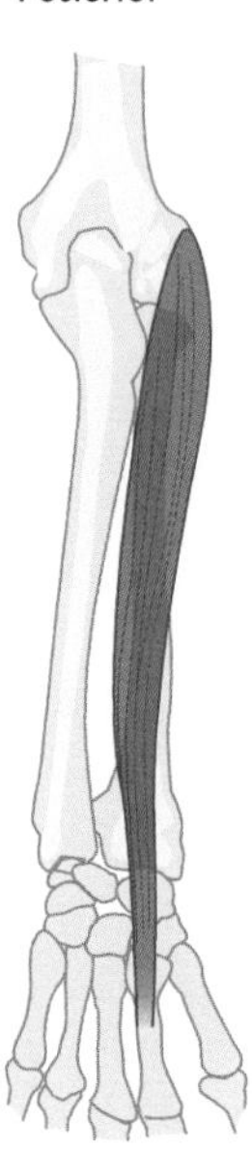

Concentric function:
Extension and radial deviation (abduction) of the hand at the wrist joint, flexion of the forearm at the elbow joint

Eccentric function:
Restrains flexion and ulnar deviation (adduction) of the hand, extension of the forearm, and pronation of the forearm at the radioulnar joint.

Isometric function:
Stabilizes wrist and elbow joints.

From:
Distal one third of the lateral supracondylar ridge of the humerus and lateral intermuscular septum

To:
Dorsal surface of the base of the second metacarpal bone on the radial side

Innervation:
Radial nerve (C5 to C6)

Major synergists:
All extensors of the hand and the flexor carpi radialis

Major antagonists:
All flexors of the hand and the extensor carpi ulnaris

Extensor carpi radialis brevis (ex-STEN-sur KAR-pee RAY-dee-AL-iss BREV-us)

Extensor means one that stretches, *carpi* means of the wrist, *radialis* means related to the radius, and *brevis* means short.

Posterior

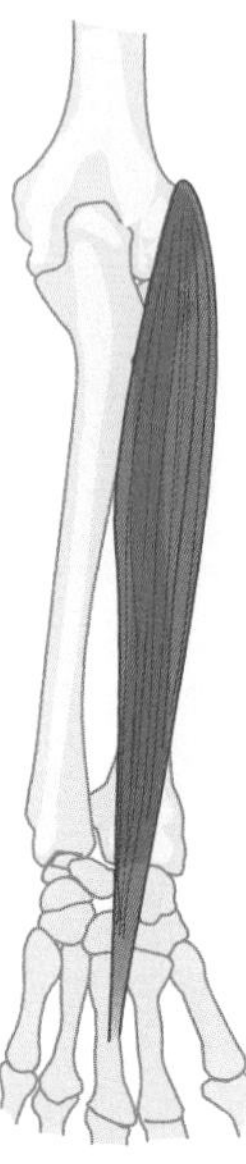

Concentric function:
Extension and radial deviation (abduction) of the hand at the wrist joint and flexion of the forearm at the elbow joint

Eccentric function:
Restrains flexion and ulnar deviation (adduction) of the hand and extension of the forearm.

Isometric function:
Stabilizes the wrist joint.

From:
Common extensor tendon from the lateral epicondyle of the humerus, radial collateral ligament of the elbow joint, and deep antebrachial fascia

To:
Dorsal surface of the base of the third metacarpal bone

Innervation:
Posterior interosseous branch of the radial nerve (C7 to C8)

Major synergists:
All extensors of the hand and the flexor carpi radialis

Major antagonists:
All flexors of the hand and the extensor carpi ulnaris

Extensor digitorum (ex-STEN-sur DIH-jih-TOR-um)

Extensor means one that stretches; *digitorum* means of the fingers or toes.

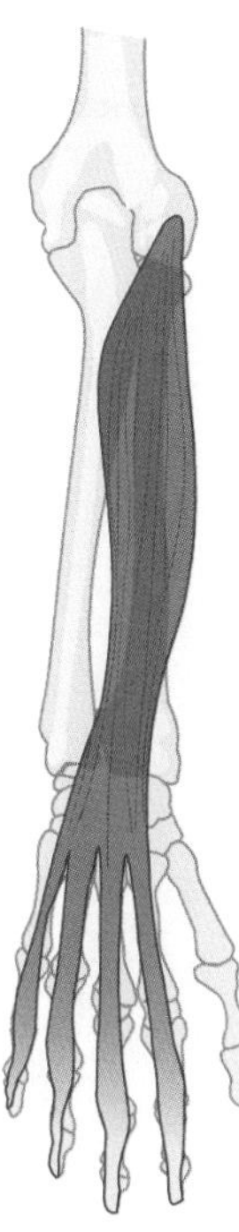

Concentric function:
Extension of fingers 2 to 5 at the metacarpophalangeal and proximal and distal interphalangeal joints and extension of the hand at the wrist joint
Eccentric function:
Restrains flexion of the fingers and flexion of the hand.
Isometric function:
Stabilizes the finger and wrist joints.
From:
Common extensor tendon from the lateral epicondyle of the humerus and intermuscular septa
To:
By four tendons to the lateral and dorsal surface of the phalanges of the second through fifth digits
Innervation:
Posterior interosseous branch of the radial nerve (C7 to C8)
Major synergists:
Extensor digiti minimi, extensor indicis, lumbricales, interossei palmares, and interossei dorsales manus
Major antagonists:
Flexor digitorum superficialis and flexor digitorum profundus
The distal tendon of this muscle forms the dorsal digital expansion of fingers 2 to 5.

Extensor digiti minimi (ex-STEN-sur DIH-jih-tee MIN-ih-mee)

Extensor means one that stretches, *digiti* means of the fingers or toes, and *minimi* means smallest.

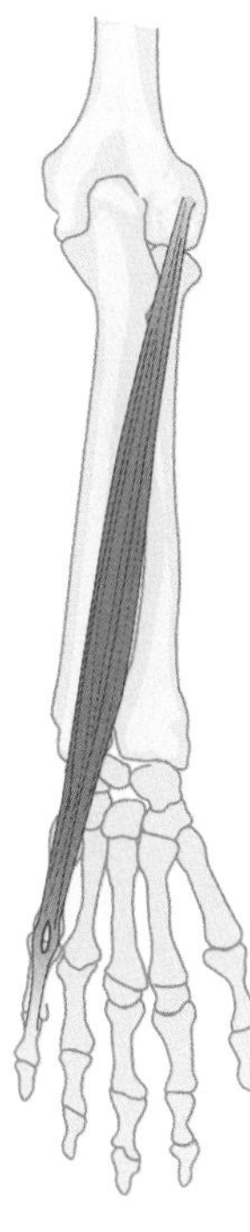

Concentric function:
Extension of the little finger at the metacarpophalangeal, proximal, and distal interphalangeal joints
Eccentric function:
Restrains flexion of the little finger.
Isometric function:
Stabilizes the little finger.
From:
Common extensor tendon from the lateral epicondyle of the humerus and intermuscular septa
To:
Into the dorsal digital expansion of the little finger with the extensor digitorum tendon
Innervation:
Posterior interosseous branch of the radial nerve (C7 to C8)
Major synergist:
Extensor digitorum
Major antagonists:
Flexor digitorum superficialis and flexor digitorum profundus

Extensor carpi ulnaris (ex-STEN-sur KAR-pee ul-NAR-iss)

Extensor means one that stretches, *carpi* means of the wrist, and *ulnaris* means related to the ulna.

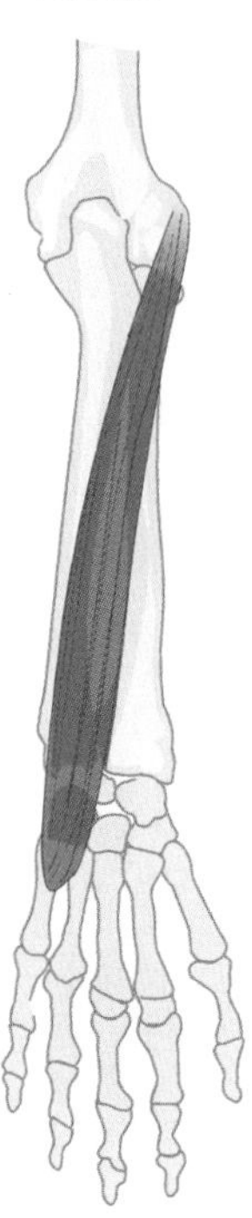

Concentric function:
Extension and ulnar deviation (adduction) of the hand at the wrist joint

Eccentric function:
Restrains flexion and radial deviation (abduction) of the hand.

Isometric function:
Stabilizes the wrist joint.

From:
Common extensor tendon from the lateral epicondyle of the humerus and the aponeurosis from the posterior border of the ulna

To:
Posterior side of the base of the fifth metacarpal bone

Innervation:
Posterior interosseous branch of the radial nerve (C7 to C8)

Major synergists:
All extensors of the hand and the flexor carpi ulnaris

Major antagonists:
All flexors of the hand and the extensor carpi radialis longus and extensor carpi radialis brevis

Posterior Extensor Group: Deep Layer

Extensor pollicis brevis (ex-STEN-sur POLL-is-iss BREV-us)

Extensor means one that stretches, *pollicis* means of the thumb, and *brevis* means short.

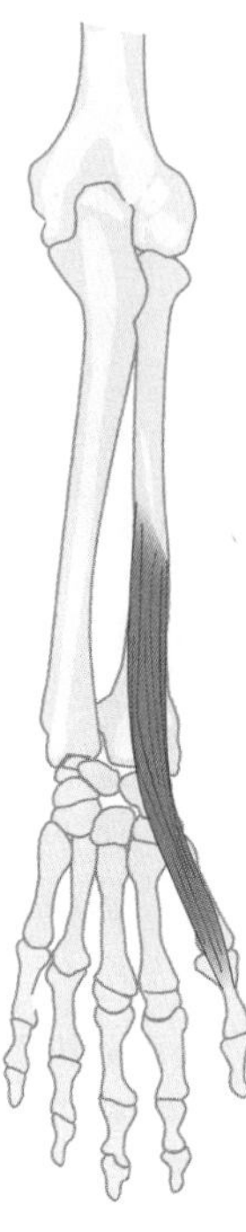

Concentric function:
Extension of the thumb at the carpometacarpal and metacarpophalangeal joints, abduction of the thumb at the carpometacarpal joint, radial deviation (abduction) of the hand at the wrist joint, and supination of the forearm at the radioulnar joints

Eccentric function:
Restrains flexion and adduction of the thumb, ulnar deviation (adduction) of the hand, and pronation of the forearm.

Isometric function:
Stabilizes the thumb.

From:
Posterior surface of the shaft of the radius distal to the origin of the abductor pollicis longus, and the interosseous membrane

To:
Base of the proximal phalanx of the thumb on the dorsal surface

Innervation:
Posterior interosseous branch of the radial nerve (C7 to C8)

Major synergists:
Extensor pollicis longus, abductor pollicis longus, and abductor pollicis brevis

Major antagonists:
Flexor pollicis longus, flexor pollicis brevis, and adductor pollicis

Abductor pollicis longus (ab-DUCK-tur POLL-is-iss LONG-us)

Abductor means one that leads away, *pollicis* means of the thumb, and *longus* means long.

Posterior

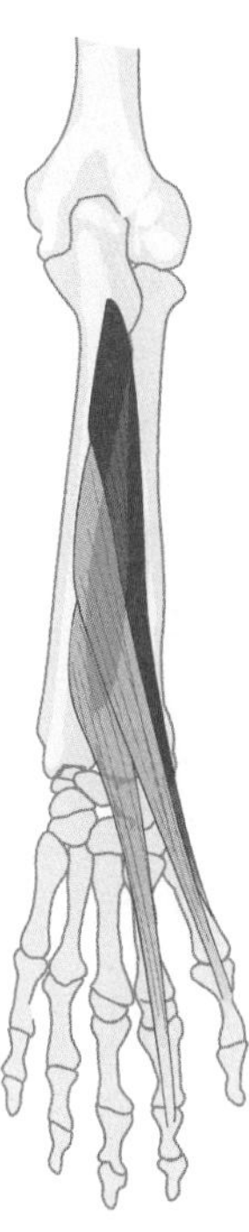

Concentric function:
Abduction and extension of the thumb at the carpometacarpal joint, radial deviation (abduction) and flexion of the hand at the wrist joint, and supination of the forearm at the radioulnar joints

Eccentric function:
Restrains adduction and flexion of the thumb, ulnar deviation (adduction) and extension of the hand, and pronation of the forearm.

Isometric function:
Stabilizes the thumb and the wrist joint.

From:
Posterior surface of the shaft of the ulna distal to the origin of the supinator, interosseous membrane, and posterior surface of the middle one third of the shaft of the radius

To:
Base of the first metacarpal bone of the thumb on the lateral side

Innervation:
Posterior interosseous branch of the radial nerve (C7 to C8)

Major synergists:
Abductor pollicis brevis, extensor pollicis longus, and extensor pollicis brevis

Major antagonists:
Adductor pollicis, flexor pollicis longus, and flexor pollicis brevis

Extensor pollicis longus (ex-STEN-sur POLL-is-iss LONG-us)

Extensor means one that stretches, *pollicis* means of the thumb, and *longus* means long.

Posterior

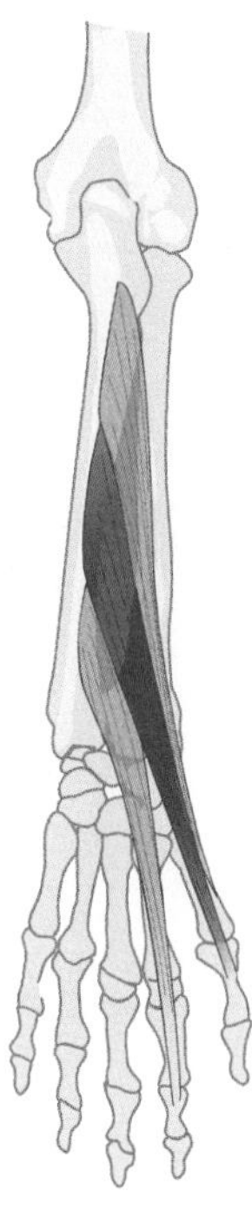

Concentric function:
Extension of the thumb at the carpometacarpal, metacarpophalangeal, and interphalangeal joints; radial deviation (abduction) of the hand at the wrist joint; and supination of the forearm at the radioulnar joints

Eccentric function:
Restrains flexion of the thumb, ulnar deviation (adduction) of the hand, and pronation of the forearm.

Isometric function:
Stabilizes the thumb and the wrist joint.

From:
Middle one third of the posterior surface of the ulna distal to the origin of the abductor pollicis longus and the interosseous membrane

To:
Dorsal surface of the base of the distal phalanx of the thumb

Innervation:
Posterior interosseous branch of the radial nerve (C7 to C8)

Major synergist:
Extensor pollicis brevis
Major antagonists:
Flexor pollicis longus and flexor pollicis brevis

Extensor indicis (ex-STEN-sur IN-dih-siss)

Extensor means one that stretches; *indicis* means of the index finger.

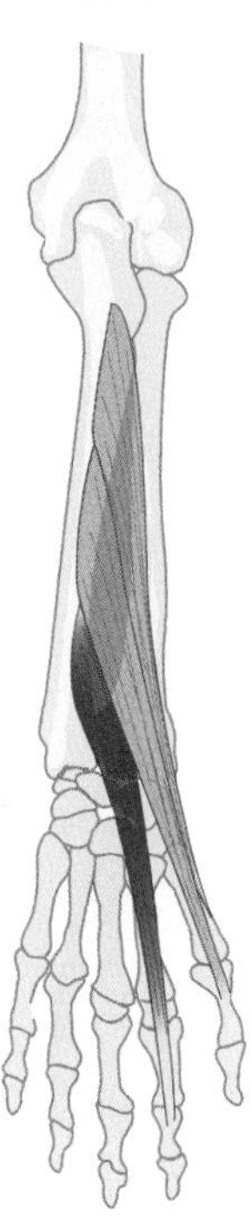

Concentric function:
Extension of the index finger at the metacarpophalangeal, proximal, and distal interphalangeal joints; adduction of the index finger at the metacarpophalangeal joint; and supination of the forearm at the radioulnar joints
Eccentric function:
Restrains flexion and abduction of the index finger and pronation of the forearm.
Isometric function:
Stabilizes the index finger.
From:
Posterior surface of the ulna and the interosseous membrane
To:
Into the dorsal digital expansion of index finger with the extensor digitorum tendon
Innervation:
Posterior interosseous branch of the radial nerve (C7 to C8)
Major synergist:
Extensor digitorum

ACTIVITY 9-63

1. Draw and color the muscles of the superficial and deep layers of the posterior extensor group in the space provided.
2. Label the proximal and distal attachment points: *P* for proximal; *D* for distal.
3. Place an X on the trigger points.
4. Palpate these muscles; identify the attachment points and the bellies of the muscles.
5. Move these muscles on yourself.

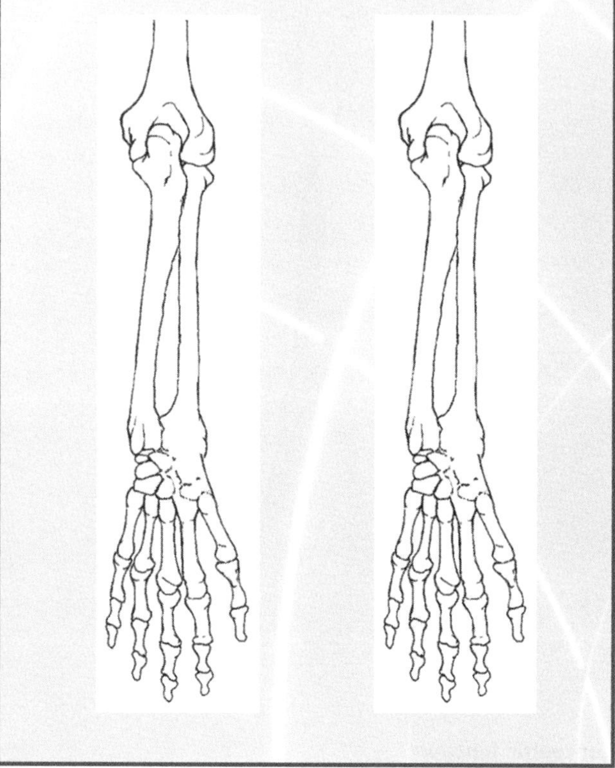

Major antagonists:
Flexor digitorum superficialis and flexor digitorum profundus
Elements common to the posterior extensor group muscles
Major synergists:
For extension, all extensors are synergistic with each other; for radial deviation of the hand, the extensor carpi radialis muscles are synergistic with the flexor carpi radialis; for ulnar deviation, the extensor and flexor carpi ulnaris muscles are synergistic
Major antagonists:
The flexor group; the ulnar deviation and radial deviation groups are antagonistic to each other
Trigger points:
Belly of each muscle, located nearer the elbow
Referred pain pattern:
From the lateral epicondyle at the elbow down the dorsum of the forearm to various parts of the hand, especially to the web of the thumb

See Activity 9-63.

Intrinsic Muscles of the Hand

Intrinsic muscles of the hand are small muscles that are located wholly within the hand (i.e., they originate and insert within the hand). The complex and intricate nature of these muscles allows for an almost limitless variety of fine hand movements. The delicacy of the muscles and the interactive pattern of their layout are unique to the human hand.

Thenar Eminence Muscles

The muscles of the thenar (THEE-nar) eminence are as follows:

Opponens pollicis (oh-PONE-ens POLL-is-iss)

Opponens means opposing; *pollicis* means of the thumb.

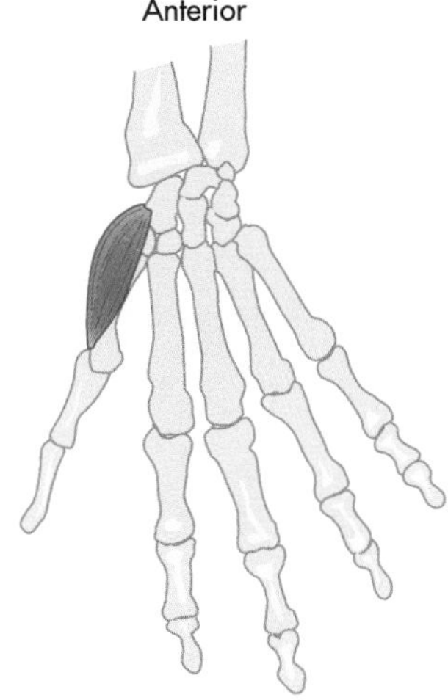

Concentric function:
Opposition of the thumb at the carpometacarpal joint (Opposition is the movement in which the thumb pad comes to meet the finger pad of any other finger; opposition of the thumb is usually considered to be a combination of abduction, flexion, and medial rotation of the thumb at the carpometacarpal joint.)

Eccentric function:
Restrains reposition of the thumb.

Isometric function:
Stabilizes the thumb.

From:
Flexor retinaculum and trapezium bone

To:
Anterior surface on the radial side of the first metacarpal bone

Innervation:
Median and ulnar nerves (C8 to T1)

Major synergists:
Flexor pollicis brevis and abductor pollicis brevis

Major antagonists:
Extensor pollicis longus, extensor pollicis brevis, adductor pollicis

Trigger points:
In the belly of the muscle

Referred pain pattern:
Into the thumb and the wrist

Abductor pollicis brevis (ab-DUCK-tur POLL-is-iss BREV-us)

Abductor means one that leads away, *pollicis* means of the thumb, and *brevis* means short.

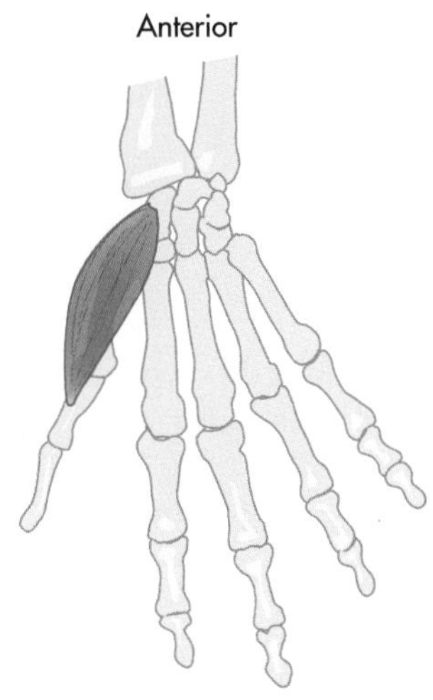

Concentric function:
Abduction of the thumb at the metacarpophalangeal joint

Eccentric function:
Restrains adduction of the thumb.

Isometric function:
Stabilizes the thumb.

From:
Flexor retinaculum, tubercle of the trapezium bone, and tubercle of the scaphoid bone

To:
Radial side of the base of the proximal phalanx of the thumb and dorsal digital expansion

Innervation:
Median nerve (C8 to T1)

Major synergist:
Abductor pollicis longus

Major antagonist:
Adductor pollicis

Trigger points:
In the belly of the muscle

Referred pain pattern:
Into the thumb and the wrist

Flexor pollicis brevis (FLEKS-or POLL-is-iss BREV-us)

Flexor means one that bends, *pollicis* means of the thumb, and *brevis* means short.

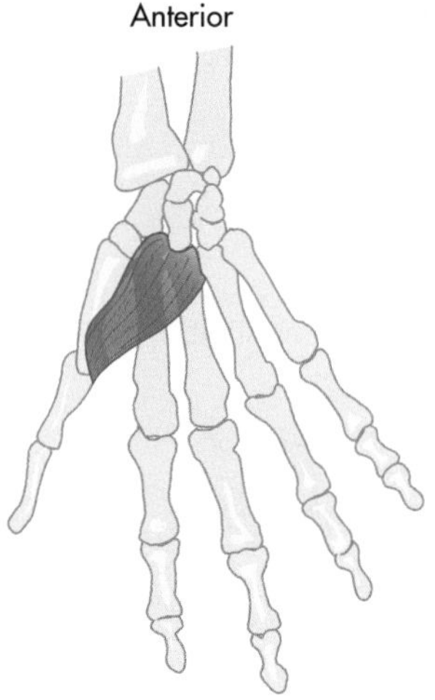

Concentric function:
Flexion of the thumb at the carpometacarpal and metacarpophalangeal joints

Eccentric function:
Restrains extension of the thumb.

Isometric function:
Stabilizes the thumb.

From:
Superficial head—Flexor retinaculum and trapezium bone
Deep head—Trapezoid and capitate bones

To:
Radial side of the base of the proximal phalanx of the thumb and dorsal digital expansion

Innervation:
Median and ulnar nerves (C8 to T1)

Major synergist:
Flexor pollicis longus

Major antagonists:
Extensor pollicis longus and extensor pollicis brevis

Trigger points:
In the belly of the muscle

Referred pain pattern:
Into the thumb and the wrist

See Activity 9-64.

Hypothenar Muscles

Opponens digiti minimi (oh-PONE-ens DIH-jih-tee MIN-ih-mee)

Opponens means opposing, *digiti* means of the fingers or toes, and *minimi* means smallest.

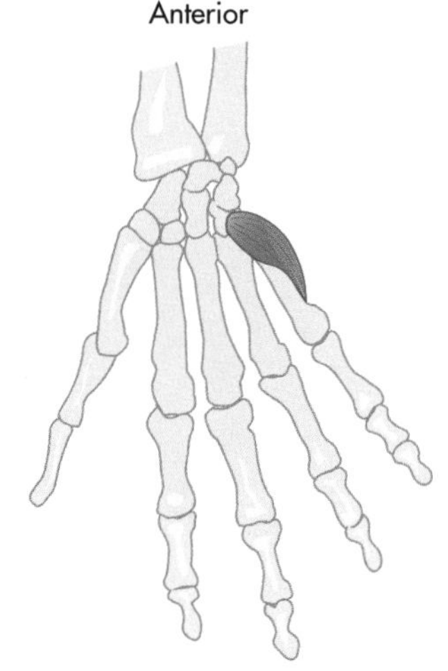

ACTIVITY 9-64

1. Draw and color the thenar muscles (the opponens pollicis, abductor pollicis brevis, and flexor pollicis brevis) in the space provided.
2. Label the proximal and distal attachment points: *P* for proximal; *D* for distal.
3. Place an X on the trigger points.
4. Palpate these muscles; identify the attachment points and the bellies of the muscles.
5. Move these muscles on yourself.

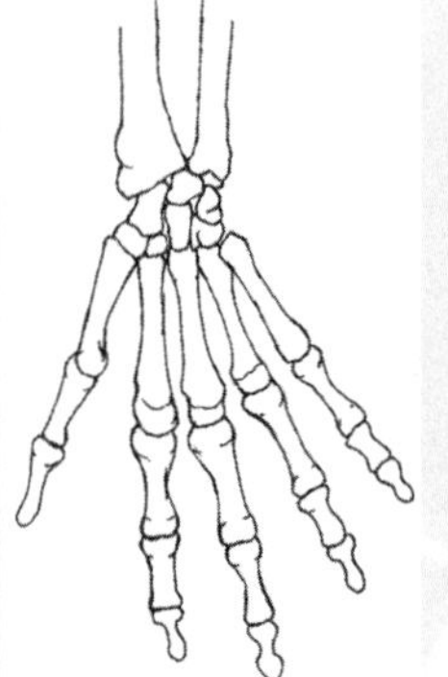
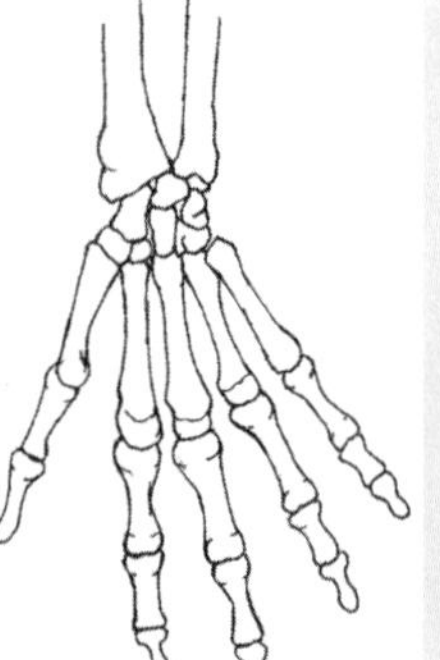
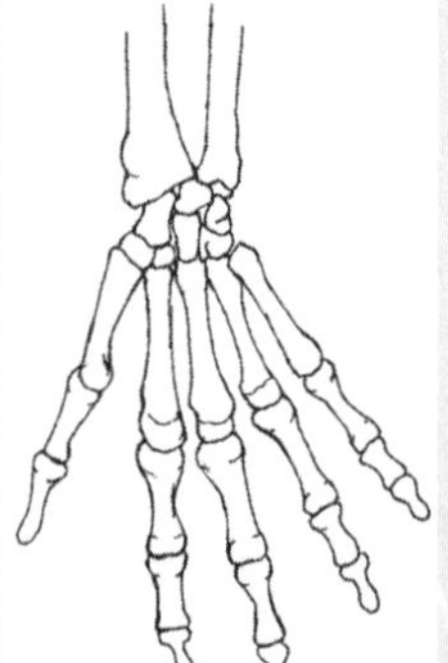

Concentric function:
Opposition of the little finger at the carpometacarpal joint (Opposition is the movement in which the finger pad of the little finger comes to meet the finger pad of the thumb. Opposition of the little finger is actually a combination of flexion, adduction, and lateral rotation of the little finger at the carpometacarpal joint.)

Eccentric function:
Restrains reposition of the little finger.

Isometric function:
Stabilizes the little finger.

From:
Flexor retinaculum and the hook of the hamate bone

To:
Entire length of the fifth metacarpal bone on the ulnar side

Innervation:
The ulnar nerve (C8 to T1)

Major synergists:
Flexor digitorum superficialis, flexor digitorum profundus, and interossei palmares (No. 3)

Major antagonists:
Extensor digitorum, extensor digiti minimi, and abductor digiti minimi manus

Trigger points:
In the belly of the muscle

Referred pain pattern:
Into the little finger and wrist

Abductor digiti minimi manus (ab-DUCK-tur DIH-jih-tee MIN-ih-mee MAN-us)

Abductor means one that leads away, *digiti* means of the fingers or toes, *minimi* means smallest, and *manus* means of the hand.

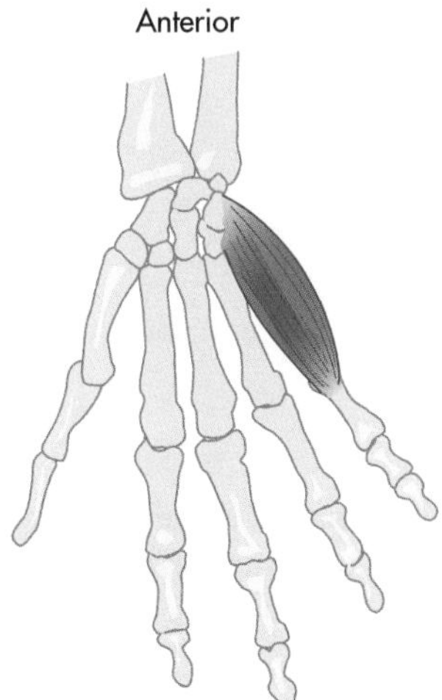

Concentric function:
Abduction of the little finger at the metacarpophalangeal joint

Eccentric function:
Restrains adduction of the little finger.

Isometric function:
Stabilizes the little finger.

From:
Tendon of the flexor carpi ulnaris and the pisiform bone

To:
Base of the proximal phalanx of the little finger on the ulnar side and dorsal digital expansion

Innervation:
Ulnar nerve (C8 to T1)

Major synergists:
No major synergists

Major antagonists:
Interossei palmares (No. 3)

Trigger points:
In the belly of the muscle

Referred pain pattern:
Into the little finger and wrist

Flexor digiti minimi manus (FLEKS-or DIH-jih-tee MIN-ih-mee MAN-us)

Flexor means one that bends, *digiti* means of the fingers or toes, *minimi* means smallest, and *manus* means of the hand.

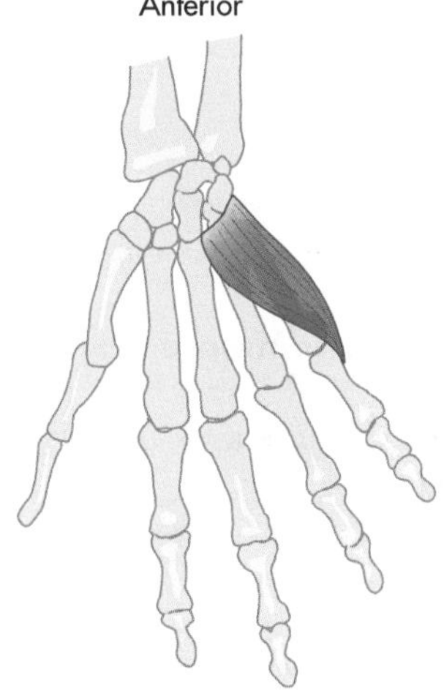

Concentric function:
Flexion of the little finger at the metacarpophalangeal joint

Eccentric function:
Restrains extension of the little finger.

Isometric function:
Stabilizes the little finger.

From:
Hook of the hamate bone and flexor retinaculum

To:
Base of the proximal phalanx of the little finger on the ulnar side

Innervation:
Ulnar nerve (C8 to T1)

Major synergists:
Flexor digitorum superficialis and flexor digitorum profundus

ACTIVITY 9-65

1. Draw and color the hypothenar muscles (the opponens digiti minimi, abductor digiti minimi manus, and flexor digiti minimi manus [brevis]) in the space provided.
2. Label the proximal and distal attachment points: *P* for proximal; *D* for distal.
3. Place an X on the trigger points.
4. Palpate these muscles; identify the attachment points and the bellies of the muscles.
5. Move these muscles on yourself.

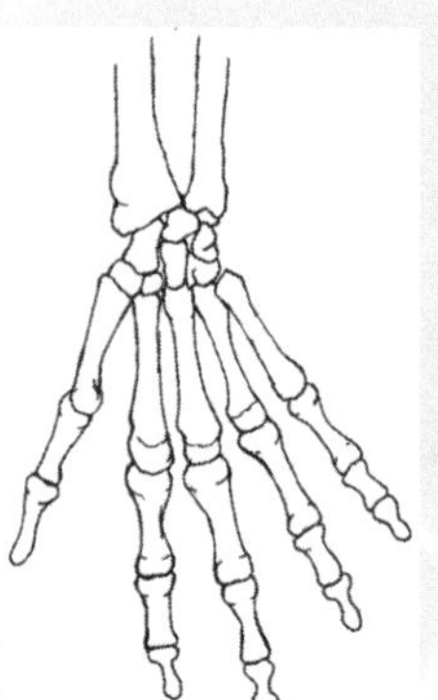
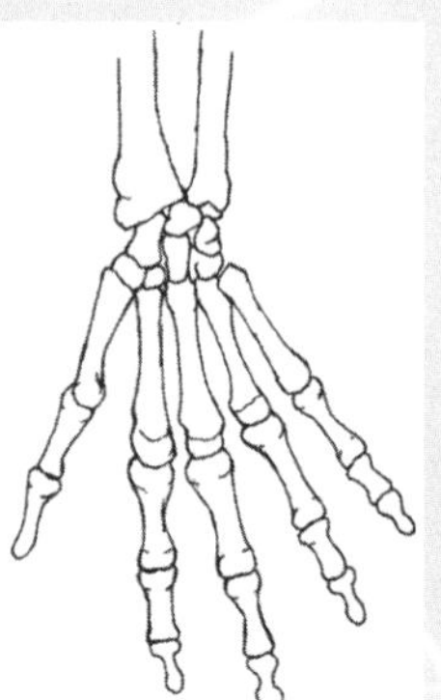
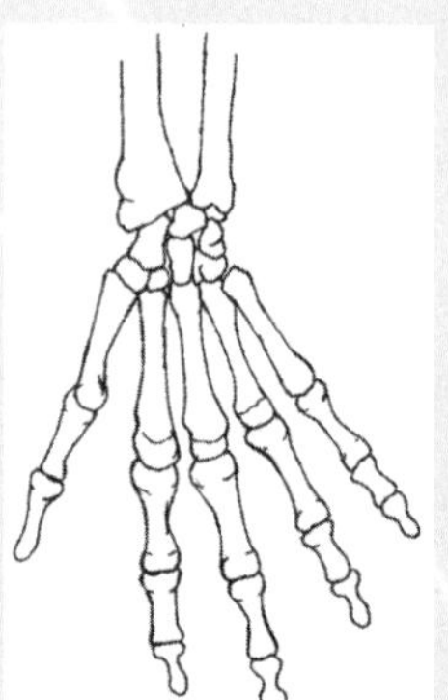

Major antagonists:
Extensor digitorum and extensor digiti minimi
Trigger points:
In the belly of the muscle
Referred pain pattern:
Into the little finger and wrist

See Activity 9-65.

Central Compartment Muscles

Adductor pollicis (ad-DUCK-tur POLL-is-iss)

Adductor means one that leads toward; *pollicis* means of the thumb.

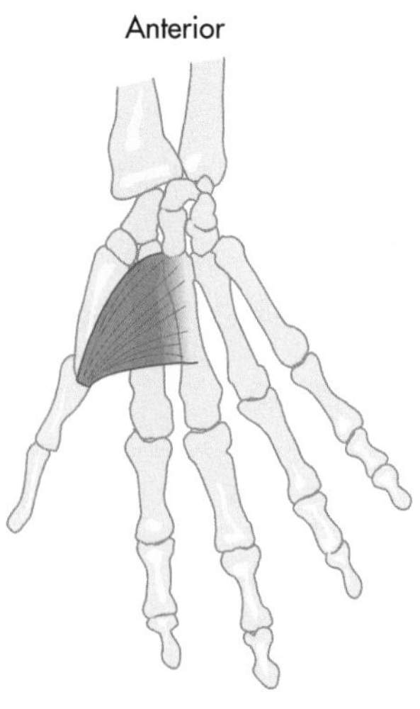

Concentric function:
Adduction of the thumb at the carpometacarpal joint
Eccentric function:
Restrains abduction of the thumb.
Isometric function:
Stabilizes the thumb.
From:
Oblique head—Trapezium, trapezoid, and capitate bones and the base of the second and third metacarpal bones
Transverse head—Palmar surface of the third metacarpal
To:
Ulnar side of the base of the proximal phalanx of the thumb
Innervation:
Ulnar nerve (C8 to T1)
Major synergists:
There are no major synergists
Major antagonists:
Abductor pollicis longus and abductor pollicis brevis
Trigger points:
In the belly of the muscle
Referred pain pattern:
Into the associated finger; commonly associated with Heberden's nodes, which develop on the dorsolateral or dorsomedial aspect of the terminal phalanx at its joint

Interossei palmares (INT-er-OSS-ee-y pal-MAR-es)

Interossei means between the bones; *palmares* means of the palm.

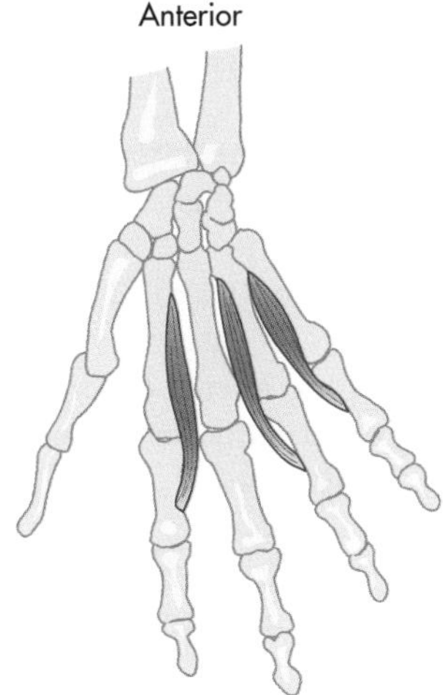

Concentric function:
Adduction of the index, ring, and little fingers (2, 4, and 5) at the metacarpophalangeal joint (adduction of a finger is a movement toward an imaginary line drawn through the middle of the middle finger); flexion of fingers 2, 4, and 5 at the metacarpophalangeal joints; and extension of fingers 2, 4, and 5 at the proximal and distal interphalangeal joints

Eccentric function:
Restrains abduction, extension, and flexion of fingers 2, 4, and 5.

Isometric function:
Stabilizes fingers 2, 4, and 5.

From:
First—Ulnar side of the base of the second metacarpal bone
Second—Radial side of the base of the fourth metacarpal bone
Third—Radial side of the base of the fifth metacarpal bone

To:
First—Ulnar side of the proximal phalanx of the index finger
Second—Radial side of the proximal phalanx of the ring finger
Third—Radial side of the proximal phalanx of the little finger

Innervation:
Ulnar nerve (C8 to T1)

Major synergists:
Lumbricales manus

Major antagonists:
Interossei dorsales

Trigger points:
In the belly of the muscle

Referred pain pattern:
Into the associated finger; commonly associated with Heberden's nodes, which develop on the dorsolateral or dorsomedial aspect of the terminal phalanx at its joint

Interossei dorsales manus (INT-er-OSS-ee-y door-SAL-es MAN-us)

Interossei means between the bones, *dorsales* means related to the back, and *manus* means of the hand.

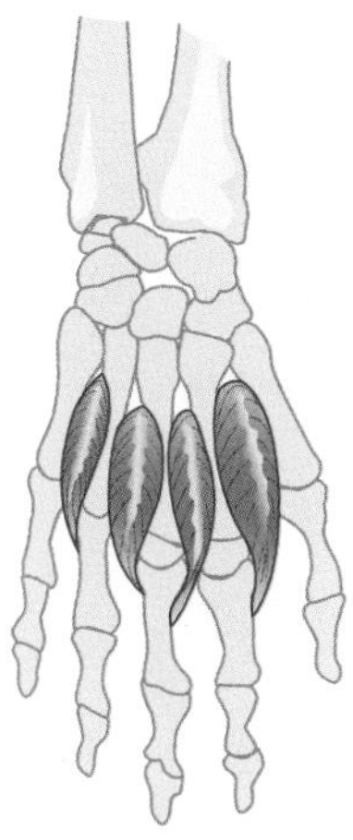

Concentric function:
Abduction of the index, middle, and ring fingers (fingers 2 to 4) at the metacarpophalangeal joint (abduction of a finger is a movement away from an imaginary line drawn through the middle of the middle finger); flexion of fingers 2 to 4 at the metacarpophalangeal joints; and extension of fingers 2 to 4 at the proximal and distal interphalangeal joints

Eccentric function:
Restrains adduction, extension, and flexion of fingers 2 to 4.

Isometric function:
Stabilizes fingers 2 to 4.

From:
First—Adjacent sides of the first and second metacarpal bones
Second—Adjacent sides of the second and third metacarpal bones
Third—Adjacent sides of the third and fourth metacarpal bones
Fourth—Adjacent sides of the fourth and fifth metacarpal bones

To:
First—Radial side of the proximal phalanx of the index finger
Second—Radial side of the proximal phalanx of the middle finger
Third—Ulnar side of the proximal phalanx of the middle finger
Fourth—Ulnar side of the proximal phalanx of the ring finger

Innervation:
Ulnar nerve (C8 to T1)

Major synergists:
Lumbricales manus
Major antagonists:
Interossei palmares
Trigger points:
In the belly of the muscle
Referred pain pattern:
Into the associated finger; commonly associated with Heberden's nodes, which develop on the dorsolateral or dorsomedial aspect of the terminal phalanx at its joint

Lumbricales manus (LUM-brih-kal-es MAN-us)

Lumbricales means earthworms; *manus* means of the hand.

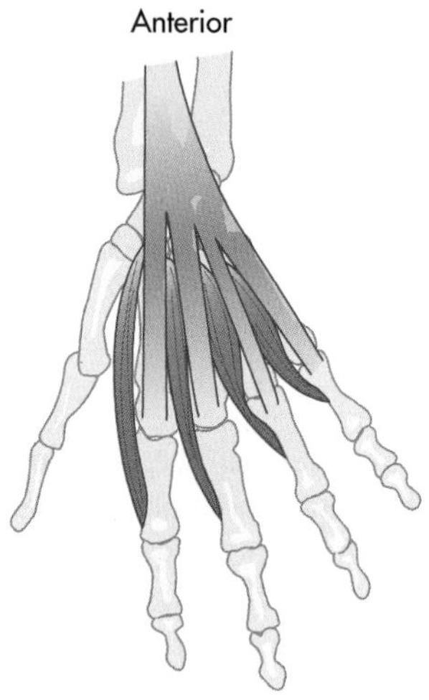

Concentric function:
Extension of the index, middle, ring, and little fingers at the interphalangeal joints and flexion of the index, middle, ring, and little fingers at the metacarpophalangeal joint

From:
First and second—Radial surface of the flexor profundus tendons of the index and middle fingers, respectively
Third—Adjacent sides of the flexor profundus tendons of the middle and ring fingers
Fourth—Adjacent sides of the flexor profundus tendons of the ring and little fingers
To:
Into the radial border of the dorsal digital expansion on the dorsal aspect of the digits
Innervation:
Median and ulnar nerves (C8 to T1)
Major synergists:
Interossei palmares and interossei dorsales manus, flexor digitorum superficialis, flexor digitorum profundus, and extensor digitorum
Major antagonists:
Flexor digitorum superficialis, flexor digitorum profundus, extensor digitorum
Trigger points:
In the belly of the muscle
Referred pain pattern:
Into the associated finger; commonly associated with Heberden's nodes, which develop on the dorsolateral or dorsomedial aspect of the terminal phalanx at its joint

See Activity 9-66.

PATHOLOGIC CONDITIONS

Mechanisms of Disease

Whenever the myofascial system (muscles and associated connective tissue) is stressed, a fairly predictable sequence of events occurs (Chaitow, 1996):

ACTIVITY 9-66

1. Draw and color the deep muscles of the hand in the space provided.
2. Label the proximal and distal attachment points: *P* for proximal; *D* for distal.
3. Place an X on the trigger points.
4. Palpate these muscles; identify the attachment points and the bellies of the muscles.
5. Move these muscles on yourself.

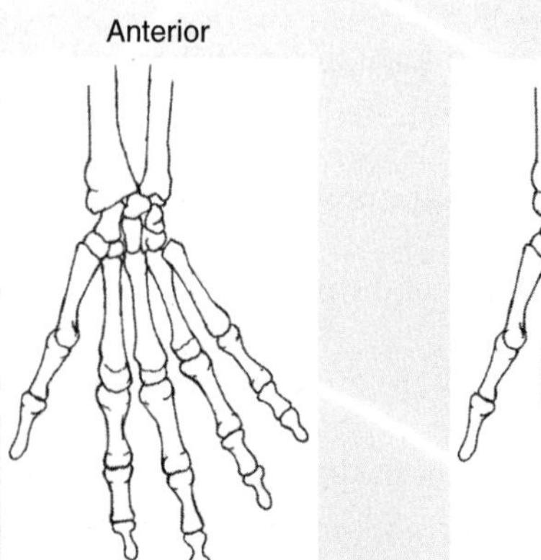

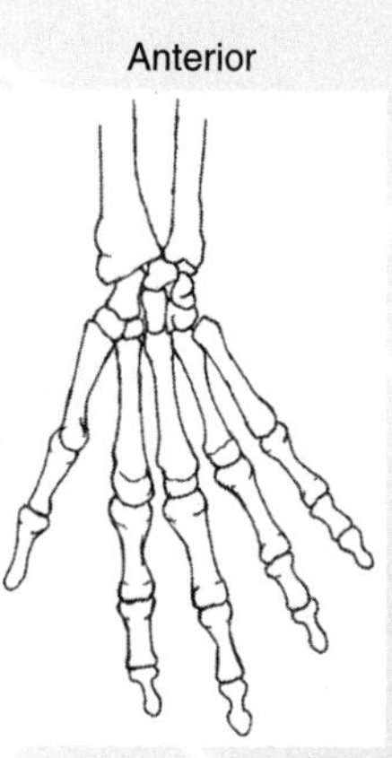

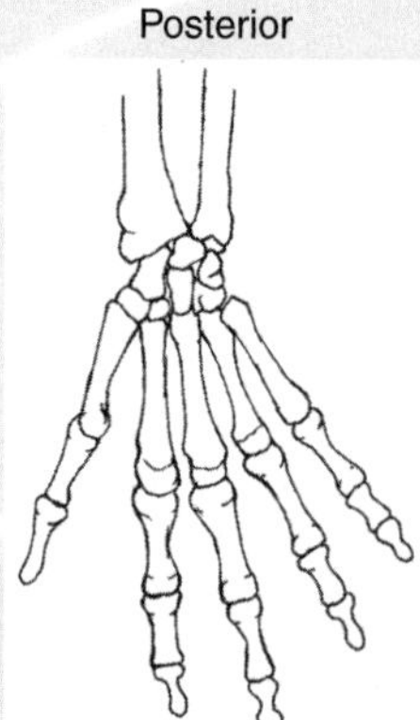

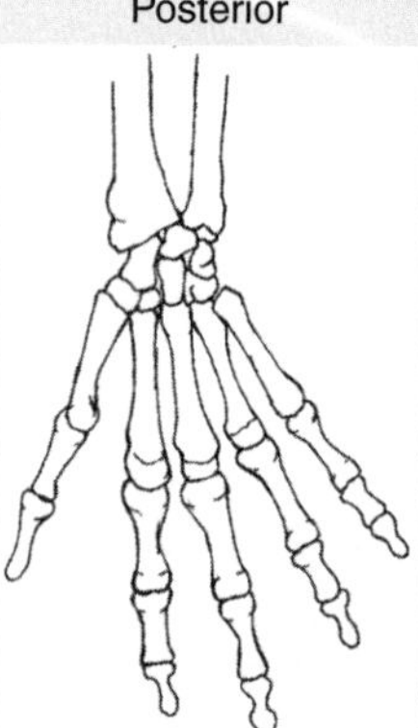

1. Causal factors (e.g., congenital factors or predisposition, overuse, misuse, abuse and disuse of the body, postural stress, and chronic stressful emotional states) and reflex factors (e.g., trigger points and dysfunctional firing patterns) can lead to increased muscle tension and retention of metabolic wastes.
2. Increased tension leads to localized ischemia and edema.
3. Pain results.
4. Pain increases tension or spasm, which increases pain.
5. Inflammation or chronic irritation may result.
6. Neurologic reporting stations in tense tissue bombard the central nervous system with information, which leads to hyperactivity.
7. Macrophages and fibroblasts are activated.
8. Connective tissue production increases, with increasing shortening of fascia.
9. Because fascia is continuous throughout the body, any distortions in one area could create distortions elsewhere, affecting structures supported by or attached to the fascia, including the nerves, muscles, lymph, and blood vessels.
10. Changes occur in the muscular tissues, leading to chronic hypertension and ultimately to fibrotic changes. Increased tension in a muscle causes inhibition of the antagonist muscles and facilitation in the synergists.
11. Chain reactions in myotatic units occur. Typically, muscles used for posture become shortened, and muscles used for motion tend to weaken. This effect alters gait reflexes, and synergists can become dominant, causing muscle firing patterns to be altered.
12. Sustained increases in muscle tension cause ischemia in tendinous areas, and areas of periosteal (bone) pain develop.
13. Abnormal biomechanics and bodywide compensatory patterns develop. Torsion patterns at the shoulder and pelvic girdle are common. Gait patterns are compromised.
14. Joint restriction or imbalance or both develop, and fascial shortening and immobility increase.
15. Trigger points develop.
16. Generalized fatigue develops as a result of wasted energy used to maintain unproductive patterns and of an interrupted sleep pattern.
17. Sympathetic arousal is heightened, generalizing the pattern.
18. Immune response is inhibited, and more serious systemic problems may develop.

Massage Intervention

Muscle dysfunction in the concentric contraction often results in short, tense muscles that do not inhibit when necessary. Trigger points often set up in the muscle belly. Concentric contraction dysfunction is an important place to begin treatment, and the muscle needs to be relaxed (inhibited and lengthened).

Muscle dysfunction in the eccentric contraction phase often results in tense but long and strained muscles that are inhibited and attempt recruitment of synergists to function. Trigger points often set up in the attachments. One should not treat any eccentric tight (long and weak) patterns with any methods that would relax (elongate) the muscle further. As the practitioner addresses concentric (tight and short) dysfunction, the inhibited muscles respond to strengthening procedures, and trigger points normalize.

Isometric muscle dysfunction usually results in agonist and antagonist patterns interacting simultaneously to stabilize a joint dysfunction (usually joint laxity, guarding an injury, or overuse). If this continues for a time, fibrosis is common, as is a reduced ability in concentric and eccentric function. Mobility and coordination decrease because stabilizing function supersedes mobility.

Intervention focuses on reversing nonproductive processes and supporting resourceful compensation patterns that develop in response to chronic problems. The goal is to support circulation, connective tissue support and pliability, and nervous system interaction. Compression and the stroking of massage supports circulation. Connective tissue responds to methods that affect the viscoelastic, plastic, and colloid properties. Muscle tension patterns respond to compression and drag that stimulates proprioceptors. Muscle energy methods systematically use contraction and relaxation of muscles combined with lengthening to restore normal length of the muscles. Trigger points respond to methods that reduce hyperactivity such as muscle energy methods and compression. Calming the sympathetic arousal is also necessary.

Medications

Pathologic conditions of the muscles are treated with antibiotics. Steroidal and nonsteroidal antiinflammatory medications ease inflammation. Muscle relaxants soothe spasm and hypertonic muscles, and analgesics treat pain. Low doses of antidepressants sometimes assist the client with sleep restoration and support of other restorative processes.

These drugs may be prescription or over-the-counter medications, herbal or homeopathic substances. Any form of medication or herbal remedy may have effects on the client that one needs to take into consideration when developing a treatment plan. One also must give consideration to the interaction between massage and the effects of medication. Many medications used to treat muscle dysfunction determine the intensity of pressure and the duration and amount of stretch one can apply to the tissues.

Any time infection is present and is being treated with antibiotics, the system already is stressed. Therapeutic methods support the healing process by promoting general relaxation but are to be performed gently so as not to place additional demand on the system to respond. When clients use antiinflammatory drugs, the practitioner should avoid methods that produce therapeutic inflammation. Muscle relaxants interfere with the normal feedback systems of the stretch and tension receptors; because these medications interrupt this protective mechanism, one must take care with any type of lengthening or stretching methods. Because analgesics interfere with the normal pain response, feedback from the client may be inaccurate. One must adjust intensity and duration.

Massage can support the use of these medications, helping to make them more effective. In some instances the dosage of medication can be reduced or the medication can be replaced by massage therapy. Ice applications can support and sometimes reduce the use of analgesics and antiinflammatory drugs. Because all medications have side effects, the ability to take smaller doses of medication for short durations is beneficial. Any change in medication use must be set in place and carefully monitored by the prescribing health care provider.

Specific Disorders

Carpal Tunnel Syndrome

Carpal tunnel syndrome is irritation of the median nerve as it passes under the transverse carpal ligament into the wrist. Carpal tunnel syndrome may cause pain, tingling, numbness, weakness in the part of the hand supplied by the median nerve, muscle connective tissue shortening, and fluid retention.

INDICATIONS CONTRAINDICATIONS

For Therapeutic Massage

Massage is indicated for the muscular connective tissue and fluid components of the condition; however, one must exercise caution around the wrist and must alter the therapy if any symptoms occur to prevent further irritation of the nerve. ■

Thoracic Outlet Syndrome

Thoracic outlet syndrome occurs because the brachial plexus and blood supply of the arm become impinged, resulting in shooting pains, weakness, and numbness. A sensation, fullness, and discoloration of the affected arm can occur from impaired circulation. The pain pattern also is referred to the shoulder and scapular region. Often the scalene muscles and pectoralis minor muscles are involved.

INDICATIONS CONTRAINDICATIONS

For Therapeutic Massage

Massage methods help relieve muscle impingement of the nerve by relaxing and lengthening the muscles. If other disorders such as spondylosis or herniated discs are the causal factors, the andela will not respond well to massage. ■

Stress-Induced Muscle Tension and Headache

Stress-induced muscle tension can result in myalgia, or muscle pain; stiffness in the neck and back often accompanies stress-induced headaches. The contracted muscles exert pressure on the nerves and blood vessels in the area, causing the pain, which is a dull, persistent ache with feelings of tightness around the head, temples, forehead, and occipital area. The headache often is less intense in the morning and worsens as the day goes on.

INDICATIONS CONTRAINDICATIONS

For Therapeutic Massage

One uses various strategies to treat stress-induced muscle tension headaches, including massage and other forms of soft tissue work, biofeedback, relaxation training, exercise, and stretching methods. Chronic patterns often indicate connective tissue shortening. Headaches respond best to whole-body therapy, which not only addresses the immediate areas but also relaxes the entire body. ■

Muscle Strain

Injury to skeletal muscles from overexertion or trauma can result in muscle strain. Muscle strains involve overstretching or tearing of muscle fibers and associated connective tissue. Although the inflammation may subside in a few hours or days, repair of damaged muscle fibers usually takes weeks, and some damaged muscle cells may be replaced by fibrous tissue, forming scars.

INDICATIONS CONTRAINDICATIONS

For Therapeutic Massage

Direct work over the area of injury is contraindicated regionally until all signs of inflammation have dissipated. The use of ice and gentle range of motion exercises can support healing. Methods to manage distortion in posture resulting from compensation in the rest of the body are helpful. ■

Contusion

Minor trauma to the muscles may cause a muscle bruise, or contusion, that involves local internal bleeding and inflammation. Severe trauma to a skeletal muscle may cause a crush injury that damages the affected muscle tissue and releases the muscle fiber contents into the bloodstream. This situation can be life-threatening, because the reddish muscle pigment myoglobin can accumulate in the blood and cause kidney failure.

INDICATIONS CONTRAINDICATIONS

For Therapeutic Massage

Direct work over the area of injury is contraindicated regionally until all signs of inflammation have dissipated. ■

Muscle Infections

Several bacteria, viruses, and parasites may infect muscle tissue, often producing local or widespread myositis (muscle inflammation). Trichinosis, which is caused by a parasite, is an example of such an infection. The muscle pain and stiffness that sometimes accompany influenza are other examples of myositis.

Poliomyelitis

Poliomyelitis is a viral infection of the nerves that control skeletal muscle movement. The disease can be asymptomatic; however, poliomyelitis often causes paralysis that may progress to death. Virtually eliminated in the United States through an effective vaccine, polio nonetheless still affects millions around the world who have not been vaccinated.

More common is the occurrence of postpolio syndrome in persons who had polio years before. The symptoms are weakness, fatigue, intolerance to cold, and general, aching pain.

INDICATIONS CONTRAINDICATIONS

For Therapeutic Massage

For postpolio syndrome, general constitutional approaches seem to work best to aid in overall pain reduction and restoration of the sleep pattern. One should avoid any form of therapy that causes therapeutic inflammation, including intense exercise and stretching programs. ■

Myositis Ossificans

Myositis ossificans involves an inflammatory process that stimulates the formation of osseous tissue in the fascial components of muscles. The disease may occur with no apparent cause or may occur following a fracture or contusion. The onset of muscle pain is gradual.

INDICATIONS CONTRAINDICATIONS

For Therapeutic Massage

Treatment is contraindicated regionally in myositis ossificans. ■

Tendonitis and Tenosynovitis

Tendonitis is the inflammation of a tendon; tenosynovitis is the inflammation of a tendon sheath. Causes include trauma, overuse, and systemic inflammatory disease such as rheumatoid arthritis. Tendonitis is most common in the tendons crossing the shoulder, elbow, hip, knee, and ankle. Calcific tendonitis is a degenerative process in the tendon associated with the deposit of calcium salts. Early diagnosis and treatment are important.

INDICATIONS CONTRAINDICATIONS

For Therapeutic Massage

Any methods that could increase the inflammatory response are contraindicated for areas of inflammation. In the acute phase the use of ice and gentle movement are indicated. Chronic conditions may benefit from methods that elongate the connective tissue structures and restore normal resting length of the muscles, relieving friction in the area. ■

Cramps/Spasms

Cramps are painful muscle spasms or involuntary twitches. Cramps involve the whole muscle; spasms involve individual motor units within a muscle. Cramps often result from mild myositis or fibromyositis, but they can be a symptom of any irritation or of an electrolyte imbalance. *Clonic spasms* alternate contraction and relaxation in the muscle. *Tonic spasms,* or tetany, are sustained muscle contractions usually caused by disorders of the central nervous system.

Cramps and spasms may seem benign, but they can be symptomatic of more severe underlying conditions. If one cannot find a logical reason for the cramps or spasms or if the cramps or spasms occur frequently, the practitioner should refer the client for a diagnosis.

INDICATIONS CONTRAINDICATIONS

For Therapeutic Massage

One can manage simple cramps or spasms by firmly pushing the belly of the muscle together or by initiating reciprocal inhibition, which involves placing the attachment of the cramping muscle close together and then contracting the antagonist. The practitioner lengthens the muscle gently after the cramp or spasm has subsided. ■

Flaccidity and Spasticity

A muscle with decreased tone is flaccid; a muscle with excessive tone is spastic.

INDICATIONS CONTRAINDICATIONS

For Therapeutic Massage

Flaccid or spastic muscles often are associated with motor neuron disorders. The reason for the change in tone determines the appropriateness of massage or movement therapy. These conditions differ from general muscle tension or weakness in that the dysfunction has a physical cause rather than a functional one. ■

Contracture

Contracture is the chronic shortening of a muscle, especially the connective tissue component. *Volkmann's ischemic contracture* occurs in the upper or lower extremity when the blood supply is cut off and can be caused by tight casts, tourniquets, fractures, dislocations, or vascular spasms. The ischemia can lead to fibroses and can result in the contracture of the muscles, tendons, and fascia.

INDICATIONS CONTRAINDICATIONS

For Therapeutic Massage

Gentle, slow intervention using connective tissue methods and stretching may improve contractures. Applying soft tissue and movement methods may prevent or slow the development of a contracture. One must consider the reason for the contracture in developing a treatment plan for managing this condition. ■

Muscular Dystrophy

The term *muscular dystrophy* encompasses a group of disorders characterized by atrophy of skeletal muscles with no malfunction of the nervous system. The muscle protein dystrophin declines or is lacking. Some forms of muscular dystrophy can be fatal.

The most common form of muscular dystrophy is Duchenne's muscular dystrophy (DMD), also called pseudohypertrophy (meaning false muscle growth) because the atrophy of muscle is masked by excessive replacement of muscle by fat and fibrous tissue. DMD usually begins with mild leg muscle weakness that progresses rapidly to include the shoulder muscles.

The first signs of DMD become apparent at about 3 years of age, and the child usually is affected severely within 5 to 10 years. Death from respiratory or cardiac muscle weakness often occurs by the time the individual is 21 years old.

Many pathophysiologists believe that DMD is caused by a missing fragment in the X chromosome, although other factors may be involved. DMD occurs primarily in boys. Because girls have two X chromosomes and boys only one, genetic diseases involving X chromosome abnormalities are more likely to occur in boys. This is true because girls with one damaged X chromosome may not exhibit an X-linked disease if the other X chromosome is normal.

Some less devastating forms of muscular dystrophy are fascioscapulohumeral dystrophy, which affects the fascia and shoulder girdle muscles, and limb-girdle dystrophy, which affects the pelvic and shoulder girdle muscles.

INDICATIONS CONTRAINDICATIONS

For Therapeutic Massage

Careful intervention may slow the atrophy. Passive and active range of motion methods not only directly affect the muscles and joints but also aid in the circulation and elimination processes. Abdominal massage may help with constipation. One should avoid methods that cause any inflammation. ■

Amyotrophic Lateral Sclerosis

Amyotrophic lateral sclerosis symptoms may include tripping; stumbling and falling; loss of muscle control and strength in hands and arms; difficulty speaking, swallowing, or breathing; chronic fatigue; and muscle twitching and cramping. Amyotrophic lateral sclerosis is characterized by upper and lower motor neuron damage. Symptoms of upper motor neuron damage include stiffness (spasticity), muscle twitching (fasciculations), and muscle shaking (clonus). Symptoms of lower motor neuron damage include muscle weakness and muscle shrinking (atrophy).

Myasthenia Gravis

Myasthenia gravis is an autoimmune disease in which the immune system attacks muscle cells at the neuromuscular junction and interferes with the action of acetylcholine. Nerve impulses from the motor neurons then are unable to stimulate the affected muscle fully.

Myasthenia gravis is a chronic disease characterized by muscle weakness, especially in the face and throat. Most forms of this disease begin with mild weakness and chronic muscle fatigue in the face and then progress to wider muscle involvement. When severe muscle weakness causes immobility in all four limbs, the condition is called a myasthenic crisis. A person in myasthenic crisis is in danger of dying of respiratory failure because of weakness of the respiratory muscles.

INDICATIONS CONTRAINDICATIONS

For Therapeutic Massage

General constitutional methods are indicated. The practitioner should avoid stressing the system and work toward general restorative processes that reduce pain, support sleep, and create an overall sense of well-being. ■

Hernia

Hernias can be subcategorized into several types. Weakness of abdominal muscles is the usual cause of a hernia, or protrusion, of an abdominal organ (commonly the small intestine) through an opening in the abdominal wall. The most common type, the inguinal hernia, occurs when the hernia extends down the inguinal canal, often into the scrotum or labia. Males experience this most often, and herniation can occur at any age. Women may experience a femoral hernia below the groin, often caused by changes that occur during pregnancy.

A reducible hernia is one in which the protruding organ can be manipulated back into the abdominal cavity naturally by lying down or by manual reduction through a surgical opening in the abdomen. A strangulated hernia is one in which the hernia is not reducible, and blood flow to the affected organ (e.g., the intestine) is blocked, which may result in obstruction and gangrene. The individual usually experiences pain and vomiting, and immediate surgical repair is required.

INDICATIONS CONTRAINDICATIONS

For Therapeutic Massage

Treatment with a hernia is contraindicated regionally, and referral is indicated for initial diagnosis or for any change in a hernia. ■

Torticollis

Torticollis, or wry neck, involves a spasm or shortening of one of the sternocleidomastoid muscles. The condition may be congenital (e.g., caused by the fetal position or by a birth injury), acute (associated with cold or flu symptoms), or chronic (resulting from emotional stress, trauma, or infection).

INDICATIONS CONTRAINDICATIONS

For Therapeutic Massage

Management of torticollis with massage therapy involves relaxing the neck, releasing trigger points, stretching the contracted muscles, and improving range of motion. Avoiding pressure on the vessels under the sternocleidomastoid muscle is important. ■

Whiplash

Whiplash is an injury to the soft tissues of the neck caused by sudden hyperextension or flexion (or both) of the neck. The most common cause is an automobile accident, resulting in pain, swelling, stiffness, and spasm in the shoulders and neck. In extension injuries, the muscles most likely to be injured are the sternocleidomastoid, scalenes, infrahyoids, suprahyoids, levator scapulae, longus colli, suboccipitals, and rhomboids. In flexion injuries, the muscles most likely to be injured are the trapezius, splenius capitis, and semispinalis capitis. A side injury affects the sternocleidomastoid, suboccipitals, and levator scapulae, and the splenius capitis and splenius cervicis. Vestibular system damage of the inner ear may result in dizziness, nausea, vomiting, headache, and gait problems.

INDICATIONS CONTRAINDICATIONS

For Therapeutic Massage

Direct intervention during the acute phase is contraindicated unless closely supervised by a physician or other qualified health professional. Massage is valuable as part of rehabilitation in the subacute phase and can help restore function if the condition is chronic. Extension injury is the more severe and requires careful intervention. ■

Dupuytren's Contracture

The first sign of a Dupuytren contracture is a thickened plaque overlying the tendon of the ring finger and occasionally the little finger at the level of the distal palmar crease. The skin in this area puckers, and a thickened, fibrotic cord develops between the palm and the finger. Flexion contracture of the fingers may increase gradually.

INDICATIONS CONTRAINDICATIONS

For Therapeutic Massage

Treatment is contraindicated regionally if methods increase symptoms. ■

Rotator Cuff Tear

Repeated impingement, overuse, or other conditions may weaken the rotator cuff and eventually cause partial or complete tears. The condition is more common after age 40. Prior injury may increase the likelihood of a tear. Symptoms include weakness, atrophy of the supraspinatus and infraspinatus muscles, pain, and tenderness. A complete tear of the supraspinatus tendon severely impairs active abduction at the glenohumeral joint. An attempt to abduct the arm instead produces a characteristic shoulder shrug.

INDICATIONS CONTRAINDICATIONS

For Therapeutic Massage

Work on acute myofascial tears is contraindicated. However, massage therapy may be indicated in the rehabilitative process and as part of a supervised treatment protocol. One can manage or improve compensatory patterns with massage. ■

Shin Splints

Shin splints are an inflammation of the proximal portion of any of the musculotendinous structures originating from the lower part of the tibia. Pain is associated with movement, and stress fractures are a common cause.

INDICATIONS CONTRAINDICATIONS

For Therapeutic Massage

Massage approaches may be beneficial as long as they do not increase inflammation and a stress fracture has been ruled out. ■

Anterior Compartment Syndrome

The anterior compartment of the leg is surrounded by a tough fascial sheath containing the tibialis anterior, the extensor digitorum longus, the extensor hallucis longus, and the peroneus (fibularis) tertius muscles, as well as nerves and blood vessels. Any condition that increases pressure in this compartment interferes with blood flow and compresses the nerves. The person usually has a tight feeling in the calf, as well as pain, numbness, and tingling. Overuse, repetitive stress, and accelerated growth of the muscles are common causal factors.

INDICATIONS CONTRAINDICATIONS

For Therapeutic Massage

Treatment is contraindicated regionally unless supervised by the diagnosing or treating health care provider. Massage methods may soften the connective tissue sheath, relieving some of the pressure, but they also could aggravate the inflammatory process. They also can relieve fluid congestion, but by enhancing circulation, they also could increase blood flow to the area, thus increasing the pressure. Elevation and ice may help. ■

Plantar Fasciitis

Plantar fasciitis is an inflammation of the plantar fascia and surrounding myofascial structures. The disorder is caused by excessive stress on the foot, especially near the attachment of the fascia to the calcaneus. The stress causes calcium to be deposited at the site, and often a spur forms. Pain in the heel is worse when the person is moving, and dorsiflexion increases the pain.

INDICATIONS CONTRAINDICATIONS

For Therapeutic Massage

Acute-phase plantar fasciitis responds to rest and ice. After the inflammation has diminished, massage of connective tissue and judicial use of stretching are beneficial. (If the client is taking antiinflammatory or pain medication, feedback mechanisms will be inaccurate.) ■

Fibromyalgia

Fibromyalgia is a syndrome with symptoms of widespread pain or aching, persistent fatigue, generalized morning stiffness, nonrestorative sleep, and multiple tender points. The symptoms often are found with headaches, irritable bladder, dysmenorrhea, cold sensitivity, Raynaud's phenomenon, restless legs, atypical patterns of numbness and tingling, and complaints of weakness. The onset usually is gradual, often following prolonged exposure to damp cold, a bacterial or viral infection, or prolonged physical or emotional stress. *Chronic fatigue syndrome* also may be present.

A disrupted sleep pattern, coupled with the dysfunction of myofascial repair mechanisms, seems to be a factor. Treatment protocols aim at sleep restoration and a gradual rebuilding of the myofascial system. Diet and lifestyle changes, moderate exercise, and various forms of complementary therapies and mind/body approaches are beneficial. If necessary, low doses of antidepressants often can help restore sleep patterns.

INDICATIONS CONTRAINDICATIONS

For Therapeutic Massage

General constitutional approaches seem to work best to aid in symptomatic pain reduction and restoration of the sleep pattern. The practitioner should avoid any form of therapy that causes therapeutic inflammation, including intense exercise and stretching programs, until healing mechanisms in the body are functioning. When one introduces exercise programs, the process needs to be gentle and slow. If tender points have been injected with antiinflammatory medications, anesthetics, or other substances, one should not massage over the area. ■

Acquired Metabolic and Toxic Myopathies

Acquired metabolic myopathies often occur following disorders of the endocrine system. Nutritional and vitamin deficiency, especially protein deficiency and lack of vitamins C, D, and E, may lead to myopathy.

Toxic myopathies are related to certain drugs and chemicals. Corticosteroid therapy may cause steroid-induced muscle weakness. An excessive alcohol intake can result in breakdown of striated muscles, which can affect the skeletal and other muscles.

INDICATIONS CONTRAINDICATIONS

For Therapeutic Massage

Treatment for these types of myopathy usually is not contraindicated, as long as the therapeutic approaches are general and focus on supporting body restoration and the healing processes. Regional avoidance of steroid injection sites is indicated. ■

Massage can support detoxification efforts, because these methods enhance circulation. One must take care in toxic conditions not to tax an already overloaded system. A general therapeutic approach over a longer period is indicated.

SUMMARY

Just as muscles are able to contract concentrically, eccentrically, and isometrically, massage professionals play various roles. You, the massage professional, are the one who provides the massage application, education to the client in wellness strategies, supports other professions in multidisciplinary teams, and maintains stability in scope of practice and ethical boundaries in the professional relationship. Just like muscles, your job requires a specific function depending on the demands and most of the time is an ever-changing dynamic process. Competency is measured by how you are able to take information and use it in a multidimensional way and in functional units. This chapter presents functional patterns of interaction of the muscles. This information is used functionally in the massage practice in multiple ways as well. Understanding the location and various actions of muscles and their relationship to the rest of the body influences skilled assessment, clinical reasoning, decision making on appropriate methods to achieve outcomes for the session, charting and other forms of written documentation, and interaction with other health and training professionals.

This chapter has taken an in-depth look at the muscular system. We have explored individual muscles and have mapped the interdependent nature of muscular action in the synergist and antagonist pattern of each muscle. We identified common trigger points and their referred pain patterns. We discussed the progression of pathologic conditions in muscle dysfunction along with the indications and contraindications for massage for specific muscle-related dysfunctions.

We explore the larger picture of dynamic movement in the next chapter, where we see all the parts—bones, joints, and muscles—as a functioning unit, which is more than the sum of its parts.

evolve

Several activities on the Fritz EVOLVE site reinforce the anatomy lessons taught in Chapter 9. Log on to your student account, and explore the dissection atlas as well as the anatomy weblinks that are located under the Chapter 9 Course Material section.

Workbook Section

1. List and describe the functions of muscles.

2. List and describe the three types of muscles.

3. List and describe the three types of skeletal muscle fibers.

4. List and describe the four components of myotatic units.

Fill in the Blank

An agonist is a muscle that causes or controls joint motion through a specified plane of motion and also is known as a primary or (1) ______________ mover.

The (2) ______________ occurs when a muscle contraction is initiated and all the muscle fibers contract to their full ability, or they do not contract at all.

A(n) (3) ______________ is a muscle that usually is located on the opposite side of the joint from the agonist and that has the opposite action. (4) ________________ and antagonist muscles can contract together at the same time in what is called a (5) ________________.

Contractility is the ability of a muscle to (6) ________ forcibly with adequate stimulation.

(7) ________________ forms a coarse sheet of fibrous connective tissue that binds muscles into functional groups and forms partitions, called intermuscular septa, between muscle groups.

Dynamic force produces (8) ________________ in or of an object.

Elasticity is the ability of a muscle to recoil and resume its original resting length after being (9) ________________. Applying force is called (10) ________________, and releasing force is called unloading.

(11) ________________ is the ability of a muscle to receive and respond to a stimulus.

(12) ________________ is the ability of a muscle to be stretched or extended.

A(n) (13) ________________ is a stabilizing muscle located at a joint that contracts to fixate, or stabilize, an area, enabling another limb or body segment to exert force and move.

The insertion is the most movable part of a muscle, or the part that attaches (14) ________________ from the midline or center of the body.

Maximal stimulus is the point at which all the motor units of a muscle have been recruited and the muscle is unable to (15) ________________ in strength.

A (16) ________________ consists of the muscle fibers innervated by a single motor neuron.

The (17) ________________ is the part of a muscle considered the least movable, or the part that attaches closest to the midline or center of the body.

Oxygen debt is the extra amount of oxygen that must be taken in to convert (18) ________________ to glucose or glycogen.

(19) ________________ force applied to an object does not produce movement.

Synergist muscles aid or assist the action of the agonists but are not primarily responsible for the action; synergists are also known as (20) ________________ muscles.

The (21) ________________ is the stimulus at which the first observable muscle contraction occurs.

Tone is a state of slight (22) ________________ in all skeletal muscle that enables the muscle to respond to stimulation.

A trigger point, as described by Janet Travell, is a (23) ________________ locus within a taut band of skeletal muscle, located in the muscular tissue or its associated fascia or both. The spot is painful on compression and can evoke characteristic (24) ________________ pain and autonomic phenomena. (25) ________________ involves neurochemical responses of the muscle fiber. Stretching involves a (26) ________________ force directed to altering connective tissue structure.

According to Myers, (27) ________________ refers to structures that maintain their integrity primarily because of a balance of continuous tensile forces through the structure.

PROBLEM SOLVING

Read the problem presented. There is no correct answer; rather the exercise is intended to assist the student in developing the analytic and decision-making skills necessary in a professional practice. After reading the problem, follow the next six steps:

1. Identify the facts presented in the information.
2. Identify the possibilities ("what if" statements) or develop your own possibilities that relate to the facts.
3. Evaluate each possibility in terms of the logical cause and effect and pros and cons.
4. Consider the effect on the persons involved.
5. Write each answer in the space provided.
6. Develop your solution by answering the question posed.

Problem

Massage professionals focus on the muscular system as they work with clients. Therefore thinking in terms of individual muscles certainly seems logical when working with assessment ... or is it? This chapter described the way muscles work in functional units. The nervous system controls muscles. Connective tissue is a huge component of muscles. Muscle tension increases with sympathetic arousal, as in the fight-or-flight response. Is it possible that therapeutic massage really has little to do with muscle tissue?

Many testing processes focus extensively on the functional aspect of individual muscles and little on the more systemic effects of massage. This situation may influence the curriculum at schools that teach massage therapies. One wonders if such an education may overemphasize the study of individual muscles and underemphasize the nervous system, endocrine system, and systemic homeostatic processes. The study of muscles is important. The truth is that the massage practitioner really understands functional patterns of movement only when he or she has a solid comprehension of the components of movement—the bones, the joints, the connective tissue, and the muscles. Also true is that the major benefits of massage are based in the systems of control and support of connective tissue structures.

Question

In this age of "too much to know," what learning is necessary to function as a competent health professional?

Facts

1. Massage professionals focus on the muscular system.
2. ______________________________

____
3. ______________________________

____

Possibilities

1. Curricula at schools that teach massage therapies may be influenced by examination requirements.
2. ______________________________

____
3. ______________________________

____

Logical Cause and Effect

1. Important areas of study are not covered effectively because of lack of time.
2. ______________________________

____
3. ______________________________

____

Effect

1. Students may be frustrated with studying information that seems less important.
2. ______________________________

____
3. ______________________________

____

In this age of "too much to know," what learning is necessary to function as a health professional?

____

____

____

____

Professional Application

What additional knowledge base would one need to work with stress-induced muscle tension and headache for therapeutic massage? Where might a massage practitioner find this information and get additional training?

____

____

____

____

____

____

____

____

____

____

____

____

____

____

____

____

____

____

WORKBOOK SECTION

FURTHER STUDY

Using additional resource material (see the Works Consulted list at the back of this book), find the chapter that pertains to the information presented in this chapter. As a study guide, locate the information presented in this text and then elaborate by writing a paragraph of additional information on each of the following topics.

1. Force

2. Motor points

3. Repair of muscle

4. Cardiac muscle

5. Smooth muscle

Answer Key

1. Muscles produce movement, generate heat, maintain posture, and stabilize joints.

   All three types of muscle tissue provide the movement necessary for survival. Skeletal muscle moves the limbs. Skeletal, cardiac, and smooth muscle produce movements such as those involved in breathing, heartbeat, digestion, and elimination.

   The relative constancy of the internal temperature of the body could not be maintained in a cool external environment if not for the "waste" heat generated by muscle tissue during contraction.

   Maintenance of a stable body posture is the primary function of the muscular skeletal system. The dynamic tension of muscle contraction opposes the forces of gravity.

   Stability of the joint structures is an often overlooked function of muscle. Especially in the more mobile joints, which by nature have a loose structural design, the dynamic and static contraction of muscles surrounding the joint provides external stability, supporting the structures of the joint proper.
2. Skeletal, cardiac, and smooth muscle

   Skeletal muscle fibers are long, cylindric, tapered cells that have cross-striations caused by the contractile structure inside. Skeletal muscles contain white, red, and intermediate muscle fibers. Each muscle fiber is wrapped by several different layers of connective tissue.

   Cardiac muscle is found in only one organ of the body, the heart. Cardiac muscle fiber does not taper, as does skeletal muscle fiber, but instead forms strong, electrically coupled junctions (intercalated disks) with other fibers. Cardiac muscles form a continuous contractile band around the heart.

Smooth muscle comprises small, tapered cells with single nuclei. Because the myofilaments are not organized into sarcomeres, they have more freedom of movement and can contract a smooth muscle fiber to shorter lengths than can be done in skeletal and cardiac muscle.

3. Fast-twitch (white) fibers contract more rapidly and forcefully, are larger than red fibers, and belong to larger motor units that activate when the nervous system demands rapid, powerful motion. They do not require much oxygen to contract and are considered anaerobic. White fibers fatigue quickly.

   Red (slow-twitch) fibers are smaller, contract more slowly and weakly, and belong to smaller motor units that respond during slower, delicate movements. Red fibers contain much larger quantities of myoglobin, require the presence of oxygen for contraction, and are considered aerobic. They do not fatigue quickly and can hold a contraction for a long period, making them highly efficient in muscles that maintain posture.

   Intermediate fibers combine the qualities of red and white fibers, allowing a rapid, moderately forceful contraction and providing moderate fatigue resistance.

4. Agonists: Muscles that use concentric contraction and cause or control joint motion through a specified plane of motion

   Synergists: Muscles in concentric contraction that aid or assist the action of the agonists

   Antagonists: Muscles that usually are located on the opposite side of the joint from the agonist and have the opposite action

   Fixators (stabilizers): Muscles that surround the joint or body part and isometrically contract to fixate or stabilize the area to enable another limb or body segment to exert force and move

Fill in the Blank

1. prime
2. all-or-none response
3. antagonist
4. Agonist
5. co-contraction
6. shorten
7. Deep fascia
8. movement
9. stretched
10. loading
11. Excitability
12. Extensibility
13. fixator
14. farthest
15. increase
16. motor unit
17. origin
18. lactic acid
19. Static
20. guiding
21. threshold stimulus
22. contraction
23. hyperirritable
24. referred
25. Lengthening
26. mechanical
27. tensegrity

CHAPTER 10

Biomechanics Basics

▼ CHAPTER OBJECTIVES

After completing this chapter, the student will be able to perform the following:

- Explain the basic principles of biomechanics.
- Identify and describe the three main biomechanical dysfunctional patterns.
- Assess biomechanical function for the regions of the body.

▼ CHAPTER OUTLINE

▼ KEY TERMS

Center of gravity An imaginary midpoint or center of the weight of a body or object, where the body or object could balance on a point.

Effort The force applied to overcome resistance.

Gait The rhythmic and alternating motions of the legs, trunk, and arms resulting in the propulsion of the body.

Gait cycle Subdivided into the stance phase and swing phase, this cycle begins when the heel of one foot strikes the floor and continues until the same heel strikes the floor again.

Kinesiology (ki-NE-SE-ol-O-JE) Combines the fields of anatomy, physiology, physics, and geometry and relates them to human movement.

Kinetic chain An integrated functional unit. The kinetic chain is made up of the myofascial system (muscle, ligament, tendon, and fascia), articular (joint) system, and nervous system. Each of these systems works interdependently to allow structural and functional efficiency in all three planes of motion: sagittal, frontal, and transverse.

Lever A solid mass such as a crowbar or a person's arm that rotates around a fixed point called the fulcrum. The rotation is produced by a force applied to a lever at some distance from the fulcrum.

Vector The direction of the force.

Biomechanics

Because a variety of forces may act on the human body and lead to movement, rest, or stress, the massage therapist must have a basic understanding of biomechanical principles. Understanding these principles helps us in assessing and observing the body and in clinical reasoning methods used to develop treatment plans.

Biomechanics is the study of mechanical principles and actions applied to living bodies. This may involve looking at the static (nonmoving) or dynamic (moving) systems associated with various activities. ***Kinesiology*** is the study of movement that emerges and blends the knowledge of anatomy, physiology, physics, and geometry and relates them to human movement. Dynamic systems can be divided into kinetics and kinematics. *Kinetics* are those forces causing movement, whereas *kinematics* are those time, space, and mass aspects of a moving system.

Physical therapists, occupational therapists, exercise physiologists, and athletic trainers deal with the performance-specific and rehabilitative analysis of human movement and undertake extended studies to address problems with biomechanics or to develop specific training and exercise protocols. One should refer clients to these professionals after identifying movement problems during assessment. Therapeutic massage can be a valuable adjunct modality to the rehabilitation programs developed by these health care specialists.

Movement is a fundamental characteristic of human behavior and is accomplished by contraction of skeletal muscles acting within a system of **levers** and pulleys formed by bones, tendons, and ligaments that network into the unified tensegric system of the body.

Muscles have properties permitting a large range of function to meet various demands; these demands may require the coordination of complex interactions. Sometimes muscles are required to function for long periods without fatiguing, and at other times muscles must provide maximal **effort** for only a few seconds. Muscles must shorten and lengthen to provide range of motion at joints, yet they must generate enough power to move a load at each end of the range. They must be able to hold a static position to provide stability. The nervous system accomplishes the fine control of muscle contraction over a wide range of lengths, tensions, speeds, and loads.

As discussed in Chapter 9, muscles differ in fiber type depending on the function of the muscle. *White fast-twitch* fibers contract rapidly and forcefully, are large, and belong to larger motor units that fire when the nervous system demands rapid, powerful motion. They do not require much oxygen to contract, are considered anaerobic, and fatigue quickly. *Red slow-twitch* fibers are smaller, contract more slowly and with less strength, and belong to smaller motor units that respond during slower, delicate movements. Red fibers contain much larger quantities of mitochondria, which produce adenosine triphosphate, therefore providing energy for cell activity. Red fibers also have myosin, which contains proteins, and myoglobin, which stores oxygen within the muscle cell. Red fibers require the presence of oxygen for contraction and are considered aerobic. They do not fatigue quickly and can hold a contraction for a long period. Red fibers often are found in postural muscles. *Intermediate fibers* combine the qualities of red and white fibers to allow a rapid, moderate force contraction and moderate fatigue resistance. Muscles also have three major contraction types: isometric, concentric, and eccentric. Chapter 9 describes and lists these functions for most of the individual muscles discussed.

Center of Gravity

The concept of *center* has many meanings. In Eastern thought, the importance of being centered often is expressed as being present in the moment and responding resourcefully to each unfolding second of life.

In biomechanical terms, the concept of center refers to the **center of gravity,** the midpoint, or center, of the weight of a body or object. The center of gravity is where the body or object would balance on a point.

No anatomic center of gravity exists. The position of the center of gravity depends on the arrangement of the body segments and changes with every movement. In terms of Eastern thought, the principles are similar, and being centered is just as situational as the center of gravity. When centered in biomechanical terms or life in general, we have the ability to respond resourcefully to each event as it happens. Any loss of biomechanical stability, such as occurs with a missing limb or altered posture, alters not only the total body weight distribution but also the center of gravity. On a mental and emotional level, most of us can understand the way losses in life change our sense of center and reveal our human potential to alter, accommodate, and adjust to change just as our body does on a physical level.

Accumulated postural or movement alterations can stress the entire system, initiating a change process that can progress toward dysfunction. Although each alteration may seem to be appropriate to the moment, the accumulated chain reaction of change can become too much and the system breaks under the inefficient function. The sense of center is lost. Understanding biomechanics helps us to be able to reverse the degeneration process and move toward efficient functioning.

Force

Force causes change. *Forces* push or pull on an object in an attempt to affect motion or shape. The human body moves under this influence, and internal and external forces affect it. Within the body, the contraction of muscles primarily produces force. External forces acting on the body include gravity and forces generated by the interaction with external objects such as lifting a box or managing an umbrella in the wind. Therapeutic massage attempts to alter body function by exerting external force to generate internal forces that then effect change in the homeostatic mechanisms of the body. Forces generated by massage include tension, torsion, bend, shear, and compression. Chapter 8 defined these forces in detail.

Technically, force is the product of mass multiplied by acceleration. A **vector** is the direction of the force. Mass is the amount of matter or material substance that forms or composes a body. For our purposes, weight and mass are the same. The weight times the speed or acceleration determines the amount of force. A light feather floating softly down to touch our arm exerts less force than a bowling ball thrown down an alley.

The following elements influence or are related to force:

Pressure: Pressure is the amount of force on a specific area.

Inertia: Inertia is the reluctance of matter to change its state of motion and can be understood as the lack of desire to shut off the TV and begin doing the reading in this text. Many of us waste energy going to the refrigerator, looking out the window, or listening to the conversations of others as we try to study. Because force is required to change inertia, any activity that is carried out at a steady pace, in a consistent direction, conserves energy. Any irregularly paced or multidirectional activity is costly to energy reserves. A movement example is handball, which is more fatiguing than dancing. A pearl of wisdom exists in the understanding of force acting on matter to change motion. Starts and stops and juggling many different tasks at one time is fatiguing and stressful. Life lived at a steady pace with a sense of direction (vector) or purpose supports effectiveness.

Acceleration: Acceleration is the rate of change in speed. To begin to move the body and attain speed generally requires a strong muscular force. Weight (mass) coupled with the influence of gravity affects speed and acceleration during physical movements. Accelerating a 200-lb adult takes more muscle force than accelerating a 100-lb child. Acceleration occurs in the same direction as the force that caused it. The change in acceleration is directly proportional to the force causing it and inversely proportional to the mass of the body. This means that a large force provides a greater degree of acceleration than a small force. Given the same amount of force, more acceleration occurs on a light body than on a heavy one.

Newton's law of reaction says that for every action, there is an opposite and equal reaction. As we place force on the floor by walking over it, the floor provides an equal resistance back in the opposite direction to the soles of our feet. Walking on a wood floor is easier than walking on a sandy beach because of the difference in the reaction of the two surfaces. The wood floor resists the weight and pushes back, making walking easier, whereas the sand dissipates the force and requires more effort with each step.

As a muscle contracts through its range of motion, the amount of moving or stabilizing force changes. As the muscle increases moving force, it decreases its stabilizing force, and vice versa. Muscles that span a long distance, such as the biceps brachii of the arm, are most efficient supplying movement through a longer range of motion. Other muscles are more effective at stabilizing the joint than moving it. The coracobrachialis of the shoulder joint is a good example; its line of pull is mostly vertical and close to the axis of the shoulder joint. Therefore the coracobrachialis has a short range of motion, which makes this muscle more effective at stabilizing than flexing the shoulder joint. Opposing muscle groups generate parallel forces to provide stability. This is achieved through co-contraction mechanisms (Figures 10-1 and 10-2).

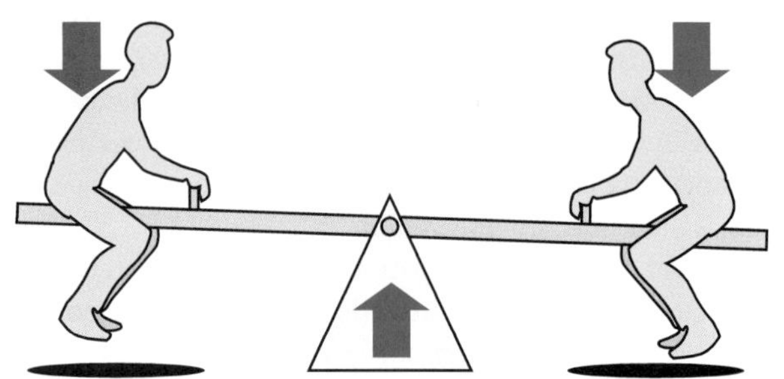

Figure 10-1
Parallel forces demonstrated by the seesaw with counterforce in the middle.

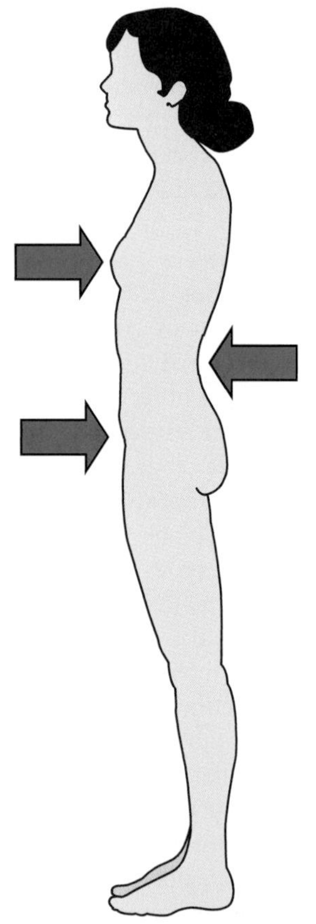

Figure 10-2
Core muscles of the torso use parallel forces to stabilize the torso, acting like a body brace and functioning like the balanced seesaw in Figure 10-1.

Levers and Fulcrums

We need force to generate a motion in a straight line and produce rotation or angular motion. We often achieve force using a lever, which helps a given effort move a heavier load or move a load farther than could otherwise be done. A lever is a rigid bar or mass that rotates around a fixed point called the axis of rotation or fulcrum. One then produces rotation by applying force to a lever at some distance from the fulcrum. The locomotion system of the human body may be considered a series of interconnected levers. In the forearm the radius and ulna act as a lever, with the elbow joint as the fulcrum (Figure 10-3).

A force applied to a lever to overcome resistance is called the *effort.* In the forearm during elbow flexion against resistance, the effort is the force exerted by the muscles. One can use the applied force, or effort, to move a resistance or load such as when lifting a box.

In the body, joints are the fulcrums and bones are the levers. Muscle contraction provides the effort and applies it at the muscle attachment points on a bone. The load that is moved includes the bone, the overlying tissues, and anything else one tries to move with that particular lever, such as a book bag.

Mechanical Advantage and Disadvantage

Mechanical advantage means that less force is required to move an object, and mechanical disadvantage requires more force to move the same object (Figure 10-4).

Regardless of the type, all levers follow the same basic principles:

- Effort closer to the load than to the fulcrum produces mechanical disadvantage.
- Effort farther from the load than from the fulcrum produces mechanical advantage.

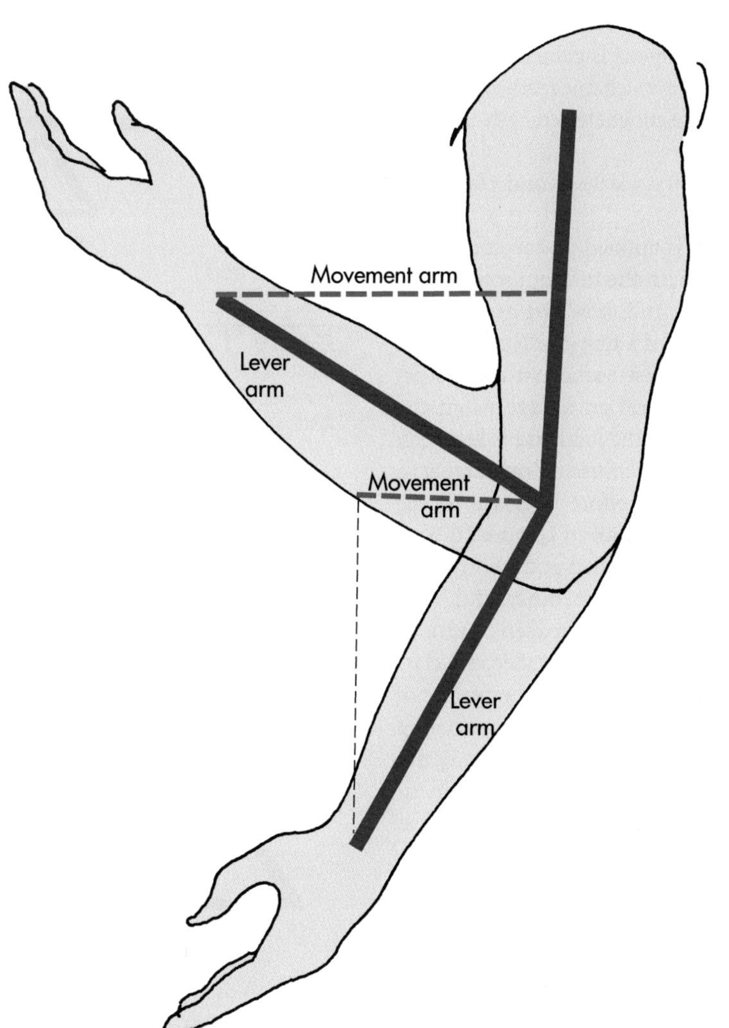

Figure 10-3
A lever is a rigid body that moves around a fixed axis. The lever arm remains the same throughout the movement, but the movement arm for the lever may change as the lever moves. (From Roberts SL, Falkenburg SA: *Biomechanics: problem solving for functional activity,* St Louis, 1992, Mosby.)

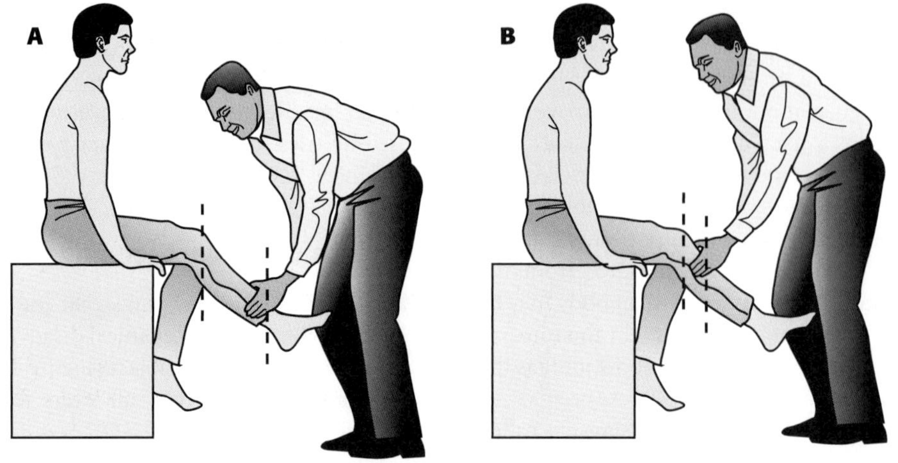

Figure 10-4
Longer force arm in **A** (mechanical advantage) requires less force than in **B** (mechanical disadvantage).

- In lever systems that operate at a mechanical disadvantage, force is lost but speed is gained.
- Lever systems that operate at a mechanical advantage are slower, more stable, and are used where strength is a priority.

Three types of levers exist: first class, second class, and third class.

In *first-class levers* the effort is applied at one end of the lever and the load at the other, with the fulcrum somewhere between them. Seesaws, scissors, and crowbars are familiar examples of first-class levers. Use of a first-class lever occurs when you lift your head off your chest. Some first-class levers in the body operate at a mechanical advantage when the effort is farther from the joint than the load and is less than the load to be moved. But other muscles operate at a mechanical disadvantage when the effort is closer to the joint and greater than the load to be moved (Figure 10-5).

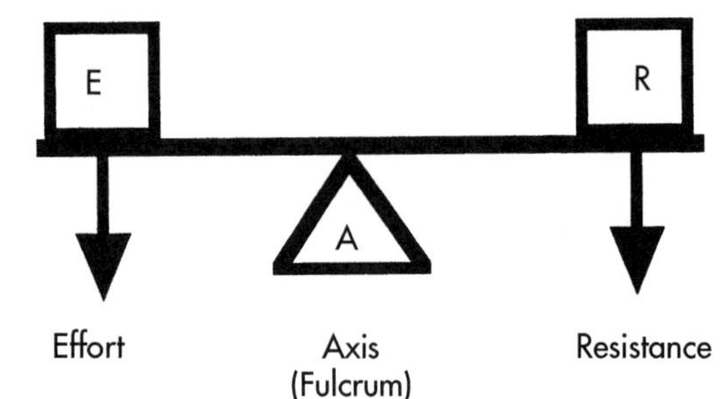

Figure 10-5
A first-class lever has its axis of motion between the force of effort and the force of resistance. (From Roberts SL, Falkenburg SA: *Biomechanics: problem solving for functional activity,* St Louis, 1992, Mosby.)

In *second-class levers* the effort is applied at the end of the lever and the fulcrum is located at the other end with the load at some intermediate point between them. A wheelbarrow is an example of this type of lever. Second-class levers are uncommon in the body, and the best example of their use is standing on your toes. Joints forming the ball of the foot act together as the fulcrum. The load is the entire body weight. The calf muscles inserted into the calcaneus exert the effort, pulling the heel upward. All second-class levers in the body work at a mechanical advantage because the muscle insertion is always farther from the fulcrum than is the load to be moved. Second-class levers are levers of strength, with speed and range of motion sacrificed (Figure 10-6).

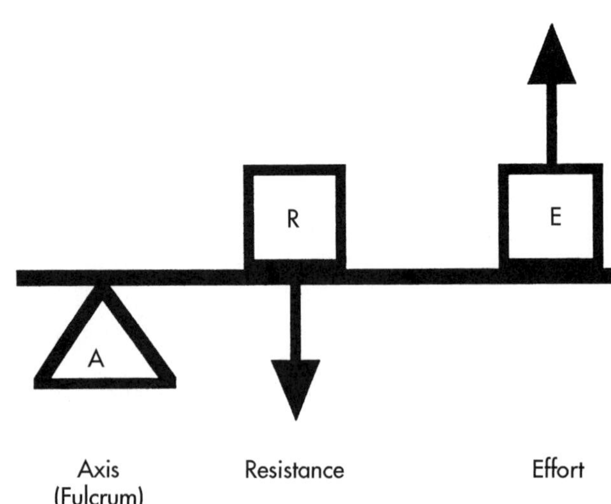

Figure 10-6
In a second-class lever the force of resistance lies between the axis of movement and the force of effort. (From Roberts SL, Falkenburg SA: *Biomechanics: problem solving for functional activity,* St Louis, 1992, Mosby.)

In *third-class levers* the effort is applied at a point between the load and the fulcrum. These levers operate with greater speed and always at a mechanical disadvantage. Tweezers or forceps provide this type of leverage. Most of the body operates with a third-class lever system that permits a muscle

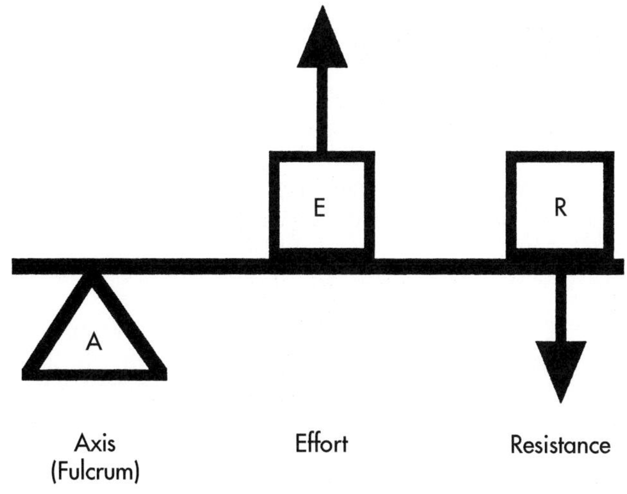

Figure 10-7
A third-class lever has its force of effort lying between the axis and the force of resistance. (From Roberts SL, Falkenburg SA: *Biomechanics: problem solving for functional activity,* St Louis, 1992, Mosby.)

to be inserted close to a joint, allowing rapid extensive movement with little shortening of the muscle. As an example, the biceps muscle of the arm provides the effort, the fulcrum is the elbow, and the force is exerted on the proximal radius. The load to be lifted is the distal forearm and anything carried in the hand or over the forearm (Figure 10-7).

Balance, Equilibrium, and Stability

Balance is the ability to control equilibrium. The two types of balance are *static* or still balance and dynamic or moving balance. Equilibrium means that all forces acting on an object are equal. Equilibrium may be static or dynamic. A body at rest or completely motionless is in *static equilibrium. Dynamic equilibrium* occurs when all of the applied and internal forces acting on the moving body are in balance, resulting in movement with no change in speed or direction. For us to control equilibrium to achieve balance, we need to maximize stability.

Stability is the resistance to change in the acceleration of the body or the resistance to the disturbance of the equilibrium of the body. Determining the center of gravity of the body and changing it appropriately may enhance stability. The center of gravity is the point at which all of the mass, or weight, of the body is balanced equally or distributed equally in all directions.

Kinesthetic physiologic functions contribute to balance. The tonic neck reflex is a reflex pattern stimulated by head movement that stimulates flexion and extension of the limbs, arms, and neck. The semicircular canals of the inner ear, vision, touch, pressure, and proprioceptive sense provide balance information. The body is in a constant dynamic state of adjustment to maintain balance, reflecting dynamic homeostasis.

Balance Principles

Basic principles of balance have broad application. The following principles speak not only of a body in balance but also of a balanced life, if applied to a social or personal realm:

- A person is balanced when his or her center of gravity falls within the base of support.
- A person is balanced in direct proportion to the size of the base of support. The larger the base of support, the more balance.
- A person is balanced depending on his or her weight, or mass. The greater the weight, the more balance.
- A person's balance depends on the height of the center of gravity. The lower the center of gravity, the more balance.
- A person's balance depends on where his or her center of gravity is in relation to the base of support. If the center of gravity is near the edge of the base, less balance is present. However, in anticipation of an oncoming force, one may improve stability by placing the center of gravity closer to the side of the base of support expected to receive the force.
- In anticipation of an oncoming force, one may increase stability by enlarging the size of the base of support in the direction of the anticipated force.
- A person may enhance equilibrium by increasing the friction between the body and the surface it contacts.
- Rotation around an axis is easier to balance. A bike that is moving is easier to balance than a bike that is stationary (Thompson and Floyd, 1994) (Activity 10-1).

Posture

The postural muscles help us to maintain our upright position in gravity. This task is awesome because the center of gravity constantly changes with each movement. When we lie down, we relieve the postural muscles of this task.

Good posture is important because it decreases the amount of stress placed on ligaments, muscles, and tendons and improves function and decreases the amount of muscle energy needed to keep the body upright.

Vertebral Alignment

The vertebral column is a column of block-shaped bones stacked in counterbalancing anterior-posterior curves. At birth the entire vertebral column is concave anteriorly and called the *primary curve.* As the child grows, anteriorly convex curves of the cervical and lumbar regions develop. These curves are maintained during rest and activity and function as shock absorbers. The thoracic and sacral curves counter the cervical and lumbar curves. The thoracic and sacral curves are concave anteriorly and convex posteriorly. Conversely, the lumbar and cervical curves are convex anteriorly and concave posteriorly. Any change of these vertebral curves, such as an increase or decrease, results in poor posture. For example, a sway back is an increased lumbar curve, called *lordosis,* whereas a flat back is a decreased thoracic curve. No lateral curves should exist. Any

ACTIVITY 10-1

Draw a picture to illustrate each of the principles of balance.

A person is balanced when his or her center of gravity falls within the base of support.

A person is balanced in direct proportion to the size of the base of support. The larger the base of support, the more balance.

A person is balanced depending on his or her weight or mass. The greater the weight, the more balance.

A person's balance depends on the height of the center of gravity. The lower the center of gravity, the more balance.

A person's balance depends on where his or her center of gravity is in relation to the base of support. A center of gravity that is near the edge of the base provides less balance. However, when anticipating an oncoming force, stability may be improved by placing the center of gravity closer to the side of the base of support expected to receive the force.

In anticipation of an oncoming force, stability may be increased by enlarging the size of the base of support in the direction of the anticipated force.

Equilibrium may be enhanced by increasing the friction between the body and the surface it contacts.

Rotation around an axis is easier to balance. A bike that is moving is easier to balance than a bike that is stationary.

lateral curvature of the spine is a pathologic condition called *scoliosis.*

The pelvis should be in a neutral position, defined as (1) when the anterior superior iliac spine and posterior superior iliac spine are level with each other in a transverse plane and (2) when the anterior superior interior spine is in the same vertical plane as the symphysis pubis. When the pelvis is in a neutral position, the lumbar curve has the desired amount of curvature. When the pelvis is tilted anteriorly, the amount of lumbar curvature increases, causing lordosis. When the pelvis is tilted posteriorly, the amount of curve decreases, causing flat back.

When weight is distributed evenly on both legs, the pelvis should remain level from side to side, with the anterior superior iliac spine and anterior superior interior spine being at the same level. During the normal walking **gait,** the pelvis dips from side to side as weight shifts from stance to swing phase. This lateral pelvic tilt is controlled by the hip abductors, mainly the gluteus medius and gluteus minimus, and the trunk lateral flexors, primarily the erector spinae and quadratus lumborum.

In the upright position, posture depends primarily on muscle contractions and fascial support to remain upright in gravity. The muscles most involved are called antigravity muscles. The antigravity muscles are primarily the hip and knee extensors and the trunk and neck extensors. Other muscles maintaining the upright position are the trunk and neck flexors and lateral flexors, hip abductors and adductors, and the ankle pronators (everters) and supinators (inverters). If all of these muscles were to relax, the body would collapse.

The ankle plantar flexors and dorsiflexors are important in controlling postural sway. Postural sway is anterior-posterior motion of the upright body caused by motion occurring primarily at the ankles. This sway results from the constant displacement and correction of the center of gravity within the base of support.

One can assess a person's posture most accurately using a plumb line suspended from the ceiling or a posture grid behind the person as a point of reference (Figure 10-8). A plumb line is a string or cord with a weight attached to the lower end. Because the string is weighted, it makes a perfectly straight vertical line in gravity.

Lateral view. In the standing position and viewed from the lateral position, the plumb line should be aligned so that it passes slightly in front of the lateral malleolus. For ideal posture, the body segments should be aligned so that the plumb line passes through the landmarks listed below as follows:

Head	Through the ear lobe
Shoulder	Through the tip of the acromion process
Thoracic spine	Anterior to the vertebral bodies
Lumbar spine	Through the vertebral bodies
Pelvis	Level
Hip	Through the greater trochanter (slightly posterior to the hip joint axis)
Knee	Slightly posterior to the patella (slightly anterior to the knee joint axis) with the knees in extension
Ankle	Slightly anterior to the lateral malleolus with the ankle joint in a neutral position between dorsiflexion and plantar flexion

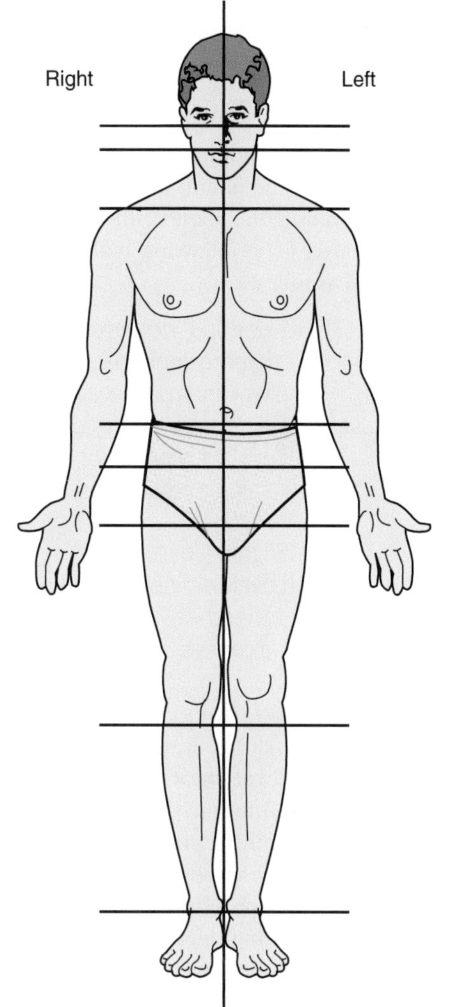

Figure 10-8
Posture grid. Gridlines identify symmetry or deviations in symmetry.

Anterior view. In the standing position and viewed from the anterior position, the plumb line should be aligned to pass through the midsagittal plane of the body, thus dividing the body into two halves. The following body segments listed below should be aligned as follows:

Head	Extended and level, not flexed or hyperextended
Shoulders	Level and not elevated or depressed
Sternum	Centered in the midline
Hips	Level with the anterior superior iliac and anterior superior interior spines in the same plane

Legs	Slightly apart
Knees	Level and not bowed or knock-kneed
Ankles	Normal arch in feet
Feet	Slight toeing outward

Posterior view. In the standing position and viewed from the posterior position, the plumb line should be aligned to pass through the midsagittal plane of the body, dividing the body into two halves. The following body segments listed should be aligned as follows:

Head	Extended, not flexed or hyperextended
Shoulders	Level and not elevated or depressed
Spinous processes	Centered in the midline
Hips	Level with posterior superior iliac spine and in the same plane with ASIS
Legs	Slightly apart
Knees	Level and not bowed or knock-kneed
Ankles	Calcaneus should be straight

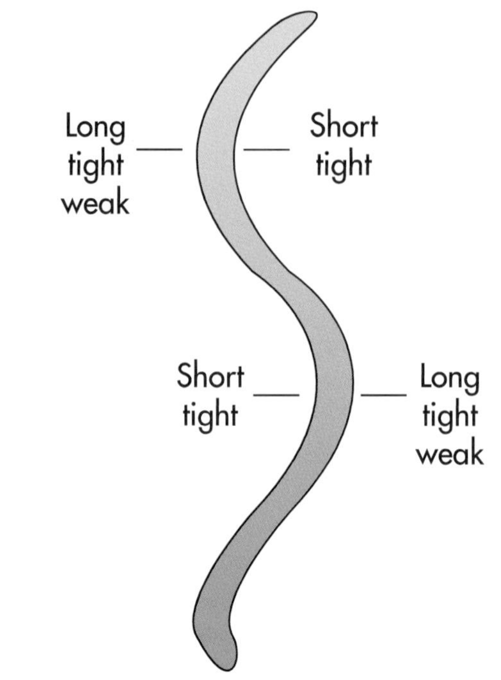

Figure 10-9
First, massage application with stretching lengthens the short, tight areas. Coupled with therapeutic exercise, massage then stimulates the long, tight, and weak areas.

Common Postural Deviations

Because standing is a closed **kinetic chain** activity (see Chapter 8) and because of the tensegric nature of body form, the position or motion of one joint affects the positions or motions of other joints.

This book does not describe the individual causes and effects of postural problems. However, one can make some general statements regarding cause and effect.

Poor posture can result from structural problems that may be caused by congenital malformation or acquired by trauma such as a compression fracture. Postural deviations also may result from neurologic conditions causing paralysis or spasticity. Most postural problems are functional, or nonstructural. For example, a person who sits or stands for long periods of time tends to slouch, resulting in a muscle imbalance, which causes positional strain.

Generally, if a person tends to maintain a posture in which a curve is increased, the muscles on the concave side tend to shorten and tighten, whereas the muscles on the convex side tend to become long and weak but still feel tight. For example, one would expect a person with a lumbar lordosis to have tight and short back extensors and weak and long abdominal muscles. Massage application helps reverse the functional strain by addressing the shortening on the concave side and stimulating the inhibited muscles on the convex side of the curve. Stretching is required for the short areas and appropriate exercise for the long areas (Figure 10-9).

Walking/Gait

Walking is an activity in which a person moves his or her body into and out of balance with each step. When standing and while walking, our center of gravity is located in our pelvis at the upper sacral region anterior to the second sacral vertebra. Our head is balanced on top of the spine, and the center of gravity for the head is in front of the ear by the cheek.

The pivot point for movement of the head is behind the center of gravity, which means that posterior occipital and cervical muscles must exert force to hold the head up. The benefit to this is that to begin forward movement, all a person has to do is relax the muscles at the back of the head. The head moves forward and, because of its weight, this movement takes the whole body with it. Beginning an action requires effort. Once started, movement takes on a momentum of its own. The same principle can be applied to a moving car. A car needs the most power when it starts off from a stationary position and little energy to keep it going at a constant speed. Our amazing bodies help us move, not by requiring increased force but by using our head to initiate the movement. "Lead all movement with your head" can be more than just a biomechanically correct statement (Figure 10-10).

Locomotion, or walking, is the act of moving from one place to another. Gait is the means of achieving this action. Despite years of scientific study we still do not know exactly how we stand upright and walk. The question remains as to how much of locomotion is innate and how much is learned. Humans certainly are driven to walk. Most authorities agree that the urge and the "hardwiring" for bipedal (two-legged) locomotion is born in us and the coordination of all the components necessary to accomplish the task is learned.

Controlling bipedal locomotion is not an easy task. Reflexive coordination by the central nervous system is an essential part of the walking pattern. The central nervous system coordinates muscles to generate the locomotion pattern through the following actions:

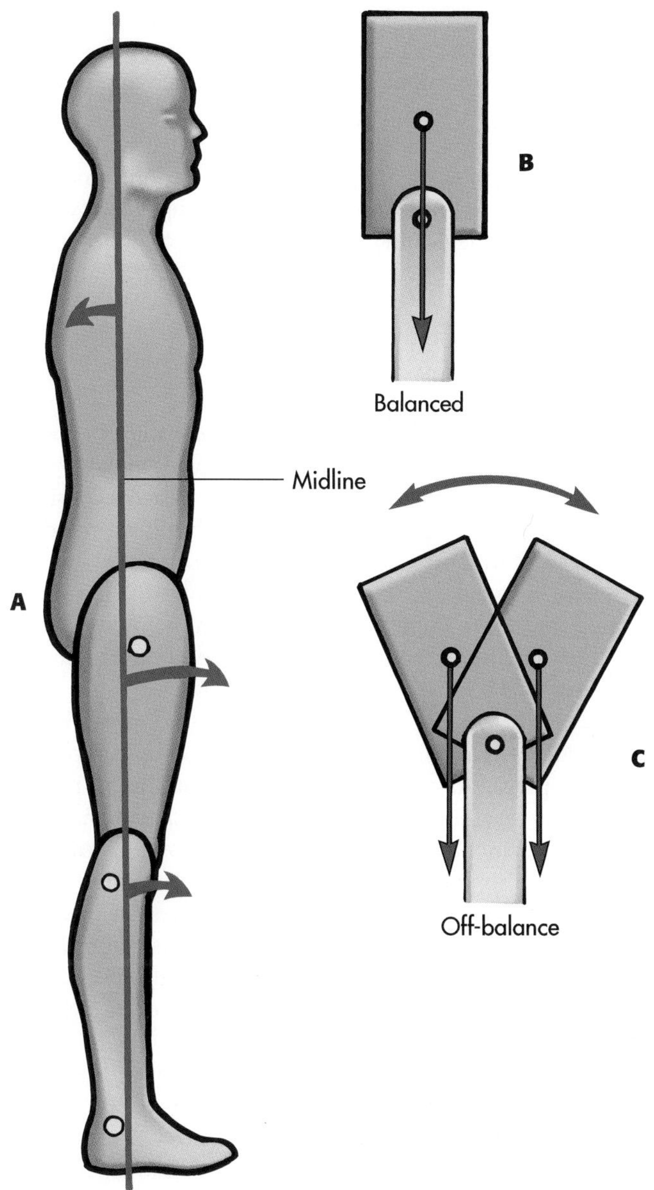

Figure 10-10
A, In normal relaxed standing the leg and trunk tend to rotate slightly off the midline of the body but maintain a counterbalance force. Balance is achieved in **B** and not in **C.** Anytime the trunk moves off this midline balance point, the body must compensate. (From Fritz S: *Mosby's fundamentals of therapeutic massage,* ed 3, St. Louis, 2004, Mosby.)

- Producing appropriate propulsive forces
- Modulating changes in the center of gravity
- Coordinating multilimb trajectories
- Adapting to changing conditions and joint positions
- Coordinating visual, auditory, vestibular, and peripheral afferent information

Understanding reflex patterns is an important part of understanding how we walk. Because most reflex actions involve a great many reflex arcs, local stimulation of a small number of receptors leads to a large number of outgoing impulses to muscles and glands. The result is a widespread and generalized reflex response. Most reflexes are polysynaptic, using many sensory neurons, interneurons, and motor neurons. Breaking down these complex functional patterns is often difficult but can be a clinical necessity if we are to understand the automatic and sometimes perpetuating responses of dysfunctional reflex patterns that interact in the ongoing attempt by the body to maintain homeostasis. One can simplify this process for understanding gait and posture. The interplay of posture and gait often is referred to as a kinetic chain, which we discuss in detail later in the chapter.

When we walk, peripheral receptors in our joints and muscles detect changes in muscle length and force, joint position, and weight-bearing status of the limbs. Righting reflexes involving the eyes and ears, together with tonic neck reflexes, maintain an upward, level, and forward head position while ocular/pelvic reflexes balance the head and pelvis position. Pressure receptors (baroreceptors) on the soles of the feet relay postural information about weight distribution. The relationship between the movement of the legs when walking and the independent use of the arm/hand complex depends on the task and environment.

Watching toddlers as they start to walk clearly reveals that from the beginning, walking is counterbalanced by activity of the arms, hands, head, and pelvis. This counterbalancing action becomes important in understanding the complex system of reflex control of gait patterns.

Normal Adult Walking Cycle

Simply stated, we walk around on two legs comprised of three segments each: the thigh, shank (lower leg), and the foot. On top of our legs are the trunk, head, and arms. The whole arm unit is used as a counterbalance and for momentum and moves opposite the leg movement. This pattern is linked by the contralateral reflex arc mechanism.

Flexion and extension of the hip joints cause some rotation in the lumbar spine, and to keep the head facing forward and the eyes level, the thorax and cervical spine rotate in the opposite direction. The same reflex patterns that coordinate this action also coordinate upright posture in gravity and righting reflexes that keep the eyes on a level plane and the head oriented to the trunk. Reciprocal movements of the upper and lower limbs occur with the right upper limb flexing at the shoulder joint simultaneous with flexion at the left hip joint. Normally, the shoulder joint starts to flex or extend slightly before the same movement occurs in the elbow joint. These movements again serve to keep the head and trunk oriented and to counterbalance the body weight in gravity.

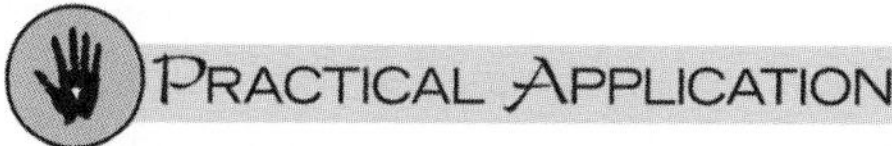

The practitioner often can trace dysfunctional patterns through these basic reflex principles. For example, a client complains of a stiff left shoulder but cannot remember how the pain began but can remember walking around an amusement park with a blister on the right heel. This dysfunctional pattern may result from a change in gait, developed from an alteration in the reciprocal counter-balancing pattern, which eventually led to the shoulder pain. One may relieve the shoulder difficulty by addressing neuromuscular tension patterns in the right leg and hip. Many such patterns could develop. A massage practitioner, paying attention to the reflex pattern operating in the body, could manage this type of soft tissue dysfunction more effectively by understanding the gait cycle and the kinetic chain. ■

Gait Cycle

Gait is defined as the rhythmic and alternating movement of the legs along with the trunk and the arms, which results in the propulsion of the body mass. Gait is an automatic function coordinated by innate and learned reflexes. Muscles certainly work together to produce movement, but an interesting note is that in large portions of the gait cycle, little or no muscle activity occurs in most of the muscle groups, pointing to the energy-efficient nature of walking.

A **gait cycle** is the period during which a complete sequence of events takes place; it begins when the heel of one foot strikes the floor. The gait cycle is subdivided into the *stance phase* and *swing phase.* The stance phase occurs when the limb under consideration is in contact with the floor. In walking a period of time always occurs when both feet are in contact with the floor; this is called *double stance.* The swing phase occurs when the foot is not in contact with the floor.

In the average walking pattern the stance phase takes about 60% of the gait cycle and the swing phase about 40%. As the speed of walking, or cadence, increases, the length of time in the stance phase decreases. Double stance time increases with slow walking.

The components of the stance phase are heel strike, foot flat, midstance, heel-off, and toe-off (Figure 10-11, *A* to *E*).

The components of the swing phase are acceleration, midswing, deceleration, and arm swing (Figure 10-12, *A* to *F*).

KINETIC CHAIN

The kinetic chain is an integrated functional unit (Figure 10-13). The kinetic chain is made up of the myofascial system (muscle, ligament, tendon, and fascia), articular (joint) system, and nervous system. Each of these systems works interdependently to allow structural and functional efficiency in all three planes of motion: sagittal, frontal, and transverse. If one or more of the systems do not work efficiently, compensations and adaptations occur in the remaining systems, leading to stress in the body and eventually resulting in the development of dysfunctional patterns.

All functional movement patterns involve acceleration provided by concentric contractions, stabilization provided by isometric contractions, and deceleration provided by eccentric contractions. All three actions occur at every joint in the kinetic chain and in all three planes of motion with each movement pattern. Muscles also must react proprioceptively to gravity, momentum, external forces, and forces created by other functioning muscles.

Muscles function cooperatively in integrated groups to provide neuromuscular control during functional movements and can be divided into two main groups (each with multiple names depending on the resource): the inner unit (stabilizers/postural muscles) and the outer unit (movers/phasic muscles).

Inner Unit

The inner unit primarily consists of intrinsic muscles that function at only one joint and are involved predominately in joint support or stabilization. Joint support systems consist of muscles that are not movement specific but that provide stability to allow movement of a joint. Joint support systems also have a broad spectrum of attachments to the joint capsule that make them ideal for increasing joint stiffness and thus stability. This group provides stability to the core and peripheral joints.

The postural/core/stabilization portion of the inner unit of the kinetic chain consists of the lumbo-pelvic-hip complex, thoracic spine, and cervical spine and operates as an integrated functional unit to stabilize the kinetic chain dynamically during functional movements of the limbs and head.

The joint support system of the core is muscles that originate or insert (or both) into the spine. The major muscles include the deep erector spinae, deep cervical muscles, transverse abdominis, abdominal obliques, diaphragm, lumbar multifidus, and the muscles of the pelvic floor.

Heel strike = Initial contact

Hip	25° Flexion	Hip extensors eccentric
Knee	0°	Quadriceps concentric
Ankle	0°	Tibials concentric

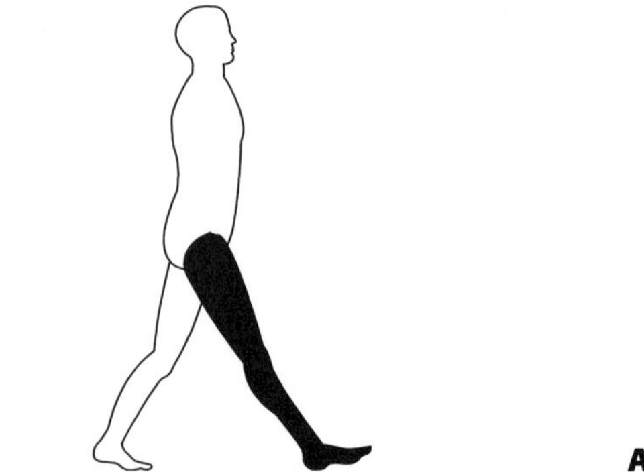

Figure 10-11
A to E, Components of the stance phase.

Foot Flat = Loading Response

Hip	26° Flexion	Hip extensors eccentric and hip abductors isometric
Knee	15° Flexion	Quadriceps eccentric
Ankle	10° Plantar flexion	Pretibials eccentric

B

- The body (center of gravity) reaches its highest point in the gait cycle

Hip	0°	Hip abductors isometric
Knee	0°	Quadriceps concentric initially, then no muscle activity
Ankle	0°	Plantar flexors (calf) eccentric

C

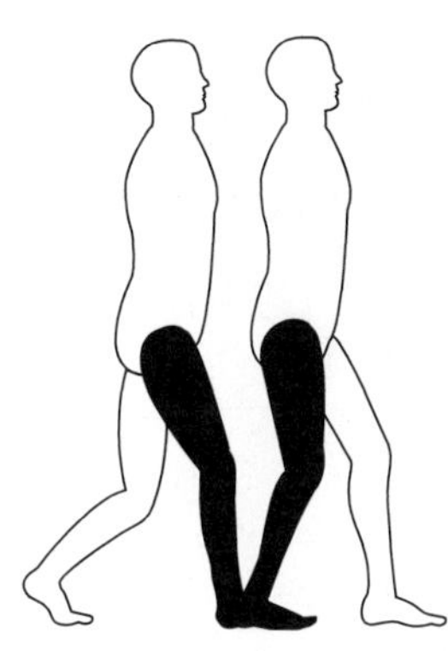

Heel-Off = Terminal Stance

Hip	20° Hip hyperextension	No muscle activity
Knee	0°	No muscle activity
Ankle	10° Dorsiflexion	Plantar flexors (calf) eccentric

D

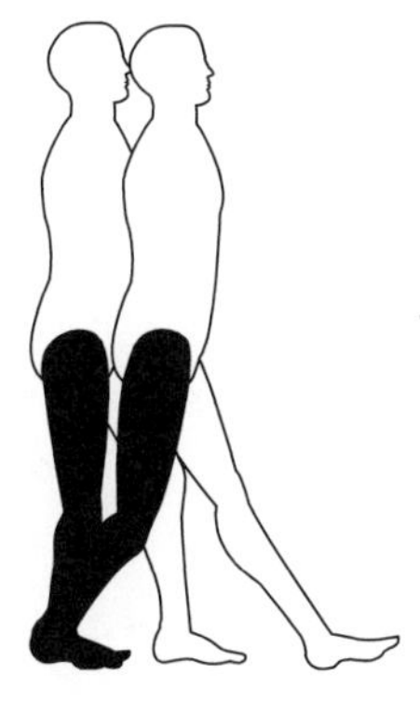

Toe-Off = Preswing

Hip	0°	Adductor longus
Knee	40° Knee flexion	No muscle activity
Ankle	20° Plantar flexion	Plantar flexors concentric initially, then no muscle activity

E

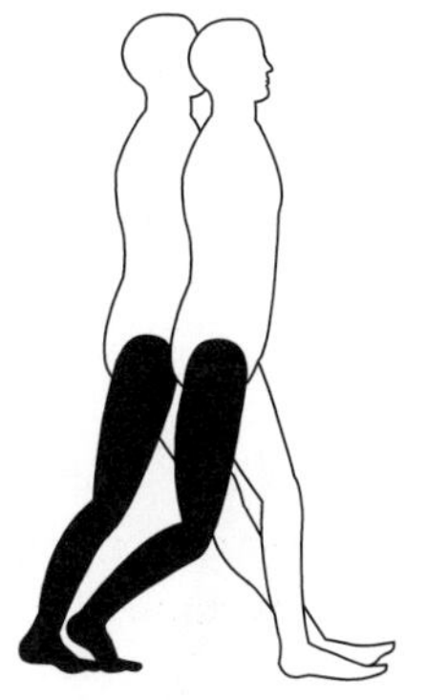

Figure 10-11—cont'd.

The peripheral joints in the shoulders, pelvic girdle, and the limbs also contain inner units of muscles. An example of a peripheral joint support system is the rotator cuff for the glenohumeral joint that provides dynamic stabilization for the humeral head in the glenoid fossa during movement.

Outer Unit

The outer unit muscles are predominately responsible for movement and typically consist of more superficial extrinsic muscles that attach from the limbs and shoulder and pelvic

Acceleration = Initial swing

Hip	15° Hip flexion	Hip flexors concentric
Knee	60° Knee flexion	Knee flexors concentric
Ankle	10° Plantar flexion	Tibials concentric

A

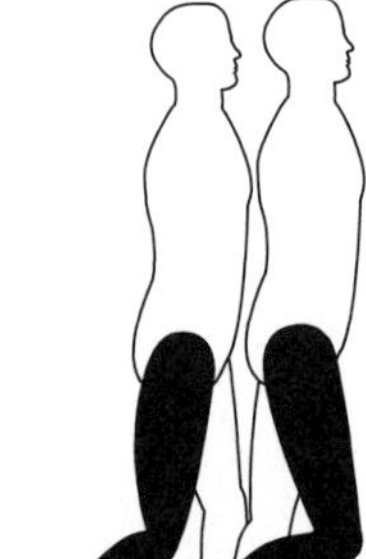

Midswing = Midswing

Hip	25° Hip flexion	Hip flexors concentric initially, then hamstrings eccentric
Knee	25° Knee flexion	Knee extension is created by momentum and gravity and short head of biceps femoris control rate of knee extension through eccentric control
Ankle	0°	Tibials concentric

B

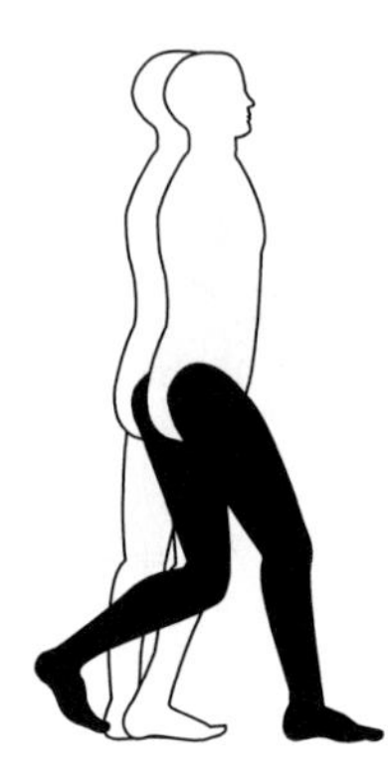

Deceleration = Terminal swing

Hip	25° Flexion	Hamstrings eccentric
Knee	0°	Quadriceps concentric to insure knee extension and hamstrings are active eccentrically to decelerate the leg
Ankle	0°	Tibials concentric

C

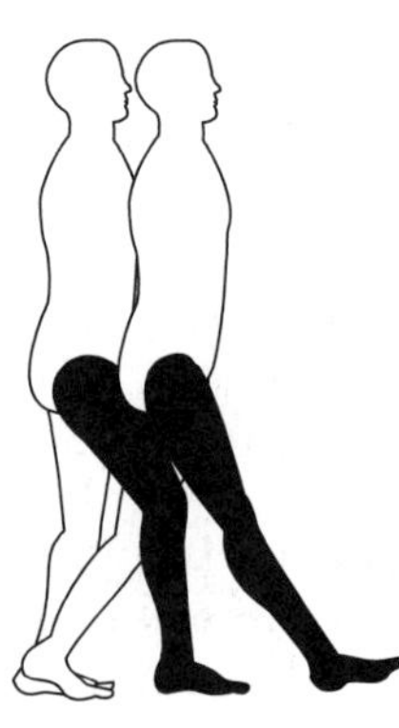

Arm swing

- The upper extremities serve an important role in counterbalancing the shifts of the center of gravity.
- A reciprocal arm swing is seen in a mature gait (e.g., the left arm swings forward as the right leg swings forward and vice versa).
- As the shoulder girdle advances, the pelvis and limb trail behind. With each step, this is reversed.

D

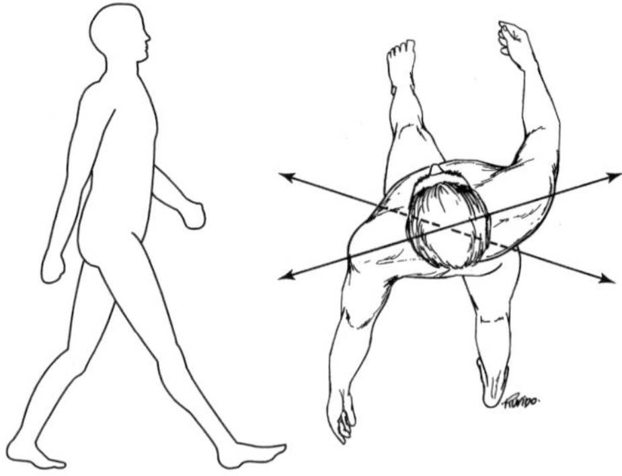

Figure 10-12
A to **F,** Components of the swing phase.

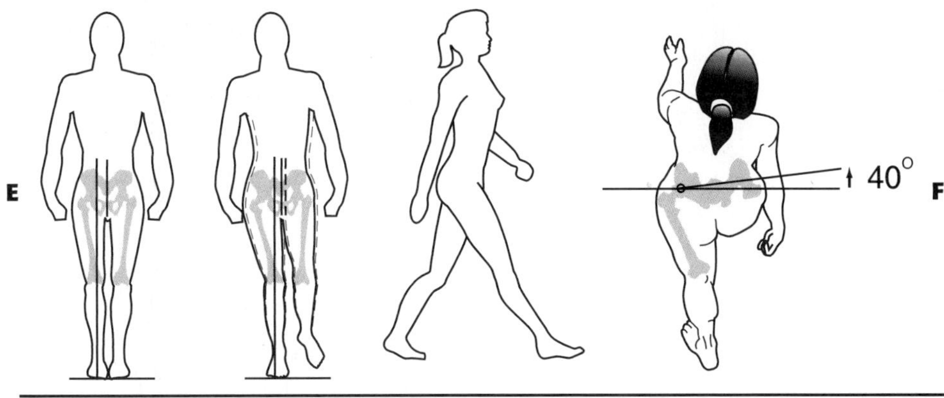

Figure 10-12—cont'd.

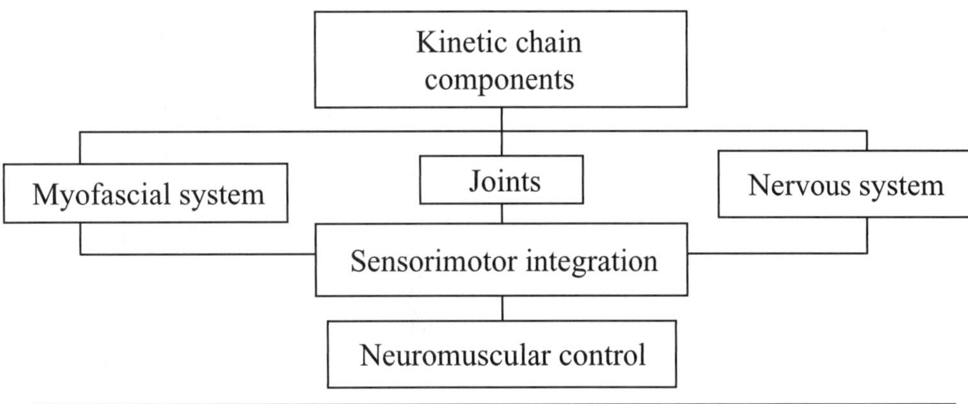

Figure 10-13
Kinetic chain components.

girdles to the trunk (core). Examples of these muscles include the rectus abdominis, external obliques, erector spinae, latissimus dorsi, hamstrings, gluteus maximus, adductors, and quadriceps. The outer unit muscles are usually larger than the inner unit and are associated with movement of the trunk and limbs.

Other ways to classify functional movement groups exist. Other groupings of muscles and connective tissue that are interactive during specific functional patterns are these:

- The erector spinae, thoracolumbar fascia, sacrotuberous ligament, and biceps femoris assist in stabilizing the sacroiliac joint. Dysfunction in these structures can lead to sacroiliac joint pain.
- The superficial erector spinae, psoas, deep erector spinae, transverse abdominis, abdominal obliques, diaphragm, lumbar multifidus, and the muscles of the pelvic floor provide intersegmental stabilization of the trunk during functional movement. Dysfunction in any of these structures can lead to sacroiliac joint instability and low back pain.
- Internal oblique, external oblique, adductor group, external rotator hip group, contralateral gluteus maximus and latissimus dorsi, anterior and posterior tibialis, soleus and gastrocnemius, and fibularis group creates a stabilizing force for the sacroiliac joint function, aid in the stability and rotation of the pelvis, and contribute to leg swing. Dysfunction in this group often leads to sacroiliac joint dysfunction and rotational strain in the lumbar spine, pelvic area, and knee and also can affect the ankle. The weakening of the gluteus maximus and/or latissimus dorsi also may lead to increased tension in the hamstrings and therefore cause recurring hamstring strains.
- Gluteus medius, tensor fascia latae, adductor group, and the quadratus lumborum are responsible for pelvofemoral stability. During single leg functional movements such as in walking, lunges, or stair climbing, the ipsilateral gluteus medius, tensor fasciae latae, and adductors combine with the contralateral quadratus lumborum to control the pelvis and femur. Dysfunction can create instability and strain during walking, running, and jumping activities.

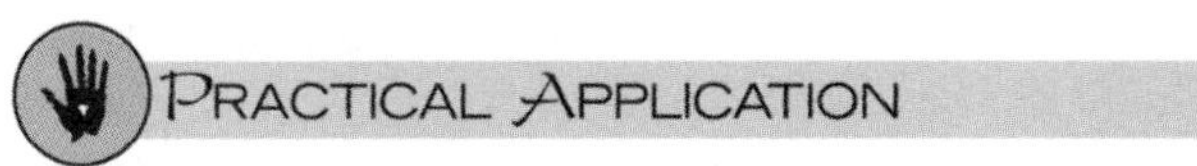

The body must be balanced in three dimensions against the forces of gravity to provide stability in the upright position and for locomotion. Balanced daily against the forces of gravity, the body reacts to pain, injury, and other stimuli through complex compensations involving many polysynaptic reflex arcs. Some compensation patterns are resourceful, such as when the body is required to adapt to a trauma or repetitive use pattern. Massage application should support these changes. Some compensation patterns become pathologic or maladaptive and increase strain in the system. Therapeutic massage can assist in reversing some of these nonproductive patterns. Any form of compensation can yield a confusing combination of signs and symptoms. Symptoms may range from clients complaining of left scapular pain after a right quadriceps injury, or pain on front left side of neck after sustaining injury to right calf (gastrocnemius/soleus). Signs such as decreased movement of extremities, splinting, and lack of bilateral symmetry also may be observable. One can derive a systematic application of assessment intervention to help understand and address this array of signs, symptoms, and compensations. Such a system is developed in this text as the *kinetic chain protocol*. Part One assesses and gives recommendations for treating postural patterns, and Part Two assesses and gives recommendations for gait patterns. ■

Stabilization of the body during normal function occurs in soft tissues between movement segments (Box 10-1). For example, the muscles located between the base of the skull and the top of the shoulders or the muscles located between the last thoracic vertebrae and the top of the hips are considered segments. These patterns balance each other to provide postural stability in a diagonal counterbalancing function. Compensation and dysfunction can occur as well. For example, if the right hip is elevated from muscles tensing in the back, typically one finds a compensation tension pattern in the anterior muscles on the left between vertebrae C7 and T12. Another example is pain in the quadriceps on the left that shows a compensation pattern in the calf on the right and the tissue between the hips and S1 on the right posterior. Tension also may develop in the tissues on the top of the left foot. The possible combination of these neurologic patterns is almost endless, yet one can assess for and treat these by applying the following principles:

1. Identify the most prominent symptom, from pain or positional distortion.
2. Methodically assess the tissues diagonally from right to left and front to back in each segment, above and below the targeted area for related tension and pain. If a symptom is on the back left, begin assessment in segments above and below the segment with the symptom, on the opposite side (in this example, right) and in the front. Continue to the next segments above and below the area just checked using diagonal patterns until all areas are covered.
3. Provide intervention. Use any massage method to reduce tension and pain in each segment before addressing main symptom, and then reassess the original symptom pattern, which should be reduced (Boxes 10-2 and 10-3; Activity 10-2).

BOX 10-1

Kinetic Chain Protocol: Posture-Movement Segments (Part 1)

The trunk moves and is balanced in the following areas:

Top of head and atlas/axis
Atlas/axis and C6/C7 vertebrae
C6/C7 and T12 (thoracolumbar junction)
T12 and S1 (sacrolumbar junction)
S1 and hips (acetabula)
Hips and knees
Knees and ankles
Ankles and tips of toes

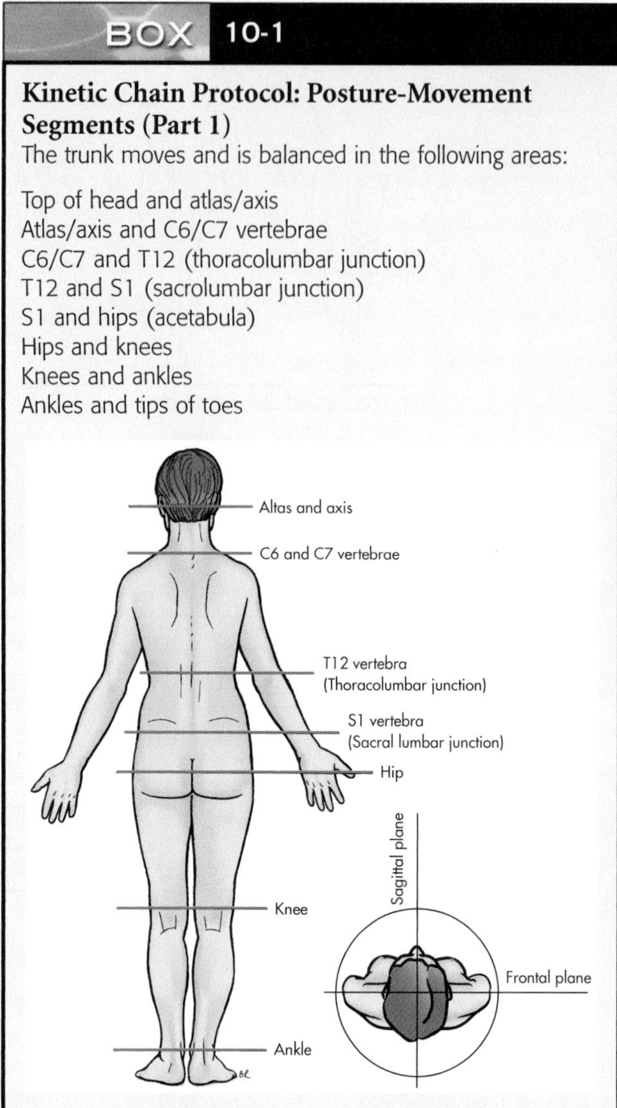

The kinetic chain also involves movement, particularly walking and running—called *gait*. Assessment and treatment of gait patterns are described in Box 10-2 and Activity 10-2 beginning on p. 497.

SITTING, STANDING, AND BENDING

One also needs to consider moving from a seated to standing position and bending to pick up an object on the floor. An important point is to squat down to pick up an object as opposed to bending over at the hip joint and then lifting up. Bending over puts an enormous strain on the back. Half the body weight is being moved in addition to the weight of the object being lifted. When squatting down and then moving from a squat to a standing position, one should keep the weight distributed over the entire bottom of the foot, particularly the heels. The tendency is to bear weight on the ball of the foot and toes. This position causes instability in the ankle and knee.

BOX 10-2

Kinetic Chain Protocol: Gait (Part 2)

Think of the two main actions involved with gait:

1. On opposite sides: Right arm flexors concentrically contract with left leg flexors.
2. On the same side: Right arm flexors concentrically contract with right leg extensors

The reciprocal is then also true:

1. On opposite sides: Left arm extensors concentrically contract with right leg extensors.
2. On the same side: Left arm extensors concentrically contract with left leg flexors.

Muscle Contraction

Muscles that concentrically contract together in these patterns should maintain a strong, steady contraction simultaneously during muscle testing. Weakness in the muscle being tested would indicate dysfunction.

One should test muscles (antagonists) that are inhibited in these patterns. The antagonist patterns should not hold easily against a force of resistance. One should not confuse this response with a dysfunctional, weak muscle. Instead, reciprocal inhibition from the prime mover produces an appropriate "letting go" sensation. If a muscle that should be inhibited remains locked in concentric contraction as indicated by "testing strong," a dysfunction in the reflex arc is present.

How to Assess

1. Isolate muscle groups. Ask client to apply force (10% to 20%) or to hold against your opposing pressure with the muscles of the control group.
2. Test the desired muscle group for strong, steady contraction in the concentric pattern or inhibition in the eccentric pattern. See Activity 10-2 on p. 497.

When in the seated position, moving to a standing position begins by leaning forward at the hips and leading with the head. The momentum carries the body forward into a semisquat. The leg muscles then lift the body into a standing position (Figure 10-14).

Muscle Firing Patterns

The central nervous system recruits the appropriate muscles in specific firing patterns to generate the appropriate muscle functions of acceleration, deceleration, or stability. Firing patterns that become abnormal, with the synergist becoming dominant, compromise efficient movement and strain the joint position. The general firing pattern is the prime movers, stabilizers, and synergists. If the stabilizer also has to move the area (acceleration) or control movement (deceleration), it typically becomes short and tight. If the synergist fires before the prime mover, then the movement is awkward and labored.

If one muscle is tight and short, reciprocal inhibition occurs; that is, a tight muscle causes decreased nervous stimulation to its functional antagonist, causing it to decrease activity. For example, a tight and short psoas decreases the function of the gluteus maximus. The activation and force production of the prime mover (gluteus maximus) decreases, leading to compensation and substitution by the synergists (hamstrings) and stabilizers (erector spinae) creating an altered firing pattern.

The most common firing pattern dysfunction is synergistic dominance, in which a synergist compensates for a prime mover to produce the movement. For example, if a client has a weak gluteus medius, then synergists

text continued on p. 504

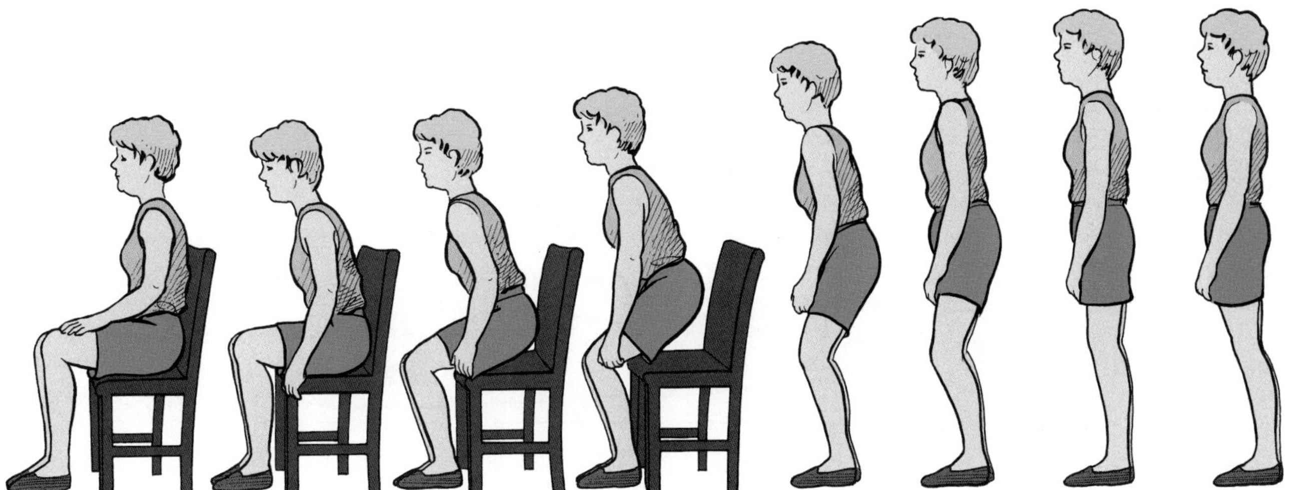

Figure 10-14
Sit-to-stand viewed laterally. (From Gillen G, Burkhardt A: *Stroke rehabilitation: a function-based approach,* St Louis, 1998, Mosby.)

BOX 10-3

Common Firing Patterns

Trunk Flexion

1. Normal firing pattern
   a. Transverse abdominis
   b. Abdominal obliques
   c. Rectus abdominis
2. Assessment
   a. Client is supine with knees and hips at 90 degrees.
   b. The client is instructed to perform a normal curl up.
   c. The massage practitioner assesses the ability of the abdominal muscles functionally to stabilize the lumbo-pelvic-hip complex by having the client draw the abdominal muscle in as when bringing the umbilicus toward the back and then doing a curl just lifting the scapula off the table while keeping both feet flat.

The inability to maintain the drawing in position or to activate the rectus demonstrates altered firing of the abdominal stabilization mechanism.

3. Altered firing pattern
   a. Weak agonist: Abdominal complex
   b. Overactive antagonist: Erector spinae
   c. Overactive synergist: Psoas or rectus abdominis
4. Symptoms
   a. Low back pain
   b. Buttock pain
   c. Hamstring shortening

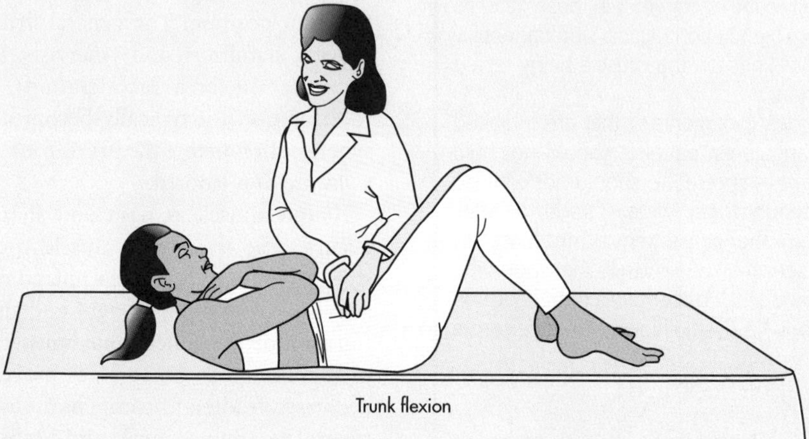

Trunk flexion

Hip Extension

1. Normal firing pattern
   a. Gluteus maximus
   b. Opposite erector spinae
   c. Same-side erector spinae and hamstring

   Or

   a. Gluteus maximus
   b. Hamstring
   c. Opposite erector spinae
   d. Same-side erector spinae
2. Assessment
   a. With the client prone the massage practitioner palpates the erector spinae with the thumb and index finger of one hand and palpates the muscle belly of the gluteus maximus and hamstring with the little finger and the thumb of the opposite hand.
   b. The practitioner instructs the client to extend the hip more than 15 degrees from the table.
3. Altered firing pattern
   a. Weak agonist: Gluteus maximus
   b. Overactive antagonist: Psoas
   c. Overactive stabilizer: Erector spinae
   d. Overactive synergist: Hamstring
4. Symptoms
   a. Low back pain
   b. Buttock pain
   c. Recurrent hamstring strains

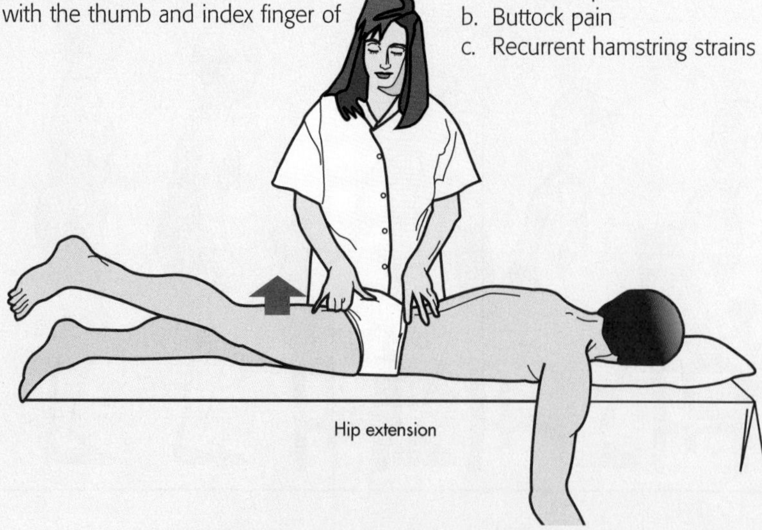

Hip extension

BOX 10-3—cont'd

Hip Abduction

1. Normal firing pattern
   a. Gluteus medius
   b. Tensor fasciae latae
   c. Quadratus lumborum
2. Assessment
   a. With the client side-lying the massage practitioner stands next to the client and palpates the client's quadratus lumborum with one hand and the tensor fasciae latae and gluteus medius with the other hand.
   b. The practitioner instructs the client to abduct the leg from the table.
3. Altered firing pattern
   a. Weak agonist: Gluteus medius
   b. Overactive antagonist: Adductors
   c. Overactive synergist: Tensor fasciae latae
   d. Overactive stabilizer: Quadratus lumborum
4. Symptoms
   a. Low back pain
   b. Sacroiliac joint pain
   c. Buttock pain
   d. Lateral knee pain
   e. Anterior knee pain

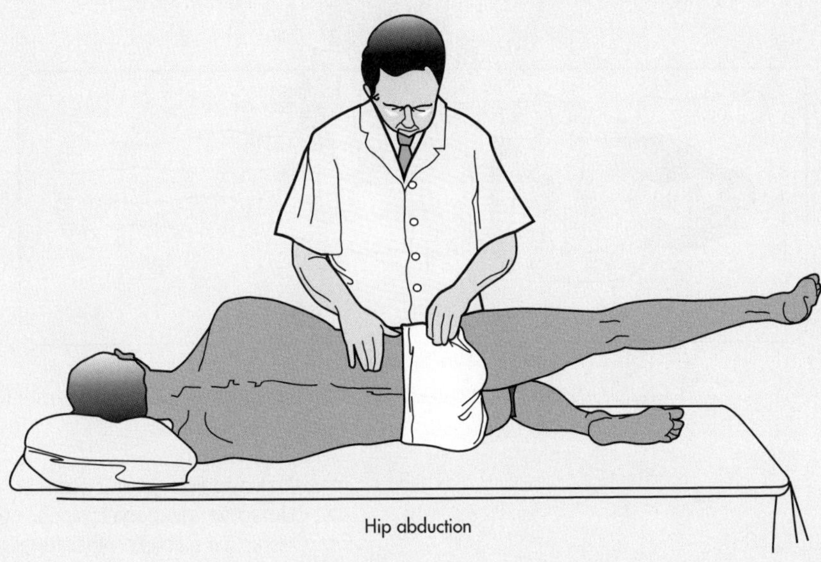

Hip abduction

Knee Flexion

1. Normal firing pattern
   a. Hamstring
   b. Gastrocnemius
2. Assessment
   a. With client lying prone the massage practitioner places fingers on the hamstring and gastrocnemius.
   b. The client flexes the knee.
3. Altered firing pattern
   a. Weak agonist: Hamstrings
   b. Overactive synergist: Gastrocnemius
4. Symptoms
   a. Pain behind the knee
   b. Achilles' tendonitis

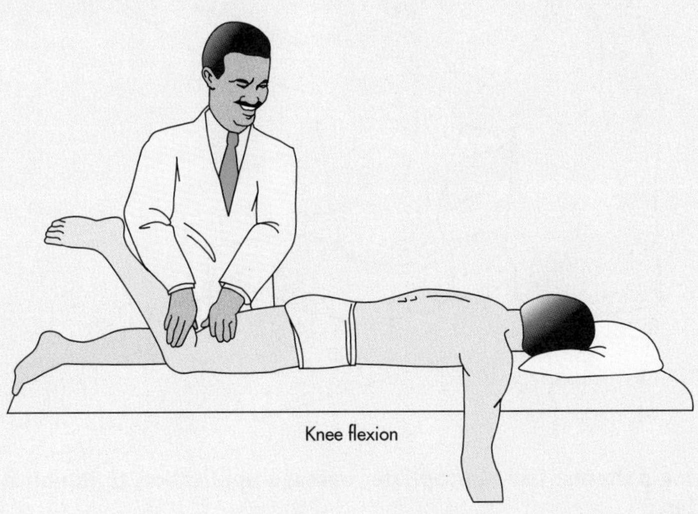

Knee flexion

Continued

BOX 10-3—cont'd

Knee Extension

1. Normal firing pattern
   a. Vastus medialis
   b. Vastus intermedialis and vastus lateralis
   c. Rectus femoris
2. Assessment
   a. Client lies supine with leg extended. The practitioner asks the client to pull the patella cranially (up). This is done by fully extending the knee. The massage practitioner places fingers on vastus medialis oblique, vastus lateralis, and rectus femoris.
3. Altered firing pattern
   a. Weak agonist: Vastus medialis, primarily the oblique portion
   b. Overactive synergist: Vastus lateralis
4. Symptoms
   a. Knee pain under patella
   b. Patellar tendonitis

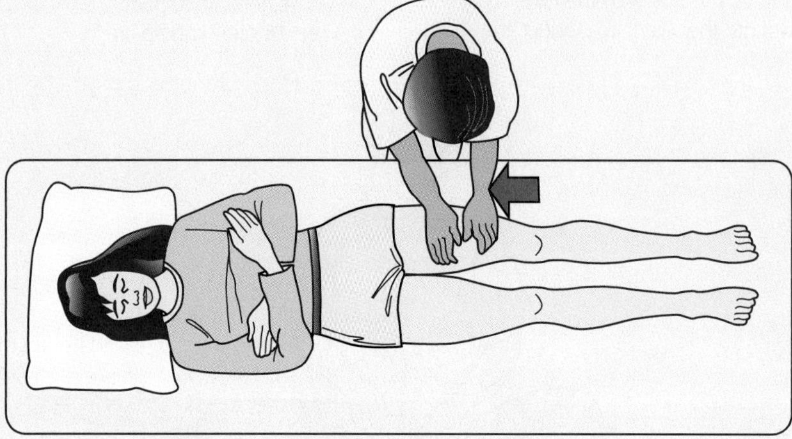

Knee extension

Shoulder Flexion

1. Normal firing pattern
   a. Supraspinatus
   b. Deltoid
   c. Infraspinatus
   d. Middle and lower trapezius
   e. Contralateral quadratus lumborum
2. Assessment
   a. Massage practitioner stands behind seated client with one hand on shoulder and the other on the contralateral quadratus area.
   b. The practitioner asks the client to abduct shoulder to 90 degrees.
3. Altered firing pattern
   a. Weak agonist: Levator scapula
   b. Overactive antagonist: Upper trapezius
   c. Overactive stabilizer: Ipsilateral quadratus lumborum
4. Symptoms
   a. Shoulder tension
   b. Headache at base of skull
   c. Upper chest breathing
   d. Low back pain

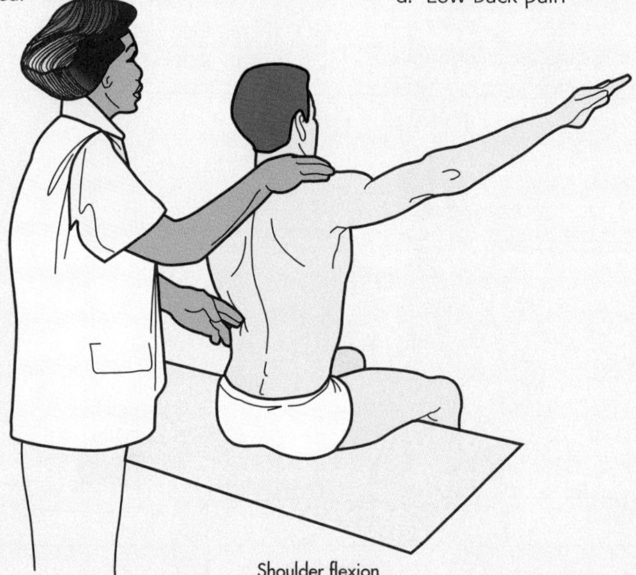

Shoulder flexion

Intervention for altered firing patterns: Use appropriate massage application to inhibit dominant muscle and then strengthen the weak muscles.

ACTIVITY 10-2

Kinetic Chain Protocol Testing

Control group: Serves as standard or reference for comparison with a test group and is the group of muscles that initiates the reflex response.

Test group: The muscle group that responds to the stimulus from the control group.

Many gait-related kinetic chain patterns exist. We will concentrate on the main patterns involved in flexion, extension, abduction, and adduction at the shoulder and pelvic girdle. For testing the arm flexors/extensors, one should stabilize the humerus superior to elbow joint and the femur above the knee.

The control group is activated first, the test group is next, and then both contractions are held simultaneously. Both groups should hold strong and steady during the test. One should chart the data to show any inhibitions.

The antagonist pattern should be inhibited during the test. The antagonists should let go. If they do not let go, the contraction maintained is concentric instead of eccentric. One should chart the data.

I. Contralateral Flexors

A. Left Arm Flexor Test (pictured)
1. Isolate and stabilize left arm and right leg in supine flexion.
2. Control group: Use right leg as control and have client hold right leg position against therapist's inferior/caudal pressure.
3. Test group: Test left arm flexors by having client hold left arm position against practitioner's inferior/caudal pressure.
4. Both groups should hold equally strong and steady. If test group is inhibited, chart the data.

Antagonist Test: Test left arm extensors by having client hold against practitioner's superior/cranial pressure. These muscles should inhibit (let go). If test group remains concentrically contracted and holds, one should chart data.

B. Right Arm Flexor Test
1. Isolate and stabilize left leg and right arm in supine flexion.
2. Control group: Use left leg as control and have client hold left leg position against practitioner's inferior/caudal pressure.
3. Test group: Test right arm flexors by having client hold right arm position against practitioner's inferior/caudal pressure.
4. Both groups should hold equally strong and steady. If test group is inhibited, chart data.

Antagonist test: Test right arm extensors by having client hold right arm position against practitioner's superior/cranial pressure. These muscles should inhibit (let go). If test group remains concentrically contracted and holds, chart data.

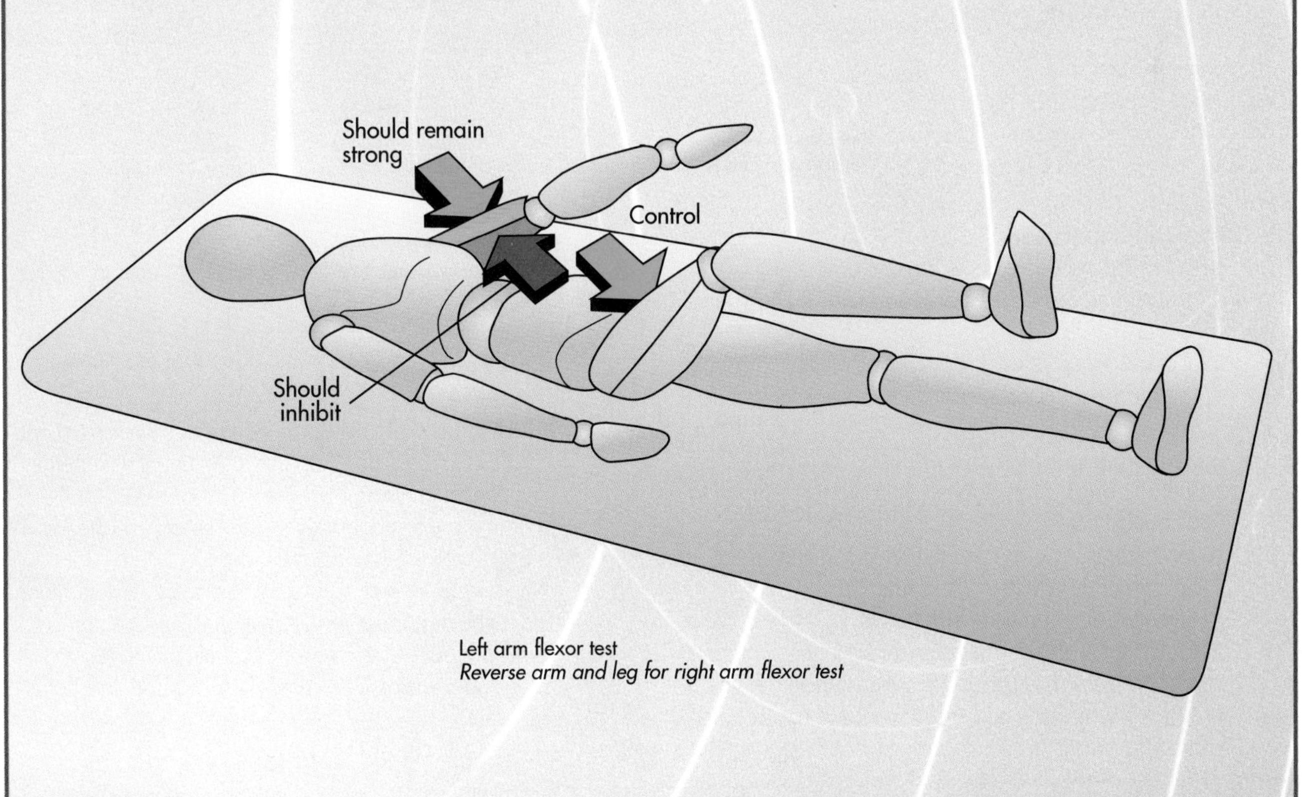

Left arm flexor test
Reverse arm and leg for right arm flexor test

Continued

ACTIVITY 10-2—cont'd

C. Left Leg Flexor Test
1. Isolate and support/stabilize left leg and right arm in supine flexion.
2. Control group: Use right arm as control and have client hold right arm position against therapist's inferior/caudal pressure.
3. Test group: Test left leg flexors by having client hold left leg position against practitioner's inferior/caudal pressure.
4. Both groups should hold equally strong and steady. If test group is inhibited, chart data.

Antagonist Test: Test left leg extensors by having client hold against practitioner's superior/cranial pressure. These muscles should inhibit (let go). If test group remains concentrically contracted and holds, chart data.

D. Right Leg Flexor Test (pictured)
1. Isolate and stabilize left arm and right leg in supine flexion.
2. Control group: Use left arm as control and have client hold left arm position against practitioner's inferior/caudal pressure.
3. Test group: Test right leg flexors by having client hold right leg position against practitioner's inferior/caudal pressure.
4. Both groups should hold equally strong and steady. If test group is inhibited (let go), chart data.

Antagonist test: Test right leg extensors by having client hold right leg position against practitioner's superior/cranial pressure. These muscles should inhibit (let go). If test group remains concentrically contracted and holds, chart data.

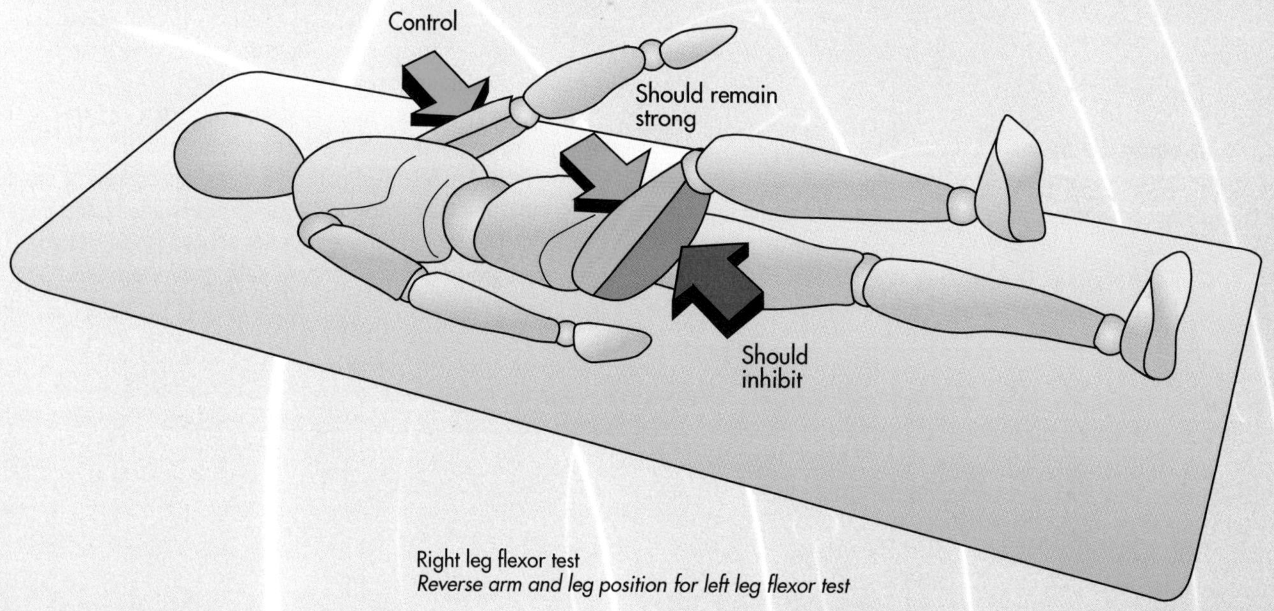

Right leg flexor test
Reverse arm and leg position for left leg flexor test

II. Contralateral Extensors

A. Left Arm Extensor Test (pictured)
1. Isolate and stabilize left arm and right leg in supine flexion.
2. Control group: Right leg is control. Have client hold leg position against practitioner's superior/cephalad pressure.
3. Test group: Test left arm extensors by having client hold arm position against practitioner's superior/cephalad pressure.
4. Both groups should stay equally strong and steady. If test group is inhibited, chart data.

Antagonist test: Test left arm flexors by having client hold left arm position against practitioner's inferior/caudal pressure. These muscles should inhibit (let go). If test group remains concentrically contracted and holds, chart data.

B. Right Arm Extensor Test
1. Isolate and stabilize left leg and right arm in supine flexion.
2. Control group: Left leg is control. Have client hold leg position against practitioner's superior/cephalad pressure.
3. Test group: Test right arm extensors by having client hold arm position against practitioner's superior/cephalad pressure.
4. Both groups should stay equally strong and steady. If test group is inhibited, chart data.

Antagonist test: Test right arm flexors by having client hold right arm position against practitioner's inferior/caudal pressure. These muscles should inhibit (let go). If test group remains concentrically contracted and holds, chart data.

ACTIVITY 10-2—cont'd

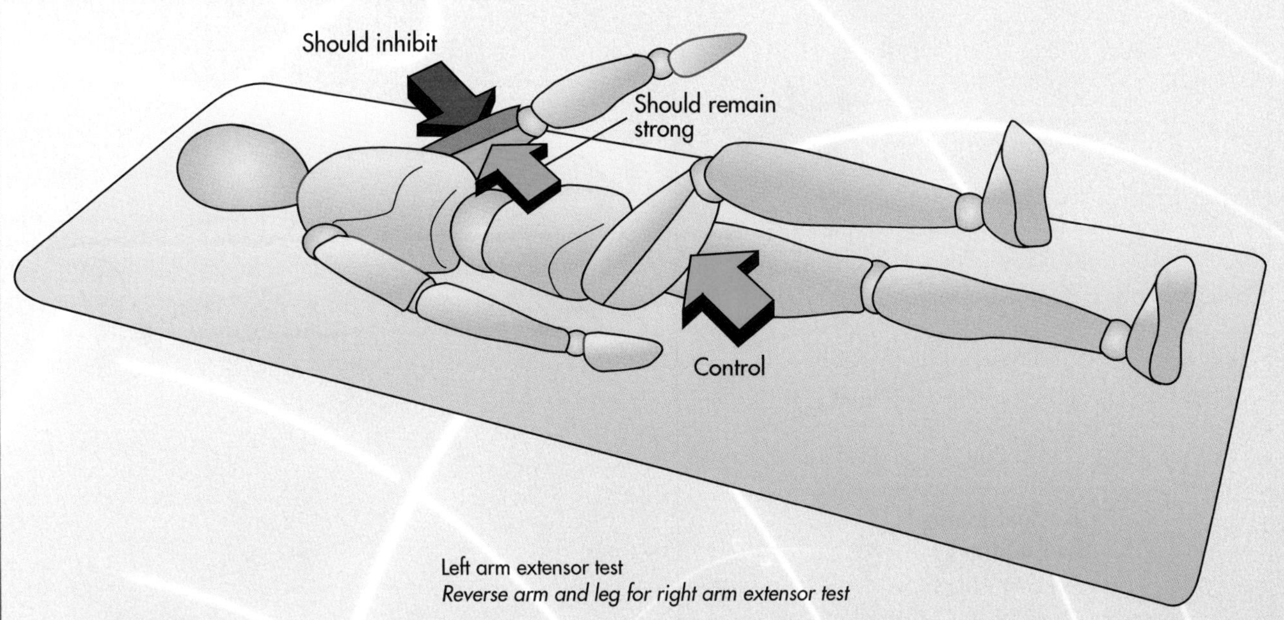

Left arm extensor test
Reverse arm and leg for right arm extensor test

C. Left Leg Extensor Test
1. Isolate and stabilize left leg and right arm in supine flexion.
2. Control group: Right arm is control. Have client hold arm position against practitioner's superior/cephalad pressure.
3. Test group: Test left leg extensors, have client hold leg position against practitioner's superior/cephalad pressure.
4. Both groups should stay equally strong and steady. If test group is inhibited, chart data.

Antagonist test: Test left leg flexor by having client hold left leg position against practitioner's inferior/caudal pressure. These muscles should inhibit (let go). If test group remains concentrically contracted and holds, chart data.

D. Right Leg Extensor Test (pictured)
1. Isolate and stabilize left arm and right leg in supine flexion.
2. Control group: Left arm is control. Have client hold arm position against practitioner's superior/cephalad pressure.
3. Test group: Test right leg extensors by having client hold leg position against practitioner's superior/cephalad pressure.
4. Both groups should stay equally strong and steady. If test group is inhibited, chart data.

Antagonist test: Test right leg flexors by having client hold right leg position against practitioner's inferior/caudal pressure. These muscles should inhibit (let go). If test group remains in a concentrically contracted pattern and holds, chart data.

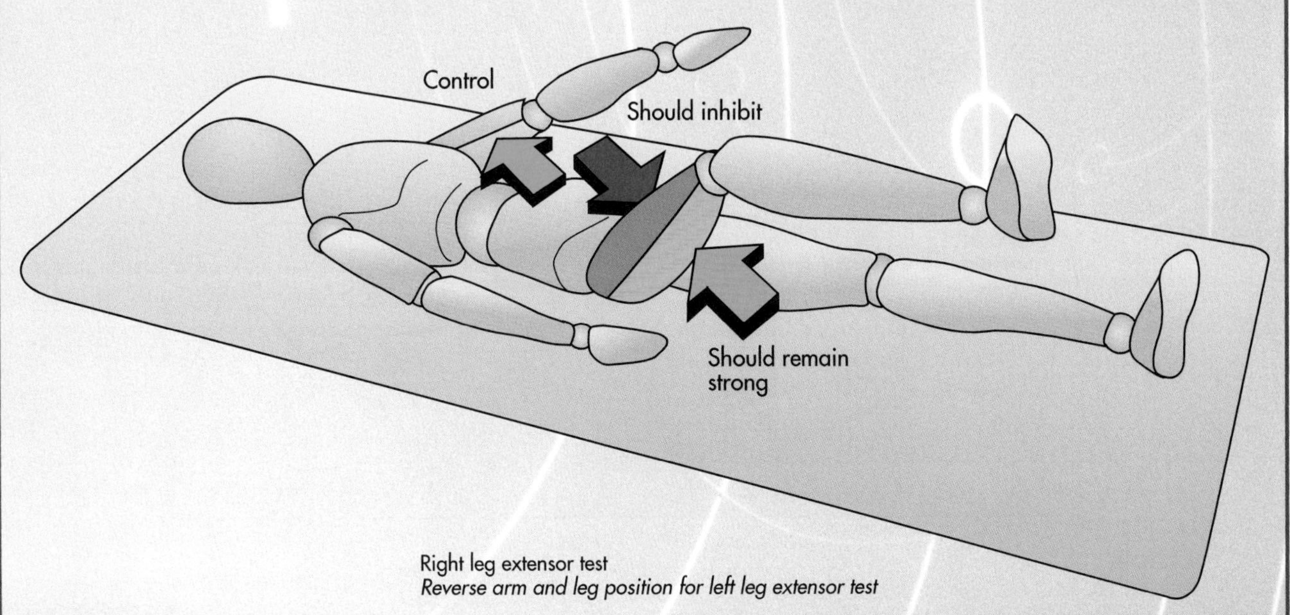

Right leg extensor test
Reverse arm and leg position for left leg extensor test

Continued

ACTIVITY 10-2—cont'd

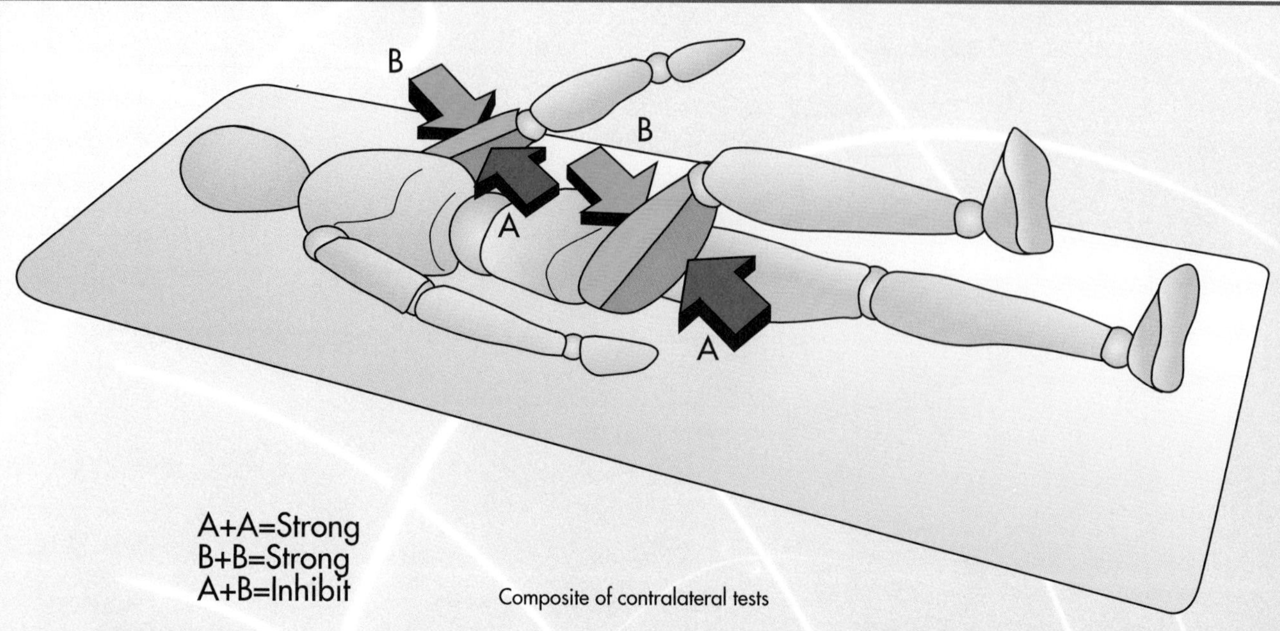

Composite of contralateral tests

III. Unilateral Flexors

A. Left Arm Flexor Test (pictured)
1. Isolate and stabilize left arm and left leg in supine flexion.
2. Control group: Left leg is control. Have client hold leg position against practitioner's superior/cephalad pressure (contracting extensors).
3. Test group: Test left arm flexors by having client hold arm position against practitioner's inferior/caudal pressure.
4. Both groups should stay equally strong and steady. If test group is inhibited, chart data.

Antagonist test: Test left arm extensors by having client hold left arm position against practitioner's superior/cranial pressure. These muscles should inhibit (let go). If test group remains concentrically contracted and holds, chart data.

B. Right Arm Flexor Test
1. Isolate and stabilize right arm and right leg in supine flexion.
2. Control group: Right leg is control. Have client hold leg position against practitioner's superior/cephalad pressure (contracting extensors).
3. Test group: Test right arm flexors by having client hold arm position against practitioner's inferior/caudal pressure.
4. Both groups should stay equally strong and steady. If test group is inhibited, chart data.

Antagonist test: Test right arm extensors by having client hold right arm position against practitioner's superior/cranial position. These muscles should inhibit (let go). If test group remains concentrically contracted and holds, chart data.

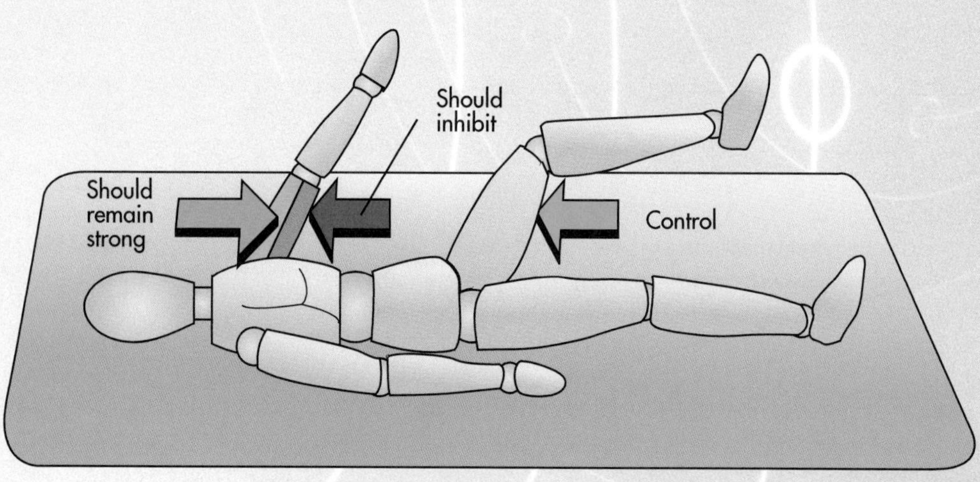

Left arm flexor test
Reverse arm and leg position for right arm flexor test

ACTIVITY 10-2—cont'd

C. Left Leg Flexor Test
1. Isolate and stabilize left arm and left leg in supine flexion.
2. Control group: Left arm is control. Have client hold arm position against practitioner's superior/cephalad pressure (contracting extensors).
3. Test group: Test left leg flexors by having client hold leg position against practitioner's inferior/caudal pressure (testing flexors).
4. Both groups should stay extensors strong and steady. If test group is inhibited, chart data.

Antagonist test: Test left leg extensors by having client hold left leg position against practitioner's, superior/cranial pressure. These muscles should inhibit (let go). If test group remains concentrically contracted and holds, chart data.

D. Right Leg Flexor Test (pictured)
1. Isolate and stabilize right arm and right leg in supine flexion.
2. Control group: Right arm is control. Have client hold arm position against practitioner's superior/cephalad pressure (contracting extensors).
3. Test group: Test right leg flexors by having client hold leg position against practitioner's inferior/caudal pressure (testing flexors).
4. Both groups should stay equally strong and steady. If test group is inhibited, chart data.

Antagonist test: Test right leg extensors by having client hold leg position against practitioner's superior/cranial pressure. These muscles should inhibit (let go). If test group remains concentrically contracted and holds, chart data.

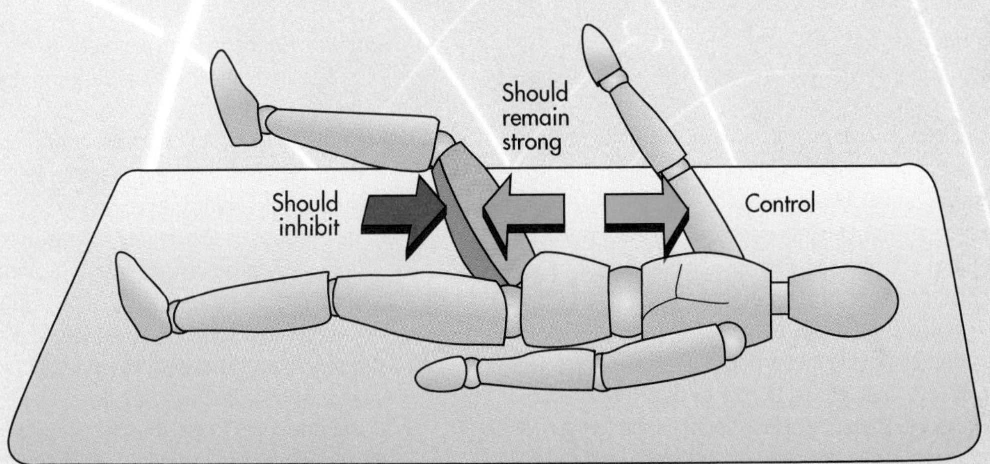

Right leg flexor test
Reverse arm and leg position for left leg flexor test

IV. Unilateral Extensors

A. Left Arm Extensor Test (pictured)
1. Isolate and stabilize left arm and left leg in supine flexion.
2. Control group: Left leg is control. Have client hold leg position against practitioner's inferior/caudal pressure (contracting flexors).
3. Test group: Test left arm extensors by having client hold arm position against practitioner's superior/cephalad pressure (testing extensors).
4. Both groups should stay equally strong and steady. If test group is inhibited, chart data.

Antagonist test: Test left arm flexors by applying inferior/caudal pressure. These muscles should inhibit (let go). If test group remains concentrically contracted and holds, chart data.

B. Right Arm Extensor Test (pictured)
1. Isolate and stabilize right arm and right leg in supine flexion.
2. Control group: Right leg is control. Have client hold leg position against practitioner's inferior/caudal pressure (contracting flexors).
3. Test group: Test right arm extensors by having client hold arm position against practitioner's superior/cephalad pressure (testing extensors).
4. Both groups should stay equally strong and steady. If test group is inhibited, chart data.

Antagonist test: Test right arm flexors by applying inferior/caudal pressure. These muscles should inhibit (let go). If test group remains concentrically contracted and holds, chart data.

Continued

ACTIVITY 10-2—cont'd

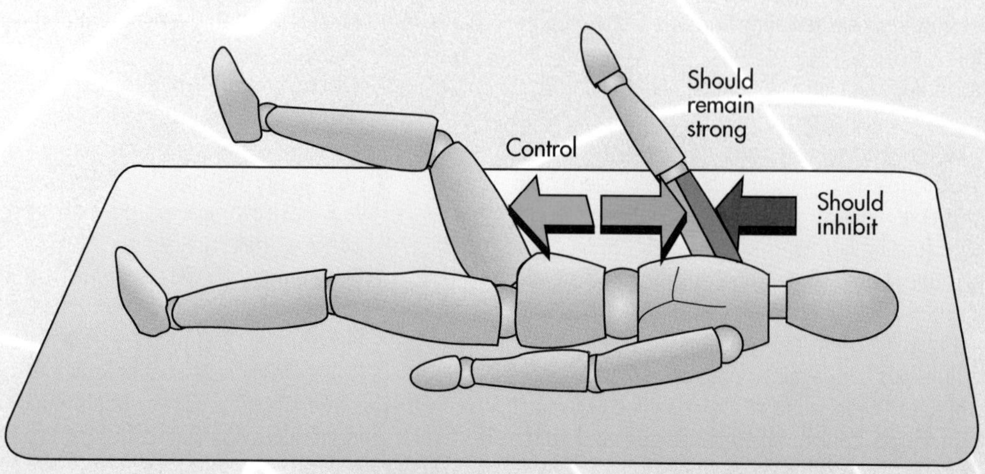

Right arm extensor test
Reverse arm and leg position for left arm extensor test

C. Left Leg Extensor Test
   1. Isolate and stabilize left arm and left leg in supine flexion.
   2. Control group: Left arm is control. Have client hold arm position against practitioner's inferior/caudal pressure (contracting flexors).
   3. Test group: Test left leg extensors by having client hold leg position against practitioner's superior/cephalad pressure (testing extensors).
   4. Both groups should stay equally strong and steady. If test group is inhibited, chart data.

   Antagonist Test: Test left leg flexors by applying inferior/caudal pressure. These muscles should inhibit (let go). If test group remains in concentric contraction and holds, chart data.

D. Right Leg Extensor Test (pictured)
   1. Isolate and stabilize right arm and right leg in supine flexion.
   2. Control group: Right arm is control. Have client hold arm position against practitioner's inferior/caudal pressure (contracting flexors).
   3. Test group: Test right leg extensors by having client hold leg position against practitioner's superior/cephalad pressure (testing extensors).
   4. Both groups should stay equally strong and steady. If test group is inhibited, chart data.

   Antagonist test: Test right leg flexors by applying inferior/caudal pressure. These muscles should inhibit (let go). If test group remains concentrically contracted, chart data.

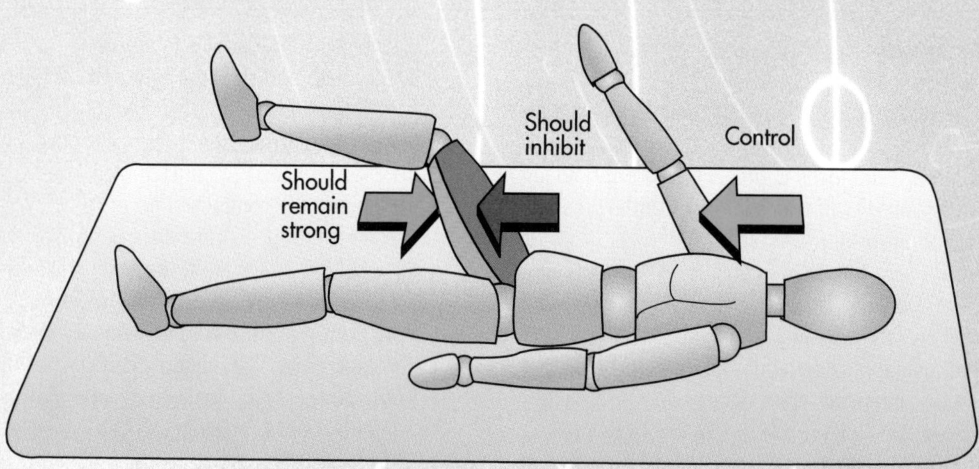

Right leg extensor test
Reverse arm and leg position for left leg extensor test

ACTIVITY 10-2—cont'd

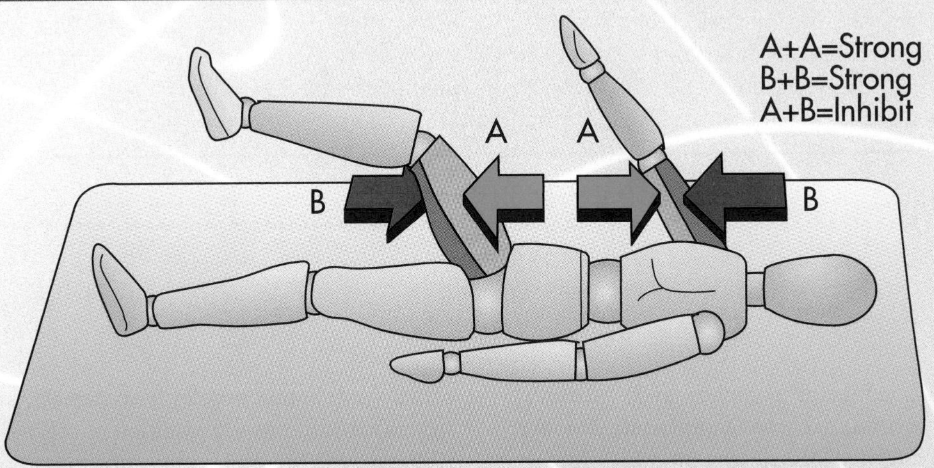

Composite of unilateral patterns

V. Medial/Lateral Symmetry

A. Bilateral Arm Adductor Test

1. Isolate and stabilize arms bilaterally in supine 90 degree flexion and legs bilaterally in flexion.
2. Control group: Bilateral legs are control. Have client hold position against practitioner's lateral pressure or squeeze a ball (contracting adductors).
3. Test group: Test bilateral arm adductors by having client hold position against practitioner's lateral pressure (testing adductors).
4. Both groups should be equally strong and steady. If test group is inhibited, chart data.

Antagonist test: Test bilateral arm abduction by having client hold arm position against medial pressure. These muscles should inhibit (let go). If test group remains concentrically contracted, chart data.

B. Bilateral Leg Adductor Test

1. Isolate and stabilize arms bilaterally in supine 90 degree flexion and legs bilaterally in flexion.
2. Control group: Bilateral arms are controls. Have client hold position against practitioner's lateral pressure or have client press palms together (contracting adductors).
3. Test group: Test bilateral leg adductors by having client hold position against practitioner's (testing adductors).
4. Both groups should be equally strong and steady. If test group is inhibited, chart data.

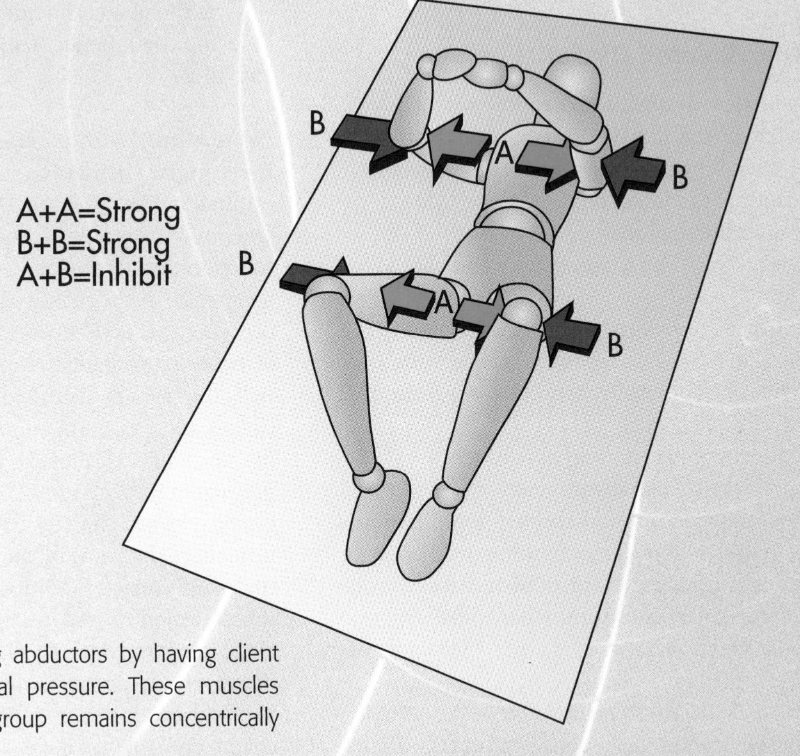

Antagonist test: Test bilateral leg abductors by having client hold against practitioner's medial pressure. These muscles should inhibit (let go). If test group remains concentrically contracted, chart data.

Continued

ACTIVITY 10-2—cont'd

Intervention: Use any massage method to inhibit muscles that test too strong by remaining in concentric contraction patterns. Appropriate methods are slow compression, kneading, gliding, and shaking. Strengthen muscles that inhibit when they should hold strong. Appropriate methods are tapotement and rhythmic tensing of inhibited muscles. Then retest pattern; it should be normal.

(tensor fasciae latae, adductor complex, and quadratus lumborum) become dominant to compensate for the weakness. This alters normal joint alignment, which further alters the normal length-tension relationships of the muscles around the joint. Box 10-3 gives more information on the most common assessment and intervention for firing patterns.

BIOMECHANICAL DYSFUNCTION

Differential diagnosis to determine the causal factors of biomechanical dysfunction is beyond the scope of this text. The modalities studied in the specific application of massage therapy have much to offer in the normalization of some types of movement dysfunction. The three areas most effectively addressed by these methods are neuromuscular, myofascial, or joint-related dysfunction.

Neuromuscular-Related Dysfunction

Neuromuscular-related dysfunction manifests as a breakdown or confusion in the nervous system interaction with muscle activity. Neuromuscular dysfunction can develop in many forms, including the following:

- Neurotransmitter fluctuations
- Hypermuscular or hypomuscular activity and altered firing patterns
- Increased tension in individual motor units or the entire muscle
- Hypersensitivity or hyposensitivity in the proprioceptive feedback loop and reflex arcs
- Central nervous system processing difficulties
- Gait reflex and kinetic chain disturbance

The myotonic unit becomes disrupted with patterns of overly tense muscles and corresponding weakened or reciprocally inhibited muscles. All of these patterns can be reduced to two: regional postural muscular imbalance and nonoptimal motor function.

Regional Postural Muscular Imbalance

Muscles and muscle groups have constant muscular tone that is defined neurologically by related segments of the spinal cord. Some muscles have higher tone, such as those that support the vertical position of the body, and others are necessary for the most important functions such as eating and breathing. The central nervous system regulates the balance of tone between muscle groups. Different pathologic processes disrupt this regulation. Most often the tone of postural muscles, which have greater tone to begin with, increases and so the imbalance appears. The muscles tense and shorten, inhibiting muscles that function toward movement and causing sensations of fatigue and heaviness in the limbs.

Postural stress, pattern overload, repetitive movement, lack of core stability, and lack of neuromuscular efficiency cause biomechanical neuromuscular imbalances.

Predictable neuromuscular chain reactions can occur. As described by Vladimer Janda, these chain reactions can be divided into two patterns: the upper and lower crossed syndromes (Chaitow L, DeLany J, 2001) (Figures 10-15, *A* and *B*, and 10-16, *A* and *B*).

One can assess and address these patterns of dysfunction by using the kinetic chain protocol, as given in Boxes 10-1 and 10-2.

Nonoptimal Motor Function

Every human being, as a result of individual form, creates an optimal motor function and carriage (how the body is held and moves) unique to that person's body. Optimal motor function defines the degree of mobility that the body needs to operate in the most economical way. When all goes well, movement usually proceeds normally. With the appearance of pathologic changes, however, motor function changes as well. Carriage is disturbed, joint mobility becomes limited, tissues and joints are altered, and the tone-strength balance in the tissues is altered. This person spends more energy performing normal movements, which causes fatigue more quickly. The change of the optimal motor function influences the work of the viscera, which in turn influences the condition of the muscles and joints and in turn alters motor function and carriage even further. Thus a vicious circle appears, in which the worsening of different processes negatively contributes to each process. One can assess and address this pattern of dysfunction by using the kinetic chain protocol (see Boxes 10-1 and 10-2) and firing patterns (see Box 10-3).

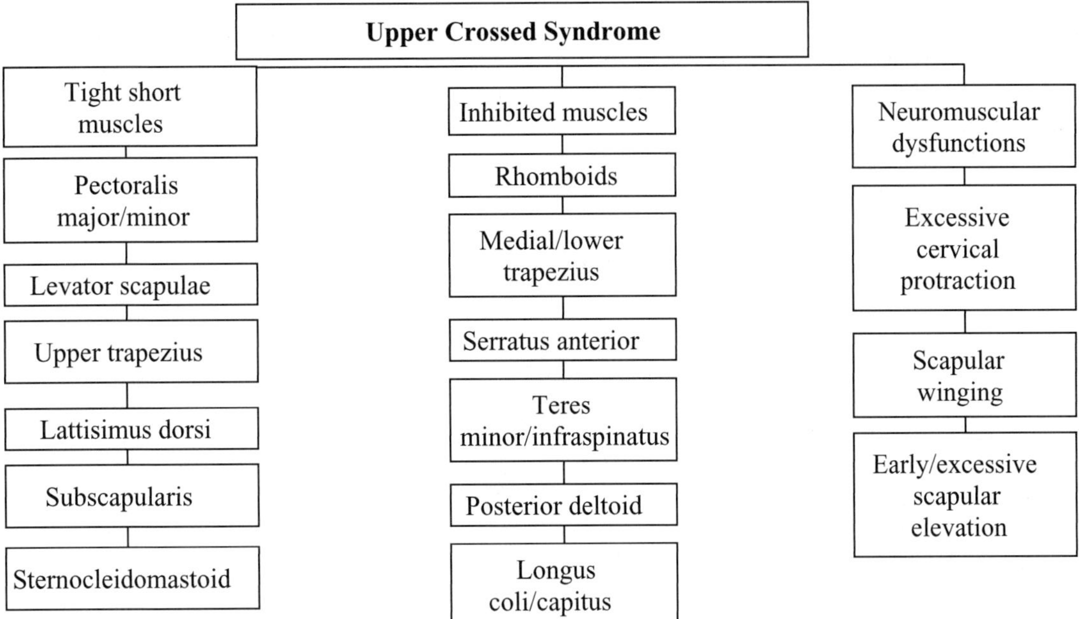

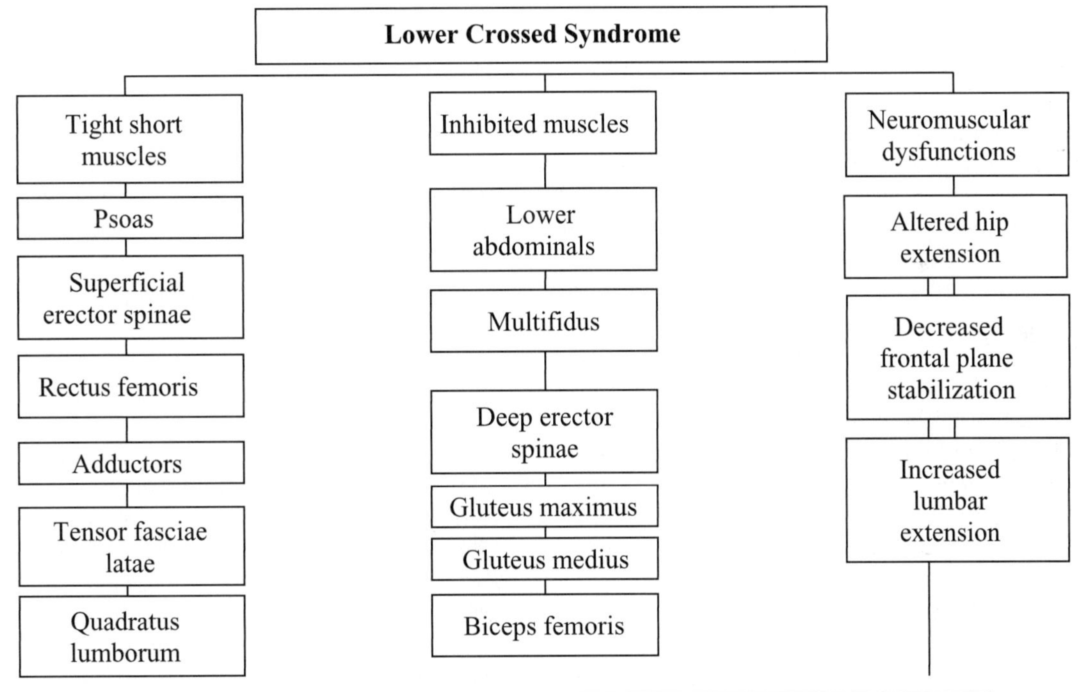

Figure 10-15
A, Upper crossed syndrome flow chart. **B,** Lower crossed syndrome flow chart. (From Chaitow L, DeLany J: *Clinical applications of neuromuscular techniques,* vol 1, *The upper body,* Edinburgh, 2001, Churchill Livingstone.)

Myofascial-Related Dysfunction

Connective tissue changes occur as function is altered or as the result of trauma, including microtrauma from accumulated overuse. Most often connective tissue loses hydration, which affects the viscous and plastic qualities resulting in shortening and reduced pliability. Connective tissues also can become overstretched and lax, reducing their ability to function as dynamic elements of stabilization. One can assess these patterns of dysfunction with various applications of massage that influence the connective tissues.

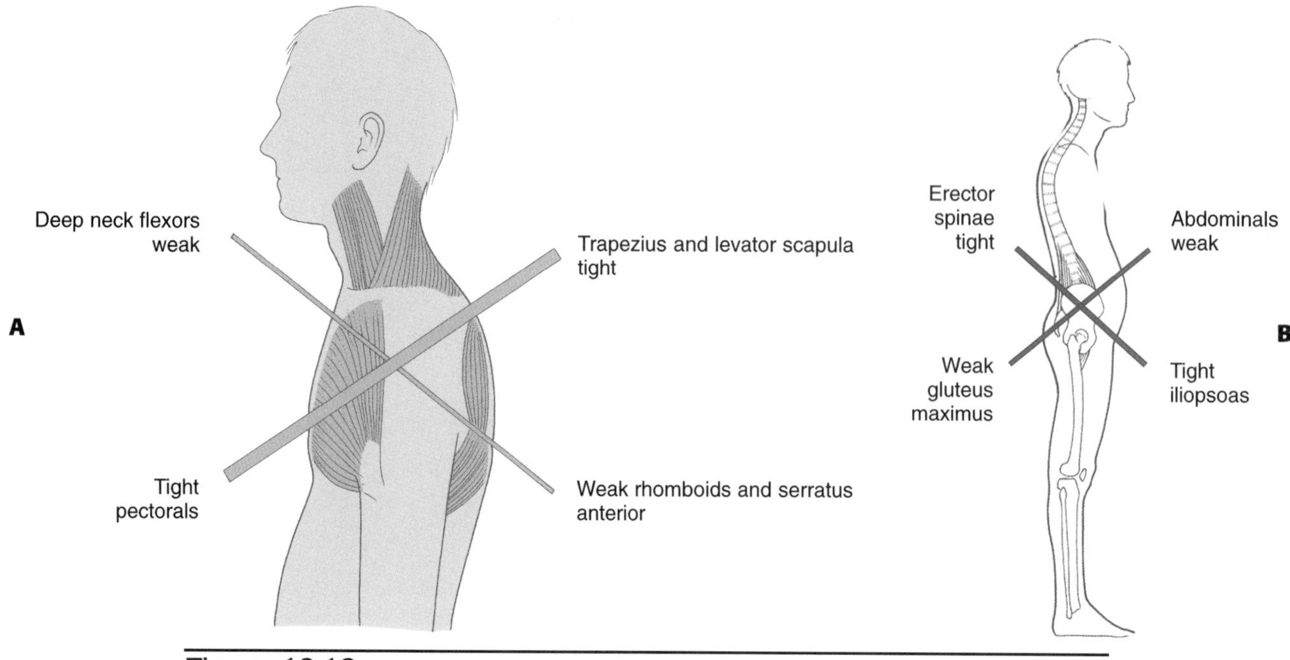

Figure 10-16
A, Upper crossed syndrome (after Janda). **B,** Lower crossed syndrome (after Janda). (From Chaitow L, DeLany J: *Clinical applications of neuromuscular techniques,* vol 1, *The upper body,* Edinburgh, 2001, Churchill Livingstone.)

Joint-Related Dysfunction

Joint-related dysfunction can be capsular (in the capsule itself) or noncapsular. The most common noncapsular pattern is the *functional block,* which is the reversible limitation of range of movement that occurs because of change in connective tissue after long-term muscle spasms. The muscle spasm first appears as a reflex defense mechanism against painful movement in an affected jointed area. Immobility of the joint increases stagnation of tissues, which leads to more pain, resulting in the development of the pain-spasm-pain cycle.

Contributing factors to functional block development include the following:

- Holding a weight that is too heavy for too long
- Constant loading on the spine such as occurs during work situations that demand long-term sitting
- Powerful effort such as used in lifting during sport or work
- Passive overstretching such as holding a heavy weight in the hand, causing development of functional block in the shoulder joint
- Reflex influences on muscles near joints
- Long-term immobility such as when wearing a cast or when bedridden

The appropriate medical professional needs to assess, diagnose, and treat specific joint dysfunction. Massage application can complement the intervention of professionals such as orthopedic physicians, osteopathic physicians, chiropractors, physical therapists, and athletic trainers.

Functional block may be treated successfully by massage (relaxation and pain management), mobilization (repeated passive movement and traction), muscle energy techniques (various forms of active muscle contraction followed by muscle lengthening), and stretching programs.

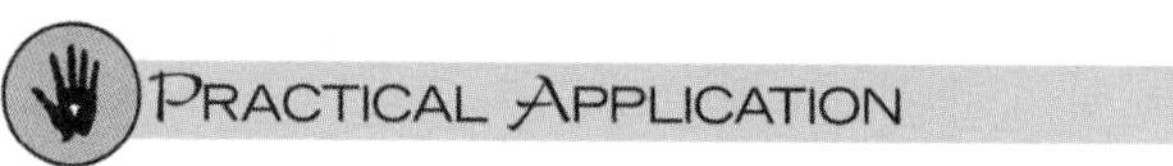

The powerful influences of massage modalities accelerate complex self-regulating processes in the direction of normalization and balance. Any massage modality influences the systems, tissues, and viscera of the body mechanically and reflexively. Massage modalities improve blood circulation, decrease chronic muscle tension, normalize range of motion of the joint, and rebuild proper proprioception.

The body perceives any technique first as a tactile perception because the surface of the skin is altered by various degrees, depending on the character of the methods. Second, massage modalities alter the degree of muscle tension. Proprioceptors of the deep tissues report to the central nervous system regarding the condition of muscle tension, capillary pressure, and blood pressure of muscles and vessels.

The tissues produce warmth. This heat acts as a thermal stimulant that signals the sympathetic and parasympathetic systems to cause vasodilation or vasoconstriction.

Chemical substances such as histamine and acetylcholine are formed in the tissues. Histamine stimulates the discharge of adrenaline. These substances are carried with the blood throughout the body, altering circulation, influencing the functions of inner organs (viscera), speeding up nerve impulses, mobilizing the immune system, normalizing blood pressure, and stimulating muscle activity.

All these signals create the reaction of the central nervous system. The goal is to generate, through massage methods, the stimulation required to generate self-regulating mechanisms, allowing the body to self-correct and restore dynamic balance or homeostasis. ■

Biomechanical Assessment

Before making decisions about referral or to determine the type or combination of modalities to use to restore balance in the biomechanical mechanisms, one must gather information.

Assessment defines mobility through active and passive movements of the affected parts and observation of a distortion in these movements. In addition, one performs muscle testing and defines the functional relationships of the muscles. One investigates any changes in body movement patterns during the client interview.

In postural imbalance some postural muscles are shortened and their antagonists are weakened. Motor function is altered as a result. Postural imbalance often manifests itself as lumbar and cervical hyperlordosis but also could lead to other changes in the spine and joints of the limbs. These changes often play a pathogenic role in movement.

Three degrees of postural imbalance of muscles may occur:

First degree: Shortening or weakening of some muscles or the formation of local changes in tension or connective tissue in these muscles

Second degree: Moderately expressed shortening of postural muscles and weakening of antagonist muscles

Third degree: Clearly expressed shortening of postural muscles and weakening of antagonist muscles with the appearance of specific, nonoptimal movement

To determine appropriate therapeutic intervention, defining which muscles are shortened and which are inhibited is important. The assessment procedures of the kinetic chain and firing pattern assessment (see Boxes 10-1 to 10-3 and Activity 10-2), along with individual muscle testing include the following: local functional block, local hypermobility or hypomobility, altered firing patterns, and postural imbalance, which all lead to changes in motor function and are accompanied by temporary or chronic joint, muscular, and nervous system disorders. Three degrees of distorted motor function exist:

First degree: For usual and simple movements, a person has to use additional muscles from different parts of the body. As a result, movement becomes uneconomical and labored.

Second degree: Moderately peculiar postures and movements of some parts of the body are present. Postural and movement distortion, such as altered firing patterns, begin to occur.

Third degree: Significantly expressed peculiarity in postures and movement occurs. Increased postural and movement distortions result.

These pathobiomechanical disturbances may occur in all age groups. On the basis of the three degrees of distorted motor function, three stages exist in the development of postural and movement pathology:

Stage 1, functional tension: At this stage, a person tires more quickly than normal. This fatigue is accompanied by some functional block in the first- or second-degree limitation of mobility, painless local myodystonia (changes in the muscle tension/length relationship), postural imbalance in the first or second degree, and nonoptimal motor function of the first degree.

Stage 2, functional stress: This stage is characterized by a feeling of fatigue from moderate activity, discomfort, slight pain, and the appearance of singular or multiple functional blocks and any degree of limited mobility. Functional block may be painless or result in first-degree pain; it may be accompanied by local hypermobility. Functional stress also is characterized by reflex vertebral-sensory dysfunction, fascial/connective tissue changes, and regional postural imbalance and by distortion of motor function in the first or second degree.

Stage 3, connective tissue changes in the musculoskeletal system: The reasons for connective tissue changes are overloading, disturbances of tissue nutrition, microtraumas, microhemorrhages, unresolved edema, and other endogenous (inside the body) and exogenous (outside the body) factors. Hereditary predisposition is also a consideration. In the third stage, osteochondrosis of the spine and weight-bearing joints may appear as single or multiple functional blocks, local hypermobility and instability of several vertebral motion segments, hypomobility, widespread painful muscle tension and fascial and connective tissue changes in the muscles, regional postural imbalance in the second or third degree in many joints, and temporary nonoptimal motor function with second- or third-degree distortion. Visceral disturbances may be present (Gurevich, 1992).

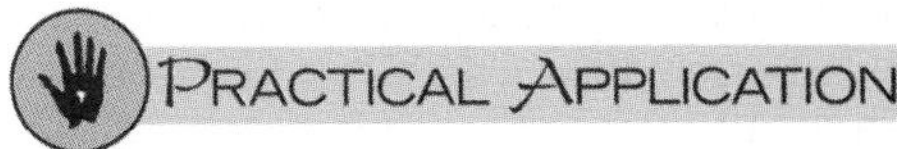

One often can manage stage 1 functional tension effectively by massage modalities and with training equivalent to 500 to 1000 hours that includes an understanding of the information presented in this text and technical training in one's chosen modality. Working with stages 2 and 3 functional stress and connective tissue changes usually requires more training and proper supervision within a multidisciplinary approach. ■

Regional Biomechanical Assessment

The clinical reasoning process is essential when assessing for biomechanical function and developing intervention (treatment) plans. For review of the clinical reasoning process, the student should refer to Chapter 3.

Intervention plans should work toward the client's goals. Relating benefit derived from the modalities to daily function is important. For example, a plan based on the client goal of more effective shoulder movement would read as follows: Improved shoulder movement would be encouraged with the use of weekly therapeutic massage and daily yoga practice. Client indicates that more effective shoulder movement could result in increased golf performance and the reduction of shoulder stiffness after the game.

A plan based on efficient biomechanical movement would focus on reestablishing or supporting effective movement patterns.

Biomechanically efficient movement is smooth, bilaterally symmetric, and coordinated, with an easy, effortless use of the body. During assessment, one should consider noticeable variations.

Each jointed area has a movement pattern. The movement is a product of the entire mechanism, including bones; joints; ligaments; capsular components and design; tendons; muscle shapes and fiber types; interlinked fascial networks; nerve distribution; myotatic units of prime movers, antagonists, synergists, fixators, and kinetic chain interactions; bodywide influence of reflexes, including positional and righting reflexes of vision and the inner ear; circulatory distribution; general systemic balance; and nutritional influences. When one assesses a movement pattern as normal, the assessment indicates that all parts are functioning in a well-orchestrated manner. If one identifies a dysfunction, causal factors can be from any one or a combination of these elements. Often a multidisciplinary diagnosis is necessary to identify clearly the interconnected nature of the pathologic condition.

Assessment also identifies areas of resourceful and successful compensation. These compensation patterns occur when the body has been required to adapt to some sort of trauma or repetitive use pattern. Permanent adaptive changes, although not as efficient as optimal functioning, are the best pattern the body can develop in response to an irreversible change in the system. One should not eliminate resourceful compensation but instead support it.

The following sections of this chapter explore movement assessments for individual jointed areas by applying a force to load the muscles to determine a response in the jointed area.

For the therapeutic massage student now, finally, all that has been studied begins to come together in a functional process. The student should remember that each joint movement pattern is part of an interconnected aspect of the kinetic chain and the tensegric nature of the design of the body. One must assess posture and movement dysfunction identified in an individual joint pattern and treat it in broader terms of kinetic chain interactions, muscle tension/length relationships, and the effects of stress and strain on the entire system.

When one assesses a movement pattern, one obtains two types of information: First, when a jointed area moves into flexion and the joint angle decreases, the prime mover and synergists concentrically contract and antagonists eccentrically contract while lengthening and the fixators isometrically contract and stabilize. Bodywide stabilization patterns also come into play to assist in allowing the motion. During assessment, one applies resistance to load the prime mover groups and synergists to assess for neurologic function of strength and, to a lesser degree, endurance as the contraction is held for a period of time.

At the same time, one can assess the antagonist pattern of the tissues that are lengthened when positioned for the functional assessment for increased tension patterns or connective tissue shortening. Dysfunction shows itself in limited range of motion by restricting the movement pattern. Therefore when placing a jointed area into flexion, one should assess the extensors for increased tension or shortening. When the jointed area moves into extension, the opposite becomes the case. The same holds for adduction and abduction, internal and external rotation, plantar and dorsal flexion, and so on.

Resistance (pressure against) applied to the muscles is focused at the end of the lever system for mechanical advantage. For example, when assessing the function of the shoulder, one focuses resistance at the distal end of the humerus, not at the wrist. When assessing extension of the hip, one places resistance at the end of the femur. When assessing flexion of the knee, one places resistance at the distal end of the tibia.

The practitioner applies resistance slowly, smoothly, and firmly at an appropriate intensity determined by the size of the muscle mass. Stabilization is essential to assess movement patterns accurately. One allows only the area being assessed to move. Movement in any other part of the body needs to be stabilized. The massage therapist usually applies a stabilizing force. As one hand applies resistance, the other provides the stabilization. Sometimes the client can provide the stabilization. Some modalities use straps to provide stabilization. The easiest way to identify the area to be stabilized is to move the area to be assessed through the range of motion. At the end of the range some other part of the body will begin to move: this is the area of stabilization. One should return the body to a neutral position, provide the appropriate stabilization to the area identified, and begin the assessment procedure.

Range of motion of a joint is measured in degrees. A full circle is 360 degrees. A flat horizontal line is 180 degrees. Two perpendicular lines (as in the shape of a capital L) create a 90-degree angle. Various ranges of motion are possible. For example, when the range of motion of a joint allows 0 to 90 degrees of flexion, anything less is hypomobile and anything more is hypermobile. A great degree of variability exists

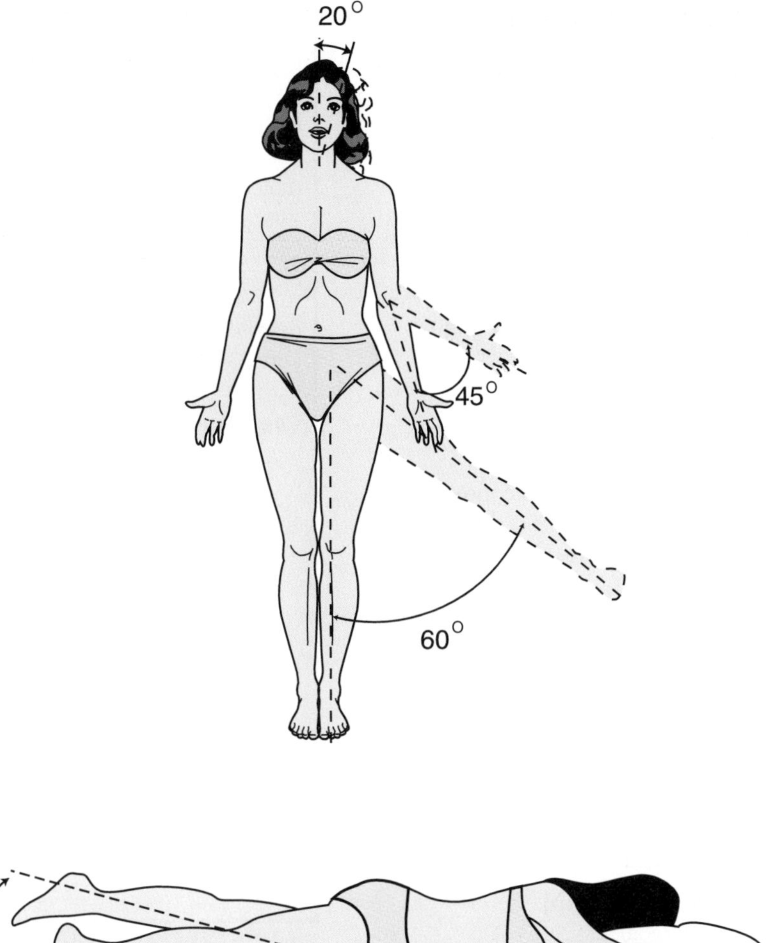

Figure 10-17
Degrees of range of motion.

among individuals as to the actual normal range of motion; the degrees provided are general guidelines (Figure 10-17). Range of motion is measured from the anatomic position. Regardless if the client is standing, supine, or side lying, anatomic position is considered 0 degrees of motion.

The section Biomechanics by Region provides specific assessment protocols for the body. In actual professional practice, the practitioner picks and chooses which assessments to perform on the basis of the client's goals and intervention processes. The activities are arranged to represent (agonist/antagonist) myotonic units; for example, trunk extension/trunk flexion and hip adduction/hip abduction.

During assessments, muscles should be able to hold against appropriate resistance without strain or pain from the pressure and without recruiting or using other muscles. One applies appropriate resistance slowly and steadily and with just enough force for the muscles to respond to the stimulus. Large muscle groups require more force than small ones. The position should be easy to assume and comfortable to maintain for a short duration, from 10 to 30 seconds. Contraindications to this type of assessment include joint and disk dysfunction, acute pain, recent trauma, and inflammation.

Results of the assessment identify appropriate function of each area or dysfunction in one, two, or three degrees. Once one completes all assessments, one describes the overall result as normal or stage 1, 2, or 3 dysfunction, as mentioned. One usually can manage first-degree and stage 1 dysfunction by general massage application. One should refer clients with stage 2 and 3 dysfunction to the appropriate health care professional and develop cooperative multidisciplinary treatment plans.

General Guidelines to Assist the Clinical Reasoning Process

Guidelines include the following:

- If an area is hypomobile, one should consider tension or shortening in the antagonist pattern as a possible cause.
- If an area is hypermobile, one should consider instability of the joint structure or muscle weakness in the fixation pattern or problems with antagonist/agonist co-contraction function.

- If an area cannot hold against resistance, one should consider weakness from reciprocal inhibition of the muscles of the prime mover and synergist pattern and tension in the antagonist pattern as possible causes.
- If pain occurs on passive movement, one should consider joint capsular dysfunction and nerve entrapment syndromes as possible causes.
- If pain occurs on active movement, one should consider muscle and fascial involvement as a possible cause.
- One always should consider bodywide reflexive patterns, as discussed in the section on posture and gait and kinetic chain, as possible causes.

The following guidelines also are important:

- The ability to resist the applied force easily should be the same or similar bilaterally.
- The client should be able to assume opposite movement patterns easily.
- Bilateral asymmetry, pain, weakness, inability to assume the isolation position or to move into the opposite position, or fatigue or a heavy sensation may indicate dysfunction.
- Intervention or referral depends on the severity of the condition (stage 1, 2, or 3) and whether the dysfunction is related to the joints, neuromuscular system, or myofascial tissues.

ACTIVITY 10-3

From a standing position, slowly move your head into flexion. Then follow with your cervical region, thoracic region, and lumbar region, each moving into flexion. Pay attention to the limitation of each region and notice the increased range of motion as each area is brought into play. Now move into extension following the same pattern. Repeat this activity for lateral flexion and rotation on both sides. In the space provided describe the experience.

Example
I noticed that it was difficult to isolate head flexion by itself.

Your Turn

BIOMECHANICS BY REGION

Trunk and Thorax Region

Biomechanics of the trunk and thorax are unique because of the complexity of the vertebral column, composed of 24 intricate and complex articulating vertebrae and 31 pairs of spinal nerves. Vertebral motion is greatest where the articulating surfaces and disks are large.

Spinal or Vertebral Movements

Movement depends on a finely integrated system of muscles that are deep—composed of numerous small bundles that attach from vertebra to vertebra—or superficial—arranged in large broad sheets.

The name given to the region of movement often precedes the descriptions of spinal or vertebral movements. For example, flexion of the trunk at the lumbar spine is known as lumbar flexion, and extension of the neck often is referred to as cervical extension. Movement of the head between the cranium and the first cervical vertebra is called capital movement. Movements occurring among the other cervical vertebrae are called cervical movements. These motions usually occur together.

The five spinal movements are as follows (Activity 10-3):

Spinal flexion: Spinal flexion is anterior movement of the spine in the sagittal plane. In the cervical region the head moves toward the chest. In the thoracic and lumbar regions the thorax moves toward the pelvis.

Spinal extension: Spinal extension is posterior movement of the spine in the sagittal plane to return from flexion. In the cervical spine the head moves away from the chest. The thorax moves away from the pelvis.

Lateral flexion (side bending): Lateral flexion in the frontal plane occurs in the cervical region when the head moves laterally toward the shoulder. In the thoracic and lumbar regions the thorax moves laterally toward the pelvis. Movement can be to the left or right.

Reduction: Reduction is the return movement from lateral flexion to neutral.

Spinal rotation (left or right): Spinal rotation in the transverse plane is the rotary or twisting movement of the spine. In the cervical region the chin rotates from neutral toward the shoulder. In the thoracic and lumbar regions the thorax rotates to one side.

As explained previously, each pair of vertebrae constitutes a vertebral motion segment, the basic movable unit of the back. Except for the atlantoaxial joint formed by the first two cervical vertebrae, little movement is possible between any two vertebrae. The amount of movement varies depending on the shape of the vertebrae, the thickness of the intervertebral disk—with thicker disks providing greater mobility—and any rib articulations. However, the cumulative effect of the movements from several adjacent vertebrae allows for substantial movements within a given area. Most of the spinal column movement occurs in the cervical and lumbar regions. Of course, some thoracic movement occurs but is slight compared with that of the neck and low back.

Rotation screws the superior vertebra down into the adjacent vertebra, compressing the disk. Prime mover muscles contract, while the contralateral muscles lengthen. Ligament structures are twisted.

In flexion the anterior muscles contract, the posterior muscles lengthen, the superior vertebra tilts toward the front, and the disks are compressed anteriorly and expand posteriorly while the nucleus moves slightly to the back. The superior articular facets slide forward on the inferior ones. The posterior ligaments are stretched and the anterior ligaments are slack.

In extension, just the opposite occurs. The posterior muscles contract and anterior muscles lengthen. The superior vertebra tilts toward the back. The disk is compressed posteriorly and expands anteriorly, and the nucleus moves slightly to the front. The articular facets are pressed together. The anterior ligaments are stretched, and the posterior ligaments slacken. Lateral flexion follows the same pattern (Figure 10-18; Activity 10-4).

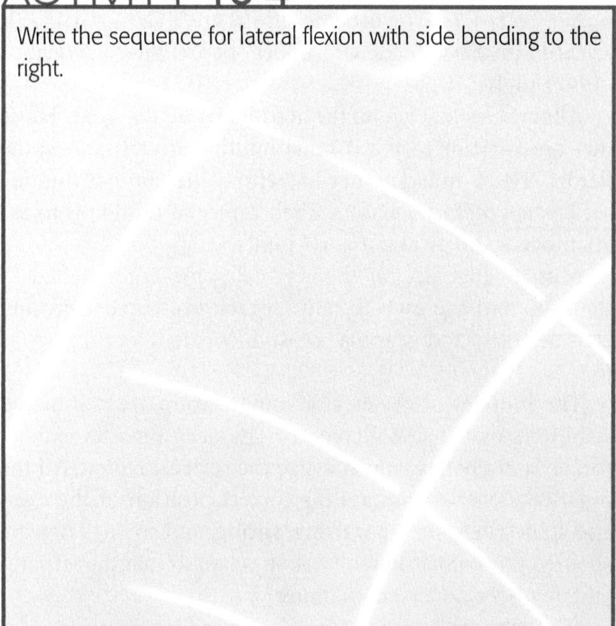

Head/Neck Region

That the neck, a small portion of our body, can be so complex and have such precise performance is hard to believe.

The neck connects to the head in the thorax and contains the C1 to C7 cervical vertebrae, spinal cord, 32 muscles, ligaments, pharynx, larynx, trachea, thyroid, esophagus, lymph glands, hyoid bone, blood vessels, and spinal nerves.

The cervical vertebrae allow the head and neck to be moved into flexion, extension, lateral flexion, and rotation. Combinations of these movements are also possible. The small bodies and thick disks of the cervical vertebrae tend to increase mobility. Side bending is somewhat restricted by the rectangular shape of the vertebral bodies. The atlas and axis (C1 and C2) form a pivot joint that allows the head and C1 to rotate almost 90 degrees, such as in a "no" motion. The short spinous processes of C3 to C6 allow for good extension of the head and neck.

Intervertebral disks make up approximately 25% of the height of the cervical spine. The ligaments connecting the occiput to the atlas are dense and broad. These ligaments protect the entrance of the spinal cord through the foramen magnum into the skull. The atlantoaxial (C1 and C2) joint almost totally depends on ligamentous structure. The cervical spine from C2 to C7 is reinforced by anterior and posterior longitudinal ligaments. These ligaments limit the amount of flexion and extension.

The body moves and is balanced at certain points throughout our form. Two of these movement segments fall

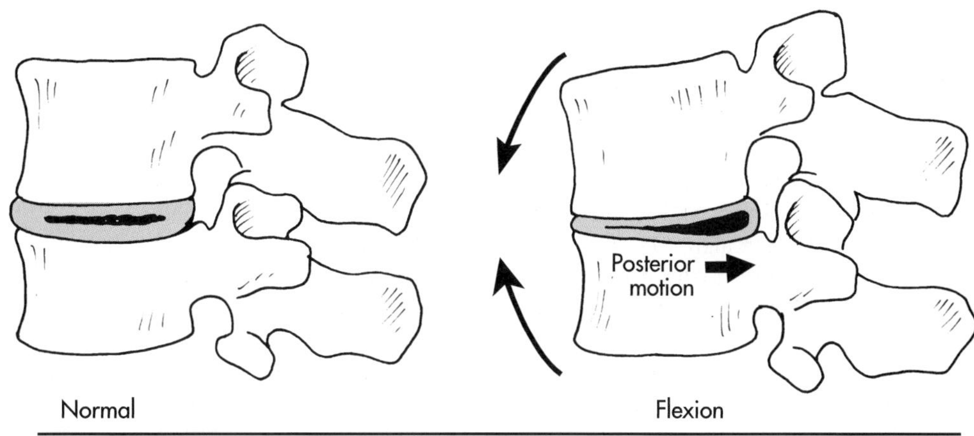

Figure 10-18
Movement of the spine from a position of extension into flexion causes the nucleus to move in a posterior direction. (From Shankman GA: *Fundamental orthopedic management for the physical therapist assistant,* St Louis, 1997, Mosby.)

within the head/neck area: one at the atlas and skull and one at C6 to C7. (The other locations are T12/L1, L4/L5/S1, acetabulum/hips, knees, and ankles (as previously described in Box 10-1.)

All muscles that act on the head insert on the skull. Those that are anterior to the coronal midline are termed *capital flexors.* Those muscles that lie behind the coronal midline are termed *capital extensors.* Their center of motion is in the atlantooccipital or atlantoaxial joints.

Muscles that act on the cervical spine are attached to the skull and the cervical and thoracic vertebrae, sternum, clavicle, ribs, and scapula. Most movement occurs at C6 to C7.

The muscles of the erector spinae group are considered stabilizers of the spinal column. The deep muscles extend, rotate, laterally flex, and stabilize the cervical region. All the muscles serve to maintain the correct position of the head and spine while we are walking, sitting, and so on. They are adapted physiologically to work in relays so that they do not fatigue under normal conditions.

The sternocleidomastoid is primarily responsible for flexion and rotation of the head and neck. Extension, particularly extension and rotation, involves the splenius muscles together with the erector spinae and the upper trapezius muscles. The neck extensors, trapezius, scalenes, sternocleidomastoid, and levator scapulae are considered major postural muscles in the body. The responsibility of these muscles is taxing even when the body has good posture and no pathologic condition is present. Many muscles of the neck are called on to assist in breathing if incorrect breathing patterns exist.

Thoracic Vertebral Column Region

The thoracic vertebrae are structured to articulate with the ribs, with stability as the main function of this outer unit region. This area does not move extensively, but small movements at the facet joints are ongoing with the breathing process.

A few large extrinsic muscles and numerous small intrinsic muscles are found in this area. *Extrinsic muscles* are defined as muscles that link a limb to the trunk of the body. Intrinsic muscles are muscles that are entirely within the body part or segment (inner unit). The largest muscle is the erector spinae (sacrospinalis), which extends on each side of the spinal column from the pelvic region to the cranium.

The erector spinae muscles function best when the pelvis is held up in front, thus pulling them down slightly in back. This lowers the origin of the erector spinae and makes them more effective in keeping the spine straight. As the spine is held straight and the ribs are raised, the chest raises and consequently makes the abdominal muscles more effective in holding the pelvis up in front and flattening the abdominal wall.

Lumbar Vertebral Column Region

The five lumbar vertebrae are the most massive of the spinal column. They carry a large share of the upper body weight, balancing the torso on the sacrum. The combined unit of the vertebrae and disks in the upright position forms the lumbar spinal curve. The lumbar vertebral disks are strong, short, and thick. The ligaments provide stability in all directions. This is the most frequently injured area of the back.

The lumbar vertebral group has less mobility than the cervical region but more than the thoracic region. Because of the absence of ribs and the shape of the spinous processes, the lumbar spine is freer in flexion and extension. Rotation, however, is limited by the amount of tension created in the surrounding ligaments and annulus fibrosus of the disks.

Motions of the lumbar spine include flexion, extension, lateral flexion, and rotation. More motion takes place at L5/S1 (the lumbosacral junction) than at L1/L2.

The angle formed between L5 and S1 is called the lumbosacral angle. This angle is approximately 41 degrees in the normal individual. This is typically a neutral position in that no erector spinae force needs to be exerted as a counterbalance. When special conditions exist such as obesity, pregnancy, abdominal muscle weakness, wearing high heels, foot pronation, and poor posture, this angle increases undesirably, which can lead to lumbar pain and dysfunction (Figure 10-19).

Abdominal muscles initiate flexion, whereas the erector spinae resist flexion. Intrinsic muscles of the back provide extension, whereas the abdominal muscles (mainly the rectus abdominis) resist. Lateral bending occurs with spinal rotation. Ipsilateral structures tend to relax, whereas contralateral structures resist. Lumbosacral rotation takes place with a variety of complex tension and relaxation

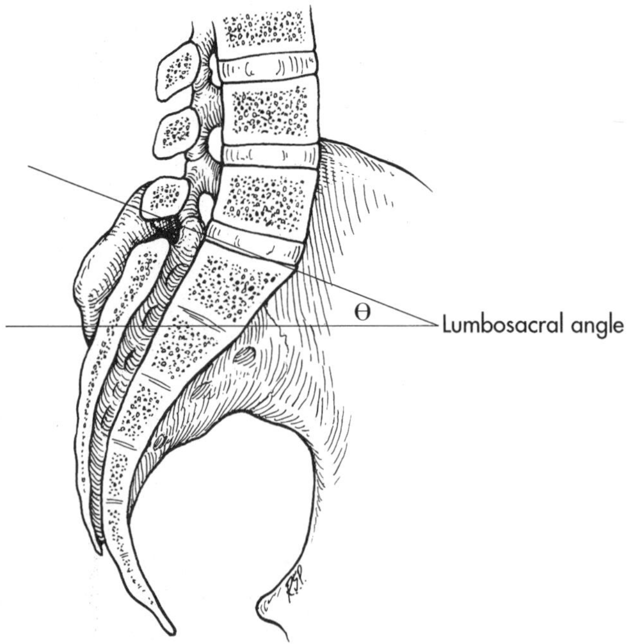

Figure 10-19
The lumbosacral angle. (From Malone TR, McPoil T, Nitz AJ: *Orthopedic and sports physical therapy,* ed 3, St Louis, 1997, Mosby.)

patterns. Rotation is limited by the straight, posteriorly oriented spinous processes.

Abdomen Region

Abdominal muscles do not extend from bone to bone, but attach into tendinous bands and an aponeurosis (fascia) around the rectus abdominis area. The abdominal muscles are the rectus abdominis, external oblique, internal oblique, and transversus abdominis.

The rectus abdominis muscle controls the tilt of the pelvis and the consequent curvature of the lower spine. Holding the pelvis up in front makes the erector spinae muscle more effective as an extensor of the spine and makes the hip flexors such as the iliopsoas more effective.

The internal oblique muscles run diagonally in the direction opposite to that of the external oblique muscles. The left internal oblique muscle causes rotation to the left, and the right internal oblique muscle causes rotation to the right. In rotary movements the internal oblique muscle and the opposite side external oblique muscle always work together.

The transversus abdominis is the chief muscle of forced expiration. Together with the external oblique and internal oblique muscles they are effective in helping to hold the abdomen flat.

Thorax Region

As covered in Chapter 7, the skeletal foundation of the thorax is formed by 12 pairs of ribs, the manubrium, the body of the sternum, and the xiphoid process. Breathing is a major function of the thorax. Breathing involves inspiration, or inhaling, and expiration, or exhaling. The primary muscles of inspiration are the diaphragm and the external intercostals.

During quiet respiration, the diaphragm may act alone, or a slight rhythmic activity may occur in the scalenus anterior and scalenus medius and in the intercostals. In deep inspiration the action of the primary muscles increases, and the sternocleidomastoid and scalenes assist in raising the ribs. Forced inspiration involves any muscles that stabilize or elevate the shoulder girdle to elevate the ribs directly or indirectly.

Expiration is primarily passive as relaxation of the prime movers and the weight of gravity pulls the rib cage down. The primary muscles of expiration are the internal intercostals. Forced expiration involves muscles that force the rib cage down (quadratus lumborum) or compress the abdominal cavity (oblique and transverse abdominals), forcing the diaphragm upward.

Two different types of breathing patterns exist: diaphragmatic and thoracic. Diaphragmatic, or abdominal, breathing is the natural way to breathe and occurs in infants and sleeping adults. Inhalation deep into the lungs occurs by the contraction of the diaphragm, flattening its dome shape and resulting in negative pressure in the lungs, which fill with air to equalize the pressure. The diaphragm then relaxes, expelling the air by its upward movement. Diaphragmatic breathing is even and relaxed.

Thoracic, or chest, breathing is common in persons with anxiety or other emotional distress. Anxious persons may experience breath holding, hyperventilation syndrome, constricted breathing, shortness of breath, or fear of passing out. Thoracic breathing occurs in persons who wear restrictive clothing, actively hold in their abdominal muscles, or lead sedentary or stressful lives. Chest breathing is often shallow, irregular, and rapid. On inhalation the chest expands and the shoulders rise to take in air. Dysfunctional patterns can develop if the accessory muscles of respiration (scalenes, sternocleidomastoid, serratus posterior superior, levator scapulae, rhomboids, abdominals, and quadratus lumborum) are used constantly for regular breathing when forced inhalation and expiration are not required (Activity 10-5).

Shoulder Region

Remarkably, the complicated framework of the shoulder not only is extremely mobile but also provides a secure and stable immovable point for specific actions such as lifting, thrusting, shoving, and pushing heavy objects. This region consists of the shoulder girdle and the shoulder, or glenohumeral joint.

Shoulder Girdle Region

The shoulder girdle is made up of the scapula and clavicle (which generally move as a unit) and associated soft tissues. The clavicle has two synovial gliding joints. The sternoclavicular joint is medial, and the acromioclavicular joint is lateral. When analyzing scapulothoracic movements, one should realize that the scapula moves on the rib cage because the joint motion actually occurs at the sternoclavicular joint and to a lesser extent at the acromioclavicular joint.

The movements of the sternoclavicular joint include elevation, depression, rotation, protraction, and retraction. For full abduction to occur, the clavicle must rotate 50 degrees posteriorly. Movement at the joint occurs indirectly as a result of scapular movement. The characteristics of the joint are influenced indirectly by the movement of the glenohumeral joint. Although no direct muscular attachments cross this joint, several muscles have indirect influence on the movement, especially the pectoralis major, subclavius, sternocleidomastoid, sternothyroid and sternohyoid, scalenus medius and scalenus posterior, and upper trapezius.

The acromioclavicular joint contributes little to scapular movement because its joint surfaces do not allow much angular movement. A rotary and hingelike motion takes place at this joint chiefly with elevation of the arm above 90 degrees. The S shape of the clavicle provides the extra motion during elevation of the arm.

The scapulae rotate at the acromioclavicular joint at the beginning of scapular movement. Of the approximately 60 degrees that scapular movement contributes to the elevation of the arm, about 30 degrees occurs at the sternoclavicular joint and the remaining 30 degrees occurs from the combined effects of clavicular rotation, which causes the

text continued on p. 518

ACTIVITY 10-5

In this activity, you will be working with a partner to assess individual movement patterns, normal function, and possible dysfunction in each other. One of you is first to isolate the specified movement patterns on each side of your partner, one side at a time, and assess for normal function by applying a gentle pressure opposite to the action of the isolation position. The body should be stabilized so that only the isolated area is moving. In some instances the ability to assume the position and maintain it indicates normal function. Muscles should be able to hold against gravity or the applied pressure without strain or pain. The position itself should be easy to assume and comfortable to maintain for a short duration, from 10 to 30 seconds. The bilateral movement patterns should be the same. The opposite movement pattern also should be able to be done easily.

Dysfunction may be indicated by bilateral asymmetry, pain, weakness, fatigue, a heavy sensation (binding), and inability to assume the isolation position or move into the opposite position. Intervention or referral depends on the severity of the condition and whether the dysfunction is neuromuscular, myofascial, or joint related.

Note: Do not perform these assessments if contraindications exist. Contraindications to this type of assessment include joint and disk dysfunction, acute pain, recent trauma, and inflammation.

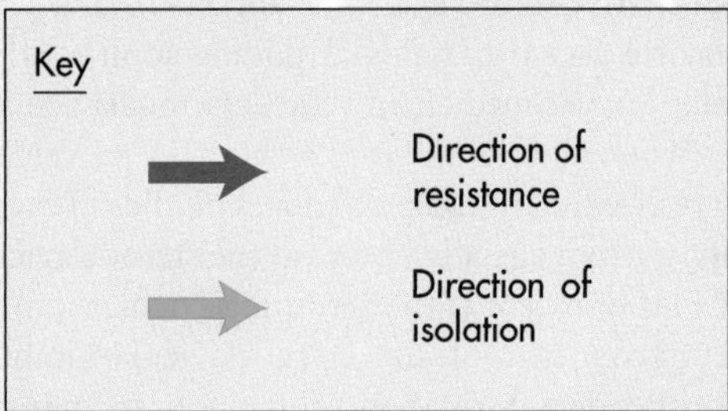

Trunk Extension

Assesses for strength and endurance in the isolation position and tension or shortening in the flexion pattern.

Muscles involved
Erector spinae (sacrospinalis) group: iliocostalis, longissimus, and spinalis
Splenius (cervicis and capitis)
Semispinalis
Multifidus

Range of motion
Thoracic spine: No range of motion
Lumbar spine: 0 to 25 degrees

Position of client
Prone, with hands clasped behind head; client may hold hands behind back.

Isolation and assessment
Client extends the lumbar spine until the head and chest are raised from the table. Ability to perform test indicates normal function. No resistance is required.

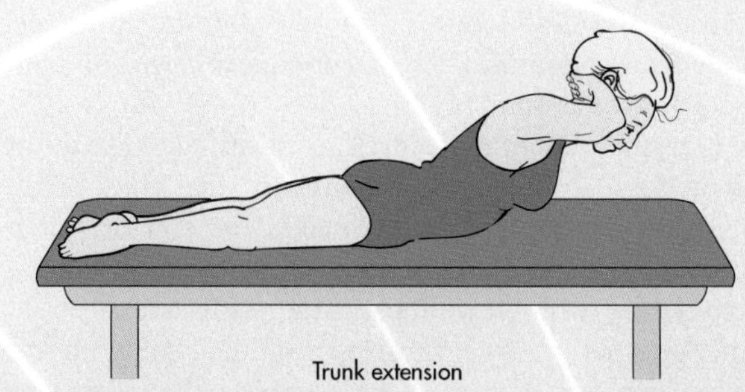
Trunk extension

Trunk Flexion

Assesses for strength and endurance in the isolation position and tension or shortening in the extension pattern.

Muscles involved
Rectus abdominis
Internal and external obliques
Psoas major and psoas minor

Range of motion
0 to 50 degrees (beyond 50 degrees, any additional flexion comes from pelvic rotation)

Position of the client
Supine, with hands clasped behind head or crossed in front and placed on shoulders, knees bent, feet flat
Note: Client is not to lift head with hands.

Isolation and assessment
Client tucks chin to chest and brings shoulders toward thighs. Ability to clear scapulae from the table indicates good function. No resistance is required.

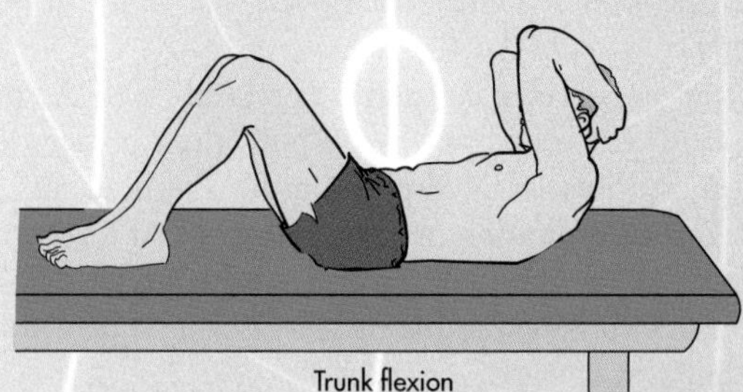
Trunk flexion

Trunk Rotation

Assesses for strength and endurance in the isolation position and tension or shortening in the contralateral pattern.

Muscles involved
External obliques
Internal obliques

ACTIVITY 10-5—cont'd

Latissimus dorsi
Rectus abdominis
Deep back muscles (unilateral test)

Range of motion
0 to 45 degrees

Position of client
Supine, with knees bent and feet flat, hands clasped across chest or held beside ears
Note: Client is not to lift head with hands.

Isolation and assessment
Client slowly flexes and rotates trunk to one side. After returning to supine position, movement is repeated on opposite side. Ability to clear scapulae from the table indicates good function. Right shoulder to left knee tests right external obliques and left internal obliques. Left shoulder to right knee tests the left external obliques and right internal obliques.

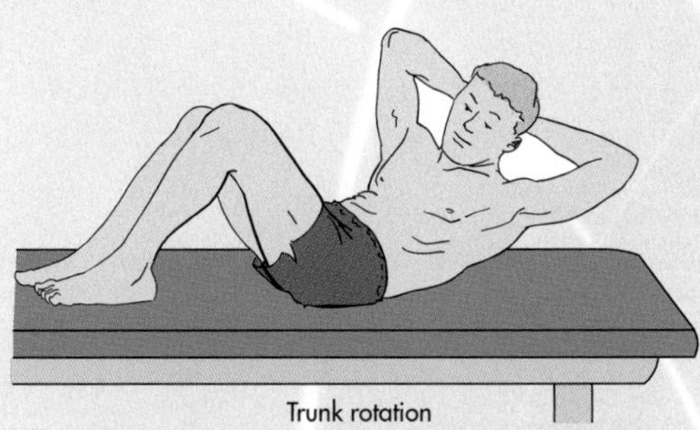
Trunk rotation

Elevation of the Pelvis (More Correctly Known as Lateral Tilt)

Assesses for strength and endurance in the isolation position and tension or shortening in the contralateral pattern.

Muscles involved
Quadratus lumborum
Latissimus dorsi
Internal abdominal obliques
Iliocostalis lumborum

Range of motion
Not applicable

Position of client
Prone with hip and lumbar spine in extension, hip slightly abducted, feet off end of table; the client grasps the edges of the table to provide stabilization during resistance.

Isolation and assessment
Client brings iliac crest toward ribs on one side while examiner applies resistance to lower leg to pull hip down.

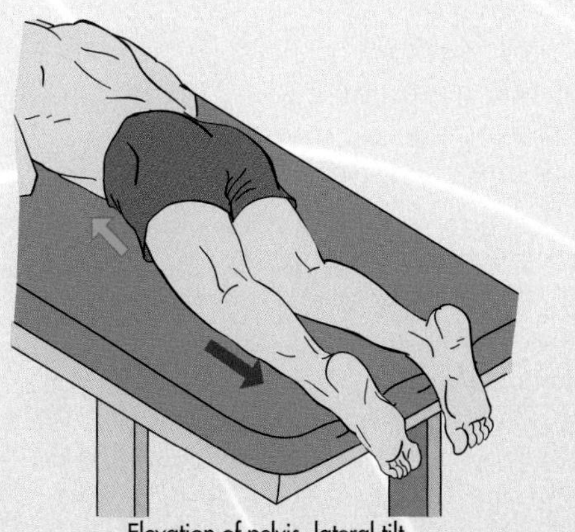
Elevation of pelvis, lateral tilt

Capital Extension

Assesses for strength and endurance in the isolation position and tension or shortening in the flexion pattern.

Muscles involved
Rectus capitis posterior major
Rectus capitis posterior minor
Longissimus capitis
Obliquus capitis superior
Obliquus capitis inferior
Splenius capitis
Semispinalis capitis

Range of motion
0 to 25 degrees

Position of client
Prone with head off end of table, arms at sides
Note: Do not do this test if client has cervical disk problems.

Isolation and assessment
Client lifts chin up away from chest, as if beginning to nod "yes"; cervical spine is not extended. Examiner applies resistance to the back of the head.

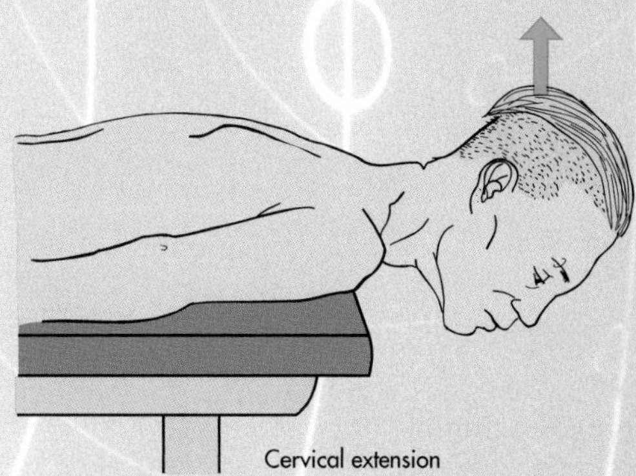
Cervical extension

Cervical Extension

Assesses for strength and endurance in the isolation position and tension or shortening in the flexion pattern

Continued

ACTIVITY 10-5—cont'd

Muscles involved
Longissimus cervicis
Semispinalis cervicis
Iliocostalis cervicis
Splenius capitis and splenius cervicis

Range of motion
0 to 25 degrees

Position of client
Prone, with head off end of table, arms along sides
Note: Do not do this test if client has cervical disk problems.

Isolation and assessment
Client extends neck by lifting head toward ceiling. No resistance is required. Ability to hold head up against gravity indicates normal function.

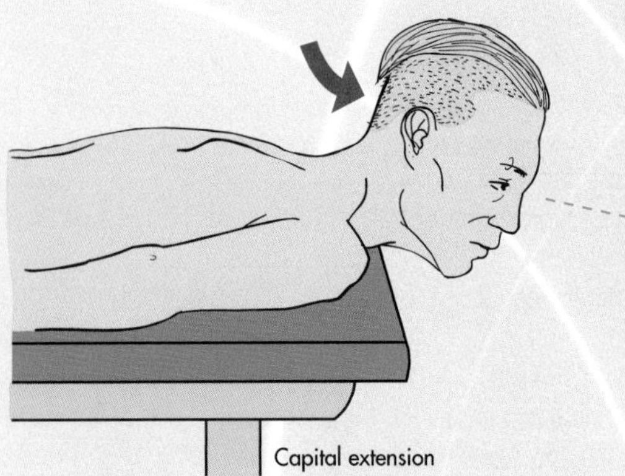
Capital extension

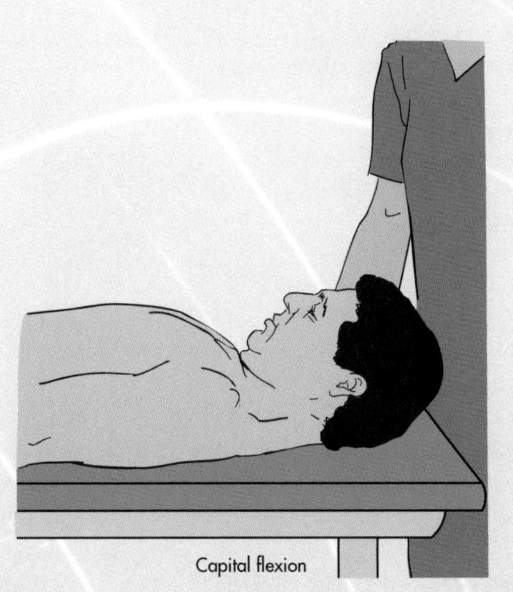
Capital flexion

Capital Flexion
Assesses for strength and endurance in the isolation position and tension or shortening in the extension pattern.

Muscles involved
Rectus longus
Capitis anterior

Range of motion
0 to 10 or 15 degrees

Position of client
Supine
Note: Do not do this test if client has cervical disk problems.

Isolation and assessment
Client tucks chin into neck as in nodding "yes." Head remains on table. No motion should occur at the cervical spine. No resistance is required.

Cervical Flexion
Assesses for strength and endurance in the isolation position and tension or shortening in the extension pattern.

Muscles involved
Scalenus anterior, scalenus medius, and scalenus posterior
Sternocleidomastoid
Longus colli

Range of motion
0 to 35 or 45 degrees
Note: Women usually have greater cervical lordosis than men, so they likely could have a greater arc of motion.

Position of client
Supine, with arms at sides and head supported on table
Note: Do not do this test if client has cervical disk problems.

Isolation and assessment
Client lifts head off table and tucks chin. This is a weak muscle group, so no resistance is required.

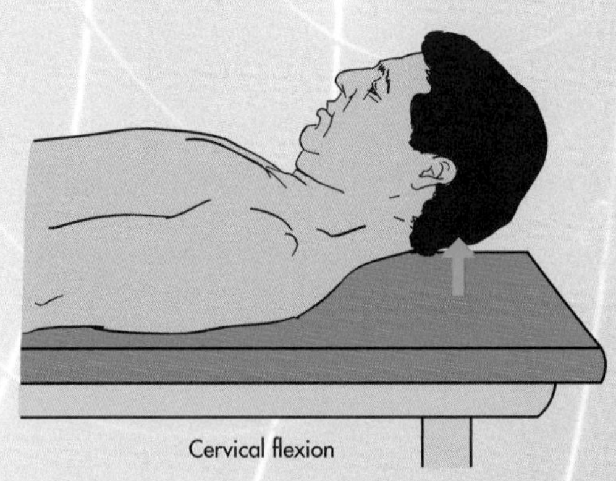
Cervical flexion

ACTIVITY 10-5—cont'd

Cervical Rotation

Assesses for strength and endurance in the isolation position and tension or shortening in the contralateral pattern.

Muscles involved
Sternocleidomastoid
Rectus capitis posterior major
Obliquus capitis inferior
Longissimus capitis

Range of motion
0 to 45 or 55 degrees
Two separate actions will be tested.

Position of client
Supine
Begin with head supported on table and turned to one side.

Isolation and assessment
Client lifts head off table without any additional rotation, returns to start position, and repeats on other side. No resistance is required.

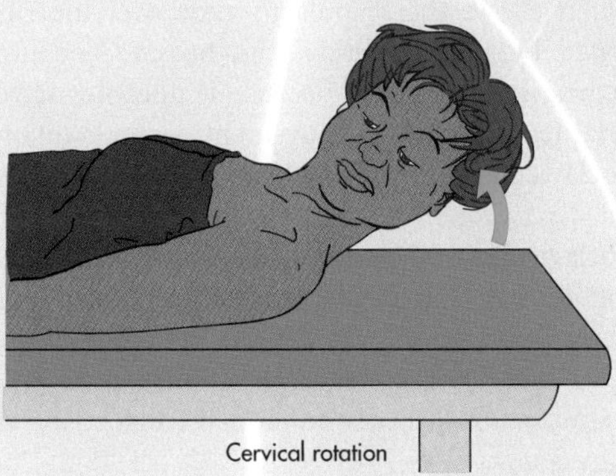
Cervical rotation

Position of client
Supine, with cervical spine in neutral flexion and extension
Begin with head supported on table and turned to one side.

Isolation and assessment
Client rotates head to neutral (nose facing ceiling) against resistance. Make sure client does not lift head off table. Repeat on opposite side.

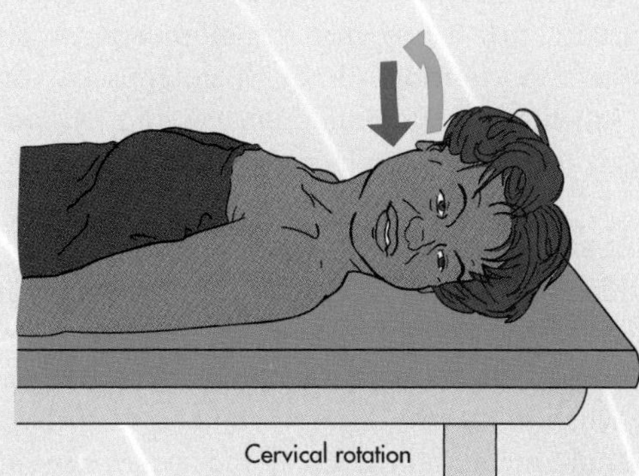
Cervical rotation

Muscles of Quiet Inspiration

Muscles involved
Diaphragm
Intercostals

Position of client
Supine

Isolation and assessment
Client inhales with maximal effort and holds maximal inspiration. Then examiner applies pressure to abdomen just below the rib cage (avoid pressure on xiphoid process).

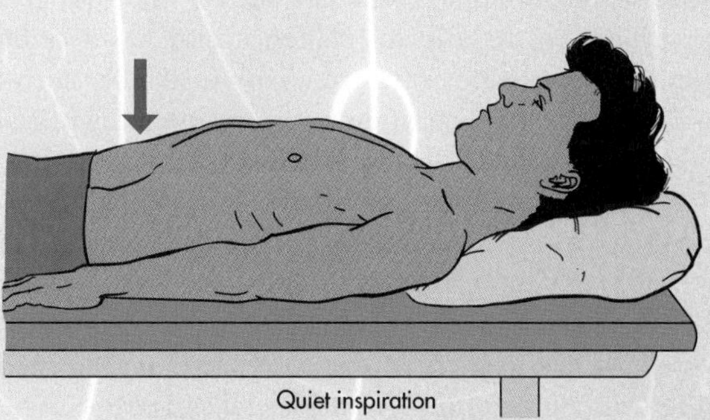
Quiet inspiration

clavicular joint surfaces to face upward, and the acromioclavicular movement that occurs at the acromioclavicular joint.

The acromioclavicular joint allows widening and narrowing of the angle between the clavicle and the scapula (from above). Narrowing occurs during protraction; widening occurs during retraction. The joint also allows for rotation of the scapula upward when the inferior angle moves away from the midline, and rotation of the scapula downward when the inferior angle moves toward the midline. The acromioclavicular joint also allows rotation of the scapula in such a way that the inferior angle swings anteriorly and posteriorly. Although no muscles directly cause movements of the acromioclavicular joint, the deltoid, upper trapezius, and subclavius muscles indirectly affect it.

Glenohumeral Joint

The shoulder, or glenohumeral joint, includes the scapula, humerus, and associated soft tissues. The only attachment of the shoulder joint to the axial skeleton is the clavicle at the sternoclavicular joint.

The glenohumeral joint is a ball-and-socket joint and is the articulation between the glenoid fossa of the scapula and the head of the humerus. Movements of the shoulder joint are many and varied. This mobile joint allows adduction, abduction, flexion, extension, hyperextension, horizontal adduction and abduction, and lateral and medial rotation of the humerus in all planes: sagittal, frontal, and transverse.

Movement of the humerus without scapular movement is unusual. Much of the movement of the scapula is related to movement at the glenohumeral joint. Flexion and abduction of the humerus elevates and abducts the scapula with upward rotation. Adduction and extension of the humerus results in depression, rotation downward, and adduction of the scapula. The scapula is abducted with humeral internal rotation and horizontal adduction. Scapular adduction accompanies external rotation and horizontal abduction of the humerus.

Because the shoulder joint has such a wide range of motion in so many different planes, it also has a certain amount of laxity, which often results in instability such as rotator cuff impingement or dislocations. Often the price of mobility is instability. The concept that the more mobile a joint is, the less stable it is, and that the more stable it is, the less mobile it is applies generally throughout the body but especially in the shoulder joint.

An important, protective fibroosseous arch over the glenohumeral joint is formed by the coracoacromial ligament, together with the acromion (or the lateral end of the clavicle articulating directly with the acromion and indirectly with the coracoid process through the coracoclavicular ligaments) and coracoid process. This arch forms a secondary restraining socket for the humeral head, preventing superior dislocation or displacement of the humeral head.

At the brim of the glenoid fossa is a fibrocartilaginous ring called the glenoid labrum that adds stability and substance to this shallow and mobile articulation.

The glenoid labrum merges with several ligaments and tendons to form the joint capsule of the glenohumeral joint. Tendons that connect at this joint are from the muscles of the subscapularis, infraspinatus, teres minor, and the supraspinatus, also known as SITS, or rotator cuff muscles, because they contribute to the rotation of the humerus. In reality, numerous muscles and tendons intersect the glenohumeral joint, and because of their attachment points, they contribute to the stability of the joint through their tension lines of pull. The deltoid forms a hood over the small muscles that closely surround the joint and acts as a shock absorber to protect the joint from impact.

The deep fascia covering the deltoid, known as the deltoid aponeurosis, is a fibrous layer that covers the outer surface of the muscle. The deep fascia is thick and strong behind, where it is continuous with the infraspinatus fascia, and thinner over the rest of the muscle. In front, the deltoid aponeurosis is continuous with the fascia covering the pectoralis major. Above, the deltoid aponeurosis is attached to the clavicle, the acromion, and spine of the scapula; below, it is continuous with the deep fascia of the arm. This extensive fascial network provides dynamic stability.

Scapulothoracic Junction

The scapulothoracic junction meets the criteria of a joint in that it allows the scapula to glide over the ribs and is separated by muscle, fascia, and bursae. The junction is not a true synovial joint because it does not have regular synovial features and its movement depends totally on the sternoclavicular and acromioclavicular joints. Even though scapular movement occurs as a result of motion at the sternoclavicular and acromioclavicular joints, the scapula can be described as having a total range of 25 degrees of abduction-adduction, 60 degrees of upward-downward rotation, and 55 degrees of elevation-depression. A large subscapular bursal sheet and fat pad enhance the gliding of this junction.

In analyzing shoulder girdle movements, focusing on a specific bony landmark such as the inferior angle (posteriorly), glenoid fossa (laterally), and acromion process (anteriorly) often is helpful. All of the following movements have their pivotal point where the clavicle joins the sternum at the sternoclavicular joint. Movements of the shoulder girdle can be described as movements of the scapula.

Movements of the Scapula

The following movements involve the scapula:

Abduction (protraction): Movement of the scapula laterally away from the spinal column

Adduction (retraction): Movement of the scapula medially toward the spinal column

Upward rotation: Turning the glenoid fossa upward and moving the inferior angle superiorly and laterally away from the spinal column

Downward rotation: Returning the inferior angle medially and inferiorly toward the spinal column and the glenoid fossa to its normal position

Elevation: Upward or superior movement, as in shrugging the shoulders
Depression: Downward or inferior movement, as in returning to normal position

Movements of the Glenohumeral Joint

The glenohumeral joint allows the following movements:

Abduction: Lateral movement of the humerus out to the side and away from the body

Adduction: Movement of the humerus medially toward the body from abduction

Flexion: Movement of the humerus anteriorly

Extension: Movement of the humerus posteriorly

Horizontal adduction (flexion): Movement of the humerus in a horizontal or transverse plane toward and across the chest

Horizontal abduction (extension): Movement of the humerus in a horizontal or transverse plane away from the chest

External rotation: Movement of the humerus laterally around its long axis away from the midline

Internal rotation: Movement of the humerus medially around its long axis toward the midline

The shoulder joint and shoulder girdle work together in carrying out upper extremity activities. Table 10-1 shows a pairing of shoulder girdle and shoulder joint movements (Activity 10-6).

Shoulder Girdle Muscles

Five muscles are involved primarily in shoulder girdle movements: trapezius, levator scapulae, rhomboids, serratus anterior, and pectoralis minor. Grouping the muscles of the shoulder girdle separately from the shoulder joint is helpful to avoid confusion. All five shoulder girdle muscles have their origin on the axial skeleton, with their insertion located on the scapula or clavicle. Shoulder girdle muscles do not attach to the humerus, nor do they cause actions of the shoulder joint. The shoulder girdle muscles are essential in providing dynamic stability of the scapula so that it can serve as a base of support for shoulder joint activities. A force couple occurs when muscles work in conjunction, pulling in different directions, to accomplish a specific movement (Figure 10-20).

The trapezius muscle fixates the scapula for deltoid action by preventing the glenoid fossa from being pulled down when the arms lift objects. The muscle is used strenuously when lifting with the hands, as in picking up a heavy wheelbarrow. The trapezius must prevent the scapula from being pulled downward such as when an object is held overhead or a person is carrying an object that is resting on the tip of his shoulder.

Shrugging the shoulder calls the levator scapulae muscle into play, along with the upper trapezius muscle.

The rhomboid muscle fixes the scapula in adduction/retraction when the muscles of the shoulder joint adduct or extend the arm. The trapezius and rhomboid muscles work together to produce adduction, with slight elevation of the scapula. To prevent this elevation, the latissimus dorsi muscle is called into play. The serratus anterior muscle acts in movements drawing the scapula forward with slight upward rotation and works along with the pectoralis major muscle in actions such as throwing a baseball. A winged scapula condition indicates a definite weakness of the serratus anterior.

The pectoralis minor muscle is used, along with the serratus anterior muscle, in true abduction (protraction) without rotation. When true abduction of the scapula is necessary, the serratus anterior draws the scapula forward

ACTIVITY 10-6

Slowly and deliberately move your scapula and glenohumeral joint through each of the movement patterns just described. Identify the interplay between the shoulder girdle movements and the shoulder joint movements. Pay attention to the limitation of each region and notice the increase in range of motion as each area is brought into play. In the space provided describe the experience.

Example
I noticed that it was confusing to attempt to isolate scapular movements by themselves.

Your Turn

TABLE 10-1
Shoulder Joint

Shoulder Joint	Shoulder Girdle
Abduction	Upward rotation
Adduction	Downward rotation
Flexion	Elevation, upward rotation, protraction
Extension	Depression, downward rotation, retraction
Internal rotation	Abduction (protraction)
External rotation	Adduction (retraction)
Horizontal abduction	Adduction (retraction)
Horizontal adduction	Abduction (protraction)

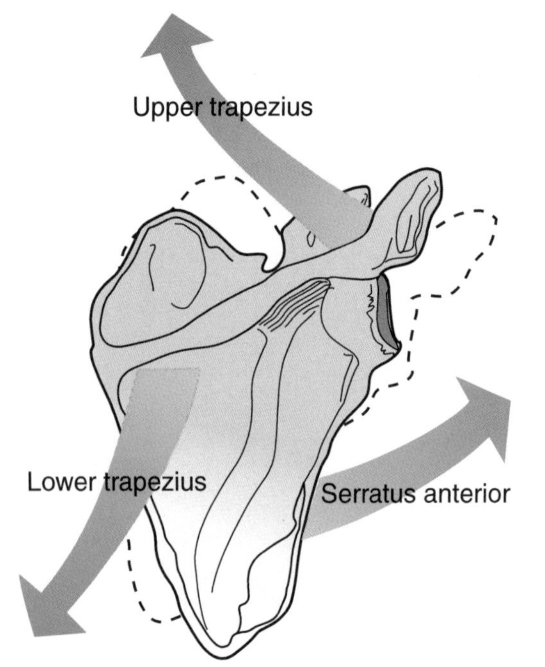

Figure 10-20
The upper trapezius, lower trapezius, and serratus anterior pull in three different directions to achieve one type of motion—upward rotation of the scapula. This is called a force couple.

with a slight upward rotation and the pectoralis minor pulls forward with slight downward rotation. The two pulling together give true abduction. These muscles work together in most movements of pushing with the hands.

Glenohumeral Joint Muscles

Muscles of the glenohumeral joint contribute to more than one action when the humerus is in a sequence of movement. The muscles involved in flexion of the shoulder and glenohumeral joint cross the joint anteriorly. The primary flexors are the pectoralis major, anterior deltoid, and coracobrachialis. Synergists to flexion are the biceps brachii and the subscapularis.

In extension of the glenohumeral joint, when movement meets no resistance, gravity is the prime mover, with the flexor muscles eccentrically contracting to control the action of extension. When resistance occurs, the posterior muscles of the glenohumeral joint go to work, specifically the teres major, latissimus dorsi, and sternocostal pectoralis. Synergists for extension are the posterior deltoid, particularly when the humerus is rotated externally, and the triceps brachii (long head) when the elbow is flexed.

Two primary movers are involved in abduction of the glenohumeral joint: the middle deltoid and supraspinatus. Both muscles intersect the shoulder superior to the glenohumeral joint. The supraspinatus begins the movement of abduction for approximately the first 110 degrees. The middle deltoid is active from approximately 90 degrees to 180 degrees. To counteract superior dislocation, the infraspinatus, subscapularis, and teres major contract to control the action of the middle deltoid.

Adduction of the glenohumeral joint is another movement in which, if no resistance occurs, gravity is the prime mover, with the abductors as the antagonist controlling the speed of the motion. With resistance, the principal adductors are the latissimus dorsi, teres major, and pectoralis major sternal, all positioned inferior to the glenohumeral joint. The synergists are the biceps (short head) and triceps (long head).

Medial rotation of the humerus results from the subscapularis and teres major as the prime movers. Both insert to the anterior aspect of the humerus. Synergists to medial rotation are the pectoralis major, anterior deltoid, latissimus dorsi, and biceps brachii (short head).

Muscles inserting into the posterior aspect of the humerus generate the lateral rotation, specifically the infraspinatus and teres minor.

Horizontal adduction results from the actions of anterior muscles, which include the anterior deltoid, pectoralis major, and coracobrachialis. The synergist to horizontal adduction is the biceps brachii (short head).

Horizontal abduction is affected by the middle and posterior deltoid, infraspinatus, and teres minor, muscles located on the posterior aspect of the joint. The synergists to horizontal abduction are the teres major and latissimus dorsi (Activity 10-7).

Elbow Region

The elbow is considered a stable joint with firm osseous support and is composed of three articulations: the humeroulnar joint, humeroradial joint, and radioulnar joint. The elbow is a uniaxial hinge joint that moves only in one plane along a single axis. Its action is flexion/extension. The elbow is capable of moving from 0 degrees of extension to approximately 145 to 150 degrees of flexion.

After the elbow flexes beyond 20 degrees, its bony stability is somewhat unlocked, allowing for more side-to-side laxity. In flexion, the stability of the elbow depends on the lateral or radial collateral ligament with most of the work by the medial or ulnar collateral ligament.

The radioulnar joint is classified as a trochoid or pivot-type joint. The radial head rotates around its location at the proximal ulna. This rotary movement is accompanied by the distal radius rotating around the distal ulna. The radial head is maintained in its joint by the annular ligament. The radioulnar joint can supinate approximately 80 to 90 degrees from the neutral position. Pronation varies from 70 to 90 degrees.

Practically any movement of the upper extremity involves the elbow and radioulnar joints. Often these joints are grouped together because of their close anatomic relationship. Radioulnar joint motion may be attributed incorrectly to the wrist joint because it appears to occur there. However, with close inspection, the elbow joint and its movements may be distinguished clearly from those of the radioulnar joints, just as the radioulnar movements may be distinguished from those of the wrist.

ACTIVITY 10-7

In this activity, you will be working with a partner to assess individual movement patterns, normal function, and possible dysfunction in each other. One of you is first to isolate the specified movement patterns on each side of your partner, one side at a time, and assess for normal function by applying a gentle pressure opposite the action of the isolation position. The body should be stabilized so that only the isolated area is moving. In some instances the ability to assume the position and maintain it indicates normal function. Muscles should be able to hold against gravity or the applied pressure without strain or pain. The position itself should be easy to assume and comfortable to maintain for a short duration, from 10 to 30 seconds. The bilateral movement patterns should be the same. The opposite movement pattern also should be able to be done easily.

Dysfunction may be indicated by bilateral asymmetry, pain, weakness, fatigue, a heavy sensation, binding, and the inability to assume the isolation position or move into the opposite position. Intervention or referral depends on the severity of the condition and whether the dysfunction is neuromuscular, myofascial, or joint related.

Note: Do not perform these assessments if contraindications exist. Contraindications to this type of assessment include joint and disk dysfunction, acute pain, recent trauma, and inflammation.

Before starting scapular motion assessments, do a visual assessment of your partner to check for variations in position and symmetry. Asymmetry often shows with one shoulder or scapula higher, especially in those who carry briefcases, purses, or babies on one side.

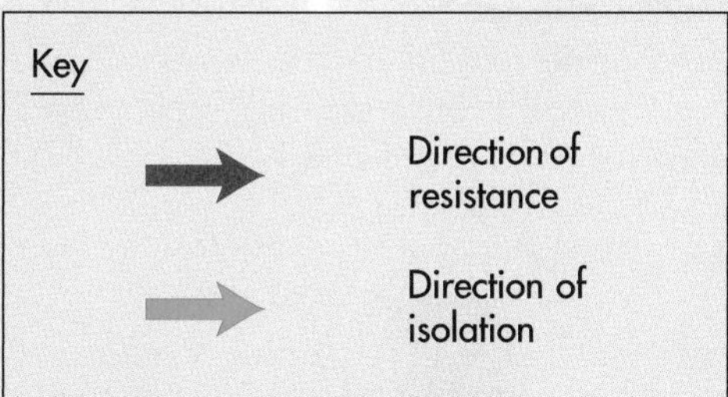

Working with your partner, determine the position of the scapulae at rest and whether the two sides are symmetric. The normal scapula lies close to the rib cage with the vertebral border nearly parallel and from 1 to 3 inches lateral to the spinous processes. The inferior angle is tucked in. If the inferior angle of the scapula is tilted away from the rib cage, check for tightness of the pectoralis minor and weakness of the trapezius.

The most prominent abnormal posture of the scapula is "winging," in which the vertebral border tilts away from the rib cage, a sign of serratus weakness.

Within the total arc of 180 degrees of shoulder forward flexion, 120 degrees is glenohumeral motion and 60 degrees is scapular motion. Because these movements are not isolated, saying that the glenohumeral and scapular motions coexist after 60 degrees and up to 150 degrees is more correct.

Passively raise your partner's test arm in forward flexion completely above his or her head to determine scapular mobility. The scapula should start to rotate at about 60 degrees, although considerable individual variation exists.

Check that the scapula basically remains in its rest position at ranges of shoulder flexion less than 60 degrees, with some variation among individuals. If the scapula moves as the glenohumeral joint moves below 60 degrees, that is, within this range they move as a unit, limited glenohumeral motion is evident, but the scapula may move through a complete or even excessive range.

From greater than 60 degrees and to about 150 or 160 degrees in active and passive motion, the scapula moves in concert with the humerus.

Scapular Abduction (Protraction)

Assesses for strength and endurance in the isolation position and tension or shortening in the scapular adduction pattern.

Muscles involved
Serratus anterior
Pectoralis minor

Range of motion
Reliable values are not available.

Position of client
Seated, with legs over end or side of table, and hands at sides on top of table

Isolation and assessment
Client flexes the straight arm to approximately 130 degrees and reaches forward to protract the scapula. The examiner palpates the medial border of the scapula and applies resistance to the arm.

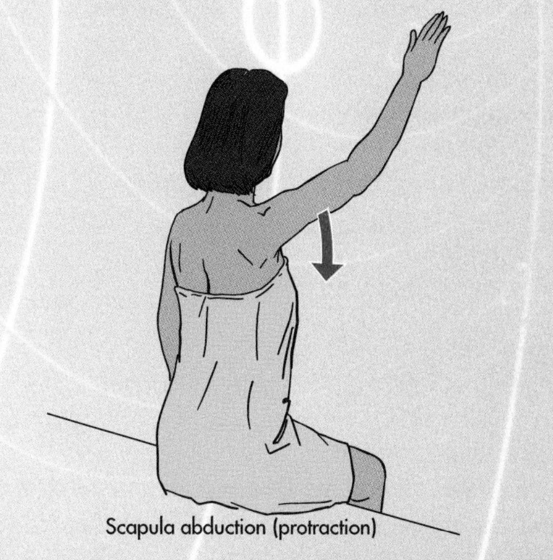

Scapula abduction (protraction)

Continued

ACTIVITY 10-7—cont'd

Scapular Adduction (Retraction)

Assesses for strength and endurance in the isolation position and tension or shortening in the scapular abduction pattern.

Muscles involved

Trapezius (middle fibers)
Rhomboideus major and rhomboideus minor
Latissimus dorsi

Range of motion

Reliable values are not available.

Position of client

Seated with legs over edge of table
Shoulder is abducted to 90 degrees and externally rotated.
Elbow is flexed to a right angle and held at shoulder level.

Isolation and assessment

Client horizontally abducts arm to adduct the scapula while examiner applies resistance to the posterior arm above the elbow to push the arm into horizontal adduction.

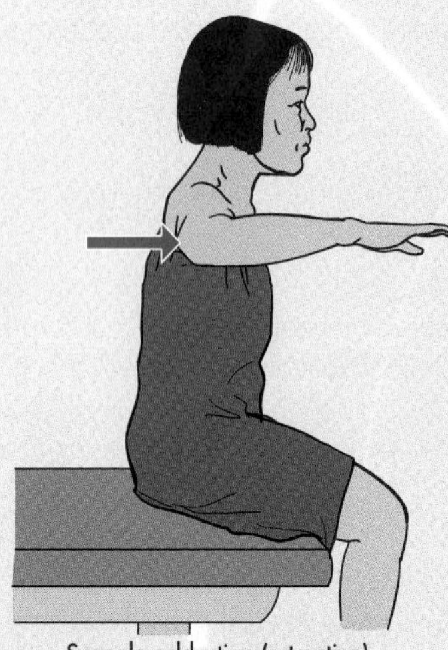

Scapula adduction (retraction)

Scapular Elevation

Assesses for strength and endurance in the isolation position and tension or shortening in the scapular depression pattern.

Muscles involved

Trapezius (upper fibers)
Levator scapulae
Rhomboideus major and rhomboideus minor

Range of motion

Reliable values are not available.

Position of client

Seated, with legs over side of table and arms relaxed

Isolation and assessment

Client lifts shoulders toward ears, as in shrugging, while examiner applies resistance to push the shoulders down.

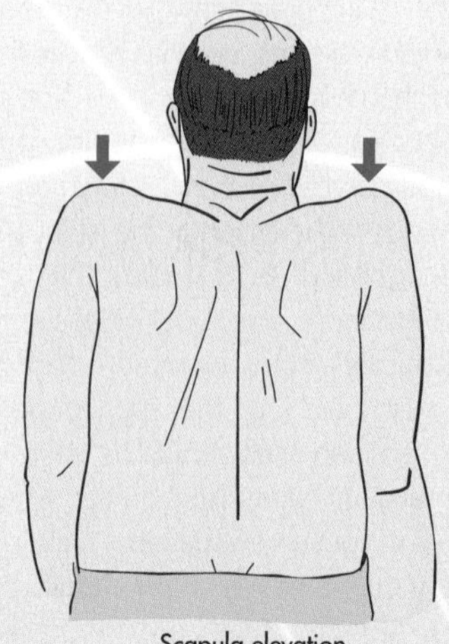

Scapula elevation

Scapular Upward Rotation with Abduction

Assesses for strength and endurance in the isolation position and tension or shortening in the scapular downward rotation pattern.

Muscles involved

Upper and lower trapezius
Anterior serratus
Pectoralis minor

Range of motion

Reliable values are not available.

Position of client

Seated, with legs over side of table, arms resting at sides

Isolation and assessment

Client flexes shoulder forward to 120 degrees with no rotation or horizontal movement while examiner applies resistance to arm just above elbow to push it down.

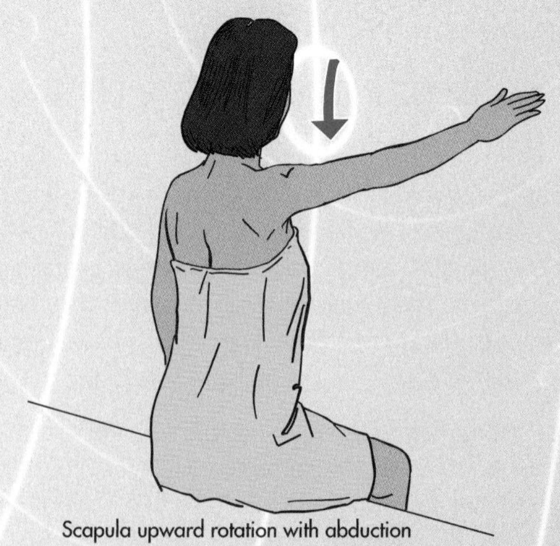

Scapula upward rotation with abduction

ACTIVITY 10-7—cont'd

Scapular Depression with Adduction and Downward Rotation

Assesses for strength and endurance in the isolation position and tension or shortening in the scapular elevation and upward rotation pattern.

Muscles involved
Lower trapezius
Lower anterior serratus
Levator scapula
Rhomboideus major and rhomboideus minor
Latissimus dorsi

Range of motion
Reliable values are not available.

Position of client
Prone
Head may be turned to either side for comfort.
Internally rotate shoulder, flex elbow, and adduct arm across back.
Hand rests on low back near waist.

Isolation and assessment
Client further adducts arm by attempting to touch the opposite side. Examiner applies resistance to the medial side of upper arm to pull it away from the body.

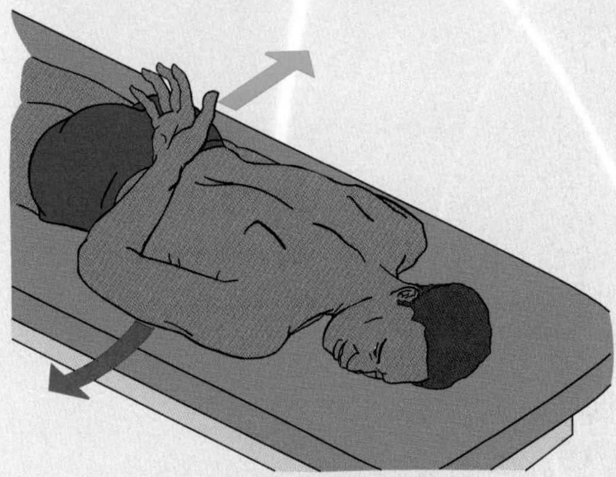

Scapular despression with adduction and downward rotation

Shoulder Flexion

Assesses for strength and endurance in the isolation position and tension or shortening in the shoulder extension and adduction pattern.

Muscles involved
Deltoid (anterior and middle)
Supraspinatus
Pectoralis major (upper)
Coracobrachialis
Biceps brachii
Subscapularis

Range of motion
0 to 180 degrees

Position of client
Seated with knees bent off table, arms at sides, elbows slightly flexed, and forearm pronated

Isolation and assessment
Client flexes shoulder to 90 degrees without rotation or horizontal movement while examiner applies resistance to upper arm above elbow to push arm down.

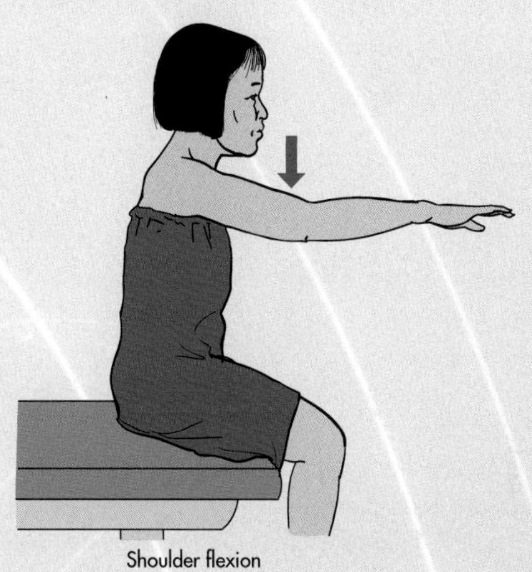

Shoulder flexion

Shoulder Extension

Assesses for strength and endurance in the isolation position and tension or shortening in the shoulder flexion pattern.

Muscles involved
Latissimus dorsi
Deltoid (posterior)
Teres major
Triceps brachii (long head)

Range of motion
0 to 45 degrees

Position of client
Prone, with arms at sides and shoulder internally rotated (palm up)
Elbow remains extended throughout isolation.

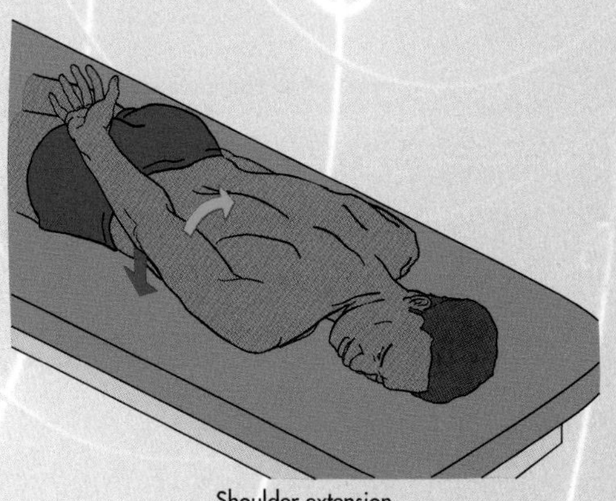

Shoulder extension

Continued

ACTIVITY 10-7—cont'd

Isolation and assessment
Client lifts arm off table and holds while examiner applies resistance to posterior arm above elbow to push it down.

Shoulder Horizontal Abduction
Assesses for strength and endurance in the isolation position and tension or shortening in the shoulder horizontal adduction pattern.

Muscles involved
Deltoid (posterior fibers)
Infraspinatus
Teres minor

Range of motion
0 to 90 degrees (beginning at 90 degrees flexion)

Position of client
Prone with shoulder abducted to 90 degrees, elbow flexed, upper arm supported on table, and forearm off edge of table

Isolation and assessment
Client horizontally (posteriorly) abducts shoulder (lifts elbow toward ceiling) while examiner applies resistance to the posterior arm above elbow to push arm down.

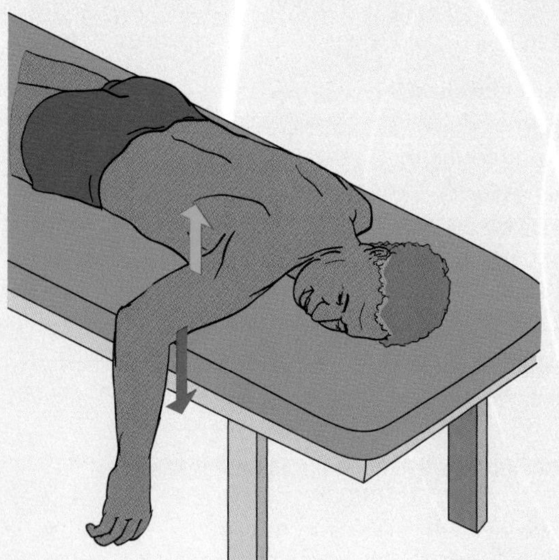

Shoulder horizontal abduction

Shoulder Horizontal Adduction
Assesses for strength and endurance in the isolation position and tension or shortening in the shoulder horizontal abduction pattern.

Muscles involved
Pectoralis major
Deltoid (anterior fibers)

Range of motion
0 to 40 degrees when starting from a position of 90 degrees of forward flexion

Position of client
Supine
Shoulder abducted to 90 degrees, upper arm supported on table, and elbow flexed to 90 degrees

Isolation and assessment
Client horizontally adducts arm to move it across the chest while examiner applies resistance to medial side of upper arm above elbow to push it down.

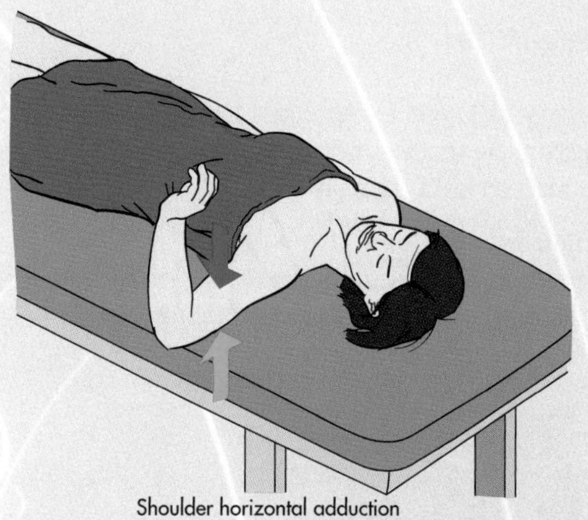

Shoulder horizontal adduction

Shoulder External or Lateral Rotation
Assesses for strength and endurance in the isolation position and tension or shortening in the shoulder internal or medial rotation pattern.

Muscles involved
Infraspinatus
Teres minor
Deltoid (posterior)

Range of motion
0 to 90 degrees

Position of client
Prone, with head turned toward test side
Shoulder is abducted to 90 degrees with upper arm fully supported on table, elbow flexed, and forearm hanging over edge of table.

Isolation and assessment
Client moves forearm upward toward the level of the table, keeping upper arm on table, while examiner applies resistance to distal forearm above wrist to push it down.

ACTIVITY 10-7—cont'd

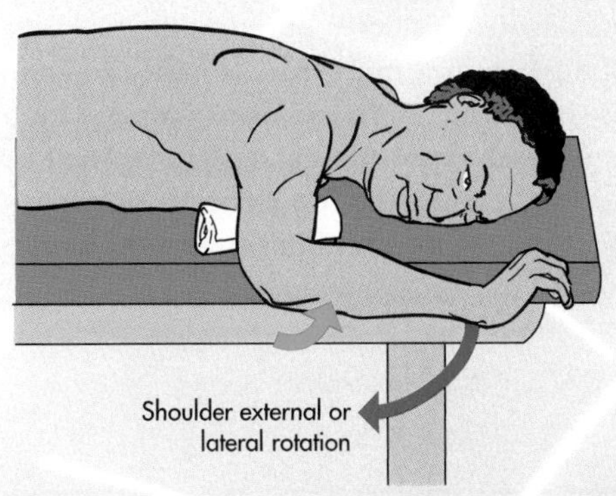

Shoulder Internal Rotation

Assesses for strength and endurance in the isolation position and tension or shortening in the shoulder external or lateral rotation pattern.

Muscles involved
Subscapularis
Pectoralis major
Latissimus dorsi
Teres major
Deltoid (anterior)

Range of motion
0 to 80 degrees

Position of client
Prone with shoulder abducted to 90 degrees, upper arm supported on table, elbow flexed, and forearm hanging over edge of table
Examiner stabilizes upper arm.

Isolation and assessment
Client moves forearm through internal rotation (backward and upward) while examiner applies resistance to forearm above wrist to push it down.

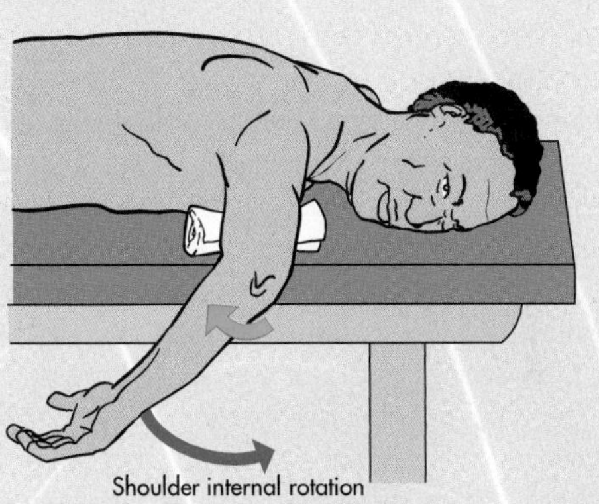

When the arm is in an anatomic extended position, the longitudinal axes of the upper arm and forearm form a valgus angle at the elbow joint known as the carrying angle; this angle approximates 5 degrees in men and between 10 and 15 degrees in women. Anatomically, the carrying angle is designed to fit closely into the waist depressions immediately superior to the iliac crest. The carrying angles should be bilaterally symmetric.

The olecranon fossa of the humerus, which receives the olecranon process of the ulna during extension, is filled with fat and covered by a portion of the triceps muscle and aponeurosis.

The cubital fossa is defined by the brachioradialis laterally and the pronator teres medially with the biceps tendon, brachial artery, and median and musculocutaneous nerves passing through this area. The biceps tendon is a taut, long structure that is medial to the brachioradialis muscle, and one can palpate the pulse of the brachial artery medial to the biceps tendon.

Movements of the Elbow

The elbow allows the following movements (Activity 10-8):

Flexion: Movement of the forearm to the shoulder by bending the elbow to decrease its angle

Extension: Movement of the forearm away from the shoulder by straightening the elbow to increase its angle

Pronation: Internal rotary movement of the radius on the ulna that results in the hand moving from the palm up to the palm down position

Supination: External rotary movement of the radius on the ulna that results in the hand moving from the palm down to the palm up position

Elbow Muscles

The elbow flexors are the biceps brachii, brachialis, and brachioradialis. The triceps brachii is the primary elbow extensor, assisted by the anconeus. The pronator group consists of the pronator teres, pronator quadratus, and brachioradialis. The brachioradialis also assists with

ACTIVITY 10-8

Slowly and deliberately move your humeroulnar joint, humeroradial joint, and radioulnar joint through each of the movement patterns described. In the space provided describe the experience.

Example
I noticed that it took less effort to pronate than to supinate.

Your Turn

supination, which is controlled mainly by the supinator muscle and the biceps brachii (Activity 10-9).

Wrist and Hand Region

The joints of the wrist, hand, and fingers often are taken for granted, even though the fine motor characteristics of this area are essential in skilled activities requiring precise functioning of the wrist and hand. Anatomically and structurally the human wrist and hand have highly developed, complex mechanisms capable of a variety of movements. The amazing diversity of motion results from the arrangement of the 29 bones, more than 25 joints, and more than 30 muscles (of which 15 are intrinsic muscles with origin and insertion found inside the hand). This complexity may be simplified by relating the functional anatomy to the major actions of the joints: flexion, extension, abduction, and adduction of the wrist and hand.

ACTIVITY 10-9

In this activity you will be working with a partner to assess individual movement patterns, normal function, and possible dysfunction in each other. One of you is first to isolate the specified movement patterns on each side of your partner, one side at a time, and assess for normal function by applying gentle pressure opposite to the action of the isolation position. The body should be stabilized so that only the isolated area is moving. In some instances the ability to assume the position and maintain it indicates normal function. Muscles should be able to hold against gravity or the applied pressure without strain or pain. The position itself should be easy to assume and comfortable to maintain for a short duration, from 10 to 30 seconds. The bilateral movement patterns should be the same. The opposite movement pattern also should be able to be done easily.

Dysfunction may be indicated by bilateral asymmetry, pain, weakness, fatigue, a heavy sensation, binding, and inability to assume the isolation position or move into the opposite position. Intervention or referral depends on the severity of the condition and whether the dysfunction is neuromuscular, myofascial, or joint related.

Note: Do not perform these assessments if contraindications exist. Contraindications to this type of assessment include joint and disk dysfunction, acute pain, recent trauma, and inflammation.

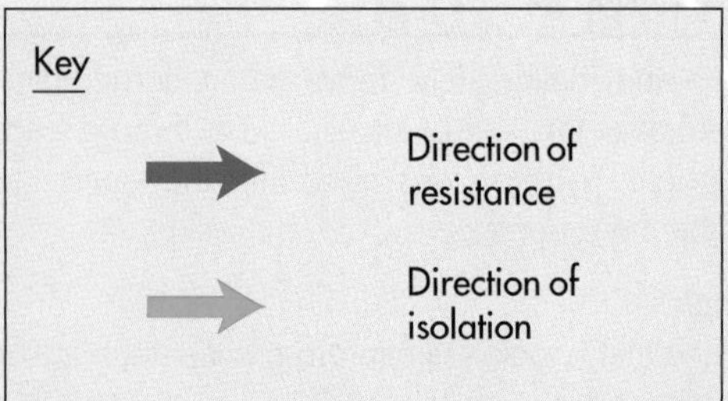

Elbow Flexion

Assesses for strength and endurance in the isolation position and tension or shortening in the elbow extension pattern.

Muscles involved
Biceps brachii (short head)
Brachialis
Brachioradialis
Pronator teres

Range of motion
0 to 150 degrees

Position of client
Seated, with arms at sides
Three separate muscles can be isolated depending on position of forearm:
Biceps brachii: forearm in supination
Brachialis: forearm in pronation
Brachioradialis: forearm in midposition between pronation and supination
Client's forearm is flexed to 90 degrees and examiner stabilizes it at the elbow.

Isolation and assessment (all three forearm positions)
Client flexes elbow through range of motion while examiner applies resistance to distal forearm.

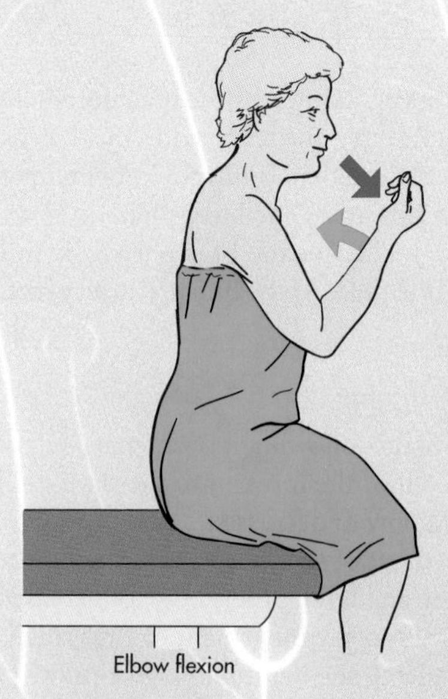

ACTIVITY 10-9—cont'd

Elbow Extension

Assesses for strength and endurance in the isolation position and tension or shortening in the elbow flexion pattern.

Muscles involved
Triceps brachii
Anconeus

Range of motion
No range of motion

Position of client
Standing or seated with arm to be tested able to extend without touching table
Forearm is flexed and examiner stabilizes it at the elbow.

Isolation and assessment
Client extends elbow to end of available range without extending shoulder. Examiner applies resistance at wrist to prevent the action.

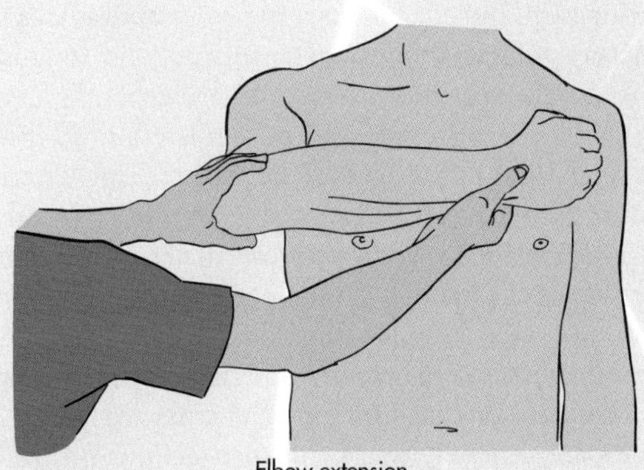

Elbow extension

Forearm Supination

Assesses for strength and endurance in the isolation position and tension or shortening in the pronation pattern.

Muscles involved
Supinator
Biceps brachii

Range of motion
0 to 90 degrees

Position of client
Seated, arm at side and elbow flexed to 90 degrees, and forearm in neutral or midposition
Examiner stabilizes at elbow with one hand and grasps forearm above wrist with other hand.

Isolation and assessment
Client supinates the forearm until the palm faces the ceiling while examiner resists the motion.

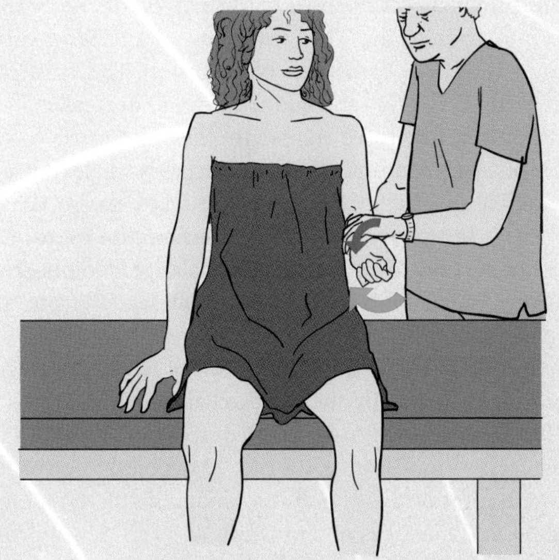

Forearm supination

Forearm Pronation

Assesses for strength and endurance in the isolation position and tension or shortening in the supination pattern.

Muscles involved
Pronator teres
Pronator quadratus
Flexor carpi radialis

Range of motion
0 to 80 degrees

Position of client
Seated, with arm at side and elbow flexed to 90 degrees, and forearm in neutral position
Examiner stabilizes at elbow with one hand and grasps forearm at wrist with other hand.

Isolation and assessment
Client pronates the forearm until the palm faces downward while examiner resists the motion.

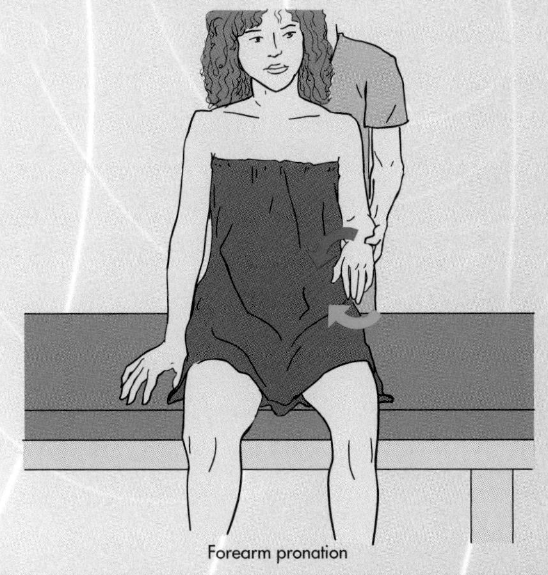

Forearm pronation

Wrist motion occurs primarily between the distal radius and the proximal carpal row, consisting of the scaphoid, lunate, and triquetrum. The joint allows 70 to 90 degrees of flexion and 65 to 85 degrees of extension. The wrist can abduct 15 to 25 degrees and adduct 25 to 40 degrees.

Each finger has three joints. In these joints, 0 to 40 degrees of extension and 85 to 100 degrees of flexion are possible. The proximal interphalangeal joint, classified as a hinge joint, can move from full extension to 90 to 120 degrees of flexion. The distal interphalangeal joints, also classified as hinge joints, can flex 80 to 90 degrees from full extension.

The thumb has only two joints, both of which are classified as hinge joints. The metacarpophalangeal joint moves from full extension into 40 to 90 degrees of flexion. The interphalangeal joint can flex 80 to 90 degrees. The carpometacarpal joint of the thumb is a unique saddle-type joint having 50 to 70 degrees of abduction and can flex approximately 15 to 45 degrees and extend 0 to 20 degrees. Numerous ligaments support and provide static stability to many joints of the wrist and hand.

Movements of the Wrist and Hand

The following are movements of the wrist and hand (Activity 10-10):

Flexion: Moving the palm of the hand or the phalanges toward the anterior or volar aspect of the forearm

Extension: Moving the back of the hand or the phalanges toward the posterior or dorsal aspect of the forearm

Abduction (radial flexion or deviation): Movement of the thumb side of the hand toward the lateral aspect or radial side of the forearm

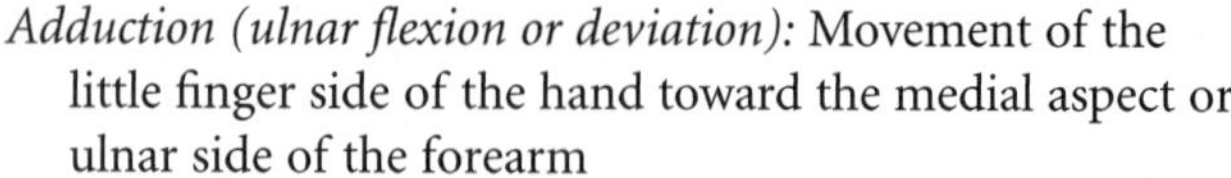

Adduction (ulnar flexion or deviation): Movement of the little finger side of the hand toward the medial aspect or ulnar side of the forearm

Opposition: Movement of the thumb across the palmar aspect to oppose any or all of the phalanges

ACTIVITY 10-10

Slowly move your wrist and fingers through the movement patterns described. Isolate wrist action from finger action. Combine as many different wrist, finger, and thumb actions as possible and notice the endless combinations. In the space provided describe the experience.

Example

I can make my hand dance.

Your Turn

Muscles of the Wrist and Hand

The extrinsic muscles of the wrist and hand may be grouped according to function and location. The wrist flexor-pronator muscle group includes the pronator teres, flexor carpi radialis, flexor carpi ulnaris, and palmaris longus. All the wrist flexors generally have their origins on the anteromedial aspect of the proximal forearm and medial epicondyle of the humerus, whereas their insertions are on the anterior aspect of the wrist and hand.

The wrist extensors include the extensor carpi radialis longus, extensor carpi radialis brevis, and extensor carpi ulnaris muscles. The wrist extensors generally have their origins on the posterolateral aspect of the proximal forearm and lateral humeral epicondyle, and their insertions are located on the posterior aspect of the hand and wrist.

The wrist abductors include the flexor carpi radialis, extensor carpi radialis longus, extensor carpi radialis brevis, abductor pollicis longus, extensor pollicis longus, and extensor pollicis brevis. These muscles generally cross the wrist joint anterolaterally and posterolaterally to insert on the radial side of the hand. The flexor carpi ulnaris and extensor carpi ulnaris adduct the wrist and cross the wrist joint anteromedially and posteromedially to insert on the ulnar side of the hand.

Another nine muscles function primarily to move the phalanges but also are involved in wrist joint actions because they originate on the forearm and cross the wrist. These muscles are generally weaker in their actions on the wrist. The flexor digitorum superficialis and flexor digitorum profundus are finger flexors, and they also assist in wrist flexion along with the flexor pollicis longus, which is a thumb flexor. The extensor digitorum, extensor indicis, and extensor digiti minimi are finger extensors and also assist in wrist extension, along with the extensor pollicis longus and extensor pollicis brevis, which extend the thumb. The abductor pollicis longus abducts the thumb and assists in wrist abduction.

Intrinsic hand muscles have their origin and insertion within the hand. They are primarily responsible for fine and precise movements of the fingers and thumb. Those acting on the thumb, located in the thenar eminence, include the opponens pollicis, abductor pollicis brevis, and flexor pollicis brevis. Those acting on the little finger are the opponens digiti minimi, abductor digiti minimi, and flexor digiti minimi brevis. These muscles are located in the hypothenar eminence. Acting with the thenar muscles, they function in opposition, allowing effective grasping movements.

The lumbricales flex the metacarpophalangeal joint and extend the interphalangeal joints. The dorsal and palmar interossei muscles are involved with adduction and abduction of the fingers. The adductor pollicis and abductor pollicis muscles adduct and abduct the thumb. With these actions the hand is able to hold and manipulate small objects such as a pencil (Activity 10-11).

Pelvic Girdle and Hip Joint Region

The pelvis consists of three bones and three joints. The bones are the two fused coxal bones (made up of the ilium, ischium and pubis) and the sacrum. The three joints are the two sacroiliac articulations and the symphysis pubis.

Motion in the Pelvic Girdle

The pelvic girdle functions as one unit with all three bones moving at all three joints. The lower extremities, the vertebral column, and the trunk influence the pelvic girdle. The unit moves around a vertical axis. In a movement to the left, the symphysis turns left of the midline, the right coxal turns forward, the left coxal turns backward, and the sacrum turns a little to the left. The reverse happens when rotating to the right.

The pelvic girdle moves back and forth within three

ACTIVITY 10-11

In this activity, you will be working with a partner to assess individual movement patterns, normal function, and possible dysfunction in each other. One of you is first to isolate the specified movement patterns on each side of your partner, one side at a time, and assess for normal function by applying a gentle pressure opposite to the action of the isolation position. The body should be stabilized so that only the isolated area is moving. In some instances the ability to assume the position and maintain it indicates normal function. Muscles should be able to hold against gravity or the applied pressure without strain or pain. The position itself should be easy to assume and comfortable to maintain for a short duration, from 10 to 30 seconds. The bilateral movement patterns should be the same. The opposite movement pattern also should be able to be done easily.

Dysfunction may be indicated by bilateral asymmetry, pain, weakness, fatigue, a heavy sensation, binding, and inability to assume the isolation position or move into the opposite position. Intervention or referral depends on the severity of the condition and whether the dysfunction is neuromuscular, myofascial, or joint related.

Note: Do not perform these assessments if contraindications exist. Contraindications to this type of assessment include joint and disk dysfunction, acute pain, recent trauma, and inflammation.

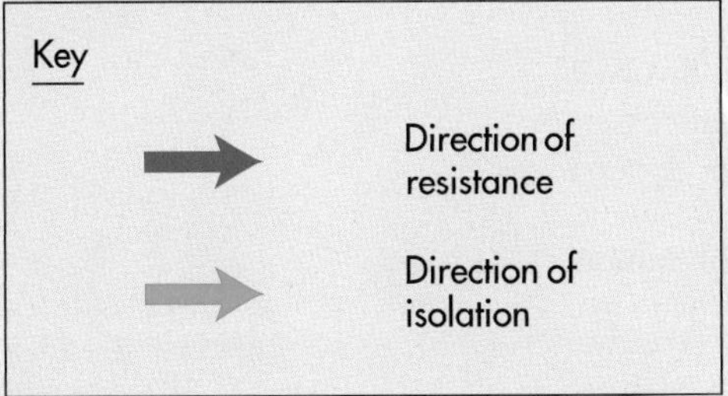

Wrist Flexion

Assesses for strength and endurance in the isolation position and tension or shortening in the extension pattern.

Muscles involved

Flexor carpi radialis
Flexor carpi ulnaris
Palmaris longus
Abductor pollicis longus
Flexor digitorum superficialis
Flexor pollicis longus
Flexor digitorum profundus

Range of motion

0 to 80 degrees

Position of client

Seated with elbow flexed if needed and the forearm supinated while supported on its dorsal surface on a table
Wrist position is neutral.

Isolation and assessment

Client flexes the wrist while examiner resists action. Make sure client's thumbs and fingers are relaxed.

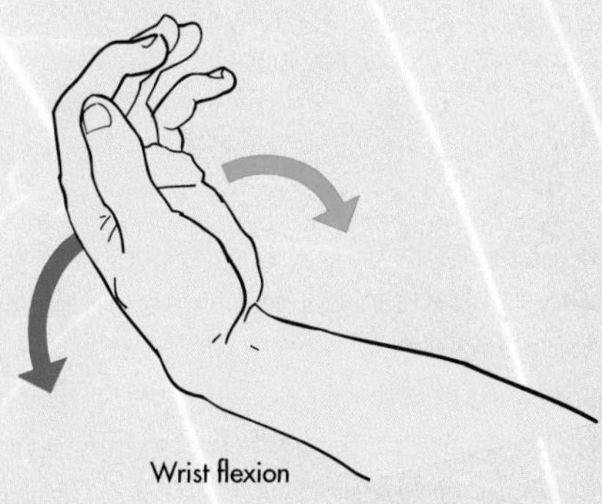

Wrist flexion

Wrist Extension

Assesses for strength and endurance in the isolation position and tension or shortening in the flexion pattern.

Muscles involved

Extensor carpi radialis longus
Extensor carpi radialis brevis
Extensor carpi ulnaris
Extensor digitorum
Extensor digiti minimi
Extensor indicis
Extensor pollicis longus

Range of motion

0 to 85 degrees

Continued

ACTIVITY 10-11—cont'd

Position of client
Seated, with elbow flexed as needed, and forearm pronated while arm is supported on table

Isolation and assessment
Client hyperextends wrist while examiner resists action. Client's thumb and fingers stay relaxed.

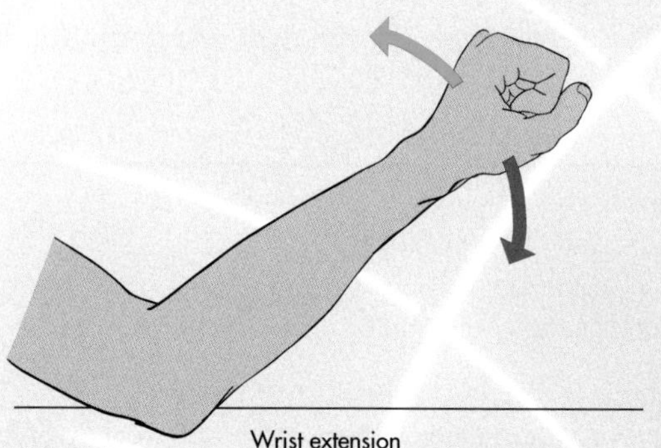
Wrist extension

Flexion of Fingers
Assesses for strength and endurance in the isolation position and tension or shortening in the finger extension pattern.

Muscles involved
Lumbricales
Dorsal interossei
Palmar interossei
Flexor digitorum superficialis
Flexor digitorum profundus

Range of motion
0 to 100 degrees

Position of client
Seated, with elbow flexed and forearm supinated and supported on a table
Wrist is maintained in neutral position.
Begin with metacarpophalangeal joints fully extended and interphalangeal joints flexed.
Each finger is to be isolated separately.

Isolation and assessment
Client flexes the metacarpophalangeal joint (bends knuckles) and extends the interphalangeal (finger) joints while examiner resists metacarpophalangeal flexion. Make sure client does not flex interphalangeal joint.

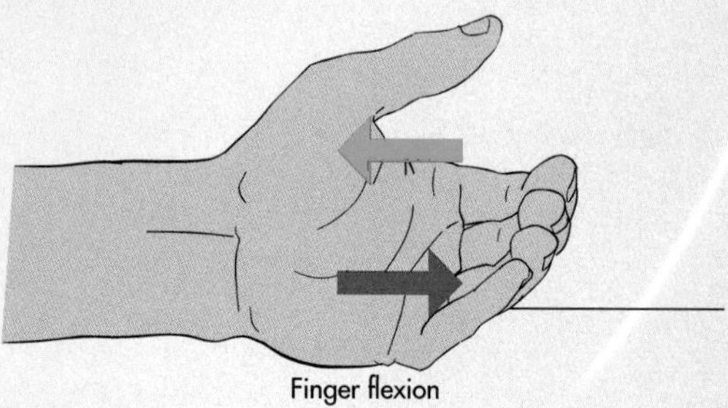
Finger flexion

Finger Extension
Assesses for strength and endurance in the isolation position and tension or shortening in the finger flexion pattern.

Muscles involved
Extensor digitorum
Extensor indicis
Extensor digiti minimi

Range of motion
0 to 15 degrees

Position of client
Seated, with forearm in pronation and supported on a table and wrist in neutral

Isolation and assessment
No resistance is required. Ability to perform isolation indicates normal function.
Extensor digitorum: Client extends metacarpophalangeal joints (all fingers simultaneously), allowing the interphalangeal joints to be in slight flexion
Extensor indicis: Client extends the metacarpophalangeal joint of the index finger.
Extensor digiti minimi: Client extends the joint of the fifth digit.

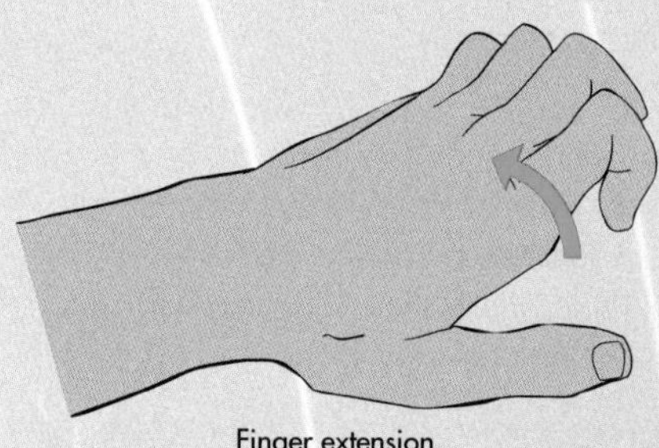
Finger extension

Finger Abduction
Assesses for strength and endurance in the isolation position and tension or shortening in the finger adduction pattern.

Muscles involved
Dorsal interossei
Abductor digiti minimi

Range of motion
0 to 20 degrees

Position of client
Seated, with forearm pronated and supported and wrist in neutral position
Fingers are abducted (separated) and metacarpophalangeal joints remain neutral.

Isolation and assessment
Each finger is isolated separately against resistance given near distal end of finger to push it together with other fingers.

ACTIVITY 10-11—cont'd

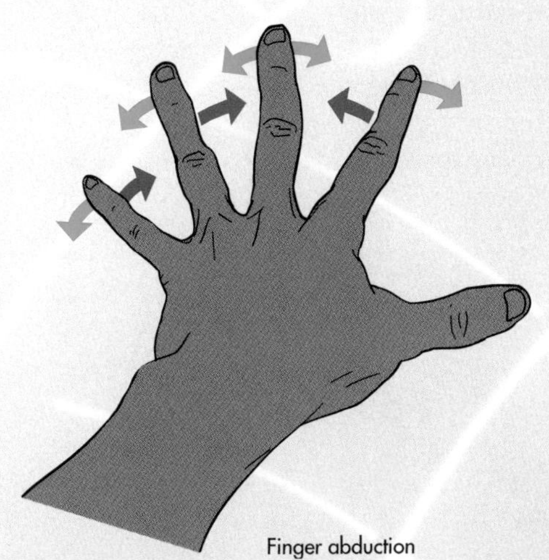
Finger abduction

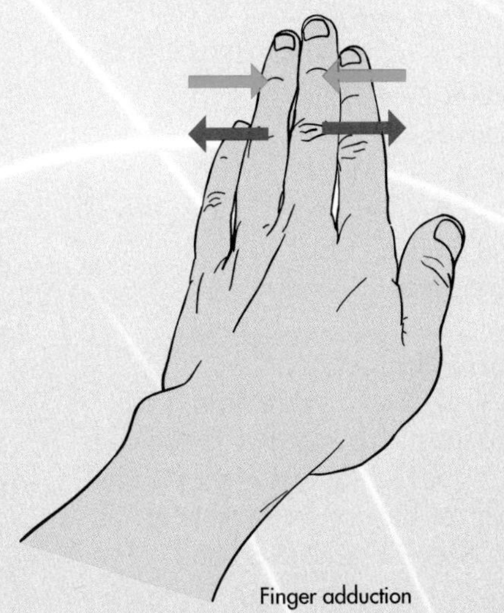
Finger adduction

Dorsal interossei:
Abduction of ring finger toward little finger (includes abductor digiti minimi)
Abduction of middle finger toward ring finger
Abduction of middle finger toward index finger
Abduction of index finger toward thumb

Finger Adduction

Assesses for strength and endurance in the isolation position and tension or shortening in the finger abduction pattern.

Muscles involved
Palmar interossei

Range of motion
0 to 20 degrees

Position of client
Seated, with elbow flexed, forearm pronated and supported, wrist in neutral, and fingers extended and adducted (together) Metacarpophalangeal joints are neutral.

Isolation and assessment
Fingers are tested separately; middle finger is not tested because it has no palmar interossei muscle. Examiner applies resistance near distal end of finger to pull it away from other fingers. Adduction of little finger is toward ring finger. Adduction of ring finger is toward middle finger. Adduction of index finger is toward middle finger. Adduction of thumb is toward index finger.

Thumb Adduction, Flexion, and Medial Rotation

Assesses for strength and endurance in the isolation position and tension or shortening in the thumb extension pattern.
Thumb extensors are extrinsic muscles.
The thumb has 0 to 20 degrees of extension.

Muscles involved
Flexor pollicis brevis
Flexor pollicis longus
Adductor pollicis

Range of motion
Metacarpophalangeal flexion: 0 to 50 degrees
Interphalangeal flexion: 0 to 80 degrees
Adduction: 0 to 70 degrees

Position of client
Seated, with forearm supinated and supported and wrist in neutral position
Carpometacarpal joint and interphalangeal joints are neutral.
Thumb is in adduction.

Isolation and assessment
Client flexes the metacarpophalangeal joint of the thumb to slide thumb across palm while examiner applies resistance to pull thumb back between carpometacarpal and interphalangeal joints. Interphalangeal joint does not flex.

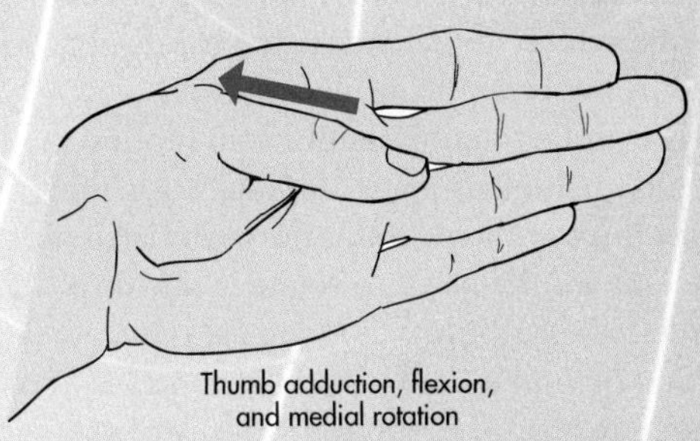
Thumb adduction, flexion, and medial rotation

Continued

ACTIVITY 10-11—cont'd

Thumb Opposition

Muscles involved
Opponens pollicis
Opponens digiti minimi

Range of motion
0 to 70 degrees

Position of client
Seated, with forearm supinated and supported, wrist in neutral position, and thumb in palmar abduction
Opponens pollicis: Apply resistance for the opponens pollicis at the head of the first metacarpal in the direction of lateral rotation, extension, and adduction.

Isolation and assessment
Client medially rotates and flexes thumb toward little finger while little finger flexes and rotates toward thumb so pads of digits touch (not tips of digits).
The examiner applies resistance on palmar surface of thumb and fifth metacarpal to bring them apart.

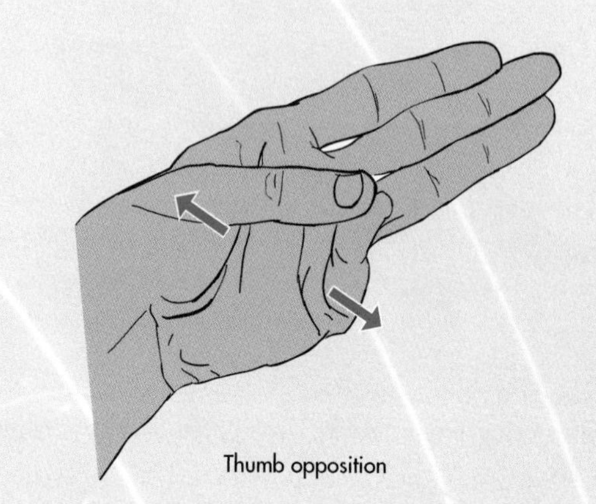
Thumb opposition

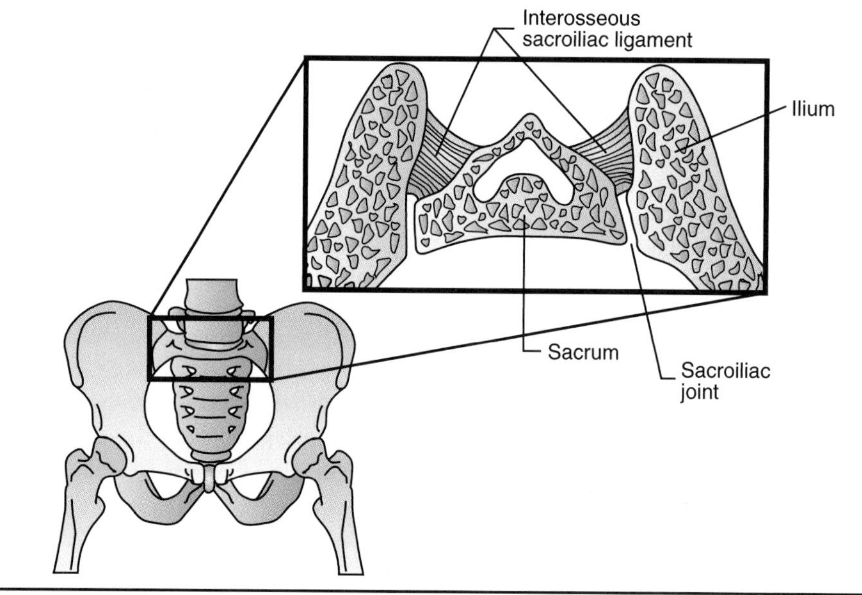

Figure 10-21
Cross section of the sacroiliac joints.

planes for a total of six different movements. Analyzing the pelvic girdle activity to determine the exact location of the movement is important to avoid confusion.

All pelvic girdle rotation results from motion at the right hip, left hip, or lumbar spine. Although for movement to occur in all three of these areas is not essential, it must occur in at least one for the pelvis to rotate in any direction. Even though the sacroiliac joints are synovial joints, they permit little movement and even fuse in many persons later in life. This general reduction of motion is related to degenerative changes such as osteoarthritis (Figure 10-21).

Four groups of ligaments form the main bond that keeps the ilium and sacrum in close approximation. Stability of the sacroiliac joints is crucial because they maintain support for a large portion of the body weight. More movement (therefore less stability) is present in the sacroiliac joints of women, who have smaller and flatter surfaces involving only the first two sacral vertebrae, than in men, who have longer, more concave surfaces involving the first three sacral vertebrae.

When weight shifts from one leg to the other while standing, the symphysis may show an upward/downward motion of 2 mm. During pregnancy the symphysis may separate from 5 to 9 mm.

During normal walking, motions involve the entire pelvic girdle and both hip joints. When the pelvic girdle rotates forward, hip flexion occurs; when it rotates backward, hip extension occurs. The symphysis pubis serves as the axis for the rotation. Jogging and running result in faster and greater range of these movements.

Muscular attachments to the pelvic girdle are extensive, but no muscles directly influence the sacroiliac joint. Indirect actions come from the abdominal muscles, which insert on the superior aspect of the pelvic girdle, and are joined by the quadratus lumborum.

Six groups of hip and thigh muscles are attached to the pelvic girdle and lower extremities. These hip muscles highly influence the movement of the two coxal bones within the pelvic girdle. Anterior to the sacroiliac joint are two important muscles, the psoas and piriformis.

The psoas crosses over the anterior aspect of the sacroiliac joint and goes from the lumbar region to insert into the lesser trochanter of the femur. The right and left piriformis muscles originate from the anterior surface of the sacrum, pass through the sciatic notch, and insert into the greater trochanter of the femur. Muscle imbalance of any of these groups can affect pelvic function adversely.

The pelvic girdle is thought to be of importance within the craniosacral system. Theory indicates that the sacrum has a mobility between the two coxals as part of the craniosacral rhythm. Any changes or alteration in biomechanical function of the pelvic girdle can influence the craniosacral mechanism negatively; the reverse is also true.

Because the pelvis is the supporting base of the spine, dysfunctions in its joints have a great effect on the lumbar spine. One usually feels sacroiliac pain as a dull ache, usually in the bones above the buttock on one side. Because the nerves in that region are not specific, one can feel pain caused by the sacroiliac joint in the groin, back of the thigh, and lower abdomen.

One of the most common dysfunctions occurs when one leans forward to lift some heavy object instead of going into the bent-knee position. If the abdominals are strong and support the anterior pelvis, stabilizing the trunk to maintain a more or less constant balance between the trunk and the pelvis, no dysfunction happens. But if the abdominal muscles and the sacrotuberous ligaments are weak, dysfunction and pain could occur.

Hip Joint

Except for the glenohumeral joint, the hip joint is one of the most mobile joints of the body, largely because of its multiaxial arrangement. Unlike the glenohumeral, the bony architecture of the hip joint provides a great deal of stability, resulting in few hip joint dislocations. An extremely strong and dense ligamentous capsule reinforces the joint, especially the anterior portion (Figure 10-22).

Because of individual differences, some disagreement exists about the exact range of each movement in the hip joint, but the ranges are generally 0 to 130 degrees of flexion, 0 to 30 degrees of extension, 0 to 35 degrees of abduction, 0 to 30 degrees of adduction, 0 to 45 degrees of internal rotation, and 0 to 50 degrees of external rotation.

Movements of the Pelvis and Hip Joints

Anterior and posterior pelvic rotations occur in the sagittal plane, whereas right and left lateral rotation occurs in the frontal plane. Right transverse (clockwise) rotation and left transverse (counterclockwise) rotation occur in the

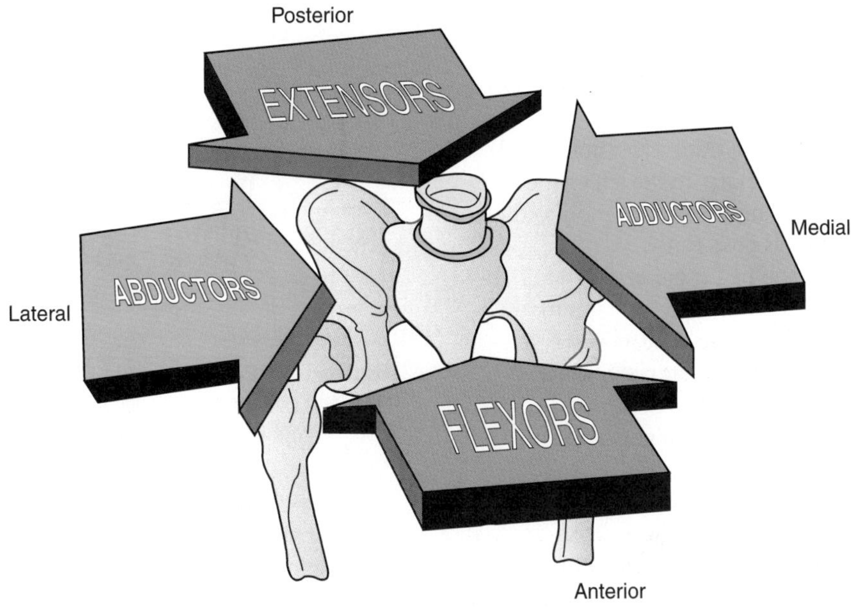

Figure 10-22
Position and function of hip and pelvic muscles.

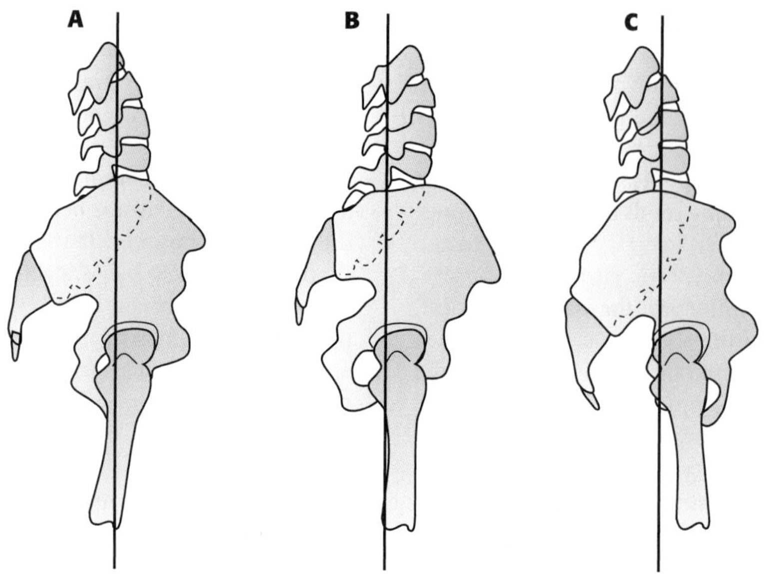

Figure 10-23
Sagittal plane pelvic movement. **A,** In the neutral position the anterior superior iliac spine and the pubic symphysis are in the same vertical plane. **B,** Anterior rotation. Pelvis tilts backward, moving the anterior superior iliac spine posterior to the pubic symphysis. **C,** Posterior rotation. Pelvis tilts forward, moving the anterior superior iliac spine anterior to the pubic symphysis.

horizontal or transverse plane of motion (Figures 10-23 to 10-25). The movements are as follows:

Anterior pelvic rotation: Anterior movement of the upper pelvis; the iliac crest tilts forward in a sagittal plane (Figure 10-23).

Posterior pelvic rotation: Posterior movement of the upper pelvis; the iliac crest tilts backward in a sagittal plane.

Left lateral pelvic rotation (tilt): In the frontal plane the left pelvis moves superiorly in relation to the right pelvis; the left pelvis rotates upward or the right pelvis rotates downward.

Right lateral pelvic rotation (tilt): In the frontal plane the right pelvis moves superiorly in relation to the left pelvis; the right pelvis rotates upward or the left pelvis rotates downward (Figures 10-24).

Left transverse pelvic rotation: In a transverse (horizontal) plane of motion the pelvis rotates to the left of the body; the right iliac crest moves anteriorly in relation to the left iliac crest, which moves posteriorly.

Right transverse pelvic rotation: In a transverse (horizontal) plane of motion the pelvis rotates to the right of the body; the left iliac crest moves anteriorly in relation to the right iliac crest, which moves posteriorly (Figures 10-25).

Hip flexion: Movement of the femur straight anteriorly toward the pelvis

Hip extension: Movement of the femur straight posteriorly away from the pelvis

Hip abduction: Movement of the femur laterally to the side away from the midline

Hip adduction: Movement of the femur medially toward the midline

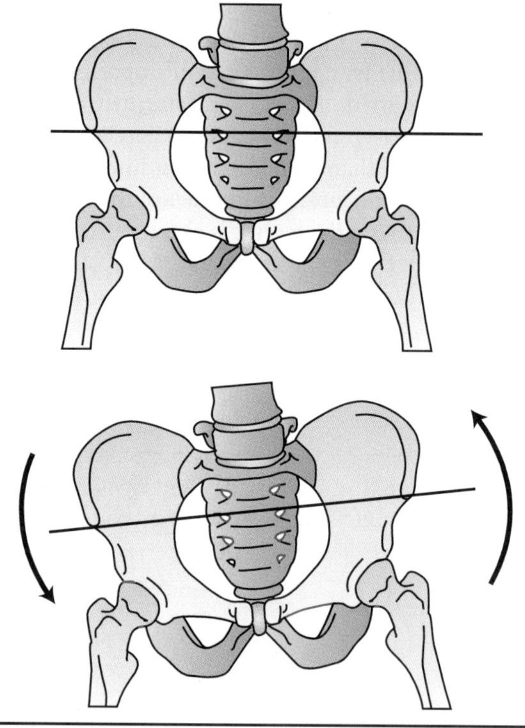

Figure 10-24
Frontal plane pelvic movement tilt. When standing upright, the iliac crests should be level in the frontal plane, and anterior superior iliac spines on the left and right should be level.

Hip external rotation: Rotary movement of the femur laterally around its longitudinal axis away from the midline

Hip internal rotation: Rotary movement of the femur medially around its longitudinal axis toward the midline

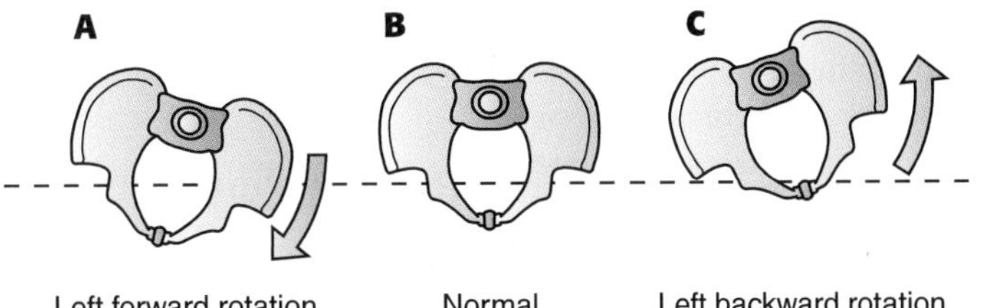

Figure 10-25
A superior view of transverse rotation of the pelvis in the transverse plane. **A,** Forward rotation. **B,** Neutral position of the pelvis. **C,** Backward rotation of the pelvis .

TABLE 10-2
Pelvic Girdle, Lumbar Spine, and Hip Joint Movements

Pelvic Rotations	Lumbar Spine Motion	Right Hip Motion	Left Hip Motion
Anterior rotation	Extension	Flexion	Flexion
Posterior rotation	Flexion	Extension	Extension
Right lateral rotation	Right lateral flexion	Adduction	Abduction
Left lateral rotation	Left lateral flexion	Abduction	Adduction
Right transverse rotation	Left lateral rotation	Internal rotation	External rotation
Left transverse rotation	Right lateral rotation	External rotation	Internal rotation

The lumbar spine, hip joint, and pelvic girdle work together in carrying out lower extremity activities. Table 10-2 shows a comparison of pelvic girdle, lumbar spine, and hip joint movements (Activity 10-12).

Muscles of the Hip Joint

At the hip joint are six two-joint muscles that have one action at the hip and another at the knee. The muscles usually involved in hip and pelvic girdle motions depend largely on the direction of the movement and the position of the body in relation to the earth and its gravitational forces. In addition, one should note that the body part that moves the most is the part least stabilized. For example, when standing on both feet and contracting the hip flexors, the trunk and pelvis flex anteriorly; but when lying supine and contracting the hip flexors, the thighs move forward into flexion on the stable pelvis. In another example, the hip flexor muscles are used in moving the legs toward the trunk, but the extensor muscles are used eccentrically when the pelvis and trunk move downward slowly on the femur and concentrically when the trunk is raised on the femur such as rising to the standing position.

In the downward phase of the knee-bend exercise, the movement at the hips and knees is flexion. The muscles involved primarily are the hip and knee extensors in eccentric contraction to control the trunk.

The iliopsoas muscle provides stabilization and powerful actions such as raising the legs from a supine position on the floor. Its origin in the lower back tends to move the lower back anteriorly, or, in the supine position, pulls the lower back up as it raises the legs. For this reason, one often feels lower back problems with this activity because leg raising is primarily hip flexion, not abdominal action. Strong

ACTIVITY 10-12

Slowly and deliberately move your joints through each of the movement patterns described. Identify the interplay between the hip movements and the pelvic girdle movements, paying close attention to the secondary movement of the pelvic girdle during hip movement. In the space provided, describe the experience.

Example
I could feel the rotation at the symphysis pubis when I walked if I placed my fingers on the joint.

Your Turn

abdominals prevent lower back strain by pulling up on the front of the pelvis and thus flattening the back.

The sartorius, a two-joint muscle, is effective as a hip or knee flexor and is weak when both actions occur at the same time. When the knees are extended, the sartorius becomes a more effective hip flexor.

The rectus femoris muscle pulls from the anterior inferior iliac spine of the ilium to rotate the pelvis anteriorly. Only the abdominal muscles, particularly the rectus abdominis, can prevent this from occurring. In older adults the pelvis may be tilted forward permanently. The relaxed abdominal wall does not hold the pelvis up, and therefore an increased lumbar curve results. The rectus femoris muscle is a powerful extensor of the knee when the hip is extended but is weak when the hip is flexed.

The pectineus tends to rotate the pelvis anteriorly. The abdominal muscles pulling up on the pelvis in front counteract this tilting.

The tensor fasciae latae muscle is used when flexion and internal rotation take place. This muscle also aids in preventing external rotation of the femur as it is flexed by other flexor muscles.

Typical action of the gluteus medius and gluteus minimus muscles occurs in walking. As the weight of the body shifts to one leg, these muscles prevent the opposite hip from sagging. Weakness in the gluteus medius and gluteus minimus can result in what is known as the Trendelenburg gait. With this weakness, the individual's opposite hip sags on weight bearing because the hip abductors cannot maintain proper alignment. As the body ages, the gluteus medius and gluteus minimus muscles tend to lose their effectiveness. Walking loses its easy spring and becomes more labored.

The gluteus maximus muscle comes into action when movement between the pelvis and the femur approaches and goes beyond 15 degrees of extension. As a result, the gluteus maximus is not used extensively in ordinary walking but is important in extension of the thigh with external rotation and stabilization between the lumbar dorsal fascia and iliotibial band.

The six deep lateral rotator muscles—piriformis, gemellus superior, gemellus inferior, obturator externus, obturator internus, quadratus femoris—provide powerful movements of external rotation of the femur. Standing on one leg and forcefully turning the body away from that leg is accomplished by contraction of these muscles.

The hamstrings (semitendinosus, semimembranosus, and biceps femoris), together with the gluteus maximus muscle, act in extension of the thigh when the knees are straight. These muscles are used in ordinary walking as extensors of the hip and allow the gluteus maximus to stabilize the movement. When the trunk is bent forward with the knees straight, the hamstring muscles have a powerful pull on the rear pelvis and tilt it down in back. If the knees are flexed when this movement takes place, the gluteus maximus chiefly does the work.

The adductor brevis, adductor longus, adductor magnus, and gracilis provide powerful movement of the thighs toward each other and are important postural muscles (Activity 10-13).

Knee Region

The knee joint is the largest and most complex joint in the body and is primarily a hinge joint. The combined functions of weight bearing and locomotion place considerable stress and strain on the knee joint. The ligaments provide static stability to the knee joint, and contractions of the quadriceps and hamstrings produce dynamic stability.

The knee includes the articulation of the femur and tibia and the patella, which covers it anteriorly. The knee acts as part of a closed kinematic chain with the lumbar spine, hip, and ankle. Weight-bearing forces normally bisect the knee even though it has a slight valgus angulation. A slight hyperextension of both knees when standing is normal (more in females). The extension ends when the capsule and ligaments twist and draw tight, locking the joint in its close-packed position. The range of motion of the knee is 5 to 10 degrees hyperextension, 135 to 150 degrees flexion with soft tissue of the calf and thigh limiting flexion, and 10 degrees internal or external tibial rotation. With the knee flexed 30 degrees or more, approximately 30 degrees of internal rotation and 45 degrees of external rotation can occur. The external rotation of the tibia toward the end of extension and internal rotation during beginning of flexion is automatic because of the shape of the articulating bones.

The quadriceps pull the patella in line with the femur. The patellar tendon pulls the patella in line with the tibia. The quadriceps (Q) angle is the angle formed by these two pulls. The tension from the quadriceps and patellar tendon plus the anterior projection of the lateral femoral condyle and the deep patellar groove in the femur hold the patella in place during flexion. As the muscle contracts, the patella moves out of the groove and lateral, and the Q angle decreases. The lateral femoral condyle and the contraction of the vastus medialis muscle (oblique pattern) help prevent lateral dislocation of the patella. This is particularly important for a female because the broader pelvis causes a greater Q angle and a stronger lateral pull (Figure 10-26 on p. 540).

The superior tibiofemoral joint aids the knee in supporting one sixth of the body weight. The joint glides anteriorly during knee flexion and rotates with ankle dorsiflexion. Joint dysfunctions such as hypomobility can lead to lateral knee, leg, or ankle pain.

Other Major Knee Components

Two cartilaginous menisci partially fill the space between the articulating surfaces of the tibia and femur. Both menisci are thicker on the periphery than in the center margin. They move with the tibia during flexion or extension and with the femur in rotation. Menisci improve weight distribution by increasing the contact area between the two long bones. They act as shock absorbers by spreading the stress over the

ACTIVITY 10-13

In this activity, you will be working with a partner to assess individual movement patterns, normal function, and possible dysfunction in each other. One of you is first to isolate the specified movement patterns on each side of your partner, one side at a time, and assess for normal function by applying gentle pressure opposite to the action of the isolation position. The body should be stabilized so that only the isolated area is moving. In some instances the ability to assume the position and maintain it indicates normal function. Muscles should be able to hold against gravity or the applied pressure without strain or pain. The position itself should be easy to assume and comfortable to maintain for a short duration, from 10 to 30 seconds. The bilateral movement patterns should be the same. The opposite movement pattern also should be able to be done easily. Dysfunction may be indicated by bilateral asymmetry, pain, weakness, fatigue, a heavy sensation, binding, and the inability to assume the isolation position or move into the opposite position.

Intervention or referral depends on the severity of the condition and whether the dysfunction is neuromuscular, myofascial, or joint related.

Note: Do not perform these assessments if contraindications exist. Contraindications to this type of assessment include joint and disk dysfunction, acute pain, recent trauma, and inflammation.

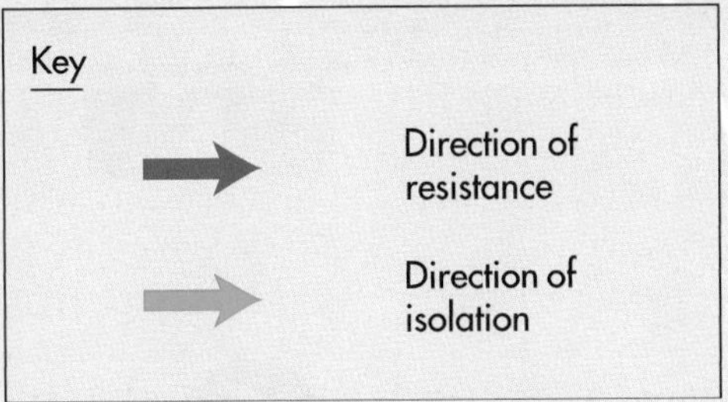

Hip Flexion

Assesses for strength and endurance in the isolation position and tension or shortening in the hip extension pattern.

Muscles involved
Psoas major
Iliacus
Rectus femoris
Sartorius
Tensor fasciae latae
Pectineus
Adductor brevis
Adductor longus
Adductor magnus

Range of motion
0 to 130 degrees

Position of client
Seated, knees bent with thighs fully supported on table and feet hanging over the edge
Client may use arms for stability.

Isolation and assessment
Client flexes hip through full range while examiner applies resistance on anterior thigh above knee to push leg down.

Hip Extension

Assesses for strength and endurance in the isolation position and tension or shortening in the hip flexion pattern.

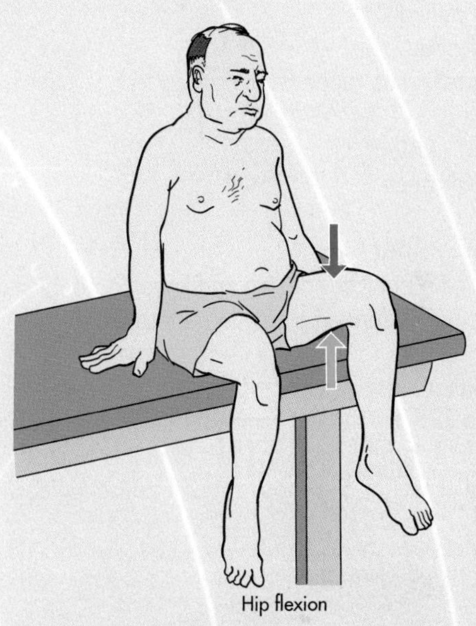
Hip flexion

Muscles involved
Gluteus maximus
Semitendinosus
Semimembranosus
Biceps femoris (long head)

Range of motion
0 to 30 degrees

Position of client
Prone, with arms overhead or abducted to hold sides of table
Place pillows under hips to help flex hips for start position.

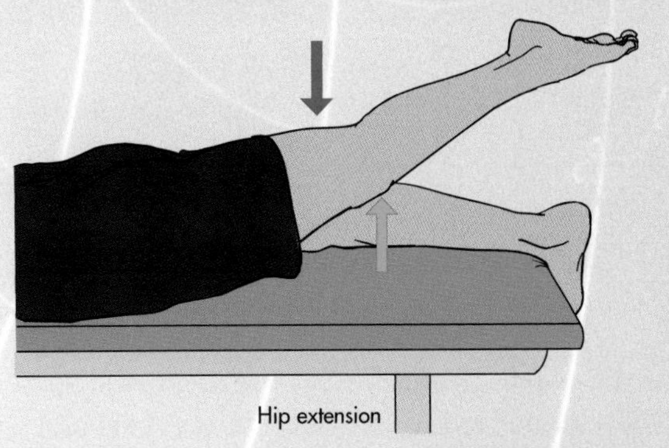
Hip extension

Continued

ACTIVITY 10-13—cont'd

Isolation and assessment
Client extends hip through entire available range of motion while knee is extended. The entire leg should clear the table. Examiner applies resistance to posterior thigh above knee to push leg down.

Hip Abduction

Assesses for strength and endurance in the isolation position and tension or shortening in the hip adduction pattern.

Muscles involved
Gluteus medius
Gluteus minimus
Tensor fasciae latae
Gluteus maximus (upper fibers)

Range of motion
0 to 35 degrees

Position of client
Side-lying on nontest side, hip and knee flexed for stability
Hip is slightly extended on leg to be tested.

Isolation and assessment
Client abducts hip through range of motion leading with heel to prevent flexing or rotating the hip. Examiner applies resistance to lateral aspect of thigh above knee to push leg down.

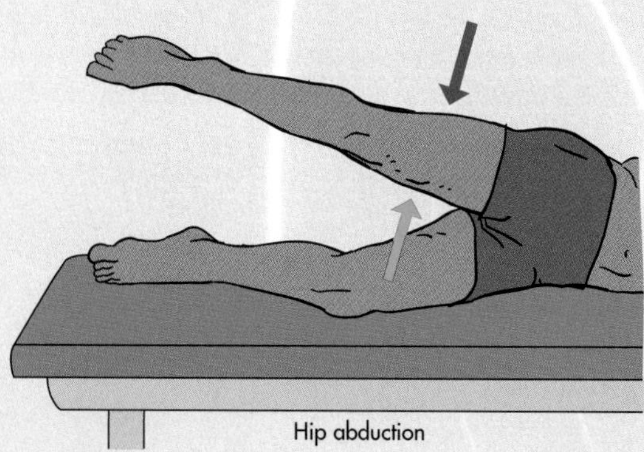

Hip abduction

Hip Adduction

Assesses for strength and endurance in the isolation position and tension or shortening in the hip abduction pattern.

Muscles involved
Adductor magnus
Adductor brevis
Adductor longus
Pectineus
Gracilis

Range of motion
0 to 15 to 30 degrees

Position of client
Side-lying on test side with uppermost limb in 25 degrees of abduction, supported by the examiner
The therapist cradles the leg with the forearm, the hand supporting the limb on the medial surface of the leg.

Isolation and Assessment
Client adducts hip until the lower limb contacts the upper one. No resistance is required.

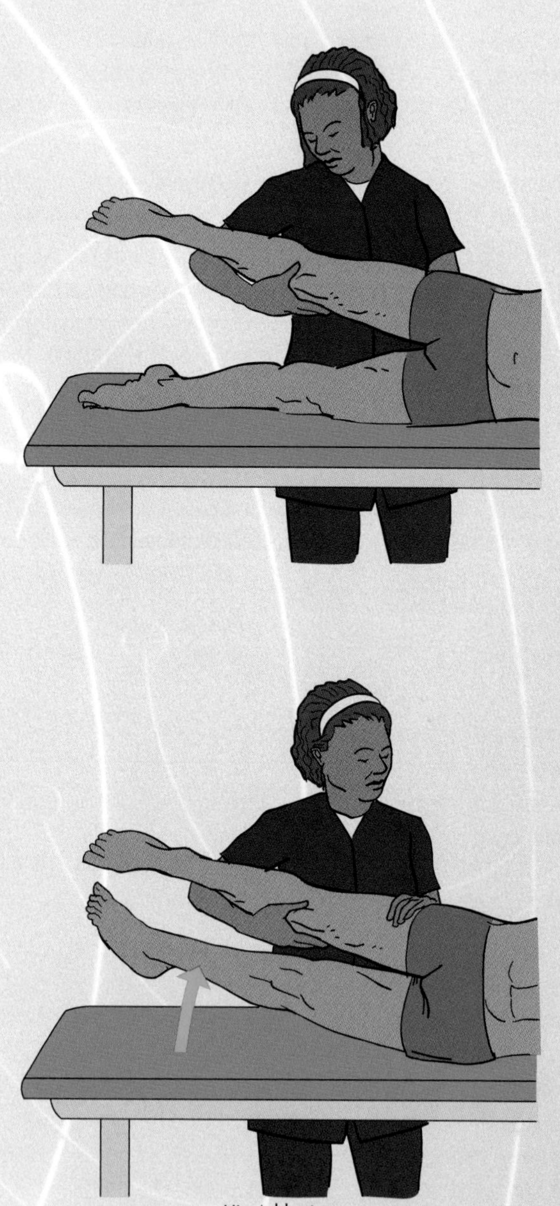

Hip Adduction

ACTIVITY 10-13—cont'd

Hip External or Lateral Rotation

Assesses for strength and endurance in the isolation position and tension or shortening in the hip internal or medial rotation pattern.

Muscles involved
Obturator externus
Obturator internus
Quadratus femoris
Piriformis
Gemellus superior
Gemellus inferior
Gluteus maximus
Sartorius

Range of motion
0 to 45 degrees

Position of client
Seated, with hips flexed but not rotated
Patella in line with anterior superior interior spine
Examiner stabilizes outer thigh above knee
Trunk is supported by placing hands at sides

Isolation and assessment
Client externally rotates hip by bringing the sole of the foot toward the opposite calf while examiner applies resistance to inner ankle. One must take care to avoid knee stress with resistance.

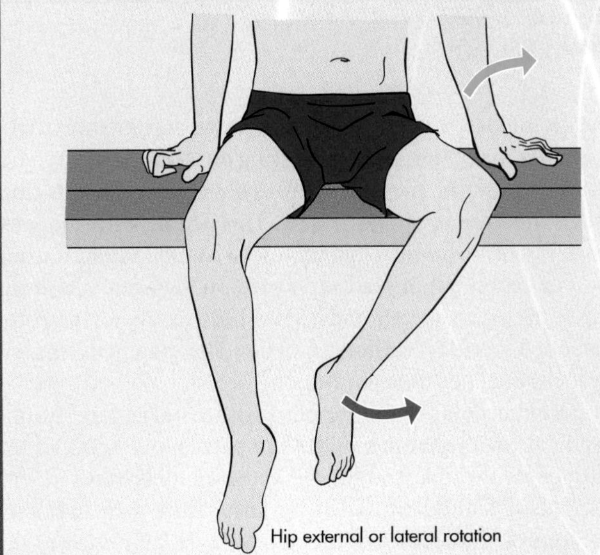

Hip external or lateral rotation

Hip Internal or Medial Rotation

Assesses for strength and endurance in the isolation position and tension or shortening in the lateral or external hip rotation pattern.

Muscles involved
Gluteus minimus
Gluteus medius
Tensor fasciae latae

Range of motion
0 to 50 degrees

Position of client
Seated, with hips flexed, patella in line with anterior superior iliac spine
Arms at sides to support the trunk
Examiner stabilizes medial thigh just above knee.

Isolation and assessment
Client internally rotates hip, turning sole of foot to the side and bringing the knee toward the opposite leg while examiner applies resistance to outer ankle, avoiding knee strain.

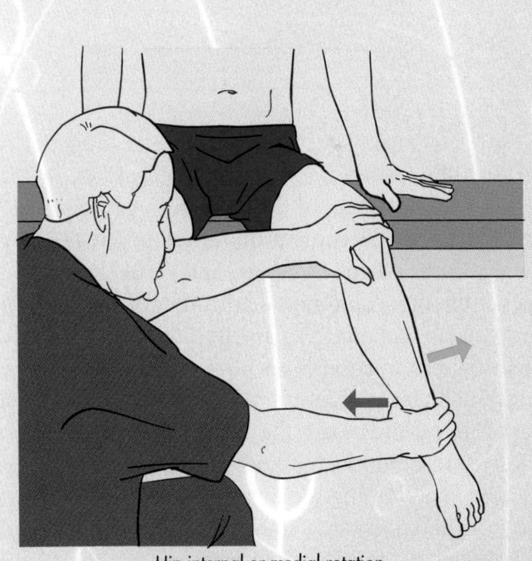

Hip internal or medial rotation

articulating surfaces, decreasing friction and cartilage wear. They are part of the locking mechanism of the knee, which prevents hyperextension by directing the movement of the articulating condyles.

The medial (tibial) collateral ligament is a strong, broad, triangular strap that attaches to the medial epicondyle of the femur. The ligament helps prevent anterior tibial displacement on the femur. The lateral collateral ligament is shorter and more rounded than the medial collateral ligament and is located between the biceps femoris tendon externally and the popliteus tendon internally. The lateral collateral ligament does not attach to the lateral meniscus. Its fibers are

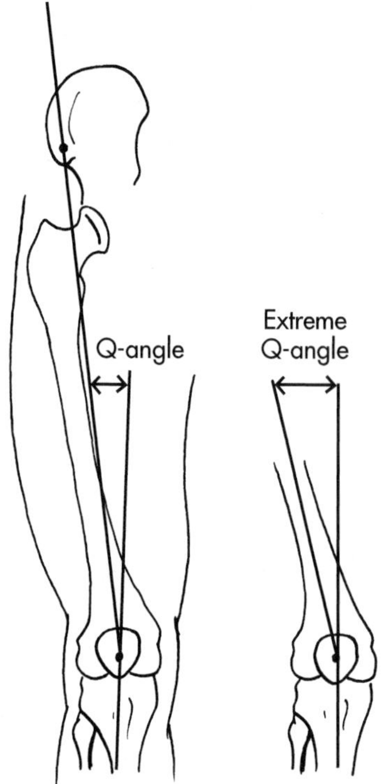

Figure 10-26
The quadriceps angle (Q angle) is measured from the anterior superior iliac spine through the axis of the patella and distally to the insertion of the patellar tendon on the tibial tuberosity. (From Shankman GA: *Fundamental orthopedic management for the physical therapist assistant,* St. Louis, 1997, Mosby.)

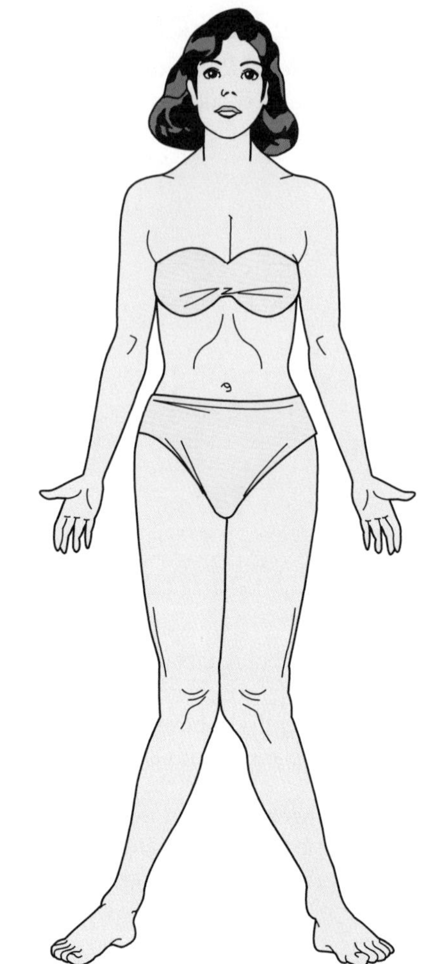

Figure 10-27
Excessive varus angulation.

tight, especially during knee extension, tibial adduction, and lateral rotation. The lateral collateral ligament helps to protect the lateral aspect of the knee from varus stress. The valgus angle is usually more pronounced in females (Figure 10-27). Excessive valgus (bowlegs) and varus (knock-knees) are two of the more common deformities of the knee joint.

The medial collateral ligament and lateral collateral ligament twist in relationship with each other to protect the knee externally from excessive tibial rotation and extension. The cruciate ligaments are the main rotary stabilizers and cross each other within the knee capsule. These ligaments are vital in maintaining the anterior, posterior, and rotary stability of the knee joint. They aid the rolling and gliding movements of the tibia on the femur and are rotary guides for the screw-home locking mechanism of the knee.

The *screw-home mechanism* occurs with rotary movement of the knee (Figure 10-28). This rotary motion occurs not as a result of muscle action but from joint and menisci structure. The articular surface of the medial femoral condyle is longer than that of the lateral condyle. In addition, the C shape of the medial meniscus allows the medial tibial condyle to rotate around the femoral condyle. The lateral meniscus is shaped like an O and holds the lateral tibial condyle more securely against the femoral condyle and does not allow motion. As a result of these structural features the medial condyle of the tibia rotates on the femur during the last 15 degrees of knee extension in an external direction in the non–weight-bearing position. In the weight-bearing position the femur medially rotates on the tibia when the knee is extended fully. This action locks the knee into extension, which allows us to stand without using muscle action but instead supported on the ligaments at the hip. This saves energy and allows individuals to stand for extended periods without fatigue. The popliteus muscle unlocks the knee to begin flexion.

The knee joint is well supplied with synovial fluid from a synovial cavity that lies under the patella and between the surfaces of the tibia and the femur. Commonly, this synovial cavity is called the capsule of the knee. More than 10 bursae are located in the knee, some of which are connected to the synovial cavity. Bursae are located where they can absorb shock or prevent friction.

Movements of the Knee

Flexion and extension of the knee occurs in the sagittal plane, whereas internal and external rotation occurs in the horizontal plane (Activity 10-14):

Flexion: Bending or decreasing the angle of the knee, characterized by the heel moving toward the buttocks

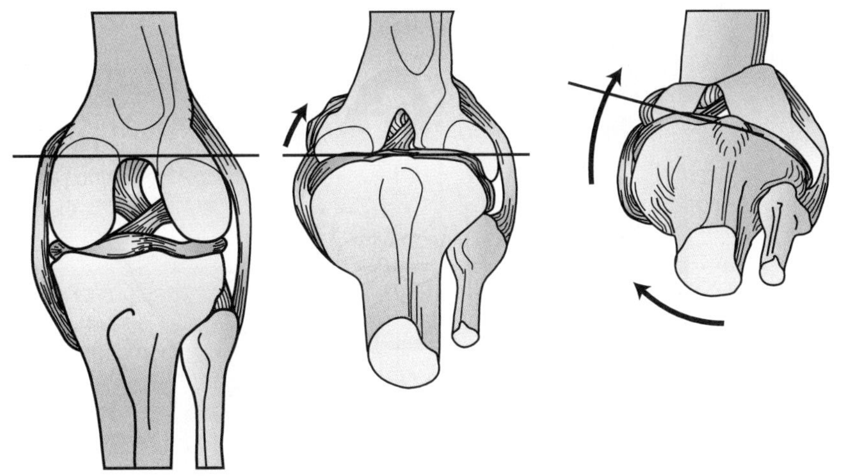

Figure 10-28
The screw-home motion of the knee. In the non–weight-bearing position the tibia laterally rotates on the femur as the knee moves into the last few degrees in extension.

ACTIVITY 10-14

Slowly and deliberately move your joints through each of the movement patterns described. In the space provided, describe the experience.

Example
I could feel the rotation of my knee during the last phase of extension and noticed how solid it felt when the screw-home mechanism kicked in.

Your Turn

Extension: Straightening or increasing the angle of the knee
External rotation: Rotary motion of the lower leg laterally away from the midline
Internal rotation: Rotary motion of the lower leg medially toward the midline

Muscles of the Knee

The muscles that flex and medially rotate the knee are the hamstrings, sartorius, gracilis, gastrocnemius, and popliteus. The popliteus muscle is the only flexor of the leg found only at the knee. All other flexors are two-joint muscles. Two-joint muscles are most effective when the origin or insertion is fixed by the contraction of the muscles that prevent movement in the direction of the pull.

The popliteus provides posterolateral stability to the knee and assists the medial hamstrings in internal rotation of the lower leg at the knee. The plantaris and gastrocnemius assist flexion.

The quadriceps extend the knee. All quadriceps muscles attach to the patella and by the patellar tendon to the tibial tuberosity. All these muscles are superficial and palpable except the vastus intermedius, which is under the rectus femoris. The quadriceps muscles generally are desired to be 25% to 33% stronger than the hamstring muscle group (knee flexors). Proper tracking of the patella is provided by the relationship between the vastus medialis (primarily oblique portion) and vastus lateralis.

The tensor fasciae latae assists with flexion and extension. The semimembranosus and semitendinosus (medial hamstrings) muscles are assisted by the popliteus to internally rotate the knee, whereas the biceps femoris (lateral hamstrings) is responsible for knee external rotation (Figure 10-29; Activity 10-15). The pes anserinus is the tendinous expansions of the sartorius, gracilis, and semitendinosus muscles at the medial border of the tibial tuberosity.

Ankle and Foot Region

The ankle joint is made up of the talus, distal tibia, and distal fibula. The ankle joint allows approximately 50 degrees of plantar flexion and 15 to 20 degrees of dorsiflexion. Greater range of dorsiflexion is possible when the knee is flexed, which reduces the tension of the biarticular gastrocnemius muscle.

Inversion and eversion, although commonly thought to be ankle joint movements, technically occur in the subtalar and transverse tarsal joints. These joints combine to allow approximately 20 to 30 degrees of inversion and 5 to 25 degrees of eversion. Minimal movement occurs within the remainder of the intertarsal and tarsometatarsal arthrodial joints.

The complexity of the foot is evidenced by the 26 bones, 19 large muscles, many small (intrinsic) muscles, and more than 100 ligaments that make up the structure of the foot. The bones of the foot connect with the upper bony structure

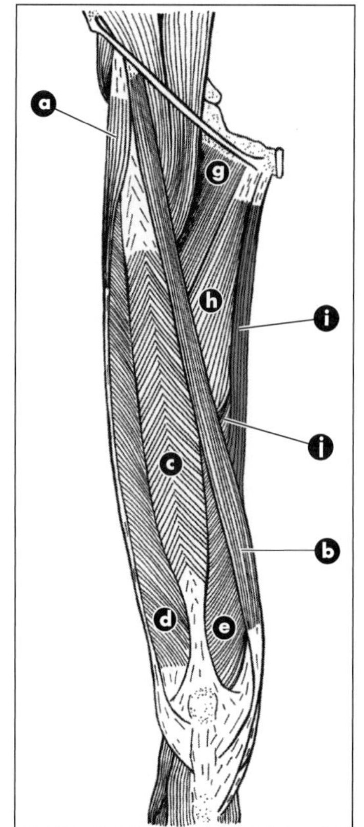

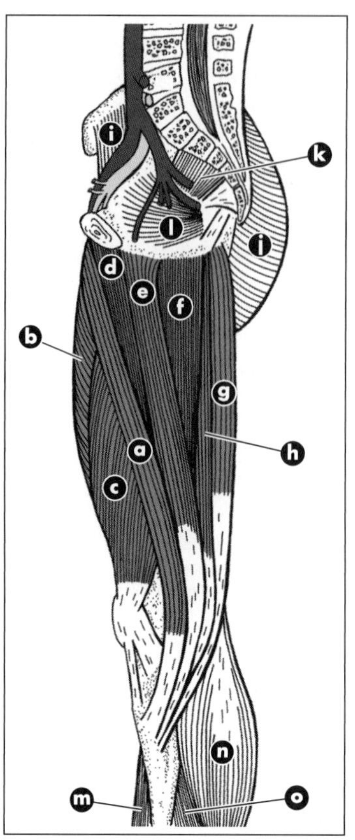

Figure 10-29
A, Anterior view of the right thigh (superficial). *a*, Tensor fasciae latae. *b*, Sartorius. *c*, Rectus femoris. *d*, Vastus lateralis. *e*, Vastus medialis. *f*, Vastus intermedius (not seen). *g*, Pectineus. *h*, Adductor longus. *i*, Gracilis. *j*, Adductor magnus. **B**, Medial view of the right thigh (superficial). *a*, Sartorius. *b*, Rectus femoris. *c*, Vastus medialis. *d*, Adductor longus. *e*, Gracilis. *f*, Adductor magnus. *g*, Semitendinosus. *h*, Semimembranosus. *i*, Iliacus. *j*, Gluteus maximus. *k*, Piriformis. *l*, Obturator internus. *m*, Tibialis anterior. *n*, Gastrocnemius (medial head). *o*, Soleus.

of the upper body through the fibula and tibia. Body weight is transferred from the tibia to the talus and calcaneus.

Support and propulsion are the two functions of the foot. Proper functioning and adequate development of the muscles of the foot and the practice of proper foot mechanics are essential for everyone. In our modern society, foot trouble is one of our most common ailments. Poor foot mechanics begun in early life invariably lead to foot discomfort in later years.

The metatarsophalangeal joint of the great toe flexes 45 degrees and extends 70 degrees, whereas the interphalangeal joint can flex from 0 degrees of full extension to 90 degrees of flexion. The metatarsophalangeal joints of the four lesser toes allow approximately 40 degrees of flexion and 40 degrees of extension. The metatarsophalangeal joints also adduct minimally. The proximal interphalangeal joints in the lesser toes flex from 0 degrees of extension to 35 degrees of flexion. The distal interphalangeal joints flex 60 degrees and extend 30 degrees. Much variation exists from joint to joint and person to person in all of these joints (Figure 10-30).

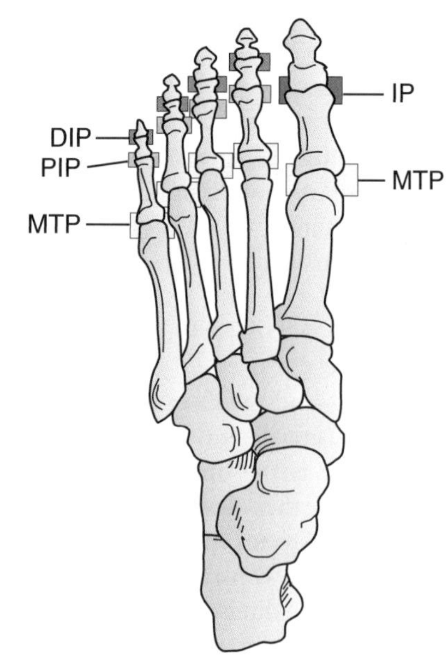

Figure 10-30
Joints of the phalanges of the foot. *DIP*, distal interphalangeal; *PIP*, proximal interphalangeal; *MTP*, metatarsophalangeal; *IP*, interphalangeal.

Ligaments in the foot and the ankle have the difficult task of maintaining the position of the arches in the foot. The

ACTIVITY 10-15

In this activity, you will be working with a partner to assess individual movement patterns, normal function, and possible dysfunction in each other. One of you is first to isolate the specified movement patterns on each side of your partner, one side at a time, and assess for normal function by applying gentle pressure opposite to the action of the isolation position. The body should be stabilized so that only the isolated area is moving. In some instances the ability to assume the position and maintain it indicates normal function. Muscles should be able to hold against gravity or the applied pressure without strain or pain. The position itself should be easy to assume and comfortable to maintain for a short duration, from 10 to 30 seconds. The bilateral movement patterns should be the same. The opposite movement pattern also should be able to be done easily.

Dysfunction may be indicated by bilateral asymmetry, pain, weakness, fatigue, a heavy sensation, binding, and the inability to assume the isolation position or move into the opposite position. Intervention or referral depends on the severity of the condition and whether the dysfunction is neuromuscular, myofascial, or joint related.

Note: Do not perform these assessments if contraindications exist. Contraindications to this type of assessment include joint and disk dysfunction, acute pain, recent trauma, and inflammation.

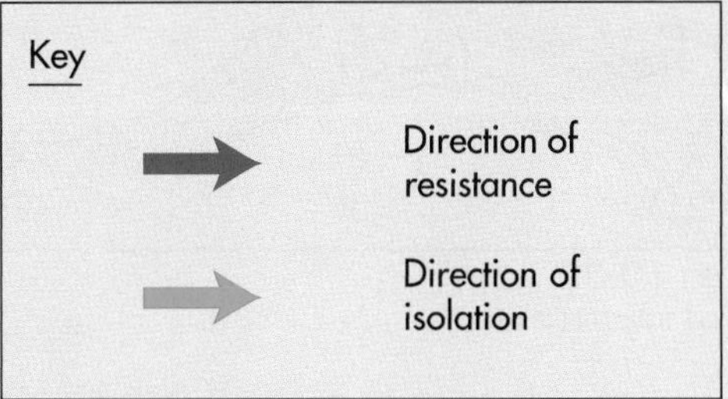

Knee Flexion

Assesses for strength and endurance in the isolation position and tension or shortening in the extension pattern.

Muscles involved
Biceps femoris
Semitendinosus
Semimembranosus
Popliteus
Gastrocnemius

Range of motion
0 to 150 degrees

Position of client
Prone, with limbs straight and toes hanging over the edge of the table
Examiner applies light to moderate counterpressure to hamstrings.

Isolation and assessment
Client flexes knee through full range, keeping thigh in contact with table. Examiner applies resistance gradually to posterior leg proximal to ankle joint after knee reaches 45 degrees to straighten leg.

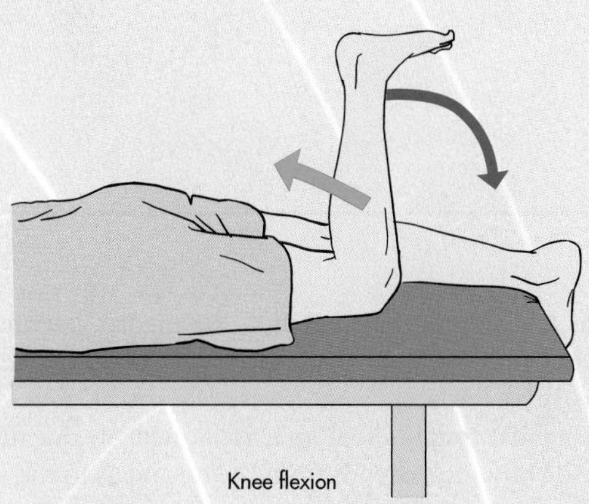
Knee flexion

Knee Extension

Assesses for strength and endurance in the isolation position and tension or shortening in the flexion pattern.

Muscles involved
Rectus femoris
Vastus intermedius
Vastus lateralis
Vastus medialis

Range of motion
0 to 135 degrees
May extend 10 degrees beyond 0 in those with hyperextension.

Position of client
Seated, with hips flexed and small pillow under thigh to maintain 90 degrees of hip flexion
Client grasps table edge for stabilization while examiner places one hand on distal anterior thigh.

Continued

ACTIVITY 10-15—cont'd

Isolation and assessment

Client extends knee through available range of motion as examiner applies resistance to distal end of anterior leg to bend it at the knee. Do not allow the client to hyperextend the knee or lift thigh off table.

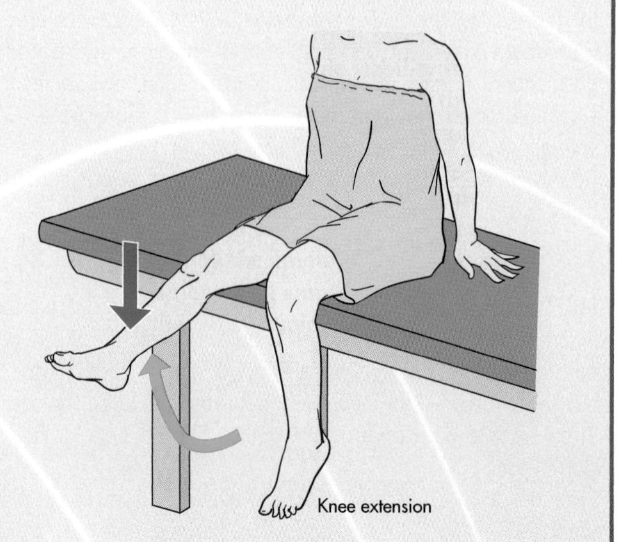

foot has three longitudinal arches: the medial, lateral, and transverse. Individual long arches vary from high, medium, and low, but a low arch is not necessarily a weak arch.

The medial longitudinal arch is located on the medial side of the foot and extends from the calcaneus to the talus, the navicular, the three cuneiforms, and the proximal ends of the three medial metatarsals. The lateral longitudinal arch is located on the lateral side of the foot and extends from the calcaneus to the cuboid and proximal ends of the fourth and fifth metatarsals. The transverse arch extends across the foot from one metatarsal bone to the other. A vast network of fascia in the sole of the foot supports the arches. Plantar fascia with the muscles provides the spring to the arch structure (Figures 10-31 and 10-32).

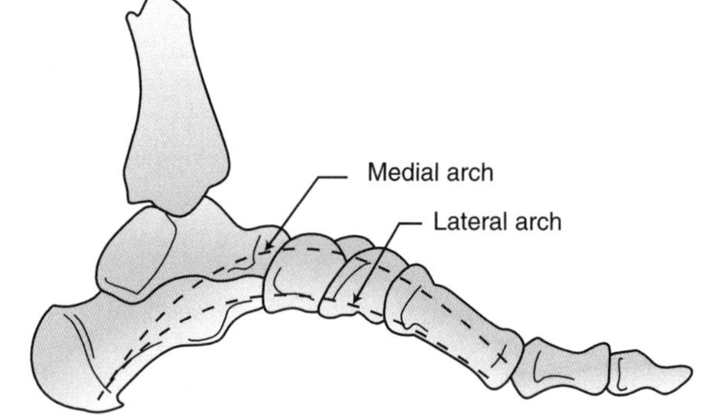

Figure 10-32
Longitudinal arches of the foot.

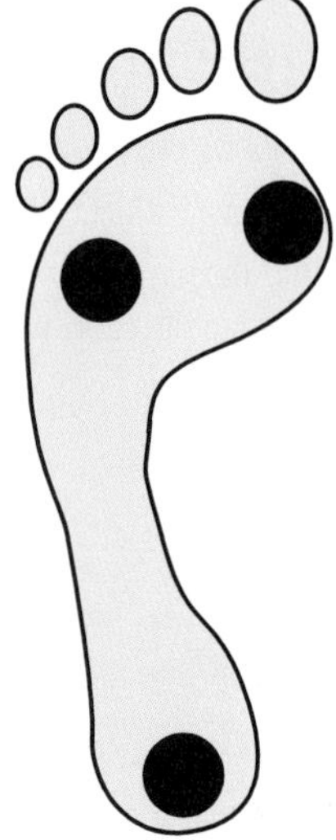

Figure 10-31
The main weight-bearing surfaces of the foot.

Movements of the Ankle and Foot

The following are movements of the ankle and foot (Activity 10-16; Figure 10-33):

Dorsiflexion: Movement of the top of the ankle and foot toward the anterior tibial bone, accomplished by the flexor muscles of the ankle

Plantar flexion: Movement of the ankle and foot away from the tibia, accomplished by the extensor muscles of the ankle

Eversion (pronation): Turning the ankle and foot outward, away from the midline, with weight on the medial edge of the foot

Inversion (supination): Turning the ankle and foot inward, toward the midline, with weight on the lateral edge of the foot

Toe flexion: Movement of the toes toward the plantar surface of the foot

Toe extension: Movement of the toes away from the plantar surface of the foot

ACTIVITY 10-16

Slowly and deliberately move your ankle and then your toes through the movement patterns. Then move the ankle and toes together and differentiate between extrinsic (muscles with attachment outside the foot proper) and intrinsic (muscles with all attachments within the foot proper) muscle activity.

In the space provided describe the experience.

Example

It was hard to isolate the intrinsic muscles.

Your Turn

Muscles of the Ankle and Foot

The large number of muscles in the ankle and foot may be grouped according to location and function. In general, the muscles located on the anterior of the ankle and foot are the dorsal flexors. Those to the posterior are plantar flexors. Muscles that are everters are located more to the lateral side, and the invertors are located medially. The muscular strength patterns are not balanced. Plantar flexion is dominant over dorsiflexion, and inversion dominates eversion.

The gastrocnemius muscle is more effective as a knee flexor if the foot is elevated and more effective as a plantar flexor of the foot if the knee is held in extension. You can observe this when someone sits too close to the wheel when driving a car. When the knees are bent, the muscle becomes an ineffective plantar flexor, and the person finds it difficult to depress the brakes.

The soleus muscle is one of the most important plantar flexors of the ankle. This is especially true when the knee is flexed. When the knee is slightly flexed, the effect of the gastrocnemius is reduced, thereby placing more work on the soleus.

The tibialis posterior muscle pulls down from the underside and contracts to invert and plantar flex the foot. Use of the tibialis posterior in plantar flexion and inversion gives support to the longitudinal arch of the foot.

Passing down the back of the lower leg under the medial malleolus and then forward, the flexor digitorum longus muscle draws the four lesser toes down into flexion toward the heel as it plantar flexes the ankle. This muscle is important in helping other foot muscles maintain the longitudinal arch.

Pulling from the underside of the great toe, the flexor hallucis muscle may work independently of the flexor digitorum longus muscle or with it.

The fibularis longus muscle passes behind and beneath the lateral malleolus and under the foot from the outside to the inner surface. Because of its line of pull, the peroneus longus is a strong everter and assists in plantar flexion. When the fibularis longus muscle is used effectively with the other ankle flexors, it helps support the transverse arch as it flexes.

The fibularis brevis muscle passes down behind and under the lateral malleolus to pull on the base of the fifth metatarsal. The fibularis brevis is a primary everter of the foot and assists in plantar flexion. In addition, the fibularis brevis aids in maintaining the longitudinal arch as it depresses the foot.

The tibialis anterior muscle holds up the inner margin of the foot. However, as it contracts, the tibialis anterior muscle dorsiflexes the ankle and is an antagonist to the plantar flexors of the ankle. The tibialis anterior is forced to contract strongly when a person ice skates or walks on the outside of the foot, and the muscle strongly supports the long arch in inversion.

Strength is necessary in the extensor digitorum longus muscle to maintain balance between the plantar and the dorsal flexors. The strength of the ankle is evident when the gastrocnemius, soleus, tibialis posterior, fibularis longus, fibularis brevis, digitorum longus, flexor digitorum brevis, and flexor hallucis longus muscles are all used effectively in walking.

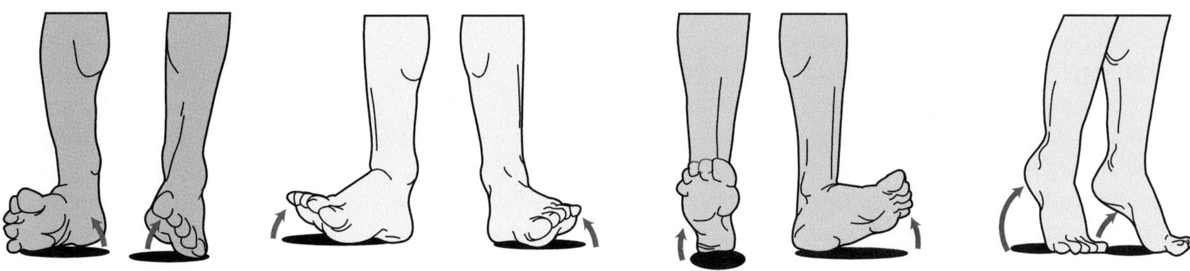

Figure 10-33
Quick tests for foot and ankle range of motion.

Intrinsic Muscles of the Foot

The intrinsic muscles of the foot have their origin and insertion on the bones within the foot. Four layers of these muscles are found on the plantar surface of the foot. These muscles are involved with dorsiflexion and plantar flexion of the toes (Activity 10-17):

First layer (most superficial): Adductor hallucis, flexor digitorum brevis, and abductor digit quinti
Second layer: Quadratus plantae and lumbricales (four)
Third layer: Flexor hallucis brevis, flexor digiti quinti brevis, and adductor hallucis
Fourth layer (deepest): Interossei (seven)

SUMMARY

This chapter has presented the basic principles of biomechanics. The kinetic chain describes three main biomechanical dysfunctional patterns, which we discussed with intervention suggestions and referral recommendations. We provided a practice assessment protocol for biomechanical function.

The concepts in this chapter may seem complex and at times difficult to understand. Comprehending how all the aspects of movement work together requires knowledge and the development of an understanding of the relationship of the pieces and how they function. Sometimes the knowledge is too great, and being able to use reference texts effectively is helpful.

Many students find themselves lost in the terminology of all the pieces: the bones, ligaments, names of the joints, actions of movement, names of the muscles, and directions for isolation. When this happens, the student should slow down and actually perform the movement while saying the words. The entire unit has been about movement. Movement is best understood by moving. The student should continue to look up the definitions of the words that are confusing. Persist in understanding biomechanical concepts. Competency in therapeutic massage is based on the integrated applications described in this chapter.

Balance and center may be the most important concepts of all. The student should remember that the importance of being centered often is expressed as being present in the moment and responding resourcefully to each unfolding second of life.

evolve

View the video clip under Course Materials Chapter 10 on the Fritz EVOLVE site for a visual demonstration of the biomechanics concepts presented in this chapter.

ACTIVITY 10-17

In this activity, you will be working with a partner to assess individual movement patterns, normal function, and possible dysfunction in each other. One of you is first to isolate the specified movement patterns on each side of your partner, one side at a time, and assess for normal function by applying gentle pressure opposite to the action of the isolation position. The body should be stabilized so that only the isolated area is moving. In some instances the ability to assume the position and maintain it indicates normal function. Muscles should be able to hold against gravity or the applied pressure without strain or pain. The position itself should be easy to assume and comfortable to maintain for a short duration, from 10 to 30 seconds. The bilateral movement patterns should be the same. The opposite movement patterns also should be able to be done easily.

Dysfunction may be indicated by bilateral asymmetry, pain, weakness, fatigue, a heavy sensation, binding, and the inability to assume the isolation position or move into the opposite position. Intervention or referral depends on the severity of the condition and whether the dysfunction is neuromuscular, myofascial, or joint related.

Note: Do not perform these assessments if contraindications exist. Contraindications to this type of assessment include joint and disk dysfunction, acute pain, recent trauma, and inflammation.

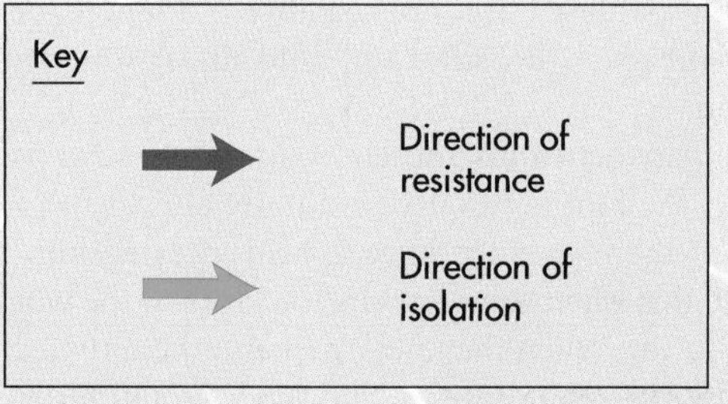

Plantar Flexion

Assesses for strength and endurance in the isolation position and tension or shortening in the dorsiflexion pattern.

Muscles involved
Gastrocnemius
Soleus
Flexor digitorum longus
Flexor hallucis longus
Plantaris
Tibialis posterior

Range of motion
0 to 50 degrees

ACTIVITY 10-17—cont'd

Position of client
Gastrocnemius: Prone, with ankle dorsiflexed off end of table and knee extended
Soleus: Prone, with knee flexed and ankle dorsiflexed

Isolation and assessment (both positions)
Client initiates plantar flexion of the ankle through the available range of motion while examiner applies resistance to posterior calcaneus or sole of foot to push foot into dorsiflexion.

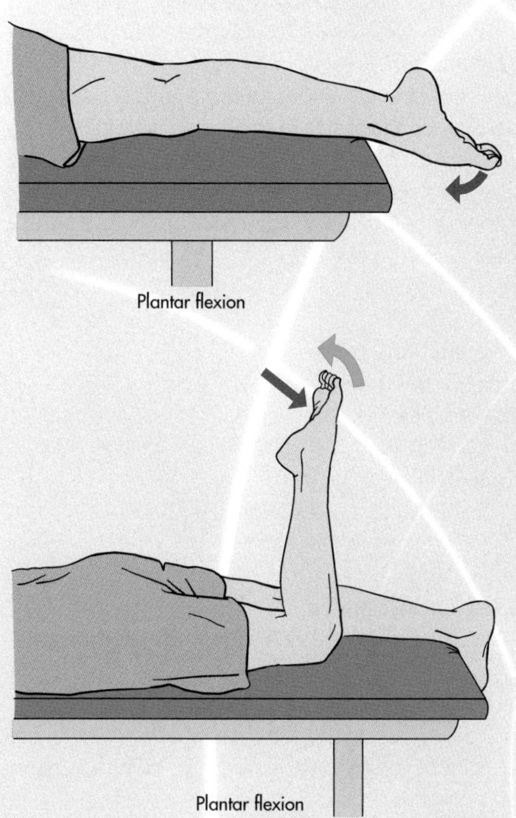

Foot Dorsiflexion
Assesses for strength and endurance in the isolation position and tension or shortening in the plantar flexion pattern.

Muscles involved
Tibialis anterior
Fibularis tertius
Extensor digitorum longus (extensor of lesser toes)
Extensor hallucis longus (greater toe extensor)

Range of motion
0 to 20 degrees

Position of client
Supine with leg straight

Isolation and assessment
Client initiates dorsiflexion of the ankle, keeping toes relaxed, and examiner applies resistance to pull foot into plantar flexion.

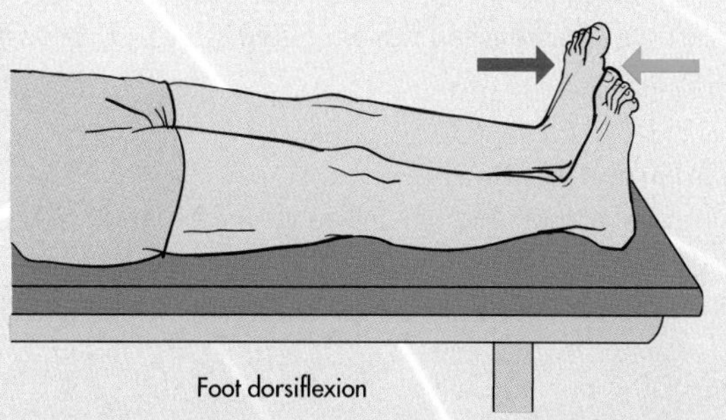

Foot Inversion
Assesses for strength and endurance in the isolation position and tension or shortening in the eversion pattern.

Muscles involved
Tibialis anterior
Tibialis posterior
Flexor digitorum longus (flexor of lesser toes)
Flexor hallucis longus (great toe flexor)
Gastrocnemius (medial head)

Range of motion
0 to 30 degrees

Position of client
Supine or side-lying on test side with ankle in neutral position

Isolation and assessment
Client inverts foot through available range of motion as examiner applies resistance to medial edge of forefoot to pull it into eversion. Client keeps toes relaxed.

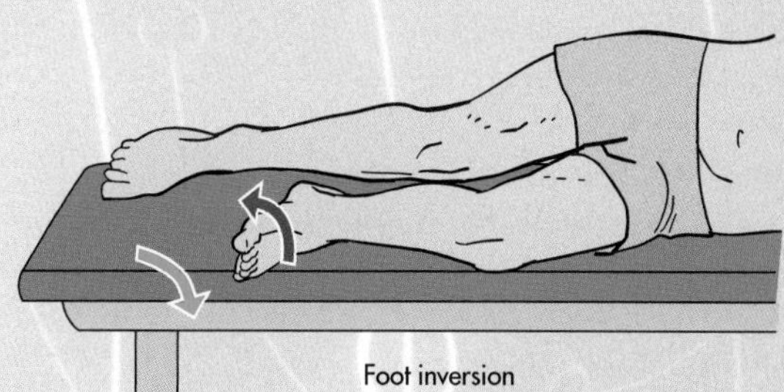

Foot Eversion
Assesses for strength and endurance in the isolation position and tension or shortening in the inversion pattern.

Muscles involved
Fibularis longus
Fibularis brevis
Fibularis tertius
Extensor digitorum longus

Range of motion
0 to 15 degrees

ACTIVITY 10-17—cont'd

Position of client
Supine or side-lying on nontest side with ankle in neutral position

Isolation and assessment
Client everts foot through full range while examiner applies resistance to lateral edge of foot to pull it into inversion.

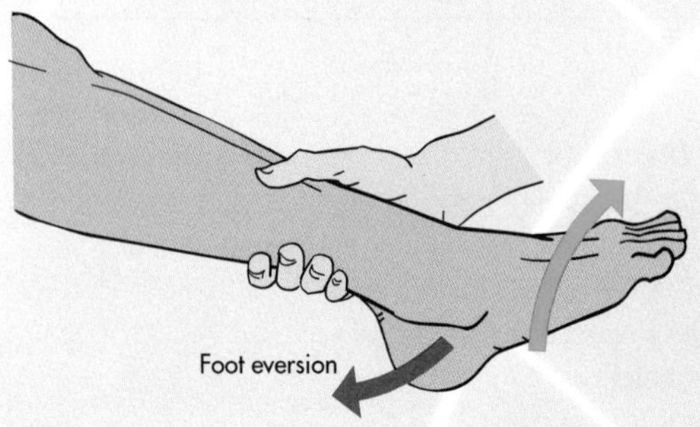

Toe Flexion
Assesses for strength and endurance in the isolation position and tension or shortening in the extension pattern.

Muscles involved
Flexor digitorum longus
Flexor digitorum brevis
Flexor hallucis longus
Flexor hallucis brevis
Flexor digiti minimi brevis
Lumbricales
Interossei (dorsal and plantar)

Range of motion
Great toe: 0 to 45 degrees
Lateral four toes: 0 to 40 degrees

Position of client
Supine with foot and ankle in neutral position
Examiner stabilizes metatarsals.

Isolation and assessment
Great toe is tested separately from lateral four toes. Client flexes great toe while examiner applies light resistance to plantar surface of proximal phalange to push it into extension. Client flexes four toes while examiner applies light resistance to plantar surface of proximal phalanges to push each toe into extension.

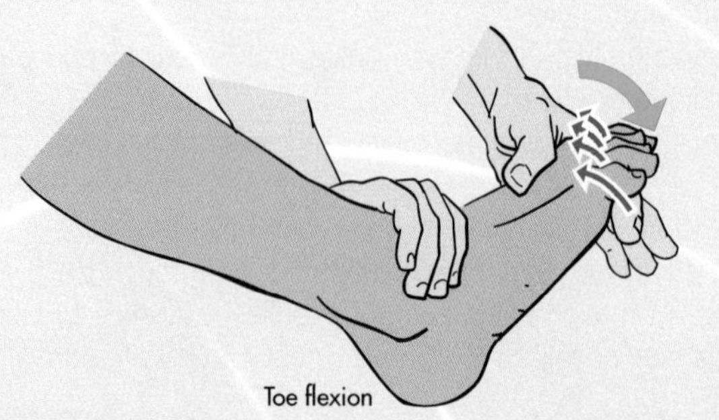

Toe Extension
Assesses for strength and endurance in the isolation position and tension or shortening in the flexion pattern.

Muscles involved
Extensor digitorum longus
Extensor digitorum brevis
Extensor hallucis longus

Range of motion
Great toe: 0 to 70 degrees
Lateral four toes: 0 to 40 degrees

Position of client
Supine with foot and ankle in neutral position
Examiner stabilizes metatarsals.

Isolation and assessment
Great toe is tested separately from lateral four toes. Client extends great toe while examiner applies light resistance to dorsal surface of proximal phalange to pull it into flexion. Client extends four toes while examiner applies light resistance to dorsal surface of proximal phalanges to pull each toe into flexion.

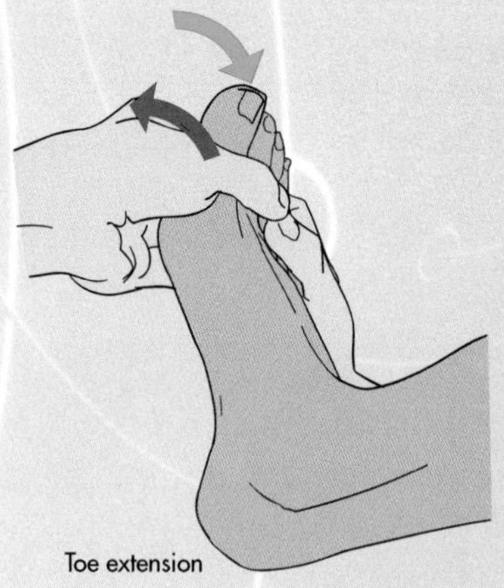

WORKBOOK SECTION

1. Explain the basic principles of balance.

___
___
___
___
___
___
___
___
___
___

2. Describe the steps in the normal adult walking cycle.

___
___
___
___
___
___
___
___
___
___

3. Identify the three main biomechanical dysfunctional patterns.

___
___
___

FILL IN THE BLANK

(1) ___ is the study of mechanical actions as applied to living bodies. (2) ___ is the study of movement that emerges and blends the knowledge of anatomy, physiology, physics, and geometry and relates them to human movement. Dynamic systems can be divided into kinetics and kinematics. Kinetics are those forces causing movement, whereas (3) ___ are those time, space, and mass aspects of a moving system.

(4) ___ is a fundamental characteristic of human behavior accomplished by the contraction of skeletal muscles acting within a system of levers and pulleys.

In biomechanical terms the concept of center refers to the (5) ___ ___, the midpoint or center of weight of a body or object. Any loss of biomechanical (6) ___, such as what occurs with a missing limb or altered posture, alters not only the total body weight distribution but also the center of gravity.

External forces acting on the body include (7) ___ and those forces generated by the interaction with (8) ___, such as lifting a box or managing an umbrella in the wind. Therapeutic massage attempts to alter body function by exerting (9) ___ forces to generate (10) ___ forces, which then effect change in the homeostatic mechanisms of the body. Forces generated by massage include tension, torsion, bend, shear, and compression.

(11) ___ is the reluctance of matter to change its state of motion. Any irregularly paced or multidirectional activity is costly to energy reserves.

(12) ___ may be defined as the rate of change in velocity and occurs in the same direction as the force that caused it.

(13) ___ is the ability to control equilibrium. Equilibrium refers to a state of zero acceleration in which no change occurs in the speed or direction of the body. (14) ___ equilibrium occurs when the body is at rest or completely motionless.

(15) ___ equilibrium occurs when all of the applied or internal forces acting on the moving body are in balance, resulting in movement with unchanging speed or direction.

(16) ___ is the resistance to change in the acceleration of a body or the resistance to the disturbance of the equilibrium of a body.

WORKBOOK SECTION

The (17) ________________ is made up of the myofascial system (muscle, ligament, tendon, and fascia), articular (joint) system, and nervous system. If one or more of the systems do not work efficiently, compensations and adaptations occur in the remaining systems, leading to stress in the body and eventually resulting in the development of dysfunctional patterns. All functional movement patterns involve acceleration provided by (18) ________________, stabilization provided by (19) ________________, and deceleration provided by (20) ________________. All three actions occur at every joint in the kinetic chain and in all three planes of motion with each movement pattern.

PROBLEM SOLVING AND PROFESSIONAL APPLICATION

Design an assessment form. On this form, list each of the activity assessments in this chapter and provide room for your responses. As you develop this form, consider how you would use it to organize the information in this chapter as you take a physical assessment. Possibilities for design of the form include a checklist or a silhouette drawing providing areas that can be marked to indicate function and dysfunction during the assessment process. You may come up with a different idea. Be creative. However, be sure to develop a comprehensive form to use as a tool that will remind you of the information in this chapter as you work professionally with a client. (The activity assessments begin with the section on Biomechanics by Region, starting with the trunk and thorax.)

FURTHER STUDY

Using additional resource material (see Works Cited list at the back of this text), identify chapters pertaining to the information presented in this chapter. As a study guide, locate the information presented in this text and then elaborate by writing a paragraph of additional information on each of the following:

Center of gravity

____
____
____
____
____
____
____
____

Levers

____
____
____
____
____
____
____
____
____
____

Gait

____
____
____
____
____
____
____
____
____
____

Answer Key

1. A person has balance when the center of gravity falls within the base of support. A person has balance in direct proportion to the size of the base of support. The larger the base of support, the more balance. A person has balance depending on the weight or mass. The greater the weight, the more balance.

   A person has balance depending on the height of the center of gravity. The lower the center of gravity, the more balance. A person has balance depending on where the center of gravity is in relation to the base of support. The balance is less if the center of gravity is near the edge of the base. However, when anticipating an oncoming force, one may improve stability by placing the center of gravity closer to the side of the base of support expected to receive the force. In anticipation of an oncoming force, one also may increase stability by enlarging the size of the base of support in the direction of the anticipated force. Equilibrium may be enhanced by increasing the friction between the body and the surface it contacts. Rotation about an axis is easier to balance. A bike that is moving is easier to balance than a bike that is stationary.

2. Human beings move about on two legs composed of three segments each: the thigh, shank, and foot. Atop the two legs is the trunk, head, and arm unit. The arm unit is used as a counterbalance and for momentum and moves opposite the leg movement. This pattern is linked in the contralateral reflex arc mechanism. Flexion and extension of the hip joints cause some rotation in the lumbar spine; to keep the head facing forward and the eyes level, the thorax and cervical spine rotate in the opposite direction. This action is coordinated by reflex patterns that coordinate upright posture in gravity and righting reflexes that keep the eyes on a level plane and the head oriented to the trunk. Reciprocal movements of the upper and lower limbs occur with the right upper limb flexing at the shoulder joint simultaneous with flexion at the left hip joint. Normally the shoulder joint starts to flex or extend slightly before the same movement occurs in the elbow joint. These movements again serve to keep the head and trunk oriented and to counterbalance the body weight in gravity.
3. Neuromuscular, myofascial, or joint related.

Fill in the Blank

1. Biomechanics
2. Kinesiology
3. kinematics
4. Movement
5. center of gravity
6. stability
7. gravity
8. external forces
9. external
10. internal
11. Inertia
12. Acceleration
13. Balance
14. Static
15. Dynamic
16. Stability
17. kinetic chain
18. concentric contractions
19. isometric contractions
20. eccentric contractions

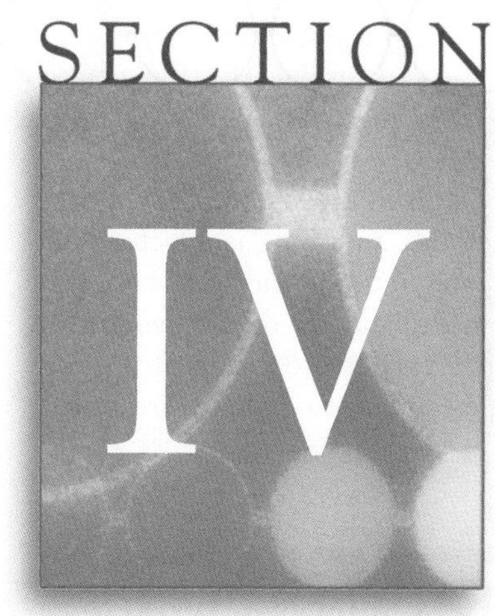

Remaining Body Systems

Any health care professional must have a comprehensive knowledge of the body to understand the ways in which the mechanisms of health and disease function and support or disrupt the homeostatic balance of a well-tuned organism. However, just as with any discipline, such study involves specialized knowledge and general knowledge.

Although all parts of the body are important, to the massage practitioner the areas of principal concern are the systems of control and movement. The first three sections covered this specialized knowledge. This last section discusses general information about the rest of the body systems with attention to specific detail for the massage professional. Chapter 11 presents pertinent information for the integumentary system, cardiovascular, and lymphatic systems and the functions of immunity. Chapter 12 presents the respiratory, digestive, urinary, and reproductive systems and deals in detail with the areas of most concern to the therapeutic massage process. Because learning does not end but evolves one layer on another, further study of these areas using a comprehensive anatomy and physiology textbook is recommended once the student has learned more basic information.

The textbook *Basic Health Care Terminology* by R.W. Williams (see Works Consulted) provided the pattern for this section. The textbook contains clear, concise descriptions of the body systems. Although the information has been adapted, paraphrased, and focused to serve the particular audience of therapeutic massage students, the text is recommended as a useful adjunct to this study.

This section contains two chapters, each with four main topic areas. Each topic area contains a clinical reasoning activity, described on page 554.

Clinical Reasoning Activities

At the end of each topic area, the student is asked to consider massage as a therapeutic intervention and to use the clinical reasoning model to justify the effectiveness of the massage method in supporting balanced functioning of each system involved. One can use this same approach to justify the use of therapeutic massage when dealing with disease or dysfunction. Students must be able to explain and justify the ways in which therapeutic massage is beneficial in supporting optimal function and how massage can manage an existing condition or support a return to health if a pathologic condition exists.

In completing the clinical reasoning activities, the student will need to refer to other sections of this text. Section Two, Systems of Control, is particularly useful. The student also will need knowledge of the therapeutic massage approach being justified. (See *Mosby's Fundamentals of Therapeutic Massage,* edition 3, 2004.)

These exercises, when well thought out, should help the student understand the connection between what is done (the therapeutic massage method) and what is effected (the change in physiology). Because what is done (the massage method) depends on where it is done (the anatomy), putting all the pieces together in an explanation of the benefits of massage will help the student not only to understand the process but also to educate others. This is particularly important when developing goal-oriented and outcome-based treatment plans for massage application.

THERAPEUTIC MASSAGE: CLINICAL REASONING MODEL FOR PROBLEM SOLVING AND JUSTIFICATION

1. **What are the facts?**
   a. Which system is involved, and which structures of that system can be reached directly and indirectly?
   b. Which of these structures are most affected by this massage?
   c. Which physiologic functions are affected by massage?
   d. When the treatment is applied, what changes in function will result in
      (1) this system
      (2) the whole body
   e. What is considered normal or balanced function?
   f. How are the functions of this system related to the homeostasis of the body?
   g. What has worked or has not worked?
   h. Where could you find information that would support the use of massage as a therapeutic intervention?
   i. What research is available to support the use of therapeutic massage?
   j. How does the massage support a healthy state?
   k. Under which pathologic or dysfunctional conditions is therapeutic massage most likely to be beneficial?
2. **What are the possibilities?**
   a. What do the data suggest?
   b. List at least three applications of massage that would affect the structure and function of the system involved.
   c. What are other ways to look at the situation?
   d. What other methods could provide similar benefits?
3. **What is the logical outcome of the therapeutic intervention?**
   a. What would be the logical progression of the symptom pattern, contributing factors, and current behavior?
   b. What are the benefits and drawbacks of using therapeutic massage as suggested?
   c. What are the costs in terms of time, resources, and finances?
   d. What is likely to happen if massage is not used?
   e. What is likely to happen if massage is used?
4. **What would be the effect on the persons involved if massage intervention was used, specifically the client, the practitioner, and other professionals working with the client?**
   a. How does each person involved (including, besides the foregoing, the client's family and support system) feel about therapeutic massage?
   b. Does the practitioner feel qualified to work with the situation and apply massage to the particular person?

c. Does a feeling of cooperation and agreement exist among all those involved? How would the practitioner recognize this feeling?

JUSTIFICATION

Using the information developed in the clinical reasoning model, present a clear, concise, valid statement of how massage would be beneficial in supporting the particular body system in a healthy condition or as part of a treatment plan for a pathologic or dysfunctional condition.

EXAMPLE OF THE CLINICAL REASONING PROCESS USED TO CREATE A JUSTIFICATION STATEMENT

The following example applies this process to the muscular system.

1. What are the facts?

a. Which system is involved, and which structures of that system can be reached directly and indirectly?

The muscles and associated connective tissue are involved, along with various nerves and sensory receptors. The circulation to the muscles is affected as well.

b. Which of these structures are most affected by this massage?

c. Which physiologic functions are affected by massage?

d. When the treatment is applied, what changes in function will result in

(1) this system

(2) the whole body

Muscle tension patterns and reflexes may be restored to balanced function if imbalances exist. Connective tissue may normalize, usually by becoming more pliable, although specific methods can be used to firm lax connective tissue. Circulation will be normalized.

e. What is considered normal or balanced function?

The muscles maintain posture, produce movement, stabilize joints, and generate heat efficiently without wasting energy. The muscles should be able to respond to activation of the sympathetic portion of the autonomic nervous system and then return to a relaxed state.

f. How are the functions of this system related to the homeostasis of the body?

The pumping action of muscle contraction supports blood and lymph circulation. Maintenance of a constant internal heat is an important part of muscle action. Support of posture and joint stability provides space for internal organs and efficient operation without restriction. Movement is used to obtain air and food and to ensure survival.

g. What has worked or has not worked?

Many different forms of massage produce beneficial results for the muscles. The basic approaches include compression, lifting, kneading, tapping, and horizontal gliding, along with various forms of active and passive movement and muscle contraction methods. The intensity, duration, and rhythm of massage applications depend on the desired results. Therapeutic massage could relax the muscles, reduce pain, increase blood and lymph circulation, increase nutrition to the muscles, and encourage repair of muscles. However, the benefits of extremely painful massage application may be diminished by activation of the defensive mechanisms of the body.

h. Where could you find information that would support the use of massage as a therapeutic intervention?

Textbooks; research institutes; various medical, nursing, physical therapy, chiropractic, and bodywork journals; professional organizations; clinical application by other professionals; and the Internet

i. What research is available to support the use of therapeutic massage?
- American Massage Therapy Association (AMTA) Data Base: *www.amtamassage.org*
- Field T: *Touch therapy,* Edinburgh, 2000, Churchill Livingstone
- Greenman P: *Principles of manual medicine,* ed 2, Baltimore, 1996, Williams & Wilkins
- MedLine: *http://www.medline.com*
- Yates J: *Physiological effects of therapeutic massage and their application to treatment,* ed 2, Vancouver, 1999, British Columbia Massage Therapist Association
- Leon Chaitow: Although not a researcher, this author effectively translates research into useful application.

j. How does the massage support a healthy state?

The various types of sensory stimulation provided by massage result in alteration of the nervous system control mechanisms toward more balanced function. The more mechanical normalization of associated connective tissue supports pliability and stability of the muscles. Massage supports circulation.

k. Under which pathologic or dysfunctional conditions is the therapeutic massage most likely to be beneficial?

Increased or decreased muscle tension from daily mechanical and emotional stress. Management of pain resulting from such alterations. Compression on nerves or vessels from increased muscle tension and the resulting pain and dysfunction.

2. What are the possibilities?

a. What do the data suggest?

The data suggest (1) normal muscle function needs support to maintain health, (2) the development of muscle problems that could be reversed readily, restoring the system to health, or (3) a serious pathologic condition that requires several interventions.

b. List at least three applications of massage that would affect the structure and function of the system involved.

Compression spreads muscle fibers, affects proprioception, and increases circulation. The "tense, relax, and lengthen" techniques affect reflex mechanisms. Tapping at the muscle tendon strengthens muscles through its effect on the tendon organ. Kneading mechanically increases connective tissue ground substance pliability.

c. What are other ways to look at the situation?

The muscle symptoms could be a reflection of a pathologic neurologic condition; medications may be influencing the muscle system; or emotional armoring in the muscles may provide effective coping patterns. A pathologic condition of the connective tissue may be present. Muscle tension patterns may be appropriate compensation patterns for joint instability or bone fragility.

d. What other methods could provide similar benefits?

Various forms of aerobic exercise; stretching programs (e.g., yoga); physical therapy; and medications

3. What is the logical outcome of the therapeutic intervention?

a. What would be the logical progression of the symptom pattern, contributing factors, and current behavior?

Increased muscle tension is a waste of energy, a common source of pain, and often interferes with sleep patterns. Any long-term sleep interference affects the restorative processes of the body. More serious pathologic conditions could result from the increased levels of stress.

b. What are the benefits and drawbacks of using therapeutic massage as suggested?

Benefits:

Massage is pleasurable, often easily accepted by the client, and effective in short-term symptom control of muscle dysfunction.

Massage can replace or reduce the use of palliative types of medication such as muscle relaxants and analgesics.

Drawback:

Massage is not curative and requires continual maintenance intervention to support benefits.

c. What are the costs in terms of time, resources, and finances?

Compared with other interventions, massage is cost-effective even for long-term intervention. Weekly or biweekly 1-hour sessions can produce sustainable results. A maintenance schedule, once goals have been achieved, can be less intensive and therefore less costly. Massage professionals are found easily in most areas. Home and office care often are available.

d. What is likely to happen if massage is not used?

Muscle tension could increase and the symptoms worsen. More serious pathologic conditions could develop.

e. What is likely to happen if massage is used?

Daily stress management and support for healthy function of the muscle system could be achieved, and use of over-the-counter or prescription medications could be reduced.

4. **What would be the effect on the persons involved if massage intervention was used, specifically the client, the practitioner, and other professionals working with the client?**

a. How does each person involved (including, besides the foregoing, the client's family and support system) feel about therapeutic massage?

Touch intervention can be nurturing to many clients; however, those who have experienced many of the various forms of touch trauma may not have predictable responses to the intense duration of touch in the form of massage. Health care professionals still are confused about the benefits and applications of massage. The practitioner may have issues of counter-transference with the client that would need to be addressed.

b. Does the practitioner feel qualified to work with the situation and apply massage to the particular person?

Depending on the practitioner's training and the client's therapeutic goals, as well as the support of other health care or training professionals, most situations can be addressed effectively with some sort of massage intervention. The more complex the situation, the more support and training are required.

c. Does a feeling of cooperation and agreement exist among all those involved? How would the practitioner recognize this feeling?

Support and cooperation depend on shared knowledge and the ability to educate in the benefits of massage. Free exchange of information with the client's permission and the client's willingness to participate would indicate cooperation.

Note: The previous questions stimulate thought processes and support more effective information gathering. The information then is evaluated, organized, and condensed to form a short, concise, and valid justification statement.

JUSTIFICATION

Therapeutic massage provides a pleasurable, easily accessible, cost-effective approach to support normal function of the muscular system. Massage increases circulation and waste removal from the muscles, maintains normal connective tissue structures, encourages appropriate neuromuscular interaction, and enhances general restorative functions.

The practitioner can manage muscle tension and pain syndromes effectively using massage as a treatment method. The general benefits listed are important in the treatment of these conditions. Massage can provide some of the same short-term benefits as medication for muscle tension and pain without the side effects.

Integumentary, Cardiovascular, Lymphatic, and Immune Systems

CHAPTER OBJECTIVES

After completing this chapter, the student will be able to perform the following:

- List and describe the components of the integumentary system.
- Describe the function of the integumentary system.
- Describe two main concerns with integumentary pathologic conditions.
- List and describe the components of the cardiovascular system.
- List and describe the components of blood.
- Describe the functions of the cardiovascular system.
- List and describe the components of the lymphatic system.
- List and describe the components of lymph.
- Describe the functions of the lymphatic system.
- Define immunity.
- Explain the difference between nonspecific and specific immunity.
- Describe and explain the implementation of Standard Precautions.
- Justify the effectiveness of therapeutic massage in supporting health maintenance for the integumentary, cardiovascular, lymphatic, and immune systems.

CHAPTER OUTLINE

KEY TERMS

Antibodies (an-ti-bod-EZ) Serum proteins of the immunoglobulin class that are secreted by plasma cells.

Arterioles (Ar-TEER-ee-olz) The smallest arteries.

Arteriosclerosis (ar-tee-ree-o-skle-RO-sis) A term meaning hardening of the arteries and referring to arteries that have become brittle and have lost their elasticity.

Artery (AR-ter-ee) A blood vessel that transports oxygenated blood from the heart to the body or deoxygenated blood from the heart to the lungs.

Atherosclerosis (ath-er-o-skle-RO-sis) A condition in which fatty plaque is deposited in medium and large arteries.

Atrium (AY-tree-um) One of the two small, thin-walled upper chambers of the heart; the right and left atria are separated by a thin interatrial septum.

Blood A thick, red fluid that provides oxygen, nourishment, and protection to the cells and carries away waste products. Whole blood consists of two components: the formed cellular elements and the liquid plasma. Blood is a form of connective tissue.

Blood pressure The measurement of pressure exerted by the heart on the walls of the blood vessels. The highest pressure exerted is called systolic pressure, which results when the ventricles are contracted. Diastolic pressure, the lowest pressure, results when the ventricles are at rest. Blood forced into the aorta during systole sets up a pressure wave that travels down the

Continued

arteries. The wave expands the arterial wall, and the expansion can be palpated by pressing the artery against tissue; the waves constitute the pulse rate.

Capillary (KAP-I-lair-ee) One of the small blood vessels found between arteries and veins that allow the exchange of gases, nutrients, and waste products. The walls of capillaries are thin, allowing molecules to diffuse easily.

Coronary arteries (KOR-o-nair-ee) The arteries that supply oxygenated blood to the heart muscle itself; they are located in grooves between the atria and ventricles and between the two ventricles.

Dermatitis (der-mah-TIE-tis) A general term for acute or chronic skin inflammation characterized by redness, eruptions, edema, scaling, and itching. The three main types are atopic dermatitis, seborrheic dermatitis, and contact dermatitis. Eczema is a form of dermatitis.

Dermis (DER-mis) The inner layer of skin that contains collagen and elastin fibers, which provide much of the structure and strength of the skin, and is much thicker than the epidermis.

Epidermis (ep-i-DER-mis) The outer or top layer of skin composed of sublayers called strata. The epidermis contains no nerves or blood vessels.

Heart The pump of the cardiovascular system; the heart is hollow, cone-shaped, and about the size of a fist and is located in the mediastinum of the thoracic cavity. The myocardium is the heart muscle itself, the endocardium is the thin inner lining, and the epicardium is the outer membrane.

Heart valves Four sets of valves that keep the blood flowing in the correct direction through the heart.

Hemorrhage (hem-OR-ej) The passage of blood outside of the cardiovascular system.

Immunity Resistance to disease provided by the body through specific or nonspecific immunity. The immune system is a functional system rather than an organ system in the anatomic sense. The most important immune cells are lymphocytes and macrophages. The key to immunity is the ability of the body to distinguish self from nonself.

Integument (in-TEG-yoo-ment) The skin and its appendages: hair, sebaceous and sweat glands, nails, and breasts.

Lymph (limf) A clear, interstitial tissue fluid that bathes the cells. Lymph contains lymphocytes, which provide immune response; returns plasma proteins that have leaked out through capillary walls; and transports fats from the gastrointestinal system to the bloodstream.

Lymph nodes Small, round structures distributed along the network of lymph vessels that provide a filtering system for removing waste products and transferring them to the bloodstream for removal to the spleen, intestines, and kidneys for detoxification. Lymph nodes are centers for lymphocyte production. Their main function is to prevent bacteria and viruses from gaining access to the bloodstream. Generally clustered at the joints for assistance in pumping when the joint moves, they are especially numerous in the axillae, groin, and neck and along certain blood vessels of the pelvic, abdominal, and thoracic cavities.

Pericardium (pair-i-KAR-dee-um) A double membranous, serous sac surrounding the heart. The pericardium secretes a lubricating fluid to prevent friction from the movement of the heart.

Plasma (PLAZ-mah) A thick, straw-colored fluid that makes up about 55% of the blood.

Standard Precautions Safety measures established by the Centers for Disease Control and Prevention. The precautions were instituted to prevent the spread of bacterial and viral infections by setting up specific methods of dealing with human fluids and waste products. Standard Precautions protect client and practitioner from pathogens.

Superficial fascia The subcutaneous tissue that composes the third layer of skin, consists of loose connective tissue, and contains fat or adipose tissue.

Tumor Also referred to as a neoplasm, a tumor is a growth of new tissues that may be benign (nonthreatening or noncancerous) or malignant (cancerous).

Veins Blood vessels that collect blood from the capillaries and transport it back to the heart. Seventy-five percent of the blood in the body is in the venous system. Larger veins often contain a set of valves that ensure that blood flows in the correct direction to the heart and also prevent backflow.

Ventricles (VEN-tri-kulz) The two large, lower chambers of the heart; they are thick walled and separated by a thick interventricular septum.

Venules (VEN-yoolz) The smallest veins.

INTEGUMENTARY SYSTEM

Physiology of Touch

The skin is the most sensitive of our organs and is the home for touch receptors of the nervous system. Touch is one of the five basic senses along with taste, vision, smell, and hearing. Touch expands on the ways we experience our world. Touch is the first sense to develop in the embryo, and the need for touch remains throughout our lives. Massage professionals touch others, and the skin is our contact point (Figures 11-1 and 11-2); therefore we must understand the effects of skin stimulation.

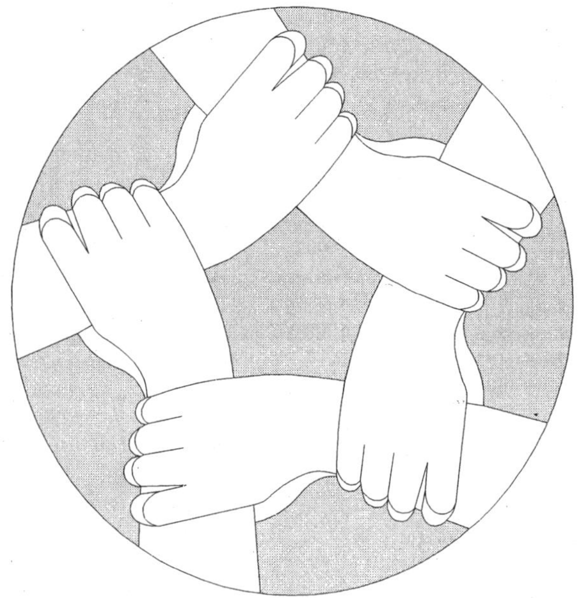

From Gillen G, Burkhardt A: *Stroke rehabilitation: a function-based approach,* St Louis, 1998, Mosby.

Touch is the most important and yet the most neglected of our senses. We can survive without sight, hearing, taste, and smell, but without the ability to feel, we are in constant danger. A complete loss of the sense of touch can cause psychotic breakdown. A lack of touch, especially in infants, the elderly, and those with weakened immune systems, can be life threatening and contribute to a condition called *marasmus* (wasting away). Sensory stimulation is essential to well-being at all stages of life, and touch is a necessary component. Touch deprivation leads to a reduced production of the neuroendocrine chemicals necessary for well-being. Touch-deprived individuals frequently develop inappropriate forms of sensory stimulation or abusive or addictive behavior (often food or drugs) in an attempt to stimulate the production of chemicals the body needs.

The ability to feel is a survival mechanism. Millions of sensory receptors in the skin alert us to danger through variations in temperature, vibration, and pressure. Touch informs us of differences in texture, shape, resistance, and tension. About one third of the 5 million or so sensory receptors are in the skin of our hands. The fingertips alone have more than 1000 nerve endings per square inch, and the lips and tongue have even more.

Different types of touch are identified by different receptors in the skin. The degree of pressure in light touch as opposed to deep touch is sensed by specific sensory receptor mechanisms and can evoke entirely different responses. A slow, light touch can relay compassion or intimacy. A deeper slow touch can evoke relaxation or security, whereas an abrupt touch startles and alerts. Touch can evoke pleasure,

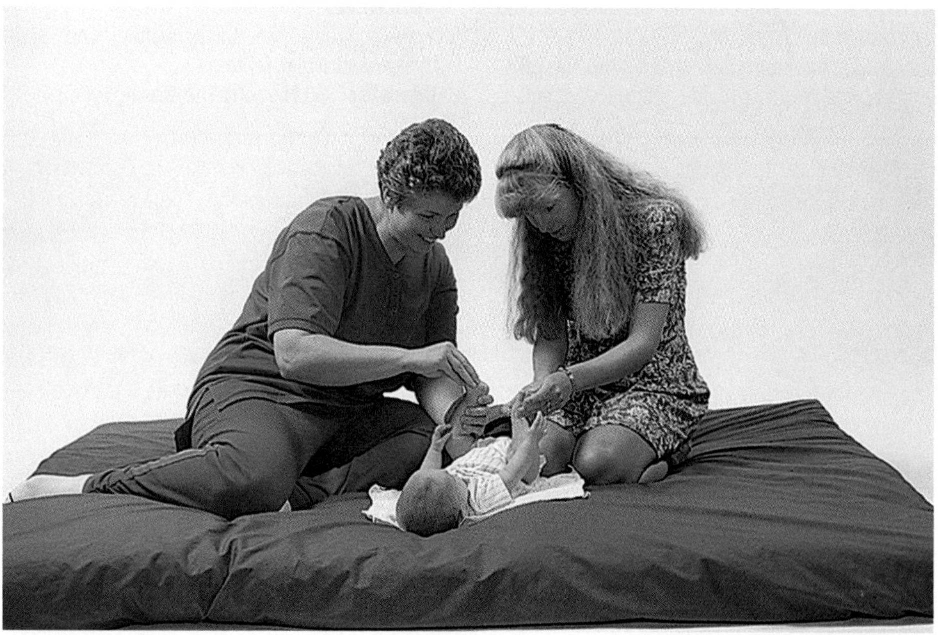

Figure 11-1
A parent being taught infant massage by a massage therapist. (From Fritz S: *Mosby's fundamentals of therapeutic massage,* ed 3, St Louis, 2004, Mosby.)

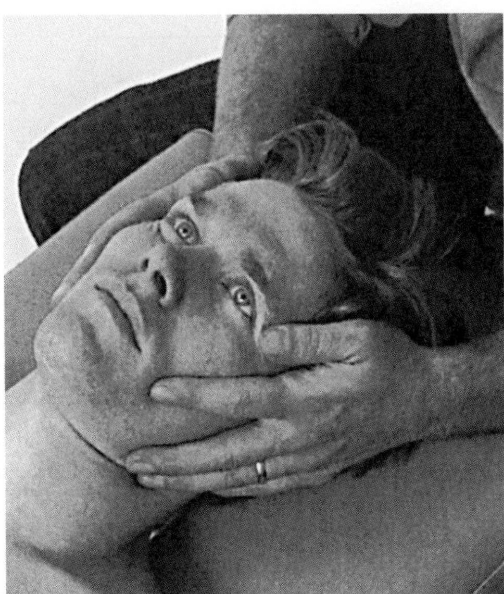

Figure 11-2
Modified from D'Ambrogio KJ, Roth GB: *Positional release therapy: assessment and treatment of musculoskeletal dysfunction,* St Louis, 1997, Mosby.

which we seek, and pain or discomfort, which we avoid. Each of these sensations triggers the manufacture and release of specific neurochemicals. (See Chapters 4 through 6.)

What more intimate form of communication is there than touch? Touch is reflected even in our language: "That was a touching experience," "What you said touched me," "You hurt my feelings," "Let's keep in touch." The various experiences of touch—nurturing, anger, parental, fearful, sexual, happy, comforting, and playful—are somehow understood by the neuropathways of the skin. How amazing (Activity 11-1).

ACTIVITY 11-1

This exercise is done with a partner. Your partner sits quietly with his or her eyes closed through the entire exercise while you think of a time when you were nurturing, angry, parental, fearful, happy, comforting, playful, and so on. Hold the thought in your mind while you touch your partner on the forearm with your hand. See if your partner can guess what emotion is being expressed.

Repeat the exercise, only this time deliberately attempt to communicate each of the emotions listed (nurturing, angry, parental, fearful, happy, comforting, playful, and so forth), using the touch of your hand on your partner's forearm. See if your partner can identify the emotion being expressed.

Then change roles. Finally, describe the experience in the space provided.

Note: Remember that the touch is limited to using your hand on your partner's forearm.

Example: Distinguishing between a nurturing touch and a comforting touch was difficult. When touching my partner, I found it easy to communicate playfulness but difficult to communicate parental feelings. I did not like keeping my eyes closed while I was touched but found it easier to touch someone else if he or she could not see me.

Your Turn

Structure of the Integument

The word ***integument*** means covering. The integumentary system, which covers our bodies, is made up of the skin and its appendages: hair, sebaceous glands, sweat glands, nails, and breasts (Figure 11-3; Activity 11-2).

Some of the major functions of the integumentary system are as follows:

- Protecting the internal organs and structures from trauma, sun exposure, chemicals, and water loss
- Assisting in immunity by preventing the entry of bacteria and viruses
- Synthesizing vitamin D when exposed to ultraviolet rays of the sun
- Detecting the sensed stimuli from touch, temperature, pain, and pressure
- Regulating body temperature
- Excreting sweat and salts and secreting sebum

Skin

The skin is the largest and heaviest organ of the body and is composed of two major layers: the **epidermis** and the **dermis.**

The epidermis, the outer layer of the skin, contains no nerves or blood vessels and consists of sublayers called strata. Most areas have four layers, but areas subject to pressure or friction such as the palms and the soles have five layers. In all areas the outermost layer is the *stratum corneum.* This layer is made up of 20 to 30 layers of flat, keratin-filled, dead cells that continuously shed and are replaced from the layer below. The innermost layer is the *stratum basale,* which produces a continuous supply of new cells. As the new cells develop and mature, they move up through the other layers until they reach the top and are shed, a process that takes about 2 to 3 weeks. This lowest layer also contains *melanocytes,* which produce *melanin,* the pigment that colors our skin.

The melanin pigment protects the skin from the harmful effects of ultraviolet radiation. The cumulative effects of exposure to ultraviolet radiation can damage fibroblasts located in the dermis, leading to faulty manufacture of connective tissue and wrinkling of the skin. Also damage to

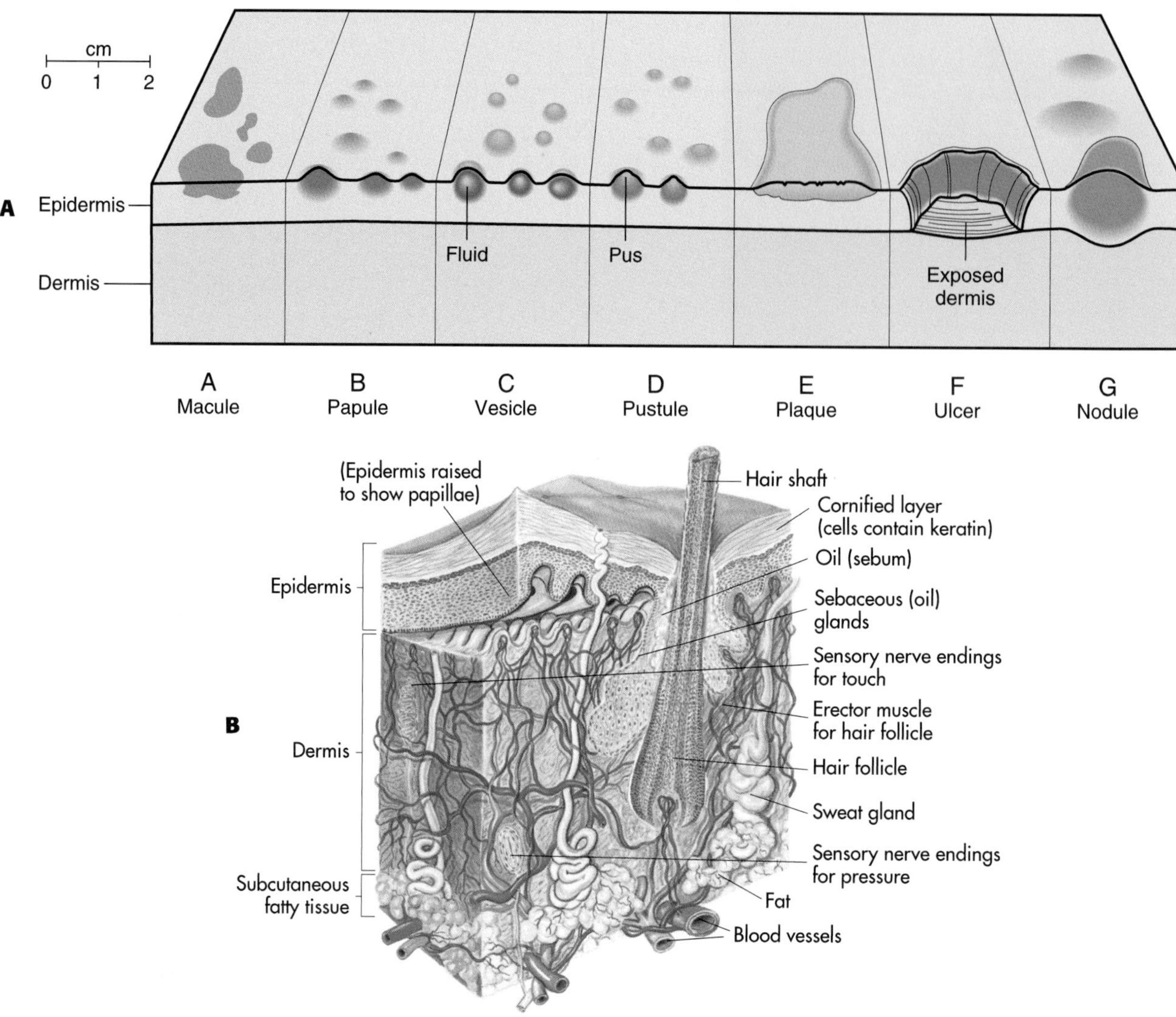

Figure 11-3
A, The appearance of various skin lesions. (From Damjanov I: *Pathology for the health-related professions,* ed 2, Philadelphia, 2000, WB Saunders.) **B,** Structures of skin. (From LaFleur Brooks M: *Exploring medical language: a student-directed approach,* ed 5, St Louis, 2002, Mosby.)

the chromosomes of multiplying cells in the stratum germinativum (basale) can cause skin cancer.

Keratin is produced in the epidermis by *keratinocytes.* Keratin is the fibrous protein that protects our skin and makes it waterproof.

The *dermis,* the inner layer of our skin, is much thicker than the epidermis. The dermis is composed of dense connective tissue that contains collagen and elastin fibers, which provide much of the structure and strength of our skin. The fibers are arranged in such a manner that the skin can be moved in many directions. Stretch marks are caused when these fibers are overstretched. The top layer of the dermis forms into ridges and presses up into the epidermis to create our fingerprints. Hair, sebaceous and sweat glands, and nails originate in the dermis and also push upward through the epidermis. Blood vessels and nerves are found in the dermis as well.

Figure 11-4 shows lines of the cleavage of the skin. This pattern of collagen and elastin fiber bundles in the dermis follows the lines of tension in the skin. The lines of cleavage are important. Injuries to the skin that are at right angles to the lines tend to gap because the cut elastin fibers recoil and pull the wound apart. Healing is slower and more scarring occurs in this kind of injury compared with injury parallel to the lines. Surgeons attempt to make surgical cuts parallel to lines of cleavage to promote healing and reduce scarring.

The *subcutaneous layer,* consisting of loose connective tissue and fat (adipose) tissue, is found below the dermis. This layer, known as the ***superficial fascia,*** sits above the muscle and bone. The subcutaneous layer is not actually a

ACTIVITY 11-2

In the figures, write the names of the integumentary structures listed below next to the matching number in the illustration. Color each part after you have labeled it.

1. Pore
2. Hair
3. Sebaceous gland
4. Fibrous tissue
5. Sweat gland
6. Nerves
7. Fat cells
8. Hair follicle
9. Blood vessels
10. Erector muscle
11. Subcutaneous layer
12. Dermis
13. Epidermis
14. Nail
15. Lunula

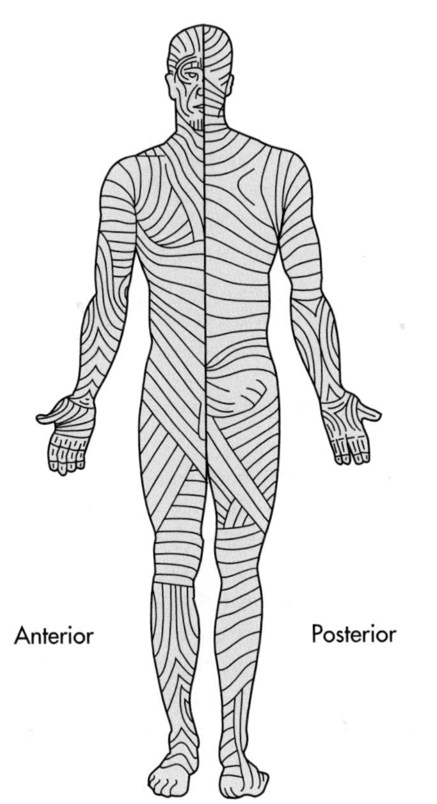

Figure 11-4
Cleavage lines.

part of the integument, but because it contains loose connective tissue that attaches to the dermis, it usually is described with the integumentary system. The adipose tissue insulates and provides padding; its distribution varies in men and women and is affected by hereditary factors.

The skin has an extensive **blood** supply and regulates heat lost from the body by altering the volume of blood flowing in the vessels of the skin. A simple assessment of circulation is to apply pressure to the nail body for 2 to 3 seconds and then release. Watch the color change as the blood refills the area. If this refilling process is longer than 2 to 3 seconds, circulation is sluggish.

The appendages of the skin are special structures that perform a variety of functions.

Hair

Hair protects the skin and orifices of the body, keeps us warm, and assists in our sense of touch. Hair is found all over the body except on the palms of the hands, the soles of the feet, the palmar and plantar surfaces of the digits, the lips, the nipples, and portions of the external genitalia. Some parts of the body appear hairless but actually have fine hair. Hair is composed of dead cells that have become keratinized, or hardened. Hair follicles, which include the hair root and connective tissue, hold the hair in place. A *root hair plexus* is a nerve that is stimulated each time the hair is moved. Tiny muscles, called *erector pili,* attach to hair follicles and cause the hair to stand on end at times. When this happens, the body is more sensitive to changes in air pressure and more alert to movement as a possible sign of danger. One reason energy forms of bodywork are thought to be effective is that the near touch and gentle movements stimulate the root hair plexus to provide sensory stimulation.

Nails

Toenails and fingernails are hard, keratinized cells that protect the ends of the digits and assist us in grasping. The *lunula* is the crescent-shaped white area at the base of the nail. The nail actually grows from the lunula, which is white because the blood vessels are covered with connective tissue and do not show. The clear, visible portion of the nail is the nail body (Figure 11-5).

Sebaceous (Oil) Glands

Most oil glands are connected to hair follicles by small ducts. They can be found over most of the body except on the palms and soles. By secreting an oily substance known as *sebum,* the oil glands prevent dehydration, soften the skin and hair, and slow the growth of bacteria. Hormones, primarily androgens, stimulate the secretion of sebum. If the sebum builds up and blocks the oil gland, a whitehead can form. If the sebum dries and makes contact with oxygen, it forms a blackhead. Acne is a bacterial inflammation of the sebaceous glands.

Sweat Glands

Known also as *sudoriferous glands,* sweat glands are found in most areas of the body. Most are located on the forehead, palms, and soles. The sweat glands are classified into types according to their structure and location; the two main types are the eccrine glands and the apocrine glands.

The *eccrine glands,* which are the most common, are responsible for the moisture that appears on the surface of the body when body temperature rises, particularly during physical activity. The functions of the eccrine glands are to cool the body and provide minor elimination of metabolic waste. Sweat is 99% water. The sympathetic division of the autonomic nervous system regulates sweating. Heat-induced sweating tends to begin on the forehead and then spreads to the rest of the body. Emotionally induced sweating, stimulated by fright, embarrassment, or anxiety, begins on the palms and in the axillae and then spreads to the rest of the body.

The *apocrine glands,* which are located in areas of body hair, discharge their secretions when a person is under stress. They begin to function during puberty. The apocrine glands differ from the eccrine glands in that the apocrine secretion is thicker and has a stronger odor. Apocrine glands are located primarily in the axillary and anogenital areas. The exact function of these glands has yet to be determined, but because they are stimulated during sexual arousal and phases of the menstrual cycle, they may be similar to the sexual scent glands in other animals.

Ceruminous glands are modified apocrine glands found in the external ear canal. They secrete a sticky substance called *cerumen,* or earwax, that prevents foreign material from entering the ear and repels insects.

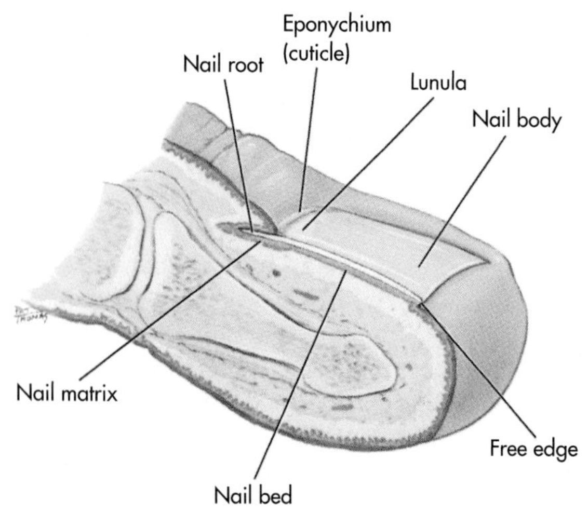

Figure 11-5
Structure of the nail. (From Jarvis C: *Physical examination and health assessment,* Philadelphia, 2002, WB Saunders.)

Mammary Glands

More commonly called breasts, mammary glands develop in the pectoral region of the chest. Developmentally, the mammary glands are modified apocrine sweat glands. The breasts are accessory reproductive structures in the female but are flat, nonfunctional organs in the male. Each mammary gland is contained within a rounded, skin-covered breast anterior to the pectoral muscles of the thorax. A ring of pigmented skin called the *areola* surrounds the nipple. Internally, each mammary gland consists of 15 to 25 lobes located around the nipple. The lobes are padded and separated from each other by fibrous connective tissue and fat. Ligaments attach the breast to the underlying muscle fascia and to the overlying skin, providing support. During lactation, glandular alveoli produce milk, which collects in lobules within the lobes and passes through lactiferous ducts to the nipple.

Skin Color

Skin color is created by combinations of pigments in the skin and in the blood flowing through the skin. These pigments are melanin, carotene, and hemoglobin.

Melanin, which is found in the epidermis, ranges in color from yellow to black. Melanin makes up most of our skin color. All of us have the same number of melanocytes, or melanin-producing cells, but the amount of melanin produced depends on genetic factors and exposure to ultraviolet light. Melanin is a natural sunscreen that protects us from ultraviolet rays by darkening our skin; this is an adaptive homeostatic function. Freckles, moles, age spots, and actinic keratoses result from increases in the melanin concentration or from changes in melanocytes.

Carotene is a yellow pigment found in the dermis that naturally gives the skin of some individuals a yellow tint. If plant foods containing carotene make up a large part of a person's diet, carotene can accumulate in the skin and adipose tissue and give the skin a temporary yellow or orange color, especially on the face and the palms.

Hemoglobin is the oxygen-carrying red pigment molecule in the blood. In persons with light skin the color of the hemoglobin shows through as pink.

The color of the skin can indicate health or a pathologic condition. For example, a blue tint to the skin can be caused by cyanosis, a condition caused by defective or deficient oxygenation of the blood. A yellow-gold color to the skin may result from jaundice or liver disorders. A bronze or metallic hue often is a sign of Addison's disease, a hypofunction of the adrenal cortex. Black and blue marks on the skin, or bruises, result from blood leaving the blood vessels and clotting in the surrounding tissues. Most commonly caused by trauma or injury, constant bruising may indicate a vitamin C deficiency or blood clotting disorder.

Emotional stimuli also influence skin color. Pallor, or whiteness of the skin, may be caused by emotional factors. One may suspect a decrease in the amount of hemoglobin, such as in anemia, in individuals who appear pale. Sometimes the lack of rosy color is caused only by opaqueness of the epidermis. The skin can contain as much as 5% of the blood in our bodies. During sympathetic autonomic activation, when the muscles need blood, the vessels of the skin contract to move the blood out. Sudden pallor may be caused by stressful situations such as those provoking anger or fear. Excessive redness may be caused by embarrassment (blushing), an increase in body temperature or fever, hypertension, inflammation, allergy, rosacea, or hormonal fluctuations.

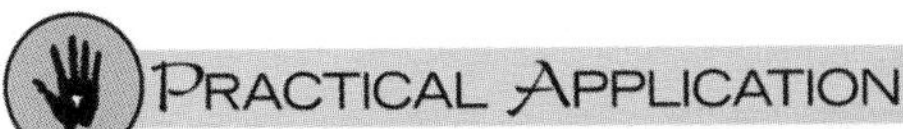

Observation of a person's skin color and changes in the appearance, texture, and suppleness of the skin and the appendages can provide information about changes in a person's health status. Because massage practitioners often touch the skin more than any other professional, they should be especially observant of the skin and its appendages, which can be indicators of dysfunction or of improved health. ■

Pathologic Conditions

Pathologic conditions of the integument give rise to two main concerns related to impairment of the structural integrity of the skin. The first concern is loss of the protection of internal structures. The second concern is loss of the ability of the skin to prevent the pathogens of contagious disease from entering the body. Observing the **Standard Precautions** guidelines established by the Centers for Disease Control and Prevention and proper sanitation methods maintains the security of the skin and its protective barriers. Pathologic conditions of the skin, especially sores, rashes, and changes in color and texture (Figure 11-6), can indicate more serious systemic disease, and the practitioner should refer the client to a physician for diagnosis.

INDICATIONS CONTRAINDICATIONS

For Therapeutic Massage

Therapeutic massage usually is not contraindicated in localized skin conditions, but local (regional) avoidance of the affected area is necessary. Localized touch can irritate most skin disorders. Massage is contraindicated if the skin is inflamed or if the condition is contagious or transmissible through touch. Malignancy is a contraindication unless the appropriate medical personnel supervise the therapy. ■

Bacterial Infections

Acne. Acne vulgaris is the common form of acne and is a chronic inflammation of the sebaceous glands and hair follicles caused by the interaction of bacteria, sebum, and sex hormones. Acne vulgaris is most common at puberty and may recur in women during menopause. The condition can produce blackheads, whiteheads, cysts, pustules, and inflamed nodules.

Boils. Boils are local staphylococcus infections similar to acne, but they are not related to adolescence or liver dysfunction. A group of interconnected boils is called a carbuncle.

Boils look like acne except that the lesions are bigger and more painful, and they usually occur singly rather than being spread over a large area.

Boils can contraindicate massage locally, and one should take care to make sure the infection is not systemic. The bacteria that cause boils are virulent and communicable. Standard precautions are indicated.

Cellulitis. Cellulitis is a rapidly spreading, acute bacterial infection of the skin usually found in the lower extremities. Bacteria enter through damaged skin or as a result of complications of diabetes or poor circulation. Symptoms include redness, heat, swelling, and pain.

Erysipelas. Erysipelas is a streptococcus infection that kills skin cells, leading to painful inflammation of the skin. Erysipelas usually occurs on the face or lower leg.

The bacterial infection can invade the lymph and circulatory systems. Massage is systemically contraindicated until the infection has passed completely.

Ecthyma. Ecthyma is a skin infection similar to impetigo but is more deeply invasive. Usually caused by a streptococcus infection, ecthyma goes through the outer layer (epidermis) to the deeper layer (dermis) of skin, possibly causing scars.

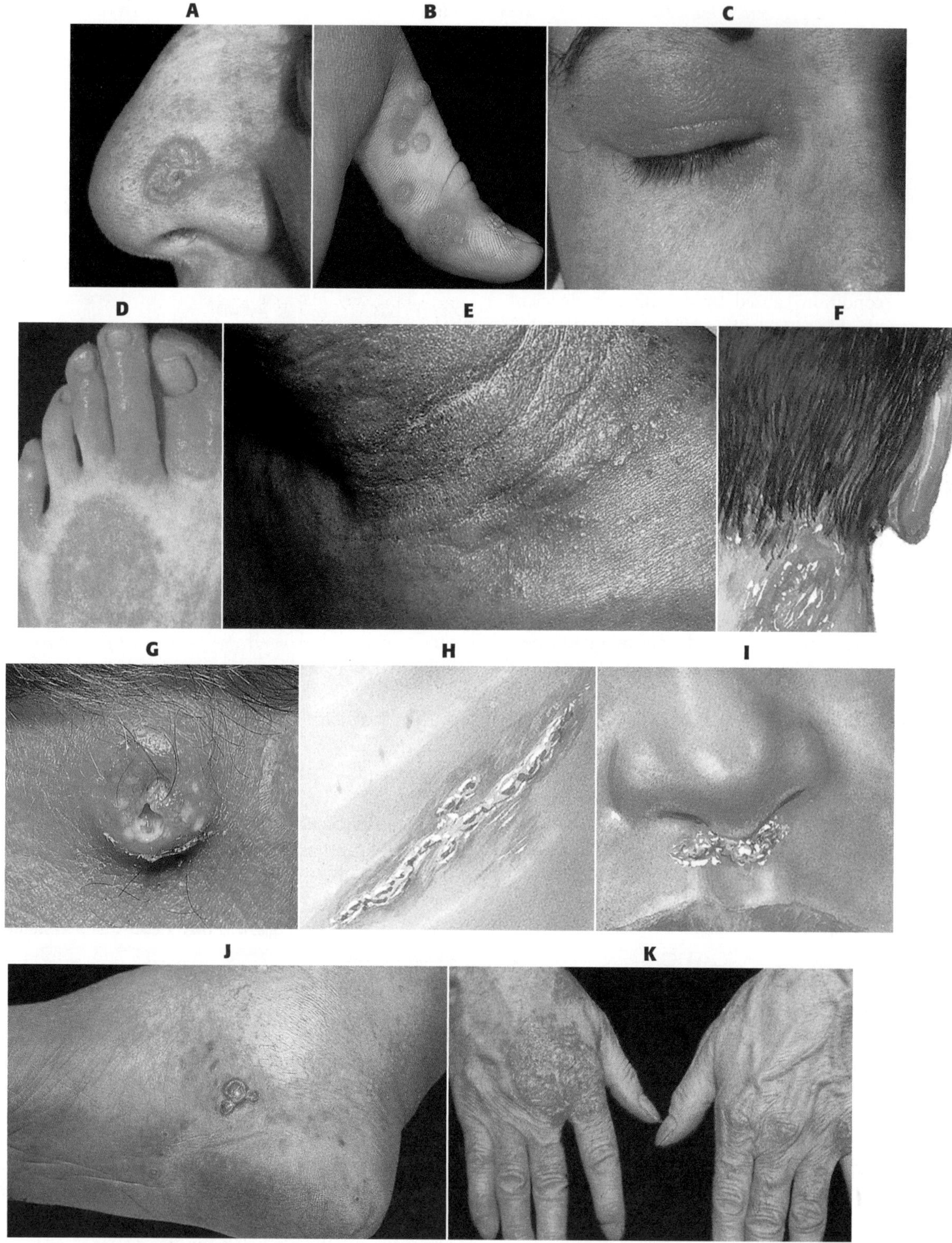

Figure 11-6

Common skin disorders. Skin problems may result from various causes such as parasitic infestations; fungal, bacterial, or viral infections; reactions to substances encountered externally or taken internally; or new growths. Many of the skin manifestations have no known cause; others are hereditary. **A,** Basal cell carcinoma. **B,** Common warts. **C,** Contact dermatitis from shampoo. **D,** Contact dermatitis from shoes. **E,** Contact dermatitis from application of Lanacaine. **F,** Dermatitis. **G,** Furuncle (boil). **H,** Herpes zoster (shingles). **I,** Impetigo contagiosa. (**P** from Barkausas VH, et al: *Health and physical assessment,* ed 3, St Louis, 2002, Mosby; **B, G,** and **M** from Thibodeau GA, Patton KT: *The human body in health and disease,* ed 3, St Louis, 2002, Mosby; **F, H, I, N,** and **O** from LaFleur Brooks M: *Exploring medical language: a student-directed approach,* ed 5, St Louis, 2002, Mosby; **A** and **J** from Habif TP: *Clinical dermatology: a color guide to diagnosis and therapy,* ed 3, St Louis, 1996, Mosby; **C, D, K, L,** and **P** courtesy American Academy of Dermatology and Institute for Dermatologic Communication and Education, Schaumberg, Illinois; and **E** from Zitelli BJ, Davis HW: *Atlas of pediatric physical diagnosis,* ed 1, 1987, Gower Medical Publishing.)

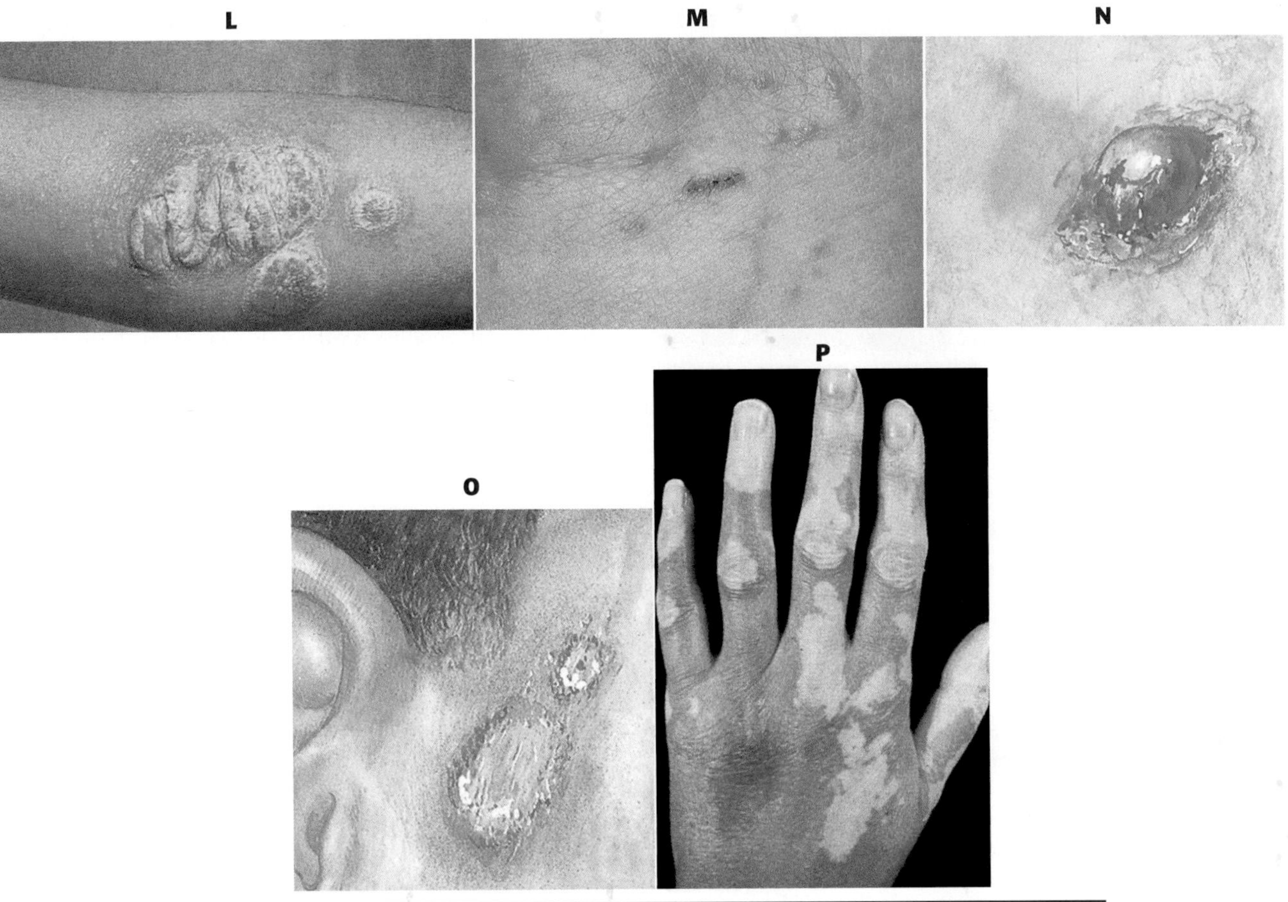

Figure 11-6—cont'd.

Impetigo. Impetigo is an acute, highly contagious, bacterial skin infection usually found on the face. Impetigo is characterized by small, red spots that develop into vesicles, which become filled with pus, burst, and develop a thick, yellow crust.

Benign Tumors and Growths

A **tumor,** also referred to as a neoplasm, is a growth of new tissue. Tumors may be benign (i.e., nonthreatening or noncancerous) or malignant (cancerous).

Angioma. An angioma is a benign tumor composed of blood or lymph vessels. Angiomata are common in newborns and usually disappear during childhood.

Lipoma. A lipoma is a benign tumor formed from mature fat cells. The tumor appears as a soft, movable, subcutaneous nodule typically found on the trunk, forearms, or neck.

Mole. A mole, or nevus, is a benign, pigmented skin growth formed of melanocytes.

Sebaceous cyst. A sebaceous cyst is a slow-growing, benign tumor caused by the blockage of a sebaceous gland. The cyst contains keratin, sebum, and hair follicle cells.

Seborrheic keratosis. A seborrheic keratosis is a slightly raised skin lesion most commonly seen on the chest, back, neck, and face. These benign growths usually appear in middle-aged and elderly individuals as light brown or black flat areas. They may grow quickly and can be mistaken for moles or warts.

Skin tag. A skin tag is a small, soft, flesh-colored or pigmented benign growth found on the neck or in the axillary or groin region.

Breast Disorders

Breast cancer. Breast cancer is the leading cause of cancer deaths in women, with the peak incidence occurring in the early menopausal age group. Most women develop a painless, firm lump, often in the upper outer quadrant. In one form of breast cancer, no lump develops. The diagnosis is made using low-voltage soft tissue radiographs called mammograms and by fine needle biopsy. The standard medical treatment is based on many factors, including the size of the lump, the patient's age and physical condition, and the involvement of lymph nodes and other tissues. Muscle tissue and lymph nodes are removed when metastasis has occurred.

Surgical intervention consists of one of the following procedures: a lumpectomy (removal of the tumor), a simple mastectomy (removal of the breast only), a radical mastectomy (removal of the breast, pectoralis major and pectoralis minor muscles, and the axillary lymph nodes), an extended radical mastectomy (in addition to the foregoing, removal of the internal mammary lymph nodes near the sternum), or a modified radical mastectomy (removal of the breast and axillary lymph nodes, preserving the pectoralis major muscle). Radiation therapy, chemical therapy (chemotherapy), and hormone therapy are other methods of intervention, which may be used alone or with surgery.

Although the number of men who develop breast cancer is small, lumps and changes in the tissues of a man's breast cannot be ignored, and one should refer such a client to a physician for examination.

Anatomic and physiologic problems after a mastectomy. With removal of the pectoralis major muscle, some flexion and adduction of the arm is lost. The client may develop the anterior part of the deltoid, as well as the coracobrachialis and the long head of the biceps, to help with flexion.

Loss of lymphatic channels in the axillae causes obstruction of lymph flow from the arm, and localized edema develops. Elevation of the arm and use of a special sleeve to provide compression are helpful. Massage may help mild cases.

Fibrocystic disease. Fibrocystic disease is the most common disorder of the breast. The condition involves the growth of small, lumpy cysts that develop because of changes in the milk-producing glands. The disease affects about 50% of women. No treatment is necessary, but because the incidence of breast cancer is higher in these women, health care providers must address recommendations on breast self-examination and the frequency of mammograms for each person.

Callus

A callus is an area of thickened, hardened skin, like a corn, that develops in an area of friction or a region of recurrent pressure. A callus involves skin that normally is thick such as the sole of the foot or the palm of the hand and usually is painless. If a callus is painful, an underlying plantar wart may be present.

Corn

A corn is a painful, conical thickening of skin over bony prominences of the feet caused by continual pressure and friction on normally thin skin. Corns located in moist areas, such as between the toes, are called soft corns.

Fungal Skin Infections

Candidiasis. Candidiasis is an infection of the skin or mucous membranes, most often caused by the organism *Candida albicans.* Red, scaly patches may appear in the creases of the axillae and groin and under the breasts, as well as between the fingers and toes. Associated candidal infections can occur in the ear, the vagina, and the mouth (thrush). *Candida albicans* is a common cause of diaper rash in infants.

Dermatophytosis: tinea (ringworm). More commonly known as ringworm, tinea is a group of common fungal infections contracted by touching contaminated items or an infected person's skin. The types of tinea are named by their location on the body. Tinea corporis appears on the nonhairy portions of the skin as fast-growing, reddish, elevated lesions surrounded by a dry and scaly or moist and crusty, raised, ringlike border, which gives it the ringworm appearance. Tinea pedis, or athlete's foot, is marked by blisters and cracking of the skin between the toes and on the ball of the foot. Tinea cruris, or jock itch, is ringworm of the pubic area.

Malignant Skin Tumors

Skin cancer is the most common of all malignancies. Most skin cancers appear on the head, neck, and other areas frequently exposed to the sun. Too much sun exposure damages the skin by causing the elastin fibers to clump, leading to leathery skin and wrinkling. Immune function may be depressed temporarily, and deoxyribonucleic acid (DNA) is altered, leading to skin cancer. Three types of malignancy can occur.

Basal cell carcinoma. Basal cell carcinoma, the most common form of skin cancer, is associated with ultraviolet light exposure. Basal cell carcinoma grows slowly and is the easiest type to treat successfully when recognized early.

Squamous cell carcinoma. Squamous cell carcinoma, also related to ultraviolet light exposure, makes up one third of all skin cancers. Like basal cell carcinoma, squamous cell carcinoma is treated best in the earlier stages, before it metastasizes. Persons with fair skin, blond or red hair, and chronic skin inflammation who are exposed to the sun or who suffered sun damage when young are more at risk for basal cell and squamous cell carcinoma.

Malignant melanoma. Malignant melanoma is the least common and the most dangerous of the skin cancers and is not connected directly to sun exposure. Because melanoma spreads rapidly, one must identify and treat it quickly. The memory device for identifying a melanoma is ABC: asymmetry, border irregularity, and color change. Most melanomata are not evenly round; rather, they have an irregular border with a white, blue, or red edge and turn color to brown or black. Moles are especially susceptible to transformation into melanomata.

Miscellaneous Skin Disorders

Alopecia. Alopecia is hair loss or baldness on parts or all of the body. Alopecia can be caused by aging, genetic predisposition, local diseases, chemotherapy, stress, or nutritional imbalances. Androgens seem to play a part in hair loss. Male-pattern baldness features hair loss on the forehead and top of the head, whereas female-pattern baldness involves thinning of the hair in the frontal and parietal regions.

Burns. The term *burn* refers to cells that are destroyed or inflamed because of heat, chemicals, radiation, or electricity. Fluid loss or secondary bacterial infection can occur as a consequence of the tissue damage. Burns are classified by the depth of damage and are identified by degree.

In a first-degree burn, only the epidermis sustains injury. Signs and symptoms can include redness, mild stinging or pain, and mild swelling. These burns usually heal within a matter of days or weeks. A mild sunburn is a first-degree burn.

In a second-degree burn the epidermis and dermis are damaged. Besides redness and moderate to intense pain and swelling, blisters usually develop. In deeper burns the tissues may be white because of damage to the vascular supply. Second-degree burns can take 6 weeks to a few months to heal and often leave scars.

In a third-degree burn the epidermis and entire dermis are damaged severely or destroyed. Damage to nerves can interrupt pain signals in the actual area of the burn. The skin may appear white, black, or charred, and no blisters form. Dehydration and infection may occur because of the loss of the protective skin barrier. A third-degree burn develops scars and may require a skin graft and a long healing period.

Dermatitis and eczema. *Dermatitis* is a general term for an acute or chronic skin inflammation characterized by redness, eruptions, edema, scaling, and itching. The term *eczema* often is used interchangeably with dermatitis, but many medical references limit the designation *dermatitis* to conditions caused by internal factors. Three major types of dermatitis have been recognized:

1. Atopic dermatitis: Atopic dermatitis is caused by an allergy or hypersensitivity, most commonly caused by pollens, cosmetics, or foods. The condition often is associated with other hypersensitivity disorders. Symptoms include inflammation, oozing and crusting, and intense itching.
2. Seborrheic dermatitis: Seborrheic dermatitis is a chronic condition that manifests with inflammation, scales, and crusting. The skin may be dry or greasy. The adult form of seborrheic dermatitis is a mild form of dandruff, most commonly seen at the eyebrows and on the scalp as a dry or greasy scaling. Cradle cap is the associated childhood form. Genetic predisposition, weather, stress, and some neurologic diseases may be risk factors.
3. Contact dermatitis: Contact dermatitis is caused by sensitivity to a substance that damages or irritates the skin such as poison ivy, a medication, cosmetics, or rubber. The condition may be marked by blisters or itchy, flaky skin.

Pseudofolliculitis barbae (razor bumps) is a common condition of the beard area occurring in African-American men and other persons with curly hair. The problem results when highly curved hairs grow back into the skin, causing inflammation and a foreign body reaction. Over time, this can cause keloidal scarring, which looks like hard bumps on the beard area and neck.

Psoriasis. Psoriasis is a common, chronic skin disease characterized by reddened skin covered by dry, silvery scales. Psoriasis most often is found on the scalp, elbows, knees, back, or buttocks.

Rosacea. Rosacea is a chronic skin problem in which the small blood vessels of the forehead, cheeks, and nose become dilated. Rosacea may affect a small area or the entire face. Eye inflammation (conjunctivitis) may develop. Rosacea may lie dormant for a time and then be activated by stress, infection, hot or spicy food, sunlight, or physical activity.

Scleroderma. Scleroderma (systemic sclerosis) is an autoimmune disorder of the connective tissue characterized by inflammation and overproduction of collagen. The resulting scarring causes the tissues to stiffen and to compress the capillaries, thus diminishing or halting blood flow. The disease usually appears in persons between 30 and 50 years of age and affects women more often than men. Characteristics include increased joint stiffness, muscle weakness, swelling of the fingers, and skin-thickening collagen deposits. Besides the integument, collagen deposits can invade many of the body systems such as the gastrointestinal tract, reducing the absorption of nutrients, and the lungs, diminishing respiratory effectiveness. Hypersensitivity to cold in the fingers, toes, ears, and nose (Raynaud's syndrome) may be present. In the most serious cases, heart and lung failure may occur.

Urticaria (hives). Urticaria, or hives, is a condition of localized skin eruptions (wheals) in the dermis caused by allergy, exposure to heat or cold, or an emotional reaction. Urticaria may be accompanied by local pruritus (itching).

Vitiligo. Vitiligo is a disease marked by loss of skin pigmentation in irregular patches. Vitiligo usually affects exposed areas of the skin in persons under 30 years of age who have a family history of the disease.

Open Wounds and Sores

Wounds include any injury to the skin that has not healed and that is vulnerable to infection if exposed to bacteria or other microorganisms. Skin injuries are vulnerable as long as a visible crust or scab remains.

Massage is contraindicated locally for any unhealed skin injury in which bleeding has occurred. When the underlying epidermis has been replaced completely, the scab falls off and the wound no longer is at risk for infection.

Massage may be contraindicated systemically if the skin injury is connected to a contraindicated underlying condition such as diabetes.

Parasitic Skin Infections

Lice. Lice are parasites, and three types affect human beings. Head lice (pediculosis capitis) are the most common type. They are found mainly on the scalp and sometimes in the eyebrows and eyelashes and cause intense itching. Outbreaks generally occur among schoolchildren. The bite of the body louse (pediculosis corporis) leaves visible, itchy, red spots primarily on the shoulders, buttocks, and abdomen. Genital lice (pediculosis pubis; crab lice) usually are found in the pubic area and are transmitted during sexual activity or contact with contaminated bedding.

Scabies. Scabies is a contagious skin disease characterized by intense itching caused by a microscopic, parasitic mite that burrows under the epidermis. Scabies can attack any area of the body, but the parts most susceptible are the finger webs, anterior wrist, elbows, axillary region, areola of the breasts, genitals, and lower buttocks. The parasite is transmitted by skin-to-skin contact with human beings or pets or by direct contact with contaminated items.

Ulcer

An ulcer is a round, open sore of the skin or mucous membrane that results from tissue damage that accompanies inflammation, infection, or malignancy.

Decubitus ulcer. A decubitus ulcer is an open sore that develops primarily over the bony areas of the heels and hips of those who are immobile, bedridden, or in a wheelchair. Continuous pressure on the skin diminishes or stops circulation, and the tissue dies.

Neurotrophic ulcer. Neurotrophic ulcers develop at pressure point areas on the feet when pain sensation is diminished or absent, as in diabetic neuropathy. Although often deep and infected, these ulcers are painless. Callus formation around the ulcer, like the ulcer itself, results from chronic pressure.

Viral Skin Infections

Chicken pox. Chicken pox is a viral infection that causes a blisterlike rash on the surface of the skin and mucous membranes. Chicken pox blisters usually appear first on the trunk and face and then spread to almost everywhere else on the body, including the scalp and penis, and inside the mouth, nose, ears, and vagina. Chicken pox blisters are about 0.2 inch to 0.4 inch (5 to 10 mm) wide, have a reddish base, and appear in crops over 2 to 4 days. Some persons have only a few blisters, although others have several hundred. As blisters itch and break, scabs form and the blisters may become infected by bacteria (a secondary bacterial infection).

Some children have a fever, abdominal pain, or a vague sick feeling along with their skin blisters. These symptoms usually last for 3 to 5 days, and temperature stays in the range of 101° to 103° F (38.3° to 39.4° C). Younger children often have milder symptoms and fewer blisters than older children or adults. Generally, chicken pox is a mild illness but can be deadly in persons who have leukemia or other diseases that weaken the immune system.

Usually a person has only one attack of chicken pox in his or her lifetime. But the virus that causes chicken pox can stay dormant in the body and can cause a different type of skin eruption, called shingles, later in life.

Herpes simplex. Herpes simplex is a viral infection resulting in cold sores or fever blisters on the face or in the mouth (type 1) or around the genitals, thighs, or buttocks (type 2).

As with all herpes viruses the virus remains dormant in the nerves of the body until resistance is low, at which time it travels down the nerve to cause the eruption. All of the herpes viruses are contagious.

Herpes outbreaks often are preceded by 2 to 3 days of tingling, itching, or pain. Blisters then appear, which gradually crust and disappear, usually within 2 weeks.

Massage is contraindicated locally for any kind of herpes in the acute stage. Herpes is contagious. One should use Standard Precautions.

Measles. Measles is a serious infection that spreads easily from person to person. Measles is caused by the measles virus.

Symptoms of measles begin 10 to 12 days after contact with an infected person. Symptoms can range from a fever (often high), fatigue, runny nose, cough, and watery red eyes. After 2 or 3 days, tiny white spots may appear in the mouth and after 2 more days, a raised, red rash starts on the face and spreads down the body and out to the arms and legs. The rash usually lasts 4 to 7 days. Symptoms usually last from 1 to 2 weeks, and measles is contagious for about 1 week before to 1 week after the rash begins. Serious complications of measles can occur.

Measles is spread from person to person by infected droplets from the mouth, nose, and throat of a person with measles. Infected droplets spread through the air or directly onto other person's hands and face through coughing and sneezing. Persons who have measles should stay away from others until at least 4 full days have passed since the time the rash first appeared.

German measles, or rubella, is a mild viral illness caused by the rubella virus. German measles causes a mild feverish illness associated with a rash, along with aches in the joints when it affects adults. The major reason for any attention being devoted to the eradication of this condition is the nasty effects that it has on the unborn baby when a pregnant woman catches it in early pregnancy.

Children usually are not affected seriously, and often the first manifestation is the rash, which is a fine, pink rash spreading from the forehead and face downward. The rash may last for 1 to 5 days. Glands (lymph nodes) often are enlarged, especially behind the ears and on the back of the head. Adults often feel more unwell before the rash appears and may have arthritic-type pain in the joints.

Molluscum contagiosum. Molluscum contagiosum is a superficial skin infection. The virus invades the skin, causing the appearance of firm, flesh-colored, doughnut-shaped bumps 2 to 5 mm in diameter. Their sunken centers contain a white, curdy-type material. The bumps can occur almost anywhere on the body including the buttocks, thighs, and external genitalia. The bumps often remain unchanged for many months, after which they disappear.

Molluscum contagiosum is caused by a virus belonging to the poxvirus family. Close physical contact is usually necessary for transmission; indirect transmission from shared towels, swimming pools, etc., also may be responsible for infection. The incubation period varies from several weeks to several months. Shaving or scratching may cause the infection to spread.

Warts. A wart is a benign growth of the keratin-producing cells of the epidermis and mucous membranes caused by the human papilloma virus. Warts are transmitted through direct contact. The common wart (verruca vulgaris) has a rough, elevated surface and is found mainly on the hands and fingers of children and young adults. Filiform warts are longer, slender growths on the face, neck, and axillae. Periungual warts are found around the nails of the fingers and toes. Flat warts are flesh colored and form when several warts spread, through scratching or shaving. Plantar warts have rough surfaces and are located in the thickened skin of the sole of the foot. They may be mistaken for calluses but often have small, dark spots that calluses do not have. Normal skin lines stop at the edge of the wart (Activity 11-3).

CARDIOVASCULAR SYSTEM

The cardiovascular system is a transport system composed of the **heart,** blood vessels, and blood. The heart is the pump that sends the oxygen and nutrient-rich blood out to the body via the **arteries** and **arterioles.** The oxygen and nutrients in the blood leave the capillaries and enter the tissues. Carbon dioxide and metabolic wastes leave the tissues, reenter the capillaries, and pass through the **venules** and **veins** on their way to the lungs, liver, and kidneys. The lungs eliminate carbon dioxide, and the liver and kidneys alter or eliminate other waste products.

Heart

The heart is the major organ of the cardiovascular system (Figure 11-7 on p. 575). The heart is a hollow, muscular pump about the size of a clenched fist that is located in the *mediastinum,* the space between the lungs. The narrow, rounded point of the cone-shaped heart lies just behind the sternum, and the broader, flat base extends slightly to the left of center, near the fifth rib. The **pericardium** is a sac that surrounds the heart and secretes a lubricating fluid that prevents friction from the movement of the heart. The pericardium also maintains the location of the heart within the thoracic cavity.

The *myocardium* is the actual heart muscle that makes up the thickest part of the heart and generates the contractions. The outer membrane of the heart is called the epicardium. The *endocardium* is the smooth, thin, inner lining of the heart. The blood actually slides along the endocardium as it flows through the heart.

The heart is divided into four chambers. The two small, thin-walled upper chambers are the atria, known separately as the left **atrium** and the right atrium, and they are separated by the interatrial septum. The two larger, lower chambers are the left and right **ventricles,** and their thick walls are separated by the interventricular septum. The atria and ventricles are separated by a fibrous structure called the skeleton of the heart.

Heart Valves

Created from the folds of the endocardium and maintained within the skeleton of the heart are the **heart valves,** four sets of valves that regulate the flow of blood through the heart. *Atrioventricular* valves allow blood to flow into the ventricles but keep it from returning to the atria. Strings of connective tissue known as chordae tendineae cordis actually connect between the ventricle wall and the valves to help close the valve without letting it collapse into the atria. The *bicuspid,* or *mitral* (left atrioventricular), valve is located between the left atrium and the left ventricle; the *tricuspid* (right atrioventricular) valve is located between the right atrium and the right ventricle.

Semilunar valves control the blood flow out of the ventricles into the aorta and pulmonary arteries and prevent any backflow of blood into the ventricles. The *aortic* valve is between the left ventricle and the aorta, and the *pulmonary* valve is between the pulmonary artery and the right ventricle. These valves open in response to pressure generated when the blood leaves the ventricle. They close when blood pools in small pockets of the cusps of the valves and pushes the valves closed (Figure 11-8 on p. 576).

Blood Vessels

The term *blood vessels* refers to the large blood vessels entering or leaving the heart that transport blood to the lungs and the rest of the body. The three great vessels are these:

Aorta: The artery that carries oxygen and nutrients away from the heart to the body

Pulmonary trunk: The artery that carries blood to the lungs to release carbon dioxide and take in oxygen

Superior vena cava: The vein that returns poorly oxygenated blood to the right atrium from the upper venous circulation

ACTIVITY 11-3

We must be able to explain and justify the therapeutic value of the work we do. The following activity will assist you in developing the skills to explain the effectiveness of therapeutic massage to clients and other health care professionals. Use the clinical reasoning model that follows to accomplish this task. The focus should be the primary massage method applied to the integumentary system. An example is provided in the section opener on p. 554.

Methods/Applications

1. What are the facts?
   a. Which system is involved, and which structures of that system can be reached directly or indirectly?
   b. What is considered normal or balanced function?
   c. How are the functions of this system related to the homeostasis of the body?
   d. Which of these structures are most affected by this massage?
   e. Which physiologic functions are affected by the massage?
   f. When the treatment is applied, what changes in function will occur in
      (1) this system
      (2) the whole body
   g. What has worked or has not worked?
   h. Where could you find information that would support the use of massage as a therapeutic intervention?
   i. What research is available to support the use of therapeutic massage?
   j. How does the intervention support a healthy state?
   k. Under which pathologic, or dysfunctional, condition is the therapeutic massage most likely to be beneficial?

ACTIVITY 11-3—cont'd

2. What are the possibilities?

   a. What do the facts suggest?

   b. List at least three applications of massage that would affect the structure and function of the system involved.

   c. What are other ways to look at the situation?

   d. What other methods could provide similar benefits?

3. What is the logical outcome of therapeutic intervention?

   a. What would be the logical progression of the symptom pattern, contributing factors, and current behaviors?

   b. What are the benefits and drawbacks of each intervention suggested?

      Benefits:

      Drawbacks:

   c. What are the costs in terms of time, resources, and finances?

   d. What is likely to happen if massage is not used?

   e. What is likely to happen if massage is used?

Continued

ACTIVITY 11-3

4. What would be the effect on the persons involved, specifically the client, practitioner, and other professionals working with the client?

a. How does each person involved (including, besides the foregoing, the client's family and support system) feel about the possible massage interventions?

b. Does the practitioner feel qualified to work with the situation and apply massage to the particular person?

c. Does a feeling of cooperation and agreement exist among all those involved, and how would the practitioner recognize this feeling?

Justification
Using the information developed in the clinical reasoning model, present a clear, concise statement of how massage would be beneficial in supporting the particular body system in a healthy condition or as part of a treatment plan for a pathologic or dysfunctional condition.

Other major blood vessels include the following:

Inferior vena cava: The vein that returns oxygen-poor blood from the lower venous circulation to the right atrium

Pulmonary veins: The four veins, two from each lung, that bring oxygen-rich blood to the left atrium

Blood Supply to the Heart

The two **coronary arteries,** which originate from the base of the aorta, supply oxygenated blood to the heart muscle. Coronary veins follow parallel to the arteries and return the blood to the right atrium via the coronary sinus. Both types of coronary vessels run in grooves between the atria and ventricles and between the two ventricles. If either of the coronary arteries is unable to supply sufficient blood to the heart muscle, a heart attack occurs. The most common site of a heart attack is the anterior or inferior part of the left ventricle.

Blood Flow through the Heart

Blood moves into and out of the heart in a well-coordinated and precisely timed rhythm. For examination purposes, the rhythm can be divided into the following stages (Figure 11-7):

Stage 1: Oxygen-poor blood from the body enters the superior and inferior venae cavae and flows into the right atrium. When the right atrium is full, it empties through the tricuspid valve into the right ventricle.

Stage 2: The right ventricle, when full, contracts and pushes blood through the pulmonary valve into the pulmonary artery. This artery divides into the left and right pulmonary arteries and takes the blood to each lung (these are the only arteries in the body that carry oxygen-poor blood). Four pulmonary veins leave the lungs carrying oxygen-rich blood back to the left atrium (these are the only veins in the body that carry oxygen-rich blood).

Stage 3: This process takes place at the same time as the process described in Stage 1. Blood leaves the left atrium and passes through to the left ventricle via the mitral valve. When full, the left ventricle contracts, using high pressure to push the blood through the aortic valve into the aorta and descending aorta and to all parts of the body except the lungs. The walls of the left ventricle are

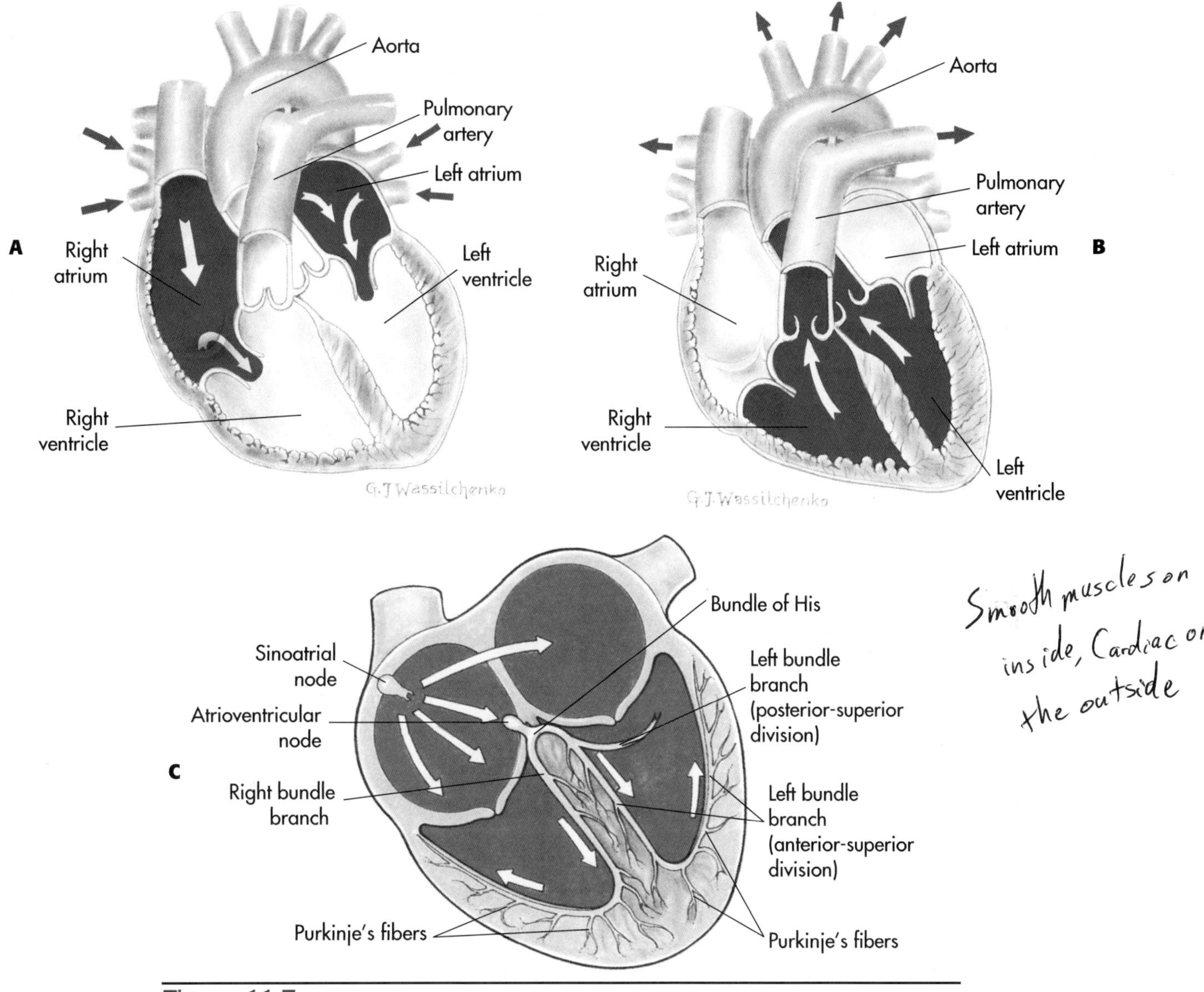

Figure 11-7
Heart and blood flow patterns. **A,** Blood flow during diastole. **B,** Blood flow during systole. **C,** Cardiac conduction. (From Canobbio MM: *Cardiovascular disorders,* St Louis, 1990, Mosby.)

thicker to provide the extra strength needed to pump blood out to the entire body.

Heart Pump

The heart has its own built-in rhythm. Not only can each cardiac cell contract without nerve stimulus, but also the heart can contract even if removed from the body. The autonomic nervous system can affect the rate of the rhythm and the force of contraction through sympathetic and parasympathetic activation.

Both atria contract while both ventricles are relaxed, and when the atria relax, the ventricles contract. This synchronization leads to the sequence of events known as the cardiac cycle. The cycle consists of one heartbeat, or diastole, which is the relaxation of the ventricles during filling, and systole, the contraction of the ventricles as they empty.

Although the heart has an atrial diastole and systole, the stronger ventricular actions are used for identification.

Our heart rate is identified by the number of cardiac cycles that occur in 1 minute. The average healthy person has 60 to 70 cycles, or beats, per minute.

The coordinated rhythm of the heart is initiated by the built-in electrical system in the sinoatrial node, which sets the pace of the heart rate. The signal originates in the right atrium and travels to the left atrium, causing the atria to contract. At the precise moment the atria have completed their contraction, the signal travels through the atrioventricular bundle to the right ventricle and into the left ventricle, causing the ventricles to contract. The rhythm can be checked through an electrocardiogram (ECG or EKG), which monitors the electric changes in the heart. A portable electrocardiogram machine, known as a Holter monitor, can

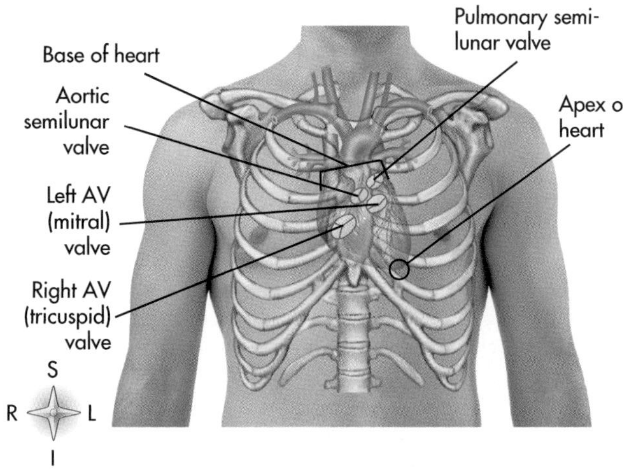

Figure 11-8
Relation of the heart to the anterior wall of the thorax. Valves of the heart are projected on the anterior thoracic wall. (From Thibodeau GA, Patton KT: *Anatomy and physiology,* ed 5, St Louis, 2003, Mosby.)

measure the heart signals over 24 hours. If difficulty with the electric system in the sinoatrial node develops, physicians can implant a device known as a pacemaker to assist or take over initiation of the signal.

Heart Sounds

Heart sounds can be heard through a stethoscope. Closure of the valves produces two main sounds. The first is a low-pitched "lubb" generated by the closing of the mitral and tricuspid valves. The second is a higher-pitched "dubb" caused by the closing of the aortic and pulmonary valves. Extra sounds such as those resulting from faulty valves are referred to as murmurs. Valves usually are quiet as they open.

Blood Volume and Flow

Cardiac output is the amount of blood pumped by the left ventricle in 1 minute. The average output under normal conditions is 5 to 6 L of blood. To pump more oxygen and nutrients to the cells during exercise and in times of stress, output may rise to 20 L or more. The speed of the blood flow is fastest in arteries and moderate in veins. The slowest blood movement is in the capillaries to allow for the exchange of nutrients and waste products between tissues and blood.

Entrainment

Entrainment is the coordination or synchronization to a rhythm and was discussed first in Chapter 2. Research at the Institute of HeartMath and other facilities indicates that the heart rhythm tends to be the guide that the other body rhythms follow. The heart rate, respiratory rate, and thalamus synchronization combine to support the entrainment process, and the other, more subtle, body rhythms follow. Most meditation processes or relaxation methods create an environment for this entrainment to occur.

The heart is considered the seat of love and the home of emotions relating to relationships. The heart is the symbol of love on Valentine's cards. We speak of how a person's heart can be broken with loss and grief. We have lost heart when we give up hope. We have a big heart when we are compassionate and nurturing. Is it possible that the strong rhythm of the heart, of which we can easily become conscious, also brings us awareness of how experience affects us? The heart rate and strength of contraction can change in a moment in response to the demands of life. Living aware of our hearts is a way to live aware of our response to experience (Figure 11-9).

Vascular System

The vascular system is the other part of the cardiovascular system and consists of blood vessels that carry blood from the heart to the lungs and body tissues and back to the heart in a continuous cycle. A blood vessel that transports blood from the heart is called an artery. Arteries eventually branch off into smaller and smaller arteries, the smallest of which are called arterioles. A **capillary** is one of the tiny blood vessels located between the arterioles and the venules, the smallest of the veins. The veins get larger and larger as they get closer to the heart. The largest veins return blood to the right atrium of the heart (Figure 11-9).

Arteries

The body has three types of arteries (Activity 11-4):

1. Elastic arteries are the large arteries capable of undergoing passive stretching. They have thick walls and recoil when the ventricles relax, which maintains pressure to move the blood. The aorta and pulmonary artery are elastic arteries.
2. Muscular arteries constitute most of the arteries in the body. These are small to medium arteries that distribute blood to all tissues by contracting or dilating to control blood flow. Located between the elastic layers are smooth muscle cells and some collagen. Although the walls of muscular arteries are distensible to a certain extent, as they become smaller and smaller with each successive branching the amount of elastic tissue decreases and the muscular component proportionately increases.

   These arteries are highly contractile, with their degree of contraction or relaxation being controlled by the autonomic nervous system and by endothelium-derived vasoactive substances. A few fine elastic fibers are scattered among the smooth muscle cells but are not organized into sheets. These are most numerous in the large muscular arteries, which are a direct continuation of the distal end of the elastic arteries.

   Muscular arteries vary in size from about 1 cm in diameter close to their origin at the elastic arteries to about 0.5 mm in diameter. Muscular arteries are composed almost entirely of smooth muscle. The larger arteries may have 30 or more layers of smooth muscle cells, whereas the smallest peripheral arteries have only 2 or 3 layers.
3. Arterioles are the smallest branches of the arterial tree. Arterioles vary in diameter ranging from 30 μm

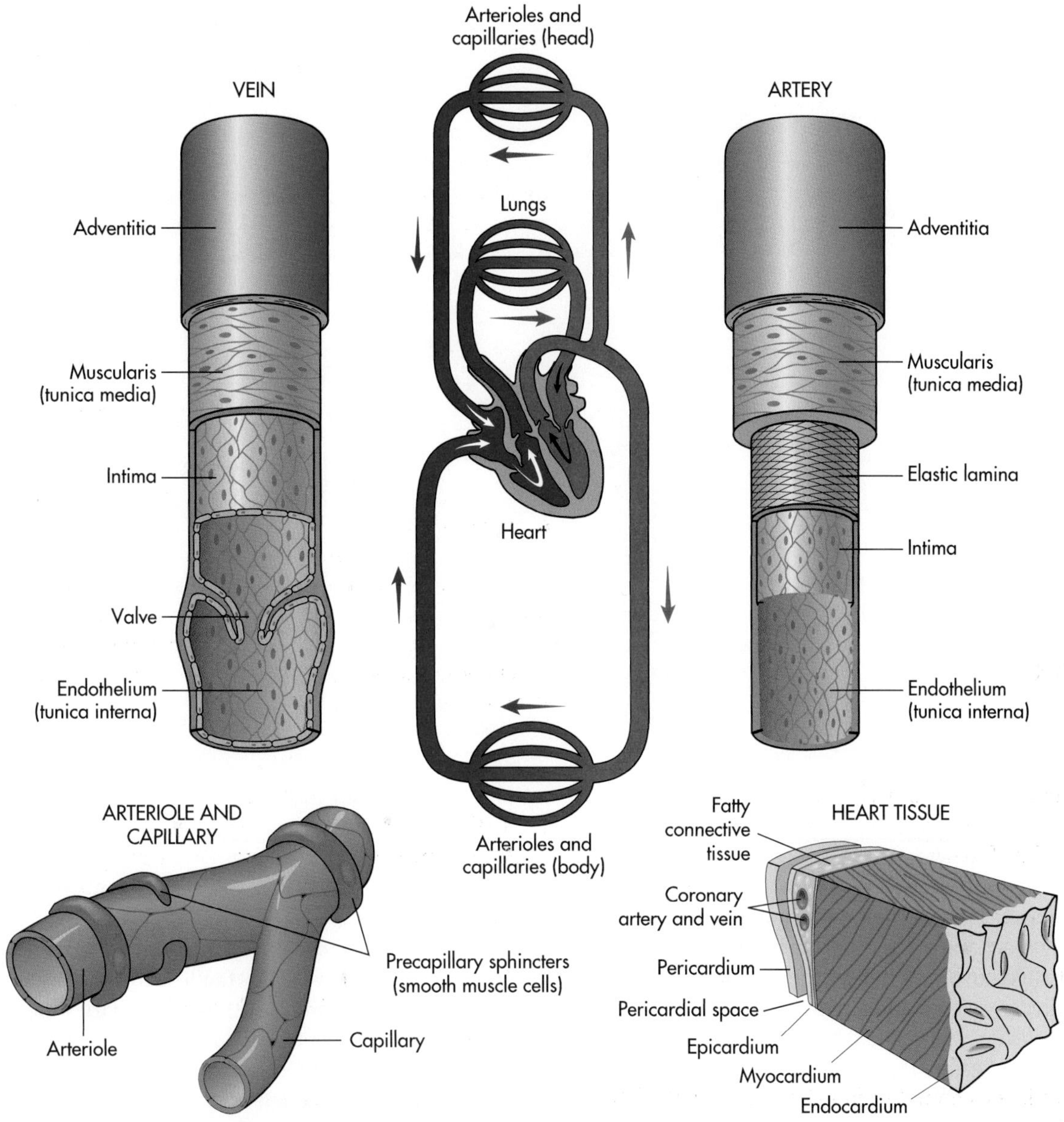

Figure 11-9

The peripheral vascular system consists of arteries, which carry oxygenated blood (red), and capillaries and veins, which carry deoxygenated blood (blue). The thick wall of the arteries is composed of distinct layers of smooth muscle cells and elastic laminae that separate these layers. In comparison, the veins have much thinner walls. The walls of the capillaries consist of a single layer of endothelium. The cross section of the heart is included for comparison. (From Damjanov I: *Pathology for the health-related professions,* ed 2, Philadelphia, 2000, WB Saunders.)

(0.03 mm) to 400 μm (0.4 mm). Any artery smaller than 0.5 mm in diameter is considered to be an arteriole.

The arterioles offer considerable resistance to blood flow because of their small radius and are the major site of resistance to flow in the vascular network. This area of high resistance to blood flow serves several functions: first, together with the elastic arteries, the resistance converts the pulsing ejection of blood from the heart into a steady flow through the capillaries; second, if no resistance were present and a high pressure persisted into the capillaries, a considerable loss of blood volume into the tissue would occur by movement of fluid across the capillary wall and around the cells. The arterioles are also important in determining the blood supply to different tissues and regions. They also constrict or dilate to control the amount of blood entering capillaries.

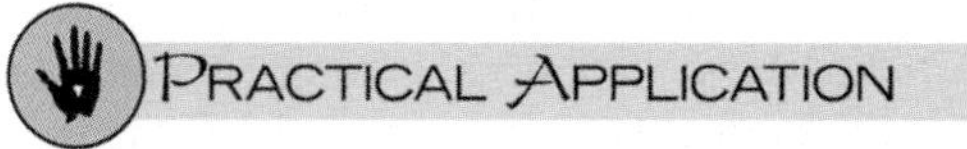

Massage therapists can increase arterial blood flow in two ways. First, by stimulating sympathetic autonomic functions, massage therapists increase the heart rate, providing more push to the blood in the arteries. The

ACTIVITY 11-4

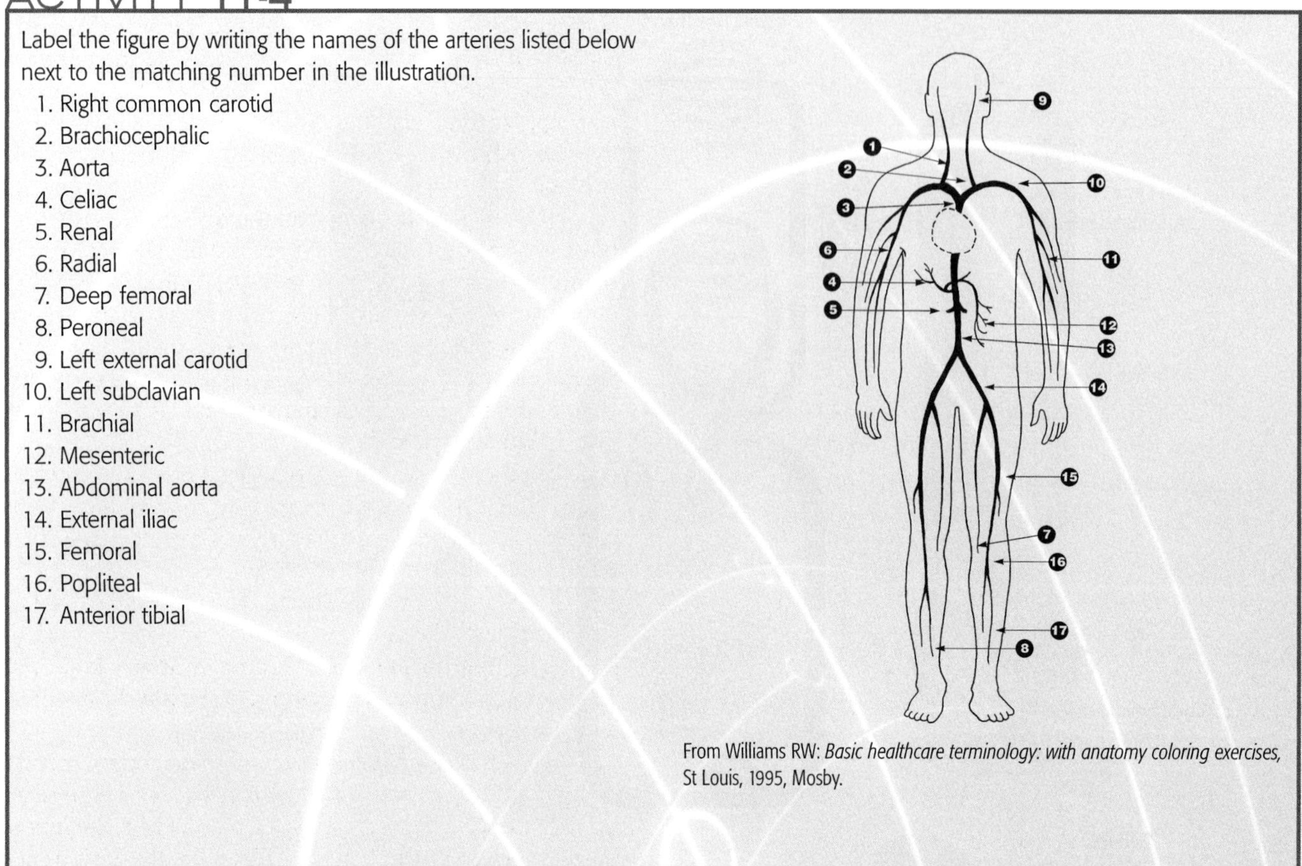

Label the figure by writing the names of the arteries listed below next to the matching number in the illustration.

1. Right common carotid
2. Brachiocephalic
3. Aorta
4. Celiac
5. Renal
6. Radial
7. Deep femoral
8. Peroneal
9. Left external carotid
10. Left subclavian
11. Brachial
12. Mesenteric
13. Abdominal aorta
14. External iliac
15. Femoral
16. Popliteal
17. Anterior tibial

From Williams RW: *Basic healthcare terminology: with anatomy coloring exercises*, St Louis, 1995, Mosby.

action is a reflexive, indirect method that involves the use of homeostatic mechanisms to maintain balance. One can structure massage to be stimulating to the sympathetic autonomic nervous system. In general, the methods used are brisk and involve active contraction of the muscles coupled with an increased respiratory rate.

Second, massage therapists can increase arterial blood flow mechanically through the pump and tube mechanism of the cardiovascular system, which functions like the fluid dynamics of hydraulics. Arteries are pliable muscular tubes that carry blood (a fluid) under pressure from the heart pump. Crimping or closing causes pressure to build up between the pump (the heart) and the barrier, like water behind a dam. With removal of the barrier the buildup of pressure provides an initial extra push to the fluid. Compression over more superficial arteries to close off the flow of blood temporarily results in the same phenomenon. Back pressure builds, and on release of the compression the blood pushes forward with more force than would have been available from the heart action alone. The massage therapist applies compression against the arteries in the legs and arms to assist peripheral circulation. The rhythm of compression and release is a rate of about 60 beats per minute, to coincide with the heart rhythm. The increase in blood flow is temporary, and in healthy individuals with adequate blood flow, the effect may be negligible (Figures 11-10 and 11-11). ■

Veins

The venous system acts as a collecting system, returning blood from the capillary networks to the heart passively down a pressure gradient (Figure 11-12). The capillaries merge to form venules, which in turn unite to form larger but fewer veins, which converge into the venae cavae. The walls of veins consist of the same three layers as arteries, but the elastic muscle components are much less prominent; the walls in general are thinner and more expandable than those of arteries.

The vessels have a large diameter (the vena cava is 2 to 3 cm in diameter) and thus offer low resistance to blood flow. Some veins, especially in the arms and legs, have internal folds of the endothelial lining that function as valves and allow blood to flow in one direction only, toward the heart. High venous pressures for long periods can damage these valves by overstretching them; for example, during pregnancy or in persons who stand for extended periods. The valves become weak, lose their function, and varicose veins develop. As a result of this, edema and varicose ulcers can develop.

A major part of the blood volume, up to 75%, is contained within the venous system, and for this reason veins sometimes are referred to as capacity vessels. The capacity of the venous system can be modified by altering the lumen size of the muscular venules and veins. The changes are caused by altering the venomotor tone, which is the degree of smooth muscle contraction in the vein.

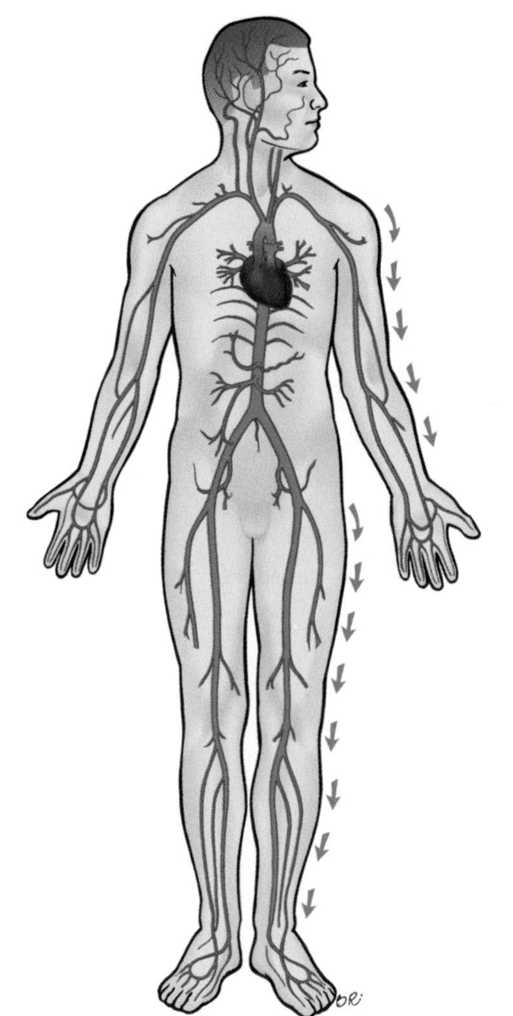

Figure 11-10
Direction of compression over arteries to increase arterial flow. (From Fritz S: *Mosby's fundamentals of therapeutic massage,* St Louis, 2004, Mosby.)

Venomotor tone is mainly under the control of the sympathetic nervous system. Changes in the venomotor tone can increase or decrease the capacity of the venous circulation and therefore can compensate partially for variations in the effective circulating blood volume.

The veins of the legs contain more valves than the veins of the arms to help fight the effects of gravity and prevent blood from pooling in the feet. Some of the more superficial veins in our hands and arms are visible. All superficial veins empty into the deeper veins that usually are found near arteries.

Venous Return

Venous blood flow occurs along small pressure gradients, and even small variations in resistance and vessel size affect the return flow.

The effect of gravity slows venous return: when one is upright, because the veins are more distended and because of the hydrostatic pressure of a column of blood in the veins below the level of the heart, blood tends to collect or pool in the feet and legs. When one is vertical, the leg veins take on a circular form that has a greater capacity; when one is horizontal, the veins take on an elliptical shape with a lower capacity. Increased venomotor tone, reducing the diameter and hence capacity of the veins, helps to reduce venous pooling. Venous pooling is not blood stagnation but indicates that the veins are accommodating a greater volume of blood.

Maintaining an adequate venous return to the heart at all times is vital because the cardiac output depends on the venous return (cardiac input). In most instances, the cardiac output equals the venous return. Thus if the venous return falls, cardiac output and blood pressure also may drop. Several mechanisms exist to help maintain the venous return at all times. Increasing the venomotor tone is an important mechanism because it decreases the capacity of the venous system and so aids venous return. After a long period of bed rest when the body is not constantly exposed to the force of gravity and the veins do not have to compensate, venomotor tone is reduced, and this method of reducing the effect of gravity is temporarily less efficient. The practitioner should remember this when helping someone up from a massage session. An essential practice is to move the client slowly and steadily and to support the person in case he or she becomes dizzy and feels faint.

Two systems sometimes referred to as the skeletal muscle pump and respiratory pump also assist venous return. Contraction of the skeletal muscles, especially in the limbs, squeezes the veins and pushes blood in the extremities toward the heart; numerous valves prevent back flow. Many communicating channels also allow emptying of blood from the superficial limb veins into the deep veins when rhythmic muscular contractions occur. Consequently, every time a person moves the legs or tenses the muscles, these actions push a certain amount of blood toward the heart. The more frequent and powerful such rhythmic contractions are, the more efficient their action. Sustained continuous muscle contractions, unlike rhythmic contractions, impede blood flow because of continuous blocking of the veins. The muscle pump mechanism is an efficient system. When an individual stands still for long periods of time, the muscle pump cannot operate and venous return decreases. The result is persons fainting from an inadequate cerebral blood flow. Thus contracting the muscles of the legs and buttocks voluntarily to aid venous return when standing still for long periods is advisable.

Respiration produces variations in intrapleural and intrathoracic pressure. Each inspiration lowers the pressure in the thorax and the right atrium of the heart and increases the pressure gradient and aids blood flow back to the heart at the same time the movement of the diaphragm into the abdomen raises the intraabdominal pressure and increases the gradient to the thorax, again favoring venous return. With expiration, the pressure gradients reverse and blood tends to flow in the opposite direction; fortunately, valves in the medium-size veins prevent this tendency.

Maintaining an adequate circulating blood volume also is necessary. If the blood volume is depleted for some reason,

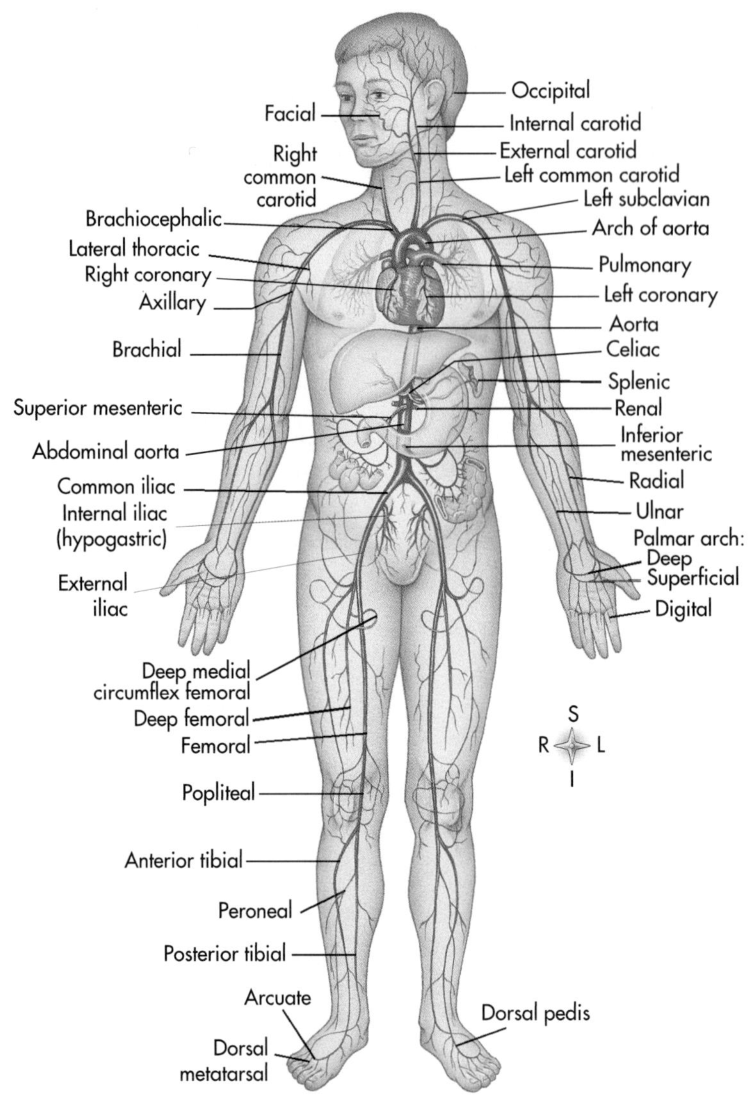

Figure 11-11
Principal arteries of the body. (From Thibodeau GA, Patton KT: *Anatomy and physiology,* ed 5, St Louis, 2003, Mosby.)

such as dehydration or **hemorrhage,** the body increases the effective circulating volume in the short term by venoconstriction and vasoconstriction in the blood reservoirs of the body such as the skin, liver, lungs, and spleen. However, restoration of the blood volume eventually requires fluid replacement. The pressures in the central regions of the venous system directly reflect the blood volume. Thus central venous pressure, or right atrial pressure, is a good indicator of blood volume, unlike arterial pressures, which are regulated and controlled reflexively (Activity 11-5; Figure 11-13).

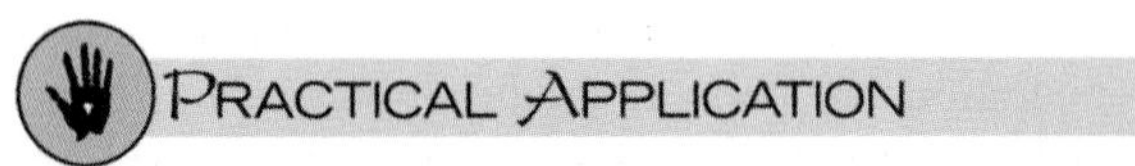

PRACTICAL APPLICATION

The practitioner can incorporate the principles affecting venous return into massage approaches to encourage venous return flow:

- Muscular pump: Rhythmic contraction and relaxation of the muscles during movement encourages venous return flow. Restoring normal muscle function and reducing muscle tension supports venous return.
- Gravity: Positioning the limbs higher than the heart passively assists venous return flow.
- Respiratory pump: Slow, deep diaphragmatic breathing with the massage modality used enhances venous return flow.
- Massage application: Stroking over the veins toward the heart passively moves blood in the veins. This method is particularly effective in the limbs. The practitioner can encourage rhythmic contraction of the muscles by having the person move his or her limbs through a complete range of motion against movement resistance in a contract-and-relax rhythm of about 60 cycles per minute. One then applies short strokes (1 or 2 inches long) over the veins toward the heart at

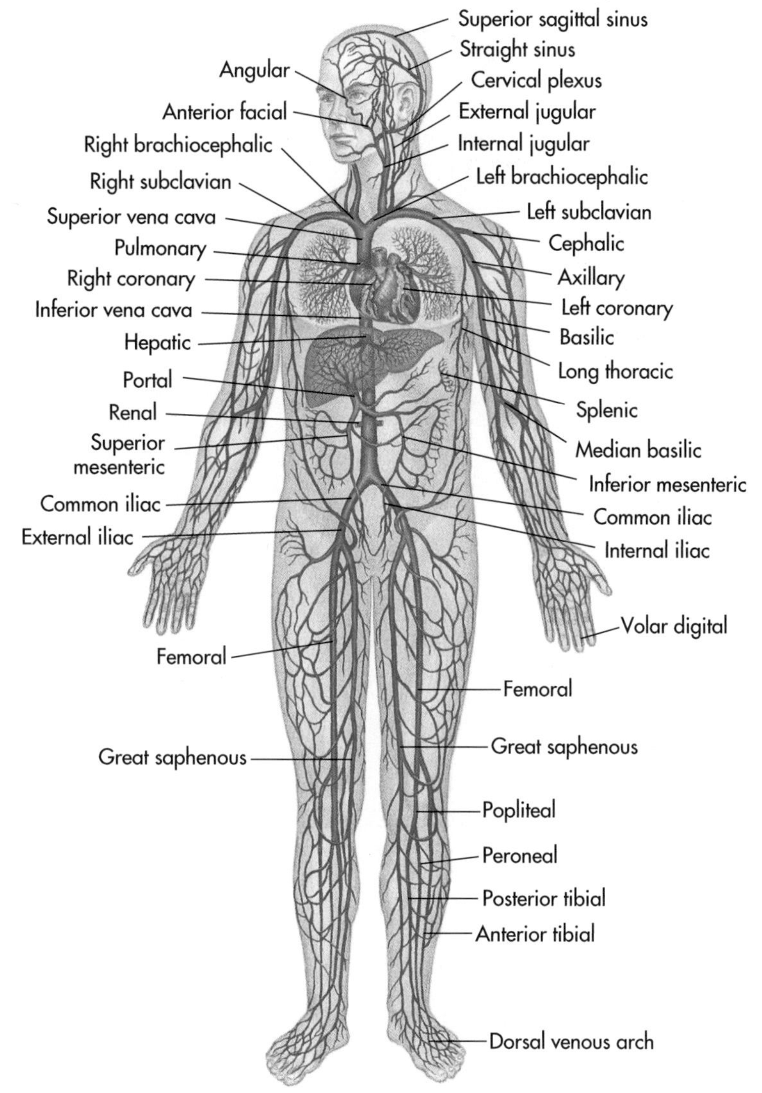

Figure 11-12
Systemic circulation: veins. (From Seidel HM, et al: *Mosby's guide to physical examination,* ed 5, St Louis, 2003, Mosby.)

sufficient pressure to push the blood in the superficial veins and places the limbs in a supported position above the heart for gravity to assist the return flow while encouraging the client to relax and breathe deeply (Figure 11-14). ■

Capillaries (Microvasculature)

Capillaries are composed of small-diameter blood vessels with partly permeable thin walls that permit the transfer of some blood components to the tissues and vice versa. Capillaries are specialized for diffusion of substances across their walls.

Capillaries are the smallest vessels of the blood circulatory system and form a complex interlinking network. Capillaries have the thinnest walls of all blood vessels and are the major site of gaseous exchange, permitting the transfer of oxygen from blood to tissues, and carbon dioxide from the tissues to the blood. Fluids containing large molecules pass across the capillary walls in both directions. Specialized regions near the junction between the terminal (smallest) arterioles and the capillaries known as precapillary sphincters consist of a few smooth muscle cells arranged circularly. Relaxed sphincters allow the capillary beds distal to the sphincters to be open and full of blood. Partially constricted sphincters reduce blood flow to the capillaries, and fully contracted sphincters allow no blood flow.

Some tissues have a much more abundant network of capillaries than others. For example dense connective tissue has a poor capillary network compared with cardiac tissue or that of the kidneys and liver.

Another modification in the structure of the microvasculature in tissues is the presence of *arteriovenous shunts* or *arteriovenous anastomoses,* which are direct connections between the arterial and venous systems that bypass the capillary beds. These short connecting vessels have strongly developed muscular control and are under sympathetic nervous control. They are found in many tissues and organs. In the skin, for example, these connections enable cutaneous

ACTIVITY 11-5

Label the figure by writing the names of the veins listed below next to the matching number in the illustration.

1. Right internal jugular
2. Right external jugular
3. Right subclavian
4. Brachial
5. Hepatic
6. Basilic
7. Renal
8. Radial
9. Ulnar
10. Femoral
11. Anterior tibial
12. Inferior vena cava
13. Mesenteric
14. Common iliac
15. Great saphenous

From Williams RW: *Basic healthcare terminology: with anatomy coloring exercises,* St Louis, 1995, Mosby.

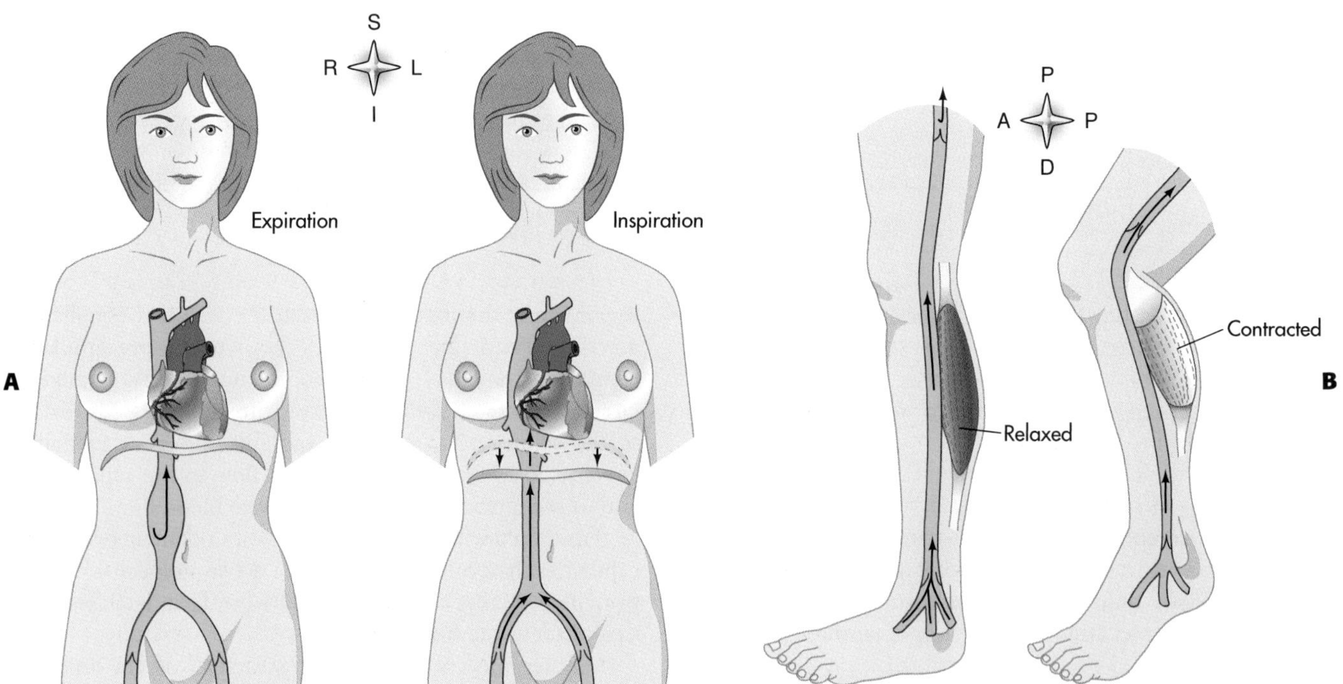

Figure 11-13

Venous pumping mechanisms. **A,** The respiratory pump operates by alternately decreasing thoracic pressure during inspiration (thus pulling venous blood into the central veins) and increasing pressure in the thorax during expiration (thus pushing central venous blood into the heart). **B,** The skeletal muscle pump operates by the alternate increase and decrease in peripheral venous pressure that normally occurs when the skeletal muscles are used for the activities of daily living. Both pumping mechanisms rely on the presence of semilunar valves in the veins to prevent backflow during the low-pressure points in the pumping cycle. (From Thibodeau GA, Patton KT: *Anatomy and physiology,* ed 5, St Louis, 2003, Mosby.)

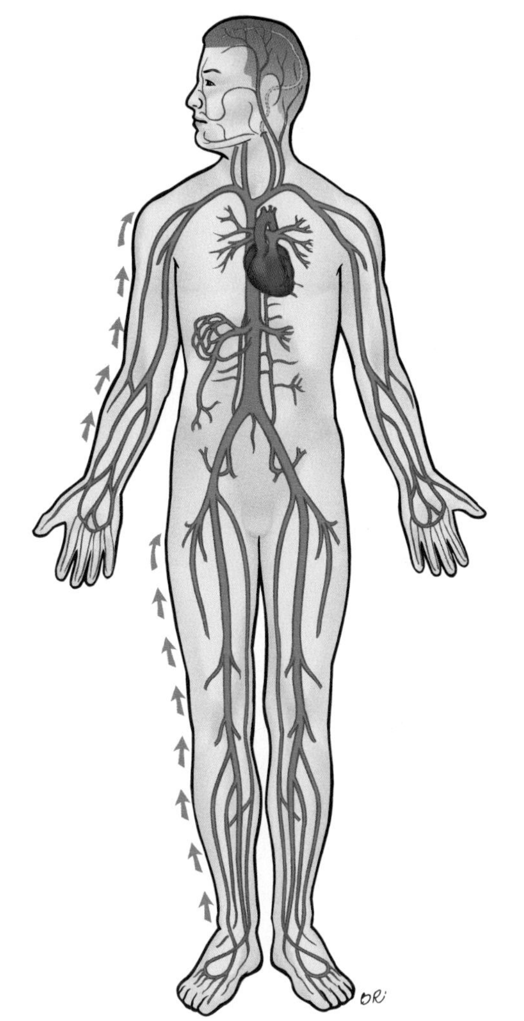

Figure 11-14
Direction of effleurage strokes to facilitate venous flow. (From Fritz S: *Mosby's fundamentals of therapeutic massage,* ed 3, St Louis, 2004, Mosby.)

blood flow to increase to allow dissipation of heat from the body surfaces when one is exercising or in high environmental temperatures.

The capillary network, whatever its form, drains into a series of vessels with increasing diameter that form venules and veins.

The capillaries are the most important vessels functionally because they transport essential materials to and from the cells. The efficient exchange between capillary blood and the surrounding tissue fluid occurs because the capillaries are so numerous and so small that blood in the capillaries flows at its slowest rate, which ensures the maximum contact time between blood and tissue. This flow of blood through the capillary bed is referred to as the microcirculation.

Practical Application

The practitioner can manipulate the network of capillaries by massage, using compression and kneading to encourage movement of blood through the capillaries. ■

Blood Pressure and Pulse

The amount of pressure exerted by the blood on the walls of the blood vessels is called **blood pressure.** The maximal pressure, called *systolic pressure,* occurs when the ventricles contract. *Diastolic pressure* occurs when the ventricles relax. Blood forced into the aorta during systole sets up a pressure wave that travels along the arteries and expands the arterial wall. One can palpate this expansion by pressing the artery against tissue. The number of waves is known as the pulse, which is a direct reflection of the heart rate.

The *pulse rate,* measured when a person is at rest, may be regular or irregular, strong or weak. An irregular pulse occurs commonly with atrial fibrillation and premature contractions. A strong pulse occurs with hyperthyroidism; a weak one with shock and myocardial infarction. A resting heart rate greater than 100 beats per minute is known as tachycardia; a heart rate less than 50 or 60 beats per minute is known as bradycardia (Figure 11-15).

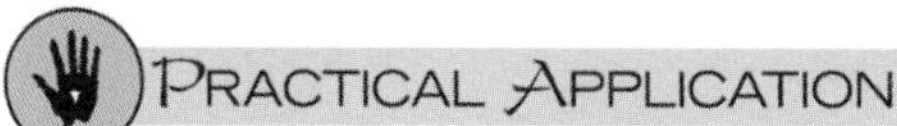

Practical Application

The practitioner can monitor the pulses during assessment. In general, the pulses should feel bilaterally equal. Should the practitioner note differences, he or she should refer the client for diagnosis. The pulse rate ranges from 50 to 70 beats per minute at rest. A rate much slower or faster indicates a need for referral. If the general intent of the therapy session is stress management focused toward relaxation with parasympathetic predomination, the pulse rate should slow somewhat over the duration of the session. The opposite is true if the goal is increased arousal of the sympathetic system to energize the client. Many Asian medical practices use the feel of the pulse in assessment of the meridian system. The pulse diagnosis takes many years to perfect. ■

Sympathetic nerves to the arterioles regulate blood pressure. Normally, arterioles are in a state of partial constriction, called arteriole tone. Stimulation of the sympathetic system causes further arteriolar constriction and an increase in blood pressure. Nonstimulation results in a decrease in blood pressure. With *hypertension,* the sympathetic system is in a state of continuous stimulation, resulting in constant high blood pressure.

Blood pressure is measured with a *sphygmomanometer,* a cloth-covered rubber bag that is wrapped around the arm over the brachial artery. Blood pressure is highest during contraction of the heart (systole), the systolic blood pressure, and is lowest when the heart is relaxed (diastole), the diastolic pressure. As the vessels become more and more remote from the heart, the systolic and diastolic pressures equalize. As the vessels change from arteries to arterioles to capillaries to venules to veins, the pressure decreases, until in the large veins the pressure may be zero or negative. For this reason, when drawing venous blood, one has to pull back on the syringe.

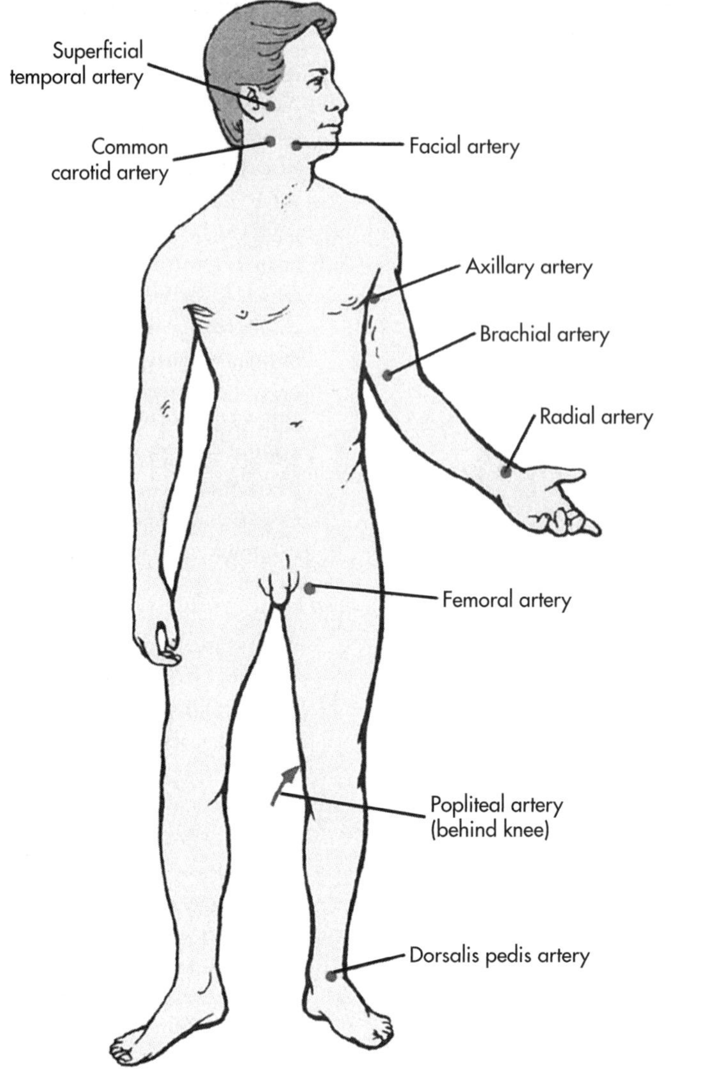

Figure 11-15
Pulse points. Each pulse point is named after the artery with which it is associated. (From Thibodeau GA, Patton KT: *The human body in health and disease,* ed 3, St Louis, 2002, Mosby.)

Blood pressure is recorded as millimeters of mercury (mm Hg), which refers to the number of millimeters of mercury displaced by the changes in pressure. The first number is the systolic pressure, and the second number is the diastolic pressure. When one records the pressure, one writes only the numbers; the unit of measure mm Hg usually is dropped.

Normal blood pressure range. Blood pressure depends on the person's size. The average newborn has a blood pressure of 90/60; at 15 years of age, the average blood pressure is about 120/60. An average, healthy young adult has a blood pressure of 120/80. Generally, a blood pressure under 100/60 is considered hypotension; a pressure above 140/90 is considered hypertension. The blood pressure changes under various conditions, and one should never use a single reading as a final determinant. A systolic increase occurs in temporary conditions such as anxiety and exercise. Hypertension involves an increase in the systolic and diastolic pressures. Hypotension is a decrease in the systolic and diastolic pressures and is an important manifestation of shock, which results from an inadequate blood supply to vital organs.

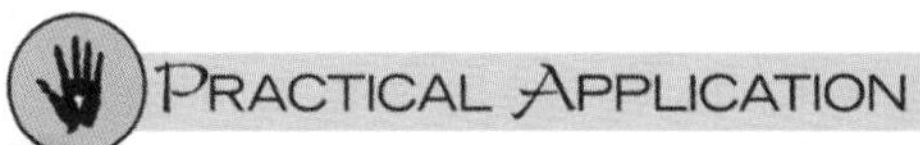

Stress management programs include methods of movement and moderate aerobic exercise, stretching programs, massage, and other forms of soft tissue methods. Although these approaches initially elevate blood pressure, when continued, they activate parasympathetic quieting responses such as slow, deep breathing and progressive relaxation and therefore tend to have a normalizing effect on the blood pressure. These methods are classified as *nonspecific constitutional approaches*; they allow the homeostatic mechanisms to reset to a more effective functional pattern after disruption. ■

Hydrostatic pressure. All fluids in a confined space exert pressure. The term *hydrostatic pressure* refers to the force that a liquid exerts against the walls of its container.

As described, the pressure that blood exerts in the vascular system is known as blood pressure. If pressure is exerted on a confined fluid, the pressure is transmitted equally in all directions, which is known as Pascal's principle. If a weak point exists in the wall of the container and the pressure exerted is great enough, the container wall may burst. This is what happens when an aneurysm bursts.

In a hypertensive individual the blood vessels harden or undergo sclerotic changes (**arteriosclerosis**) to prevent the vessels from bursting with the increased blood pressure.

The flexibility of the container such as with veins also influences the hydrostatic pressure that develops: if the container is flexible, the pressure in the fluid is less than in a rigid container.

The flow of a fluid through a vessel is determined by the pressure difference between the two ends of the vessel and also the resistance to flow. For any fluid to flow along a vessel a pressure difference must exist; otherwise, the fluid will not move. In the cardiovascular system the pumping of the heart generates the "pressure head" or force, and a continuous drop in pressure occurs from the left ventricle of the heart to the tissues and from the tissues back to the right atrium of the heart. Without this drop in blood pressure, no blood would flow through the circulatory system. Resistance is a measure of the ease with which a fluid flows through a tube: the easier flow is, the less the resistance to flow, and vice versa. In the circulatory system the resistance usually is described as the vascular resistance, because it mainly originates in the peripheral blood vessels, and also is known simply as the peripheral resistance.

Resistance is essentially a measure of the friction between the molecules of the fluid, and between the tube wall and the fluid. The resistance depends on the viscosity of the fluid and the radius and length of the tube.

The smaller the radius of a vessel, the greater the resistance to the movement of particles. This increased resistance results from a greater probability of the particles of the fluid colliding with the vessel wall. When a particle collides with the wall, some of the kinetic energy (energy of movement) of the particle is lost on impact, resulting in the slowing of the particle. Thus in a smaller-diameter vessel, a greater number of collisions occur, reducing the energy content and speed of the particles moving through the vessel. The result is a decrease in the hydrostatic pressure.

Small alterations in the size of the radius of the blood vessels, particularly of the more peripheral vessels, can influence the flow of blood. Changes in the walls of large and medium-size arteries cause narrowing of the lumen of the vessels and result in an increased vascular resistance.

Viscosity of the fluid. *Viscosity* is a measure of the tendency of a liquid to resist flow. The greater the viscosity (thickness) of a fluid, the greater the force required to move that liquid. For example, water has less viscosity than a milkshake.

Normally the viscosity of blood remains constant, but in polycythemia, in which the red cell content is high, the viscosity of the blood can be considerably greater, reducing the blood flow. Severe dehydration, in which loss of **plasma** occurs, and cooling of the blood also can lead to increased viscosity.

The nature of the lining of the tube or vessel also influences the way fluids flow. If the lining of the blood vessel is smooth, the fluid flows evenly; this is known as streamline or laminar flow. However, if the lining is rough or uneven or the fluid flows irregularly, the fluid flows turbulently. Laminar flow is characteristic of most parts of the vascular system and is silent, whereas turbulent flow is audible, such as during blood pressure measurements with a sphygmomanometer.

Medulla and Baroreceptors

In the medulla of the brain the cells of the reticular formation regulate three vital signs: heart rate, blood pressure, and respiration. They work with signals from the various nerve centers in the body. One type of nerve center in the cardiovascular system is the *baroreceptor.*

Baroreceptors are stretch receptors in the carotid arteries, the aorta, and nearly every large artery of the neck and thorax. When blood pressure increases, arteries stretch. The baroreceptors transmit signals about sudden, brief changes in blood pressure such as when we change position. When blood pressure is elevated for a long period, the baroreceptor reflex resets to the new blood pressure level.

When blood pressure suddenly drops, the frequency of signals from the baroreceptors declines. This change sets off a response in the cardioregulatory center of the medulla that increases sympathetic stimulation and decreases parasympathetic stimulation, resulting in an increase in the heart rate and blood pressure. Conversely, when blood pressure increases, the signal increases and the medulla changes its output to slow the heart rate and blood pressure by increasing parasympathetic signals. This is another example of how a negative feedback system works in the body.

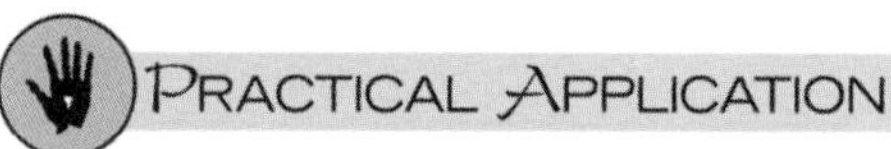

Stimulation of baroreceptors during therapeutic massage could affect blood pressure. The blood pressure could drop, and the client may be light-headed and show other signs of low blood pressure. ■

Names of Specific Arteries and Veins

The names of most arteries and veins are derived from the anatomic structure they serve. The femoral artery and the femoral vein, for example, are found close to the femur, where these blood vessels serve the tissue of the upper and lower leg. The renal artery is so named because it exits the abdominal aorta and enters the kidney. The renal vein exits the kidney and enters the inferior vena cava. Arteries and veins are found on both sides of the body and are identified as right or left (e.g., the right common carotid artery and the left common carotid artery).

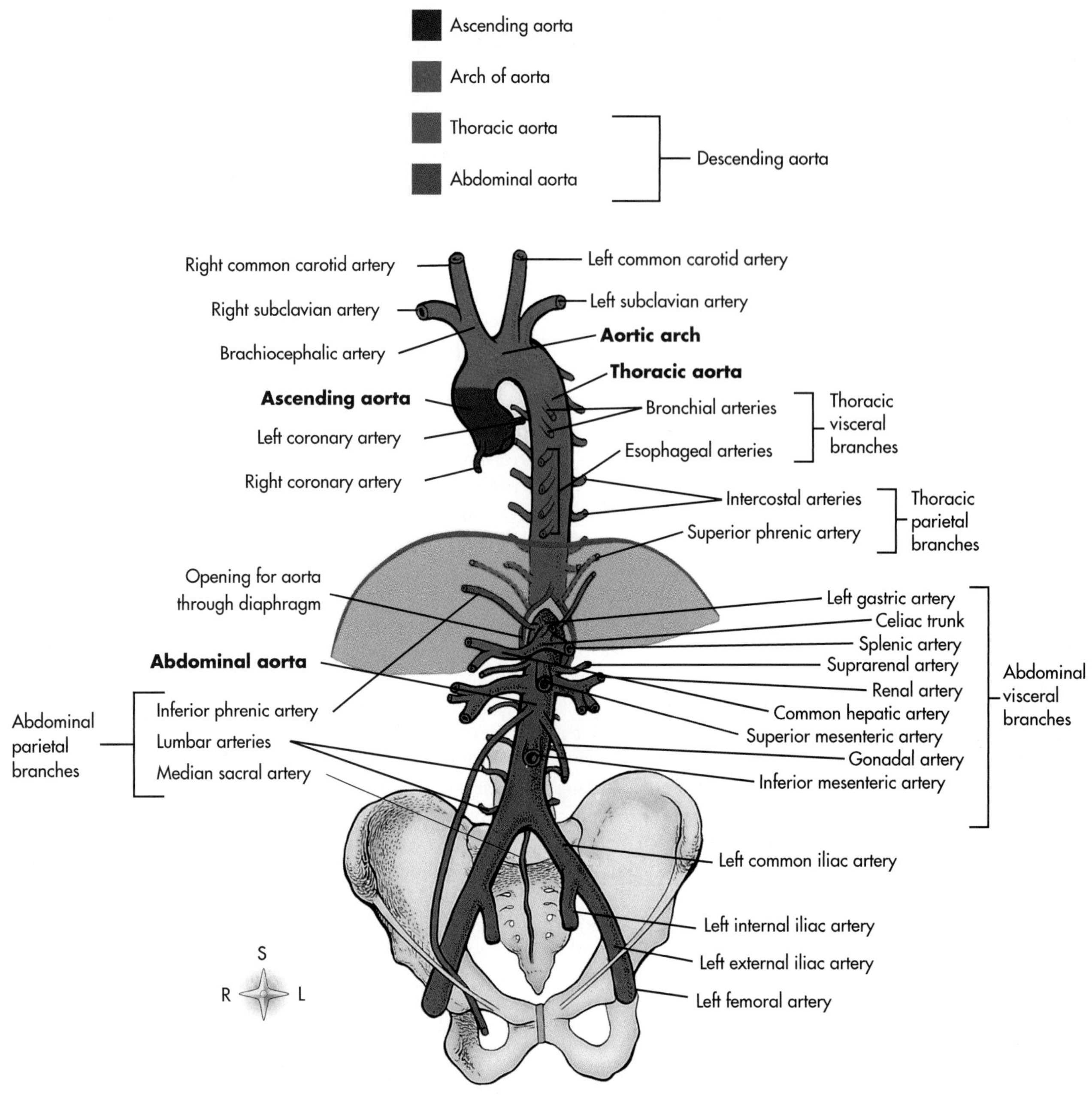

Figure 11-16
The aorta. The aorta is the main systemic artery, serving as a trunk from which other arteries branch. Blood is conducted from the heart first through the ascending aorta, then the arch of the aorta, and then through the thoracic and abdominal segments of the descending aorta. (From Thibodeau GA, Patton KT: Anatomy and physiology, ed 5, St Louis, 2003, Mosby.)

The following is a list of the main arteries and veins. Many of them change names as they enter into and pass through certain areas of the body. The student can use the illustrations to trace the location of these vessels (Figure 11-16; see Figures 11-11 and 11-12).

Arteries. The names of arteries are listed according to the body region they serve.

Main arteries of the head and neck. The arch of the *aorta* gives rise to three arteries; from right to left, they are the *brachiocephalic* (or innominate) *artery,* the *left common carotid artery,* and the *left subclavian artery.* The subclavian artery supplies the upper extremities.

The brachiocephalic artery, a short artery, becomes the right common carotid artery and the right subclavian artery.

The common carotid arteries branch at the level of the upper part of the thyroid cartilage to become the *external* and *internal carotid arteries.* The common carotid artery is an important pulse-taking artery; damage to this artery may result in a transient ischemic attack. The internal carotid artery supplies the brain; the external carotid artery supplies the face, head, and neck.

The *superficial temporal artery* is the cranial termination of the external carotid artery. The superficial temporal artery is a pulse-taking artery located superior and anterior to the ear.

The two vertebral arteries become the *basilar artery,* which helps supply the brain.

Main arteries of the upper extremity. The subclavian artery becomes the *axillary artery* at the clavicle.

Near the head of the humerus, the axillary artery becomes the *brachial artery.* The brachial artery is the main artery for measuring blood pressure and is also a pulse-taking artery.

The brachial artery divides at the elbow region into the *ulnar* and *radial arteries.*

The ulnar artery lies deep and medial. The radial artery lies more superficial and lateral. Both arteries communicate in the hand via two deep anastomoses and a superficial and deep palmar arch.

Main arteries of the trunk. After supplying the head, neck, and upper extremity, the *aorta* descends posteriorly as the *thoracic aorta,* sending branches to the intercostal muscles as the *right* and *left intercostal arteries.*

The intercostal arteries anastomose anteriorly with the left and right *internal thoracic arteries.* If the aorta is damaged, the intercostal muscles, which are important in breathing, may still receive a blood supply by way of the internal thoracic arteries.

Main arteries of the abdomen. When the thoracic aorta penetrates the diaphragm, it is known as the abdominal aorta, which supplies the abdominal organs. The following structures, listed in a cranial to caudal direction, are the main branches of the abdominal aorta:

Celiac trunk: Supplies the stomach, spleen, and liver via the gastric, splenic, and hepatic arteries.

Superior mesenteric artery: Supplies the small intestine, part of the pancreas, and half of the colon.

Renal arteries: Supply the kidneys.

Testicular or ovarian arteries: Supply the gonads.

Inferior mesenteric artery: Supplies the remaining half of the colon to the rectum.

The abdominal aorta then divides into the *left* and *right common iliac arteries.* The common iliac divides into the *internal iliac artery,* which supplies the pelvic organs, and the *external iliac artery.*

Main arteries of the lower extremity. After passing under the inguinal ligament, the external iliac artery becomes the *femoral artery.* The femoral artery lies superficially at the femoral triangle and then descends posteriorly through the adductor muscles. The femoral artery is an important pulse-taking artery. When the femoral artery emerges behind the knee in the popliteal region, it becomes the popliteal artery. The *popliteal artery* then divides to become the *anterior* and *posterior tibial arteries.*

The anterior tibial artery becomes the *dorsalis pedis artery* on the dorsal aspect of the foot. The dorsalis pedis is an important pulse-taking artery.

The posterior tibial artery descends behind the medial malleolus and is also a pulse-taking artery but usually is more difficult to find than the dorsalis pedis.

Veins. The names of the veins are listed according to the body region they serve.

Main veins of the head and neck. The following are veins of the head and neck:

Superficial: The *right* and *left external jugular veins* drain blood from the face, head, and neck. Each *external jugular vein* empties into a *subclavian vein.*

Deep: Venous drainage from the brain is accomplished by the *internal jugular veins.* Each internal jugular vein joins a subclavian vein to form a *brachiocephalic vein.*

Main veins of the upper extremity. Superficial veins originate on the dorsum of the hand as the *dorsal venous plexus.* They curve around the wrist to the ventral side as the *cephalic vein,* which runs along the lateral aspect of forearm and arm, going deep at the deltoid muscle, and the *basilic vein,* which runs along the medial aspect of forearm and arm and goes deep at the biceps muscle. The *medial cubital vein* is an anastomosis between the basilic and cephalic veins.

The deep veins form from branches in the hand and forearm. Although some individuals have a short *brachial vein,* most often the first main deep vein is the *axillary vein.* The axillary vein becomes the *subclavian vein* when it passes under the clavicle.

Main veins of the trunk. The subclavian vein joins the *internal jugular vein* to become the *brachiocephalic vein.* The subclavian vein is an important central vein for intravenous infusion.

Two brachiocephalic veins join to become the *superior vena cava,* which empties into the right atrium.

The *azygos system,* which lies on the posterior body wall, drains the intercostal veins. The azygos vein empties into the superior vena cava.

The *inferior vena cava* drains blood from the abdominal viscera into the right atrium. The digestive organs and spleen first drain into the *portal vein,* which empties into the liver. The following veins, listed from cranial to caudal, are branches of the inferior vena cava:

- *Hepatic veins* from the liver
- Right and left *renal veins* from the kidneys
- Right and left *testicular* or *ovarian veins* from the gonads
- Two common iliac veins (the continuation of the femoral veins)

Main veins of the lower extremity. Superficial veins of the leg begin as a *dorsal venous arch* on top of the foot.

The *great saphenous vein* ascends medially from the foot up the leg to the thigh and drains into the *femoral vein.* The great saphenous veins may become chronically dilated in some persons and develop into varicose veins. They then may become inflamed and form blood clots, a condition known as thrombophlebitis.

The *small saphenous vein* runs laterally from the foot along the gastrocnemius muscle and drains into the *popliteal vein.*

The *anterior tibial vein* and *posterior tibial vein* drain into the popliteal vein.

The popliteal vein becomes the *femoral vein* after it passes the knee. The deep veins of the leg may become inflamed, a condition referred to as deep vein thrombosis, which is a more serious condition than superficial thrombophlebitis. The clot may break off and travel to the heart and then lodge in the lung as a pulmonary embolism (see Figure 11-12).

Hepatic Portal System

Any portal system is defined by the fact that blood drains from one venous system to another without having arteries between the two. This occurs in the pituitary gland and in the abdomen.

The hepatic portal system begins in the capillaries of the digestive organs and ends in the portal vein. The *splenic vein* and the *superior mesenteric vein* anastomose to form the *portal vein.* The *inferior mesenteric vein* typically joins with the splenic vein at some point along its course deep to the pancreas. The *portal vein* is deep to the *proper hepatic artery* and *common bile duct* and runs within the free right edge of the lesser omentum. This set of three structures—the hepatic artery, bile duct, and portal vein—is called the hepatic triad. The portal veins again become smaller and smaller in the liver until reaching the second venous capillary bed called the sinusoids of the liver. Portal blood contains substances absorbed by the stomach and intestines. Portal blood passes through the liver, which absorbs, excretes, or converts nutrients and toxins.

Once filtered the blood passes into the *central vein,* which is the beginning of the second venous system. This venous system is filled with progressively larger and larger veins known as *hepatic veins.* The hepatic veins eventually drain the filtered blood through the three large hepatic veins. Restriction of outflow through the hepatic portal system can lead to portal hypertension. Portal hypertension most often is associated with cirrhosis.

The liver receives approximately 30% of resting cardiac output and is therefore a vascular organ. The hepatic vascular system has a considerable ability to store and release blood and functions as a reservoir within the general circulation.

In the normal situation, 10% to 15% of the total blood volume is in the liver, with roughly 60% of that in the sinusoids. With loss of blood the liver dynamically adjusts its blood volume and can eject enough blood to compensate for a moderate amount of hemorrhage. Conversely, when vascular volume increases acutely, as with rapid infusion of fluids, the hepatic blood volume expands, providing a buffer against acute increases in systemic blood volume.

Blood

Blood, the thick, red fluid in our bodies, is a form of connective tissue. Blood transports nutrients to the individual cells and removes waste products. Whole blood consists of solid formed elements and the liquid matrix, or plasma.

Red blood cells, white blood cells, and platelets are the formed elements of blood that float in the plasma, a thick, straw-colored fluid (Activity 11-6). Amino acids, carbohydrates, electrolytes, hormones, lipids, proteins, vitamins, and waste materials are the other constituents of blood. A person who weighs 140 to 150 lb has about 5 qt of blood.

In an adult, blood cells form mainly in the red marrow of the bones of the chest, vertebrae, and pelvis. Yellow marrow can convert to red marrow if the body requires increased production of blood cells. The stages of blood cell development in red marrow constitute a process called *hematopoiesis.* Blood cells originate from a common precursor cell called the stem cell. Immature blood cells are *blast cells.* When the cells are mature, they move into the bloodstream. In persons with leukemia, blast cells may be seen in peripheral blood because the body sends them out even before they are mature.

Red Blood Cells

Red blood cells, also known as erythrocytes or red blood corpuscles, make up more than 90% of the formed elements in blood. They are round and have raised edges and a flattened middle. Their function is to transport oxygen to the cells and carbon dioxide away from the cells. Men have slightly more red blood cells than women, and the cells live slightly longer in men (about 120 days) than in women (110 days). The body recycles dead red blood cells, using hemoglobin in new cells and breaking down proteins from the dead cells into amino acids to create new blood proteins.

Because red blood cells cannot divide, they must be produced frequently to replace dead cells. A red blood cell loses its nucleus and most of its organelles during development. Red bone marrow produces enough red blood cells daily to replace dead blood cells. The body needs a proper intake and assimilation of iron, vitamin B_{12}, and folic acid to produce new red blood cells.

Erythrocytes contain an iron-protein compound known as hemoglobin. Oxygen binds to *hemoglobin* in the capillaries of the lungs and is transported to all parts of the body. A lack of oxygen, or anemia, can stimulate *erythropoiesis,* the production of red blood cells. Red blood cells also transport carbon dioxide from the tissues of the body to the lungs. An abnormal increase in red blood cells is known as *polycythemia*; an abnormal decrease is called *anemia.*

A variety of chemicals are present in red blood cells. Some of these chemicals commonly are called factors and are used to identify the type of blood. The best known grouping method is the ABO system. This system has four blood groups, A, B, AB, and O, commonly called the *blood types.* The Rh system, the most complex of all the blood grouping methods, has 42 different groups.

White Blood Cells

White blood cells also are called leukocytes or white blood corpuscles. Their white color is from a lack of hemoglobin. The usual ratio of white to red blood cells is 1 to 500. The

ACTIVITY 11-6

Color the blood cells shown in the figure, parts A through G.

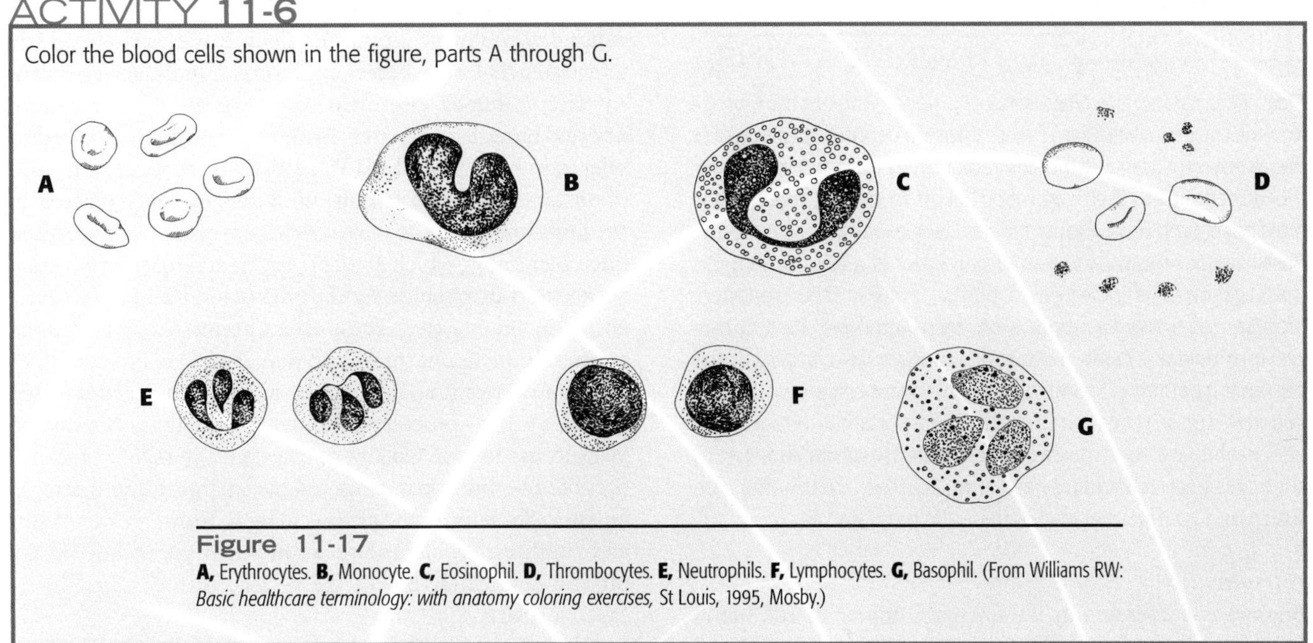

Figure 11-17
A, Erythrocytes. **B,** Monocyte. **C,** Eosinophil. **D,** Thrombocytes. **E,** Neutrophils. **F,** Lymphocytes. **G,** Basophil. (From Williams RW: *Basic healthcare terminology: with anatomy coloring exercises,* St Louis, 1995, Mosby.)

main function of the white blood cells is to protect the body from pathogens and remove dead cells and substances. White blood cells are divided into the following five groups:

Neutrophils: Neutrophils are granular leukocytes; more than half of all white blood cells are neutrophils. These cells fight disease by engulfing bacteria in a cell-eating process called *phagocytosis,* which is the ingestion and digestion of particles by a cell. Neutrophils are important in the defense of the body against bacterial infection. A buildup of neutrophils and the debris they collect is called *pus.*

Lymphocytes: Lymphocytes account for about 30% of the total number of white blood cells in the body. They produce **antibodies** and chemicals that are active in regulating disease, allergic reactions, and controlling tumors.

Monocytes: Monocytes are the largest of the white blood cells, yet they account for only about 6% of the total number. They also protect the body through phagocytosis. Monocytes are unique because when they leave the blood and enter the tissues, they can develop into large phagocytic cells called macrophages.

Eosinophils: About 3% of the total white blood cell count is made up of eosinophils. However, the number increases greatly with parasitic infections or allergic reactions (e.g., hay fever). Eosinophils are capable of phagocytic activity, and they release chemicals during the inflammatory process.

Basophils: Basophils are also granular white blood cells, and they make up about 1% of the total white blood cell count. Their exact function is not yet understood clearly.

Platelets

Thrombocytes, also called platelets, are the smallest cellular elements of the blood. They are important in the blood clotting process and are manufactured in the bone marrow.

Plasma

Plasma is the straw-colored liquid found in blood and lymph and is about 90% water; the rest is nutrients, gases, and waste products. Plasma constitutes about 55% of blood and plays a major role in the movement of water between the tissues and the blood.

Clotting

Damage to a blood vessel causes the release of chemicals. Special proteins, called clotting factors, are activated and then form additional clotting factors. A special protein called *fibrin* forms and seals the damaged blood vessels by trapping red blood cells, platelets, and fluid to form a clot. Fibrin then anchors the clot. The clotting process starts the instant the blood vessel is damaged and takes only a few minutes to complete. Calcium and vitamin K are important to the success and speed of the clotting process (see Activity 11-6).

Pathologic Conditions

Cardiovascular disease is the leading cause of death in Western societies. Cardiac arrest may occur because of a number of conditions, the most common being a heart attack (myocardial infarction).

INDICATIONS/CONTRAINDICATIONS

For Therapeutic Massage

In general, cardiovascular disease presents contraindications for therapeutic massage. If the contraindication does not arise from the disease itself, the medication taken to control the disease may pose problems. Blood thinners, for example, increase the possibility of bruising and hemorrhage. Nonetheless, therapeutic massage often is indicated as part of a supervised treatment program. The key is supervision by a qualified health care provider, because cardiovascular diseases can be complex in the presenting pathologic condition and the treatment protocols. The general stress management and homeostatic normalization effects of therapeutic massage treatments are desirable for most cardiovascular difficulties as long as the treatments are supervised as part of a total therapeutic program. ■

Anemia

Anemia is a decrease in the normal number of red blood cells or in the amount of hemoglobin or iron in the blood. The various anemias are classified according to whether the cause is a loss in the number or change in the usability of red cells or a decline in the production of red cells.

Aneurysm

An aneurysm is a permanent dilation (ballooning) of part of a vessel because of weakness or damage to its structure. Although the usual result of arteriosclerosis is an aneurysm, the condition also may be congenital or result from inflammation. The most common sites are the aorta and the arteries of the brain. Aneurysms are dangerous because they tend to burst.

Angina Pectoris

Angina pectoris is chest pain or discomfort that results when the amount of oxygen supplied to the heart declines. Angina pectoris is caused mainly by coronary artery disease but also can be a sign of heart disease, anemia, or hyperthyroidism. Symptoms most often occur during exertion, emotional upset, or cold weather. The pain begins in the center of the chest and often spreads to the arms, neck, or jaw. In severe cases, pain may occur when the person is at rest. Rest or the use of nitroglycerin usually relieves the symptoms.

Arrhythmia

Arrhythmias are conditions that affect the heart rate. The rhythm of the heart may be partly or completely irregular or may be regular but with a frequency that is too slow or too fast. Treatment may include medication, installation of a pacemaker to start the heartbeat, or use of a defibrillator to restore normal heart rhythm.

Arterial Inflammation

Endarteritis obliterans is a defect in which the artery walls become inflamed, blocking the opening of the vessel and blocking the smaller vessels.

Arteriosclerosis and Atherosclerosis

Arteriosclerosis, which means hardening of the arteries, refers to arteries that have become brittle and lost their elasticity. Arteries gradually lose elasticity as we age. If they cannot enlarge, blockage becomes more serious. Although arteriosclerosis has several causes, the most common and important is **atherosclerosis,** the deposit of fatty plaques in medium and large arteries. Often the two terms are used interchangeably, which is incorrect. In atherosclerosis, small fat deposits from cholesterol in the blood build up at stress points in the arteries. These stress points occur where the arteries branch out or incur damage. The fat combines with connective tissue sent to repair the damage and forms plaque. As this process continues, blood flow diminishes. Symptoms do not usually appear until a major blockage occurs. The body compensates by enlarging the artery, if possible. Sometimes the artery enlarges, forms an aneurysm, and ruptures. Problems also occur when the plaque breaks off and completely blocks the vessels. In the brain, this is called a stroke.

Countries with high-fat diets, particularly diets high in saturated fatty acids and cholesterol, have a higher incidence of atherosclerosis. Nonsurgical interventions such as modifying the diet and taking part in aerobic exercise may be able to enlarge an artery, increasing the blood flow. Also, collateral circulation may develop around the blockage as new vessels develop. Surgical interventions may include creating a bypass from blood vessels transferred from other parts of the body, excising the blockage, or enlarging the vessel (Figure 11-18).

Bone Marrow Suppression Anemia

Various types of anemia result from bone marrow suppression. Marrow suppression may occur in individuals undergoing chemotherapy or taking certain antibiotics, as a complication of radiation therapy, or in persons with chronic diseases. The red blood cells may be damaged or destroyed, and the body often tries to compensate by producing new ones and sending them out before they mature. Severe cases require blood transfusions, along with bone marrow transplantation.

Bradycardia

In bradycardia the resting heart rate is less than 60 beats per minute. However, healthy athletes often have a heart rate between 50 and 60 beats per minute, which in these individuals is not necessarily a pathologic condition. Primary treatment, when necessary, involves administration of atropine, a parasympathetic blocking agent.

Congestive Heart Failure

Heart failure occurs when the heart muscle weakens and cannot pump sufficient blood, when the heart valves are damaged, or because of hypertension or excessive demands on the heart. Blood pools in the veins and not enough reaches the heart. The heart compensates by pumping out more blood, causing even more pooling in the veins and

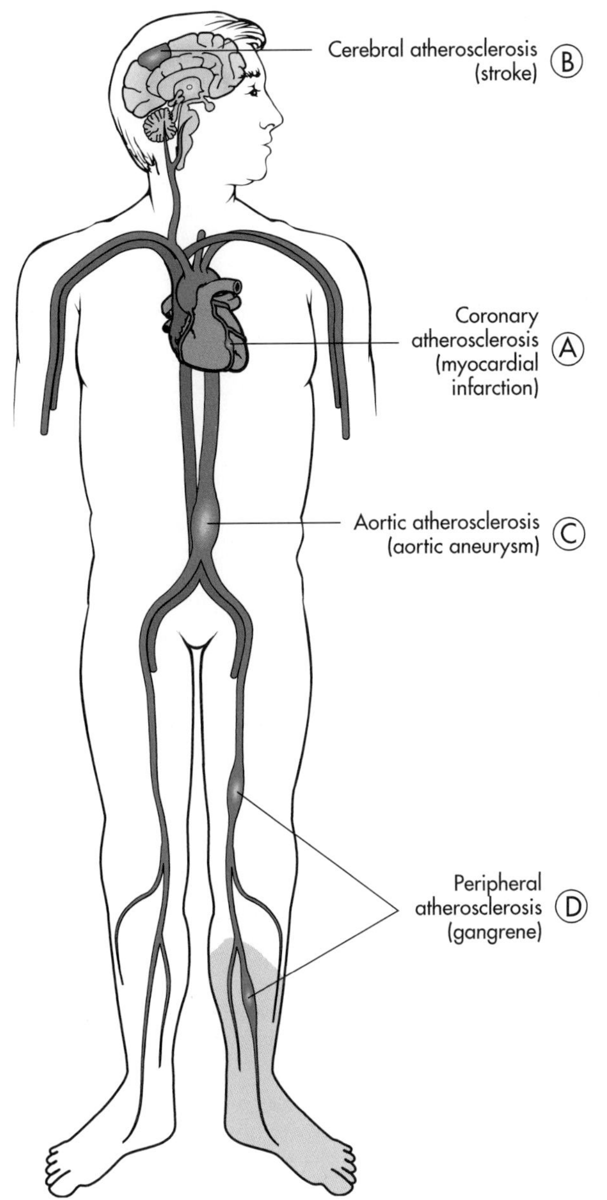

Figure 11-18
The four major forms of atherosclerosis are classified as coronary (**A**), cerebral (**B**), aortic (**C**), and peripheral vascular (**D**). (From Damjanov I: *Pathology for the health-related professions,* ed 2, Philadelphia, 2000, WB Saunders.)

organs. This buildup of fluid is called congestion; thus the condition is called congestive heart failure. Treatment usually includes use of a diuretic such as furosemide (Lasix) to eliminate excess fluid and reduce blood pressure (Figure 11-19).

Coronary Artery Disease

Coronary artery disease most often is caused by arteriosclerosis, atherosclerosis, and thrombus formation in one or more of the coronary arteries. Partial occlusion causes the transient chest and arm pain of angina. Total occlusion causes the crushing or squeezing pain of infarction. Blockage of the artery diminishes the amount of oxygen and nutrients reaching the heart tissues. Some of the many risk factors that contribute to coronary artery disease can be controlled, such as diet, weight, and avoidance of smoking. Treatment frequently includes the use of beta-blockers and calcium channel blockers to slow the heart rate and reduce the strength of the contraction. In addition to lowering the blood pressure, calcium channel blockers dilate the coronary arteries.

Edema

Edema is the accumulation of abnormal amounts of fluid in tissue spaces and often accompanies congestion, which is an increase in the volume of blood in dilated vessels. Common causes of edema are heart failure, kidney disease, and liver disease. Localized edema occurs with inflammation and lymphatic obstruction.

Embolus

An embolus is a plug in the bloodstream that may consist of a blood clot (a thrombus), plaque, air or gas, fat, tumor cells, tissue, or clumps of bacteria.

Heart and Pericardium Inflammation

Inflammation that affects the heart and pericardial sac is uncommon. Inflammation usually follows acute or chronic viral or bacterial infections or accompanies alcohol abuse or radiation therapy. The symptoms usually are mild but can lead to heart failure or arterial blockage if the condition is not treated early.

Pericarditis is an inflammation of the pericardium; *myocarditis* is an inflammation of the heart muscle. Endocarditis may affect the endocardium, heart valves, or both.

Hemophilia

Hemophilia is a bleeding disorder in which factor VIII, a vital clotting factor in the blood, is greatly diminished or lacking. In more than 75% of cases the disease is inherited. Although hemophilia is passed on by women, they usually have only minor bleeding problems or no symptoms. Men with hemophilia may have extended episodes of bleeding and may be susceptible to internal bleeding from minor trauma.

Hemorrhage

Hemorrhage refers to passage of blood outside of the cardiovascular system. Depending on the source, hemorrhage may be classified as cardiac, aortic, arterial, capillary, or venous. Clinically, hemorrhage may be of sudden onset (acute puncture wound), may be long-standing (chronic) such as from an ulcer, or may be recurrent and marked by repeated episodes of blood loss. The following are several clinical terms that describe various forms of hemorrhage:

Hemoptysis: Respiratory tract bleeding with expectoration
Hematemesis: Vomiting of blood

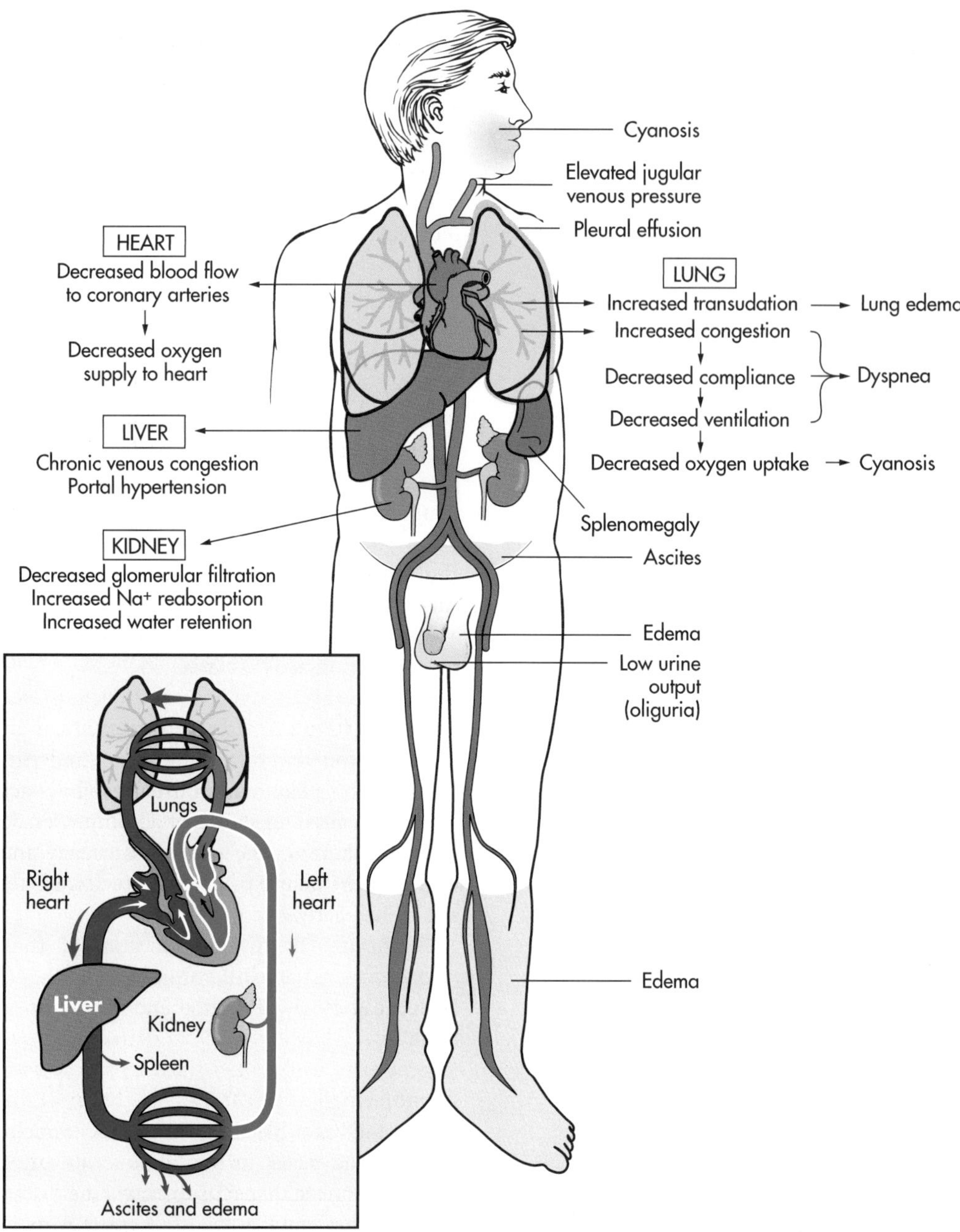

Figure 11-19
Congestion heart failure. Left heart failure leads to pulmonary edema. Right ventricular failure causes peripheral edema that is most prominent in the lower extremities. (From Damjanov I: *Pathology for the health-related professions,* ed 2, Philadelphia, 2000, WB Saunders.)

Melena: Passage of black, discolored blood in the stool. This represents upper gastrointestinal tract bleeding in which the blood is exposed to hydrochloric acid, which produces the color change.

Hematuria: Blood in the urine

Metrorrhagia: Uterovaginal bleeding. Menstrual bleeding is called *menorrhagia* (heavy menstrual bleeding).

Hypertension

Most authorities consider hypertension to be a sustained blood pressure greater than 140/90 mm Hg. Hypertension is graded as mild, moderate, borderline high, or severe, depending on the diastolic reading. In most cases the cause is unknown (essential hypertension), although kidney disease and arteriosclerosis may play a role. With hypertension, continuous sympathetic stimulation constricts arterioles. Chronic untreated hypertension leads to hypertensive heart disease. The heart becomes enlarged because of the increased work of the left ventricle against arteriolar resistance, and heart failure or infarct may result. Other important complications of untreated hypertension are stroke and kidney disease.

Nondrug therapy consists of restricting salt (which reduces fluid retention), losing weight (which reduces the resistance against which the heart must pump), reducing the consumption of alcohol, avoiding smoking, and participating in stress management and aerobic exercise programs.

Medical treatment may include a diuretic, a beta-blocker, a calcium channel blocker, an angiotensin-converting enzyme, or a combination of these medications as needed.

Ischemia

Ischemia is a temporary deficiency or diminished supply of blood to a tissue.

The student should note to take care to avoid any form of therapeutic massage over sites of thrombophlebitis or deep vein thrombosis. Systemic contraindications also may be present. The practitioner should refer any client with unexplained leg pain for diagnosis.

Mitral Valve Dysfunction

Although all valves may undergo some change in structure or function, the mitral valve is the one most commonly affected.

Mitral valve prolapse is a deformity in the mitral valves that may be congenital or may result from rheumatic fever or some other heart disease. The valve does not close completely, and blood leaks back into the left atrium. Although many persons do not notice any symptoms, others may experience chest pain, palpitation, fatigue, or shortness of breath. This condition may be a factor in anxiety-related disorders.

Mitral valve stenosis is scarring that causes the parts of the valve to stick together and gradually narrow. Blood backs up in the left atrium and pressure increases, which causes blood to back up into the pulmonary veins.

Myocardial Infarction (Heart Attack)

An infarct is an area of dead tissue that results when the blood supply to that area is cut off. Most heart attacks occur because of blockage of a coronary artery by a blood clot, especially in arteries narrowed by coronary artery disease. The blocking of blood flow damages or destroys the heart muscle. The first symptom is usually a crushing pain in the center of the chest over the sternum. Pain also may occur in the arms, neck, jaw, and upper abdomen and occasionally in the back. The person also may perspire heavily and complain of dizziness, chills, or nausea. Immediate treatment is essential.

Nutritional Anemias

Iron deficiency anemia may result from an inability to absorb sufficient iron in the small intestine or maintain iron levels in the blood. *Pernicious anemia* usually results from an inability to absorb vitamin B_{12}. Other nutritional anemias may result from folic acid deficiency or lack of intrinsic factor in the stomach.

Occlusion

An occlusion is a blockage of a vessel.

Polycythemia

Polycythemia is an increase in red cells. This condition may be normal for persons living at high altitudes, where oxygen is low, because more red cells are needed to carry what little oxygen is available. The condition also may be related directly to smoking or to taking diuretics. In rare cases actual overproduction is the problem and must be slowed to prevent serious complications.

Raynaud's Disease and Phenomenon

Raynaud's disease, a primary condition, and Raynaud's phenomenon, a secondary condition, are primarily circulatory disorders that affect the blood supply to the fingers and toes and occasionally to the nose. Temporary spasms in the small arteries reduce or stop blood flow to the area, and the skin turns pale and then blue. Tissue damage or ulceration or both may follow. The Raynaud's disorders are aggravated by cold and emotional disturbances and often occur in individuals with connective tissue disorders or other systemic or emotional disturbances.

Rheumatic Heart Disease

Rheumatic fever may occur in young children after an untreated streptococcal throat infection as an immunologic response to bacterial substances remaining in the body. Besides its signature rash, other signs and symptoms include joint pain, swelling, fever, and endocarditis. If left untreated, the endocarditis may result in rheumatic heart disease, in which the inflamed heart valves, particularly the mitral valve, become deformed.

Shock

Shock is a condition that results when the blood supply to vital organs becomes inadequate, causing diminished function of these organs. The blood vessels dilate rapidly, and blood pressure drops. The brain receives insufficient oxygen and can be damaged. Treatment usually consists of administration of intravenous fluids until the person's condition stabilizes and the cause can be determined.

The four main types of shock are *hypovolemic shock,* which results from a loss of blood or other bodily fluids; *cardiogenic shock,* which results from defective heart function, meaning the heart does not pump sufficient blood; *septic shock,* which is caused by a bacterial infection (e.g., toxic shock syndrome), and *anaphylactic shock,* which results from an allergy or overreaction of the immune system.

Sickle Cell Anemia

Sickle cell anemia is an inherited disease that affects mainly those who live in the Mediterranean region or in Africa or the descendants of these population groups. Sickle cell anemia is the most prevalent of the *hemolytic anemias,* disorders that cause premature destruction of red blood cells. In sickle cell anemia, blood cells contain hemoglobin S because of an amino acid substitution on the hemoglobin molecules. These cells collapse and, because of their abnormal shape, do not flow smoothly through the vessels and can block them. When the sickle cells block small blood vessels, multiple infarctions can result throughout the body. Common signs and symptoms are jaundice, diminished growth and development, and pain in the arms, legs, and abdomen because of lack of oxygen. Infection or a cerebrovascular accident causes death. The primary treatment is symptomatic and includes administration of oxygen, blood transfusions, and use of analgesics.

Tachycardia

In most healthy persons the heart rate increases in response to extra demands on the heart such as those imposed by exercise. In tachycardia the heartbeat increases suddenly without any increase in physical or emotional stress. Treatment ranges from no intervention to administration of sympathetic blocking agents. Interventions for persons with *paroxysmal supraventricular tachycardia* include interrupting the sympathetic signals by methods such as holding the breath or rinsing the face with cool water. Because stimulation of the vagus nerve slows the heart rate, Valsalva's maneuver (forced expiration against a closed airway) may help. A physician may massage the carotid baroreceptor or inject medication to reduce the heart rate.

Temporal Arteritis

Temporal arteritis is an inflammation of the temporal arteries, which causes pain, swelling, and tenderness. The condition also can cause a decrease or loss of vision and in severe cases stroke.

Thrombocytopenia

Thrombocytopenia is a decrease in platelets, which diminishes the ability of the blood to clot. Common causes include blood loss, infection, cancer (especially Hodgkin's disease and leukemia), and lupus. The condition also may result from radiation therapy or chemotherapy. Idiopathic thrombocytopenic purpura is an autoimmune disease in which antiplatelet antibodies are present. Common signs include easy bruising, nosebleeds, bleeding gums, and blood in the urine. Complications include cerebral hemorrhage and bleeding into nerve tissue, causing paralysis.

Thrombus

A thrombus is an intravascular clot and a type of embolus (Figures 11-20 and 11-21).

Varicose Veins

Varicose veins result when veins stretch so much that the valves cannot close sufficiently. More women than men are affected. The condition may be congenital and may result from remaining in one position (especially standing) too long or may be caused by obesity, pregnancy, or menopause. The great and small saphenous veins are affected most often.

Treatment includes rest, elevating the legs, wearing compression stockings, surgical removal of the vein, or sclerotherapy (injection of a saline solution into the vein) (Figure 11-22).

Vein Inflammation

The term *phlebitis* refers to inflammation of a vein caused by injury, infection, or swelling. These insults diminish blood flow, which may cause thrombic clots to develop, a condition known as thrombophlebitis. The superficial leg veins are the most common sites, primarily the saphenous veins. Clots also may form in the deep veins, especially in the legs and abdomen, a condition known as deep vein thrombosis. These clots can break off and travel to the lung, resulting in a pulmonary embolism (Activity 11-7).

ACTIVITY 11-7

We must be able to explain and justify the therapeutic value of the work we do. The following activity will assist you in developing the skills to explain the effectiveness of therapeutic massage to clients and other health care professionals. Use the clinical reasoning model that follows to accomplish this task. The focus should be the primary massage method applied to the cardiovascular system. An example is provided in the section opener on p. 554.

Methods/Applications

1. What are the facts?
   a. Which system is involved, and which structures of that system can be reached directly or indirectly?
   b. What is considered normal or balanced function?

ACTIVITY 11-7—cont'd

c. How are the functions of this system related to the homeostasis of the body?

d. Which of these structures are most affected by this massage?

e. Which physiologic functions are affected by the massage?

f. When the treatment is applied, what changes in function will occur in

(1) this system?

(2) the whole body?

g. What has worked or has not worked?

h. Where could you find information that would support the use of massage as a therapeutic intervention?

i. What research is available to support the use of therapeutic massage?

j. How does the intervention support a healthy state?

k. Under which pathologic, or dysfunctional, condition is the therapeutic massage most likely to be beneficial?

2. What are the possibilities?

a. What do the facts suggest?

b. List at least three applications of massage that would affect the structure and function of the system involved.

Continued

ACTIVITY 11-7—cont'd

c. What are other ways to look at the situation?

d. What other methods could provide similar benefits?

3. What is the logical outcome of therapeutic intervention?

a. What would be the logical progression of the symptom pattern, contributing factors, and current behaviors?

b. What are the benefits and drawbacks of each intervention suggested?

Benefits:

Drawbacks:

c. What are the costs in terms of time, resources, and finances?

d. What is likely to happen if massage is not used?

e. What is likely to happen if massage is used?

4. What would be the effect on the persons involved, specifically the client, practitioner, and other professionals working with the client?

a. How does each person involved (including, besides the foregoing, the client's family and support system) feel about the possible massage interventions?

b. Does the practitioner feel qualified to work with the situation and apply massage to the particular person?

ACTIVITY 11-7—cont'd

c. Does a feeling of cooperation and agreement exist among all those involved, and how would the practitioner recognize this feeling?

Justification

Using the information developed in the clinical reasoning model, present a clear, concise statement of how massage would be beneficial in supporting the particular body system in a healthy condition or as part of a treatment plan for a pathologic or dysfunctional condition.

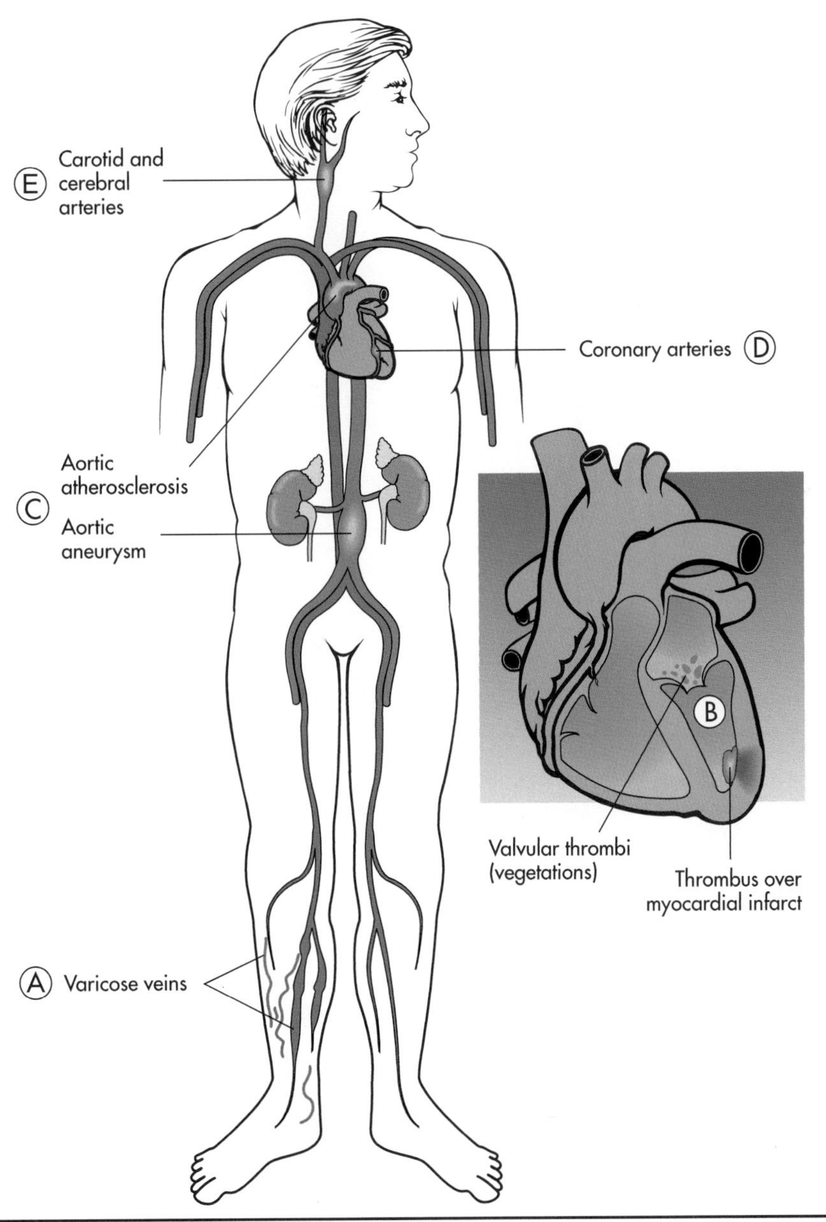

Figure 11-20

Common sites of thrombus formation. (From Damjanov I: *Pathology for the health-related professions,* ed 2, Philadelphia, 2000, WB Saunders.)

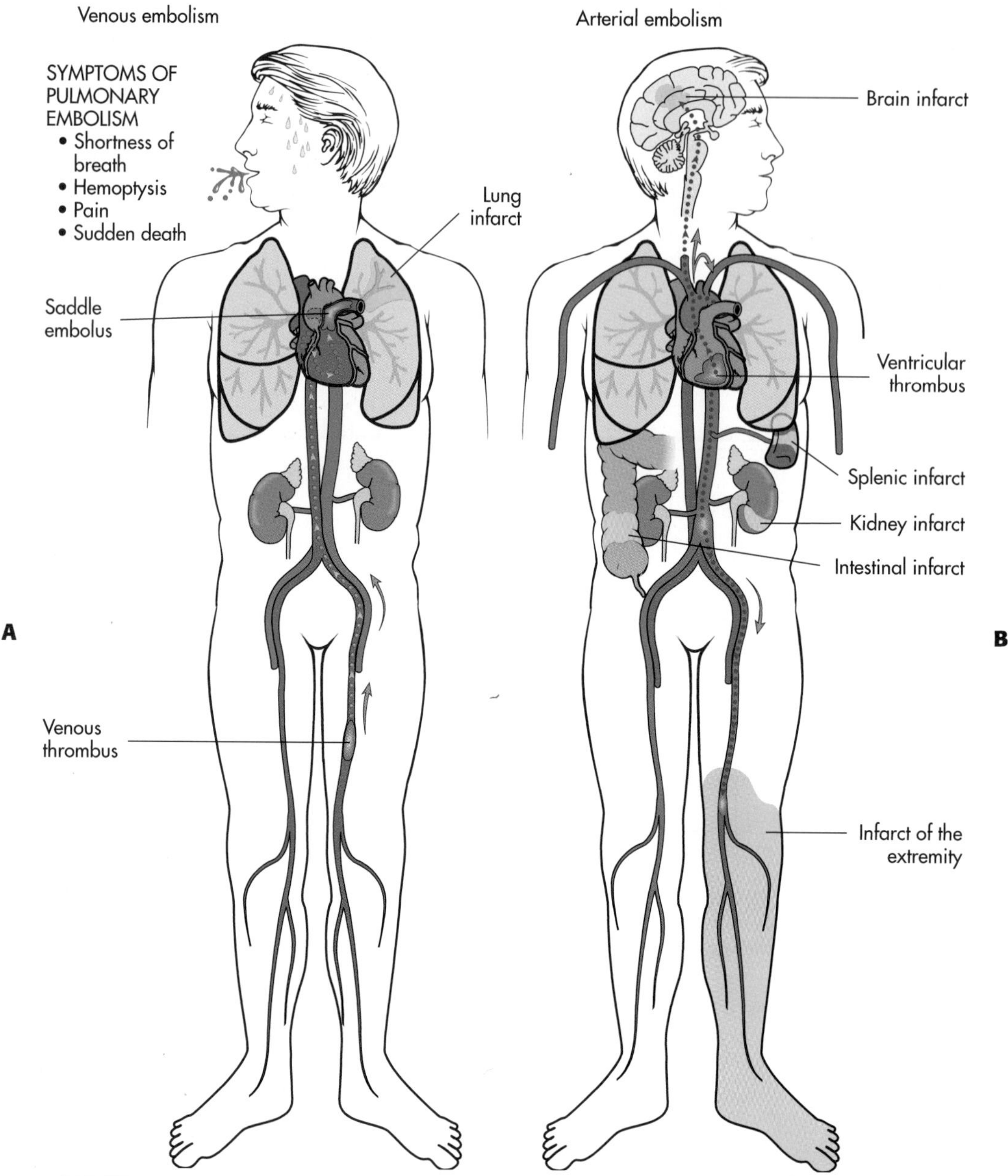

Figure 11-21
Venous and arterial emboli. **A,** Venous emboli can lodge in the lung, causing a variety of symptoms and conditions. **B,** Arterial emboli may occlude arteries in many organs. (From Damjanov I: *Pathology for the health-related professions,* ed 2, Philadelphia, 2000, WB Saunders.)

LYMPHATIC SYSTEM

The lymphatic system comprises the spleen, thymus, and lymph nodules; the lymph channels, ducts, and nodes; and lymph and lymphocytes. The lymphatic system is a one-way system that begins in the tissues and ends when it reaches the blood vessels. The system helps the body maintain homeostasis by collecting accumulated tissue fluid around the cells and returning it to the blood circulation. The lymphatics play an active part in the immune defenses of the body by filtering out and destroying foreign substances and microorganisms and also play an active role in digestion by absorbing fats from the small intestine (Figure 11-23).

Lymph

Interstitial fluid (fluid around the cells) comes from the blood as it seeps through the capillaries. Between the cells, lymph forms as interstitial fluid and becomes lymph as it moves into the lymph capillaries. Lymph contains less protein and far fewer red and white blood cells than does blood plasma. Lymph carries plasma proteins to the bloodstream and transports absorbed fats from the gastrointestinal system to the bloodstream.

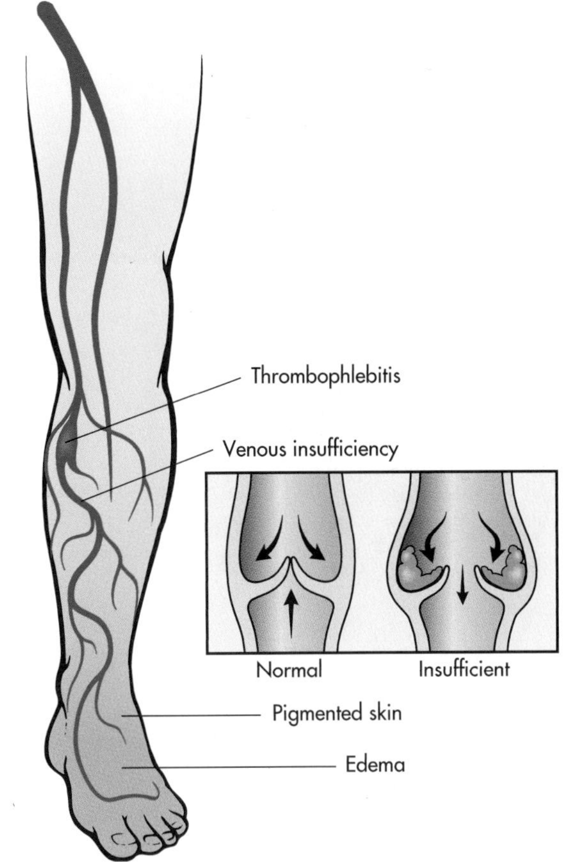

Figure 11-22
Varicose veins of the calf. The inset shows venous valvular insufficiency, which accounts for the reflux of blood. (From Damjanov I: *Pathology for the health-related professions*, ed 2, Philadelphia, 2000, WB Saunders.)

Lymph Vessels, Nodes, and Organs

Lymph Vessels

The lymph capillaries are tiny open-ended channels located in tissue spaces of the entire body except for the brain, spinal cord, and cornea (Figure 11-24). A lymphatic capillary network of vessels slightly larger than blood capillaries drains tissue fluid from nearly all tissues and organs that have a blood vascularization. The blood circulatory system is a closed system, whereas the lymphatic system is an open-ended system, beginning blind in the interstitial spaces. The moment the fluid enters a lymph capillary, a flap valve prevents it from returning into interstitial spaces. Lymph capillaries join to form larger lymph vessels that look like veins, but have thinner, more transparent walls. Like veins, they have valves to prevent back flow. The large vessels continue to merge and eventually become two main ducts called the right lymphatic duct and the thoracic duct (left lymphatic duct). The right lymphatic duct drains the upper right half of the body and empties into the right subclavian vein. The thoracic duct drains the rest of the body and empties into the left subclavian vein.

Lymph Nodes

Lymph nodes are small, round structures located along the lymph vessels. They generally are clustered at the joints, which assists in pumping lymph through the nodes when the joint moves. The superficial lymph nodes are most numerous in the groin, axillae, and neck; most of the deep lymph nodes are found alongside blood vessels of the pelvic, abdominal, and thoracic cavities. All lymph passes through one or more nodes before it enters the bloodstream and, as it passes through, can activate immune function. Lymph nodes produce mature lymphocytes, white blood cells that destroy bacteria, virus-infected cells, foreign matter, and waste materials. Production of lymphocytes increases (in nodes) when lymphatic flow increases, such as with lymphatic drainage techniques. Identification of bacteria or viruses in the lymph stimulates production of lymphocytes in the nodes. The nodes also provide a filtering system that removes waste products and transfers them for detoxification in the other systems of the body. During times of infection, the additional activity in the nodes and the buildup of the microorganisms can make the nodes swollen and painful.

The following are the locations of the lymph nodes:

- Preauricular lymph nodes are located just in front of the ear and drain the superficial tissues and skin on the lateral side of the head and face.
- Submental and submaxillary nodes are located in the floor of the mouth and drain lymph from the nose, lips, and teeth.
- Cervical lymph nodes are located at the neck.
- Superficial cubital or supratrochlear nodes are located just above the bend of the elbow and drain lymph from the forearm.
- Axillary lymph nodes located deep in the underarm and upper chest drain lymph from the arm and upper part of the thoracic wall, including the breast.
- Inguinal lymph nodes located in the groin drain lymph from the leg and external genitals.
- Popliteal lymph nodes are located behind the knee.

Spleen

The spleen, the largest of the lymphoid organs, is located near the stomach under the diaphragm. Macrophages in the spleen filter out worn-out red blood cells and destroy microorganisms in the blood. The spleen serves as a blood reservoir and can release small amounts of blood into the circulation during times of emergency or blood loss. The spleen functions with the lymphatic system by storing lymphocytes and releasing them as part of the immune response.

Thymus

The thymus gland is a triangular gland composed of lymphoid tissue and is located in the upper chest, above the superior vena cava and below the thyroid gland, where it lies against the trachea. This gland is most prominent in the newborn and begins to atrophy after puberty, becoming only a small lymphoid remnant in the adult. The thymus is

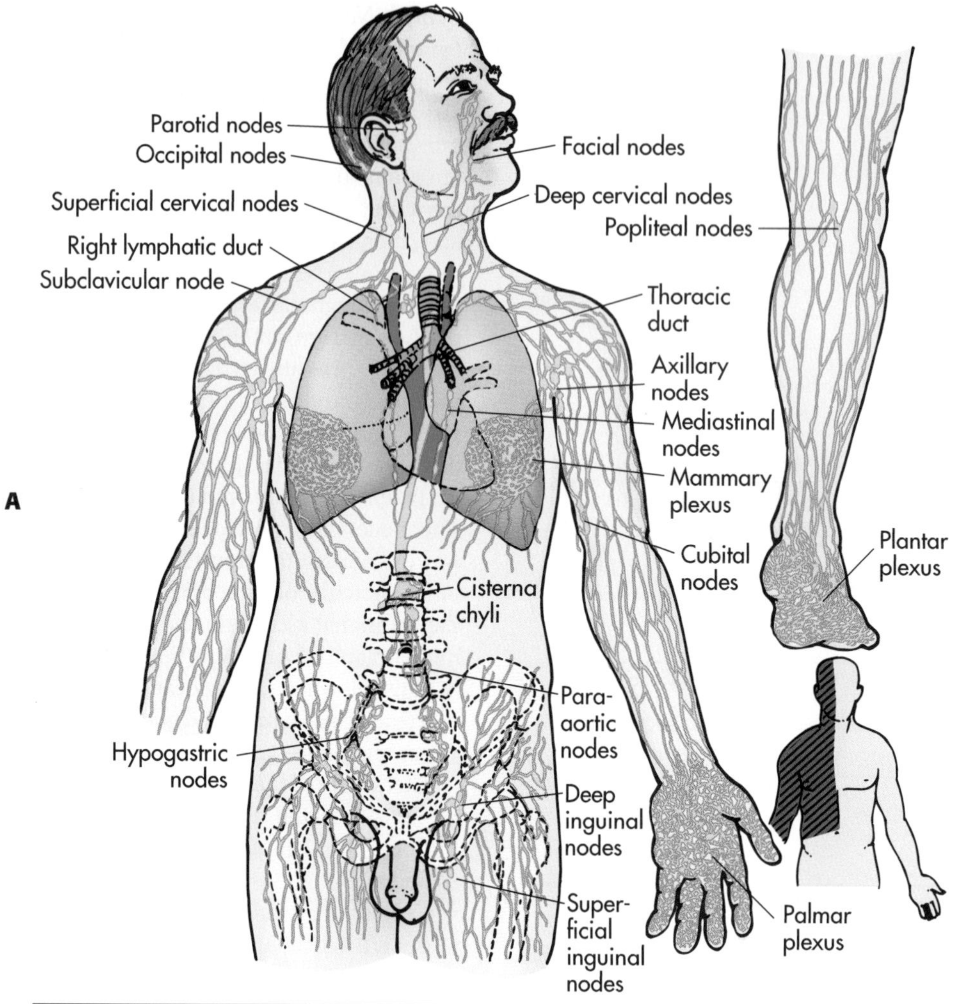

Figure 11-23
A, Principal lymph vessels and nodes. **B,** Major organs and vessels of the lymphatic system. (**A** from Birmingham JJ: *Medical terminology: a self-learning text,* ed 3, St Louis, 1999, Mosby.)

(Continued)

important in the development and maturation of certain lymphocytes and in programming them to become T cells of the immune system.

Lymph Nodules

Lymph nodules are small masses of lymph tissue (up to 1 mm or so in diameter) in which lymphocytes are produced. Collectively this tissue is referred to as *mucosa-associated lymph tissue* and along with the spleen and thymus is involved in the development of immunity. This tissue does not filter lymph but is positioned strategically to protect the respiratory and gastrointestinal tracts from microbes and other foreign material. Lymph nodules are scattered throughout loose connective tissue, especially beneath moist epithelial membranes such as those that line the upper respiratory tract, intestine, and urinary tract. Lymph nodules appear to be distributed strategically to defend the body against disease organisms that penetrate the lining of passageways that communicate with the outside of the body. A lymph nodule consists mainly of large numbers of lymphocytes enmeshed within reticular fibers. Lymph nodules do not have vessels bringing lymph to them. The periphery of the nodule is not sharply defined.

Most lymphatic nodules are small and solitary. However, some are found in large clusters. For example large aggregates of lymph nodules occur in the wall of the lower portion (ileum) of the small intestine. These large masses of lymph nodules are known as *Peyer's patches. Tonsils* are also aggregates of lymph nodules. Tonsils are located strategically under the epithelial lining of the oral cavity and pharynx to defend against invading bacteria. The tonsils therefore produce lymphocytes. The lingual tonsils are located at the base of the tongue. The single pharyngeal tonsil is located in the posterior wall of the nasal portion of the pharynx above the soft palate and often is referred to as the adenoids.

Lymph nodules include the following:

- Palatine and lingual tonsils located between the mouth and the oral part of the pharynx
- Pharyngeal tonsil located on the wall of the nasal part of the pharynx
- Solitary lymphatic follicles dispersed throughout the body

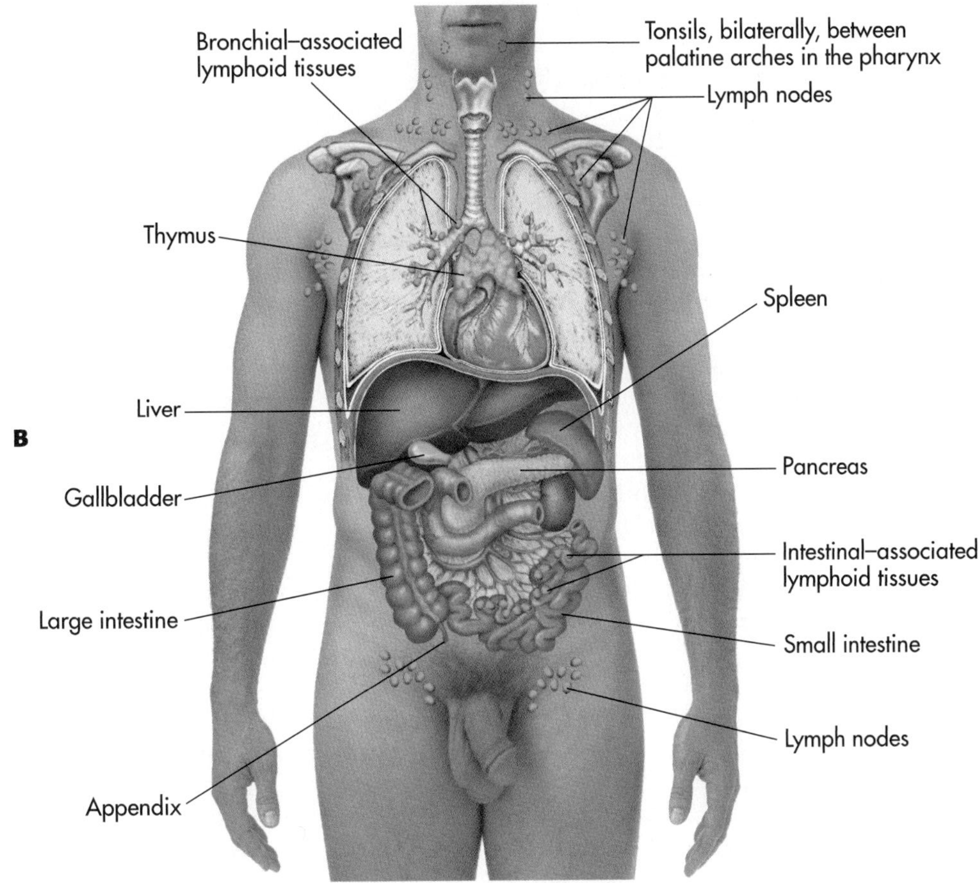

Figure 11-23—cont'd.

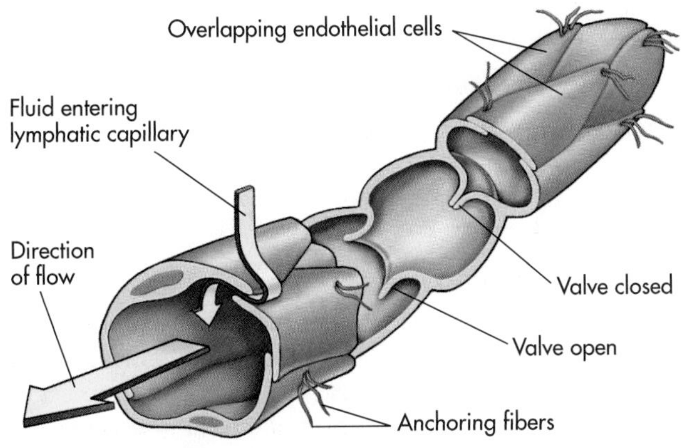

Figure 11-24
Structure of a typical lymphatic capillary. The interstitial fluid enters through clefts between overlapping endothelial cells that form the wall of the vessel. Semilunar valves ensure one-way flow of lymph out of the tissue. (From Thibodeau GA, Patton KT: *Anatomy and physiology,* ed 5, St Louis, 2003, Mosby.)

- Aggregated lymphatic follicles (Peyer's patches) located in the wall of the small intestine
- Vermiform appendix, an outgrowth from the cecum (first part of the large intestine)

Lymphatic Pump and Drainage

Collection of lymph begins in the interstitial spaces where the lymphatic system picks up a portion of fluid that has seeped from the blood capillaries around the cells for disposal. This fluid contains large waste particles and debris and other material from which the body might need to recover protein. The lymph nodes spaced along the course of the vessels screen out foreign particulate matter and pathogenic bacteria. Location of the nodes at the joints supports a pumping action. Although the lymph system has no muscular pumping organ such as the heart connected to the lymphatic vessels to force lymph onward, still lymph moves along slowly and steadily. Lymph flows through the thoracic duct and reenters the general circulation at the rate of about 3 L per day and occurs despite the fact that most of the flow is against gravity or uphill. Lymph moves through the system in the right direction because of the large number of valves that permit fluid flow only in the central direction.

Movement of lymph throughout the lymphatic system is known as lymphatic drainage, and it begins in the lymph capillaries. Lymph movement out of the interstitial spaces and into the lymph capillaries is assisted by the pressure exerted by compression of skeletal muscles against the vessels during movement, changes in internal pressure during respiration, and the opening of lymph vessels from the pull of the skin and fascia during movement. Major lymph plexuses are found on the soles and the palms, possibly because the rhythmic pumping of walking and grasping facilitate lymphatic flow. Current research suggests that the lymph vessels themselves may have an intrinsic pumping action. The vessels have valves every 6 to 20 mm that occur directly between two to three layers of spiral smooth muscles. The unit is called a *lymphangion*. The rhythmic smooth muscle contraction causes the lymph vessels to undulate almost like intestinal tract peristalsis. Some researchers think that lymphatic smooth muscle contraction produced by the lymphangions is the sensation felt by those that sense a rhythmic pulsation of the body.

The alteration of valves and smooth muscles gives a characteristic moniliform shape to these vessels, like pearls on a string.

Lymphatic circulation is separated into two layers:

1. The superficial circulation, which constitutes 60% to 70% of lymph circulation, is located just under the skin in the superficial fascia, dermoepidermic junction. The superficial circulation is not stimulated directly by exercise but is influenced by the stretching and pulling of the skin and superficial fascia during movement.
2. The deep muscular and visceral circulation, below the fascia, is activated by muscular contraction.

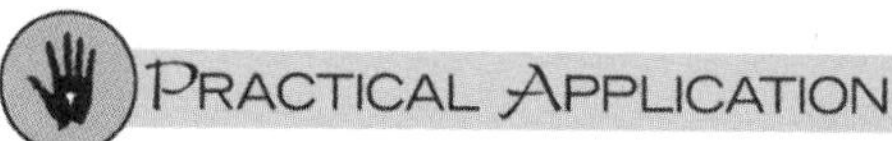

One of the extensively documented benefits of massage is stimulation of the lymphatic system. Simple muscle tension and binding of connective tissues puts pressure on the lymph vessels and may block them, interfering with efficient drainage. Therapeutic massage can normalize muscle tension and connective tissue pliability. As the muscles relax and the connective tissue has more space, the lymph vessels open.

Specialized application of massage can be effective in increasing lymph removal from stagnant or edemic tissue. Massage application using light pressure to drag the skin significantly increases superficial lymph movement by crosswise and lengthwise stretching of the anchoring filaments of the lymph vessels, which open the lymph capillaries, thus allowing the interstitial fluid to enter the lymphatic system. The practitioner applies the massage strokes along the direction of normal lymphatic drainage and speeds up lymph movement.

The lymph from the left arm flows from the fingers toward the axilla and from there flows to the neck region where it joins the thoracic duct. Lymph from the right arm does the same as the left except that it drains into the smaller right lymphatic duct. Both ducts empty into the junction of the subclavian and internal jugular veins. The lymph from the right side of the chest, face, and scalp also flows toward the right axilla and into the right lymphatic duct. The lymph from the left side of the face and scalp flows into the thoracic duct.

The lymph from the feet and legs drains upward toward the groin into the abdomen and empties into the lower end of the thoracic duct called the *cisterna chyli*.

Eighty-five percent of the lymph flow from the chest drains into the respective axillary nodes. The remaining lymph drains into nodes located behind the sternum and lymph vessels located in the pectoralis muscle. In general, move toward the groin and the axilla.

Lymphatic massage mechanically stimulates the flow of lymph by tracing the lymphatic routes with light pressure to drag the skin to pull the skin and superficial connective tissues affecting the anchoring filaments of the lymph capillaries, ultimately opening them. The focus of the pressure is on the dermis just below the surface layer of skin and the layer of tissue just beneath the skin and above the muscles (the superficial fascia). Little pressure is required to reach the area; too much pressure presses the capillaries closed and nullifies any effect.

Rhythmic, gentle, passive and active joint movement and rhythmic muscle contraction reproduces the normal way the body pumps lymph, especially the deep lymphatic circulation. During massage, the practitioner can stimulate this process by using rhythmic compression with enough depth to compress the muscles. The client helps the process by breathing slowly and deeply, which stimulates lymph flow. When possible, one should position the area being massaged above the heart so that gravity can assist the lymph flow. Because lymph capillary plexuses are present on the bottoms of the feet, rhythmic compression on the soles also enhances lymph flow. When applying lymph drainage techniques, one must take care to avoid excessive increases in the volume of lymph flow in persons who have heart and kidney conditions, for the venous system must accommodate the load once the fluid has been delivered to the subclavian veins. Significantly increasing the load could place excessive strain on the heart and kidneys (Figure 11-25). ■

Pathologic Conditions

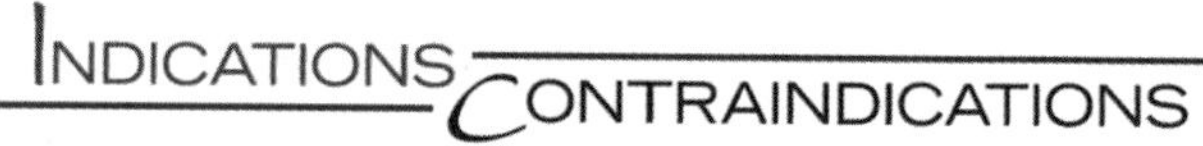

For Therapeutic Conditions

Massage is contraindicated for malignant and infectious conditions until the client's health care professional gives approval. Modification of massage application is necessary depending on the type of treatment the client is receiving and the stress and fatigue levels. Massage that relaxes the client supports well-being and is helpful.

The practitioner can manage simple edema with massage application focused to support the lymphatic system. The appropriate health professional needs to supervise massage application for clients with more complicated lymphedema. ■

Hodgkin's Disease

Hodgkin's disease is a painless swelling of the lymph nodes, primarily in the neck and groin, caused by enlarged, mutated macrophages. Radiation and chemotherapy are the primary treatment methods, and this disease has one of the highest cure rates for any form of cancer. Some individuals may require bone marrow transplantation.

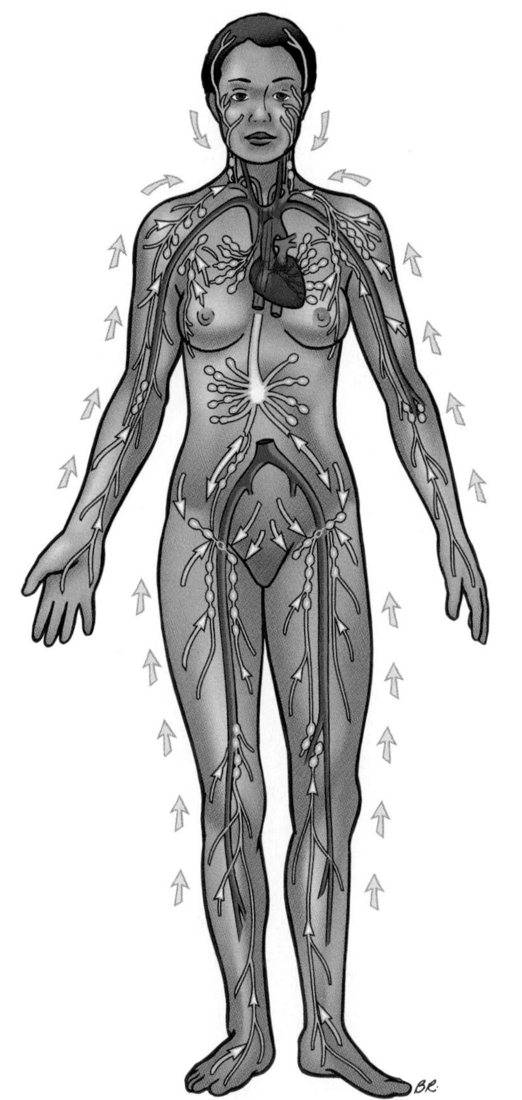

Figure 11-25
Direction of strokes for facilitating lymphatic flow. (From Fritz S: *Mosby's fundamentals of therapeutic massage,* ed 3, St Louis, 2004, Mosby.)

Infectious Mononucleosis

Infectious mononucleosis is a contagious viral infection more common in teenagers and young adults. Mononucleosis affects the lymphocytes, causing an increase in the number and a change in the structure of some of these cells. The infection is transmitted primarily by kissing, hence its nickname, the "kissing disease." Common signs and symptoms are fever, sore throat, enlarged cervical lymph nodes, a rash, and in some, anemia. Complications include a ruptured spleen, hepatitis, encephalitis, meningitis, and depression. The primary treatment is bed rest for several weeks or months.

Leukemia

Leukemia is cancer of the white blood cells. Not only does the body produce abnormal cells at a faster rate, but also these cells live longer. Because the cancerous cells do not have the same structure as healthy white blood cells, they function differently. Leukemic cells do not perform the functions of phagocytosis. They build up and invade the organs of the body, interfering with organ function. Leukemia may affect red blood cell and platelet production, which takes place in the marrow, resulting in anemia or diminished clotting ability. Brain hemorrhage and infection may follow.

Leukemia may progress rapidly (acute leukemia) or slowly (chronic leukemia). In most cases the acute forms show mostly immature blast cells, and the chronic forms show mostly mature types. Two categories of leukemia are described by the white blood cell they affect. Lymphocytic leukemia affects the cells that become lymphocytes; myelocytic leukemia is a cancer of the cells that develop into granulocytes or monocytes. The myelocytic leukemias also may be identified by the terms *granulocytic* or *monocytic leukemia.*

The common leukemias are as follows:

Acute myelogenous leukemia: Develops rapidly and demonstrates symptoms such as an increase in infections, sores in the mouth, and an increased tendency to bruise or bleed.

Chronic myelogenous leukemia: Found in young adults and most often associated with a chromosome abnormality.

Acute lymphoblastic (acute lymphocytic) leukemia: Affects children, with a peak incidence at 5 years of age; frequently can be cured with chemotherapy, and complete remission often occurs.

Chronic lymphocytic leukemia: Affects older persons; the increase in abnormal white cells reduces the number and effectiveness of the normal white blood cells, sometimes resulting in anemia and an increase in infections; often no therapy is required unless symptoms are evident.

Lymphedema

Lymphedema is an increase of tissue fluid caused by inflammation or obstruction from scar tissue, parasites, or trauma. For example, after a radical mastectomy, in which axillary lymph channels are removed, arm drainage often is blocked partly and the arm swells. The primary treatment for generalized edema is cautious use of diuretics to remove the fluid. Some forms of massage are effective for managing moderate lymphedema. External pumping sleeves that rhythmically compress the area are beneficial in chronic cases. The practitioner should refer a client with any form of edema for diagnosis because edema is symptomatic of many disease processes, particularly cardiovascular disease.

Lymphomata

A lymphoma is a tumor of the lymphatic system that is almost always malignant. Most lymphomata are first felt as enlarged, painless lymph nodes or lymphoid tissues. Lymphomata generally are divided into two categories: Hodgkin's disease and non-Hodgkin's lymphoma.

Non-Hodgkin's Lymphoma

Non-Hodgkin's lymphoma is any cancer of lymphoid tissue that is not classified as Hodgkin's disease. Most non-

Hodgkin's lymphomata involve mutation of lymphocytes, correlation with retroviruses, or T-cell leukemia. As with Hodgkin's disease, the first symptom is swollen lymph nodes, most often in the neck, axilla, or groin. But unlike Hodgkin's disease, non-Hodgkin's lymphoma is a grouping of diverse lymphomata that may manifest different primary and secondary symptoms. Non-Hodgkin's lymphoma often is subcategorized by grade and area of tumor involvement.

Some forms of leukemia may be classified as lymphomata because they involve lymphocytes. However, not all types of leukemia are disorders of the lymphoid tissues; instead, some could be classified as blood disorders (Activity 11-8).

ACTIVITY 11-8

We must be able to explain and justify the therapeutic value of the work we do. The following activity will assist you in developing the skills to explain the effectiveness of therapeutic massage to clients and other health care professionals. Use the clinical reasoning model that follows to accomplish this task. The focus should be the primary massage method applied to the lymphatic system.

Methods/Applications

1. What are the facts?
   a. Which system is involved, and which structures of that system can be reached directly or indirectly?
   b. What is considered normal or balanced function?
   c. How are the functions of this system related to the homeostasis of the body?
   d. Which of these structures are most affected by this massage?
   e. Which physiologic functions are affected by the massage?
   f. When the treatment is applied, what changes in function will occur in
      (1) this system?
      (2) the whole body?
   g. What has worked or has not worked?
   h. Where could you find information that would support the use of massage as a therapeutic intervention?
   i. What research is available to support the use of therapeutic massage?

ACTIVITY 11-8—cont'd

j. How does the intervention support a healthy state?

k. Under which pathologic, or dysfunctional, condition is the therapeutic massage most likely to be beneficial?

2. What are the possibilities?

a. What do the facts suggest?

b. List at least three applications of massage that would affect the structure and function of the system involved.

c. What are other ways to look at the situation?

d. What other methods could provide similar benefits?

3. What is the logical outcome of therapeutic intervention?

a. What would be the logical progression of the symptom pattern, contributing factors, and current behaviors?

b. What are the benefits and drawbacks of each intervention suggested?

Benefits:

Drawbacks:

c. What are the costs in terms of time, resources, and finances?

d. What is likely to happen if massage is not used?

e. What is likely to happen if massage is used?

Continued

ACTIVITY 11-8—cont'd

4. What would be the effect on the persons involved, specifically the client, practitioner, and other professionals working with the client?

   a. How does each person involved (including, besides the foregoing, the client's family and support system) feel about the possible massage interventions?

   b. Does the practitioner feel qualified to work with the situation and apply massage to the particular person?

   c. Does a feeling of cooperation and agreement exist among all those involved, and how would the practitioner recognize this feeling?

Justification

Using the information developed in the clinical reasoning model, present a clear, concise statement of how massage would be beneficial in supporting the particular body system in a healthy condition or as part of a treatment plan for a pathologic or dysfunctional condition.

IMMUNE SYSTEM

Immunity is a complex response that networks all of the systems in our bodies to eliminate any pathogen, foreign substance, or toxic material that can be damaging to the body. The immune system is not a specific structural organ system; rather, it is a functional system (Figures 11-26 and 11-27). The immune system responds in one of two ways by drawing on the structures and processes of each of the organs, tissues, and cells and the chemicals produced in them. In a *nonspecific (innate) immune response,* the body responds exactly the same way to all substances that are not identified as part of the body. Nonspecific response is programmed genetically in the human body. *Specific immunity* involves specific responses to each identified foreign substance and calls on special memory cells to help if that pathogen reappears. Specific immunity can be acquired in one of two ways: through natural immunity, which is the result of natural exposure, or through artificial immunity, in which a substance, such as a vaccine, is introduced into the body to stimulate the immune response.

The key to immunity is the ability of the body to recognize self and nonself. The recognition of self begins during fetal development and continues throughout life. In many psychologic approaches and spiritual practices, self-recognition is also a core issue—who am I? When this recognition of self breaks down, the body attacks itself or fails to defend against antigens. Life tends to do the same thing when our sense of mental or spiritual self breaks down. Psychologic approaches provide structure, methodology, and professional support for the rediscovery of the self. Spiritual healing practices often provide community, ritual, and disciplines for self-understanding and self-awareness. These same practices often are integrated into aspects of mind/body medicine. The concept that knowing the self supports health makes sense.

The body must be able to identify which substances are capable of causing a threat before initiating any kind of response. This recognition is immunologic. An *antigen* is any substance that causes the body to produce *antibodies.* Antigens are usually proteins identified as harmful or potentially dangerous to the body. Foreign antigens are those that come from outside the body, and self-antigens are those that come from within. An antibody is a specific protein produced to destroy or suppress antigens. *Microorganisms* are minute life forms that may be damaging to the body or may interfere with its function.

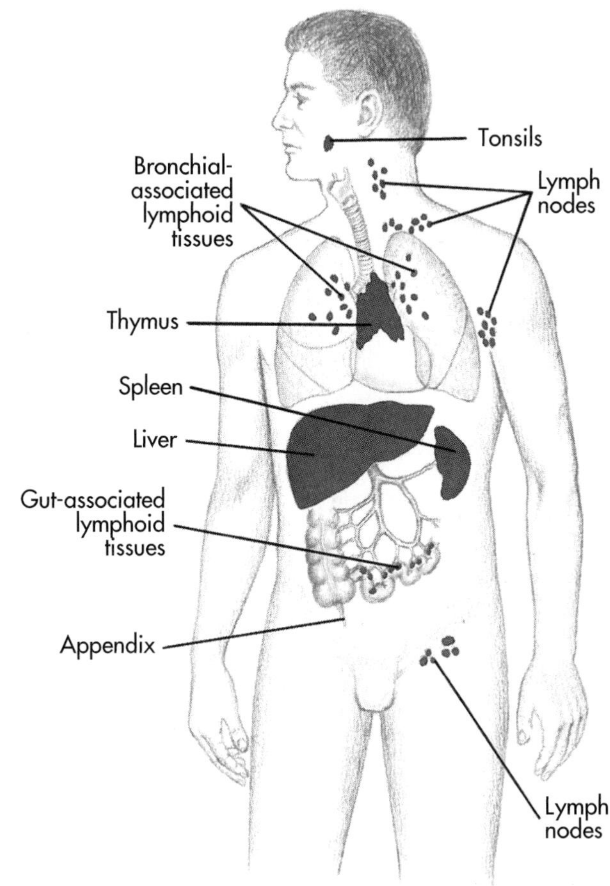

Figure 11-26
Organization of the immune system. Cellular constituents of the immune system are derived from bone marrow stem cells. When they mature, these cells are released into the peripheral blood flow and subsequently populate organized tissues of the lymphoreticular system. (From Thompson JM, et al: *Mosby's clinical nursing,* ed 5, St Louis, 2002, Mosby.)

Microorganisms share the property of being submicroscopic. Many microorganisms do not normally cause disease in human beings, existing in a state of *commensalism,* in which the organism gives little or no benefit or harm to human beings, or in *mutualism,* in which both gain some benefit. This nonharmful balance exists when the immune system works well, but these same organisms can cause infection if the immune system does not function properly. Many other microorganisms can cause infectious disease and are called *pathogens.* Pathogens, as explained in Chapter 2, fall into five main groups:

1. Viruses
2. Bacteria
3. Fungi
4. Protozoa
5. Pathogenic animals

In addition, two other classes of small agents can cause disease:

1. Ticks and mites
2. Mesozoa and leeches

These organisms cause *infestations* rather than infectious disease.

Infectious disease is by far the greatest cause of disease and death worldwide. Respiratory infections and gastrointestinal infections cause more deaths worldwide than all other diseases added together. General symptoms of infectious diseases are as follows:

- Fever
- Increased catabolism
- Malaise

Opportunistic infections occur when the normal human defenses are so weak that they allow infection to take place by organisms that generally would not be able to cause infection in a healthy human being. *Nosocomial infections* are transmitted in hospitals; some of these may be opportunistic infections or may occur because of the special nature of the hospital environment.

The time between the exposure to a pathogen and the first appearance of symptoms is called the *incubation period,* and although no symptoms are apparent, the organism may be causing substantial damage during this time. A period known as the *prodrome* may follow in which nonspecific signs and symptoms such as headache, fever, and lethargy appear before the development of the acute phase and specific symptoms. Once the acute stage has passed, a period of *resolution* occurs in which the severity of the symptoms gradually decreases. Finally, *convalescence* occurs in which the symptoms have largely disappeared, but the body is still recovering.

The time, course, and severity of the disease depends on the balance between the virulence (strength) of the infecting agent and the success with which the immune system combats the organism. Some infections may occur that are not sufficiently severe to produce clinical symptoms, and these are called *asymptomatic* or *subclinical infections. Clinical infection* has a number of outcomes covering the spectrum between death and complete recovery. *Latency* refers to a situation in which a pathogen persists in a dormant, inactive form without causing damage but may reactivate to cause problems at a later date. An example is herpes simplex virus, which lies dormant within dorsal root ganglia after the primary infection but may reactivate periodically to cause cold sores.

Microorganisms are everywhere. They are in the air we breathe and in or on the food we eat. Thus our epithelial surfaces (skin, respiratory tract, gastrointestinal tract, and genitourinary tract) are exposed continuously to microorganisms. Disease occurs when microorganisms invade epithelial surfaces. In view of our constant exposure to microorganisms, what is surprising is that we enjoy long, infection-free periods and that infections are the exception rather than the rule.

When the immune system operates effectively, it intelligently protects the body from most infectious microorganisms and any of the cells of the body that have turned against it, that is, cells that have overreacted in their response or that develop and grow at an unhealthy rate or by mutating (cancer). The immune system does this directly by cell attack and indirectly by releasing mobilizing chemicals and protective antibody molecules.

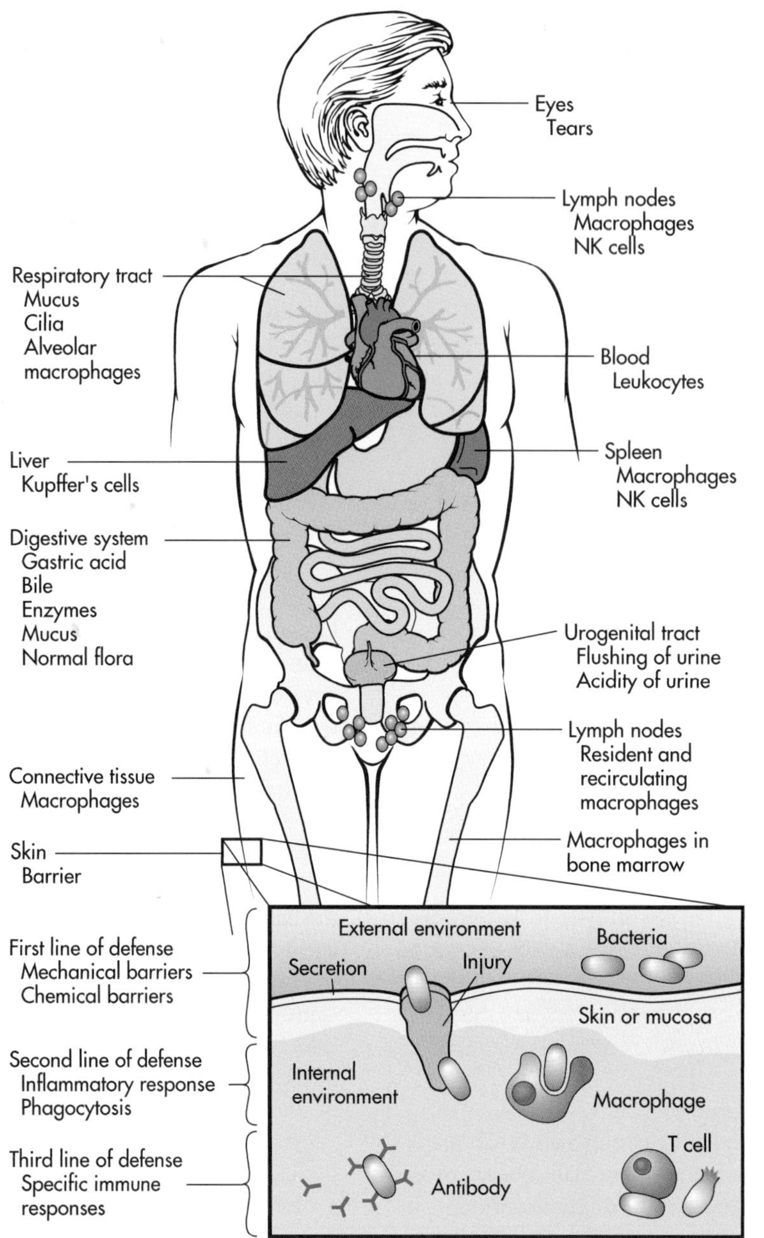

Figure 11-27

Natural protective mechanisms of the human body. *NK*, natural killer (cells). (From Damjanov I: *Pathology for the health-related professions*, ed 2, Philadelphia, 2000, WB Saunders.)

Nonspecific Defenses

Nonspecific (innate/natural) immunity can involve actions such as sneezing or coughing to remove microorganisms from the respiratory tract. Keeping the structure of the skin intact prevents potentially damaging substances from entering the body. Vomiting and diarrhea remove offending substances from the digestive tract. No matter what the substance is, the body responds in the same manner, with the same chemicals and cells mediating the actions. This general response is a preventive measure and a first response in immune function.

Cellular response is the action of the blood cells, primarily white blood cells, that deals with pathogens. Natural killer cells are a subset of lymphocytes that can eliminate virus-infected cells. Cells such as macrophages and neutrophils begin to phagocytize, or to surround and destroy, pathogens. Basophils and mast cells (from connective tissue) release chemicals that initiate inflammation. Eosinophils release chemicals that slow or stop the inflammatory response—how the body maintains homeostasis.

Chemical response includes not only the chemicals released by the previously mentioned cells but also substances found throughout the body. Our skin and mucous membranes maintain a certain degree of acidity that prevents entry of foreign pathogens. Mucus is sticky and contains enzymes that destroy these microorganisms, and saliva, tears, and urine actually wash them out of the body. *Complements* are proteins found in blood that combine to create substances that phagocytize bacteria. *Interferon* is a protein produced by cells infected by viruses. Interferon forms antiviral proteins to help protect uninfected cells.

Inflammatory response is a sequence of events involving chemical and cellular activation that destroys pathogens and aids in the repair of tissues (see Chapter 2). For example, when damage occurs to tissue, basophils and mast cells release chemicals that increase the blood flow, which brings neutrophils and macrophages to the area. The phagocytic white cells, mainly macrophages, enter the tissues to destroy any bacteria. At the same time, the chemical response changes the permeability of the blood vessel wall so that fibrin can enter the tissues to repair the damage. This process continues until the repair of the damage and removal of all bacteria is complete (Figure 11-28).

Sanitary practices such as hand washing, disinfecting, and sterilization support immunity by preventing exposure to pathogens. Each body area has a mechanical aspect of innate immunity.

Skin

Just as the husk on a fruit or berry protects it from drying up in drought or swelling up in rain, so the skin protects the body from the undue entry or loss of water. The skin contains glands known as sebaceous glands. These glands are associated with the hair follicles and are most numerous on the scalp, the face, the middle of the back, and around the genitalia. They produce a substance known as sebum, which comprises triglycerides, waxes, paraffins, and cholesterol. The main function of the sebum is to waterproof the skin, but sebum also is thought to have an antibacterial action. The skin also protects from minor mechanical blows. When intact, the skin is virtually impermeable to microorganisms and also protects from chemicals (weak acids, alkalis, etc.) and most gases, although some gases developed for use in chemical warfare can be absorbed through the skin. The integument gives some protection from physical trauma, for instance from some forms of radiation such as alpha rays and, to a lesser extent, from beta rays. The skin is totally impermeable to alpha rays, and beta rays can penetrate only a few millimeters, thus the skin protects the underlying organs from their potentially harmful effects. In addition, melanin in the skin protects it from the harmful effects of ultraviolet radiation.

Each square centimeter of skin may contain up to 3 million microorganisms, most of which are harmless. The skin does not provide a hospitable environment for bacteria unless they have become adapted through evolution to live there. The application of strong deodorants and the use of strong soaps that alter the skin pH from acid to alkaline upset the fine balance that exists between our parasites and us. These tend to kill or inhibit the normal flora, leaving the area open to potential colonization by pathogens.

Arms and legs have the fewest microorganisms (only 1000 to 10,000 per square centimeter), whereas the forehead may contain as many as 1 million per square centimeter and between the toes, up to 1 billion per square centimeter.

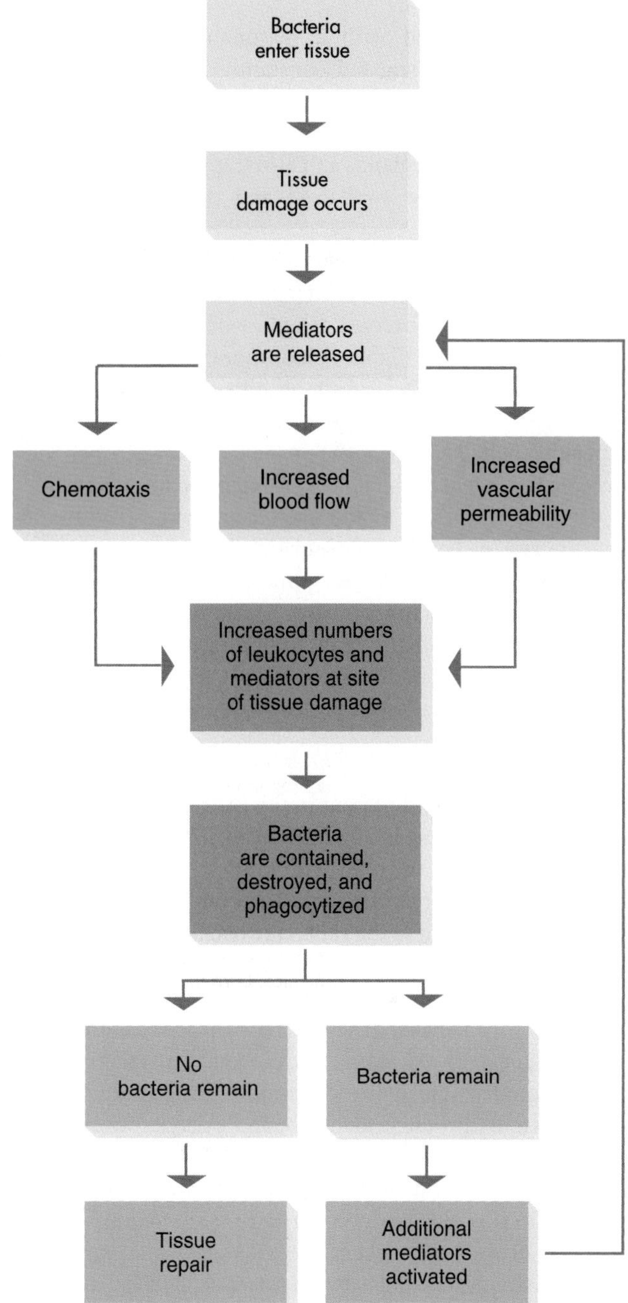

Figure 11-28
Inflammatory response. Tissue damage caused by bacteria triggers a series of events that produces the inflammatory response and promotes phagocytosis at the site of injury. These responses tend to inhibit or destroy the bacteria. (From Thibodeau GA, Patton KT: *Anatomy and physiology,* ed 5, St Louis, 2003, Mosby.)

Microorganisms thrive in moist conditions, and so the axillae (armpits) and groin provide favorable areas for their growth. The skin can never be sterilized completely. The topical application of alcohol and iodine-based lotions may cause the death of a large percentage of resident organisms, but such applications do not remove those bacteria that inhabit the hair follicles and make up at least 20% of the resident bacteria.

Mouth

The mouth is lined with a reasonably tough mucous membrane that is irrigated constantly by a back flow of saliva. This flow is directed toward the throat and has the dual purpose of preventing microorganisms from infecting the salivary glands and also trapping the organisms so that they can be swallowed and disposed of in the digestive tract.

Saliva contains an enzyme called *lysozyme* that is antibacterial and mucus that in turn contains immunoglobulin A. Persons who have become dehydrated have a reduced flow of saliva and are at a higher risk of mouth infections.

The resident bacteria of the mouth are generally harmless. Indeed, some such as alpha-hemolytic streptococcus are a positive benefit because they produce hydrogen peroxide (a bleaching agent), which helps to keep the mouth clean.

Persons who are on a prolonged course of oral antibiotics run the risk of having their normal flora (bacteria) wiped out, which can result in the opportunistic infection of the mouth by other microorganisms. A common organism that can become problematic is the unicellular fungus *Candida albicans,* which causes thrush.

The tonsils also assist in protecting the oral cavity.

Stomach

The hydrochloric acid present in the gastric juices produced by the stomach lining is of a sufficiently low pH to kill most organisms entering the body with food or drink or by being swallowed. Some organisms, however, can resist this strong acid. Examples include the tubercule bacillus, enteroviruses, salmonella, and the eggs of parasitic worms.

Milk and proteins are effective buffers against stomach acid, and organisms that enter the stomach accompanied by this type of food stand more chance of escaping the damaging effects of hydrochloric acid. Thus contaminated meat and dairy products tend to be more dangerous in terms of acquiring an infection.

One may regard vomiting as a defense mechanism because it rids the body of irritants and toxins such as alcohol, drugs, and bacterial toxins in some instances, although this protection is by no means fully effective.

Intestines

The small and large intestines rely to a great extent on the bactericidal action of the stomach.

In addition, the normal beneficial flora of the area such as *Escherichia coli,* nonhemolytic streptococci, and anaerobic bacteroides contribute to the normal functioning of the gut. The importance of their role becomes more evident when the administration of broad-spectrum antibiotics or indiscriminant use of laxatives removes them. The intestines then are open to colonization by pathogenic bacteria such as *Staphylococcus pyogenes* that may be resistant to antibiotics.

In addition, the small and large intestines are supplied liberally with lymphatic tissue throughout their length. The lymph participates in the nonspecific and acquired immune defense systems of the body.

One also may regard diarrhea, like vomiting, as a defense mechanism, although in most instances it occurs far too late in the course of an infection to be of much benefit.

Respiratory Tract

Upper respiratory tract. Hairs in the nose prevent insects and large particles from entering the upper respiratory tract. The ciliated nasal mucosa secretes a backward-flowing stream of mucus that traps smaller particles and has bactericidal and virucidal properties. Lysozyme is also present in nasal secretions.

The epithelium of the upper respiratory tract is thin and unfortunately is prone to infections by rhinoviruses and adenoviruses, which are not affected by the nasal secretions. Sneezing is a protective reflex that expels irritants.

Trachea and lungs. The trachea and bronchi are lined with a ciliated mucous membrane that serves to trap any organisms in debris that may have escaped through the upper tract. The cilia beat upward and hence shift a stream of mucus away from the lungs and toward the pharynx to be swallowed. Should any organisms reach the alveoli, alveolar macrophages phagocytose them. The lung is well supplied with lymph nodes that act as another filter.

Coughing is a defensive reflex that removes particulate matter or excess mucus in the lower tract.

Genitourinary Tract

The constant downward flow of urine through the ureter and bladder tends to protect against ascending infections. Urination irrigates the urethra. Urination is an effective response in the long male urethra but is less so in the female. The adult female urethra is only 2 or 3 cm long and forms a short and readily available entry point for organisms to invade the bladder.

Sexual activity in the female may predispose to the occurrence of cystitis (inflammation of the urethra). The most common offending organism is coliform bacillus from the perineal area.

The beneficial resident flora of the vagina, especially lactobacillus, helps to maintain an acid environment, creating an inhospitable habitat for invading pathogens. Some vaginal deodorants disturb the pH balance of the vaginal area and can result in infection, often from the opportunistic *Candida albicans.*

Eye

Tears produced by the lacrimal glands constantly irrigate the surface of the eyeball. Tears contain high levels of lysozyme, in fact the highest of any of the body secretions, and as a result this forms an effective barrier against infection. If the diet lacks in vitamin A, the production of lysozyme in the tears decreases and can predispose a person to eye infection. Blinking is a defense reflex that eliminates irritants and ensures even distribution of the tears.

In some conditions, such as facial paralysis or stroke, this reflex is lost, and preventing the eye from drying up by keeping it closed or covered and by regular irrigation becomes necessary.

Ear

Ceruminous glands located in the outer ear canal are modified sweat glands that produce cerumen or ear wax. Cerumen provides a sticky barrier to foreign agents entering the ear canal.

Specific Immunity

Specific immunity is the ability to recognize certain antigens and to destroy them (Table 11-1).

Lymphocytes are the cells of specific immunity because they can recognize and destroy specific molecules. Memory cells are the reason that, after we have had a disease such as measles, the lymphocyte pattern set up with the first infection can respond to a second exposure and prevent reinfection. Lymphocytes develop in the following three ways:

1. T cells begin in the bone marrow and grow in the thymus. They are able to recognize antigens and respond by releasing inflammatory and toxic substances. Specialized T cells also regulate immune responses. T4 cells release molecules that amplify the response, and T8 cells suppress the response of the body. Some T cells develop into memory cells and handle secondary response on reexposure to antigens that already have produced a primary response.
2. B cells grow and develop in the bone marrow. B cells contain immunoglobulin, an antibody that responds to specific antigens. Some B cells modify and become antigen nonspecific, which provides them with a greater ability to respond to bacterial and viral pathogens. Some B cells, like T cells, become memory cells and handle reexposure to antigens.
3. A few lymphocytes do not develop the same structural or functional characteristics as the T cells and B cells. These null cells are known as natural killer cells. They also develop in the bone marrow and, when mature, can attack and kill tumor cells and virus-infected cells during their initial developmental stage before the immune system is activated. Plasma cells are fully differentiated descendants of B lymphocytes.

Because of the structure of the body, specific defense responses can develop quickly. Because lymph capillaries pick up proteins and pathogens from nearly all body tissues, immune cells in lymph nodes are in a strategic position to encounter a large variety of antigens. Lymphocytes and macrophages in the tonsils act primarily against microorganisms that invade the oral and nasal cavities, and the spleen acts as a filter to trap blood antigens.

Antibodies are serum proteins of the immunoglobulin class secreted by plasma cells. Antibody production begins with contact between an antigen and the cells of the immune system. Any substance identified by the body as foreign could become an antigen and stimulate an immune response. This activation of B cells produces specific antibodies that can react with the antigen.

Lymphocytes use three ways to fight infection:

Strategy One: Elimination of extracellular microorganisms.

In response to infection, B cells mature into plasma cells that secrete soluble recognition molecules (antibodies). B cells recognize microbes because they express membrane-bound antibody that acts as an antigen receptor.

In the primary response, at the time of first infection no antibody exists in blood, and the level of antibody does not begin to increase until 7 to 10 days afterward. The level of antibody rises slowly to a low peak and then gradually declines toward baseline.

In the secondary response, on subsequent exposure to the same microorganisms the level of antibody begins to increase within 24 hours and reaches and sustains a high level.

Antibody recognizes structures on surface of microorganisms and proteins, carbohydrates, and

TABLE 11-1
Types of Specific Immunity

TYPE	DESCRIPTION OR EXAMPLE
Inherited immunity	Immunity to certain diseases develops before birth; also called inborn immunity.
Acquired immunity	
Natural immunity	Exposure to the causative agent is not deliberate.
Active (exposure)	A child develops measles and acquires an immunity to a subsequent infection.
Passive (exposure)	A fetus receives protection from the mother through the placenta, or an infant receives protection via the mother's milk.
Artificial immunity	Exposure to the causative agent is deliberate.
Active (exposure)	Injection of the causative agent, such as a vaccination against polio, confers immunity.
Passive (exposure)	Injection of protective material (antibodies) that was developed by another individual's immune system.

From Thibodeau GA, Patton KT: *Anatomy and physiology,* ed 5, St Louis, 2003, Mosby.

lipids. Thus serum from an immune individual contains many different types of antibodies, each of which recognize different structures on the surface of the membrane.

Antibodies are soluble and diffuse through tissues to target extracellular microorganisms. Binding of antibody to microorganisms activates mechanisms to eliminate the microorganisms.

Strategy Two: Elimination of microorganisms that normally survive for long periods in macrophages.

The primary response does not kill some microorganisms, but they survive and multiply in macrophages. Elimination occurs by use of a subpopulation of cells called *helper T cells.* These cells recognize macrophages containing intracellular bacteria by means of a T cell antigen receptor, which is not an antibody. They help macrophages to kill bacteria by synthesizing soluble molecules (cytokines) that stimulate bacterial-killing mechanisms of macrophages.

Strategy Three: Elimination of microorganisms that infect cells without an endogenous antimicrobial defense system.

Viruses can infect any type of cell, and most cells do not possess antimicrobial mechanisms. During intracellular replication, virus proteins appear on the surface of the infected cell. A second subset of T cells, cytotoxic T cells, recognizes these virus (foreign) antigens and secretes cytotoxic molecules that kill the infected cells.

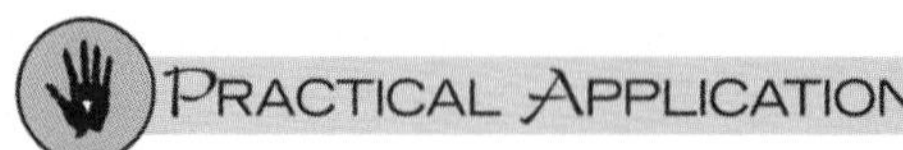

Homeopathy is a form of health care that introduces minute energetic forms of various plants and other substances into the body. The premise is that if large doses of a substance cause a particular physiologic response (e.g., vomiting), minuscule energetic tracings of the same substance would rally the defenses of the body to restore balance to whatever was causing the disruption.

The concept of vaccination is similar to and may have been based on the concept of homeopathy. The difference is the strength of the product. Vaccines are weakened or killed forms of the actual pathogen, whereas homeopathic substances are energetic forms of the actual substance. Live vaccines can cause disease, as apparent by the symptoms babies sometimes develop when they receive their immunizations. However, both systems seek to activate and teach the body to protect and heal itself. ■

Immune System Dysfunction

The organizational structure and responses of the immune system can break down (Box 11-1). The imbalances that occur are *immune deficiencies, hypersensitivity,* and *autoimmune diseases.*

Immune deficiency is a condition in which the body is unable to mount the proper immune response to a pathogen. An analogy would be an office that has too much

BOX 11-1

Four Classes of Immune Hypersensitivity Malfunction

Type I Immediate Anaphylactic Hypersensitivity

The results of this type of reaction are exemplified best by allergic asthma, atopic dermatitis (eczema), allergic rhinitis (hay fever), and acute urticaria (hives).

Type I hypersensitivity is considered to be one of the most powerful effector mechanisms of the immune system. This reaction begins rapidly. The most serious or extreme systemic form is **anaphylaxis.**

Allergies now are recognized as common, affecting 20% of all persons in the United States. Allergies are considered the most common immune disorder in the world.

Type II Antibody-Dependent Cytotoxic Hypersensitivity

Type II hypersensitivity, which involves antibody responses against antigens on cells, is also an immediate reaction such as with incompatible blood from a transfusion.

Exposure to certain medications can cause a similar process; the drug molecules probably combine with a protein in the blood before being misidentified as an antigen.

Penicillin and its derivatives are responsible for most of the recorded allergic reactions to drugs and 97% of the deaths caused each year by drug allergies.

Symptoms are typically mild: hives, some fever, chills, swelling of lymph nodes, and sometimes arthritic-like discomfort.

Type III Immune Complex–Mediated Hypersensitivity

The immune system misidentifies a protein in antiserum as potentially harmful and develops a response against the antiserum.

Type III response is similar to type I in that some of the same effects occur: blood vessel dilation, sneezing, coughing, and itching.

Type IV Cell-Mediated (Delayed Type) Hypersensitivity

Type IV hypersensitivity involves T cells and activated macrophages, not antibodies.

This type of reaction is an important part of the process of immunity to many intracellular infectious agents, and this response also is involved in graft rejection and tumor immunity.

work and not enough workers to get the job done. The work piles up, the workers get further and further behind, and eventually the office system breaks down. Some immune deficiencies are present at birth. These congenital problems affect the development of lymphocytes and result in severe inability to respond to disease. Other immune deficiencies arise later in life, such as acquired immunodeficiency syndrome (AIDS). Chronic stress also suppresses the immune system. Stress can be caused by physical mechanisms (e.g., chronic pain), other forms of chronic disease, or unresolved emotional or spiritual disturbances. When immunosuppressed, the body is more likely to be susceptible to a variety of bacterial, viral, and toxic pathogenic activity.

Hypersensitivity

The immune system also can become overactive, a condition called hypersensitivity or allergy. Few persons die from an allergy, but allergies can make life miserable. Allergy can be understood by equating the immune system response to creating mountains out of molehills. Anaphylactic shock is the exception, and although rare, it is life-threatening. *Anaphylactic shock* is a severe, usually immediate reaction to a substance that causes respiratory distress, anxiety, and weakness. In extreme cases, anaphylactic shock also can involve arrhythmia and can result in death if not treated immediately (see Box 11-1).

Autoimmune diseases occur when the body cannot distinguish self from nonself; self-antigens are treated as foreign antigens. When the recognition of self breaks down, the immune cells begin to attack the self. Some of the autoimmune diseases are multiple sclerosis, Graves' disease, rheumatoid arthritis, and juvenile diabetes.

Mind/Body Connection

The sheer power of the mind to affect the body as a whole and the general state of health is amazing. Scientists have confirmed that a witch doctor can cause death simply by telling those who believe in his powers that they are going to die. Moreover, scientists have confirmed that we can think ourselves to health.

Studies of neuroimmunomodulation have discovered that left-handed persons are more likely to suffer immune system disorders than are right-handed persons. These studies indicate that the left hemisphere most directly controls the immune cells through the T cell response, but that the right hemisphere enhances and modulates the response. Other investigations have shown that although the nervous and immune systems have different chemical languages, they seem to share a few of the more important chemical signals such as those of the opiate neuropeptides. Like neurons, many cells involved with the immune response have receptors for the opiate neuropeptides, which have long been known to influence mood and behavior. Many scientists are convinced that macrophages have receptors for these neuropeptides, which are released by pain-sensing neurons and lymphocytes. Why these cells, which are active in immunity, should respond or react to chemicals used by the nervous system to deal with pain is not understood fully. This process is thought to be an important link in the communication between the brain and body.

High levels of natural opiates or heroin suppress natural killer cell activity. During times of stress and severe depression, T cells are depressed, which weakens the immune system and increases our susceptibility to physical illness. Hormones such as corticosteroids and epinephrine also provide chemical links between the two systems.

Immune function gradually declines as we age. Scientists do not understand this process, but studies in longevity have found a link between living vitally in the advanced years and a balanced life that includes physical activity, a simple diet, a moderate lifestyle, regular sleep and wake cycles, loving relationships, a sense of purpose or reason for being, and spiritual strength. These same factors have been shown to support the immune response and the regeneration and healing capacities of the body.

Immunity is a bodywide process. The integumentary system, especially the keratinized epithelial cells, provides a mechanical barrier, and these same cells act as an alarm system, triggering responses when the integument is breached. The skeletal system provides the bone marrow as the developmental home for the lymphocytes and macrophages. Heat from the muscle system actively initiates feverlike effects. The nervous and endocrine systems directly interact, linking the mind/body effects of the immune response through a shared chemical language. The cardiovascular system provides the travel network, lymphatic system, and filtering system. The respiratory system provides oxygen needed by immune cells, and the digestive system nourishes the immune cells and secretes acids hostile to pathogens. The urinary system eliminates waste and maintains the protective acid balance. The reproductive system works with the endocrine system to influence the process through hormone function.

The immune system is truly the best example of teamwork or a multidisciplinary approach in the body, and a lesson can be learned here. When any one of us does not do our job, others are overtasked; in the body, this is immune deficiency. When we overreact, our hypersensitivities are unproductive and we feel miserable, wasting energy that could be better used in other ways. When we are unaware of our self (autoimmunity), not only do we attack ourselves, we also cannot combine efforts to support others. Again, energy for the common good is wasted, and a lack of self-recognition destroys us, little by little. The amazing multidimensional links of the immune system support the idea that we truly are what we think, eat, do, hate, love, breathe, support, and become. Living well in our own bodies and sharing space with all forms of life on this planet reflects the ancient spiritual wisdom of living in a balanced way with cooperation and respect.

Pathologic Conditions

INDICATIONS CONTRAINDICATIONS

For Therapeutic Massage

Therapeutic massage approaches support immune function by supporting balanced homeostatic functions. No specific methods are used for the immune system, yet any behavior that supports wellness, including regular massage, supports immunity. Any modality that normalizes autonomic nervous system functions supports immunity.

Any activity, including therapeutic massage, that causes the body to adapt puts stress on the system. If the client is basically healthy, he or she will be able to adapt without overstressing the body. However, if a client is immune suppressed, the reserves to adapt are already at the breakdown point. The practitioner must gauge the intensity and duration of bodywork methods against the ability of the body to adapt, so that the stress introduced supports a return to balance and is not "the straw that breaks the camel's back." The premise of "less is more" is a wise approach for individuals with immune dysfunction. Massage professionals should follow Standard Precautions.

AIDS and HIV Infection

AIDS is caused by a dysfunction in the immune system of the body. The diseases of AIDS are caused by germs encountered in everyday life. In fact, some of these germs live permanently in small numbers inside the human body. When the immune system weakens, these germs have the opportunity to multiply freely; thus the diseases these germs cause are called *opportunistic diseases.*

The human immunodeficiency virus (HIV), which may be responsible for AIDS, is a ribonucleic acid (RNA) virus. In most RNA viruses the viral RNA directly hijacks the host cell. However, HIV is different. After the virus enters the host cell, the RNA strand "writes" dual strands of viral DNA (the opposite of human cells). This backward writing is called reverse transcription. The newly written DNA strands then go on to hijack the cell and oversee the production of new RNA replicas. Reverse-writing viruses such as HIV are called retroviruses.

As a group, retroviruses can live in their hosts for a long time without causing any sign of illness. In most animals, retrovirus infections last for life. Retroviruses are not tough; they die when exposed to heat, are killed by many common disinfectants, and usually do not survive if the tissue or blood they are in dries up. However, retroviruses have a high rate of mutation and as a result tend to evolve quickly into new strains or varieties. HIV seems to share this and other traits with other known retroviruses.

HIV likes to replicate (live) in the lymphocytes, or T cells. The favorite target of the virus is the T4 cell. The T4 cell, also called the helper/inducer T-cell, performs a vital job in the immune system by finding germ invaders while circulating through the bloodstream and bumping into them. On recognizing the invading germ, the T4 cell releases a chemical alarm that triggers other parts of the immune system into action.

HIV infection of the T4 cells creates a defect in the immune system that eventually may cause AIDS. After HIV hijacks a T cell, the lymphocyte stops functioning normally, although this change is not immediately apparent. Then . . . nothing happens. Evidently, little or no viral replication takes place for an indefinite period. The HIV takeover is a quiet event.

When the T4 cell does become active, rather than functioning normally, it manufactures viral RNA strands. An infected T4 cell no longer detects invaders and triggers alarms. Eventually, the infected T4 cells begin to die, gradually reducing the T4 cell alarm network and allowing opportunistic diseases to enter and grow within the body.

HIV must travel from the inside of one person to the inside of another person, arriving with its RNA strands intact. Then the virus, or its intact RNA strands, must get into the bloodstream of the new host and find and enter a T cell. Once inside a host cell, HIV can prepare for replication. After replication, replica viruses infect other host cells, probably attaching to new host cells when the infected host cell collides with other cells in the bloodstream.

Viruses generally are not able to enter the body through intact skin. Therefore, viruses must enter the body through an open wound or one of a number of possible body openings. Most of these body openings contain mucous membranes, which protect most openings and passages in the human body. These membranes secrete mucus, which contains germicidal chemicals and keeps the surrounding tissues moist. Mucous membranes are found in the mouth, inside the eyelids, in the nose and air passages leading to the lungs, in the stomach, along the digestive tract, in the vagina, in the anus, and inside the opening of the penis. Many viruses, if placed on the surface of a mucous membrane, can travel through the membrane and enter the tiny blood vessels inside.

The danger with HIV is different. With HIV, the major infection sites are the bloodstream and central nervous system. Although HIV-carrying macrophages (roving white blood cells that engulf invaders but are susceptible to HIV infection) are found in the connective tissues of the lungs and in oral and mucous membranes, the number of viral organisms present does not seem great. Thus HIV is present in low concentrations, if at all, in saliva and sputum. Therefore coughing should not expel a large quantity of HIV, if any. Apparently, HIV cannot cross the mucous membrane easily, and large concentrations of HIV probably are necessary.

HIV can be found in any bodily fluid or substance that contains lymphocytes. Substances that contain lymphocytes include blood, semen, vaginal and cervical secretions, mother's milk, saliva, tears, urine, and feces.

The presence of HIV in a substance does not necessarily mean that the substance is capable of transmitting HIV infection. All of these substances are capable, in theory, of transmitting disease, but in reality the most dangerous substances seem to be blood, semen, cervical and vaginal secretions, and perhaps feces. Despite much looking, no one has been able to find a clear-cut case of saliva causing transmission, although kissing theoretically could.

The concentration of HIV in these substances is important when it comes to infection. The higher the concentration of viral organisms in a substance, the more likely it is that HIV can be transmitted by that substance. Below a certain concentration of organisms, the substance cannot effectively transmit HIV infection.

Hepatitis

Hepatitis is an inflammatory process and an infection of the liver caused by a virus. Hepatitis A, the less serious form, usually is transmitted by fecal contamination of food and water and does not become chronic. Once infected, a person becomes immune to future hepatitis A infections.

Hepatitis B is transmitted through routes similar to those for HIV. Hepatitis B may be acute or chronic. The acute symptoms are similar to those of hepatitis A, but hepatitis B is much more severe in the chronic and acute stages. As liver cells die, liver function is impaired, and death can result.

Two types of vaccines are available for preventing hepatitis B. More than 1 million persons in the United States are estimated to be carriers of the hepatitis B virus. Hepatitis B is 100 times more contagious than HIV.

Hepatitis C accounts for 85% of the new cases of hepatitis each year. Hepatitis C is transmitted mostly by blood transfusions or when intravenous drug users share needles. This disease usually becomes chronic.

Hepatitis D infects only those who have hepatitis B, and the symptoms are more severe than other forms of hepatitis. Vaccines do not appear to be effective for hepatitis D.

Hepatitis E is transmitted through food and water contaminated with feces and is usually a self-limited type of hepatitis that may occur after natural disasters.

The treatment for all forms of hepatitis is rest and a high-protein diet. Observance of the Standard Precautions can prevent the spread of hepatitis. Obviously, persons must avoid all behaviors that are means of transmission for HIV and HBV.

Autoimmune Disease

The inflammatory response triggered by the immune complex is the pathogenic mechanism of tissue injury in a number of autoimmune diseases, including arthritis, vasculitis, and glomerulonephritis (Table 11-2). Immune complex injury may result from activation of resident tissue inflammatory cells and the recruitment of circulating monocytes or neutrophils to various sites. A growing consensus among scientists is that common disorders such as atherosclerosis, colon cancer, and Alzheimer's disease are caused in part by a chronic inflammatory syndrome (Activity 11-9).

ACTIVITY 11-9

We must be able to explain and justify the therapeutic value of the work we do. The following activity will assist you in developing the skills to explain the effectiveness of therapeutic massage to clients and other health care professionals. Use the clinical reasoning model that follows to accomplish this task. The focus should be the primary massage method applied to the immune system.

Methods/Applications

1. What are the facts?

   a. Which system is involved, and which structures of that system can be reached directly or indirectly?

   b. What is considered normal or balanced function?

   c. How are the functions of this system related to the homeostasis of the body?

   d. Which of these structures are most affected by this massage?

Continued

ACTIVITY 11-9—cont'd

e. Which physiologic functions are affected by the massage?

f. When the treatment is applied, what changes in function will occur in

(1) this system?

(2) the whole body?

g. What has worked or has not worked?

h. Where could you find information that would support the use of massage as a therapeutic intervention?

i. What research is available to support the use of therapeutic massage?

j. How does the intervention support a healthy state?

k. Under which pathologic, or dysfunctional, condition is the therapeutic massage most likely to be beneficial?

2. What are the possibilities?

a. What do the facts suggest?

b. List at least three applications of massage that would affect the structure and function of the system involved.

c. What are other ways to look at the situation?

d. What other methods could provide similar benefits?

ACTIVITY 11-9—cont'd

3. What is the logical outcome of therapeutic intervention?

   a. What would be the logical progression of the symptom pattern, contributing factors, and current behaviors?

   b. What are the benefits and drawbacks of each intervention suggested?

   Benefits:

   Drawbacks:

   c. What are the costs in terms of time, resources, and finances?

   d. What is likely to happen if massage is not used?

   e. What is likely to happen if massage is used?

4. What would be the effect on the persons involved, specifically the client, practitioner, and other professionals working with the client?

   a. How does each person involved (including, besides the foregoing, the client's family and support system) feel about the possible massage interventions?

   b. Does the practitioner feel qualified to work with the situation and apply massage to the particular person?

   c. Does a feeling of cooperation and agreement exist among all those involved, and how would the practitioner recognize this feeling?

Justification

Using the information developed in the clinical reasoning model, present a clear, concise statement of how massage would be beneficial in supporting the particular body system in a healthy condition or as part of a treatment plan for a pathologic or dysfunctional condition.

TABLE 11-2
Types of Autoimmune Disorders

DISEASE	PRIMARY SITE/MODE OF ACTION	DESCRIPTION
Addison's disease	Surface antigens on adrenal cells	Hyposecretion of adrenal hormones, resulting in weakness, reduced blood sugar, nausea, loss of appetite, and weight loss
Cardiomyopathy	Cardiac muscle	Disease of cardiac muscle (i.e., the myocardium), resulting in loss of pumping efficiency (heart failure)
Diabetes mellitus (insulin-dependent or type I)	Pancreatic islet cells, insulin, insulin receptors	Hyposecretion of insulin by the pancreas, resulting in very high blood glucose levels (in turn causing a host of metabolic problems, even death if untreated)
Glomerulonephritis	Blood antigens form immune complexes that deposit in kidney	Disease of the filtration apparatus of the kidney (renal corpuscle), resulting in fluid and electrolyte imbalance and possibly total kidney failure and death
Graves' disease (type of hyperthyroidism)	Thyroid-stimulating hormone receptors on thyroid cells	Hypersecretion of thyroid hormone and resulting increase in metabolic rate
Hemolytic anemia	Surface antigens on red blood cells (RBCs)	Condition of low RBC count in the blood because of excessive destruction of mature RBCs (hemolysis)
Multiple sclerosis	Antigens in myelin sheaths of nervous tissue	Progressive degeneration of myelin sheaths, resulting in widespread impairment of nerve function (especially muscle control)
Myasthenia gravis	Antigens at neuromuscular junction	Muscle disorder characterized by progressive weakness and chronic fatigue
Myxedema	Antigens in thyroid cells	Hyposecretion of thyroid hormone in adulthood, causing decreased metabolic rate and characterized by reduced mental and physical vigor, weight gain, hair loss, and edema
Pernicious anemia	Antigens on parietal cells; intrinsic factor	Abnormally low RBC count resulting from the inability to absorb vitamin B_{12}, a substance critical to RBC production
Reproductive infertility	Antigens on sperm or tissue surrounding ovum (egg)	Inability to produce offspring (in this case because of destruction of gametes)
Rheumatic fever	Cardiac cell membranes (cross-reaction with group A streptococcal antigen)	Rheumatic heart disease; inflammatory cardiac damage (especially to the endocardium and valves)
Rheumatoid arthritis	Collagen	Inflammatory joint disease characterized by synovial inflammation that spreads to other fibrous tissues
Systemic lupus erythematosus	Numerous	Chronic inflammatory disease with widespread effects and characterized by arthritis, a red rash on the face, and other signs
Ulcerative colitis	Mucous cells of colon	Chronic inflammatory disease of the colon characterized by watery diarrhea containing blood, mucus, and pus

From Thibodeau GA, Patton KT: *Anatomy and physiology,* ed 5, St Louis, 2003, Mosby.

SUMMARY

The justification activities in this chapter and in Chapter 12 represent the outcomes of a competency-based education.

In fact, all of the problem-solving activities support competency. Being a competent massage therapist is much more than recall of factual data. Competence is based on how you use that data in a professional application of massage. Clinical reasoning is necessary to use information in professional practice. How do you plan and organize an effective massage session? How do you provide assessment to determine indications and contraindications for massage? How do you choose a massage application based on physiologic effects? How do you collect and analyze data to develop appropriate treatment plans and then provide informed consent? How do you know if you are functioning within your scope of practice? How do you identify the most logical approach for massage application including things such as time management, body mechanics and ergonomic practice, and type of equipment needed? How do you evaluate the behaviors, feelings, and outcomes of the professional relationship measured against the outcomes of the massage? All of this plays into ethical professional practice including principles of respect, benefits that outweigh the burden of treatment, do no harm, etc.

This chapter began with a discussion of touch, an important topic that certainly one could explore in more depth, because massage therapy depends on touch, not only for therapeutic benefit but also for the compassionate, nurturing connection between practitioner and client.

We presented basic anatomy, physiology, and pathologic conditions of the integumentary, cardiovascular, lymphatic, and immune systems.

The justification exercises began the process of explaining and validating therapeutic massage. Being able to justify the effectiveness of therapeutic massage in supporting health maintenance or as part of a multidisciplinary approach for pathologic conditions will become increasingly important as more persons use these methods. Being able to explain the benefits of therapeutic massage and the skills each professional has to offer, based on a solid foundation of anatomy and physiology, adds to professional development and supports the use of these important treatments.

For the student to find the justification activities difficult is common. Rising above the discomfort to achieve an integrated practice is necessary. The student should go back and do the activities again and again using different scenarios and conditions. The student should remember that in professional practice, clinical reasoning, problem solving, and integrating knowledge with application is the measure of a competent massage therapist.

evolve

Log on to your student account on the Fritz EVOLVE site and read the therapeutic massage case study under Course Materials Chapter 11. Then, list the reasons that justify the effectiveness of therapeutic massage in supporting health maintenance for the cardiovascular system.

WORKBOOK SECTION

SHORT ANSWER

1. What are some of the major functions of the integumentary system?

2. List the appendages of the skin.

3. What are the two main concerns with integumentary pathologic conditions?

4. List and describe the three types of arteries and give an example of each type.

5. List the four sets of heart valves and explain what each set does.

6. Why is venous blood return important? List factors that can affect it.

7. What are the five groups of white blood cells?

8. How is blood supplied to the heart? What happens if this supply is interrupted?

9. What are the normal and abnormal heart sounds, and how are they produced?

10. What are the normal ranges for blood pressure based on size, and what are the terms used for high blood pressure and low blood pressure?

____

____

____

____

____

11. What are the two main lymphatic ducts? How are they formed, and into what do they empty?

____

____

____

____

____

____

12. What are lymph nodes and where are they found?

____

____

____

____

____

13. What is the name of the defense system of the body, and in what way does it respond to threats?

____

____

____

____

____

____

____

14. How is nonspecific immunity provided?

____

____

____

____

____

FILL IN THE BLANK

The (1) _______________ is made up of the skin and its appendages: hair, sebaceous glands, sweat glands, nails, and breasts.

The (2) _______________ is the outer layer of skin; it consists of sublayers called strata. Four or five layers of strata make up the outer layer of skin, depending on the location on the body.

The (3) _______________, the inner layer of skin, is much thicker than the epidermis and is composed of dense connective tissue that contains collagen and elastin fibers. The various appendages of the skin originate in the dermis and push upward through the epidermis. Blood vessels and nerves are present in the dermis but not in the epidermis. Subcutaneous tissue, which is located below the dermis, is also called (4) _______________ _______________. It consists of loose connective tissue and contains fat (adipose) tissue.

The (5) _______________ _______________ is a transport system composed of the heart, blood vessels, and blood. It functions to bring nutrients to the tissues and remove waste products from them.

One part of the cardiovascular system, the (6) _______________, is a hollow, muscular pump about the size of a closed fist. It is located in the (7) _______________, the space between the lungs. The (8) _______________ is a sac that surrounds the heart. It secretes a lubricating fluid that prevents friction caused by the movement of the heart.

The two small, thin-walled upper chambers of the heart are the (9) _______________, known separately as the right atrium and left atrium. They are separated by the thin interatrial septum. The two large lower chambers are the left and right (10) _______________. Their thick walls are separated by the interventricular septum.

(11) _______________ _______________ is the amount of blood pumped by the left ventricle in 1 minute.

WORKBOOK SECTION

The average output is 5 to 6 L of blood under normal conditions.

The (12) ________________ ________________ is the sequence of events in one heartbeat. It consists of diastole and systole. The average person has 60 to 70 cardiac cycles per minute. The number of cardiac cycles in 1 minute is known as the (13) ________________ ________________.

The vascular system is the other part of the cardiovascular system. The vascular system consists of blood vessels that carry blood from the heart to the lungs and body tissues and back to the heart in a continuous cycle. Blood vessels that transport blood from the heart are called (14) ________________; these branch off into smaller and smaller arteries. The smallest of the arteries are called the (15) ________________.

(16) ________________ are the tiny blood vessels located between the arterioles and the veins. The function of the (17) ________________ is to collect blood from the capillaries and transport the blood back to the heart. The smallest of the veins are the (18) ________________. The veins get larger as they get closer to the heart. The largest veins return blood to the right atrium of the heart.

The amount of pressure exerted by the blood on the walls of the blood vessels is called (19) ________________ ________________. The maximal pressure is called (20) ________________ ________________; this occurs when the ventricles contract. (21) ________________ ________________ occurs when the ventricles relax. Blood pressure is measured with a (22) ________________, a cloth-covered rubber bag that is wrapped around the arm over the brachial artery. Blood pressure is highest during contraction of the heart (systole), which produces the systolic blood pressure. Blood pressure is lowest when the heart is relaxing (diastole), which gives the diastolic pressure.

The hepatic portal system begins in the capillaries of the digestive organs and ends in the (23) ________________ ________________. Portal blood contains substances absorbed by the stomach and intestines. Portal blood is passed through the (24) ________________, which absorbs, excretes, or converts nutrients and toxins. Restriction of outflow through the hepatic portal system can lead to (25) ________________ ________________.

(26) ________________, the thick, red fluid in our bodies, is a form of connective tissue. It transports nutrients to the individual cells and removes waste products.

The cellular substances in blood are red blood cells, white blood cells, and platelets. Blood cells float in a thick, straw-colored fluid called (27) ________________. Red blood cells, also called (28) ________________, or red blood corpuscles, constitute more than 90% of the formed elements in blood. Their function is to transport oxygen to the cells and carbon dioxide away from the cells.

White blood cells also are called (29) ________________, or white blood corpuscles. Their white color is due to a lack of hemoglobin.

Thrombocytes, also called (30) ________________, are the smallest cellular elements of the blood. They are important in the blood-clotting process and are manufactured in the bone marrow. A special protein, called (31) ________________, is formed to seal damaged blood vessels by trapping red blood cells, platelets, and fluid to form a clot. This protein also anchors the clot in place.

The term (32) ________________ means hardening of the arteries and refers to arteries that have become brittle and have lost their elasticity. Although the condition has several causes, the most common and important cause is (33) ________________, the deposit of fatty plaques in medium and large arteries.

The (34) ________________ ________________ collects accumulated tissue fluids from the entire body and returns them to the blood circulation. The system is one way, beginning in the tissues and ending in the blood vessels. The lymphatics work as an active part of our immunity by filtering and destroying foreign substances and microorganisms. Foreign particulate matter and pathogenic bacteria are screened out by the (35) ________________ ________________ that are spaced along the course of the vessels. They also play an active role in digestion by absorbing fats from the small intestine.

(36) ________________ is a clear interstitial tissue fluid that bathes the cells. The tiny (37) ________________ ________________ are open-ended channels found in the tissue spaces of the entire body except for the brain, spinal cord, and cornea. They join to form larger lymph vessels that look like veins but have thinner, more transparent walls. Like veins, they have valves to prevent backflow.

(38) ________________ is a complex response that networks all of the systems in the body to eliminate any pathogen, foreign substance, or toxic material that can be damaging to the body. The immune system is not a specific structural organ system, but rather a functional system. The immune system protects the body directly by cell attack and indirectly by releasing mobilizing chemicals and protective (39) ________________ ________________.

(40) ________________ are the cells of specific immunity because they recognize and destroy specific molecules and have the ability to remember that particular pathogen.

Exercise: Skin Structure

In the cross section of the skin structure pictured below, write the name of each component next to the corresponding letter. Color each part after you label it.

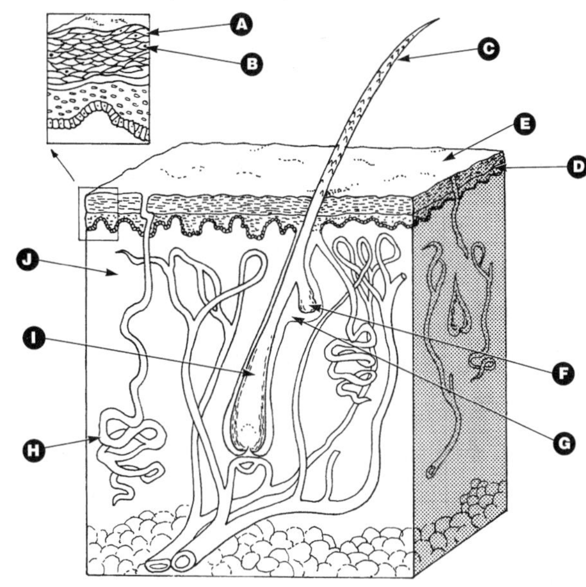

Exercise: Structures of the Heart

In the structures of the heart pictured below, write the name of each structure next to the corresponding letter. Color each part after you label it.

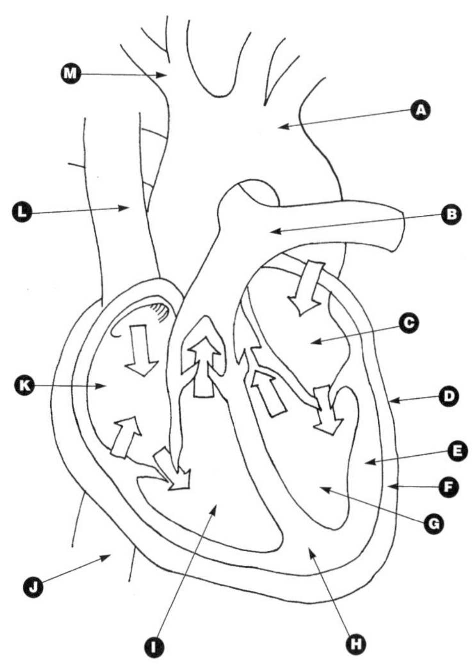

WORKBOOK SECTION

Answer Key

1. The integumentary system protects the internal organs and structures from trauma, sun exposure, chemicals, and water loss; assists the immune function by preventing the entry of bacteria and viruses; synthesizes vitamin D when exposed to the ultraviolet rays of the sun; detects the stimuli sensed as touch, temperature, pain, and pressure; regulates body temperature; excretes sweat and salts; and secretes sebum.
2. Hair, sebaceous glands, sweat glands (apocrine and eccrine), nails, and breasts (mammary glands)
3. The first concern is loss of skin protection of internal structures. The second concern is loss of the ability of the skin to prevent the pathogens of contagious disease from entering the body.
4. Elastic arteries: The large arteries capable of undergoing passive stretching. They have thick walls and recoil when the ventricles relax; this maintains pressure to move the blood. Examples include the aorta and pulmonary artery.
   Muscular arteries: The small and medium arteries that distribute blood to all tissues by contracting or dilating to control blood flow. Most of the arteries in the body are of this type.
   Arterioles: The smallest arteries. They have a diameter of less than 0.5 mm. They constrict or dilate to control the amount of blood entering capillaries.
5. Atrioventricular valves allow blood to flow into the ventricles but prevent it from returning to the atria. Semilunar valves control the blood flow out of the ventricles into the aorta and pulmonary arteries and prevent any backflow of blood into the ventricles. The aortic valve is found between the left ventricle and aorta, and the pulmonary valve is between the pulmonary artery and right ventricle. These two valves open in response to pressure generated by the blood leaving the ventricle and close when blood pools in small pockets of the cusps of the valves, pushing the valves closed.
6. If the heart is to have sufficient blood for normal cardiac output, proper venous return of blood must exist. Some factors that affect venous return include the following:
   Valves: Valves close in the veins to prevent backflow and pooling of blood. Improperly working valves can cause blood to back up and remain in the venous system.
   Muscular pump: Muscle contractions help push venous blood toward the heart.
   Gravity: Standing in one position for a long time is detrimental to venous return because blood in the veins below the heart constantly must overcome gravity to return to the heart.
   Respiratory pump: During inhalation and exhalation, movement of the diaphragm and intercostal muscles helps move blood through the venous system.
7. Neutrophils, monocytes, lymphocytes, eosinophils, and basophils
8. The two coronary arteries, which originate from the base of the aorta, supply oxygenated blood to the heart muscle. Coronary veins follow parallel to the arteries and return the blood to the right atrium via the coronary sinus. Both types of coronary vessels run in grooves between the atria and ventricles and between the two ventricles. If either of the coronary arteries is unable to supply sufficient blood to the heart muscle, a heart attack occurs. The most common site of a heart attack is the anterior or inferior part of the left ventricle.
9. Two main sounds result from the closure of the valves. The first is a low-pitched "lubb" produced by closure of the mitral and tricuspid valves. The second is a higher-pitched "dubb" caused by the closure of the aortic and pulmonary valves. Extra sounds, such as those resulting from faulty valves, are referred to as murmurs. Valves usually are quiet as they open.
10. Blood pressure depends on a person's size. The average newborn has a blood pressure of 90/60; at age 15, the average blood pressure is about 120/60. An average, healthy young adult has a blood pressure of 120/80. On average, a blood pressure greater than 140/90 is considered hypertension; a blood pressure less than 100/60 is considered hypotension. Blood pressure changes under various conditions, and one should never use a single reading as a final determinant.
11. The large lymph vessels gradually merge and eventually become two main ducts, called the right lymphatic duct and the thoracic duct (or left lymphatic duct). The right lymphatic duct drains the upper right half of the body and empties into the right subclavian vein. The thoracic duct drains the rest of the body and empties into the left subclavian vein.
12. Lymph nodes are small, round structures located along the lymph vessels. They are composed of lymphatic tissue and generally are clustered at the joints, which assists in pumping when the joint moves. The superficial lymph nodes are most numerous in the groin, axillae, and neck, whereas most of the deep lymph nodes are found beside blood vessels of the pelvic, abdominal, and thoracic cavities.
13. The defense system of the body is known as the immune system; it is not a specific structural organ system, but rather a functional system. The immune system responds in one of two ways by drawing on the structures and processes of each of the organs, tissues, cells, and chemicals produced within. In a nonspecific immune response the body responds exactly the same way to all substances that are not identified as part of the body. Nonspecific response is programmed genetically into the human body. Specific immunity produces specific responses to each identified substance and calls on special memory cells to help if that substance reappears. Specific immunity can be acquired in one of two ways: through natural immunity, which is the result of natural exposure, and through artificial immunity, which involves introducing a substance into the body to stimulate the immune response.
14. Nonspecific immunity can involve actions such as sneezing or coughing to remove microorganisms from our respiratory tract. Keeping the structure of the skin intact prevents entry of potentially damaging substances into the body. No matter the substance, the body responds in the same manner, with the same chemicals and cells mediating the actions. This general response is a prevention and a first response in immune function.

WORKBOOK SECTION

Fill in the Blank

1. integument
2. epidermis
3. dermis
4. superficial fascia
5. cardiovascular system
6. heart
7. mediastinum
8. pericardium
9. atria
10. ventricles
11. Cardiac output
12. cardiac cycle
13. heart rate
14. arteries
15. arterioles
16. Capillaries
17. veins
18. venules
19. blood pressure
20. systolic pressure
21. Diastolic pressure
22. sphygmomanometer
23. portal vein
24. liver
25. portal hypertension
26. Blood
27. plasma
28. erythrocytes
29. leukocytes
30. platelets
31. fibrin
32. arteriosclerosis
33. atherosclerosis
34. lymphatic system
35. lymph nodes
36. Lymph
37. lymph capillaries
38. Immunity
39. antibody molecules
40. Lymphocytes

Exercise: Skin Structure

A. Horny tissue
B. Melanin
C. Hair
D. Epidermis
E. Skin
F. Sebaceous gland
G. Sebum
H. Sweat gland
I. Hair follicle
J. Dermis

Exercise: Structures of the Heart

A. Aorta
B. Pulmonary artery
C. Left atrium
D. Endocardium
E. Myocardium
F. Pericardium
G. Left ventricle
H. Septum
I. Right ventricle
J. Inferior vena cava
K. Right atrium
L. Superior vena cava
M. Blood vessel

Respiratory, Digestive, Urinary, and Reproductive Systems

CHAPTER 12

▼ CHAPTER OBJECTIVES

After completing this chapter, the student will be able to perform the following:

- List and describe the components of the respiratory system.
- Describe the function of the respiratory system.
- Explain breathing pattern disorder.
- List and describe the components of the digestive system.
- Describe the process of digestion.
- List and describe the main food groups.
- List and describe the components of the urinary system.
- Describe the function of the urinary system.
- List and describe the components of the male and female reproductive systems.
- Explain the three stages of pregnancy.
- Justify the effectiveness of therapeutic massage modalities for support of health maintenance for the respiratory, digestive, urinary, and reproductive systems.

▼ CHAPTER OUTLINE

▼ KEY TERMS

Absorption The movement of food molecules from the digestive tract to the circulatory or lymphatic systems.

Basal metabolic rate (BA-sal) The rate of energy expenditure of the body under normal, relaxed activities.

Breathing pattern disorder A complex set of behaviors that leads to overbreathing without a pathologic condition present. The condition is functional in which all the parts are working effectively; therefore a pathologic condition does not exist. Instead, the breathing pattern is inappropriate for the situation, resulting in confused signals to the central nervous system, which sets up a whole chain of events.

Diaphragm A dome-shaped sheet of muscle attached to the thoracic wall that separates the lungs and thoracic cavity from the abdominal cavity. As the chest cavity enlarges, the diaphragm moves downward and flattens to create a vacuum that allows air to flow into the lungs. As the chest contracts and the diaphragm relaxes, the diaphragm arches upward, helping air to flow out of the lungs.

Digestion The mechanical and chemical breakdown of food from its complex form into simple molecules.

Elimination (egestion) Removal and release of solid waste products from food that cannot be digested or absorbed.

External respiration The exchange of oxygen and carbon dioxide between the lungs and the bloodstream.

Gestation (jes-TAY-shun) The period of fetal growth from conception until birth.

Hyperventilation (hye-per-ven-ti-LAY-shun) Abnormally deep or rapid breathing in excess of physical demands.

Continued

Ingestion (in-JEST-chun) Taking food into the mouth.

Internal respiration The exchange of gases between the tissues and blood.

Lower respiratory tract The larynx, trachea, bronchi, and alveoli.

Lungs The primary organs of respiration, the lungs are soft, spongy, highly vascular structures separated into the left and right lungs by the mediastinum. Each lung is separated into lobes. The right lung has three lobes: an upper, middle, and lower; the left, two lobes: an upper and lower.

Peristalsis (pair-I-STAL-sis) Rhythmic contraction of smooth muscles that propel products of digestion along the tract from the esophagus to the anus.

Respiration The movement of air in and out of the lungs, the exchange of oxygen and carbon dioxide between the lungs and blood, and the exchange between blood and body tissues.

Sinus (SYE-nus) Four groups of air-filled spaces that open into the internal nose. They are located in the frontal, ethmoid, sphenoid, and maxillary bones of the skull. Sinuses are lined with mucosa and function to lighten the weight of the skull, making it easier to hold the head up, and help in the production of sound.

Thorax (THOR-aks) Also known as the chest cavity, the thorax is the upper region of the torso enclosed by the sternum, ribs, and thoracic vertebrae and contains the lungs, heart, and great vessels.

Upper respiratory tract The nasal cavity and all its structures and the pharynx.

RESPIRATORY SYSTEM

Of all the basic life support systems in the body, the respiratory system is the only one under voluntary and automatic control. The respiratory system functions to obtain the oxygen necessary to create energy for body functions and to eliminate carbon dioxide produced during cellular metabolism. Persons can exercise considerable voluntary control over respiratory movements, most often in connection with speech. **Respiration** and breath are connected intimately to the expression of emotion, as in laughing or crying, the explosive burst in anger, breath holding in fear, and the sigh of relief. Breathing is a sacred act. According to biblical Scripture, "God breathed into man the breath of life, and man became a living soul." This voluntary control of breathing allows a person to regulate the autonomic nervous system. Therefore control of breathing becomes important in many relaxation and meditation practices.

In terms of vital functions the respiratory system may be considered the most important because the heart and brain require a continuous supply of oxygen to function. *Apnea*, the lack of spontaneous breathing, can cause irreversible brain damage if it continues for more than 3 or 4 minutes.

Respiration is the movement of air in and out of the **lungs,** the exchange of oxygen and carbon dioxide between the lungs and blood and between blood and body tissues. *Breathing* is a mechanical action of inhalation and exhalation that draws oxygen into the lungs and releases carbon dioxide into the atmosphere.

External respiration is the exchange of oxygen and carbon dioxide between the lungs and the bloodstream. The exchange of gases between the tissues and blood is called ***internal respiration.***

On the average, we breathe 12 to 16 times per minute. Each breath contains approximately 500 ml of air (about 2 cups), so in 1 hour we breathe about 360 L, or 82 gal, of air.

The organs of the respiratory system are divided into upper and lower regions. The **upper respiratory tract** consists of the nasal cavity, all its structures, and the pharynx; the **lower respiratory tract** consists of the larynx, trachea, and bronchi and alveoli in the lungs (Figure 12-1).

Organs of the Respiratory System

Nose and Nasal Cavity

The structure of the nose is divided into two parts: the external and internal portions. The lower two thirds of the external nose is composed mostly of cartilage. The upper third, or bridge of the nose, is formed from two small, hard nasal bones. The tip of the nose is the apex, and the nostrils are the *nares.* Air enters the external nares and passes across

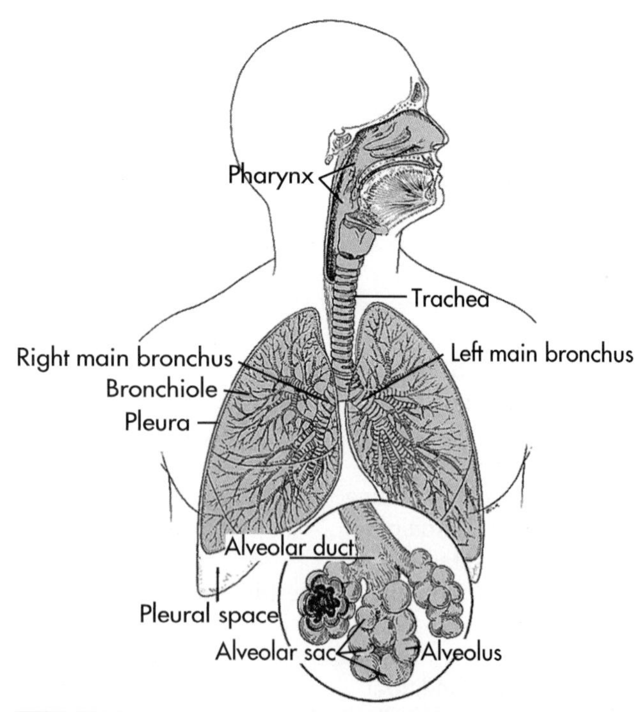

Figure 12-1
Pharynx, trachea, and lungs. Alveolar sacs in inset. (From Thibodeau GA: *Anthony's textbook of anatomy and physiology,* ed 17, St Louis, 2003, Mosby.)

internal nasal hairs that trap particles of dirt and other foreign material; the air then flows into the nasal cavity.

The internal nose is the continuation of the nose inside the skull and above the mouth and includes the **sinuses.** The roof is formed by a small portion of the frontal bone and the ethmoid and sphenoid bones, and the floor is formed by the hard palate, consisting of the maxillae and palatine bones. The internal nares are the portion of the internal nose that communicates with the throat. The nasal cavity is the actual space inside the external and internal nose structures and is separated into left and right sides by the *septum,* a partition composed of cartilage and bone. At the upper portion of the nasal cavity, three thin, curled bones, the turbinates or conchae, project inward from the two outer walls. These turbinates separate into small, grooved passageways, each called a meatus, that continue to move the air. Air that passes through the nasal cavity is warmed by small blood vessels close to the surface of the lining and moistened by the mucous membranes and secretions from the sinuses. The mucous membranes line the entire respiratory tract, and the sticky mucus traps smaller inhaled particles, helping to prevent infection. The small hairs, or cilia, that line the nasal cavity, larynx, and trachea transport these foreign particles to the throat, where they are swallowed to be destroyed in the stomach.

Nerve endings for the olfactory nerve lie on the upper third of both sides of the nasal septum, the olfactory region, and are stimulated by changes in gas consistency. Olfactory nerve fibers pass through small holes in the ethmoid bone to the olfactory bulb and then to the cortex, which interprets the impulses as smell.

Venous areas called swell bodies are located on the turbinates. About every half hour, the swell bodies on one side of the nasal cavity engorge with blood, resulting in decreased air flow on that side, with good flow on the other side. Then the process reverses. These periodic changes permit the inside of the nose to recover from drying. This same mechanism becomes important during sleep. When a person lies with his or her head to one side, the swell bodies of the lower nostril become congested. The chamber narrows and the lumen closes. When sleeping, we only breath though one nostril at a time. The closure of the nostril then initiates movement of the head from one side to the other, which in turn causes a major movement and turning of the body. This head-body moving cycle, initiated by the nose, ensures maximal rest during sleep. A poorly functioning nose may allow the body and head to remain in one position and can cause symptoms such as backaches, numbness, cramps, and circulatory dysfunction.

The nasal septum is supplied with sensory nerves and blood vessels. Nasal reflex responses and referred phenomena are well established between the nose, ears, throat, larynx, heart, lungs, **diaphragm**, nervous system, and body temperature. Contained in the coordination of these various reflex patterns is the mechanism of entrainment between heart rate, breathing rate, and synchronization of other body rhythms. Most relaxation methods and methods of ritual, meditation, and many healing practices incorporate a form of structured breathing. This practical application of ordering and coordinating body rhythms seems to be accomplished through the coordination of air flow through the nose.

A deviated septum is a condition in which the cartilage is bent, usually as the result of a blow to the nose, resulting in difficulty in breathing from one side of the nose. As simple as this seems, because of reflex patterns, any disruption of air flow through the nose can have bodywide effects such as disturbing sleep patterns.

Sinuses

The sinuses are four groups of air-filled spaces that open into the internal nose. They are located in the frontal, ethmoid, sphenoid, and maxillary bones of the skull. Sinuses are lined with mucosa and function to lighten the weight of the skull, making it easier to hold the head up, and help in the production of sound. Because the sinus mucosa communicates with the nasal cavity, sinuses are prone to the same infections as the nasal cavity.

Pharynx

The pharynx, or throat, is divided into three areas. The nasopharynx is the continuation of the nasal cavity into the throat and transports air. The eustachian tubes open into the nasopharynx and help equalize pressure in the head, nose, and pharynx. The oropharynx is the portion of the throat that you can see; it contains the tonsils and functions as a passageway for food between the mouth and the esophagus and as a passageway for air between the nose, mouth, and trachea. The laryngopharynx begins at the hyoid bone and separates into the esophagus and larynx and so functions as a pathway for respiration and digestion. At the entrance to the larynx is a small cartilaginous flap, the epiglottis. As we swallow food, the epiglottis closes over the glottis, preventing food or fluids from entering the lungs.

Larynx

The larynx, or voice box, connects the pharynx to the trachea and consists of cartilage, ligaments, connective tissue, muscles, and the vocal cords. The cartilage provides a rigid structural framework for the larynx and trachea below, making sure that the airway is open at all times. The thyroid cartilage, known as the Adam's apple, is located on the anterior portion of the larynx and is larger in men. The vocal cords and the spaces between the cords are located inside the glottis.

The function of the larynx, in addition to permitting air passage to and from the lungs, is to produce sound, or phonation. The lips and the tongue create speech. As we exhale, the vocal cords vibrate to produce high or low sounds, or pitch. In high-pitch sounds the glottis is narrower and the vocal cords are more tense, whereas in low-pitch sounds the glottis is more open and the vocal cords are more relaxed. Laryngitis is an inflammation of the vocal cords caused by overuse, infection, or irritation from substances such as cigarette smoke or tumors. Laryngitis can cause hoarseness or loss of the voice. Obstruction of the glottis, such as with food, can be fatal. Bacterial infection of the epiglottis (epiglottitis) in children is a life-threatening but rarer cause of obstruction.

Trachea

The trachea, or windpipe, is the main airway to the lungs and is a 4- to 5-inch tube that begins at the glottis and ends at the junction of the two main bronchi near the level of the sternal angle. The trachea consists of 16 to 20 horseshoe-shaped rings of cartilage that have connective tissue between them. When a foreign particle enters the trachea, mucus and cilia trap it and initiate the cough reflex.

The trachea branches off into two bronchi, which have the same structural framework, except that they have more smooth muscle than the trachea. The first branches of the bronchial tubes are the right and left primary bronchi. Each main bronchus divides into two (left lung) or three (right lung) lobar bronchi.

Lungs

The two lungs are the primary organs of respiration. These soft, spongy, highly vascular structures are separated into the left and right lungs by the *mediastinum.* Each lung is separated into lobes. The right lung has three lobes: an upper, middle, and lower; the left has two lobes: an upper and lower.

The lobar bronchi, which extend from the trachea, each divide into 10 segmental bronchi, which further divide. The amount of cartilage in each tube gradually decreases until the tubes lack cartilage. At this point the tubes are about 1 mm in diameter and are known as the bronchioles, which terminate in the air sacs, or alveoli. The alveoli are surrounded by capillaries, and this is where the internal respiration takes place.

The lungs are enclosed in a pleural cavity lined with two pleural membranes. One connects directly to the lung, and the other attaches to the mediastinum and inside chest wall. This cavity created by the membranes contains approximately 1/2 tsp of lubricating fluid that reduces friction between the two layers as we breathe. Increases in the amount of fluid often occur with diseases such as lung cancer and pulmonary edema and can make breathing difficult. Pneumothorax is a condition in which air enters the pleural cavity as a result of trauma or rupture of part of the lung. This can be caused by a penetrating injury such as from a bullet or knife or in disease processes such as emphysema. A chest tube called a thoracotomy tube inserted between the ribs and connected to a pump removes the air. In hemothorax, physicians can drain blood in the pleural space in a similar manner.

Diaphragm

The diaphragm is a dome-shaped sheet of muscle attached to the thoracic wall that separates the lungs and thoracic cavity from the abdominal cavity. As the chest cavity enlarges, the diaphragm moves downward and creates a vacuum that allows air to flow into the lungs. As the chest contracts and the diaphragm relaxes, the diaphragm arches upward, helping air to flow out of the lungs.

Thorax

The **thorax,** or chest cavity, is the upper region of the torso enclosed by the sternum, ribs, and thoracic vertebrae and contains the lungs, heart, and great vessels (Figure 12-2).

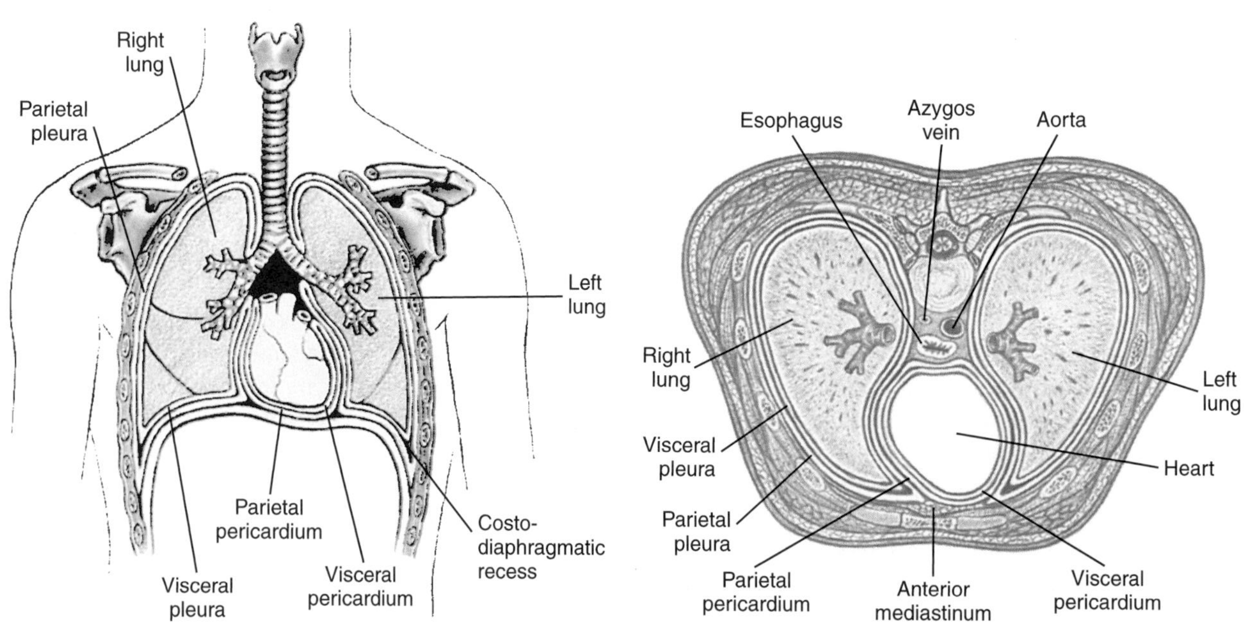

Figure 12-2
The thoracic cavity. The thoracic cavity, or chest cavity, is divided into three subdivisions (left and right pleural divisions and mediastinum) by a partition formed by a serous membrane called the *pleura.* (From Thibodeau GA, Patton KT: *Anatomy and physiology,* ed 5, St Louis, 2003, Mosby.)

Nerves and Vessels of the Lungs and Respiratory Muscles

The autonomic nervous system supplies the bronchi and bronchioles. Stimulation of the vagus nerve (parasympathetic) causes contraction of the smooth muscles and narrows the diameter of the tubes (bronchoconstriction). Stimulation of sympathetic nerves initiates smooth muscle relaxation, resulting in widening of the tubes (bronchodilation).

The nerve supply to the intercostal muscles is from spinal nerves T1 to T11. The phrenic nerve originates at C3 to C5 and innervates the diaphragm. The reason that the nerve supply originates so distant is that during fetal development, the diaphragm actually begins its growth in the neck and then descends from the neck to the abdomen. A broken neck that injures the spinal cord below C5 still allows the person to breathe because the diaphragm does most of the breathing. Injury to both phrenic nerves or a spinal cord injury above C3 to C5 severely compromises breathing.

The pulmonary arteries and veins participate in the exchange of oxygen and carbon dioxide between the capillaries and alveoli. Branches of the aorta and upper intercostal arteries supply blood to most of the lung tissue. Venous drainage is from the azygos vein on the right side of the thorax, and the first intercostal vein on the left.

Mechanics of Breathing

During the moments before we take a breath, the pressure inside the lungs and outside the body is equal, whereas the pressure inside the pleural space is slightly lower. When we begin to inhale, the external intercostal muscles between the ribs contract, lifting the lower ribs up and out. This creates a vacuum that expands the lungs, causing the pressure inside the lungs to decrease. The diaphragm moves down, increasing the volume of the pleural cavities and decreasing lung pressure even more. Elastic fibers in the alveolar walls stretch, permitting expansion of the air sacs. The lungs draw air in until the pressure is equal again.

As we exhale, the pressure inside the pleural cavity increases; the external intercostals, diaphragm, and alveolar walls relax; the volume inside the lungs decreases; and the pressure in the lungs increases until it again equals the atmospheric pressure (Figure 12-3).

In diseases such as asthma, bronchitis, and emphysema, one often uses accessory muscles of respiration. Contraction of the sternocleidomastoid and other muscles of the neck aid inspiration, whereas use of the internal intercostals and abdominal muscles aids expiration (Figures 12-4 to 12-6).

Lung Volumes

Breathing in and out changes the volume of air. One can measure four different pulmonary volumes to use as guidelines in health assessments. The *tidal volume* is the amount of air taken in or exhaled in a single breath during normal breathing, usually while the person is resting. The *inspiratory reserve volume* is the amount of air one can inhale forcefully after normal tidal volume inspiration, whereas the *expiratory reserve volume* is the amount of air one can exhale forcefully after a normal exhalation. The reserve volume is the amount of air that remains in the lungs and passageways after a maximal expiration. The *vital capacity* is the total of the tidal volume, inspiratory reserve volume, and expiratory reserve volume. In the normal, healthy adult lung, vital capacity usually varies from 3.5 to 5.5 L of air.

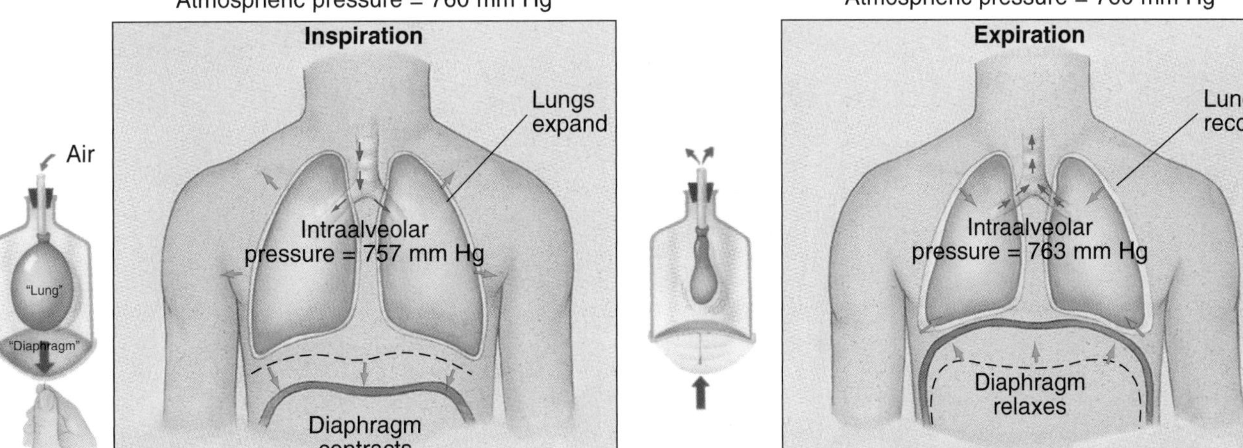

Figure 12-3
Mechanics of breathing. During *inspiration,* the diaphragm contracts, increasing the volume of the thoracic cavity. This increase in volume results in a decrease in pressure, which causes air to rush into the lungs. During *expiration,* the diaphragm returns to an upward position, reducing the volume in the thoracic cavity. Air pressure increases then, forcing air out of the lungs. Insets show the classic model in which a jar represents the rib cage, a rubber sheet represents the diaphragm, and a balloon represents the lungs. (From Thibodeau GA, Patton KT: *Anatomy and physiology,* ed 5, St Louis, 2003, Mosby.)

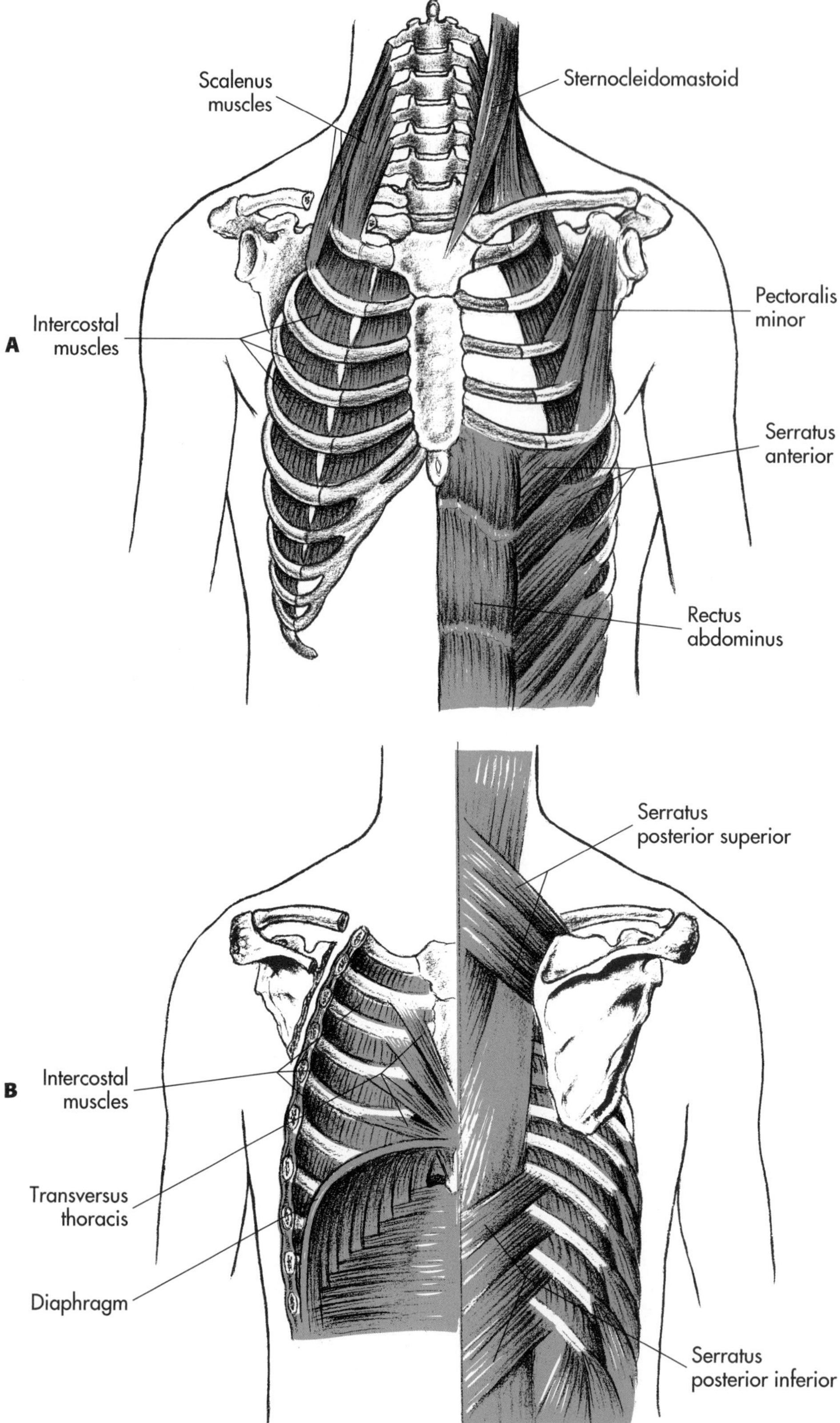

Figure 12-4

Muscles of respiration. **A,** Anterior view. **B,** Posterior view. (From Seidel HM et al: *Mosby's guide to physical examination,* ed 5, St Louis, 2003, Mosby.)

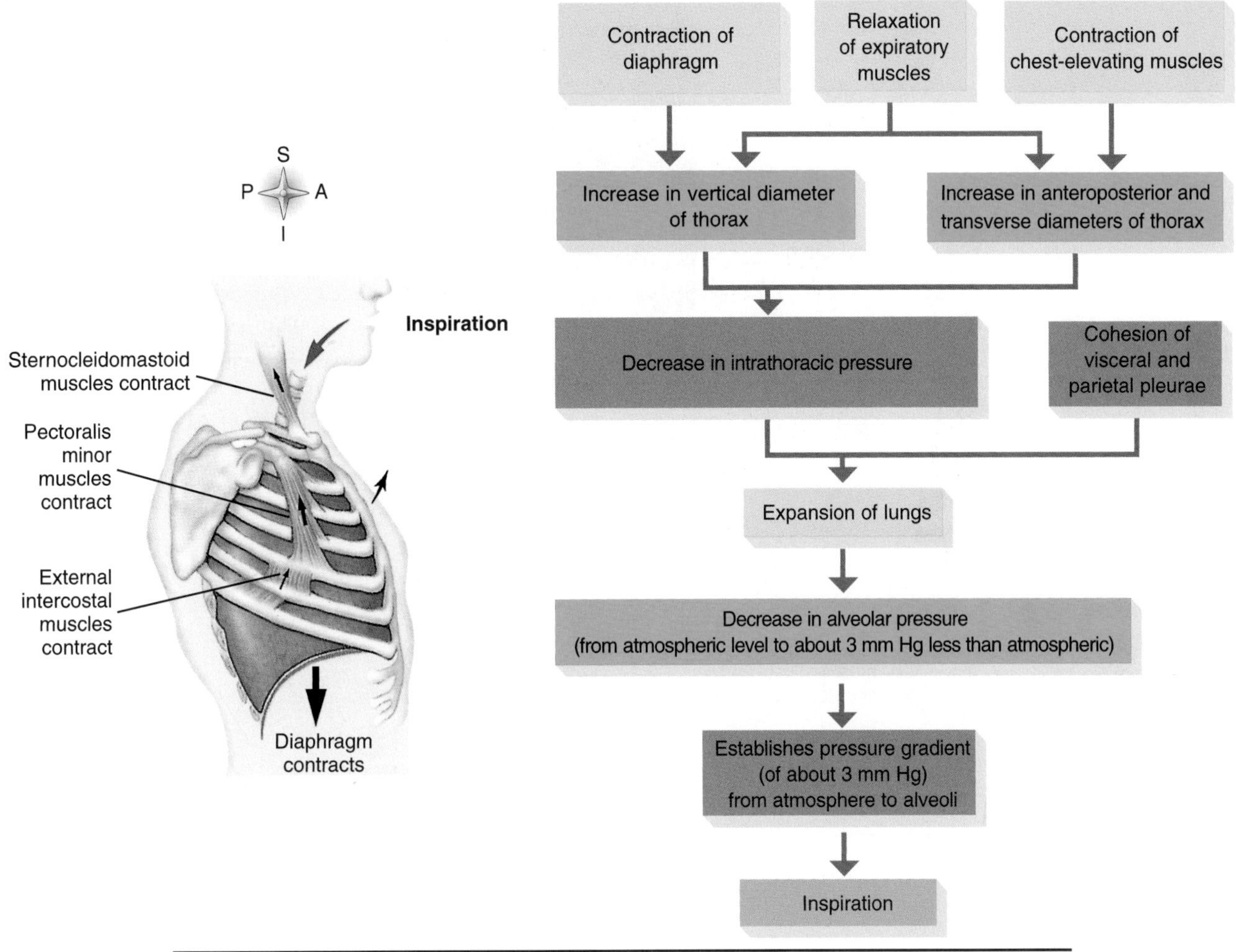

Figure 12-5
Mechanism of inspiration. (From Thibodeau GA, Patton KT: *Anatomy and physiology,* ed 5, St Louis, 2003, Mosby.)

In lungs with diseases such as asthma and emphysema the vital capacity and expiratory reserve volumes are abnormal. A person with asthma, for example, may have a normal tidal volume and vital capacity but decreased expiratory reserve volume, whereas a person with emphysema may have a normal (but often decreased) tidal volume and decreased vital capacity and expiratory reserve volume. The end result is that the person cannot exhale effectively.

Transport of Oxygen and Carbon Dioxide

The exchange of oxygen and carbon dioxide takes place by diffusion. The pulmonary arteries bring oxygen-deficient blood from the right ventricle to the lungs. Carbon dioxide diffuses from the bloodstream through the capillary and alveolar membranes for exhalation by the lungs. Oxygen diffuses in the opposite direction, from the alveoli through both membranes and into the bloodstream. The pulmonary veins return oxygen-rich blood to the left atrium.

The amount of oxygen in the blood depends on the amount of oxygen available in the atmosphere. The air in the average room is composed of the following:

Nitrogen (N_2): 79%
Oxygen (O_2): 20.96%
Carbon dioxide (CO_2): 0.04%

Red blood cells transport oxygen in the blood as oxyhemoglobin. Red blood cells move into the capillaries. At the arteriole end of the capillary, oxygen leaves the red blood cell, and then passes through the capillary membrane into the tissue fluid. Oxygen then diffuses through the tissue cell membrane to be used for cellular metabolism.

Carbon dioxide moves out of the tissue cell in the reverse direction through the same membranes into the red blood cell, where most of it is converted to bicarbonate ion (HCO_3). The plasma transports bicarbonate to the lungs, where the process reverses in the alveolus to allow exhalation of carbon dioxide.

Control of Breathing

The respiratory center is a group of nerve cells in the medulla and pons. A variety of stimuli affect the center. Impulses from the cerebral cortex under voluntary control modify respiration, as do changes in the carbon dioxide

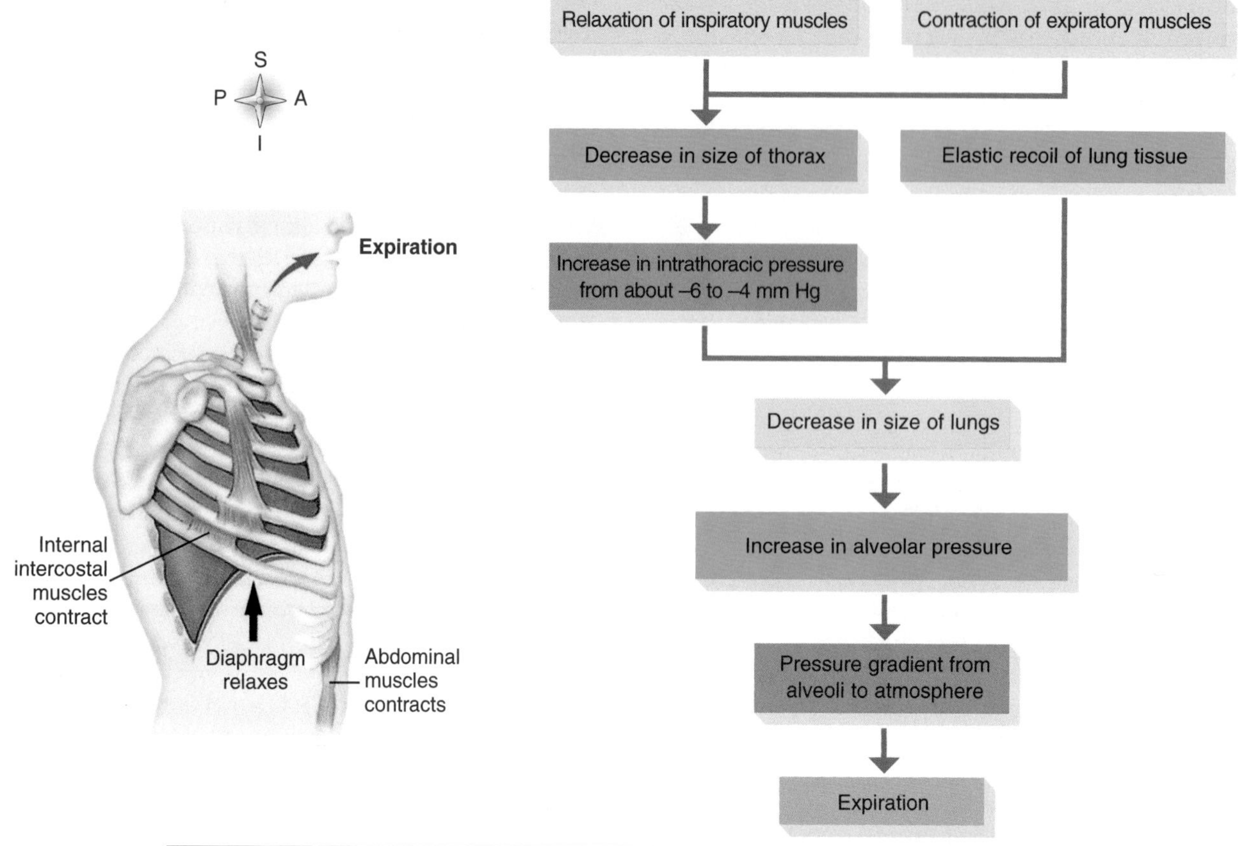

Figure 12-6
Mechanism of expiration. (From Thibodeau GA, Patton KT: *Anatomy and physiology,* ed 5, St Louis, 2003, Mosby.)

content and acidity of blood and cerebrospinal fluid. Chemoreceptors, nerve cells found near the baroreceptors, are sensitive to the oxygen level and to a lesser extent to carbon dioxide and pH (acid/base balance) levels in the bloodstream. Two chemoreceptors are located near the arch of the aorta (aortic bodies), and one is in each carotid artery (carotid bodies). The aortic bodies transmit impulses to the respiratory center in the medulla through the vagus nerve; the carotid bodies transmit by way of the glossopharyngeal nerve. A low concentration of oxygen in the body stimulates the chemoreceptors, and the respiratory rate increases.

Respiratory Rate

The respiratory rate in adults is about 12 to 16 breaths per minute and in the newborn is about 35, gradually decreasing to adult values at about age 20 (Figure 12-6). Emotions are a powerful stimulus for respiratory changes. Fear, grief, and shock slow the rate, whereas excitement, anger, and sexual arousal increase the respiratory rate.

Besides the effects of emotions, changes in breathing rates can occur as a result of increased oxygen requirement from exercise, in obesity as a result of increased vessel resistance, during infections and fever because of increased energy requirements, in heart failure from decreased oxygen flow, during pain because of increased nervous stimulation, with anemia because of decreased oxygen transport, in hyperthyroidism from an increase in metabolic rate, and during emphysema as a result of blockage of oxygen. *Hyperpnea* is fast breathing, and *tachypnea* is rapid, shallow breathing. This type of breathing can lead to acute **hyperventilation** or chronic overbreathing called **breathing pattern disorder,** which causes a variety of signs and symptoms, as discussed later in this section. *Bradypnea,* or slow breathing, occurs in alcohol and other depressant drug intoxication because of the depressant action on the brain. Bradypnea also occurs in increased intracranial pressure from pressure on the respiratory center and in diabetic coma. Periods of hyperpnea alternating with periods of *apnea* (no breathing) sometimes occur in the sleep of infants, particularly premature ones. These patterns also appear in brain injury and in the terminally ill.

Reflexes That Affect Breathing

Foreign matter or irritants in the trachea or bronchi stimulate the cough reflex. The epiglottis and glottis reflexively close, and contraction of the expiratory muscles causes air pressure in the lungs to increase. The epiglottis and glottis open suddenly, resulting in an upward force of air in a cough that removes the offending contaminants in the throat.

The sneeze reflex is similar to the cough reflex, except that contaminants or irritants in the nasal cavity provide the stimulus. A burst of air moves through the nose and mouth, forcing the contaminants out of the respiratory tract.

A hiccup is an involuntary, spasmodic contraction of the diaphragm causing the glottis to close suddenly, producing a characteristic sound.

A yawn is slow, deep inspiration through the open mouth. Scientists still have not found the actual physiologic mechanism for yawning.

Pathologic Conditions

Asthma

Asthma is the narrowing of the small airways not related to cardiovascular disease. Asthma presents itself as acute attacks that constrict and obstruct these airways. Asthma attacks may be triggered by allergic reactions, air pollutants, exercise, hypersensitivity to substances such as wood or flour, chemicals, viral infections, or an emotional upset. During an episode, the smooth muscle layer of the bronchi and bronchioles goes into spasm (constriction) and the glands of the bronchi hypersecrete mucus. The airways fill with thick mucus, and air cannot leave the lungs. Breathlessness, coughing, chest tightness, and wheezing occur as the person tries to force air out of the lungs. Arterial blood gases initially show a low amount of carbon dioxide, a condition known as respiratory alkalosis. Long-term therapy may include the use of a bronchodilator, mast cell stabilizer, or corticosteroids. Antibiotics may benefit the person if the trigger is a respiratory infection.

Carbon Monoxide Poisoning

Carbon monoxide poisoning is the leading cause of gas deaths in this country. Carbon monoxide is odorless and binds to hemoglobin 210 times more readily than oxygen. Most deaths occur from smoke inhalation during fires. Some occur from automobile exhaust fumes, poorly ventilated or defective gasoline heaters, and charcoal stoves. Poisonings also occur in machine shops in which ventilation is poor. Symptoms are headache, dizziness, weakness, and nausea and occur when the blood has about 6% to 7% carboxyhemoglobin.

Choking

Choking often happens when a person is talking while eating and inhales at the same time as swallowing. The piece of food, usually meat, obstructs the larynx. Frequently, the person also is drinking alcohol. The person starts to cough, which often dislodges the object. If not, the airway can become blocked totally. The person usually appears distressed, grasps his neck, and cannot inhale or exhale. The term *café coronary* has been applied because choking often occurs in a restaurant and superficially resembles a heart attack.

Before beginning assistance, ask the person if he or she can speak. One who can speak is not choking. First aid for choking is the Heimlich maneuver (Box 12-1).

BOX 12-1

Heimlich Maneuver

The Heimlich maneuver is an effective and often lifesaving technique one can use to open a suddenly obstructed windpipe. The maneuver uses air already present in the lungs to expel the object obstructing the trachea. Most accidental airway obstructions result from pieces of food aspirated during a meal; the condition sometimes is referred to as a "cafe coronary." Other objects such as chewing gum or balloons frequently are the cause of obstructions in children. Individuals trained in emergency procedures must be able to tell the difference between airway obstruction and other conditions such as heart attacks that produce similar symptoms. The key question they must ask the person who appears to be choking is, "Can you talk?" A person with an obstructed airway will not be able to speak, even while conscious. The Heimlich maneuver, if the victim is standing, consists of the rescuer grasping the victim with both arms around the victim's waist just below the ribcage and above the navel. The rescuer makes a fist with one hand, grasps it with the other, and then delivers an upward thrust against the diaphragm just below the xiphoid process of the sternum. The thrust compresses air trapped in the lungs, forcing the object that is choking the victim out of the airway.

Technique if victim can be lifted

1. Rescuer stands behind the victim and wraps both arms around the victim's chest slightly below the ribcage and above the navel. Rescuer allows victim to fall forward with head, arms, and chest over the rescuer's arms.
2. Rescuer makes a fist with one hand and grasps it with the other hand, pressing thumb side of fist against victim's abdomen just below the end of the xiphoid process and above the navel.
3. The rescuer uses the hands only to deliver the upward subdiaphragmatic thrusts. Each thrust is performed with sharp flexion of the elbows, in an upward rather than inward direction, and is usually repeated four times. An important precaution is not to compress the ribcage or actually press on the sternum during the Heimlich maneuver.

Technique if victim has collapsed or cannot be lifted

1. Rescuer places victim on floor face up.
2. Facing victim, rescuer straddles the victim's hips.
3. Rescuer places one hand on top of the other, with the bottom hand on the victim's abdomen slightly above the navel and below the ribcage.
4. Rescuer performs a forceful upward thrust with the heel of the bottom hand, repeating several times if necessary.

Modified from Thibodeau GA, Patton KT: *Anatomy and physiology,* ed 5, St Louis, 2003, Mosby.

Chronic Obstructive Pulmonary Disease

Although the processes involved in the evolution of emphysema and bronchitis are different, the end result is irreversible respiratory insufficiency, sometimes called chronic obstructive pulmonary disease. In emphysema the obstruction is in the alveoli; in bronchitis the obstruction is in the bronchi. A component of each appears in heavy smokers.

Acute bronchitis often occurs along with an upper respiratory infection, measles, or the flu. A virus usually causes infection, but the cause also may be bacterial infection. Symptoms include a mild fever, an increase in mucus secreted, and coughing in an attempt to loosen and remove the phlegm, which is often yellow and green. Prolonged irritation by cigarette smoke is the usual cause of *chronic bronchitis.* The person usually has a chronic cough. As in the acute stage, sputum production increases in response to the constant irritation of the tissues. The lung tissue changes, and the person becomes less able to tolerate exercise and any activity. The smoke damages the cilia, so excess mucus cannot be moved out of the airway. One may hear wheezing noises. Treatment involves the use of bronchodilators and oxygen therapy. The condition often reverses on cessation of cigarette smoking.

In *emphysema* resulting from long-term irritation of the bronchi and bronchioles, mucus and pus accumulate, and the air in the alveoli becomes trapped. When the pressure exceeds the elastic limit, the alveoli become permanently ballooned, producing the typically barrel-chested person who uses the internal intercostals as well as the abdominal and neck muscles to breathe. As emphysema progresses, the person becomes breathless with minor exertion. Inflammation brings in more white blood cells, which break down the walls of the alveoli, which merge to form larger sacs. Alveolar destruction results in less surface area for the internal exchange of gases, so oxygen in the blood decreases. Emphysema is the most common cause of respiratory failure. Bronchodilators and oxygen therapy may help.

Common Cold

More than 200 viruses can cause the common cold, which is transmitted easily. Usually affecting the nasal mucosa, the viruses may spread to the sinuses, pharynx, and down the respiratory tract. The person's temperature rises to eliminate the virus. Irritation in the nose and pharynx causes coughing and sneezing. Fluids and bed rest are recommended.

Croup

Croup is a viral infection in children that most often affects boys ages 3 months to 5 years. The larynx, trachea, and bronchi are red and swollen and may block the glottis. A "seal bark" cough is usually present. Sometimes a high-pitched whistling inhalation is present, and the child must use his neck and abdominal muscles to breathe. Humidified air often eases the symptoms; if not, oxygen therapy may help.

Cystic Fibrosis

Cystic fibrosis is a genetic disorder that causes abnormally thick and sticky mucus to be produced throughout the body. This mucus cannot be moved out by the cilia, so bacteria and viruses are held in instead of moved out of the body. Infections develop, with obstruction of the smaller airways. (See the section on the digestive system for more information.)

Drowning

In drowning the victim inhales and swallows water. In 10% of cases the larynx goes into spasm on inhalation of the first small amount of fluid, and asphyxia or suffocation (from lack of oxygen and an increase in carbon dioxide) takes place even with no fluid in the lungs. Survival depends mostly on the continued presence of a pulse and not necessarily on the time of immersion. Treatment in near-drowning consists of cardiopulmonary resuscitation, with oxygen given at the hospital and bicarbonate for the acidosis caused by the carbon dioxide levels.

Hay Fever

Hay fever is an allergic reaction in persons who have a sensitivity to pollen, house dust, and feathers, among other things. Nasal vessels engorge with blood and become congested. Fluid leaks from the capillaries into the tissue spaces and drains into the nasal cavity, causing a runny nose. The congestion and edema cause the irritation, sneezing, redness, and swelling in the allergy sufferers in the spring and summer months. Treatment is with an antihistamine and decongestant.

Hiccups

Hiccups (singultus) are a sudden involuntary contraction of the inspiratory muscles, producing the sound of inspiration with the glottis closed. Most cases involve food or alcohol, are short-lived, and resolve without therapy. The reflex is primitive, similar to yawning, coughing, sneezing, and vomiting. The reflex is designed to dislodge a foreign object. Often, sedatives and home remedies work. In prolonged cases a tranquilizer may be necessary.

Breathing Pattern Disorder

Physiologists define hyperventilation as abnormally deep or rapid breathing in excess of physical demands.

Breathing pattern disorder (previously called hyperventilation syndrome) is a complex set of behaviors that leads to overbreathing in the absence of a pathologic condition. Hyperventilation is a functional condition in which all the parts are working effectively; therefore a pathologic condition does not exist. Instead, the breathing pattern is inappropriate for the situation, resulting in confused signals to the central nervous system, which sets up a whole chain of events. Persons experiencing this difficulty often are told that nothing is wrong, which induces further puzzlement and adds to their anxiety, or they are told to take a few deep breaths, which increases their symptoms. One review indicates that as many as 28% of patients within various medical populations may experience functional breathing pattern disorder.

Increased ventilation is a common component of fight-or-flight responses, but when our breathing increases and our actions and movements are restricted, we are breathing in excess of metabolic need. Blood levels of carbon dioxide fall, and symptoms may occur. As we exhale too much carbon dioxide too quickly, our blood becomes more alkalotic. These biochemical changes can cause many of the following signs and symptoms:

Cardiovascular: Palpitations, missed beats, tachycardia, sharp or dull atypical chest pain, angina, vasomotor instability, cold extremities, Raynaud's phenomenon, blotchy flushing of blush area, and capillary vasoconstriction (face, arms, and hands)

Neurologic: Dizziness, unsteadiness or instability; faint feelings (rarely actual fainting); visual disturbance (blurred or tunnel vision); headache (often migraine); paresthesia (i.e., numbness, uselessness, heaviness, "pins and needles," burning, limbs feeling out of proportion or "not belonging"), commonly of hands, feet, or face, sometimes scalp or whole body; intolerance of light or noise; large pupils (wearing dark glasses on a dull day); and sensation of faintness or giddiness

Respiratory: Shortness of breath typically after exertion, irritable cough, tightness or oppression of chest, difficulty breathing, asthma, air hunger, inability to take a satisfying breath, excessive sighing, yawning, and sniffing

Gastrointestinal: Difficulty in swallowing, dry mouth and throat, acid regurgitation, heartburn, hiatal hernia, nausea, flatulence, belching, air swallowing, abdominal discomfort, and bloating

Muscular: Cramps, muscle pains (particularly occipital, neck, shoulders, between scapulae; less commonly, the lower back and limbs), tremors, twitching, weakness, stiffness, or tetany (seizing up)

Psychic: Tension, anxiety, "unreal feelings," depersonalization, feeling "out of body," hallucinations, fear of insanity, panic, phobias, and agoraphobia; dyspneic (no air) fear is a core factor in the cause of panic attacks.

General: Weakness; exhaustion; impaired concentration, memory, and performance; disturbed sleep, including nightmares; emotional sweating (axillae, palms, sometimes whole body); and dull mind

Cerebrovascular constriction, a primary response to breathing pattern disorder, can reduce the oxygen available to the brain by about one half. Among the resulting symptoms are dizziness, blurring of consciousness, and possibly because of a decrease in cortical inhibition, tearfulness and emotional instability. Other effects of breathing pattern disorder for which therapists should watch are generalized body tension and chronic inability to relax. In addition, those who display breathing pattern disorder are particularly prone to spasm (tetany) in muscles involved in the attack posture: they hunch their shoulders, thrust their head and neck forward, scowl, and clench their teeth.

Influenza

Influenza (flu) is a common viral infection of the entire body, resulting in fever, muscle aches and weakness, backache, and cough. Primary treatment, as with most viral infections, is bed rest and fluids.

Lung Cancer

About 90% of all cases of lung cancer are caused by tobacco. Primary tumors usually develop in the bronchi and block air passages. Cancer in the lung can spread to other parts of the body. Symptoms frequently begin with cough, blood in the phlegm, wheezing, chest pain, and fever. A large tumor may cause problems with swallowing. Diagnosis is by a physical examination, x-ray films, and computed tomography scans.

Pleurisy

Pleurisy (pleuritis) is an inflammation of the pleural membrane, usually from a lung infection such as pneumonia. The inflamed membranes rub against each other, causing stabbing pain that is worse during inhalation.

Pneumonia

Pneumonia is an acute infection of the lungs caused by bacteria or viruses, fungi, exposure to certain chemicals, or inhaled substances. Symptoms include fever, chills, chest pain, difficulty breathing, headache, loss of appetite, muscle and joint pain, a cough usually accompanied by yellow or green sputum, and rales (the sound of movement of air and fluid in the bronchial tree). One makes a diagnosis after reviewing client history and test results, most often a chest x-ray film showing an abnormal white area. Evaluation of sputum and blood tests often show an elevated white count. Primary treatment for bacterial pneumonia is an antibiotic, bed rest, and fluids. In serious cases the person must be hospitalized and given oxygen and antibiotics.

Pulmonary Embolism

In pulmonary embolism, a clot detaches from a deep vein in the leg or pelvis and travels to the right atrium, then to the right ventricle, and on to the pulmonary artery. Predisposing factors of clot formation are obesity, heart failure, surgery and immobilization, and a history of thrombophlebitis. A clot that lodges at the junction of the pulmonary trunk and the pulmonary arteries may cause death. A clot that moves into a pulmonary artery and lodges destroys lung tissue and is called a pulmonary infarction. The person suddenly becomes short of breath. Other signs and symptoms are chest pain, fever, and wheezing. One makes a diagnosis using a lung scan and pulmonary angiogram. Treatment consists of intravenous anticoagulant (heparin) therapy to prevent further clotting and the use of a clot-dissolving medication. Subsequent therapy often involves orally administered warfarin (Coumadin).

Pulmonary Edema

Pulmonary edema is the accumulation of fluid in the lungs. The most common cause is heart failure, although kidney disease, pneumonia, or other disorders may cause pulmonary edema. Treatment usually involves diuretics and oxygen therapy.

Sinusitis

Sinusitis is inflammation of the sinuses that most commonly accompanies a nasal infection. Congestion, edema, and pain are present because of irritation of the sensory nerve endings in the periosteum. Pain takes the form of a headache, particularly if the frontal sinus is involved. Congestion blocks drainage into the nasal cavity. The maxillary sinus lies over the upper teeth, and sometimes a person has difficulty telling whether the problem is a sinus attack or a toothache because of the similarity of the pain pattern. Treatment often consists of an antibiotic and a decongestant.

Sleep Apnea

In the disorder known as sleep apnea, the person stops breathing for a period of 10 seconds or more while sleeping, at least a few times per hour. Each time breathing stops, oxygen levels fall and cause the person to wake, which results in resumption of breathing. Sleep apnea most often occurs because of obstructed breathing, which is identified as obstructive sleep apnea (OSA). OSA results in drowsy episodes accompanied by snoring and apneic spells. OSA is more common in men, especially those who are overweight and are heavy drinkers. OSA also occurs in persons with enlarged tonsils, small jaws, large tongues and soft palates, and other subtle anatomic abnormalities. Persons taking medications such as sleeping pills can suffer from OSA because the upper airway muscles can relax too much. The tongue appears to fall back during the non–rapid eye movement sleep and block the airway. Infant apnea is associated with infections that obstruct the airway; sometimes the cause is not identifiable. Sudden infant death syndrome (SIDS) may be a variation. Central nervous system and obstructive problems may cause SIDS, but OSA seems to be an important component. Additional risk factors for SIDS include being male, low birth weight, decreased carotid body substance, and an upper respiratory infection.

Sore Throat

Sore throat, or pharyngitis, is an inflammation of the pharynx. If tonsils are involved, the condition is tonsillitis. The cause is usually viral, but a throat culture may show *Streptococcus,* the organism that causes rheumatic fever, rheumatic heart disease, or glomerulonephritis as complications in certain individuals. Common signs and symptoms are a red, tender throat, enlarged cervical lymph nodes, and fever. Treatment consists of rest, an analgesic, saline gargles, and an antibiotic if the culture is positive for *Streptococcus.*

Tuberculosis

Tuberculosis is an infection that develops as chronic inflammatory lesions from the bacillus *Mycobacterium tuberculosis.* Once thought to be a rare occurrence, tuberculosis is on the rise again in adults who are immunosuppressed. Although any site of the body may be affected, pulmonary tuberculosis is by far the most common. In rare cases tuberculosis also may affect the bones and kidneys. Early symptoms include listlessness and fatigue, chest pain, fever, and weight loss. The disease progresses to impair respiratory function severely and spreads to involve other body sites. This disease is contagious, spread by inhalation or ingestion of infected droplets dispersed by the infected person through coughing and nasal discharge. Treatment includes rest, nutritional support, and a medication regimen that may last more than a year. The disease is no longer infectious after the sputum tests free of bacteria, although the bacteria may lie dormant.

INDICATIONS CONTRAINDICATIONS

For Therapeutic Massage

Any of the listed disorders of the respiratory system of viral or bacterial cause usually contraindicate therapeutic massage until the disease runs its course. Whenever the body is under stress, as with respiratory infection, further stress in the system can worsen the condition. Simple palliative measures to provide comfort and encourage sleep are appropriate. The practitioner should follow all sanitary procedures and Standard Precautions.

In chronic conditions such as asthma or emphysema, general stress management and maintenance of normal function of the muscles of respiration are beneficial, again gauging the appropriate added stress levels caused by the massage stimulation. In cystic fibrosis, percussion helps loosen the phlegm but should not be attempted without medical supervision and training.

Therapeutic massage approaches and moderate application of movement therapies such as tai chi, yoga, or aerobic exercise often help breathing pattern disorder. Almost every meditation or relaxation system uses breathing patterns because they are a direct link to altering autonomic nervous system patterns, which in turn alters mood, feelings, and behavior. Other ways to modulate breathing are through singing and chanting.

The shoulders should not move during normal breathing. One should activate the accessory muscles of respiration located in the neck area only when increased oxygen is required for fight or flight. This is the pattern for sympathetic breathing. If the person does not use the additional oxygen through increased activity levels, blood gas levels change and symptoms appear. Constant activation of the accessory muscles of respiration such as the scalenes, sternocleidomastoid, serratus posterior superior, levator scapulae, rhomboids, abdominals, and quadratus lumborum for breathing when forced inhalation and expiration are not called for results in dysfunctional muscle patterns. Therapeutic massage can bring balance into these areas to encourage a more effective breathing pattern. General stress management reduces anxiety and helps to normalize the breathing pattern.

Although detailed discussion of the many meditations, breathing modulation, or retraining measures is beyond the scope of this text, two basic types of systems exist: one leading to physiologic hyperarousal and one to hypoarousal. Both processes facilitate a reestablishment of homeostasis, just as a muscle can be encouraged to relax by tensing it first and then releasing it or by using the antagonist pattern to initiate reciprocal inhibition to allow the muscle to relax. Hyperarousal systems increase sympathetic activity with a secondary parasympathetic balance. Aerobic exercise is an example. Hypoarousal systems directly activate parasympathetic responses. Examples are quiet reflection or meditative prayer combined with a chant to promote exhalation. Many resources use retraining programs to improve breathing patterns, and the recommendation is to find one that is comfortable and use it regularly.

Herbs such as eucalyptus give off a vapor that is soothing to the respiratory system. Aromatherapy uses different scents that are taken into the body through the respiratory system. Some scents have a stimulating effect, and others have a more calming effect. The efficacy of aromatherapy is valid when we understand the influence of the sense of smell on physiology. As with most forms of therapeutic massage, aromatherapy is nonspecific, supporting the body in balanced function (Activity 12-1). ■

Digestive System

Digestion is a physiologic process that involves the intake and assimilation of nutrients and the **elimination** of waste (Figures 12-7 and 12-8). The intake of food is much more than a means of gaining nutrients for growth, repair, and maintenance of the body. Eating is a pleasurable activity and social event that involves many neurochemical interactions. Food choices can have an effect on our health risks. Biologic drives for food, especially foods high in fat and simple carbohydrates or sugars, played an important part in early human survival. These foods, which are rare in nature, supply quick and sustaining energy sources. No longer rare in our society, an overabundance of fat and sugar feeds the biologic cravings we still have even though the energy required to acquire these food sources has decreased. The result is an epidemic of obesity.

Emotional eating is one type of substitution for lack of touch stimulation and loving relationships with others because the chemicals stimulated during all these processes are similar. Foods such as chocolate and other fat/carbohydrate combinations, along with some form of protein, generate serotonin and other feel-good neurochemicals just as effectively as a hug does. Food behaviors can become as addictive as any other pleasurable activity. Exercise also results in a chemical pattern similar to eating or being touched. Therefore moderate exercise programs are beneficial to weight management. Because biologic tendencies are for energy conservation, and our biologic patterns are for survival in a more primitive environment, the internal drive toward movement and activity was originally to provide for shelter, food, and protection. In society today we find ourselves needing to move for the sake of movement without an immediate survival process attached to it. This is a physiologically confusing process and may be part of the reason that some persons have difficulty finding any motivation to exercise.

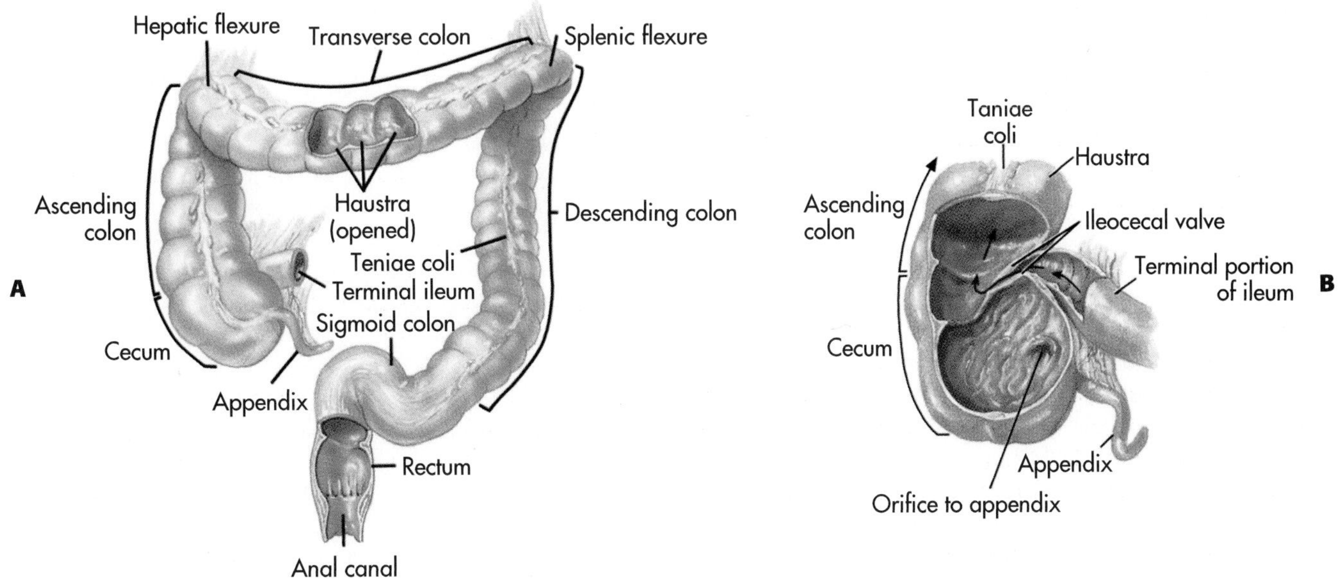

Figure 12-7
A, Anatomy of large intestine showing the junction between the large and small intestines and the entry of the ileum into the cecum. **B,** Enlarged detail of cecum and terminal ileum. (From LaFleur Brooks M: *Exploring medical language: a student-directed approach,* ed 5, St Louis, 2002, Mosby.)

ACTIVITY 12-1

We must be able to explain and justify the therapeutic value of the work we do. The following activity will assist you in developing the skills to explain the effectiveness of therapeutic massage to clients and other health care professionals. Use the clinical reasoning model that follows to accomplish this task. The focus should be the primary massage method applied to the respiratory system.

Methods/Applications

1. What are the facts?

   a. Which system is involved, and which structures of that system can be reached directly or indirectly?

   b. What is considered normal or balanced function?

   c. How are the functions of this system related to the homeostasis of the body?

   d. Which of these structures are most affected by this massage?

   e. Which physiologic functions are affected by this massage?

   f. When the treatment is applied, what changes in function will occur in

      (1) this system?

      (2) the whole body?

ACTIVITY 12-1—cont'd

g. What has worked or has not worked?

h. Where could you find information that would support the use of massage as a therapeutic intervention?

i. What research is available to support the use of the therapeutic massage?

j. How does the intervention support a healthy state?

k. Under which pathologic or dysfunctional conditions is the therapeutic massage most likely to be beneficial?

2. What are the possibilities?

a. What do the facts suggest?

b. List at least three applications of massage that would affect the structure and function of the system involved.

c. What are other ways to look at the situation?

d. What other methods could provide similar benefits?

3. What is the logical outcome of therapeutic intervention?

Continued

ACTIVITY 12-1—cont'd

a. What would be the logical progression of the symptom pattern, contributing factors, and current behaviors?

b. What are the benefits and drawbacks of each intervention suggested?

Benefits:

Drawbacks:

c. What are the costs in terms of time, resources, and finances?

d. What is likely to happen if massage is not used?

e. What is likely to happen if massage is used?

4. What would be the effect on the persons involved, specifically the client, practitioner, and other professionals working with the client?

a. How does each person involved (including, besides the foregoing, the client's family and support system) feel about the possible massage interventions?

b. Does the practitioner feel qualified to work with the situation and apply massage to the particular person?

c. Does a feeling of cooperation and agreement exist among all those involved, and how would the practitioner recognize this feeling?

Justification

Using the information developed in the clinical reasoning model, present a clear, concise statement of how massage would be beneficial in supporting the particular body system in a healthy condition or as part of a treatment plan for a pathologic or dysfunctional condition.

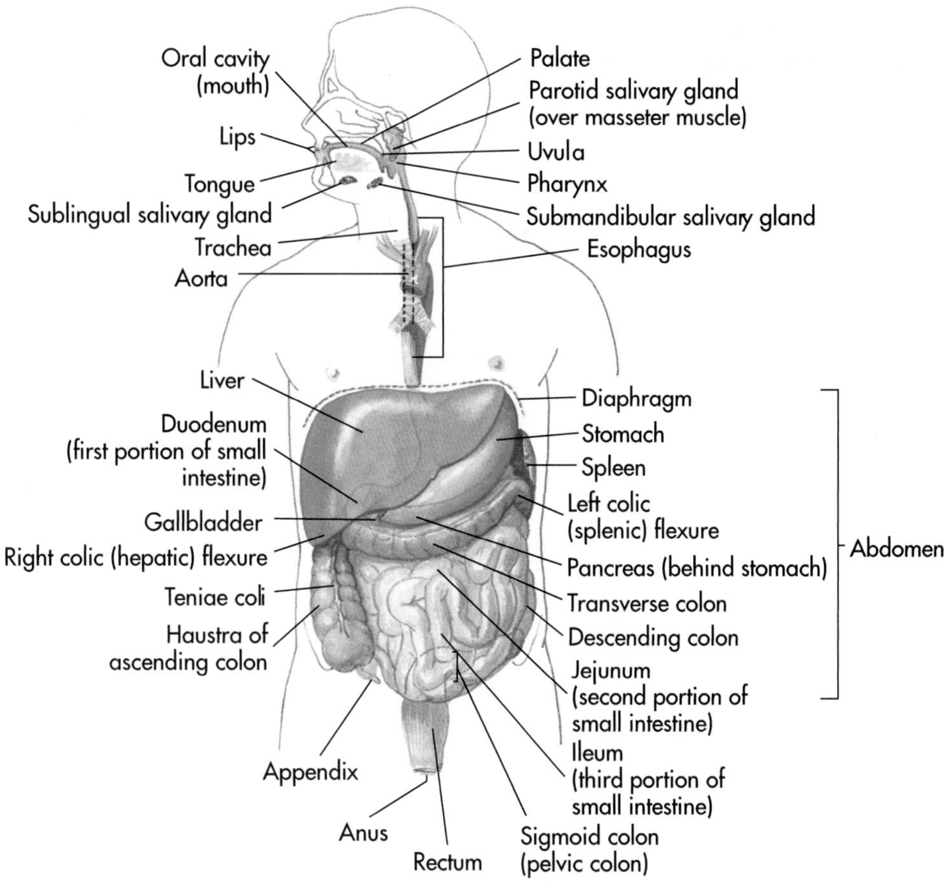

Figure 12-8
Organs of the digestive system and some associated structures. (From LaFleur Brooks M: *Exploring medical language: a student-directed approach,* ed 5, St Louis, 2002, Mosby.)

Eating food and fasting as a cleansing or purification process are often at the heart of social and religious rituals. What would a holiday be without all the food? Healing practices usually involve the ingestion of a healing herb or brew. Mating behaviors, found as we pair into couples, often involve food and feeding behaviors. Who falls in love without sharing a meal—one milkshake with two straws—and, of course, the Western ritual of feeding each other the wedding cake?

One of the first acts of parental bonding is feeding the infant. Our lips and tongue remain forever sensitive to sensory stimulation connected with soothing and pleasurable behaviors. The act of eating stimulates these areas and provides comfort and sensory stimulation, as do childhood thumb sucking and adult kissing.

Even the process of elimination and social constraints and rules about passage of intestinal gas becomes important. Is a belch rude behavior best kept in private or a compliment for a good meal? One cause of chronic constipation in Western society is the social stigma involved with the act of a bowel movement.

Food itself is interesting. Whether the food source is plant or animal, the life force is transferred from one being to another. Eating is the giving of one life for the continuation of another. "What greater gift is there than laying down your life for another?" is an inspiring quote. Human beings are at the top of the food chain. Regardless of what we eat, many lives—plant and animal—have been sacrificed so we may live. Ancient peoples and those who still attempt to live in the old ways remember this. The act of asking for a blessing on the food is the ritual of respect and honoring of the life force given so we may live.

As we explore the parts and process of the digestive system ever so briefly in this text, the student would do well to remember the bigger picture involved with the intake of food and water, and the process of receiving energy from one so that another may live.

Organs and Structures of the Digestive System

The digestive system is one long tube with accessory organs that starts at the mouth, extends through the body, and ends at the anus (Figure 12-9). This tube is known as the gastrointestinal tract, also referred to as the alimentary canal. The gastrointestinal tract is about 30 feet long and contains several special structures throughout its length. The entire lining is a mucous membrane made up of three

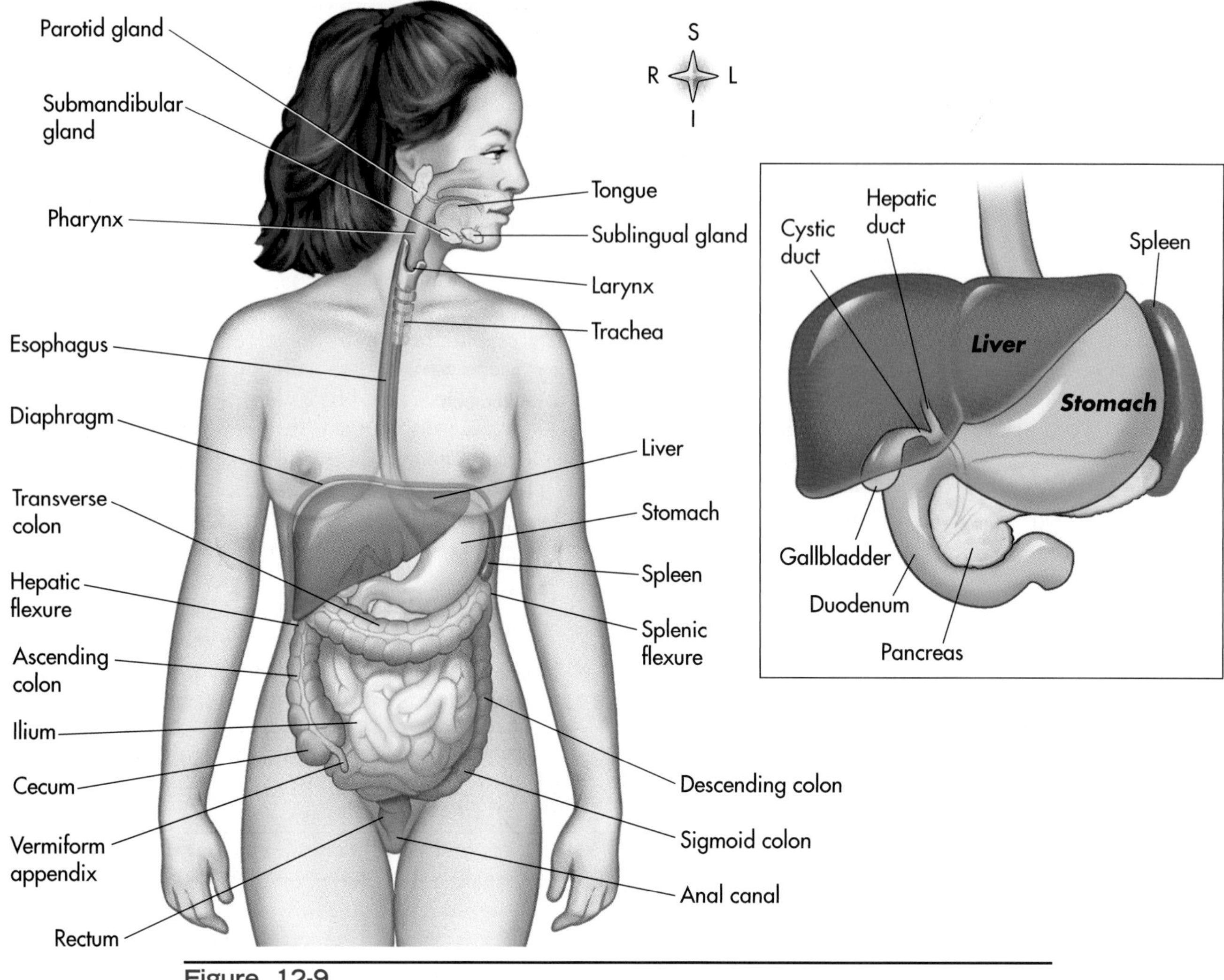

Figure 12-9
Location of digestive organs. (From Thibodeau GA, Patton KT: *The human body in health and disease,* ed 3, St Louis, 2002, Mosby.)

layers of tissues: epithelium, connective tissue, and smooth muscle.

The *digestive tract* consists of the mouth, pharynx, esophagus, stomach, small intestine, large intestine, rectum, and anus. Accessory structures include the salivary glands, pancreas, liver, and gallbladder. The stomach and 24 to 30 feet of intestines lie in the abdominal cavity.

The abdomen, or abdominal cavity, contains the major organs of digestion. The cavity is lined with a mucous membrane called the *peritoneum* that prevents friction. The portion of the peritoneum lying against the body wall is the parietal peritoneum; the portion surrounding each organ is the visceral peritoneum. The *peritoneal cavity* is defined as the fluid-filled space between the parietal and visceral peritoneum. The peritoneal cavity lubricates and allows the viscera to move. In the embryo, the peritoneum is a large sac that lines the abdominal cavity. The beginnings of viscera are outside the sac. As they develop, they push into the peritoneum in varying degrees. Some organs are covered with peritoneum on only the anterior surface (*retroperitoneal*), whereas some organs are covered completely with peritoneum except for the small area where the mesentery attaches (*intraperitoneal*). Damage to the mesothelium (single-cell layer epithelium) lining the peritoneum could result in the peritoneal layers adhering to each other, which could interfere with the normal movement of viscera. The intestines are suspended by a double layer of peritoneum: the mesentery (small intestine) and the mesocolon (transverse colon). The *greater omentum* is located from the stomach to the transverse colon. Fat stored in the greater omentum accounts for much of the girth in obesity. The *lesser omentum* runs from the stomach and duodenum to the liver. A double-layered sheet or fold of peritoneum is called the omenta. *Peritoneal ligaments* consist of double layers of peritoneum. They connect organs with other organs or the abdominal wall and may contain blood vessels or remnants of blood vessels. The greater omentum is divided into three peritoneal ligaments: *gastrocolic ligament,* the apronlike part attached to the transverse colon; *gastrosplenic ligament,* the left part that connects the spleen to the greater curvature of the stomach; and *gastrophrenic ligament,* the superior part that attaches to the diaphragm.

Mouth

The mouth is the oral cavity and makes up the first portion of the gastrointestinal tract. The mouth includes the lips, cheeks, tongue, hard and soft palates, teeth, and salivary glands.

The tongue is a large, strong muscle that mixes the food particles with saliva and helps us swallow. The tongue also contains the taste buds.

The palate forms the roof of the mouth. The anterior hard part is the partition between the oral and nasal cavities and consists of the palatine and maxillae bones. The posterior soft portion is the partition between the oropharynx and nasopharynx.

Teeth are accessory structures used to bite off and mechanically break up large pieces of food into smaller ones that can be swallowed. These bonelike structures are actually calcified connective tissue covered with enamel.

Salivary glands are located inside the mouth and provide secretions that keep the mucous membrane of the mouth moist and that moisten and lubricate food to aid in swallowing. Saliva is mainly water mixed with a small amount of salts and organic substances. One of these is the enzyme amylase, which breaks down carbohydrates. Smell, sight, taste, and the thought of food stimulate parasympathetic nerve fibers to increase the secretion of saliva. Food that is mechanically chewed, chemically broken down, and mixed with water is referred to as a bolus.

Pharynx

The pharynx is a cavity located behind the mouth that receives the bolus from the mouth.

Esophagus

The esophagus is a 10-inch, muscular, collapsible tube directly behind the trachea that extends from the pharynx to the stomach. The opening into the stomach is the esophageal hiatus, and at the point of attachment is a thickened region called the cardiac sphincter, which keeps the entrance to the stomach closed and prevents gastric regurgitation.

Stomach

The stomach is a J-shaped, saclike organ that is actually an enlargement of the gastrointestinal tract. Its widest part is located beneath the diaphragm. The narrow, distal end lies under the liver and empties into the duodenum. The stomach receives the bolus from the esophagus and continues the digestion process. With the addition of more liquids the bolus breaks down and becomes a semiliquid known as *chyme.* The stomach contains folds called *rugae* that enable the stomach to expand as one ingests food. The walls of the stomach contain gastric glands that secrete the hormone gastrin and gastric juices, including hydrochloric acid, enzymes, mucus, and water. The *pylorus* is the part of the stomach that narrows to connect with the duodenum. The stomach ends at the *pyloric sphincter,* a muscle that regulates the flow of chyme into the small intestine. Some gastric cells have histamine receptors. Irritation of the stomach appears to liberate histamine, a potent stimulator of gastric acid secretion. Cimetidine (Tagamet) competes with histamine for receptor sites, thus blocking the secretion of acid and making it an effective medication for treating ulcers.

Small Intestine

The small intestine is a coiled, muscular tube approximately 24 to 30 feet long. The small intestine receives the chyme from the stomach and continues the digestive process using intestinal juices from the small intestine and secretions from the pancreas, liver, and gallbladder. The small intestine consists of three parts:

1. The *duodenum* (DU-O-DE-num) is the shortest portion, making up the first 10 inches of the small intestine. The duodenum forms a C-shaped curve, circling the head of the pancreas, at which point it becomes the jejunum. Ducts from the liver, gallbladder, and pancreas enter this structure.
2. The *jejunum* (JE-JU-num) continues from the duodenum for the next 7 to 8 feet. The jejunum is supplied with blood vessels, lymph vessels, and nerves by a fold in the peritoneum called the mesentery. Numerous glands located in the walls of the jejunum provide secretions for the digestive process, the primary function of the jejunum. Most of the **absorption** of foodstuffs takes place in the jejunum, with some in the ileum.
3. The *ileum* (il-E-um) makes up the final 12 feet of the small intestine. The ileum connects the small intestine to the large intestine at the ileocecal valve, a sphincter. Mesenteries support the ileum and provide the means for blood vessels, lymph vessels, and nerves to supply the ileum. Absorption of food into the bloodstream and the lymphatic system is the major function of the ileum.

Pancreas

The pancreas is a long gland (about 5 inches by 1 inch) that lies behind the stomach and is connected to the duodenum by two pancreatic ducts. Most of the pancreas functions as an endocrine gland by producing digestive enzymes called pancreatic juices. About 1% of the cells of the pancreas, the islets of Langerhans, are scattered throughout the pancreas and secrete the hormones insulin, glucagon, and somatostatin.

Liver

The largest gland of the body and weighing about 3 lb, the liver lies under the diaphragm. The liver has many important functions, including the following:

1. Is active in protein metabolism.
2. Breaks down fatty acids and stores the fat we need as fuel.
3. Removes glucose from the blood and stores it as glycogen when blood sugar levels are high; converts it back to glucose when blood sugar levels are low.

4. Secretes bile, which is important in the digestion of fats.
5. Stores vitamins A, B_{12}, D, E, K, iron, and copper.
6. Detoxifies the blood by removing drugs or hormones.
7. Converts amino acids into glucose or fatty acids, depending on the needs of the body.
8. Destroys old red and white blood cells.

Gallbladder

The gallbladder is a small 3- to 4-inch sac that lies on the undersurface of the liver; its function is to store and concentrate bile. The gallbladder releases bile into the small intestine by way of the cystic duct.

Large Intestine

The large intestine is a large muscular tube, about 4 to 5 feet long and $2^1/_2$ inches in diameter. The large intestine has few digestive functions but does serve to reabsorb water and electrolytes, manufacture vitamins, and form and store the feces until defecation occurs. The large intestine, also called the colon, consists of eight parts:

1. The *cecum* begins as a blind pouch about 3 inches long and receives the digestive matter from the ileum of the small intestine.
2. The *appendix* is a narrow, twisted, close-ended tube attached to the cecum. The appendix contains lymphatic tissue, but its function has not been defined clearly.
3. The *ascending colon* goes up on the right side of the abdomen to the underside of the liver, where it curves toward the left. This curve is known as the hepatic flexure.
4. The *transverse colon* goes across the abdomen from the hepatic flexure to the spleen, where it turns downward at the splenic flexure.
5. The *descending colon* extends down the left side of the abdomen from the splenic flexure to about the top of the iliac crest.
6. The *sigmoid colon* forms an S-shaped curve beginning at the left iliac crest and continues to the middle of the abdomen, where it connects the descending colon to the rectum.
7. The *rectum* is a straight, 5- to 6-inch continuation of the sigmoid colon, beginning at about the level of S3.
8. The *anal canal* is the last inch of the rectum, and it ends at the anus, a sphincter muscle of smooth and skeletal muscle that controls the involuntary and voluntary elimination of feces.

The main function of the colon is the absorption of water and sodium.

Undigested matter passes as feces. The brown color of stool results from the breakdown products of bile pigments. The colon contains large numbers of bacteria, and they may have a role in the production of vitamins.

Medicines often are given as rectal suppositories because the colon has great absorptive capacity.

A colostomy is an artificial opening between the colon and skin of the abdomen for the evacuation of feces. Usually done to relieve tumor obstruction, physicians can perform a colostomy as a temporary measure when inflammation or trauma is present.

Nerves

Parasympathetic stimulation from the vagus and pelvic nerves (from the sacral part of the spinal cord) increases **peristalsis** and secretion of mucus, which protects the intestinal wall. Sympathetic stimulation has the opposite effect.

Digestion

The function of the digestive system is to break down foods to be assimilated by the body. Digestion begins in the mouth and ends in the small intestine (Figure 12-10) and is accompanied by digestive enzymes (protein catalysts) that

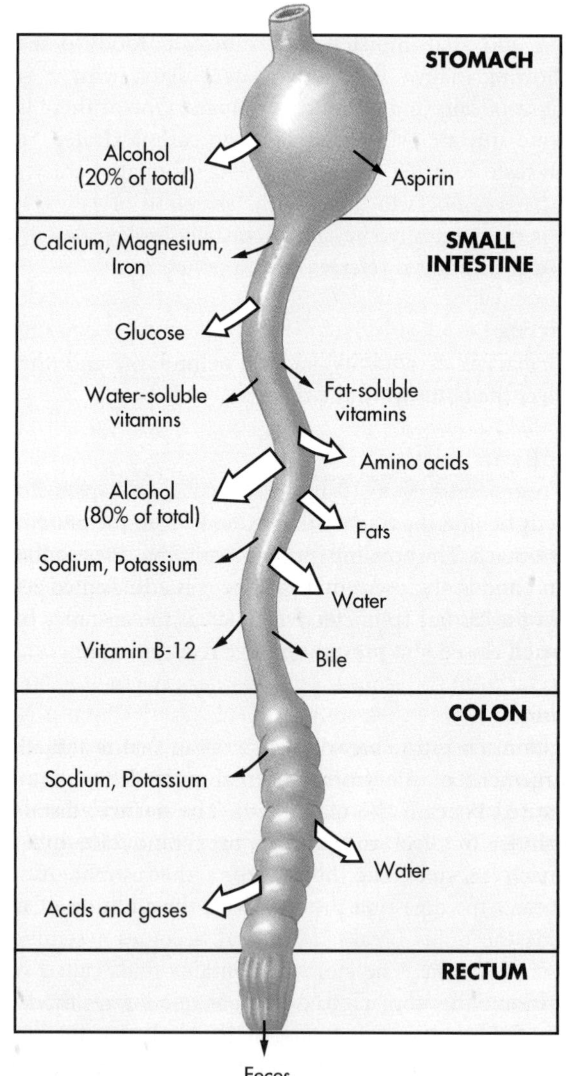

Figure 12-10
Absorption sites in the digestive tract. The size of the arrow at each site indicates the amount of absorption of a particular substance at that site. Most absorption occurs in the intestines, particularly the small intestine. (From Thibodeau GA, Patton KT: *Anatomy and physiology*, ed 5, St Louis, 2003, Mosby.)

TABLE 12-1
Chemical Digestion

Digestive Juices and Enzymes	Substance Digested (or Hydrolyzed)	Resulting Product*
Saliva		
Amylase	Starch (polysaccharide)	Maltose (a double sugar, or disaccharide)
Gastric Juice		
Protease (pepsin) plus hydrochloric acid	Proteins	Partially digested proteins
Pancreatic Juice		
Proteases (e.g., trypsin)†	Proteins (intact or partially digested)	Peptides and **amino acids**
Lipases	Fats emulsified by bile	**Fatty acids, monoglycerides,** and **glycerol**
Amylase	Starch	Maltose
Intestinal enzymes‡		
Peptidases	Peptides	Amino acids
Sucrase	Sucrose (cane sugar)	**Glucose** and **fructose**§ (simple sugars, or monosaccharides)
Lactase	Lactose (milk sugar)	**Glucose** and **galactose** (simple sugars)
Maltase	Maltose (malt sugar)	Glucose

*Substances in boldface type are end products of digestion (that is, completely digested nutrients ready for absorption).
†Secreted in inactive form (trypsinogen); activated by enterokinase, an enzyme in the intestinal brush border.
‡Brush-border enzymes.
§Glucose also is called *dextrose;* fructose also is called *levulose.*
From Thibodeau GA, Patton KT: *Anatomy and physiology,* ed 5, St Louis, 2003, Mosby.

split large substances into small ones. The gastrointestinal tract contains glands that secrete mucus and digestive enzymes (Table 12-1). The rhythmic contraction of smooth muscle called peristalsis propels products of digestion along the tract from the esophagus to the anus (Figure 12-11).

Box 12-2 shows the four essential steps in the process of digestion. Digestion secretion generally refers to the release of various substances from the exocrine glands that serve the digestive system (Table 12-2). Digestive secretion includes the release of saliva, gastric juice, pancreatic juice, bile, and intestinal enzymes.

Nutrition

Nutrition is the use of food for growth and maintenance of the body. Poor nutrition has an effect on general health, stress response, and sleeping. In the elderly, decreased ability to digest and assimilate food accounts for much of their poor nutrition. Others may have diseases that can cause nutritional deficiencies. For most of us, our nutritional problems result from not following dietary recommendations. Nutrition involves food. Food affects the mood. Mood influences feelings. Behavior supports feelings, and the whole issue of food is often an emotional topic.

The basics of good nutrition include eating a diet high in vegetables, grains, legumes, and fruit that is fresh, clean, and grown on nutrient-rich soil. Our protein requirement is moderate and may be met from animal or nonanimal sources. Fat and sugar requirements in the diet are small, but human beings have a strong urge for sweets and fats. This instinctive craving for fat and sugar causes many of our dietary problems. An ideal diet is low to moderate in unsaturated fats (avoid hydrogenated fats), sugars, and protein, with the bulk of the calories coming from complex carbohydrates. These recommendations can vary because differing genetic predisposition, age, and health can influence the ratio of fats, proteins, and carbohydrates that best suits an individual.

The food we eat is only as good as the soil on which it is grown or the food the animals were fed. Many suggest that much of the soil used in agriculture is worn out, depleted, and toxic from the continued use of artificial fertilizers and pesticides and overuse without rest time to replenish itself. If this is the condition of the soil, what is the nutritional value

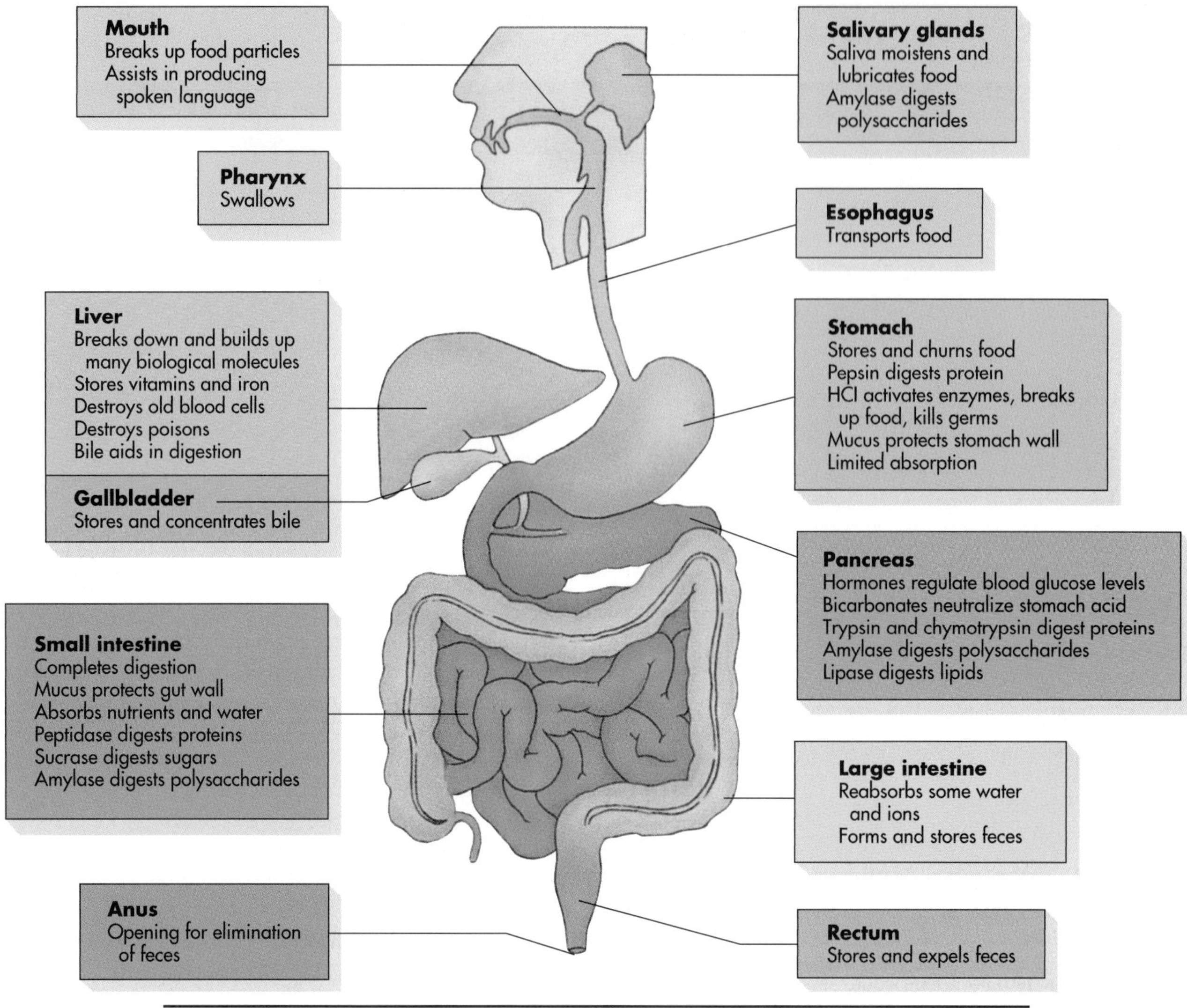

Figure 12-11
Summary of digestive function. (From Thibodeau GA, Patton KT: *Anatomy and physiology,* ed 5, St Louis, 2003, Mosby.)

of the food grown in it? Food is most nutritious when freshly harvested and ripe. Food eaten a day after harvest has lost a substantial amount of nutrients. Food, mostly fruit, picked green is not as nutritious as fruit allowed to ripen on the vine. Food preservation methods all result in loss of nutritional value in the food. Under ideal conditions, we would harvest all of our food an hour before we eat, but this is not possible for most of us. We have to make a trade-off between convenience and nutrition in many cases.

Many persons take nutritional supplements, and many opinions exist on this topic. One must remember that these are supplements to our diet and should not be expected to replace proper food intake. The closer a supplement is to a real food, the better the body is able to use it. Supplements usually are best taken with food to maximize absorption and use.

Drinking enough pure water is important to optimal body function. Recommendations are for at least 64 ounces of water per day for efficient body function.

Main Food Groups

Proteins. Proteins are large high-molecular-weight substances containing carbon, hydrogen, oxygen, and nitrogen and smaller amounts of other elements. Proteins break down into amino acids, which the body then absorbs. The body uses 24 amino acids for its metabolic requirements. Most can be manufactured in the liver from other amino acids, but eight cannot. These eight are referred to as essential amino acids: phenylalanine, valine, threonine, leucine, isoleucine, methionine, tryptophan, and lysine. In addition, histidine and arginine are required for growth and development. Dietary proteins include animal products and bean and grain combinations.

Proteins are the chief structural components of the body. Enzymes, some hormones, muscle tissue, and a substantial portion of chromosomes are proteins. Proteins are essential components of the cell membrane. Important compounds such as epinephrine and acetylcholine are derived from amino acids.

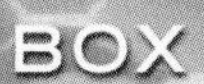
BOX 12-2

Steps in the Digestion Process

First Step
Ingestion: Food enters the mouth (i.e., eating).

Second Step
Digestion: The mechanical and chemical breakdown of food from its complex form into simple molecules.

Third Step
Absorption: The movement of the simple molecules from the digestive tract into the circulatory or lymphatic systems; vitamins and minerals are absorbed in the small intestine; amino acids, simple sugars, and small fatty acids pass through the intestinal villi into the bloodstream; larger fatty acids are reconstituted to fats in the intestinal wall and pass into the lymphatic system; capillaries of the intestinal villi become venules and then veins and finally the large portal vein carries absorbed foodstuffs to the liver; the liver converts these substances into compounds required for body functions.

Fourth Step
Elimination (egestion): Removal and release by defecation of solid waste products (feces) from food that cannot be digested or absorbed.

Carbohydrates. Carbohydrates have as basic components carbon, hydrogen, and oxygen in definite proportions. Complex carbohydrates are long chains of glucose molecules found in rice, vegetables, and so on. Animal starch or glycogen is the storage form of glucose in liver and muscle. Starch is digested in the mouth and small intestine and breaks down into monosaccharides and disaccharides, which are sugars or simple carbohydrates.

Glucose is the main fuel for the manufacture of adenosine triphosphate in the cell. The liver converts sugars to glucose.

Fats. Fats, or triglycerides, break down into fatty acids and glycerol. A fatty acid is a molecule consisting of a chain of carbons with no double bonds (saturated) or several double bonds (unsaturated). The unsaturated fats most closely resemble body fat and are more easily assimilated and used. Saturation (addition of hydrogen molecules) makes fat more solid and less desirable in the diet. Linoleic acid is an example of a fatty acid essential to human nutrition. In addition to serving as a reservoir of stored energy, fats are essential components of many hormones, the cell membrane, and the myelin sheath of the nerve fiber. Dietary fats are found in nuts, seeds, oils, and animal products.

Vitamins. Vitamins are growth factors needed in small amounts for daily body metabolism. They are classified as fat soluble or water soluble. Many vitamins act as enzyme activators (coenzymes). The fat-soluble vitamins are more toxic because excess amounts are stored in the fat tissue and are not excreted readily. Water-soluble vitamins, however, are absorbed and excreted more easily.

Citric Acid Cycle

The citric acid cycle (Krebs cycle) is the main pathway by which food energy is released by cells to manufacture their own energy-rich adenosine triphosphate. The citric acid cycle is a complex transformation process. Glycogen (from the liver) is converted to glucose and then to pyruvic acid, which then enters the citric acid cycle. The end result of many chemical reactions is energy for cellular function (Figure 12-12).

Metabolic Rate

Metabolic rate is the catabolic rate, or rate of energy release.

The ***basal metabolic rate,*** *BMR*, is not the minimum metabolic rate and does not indicate the smallest amount of energy that must be expended to sustain life. BMR does indicate, however, the smallest amount of energy expenditure that can sustain life and also maintain the waking state and a normal body temperature in a comfortably warm environment (Figure 12-13). The BMR is the rate of energy expenditure under basal conditions, that is when the individual:

- Is awake but lying down and not moving.
- Is 18 to 23 hours after the last meal.
- Is in a comfortably warm environment.

The BMR is not identical for all individuals because of the influence of the following factors:

Size: BMR is calculated from the individual's height and weight. A large individual has more surface area and a greater BMR than a small individual.

Sex: Men oxidize their food approximately 5% to 7% faster than women, so the same size male has a BMR greater than the female. This gender difference in BMR probably results from the difference in the proportion of body fat determined by sex hormones. Women tend to have a higher percentage of body fat (and thus a lower total lean mass) than men. Fat tissue is less metabolically active than lean tissues such as muscle.

Age: The younger the individual, the higher the BMR for a given size and sex.

Thyroid hormones: Thyroid hormones (T_3 and T_4) stimulate basal metabolism. Without a normal amount of these hormones in the blood, one cannot maintain a normal BMR.

Body temperature: An increase in body temperature increases BMR. A decrease in body temperature (hypothermia) has the opposite effect.

Drugs: Stimulants increase the BMR, and depressants decrease the BMR.

Other factors: Other factors, such as emotions, pregnancy, and lactation (milk production), also influence basal metabolism.

All of these factors increase the BMR.

TABLE 12-2
Digestive Secretions

DIGESTIVE JUICE	SOURCE	SUBSTANCE	FUNCTION
Saliva	Salivary glands	Mucus	Lubricates bolus of food; mixing of food.
		Amylase	Enzyme; begins digestion of starches.
		Sodium bicarbonate	Increases pH (for optimal amylase function).
		Water	Dilutes food and facilitates mixing.
Gastric juice	Gastric glands	Pepsin	Enzyme; digests proteins.
		Hydrochloric acid	Breaks down proteins; decreases pH (for optimal pepsin function).
		Intrinsic factor	Protects and allows later absorption of vitamin B_{12}.
		Mucus	Lubricates chyme; protects stomach lining.
		Water	Dilutes food and facilitates mixing.
Pancreatic Juice	Pancreas (exocrine portion)	Proteases (trypsin, chymotrypsin, collagenase, elastase, etc.)	Enzymes; digest proteins.
		Lipases (lipase, phospholipase, etc.), colipase	Enzymes; digest lipids. Coenzyme; helps lipase digest fats.
		Nucleases	Enzymes; digest nucleic acids (RNA and DNA).
		Amylase	Enzyme; digests starches.
		Water, mucus	Dilute food; facilitate mixing and lubricate.
		Sodium bicarbonate	Increases pH (for optimal enzyme function).
Bile	Liver (stored and released by gallbladder)	Lecithin and bile salts	Emulsify lipids.
		Sodium bicarbonate	Increases pH (for optimal enzyme function).
		Cholesterol	Excess cholesterol from body cells; to be excreted with feces.
		Products of detoxification	From detoxification of harmful substances by hepatic cells; to be excreted with feces.
		Bile pigments (mainly bilirubin)	Products of breakdown of heme groups during hemolysis; to be excreted with feces.
		Mucus	Lubricates
		Water	Dilutes food and other substances; facilitates mixing.
Intestinal juice	Mucosa of small and large intestines	Mucus	Lubricates.
		Sodium bicarbonate	Increases pH (for optimal enzyme function).
		Water	Small amount; carries mucus and sodium bicarbonate.

From Thibodeau GA, Patton KT: *Anatomy and physiology,* ed 5, St Louis, 2003, Mosby.

Energy Balance and Body Weight

Total metabolic rate is the amount of energy used or expended by the body in a given time. The BMR usually constitutes about 55% to 60% of the total metabolic rate. The energy used to do all kinds of skeletal muscle work contributes to the total metabolic rate. The metabolic rate increases for several hours after a meal, apparently because of the energy needed for metabolizing foods.

The body attempts to maintain a state of energy balance when its energy input equals its energy output. Energy input per day equals the total calories (kilocalories) in the food ingested per day. Energy output equals the total metabolic rate expressed in kilocalories. Energy intake versus output determines body weight.

Body weight remains constant (except for possible variations in water content) when the body maintains energy balance. Body weight increases when energy input exceeds energy output, and the body synthesizes and stores fat. Body weight decreases when energy input is less than energy output.

Mechanisms for regulating food intake still are not established clearly, but studies seem to indicate that a portion of the lateral hypothalamus functions as an appetite center (feeling hungry) and satiety center (feeling full). Many factors operate together as a complex mechanism for regulating food intake.

Pathologic Conditions

Appendicitis

Appendicitis is an inflammation of the appendix usually from bacterial infection. Signs and symptoms often begin

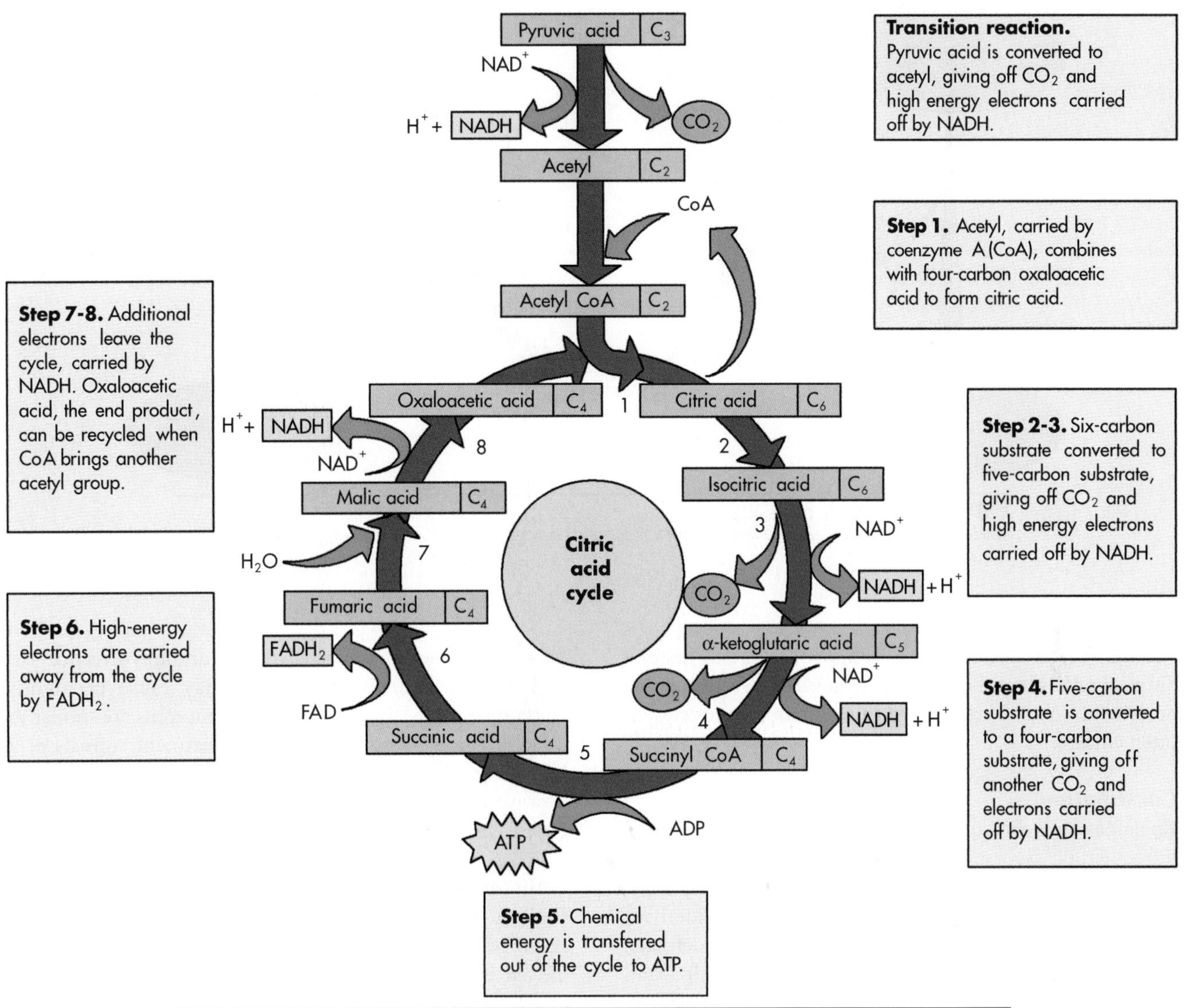

Figure 12-12
Citric acid cycle. The transition reaction prepares each pyruvic acid molecule to enter the citric acid cycle, yielding a pair of high-energy electrons and a CO_2 molecule. Coenzyme A (*CoA*) picks up the acetyl group thus formed and takes it into the citric acid cycle proper, which is described here as a recurring series of eight steps. (From Thibodeau GA, Patton KT: *Anatomy and physiology,* ed 5, St Louis, 2003, Mosby.)

with discomfort in the umbilical region that becomes painful and localized in the lower right quadrant, with fever, nausea, and vomiting. The appendix may be inflamed or abscessed or may burst. If the appendix bursts, the pain initially decreases because of the pressure release, but the bacteria spread to the abdominal cavity, resulting in peritonitis or infection of the peritoneal membrane that can be fatal.

Cirrhosis

Cirrhosis is the infiltration of connective tissue into the functioning cells of the liver that causes slow deterioration of the liver. End stage signs and symptoms include jaundice, portal hypertension, and fluid accumulation in the peritoneal cavity. The most common cause is alcoholism, although cirrhosis also occurs in hepatitis. Cirrhosis interrupts many systemic functions. If the disease is not too far advanced and causal factors can be eliminated, liver regeneration capacity is good.

Colon Cancer

Colon cancer is the most common cancer and usually affects the lowest part of the rectum. Males and females are equally susceptible. Tumors of the ascending colon (right-sided) usually cause rectal bleeding; those in the descending colon cause constipation and obstructive symptoms. Polyps and ulcerative colitis are important risk factors. Screening for blood in the stool, as well as sigmoidoscopy, detects most

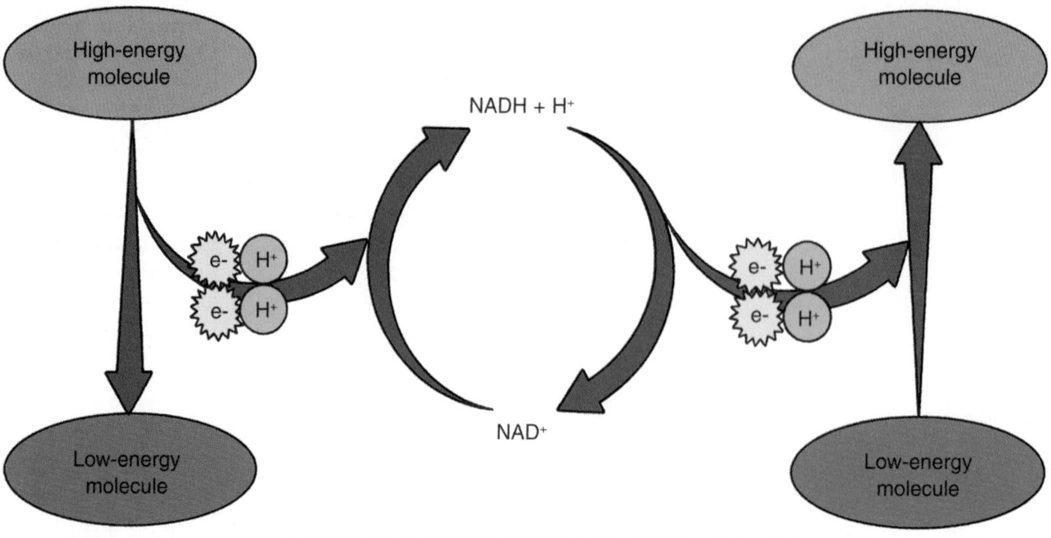

Figure 12-13
Metabolic rate. (From Thibodeau GA, Patton KT: *Anatomy and physiology,* ed 5, St Louis, 2003, Mosby.)

lesions; 70% are located in the sigmoid colon and rectum. Surgical removal of the bowel or removal of a section of the bowel with the ends reattached to maintain a passageway is often curative.

Constipation

Constipation is difficulty passing stools or an incomplete or infrequent passage of hard stool. Among the organic causes are *intestinal obstruction, diverticulitis,* and *tumors.* Functional impairment of the colon may occur in elderly or bedridden clients who fail to respond to the urge to defecate. Backache and headache may be present. Constipation and diarrhea are common side effects of many medications. Increase in fluid and dietary bulk and exercise are helpful. Stool softeners may be prescribed for the constipation. Education about regular bowel habits may be necessary.

Cystic Fibrosis

Cystic fibrosis is a genetic disease involving exocrine gland dysfunction. Secretions from the pancreas, mucous glands of the respiratory tract, and sweat glands are defective. Without production of pancreatic enzymes, the digestive tract cannot break down food and absorb fats and nutrients. Rarely does a child survive beyond the teen years; most die from pulmonary infections. Treatment is a high-protein, high-calorie diet accompanied by the replacement of pancreatic enzymes. Antibiotics and inhalation and physical therapy are useful. Continuous home pulmonary care is often necessary.

Diverticular Disease

Diverticula are small, saclike outpouchings of the intestinal wall found in weak areas of the colon near where vessels are located. Most occur in the sigmoid colon. When multiple diverticula are present, the condition is diverticulosis. If they become inflamed and infected, the condition is diverticulitis. Perforation of a diverticular sac may cause peritonitis (inflammation of the peritoneum). Symptoms are similar to irritable bowel syndrome. Primary treatment consists of a high-fiber diet, increased intake of fluids, a bulk-forming laxative such as psyllium (Metamucil), and an antibiotic. Severe cases may require hospitalization.

Gallbladder Disease

Gallbladder disease (cholelithiasis) is almost always the result of a gallstone composed of bile salts and cholesterol lodged in the cystic duct. A fatty meal often precedes an attack because the presence of fat stimulates contraction of the gallbladder. Signs and symptoms are as follows:

- Pain in the right upper quadrant of the abdomen, often radiating to the right scapula or upper back
- Nausea and vomiting
- Fever

Gallbladder colic is pain caused by a stone temporarily obstructing the cystic duct or common bile duct. Cholecystitis is inflammation of the gallbladder from obstruction of the cystic duct or common bile duct (choledocholithiasis or common bile duct stone). Cholangitis is infection of the biliary tree.

Treatment of mild cases of gallbladder disease involves using an analgesic and eliminating fatty foods from the diet. If infection is present, antibiotics are used. Surgical removal of the gallbladder may be necessary.

Gastroenteritis

Gastroenteritis is a general term for irritation, inflammation, or infection of the gastrointestinal tract. If the stomach is involved, the condition is gastritis. Hemorrhagic gastritis is characterized by bleeding erosions, also is called acute erosive gastritis or multiple gastric erosions, and can occur without any apparent reason. Hemorrhagic gastritis is associated, however, with aspirin ingestion, burns, traumatic injury, surgery, shock, liver disease, respiratory problems, and septicemia and can cause vomiting and diarrhea and lead to dehydration. Gastroenteritis can become dangerous if infectious organisms or toxic substances enter the bloodstream.

If the intestine is affected, the condition is enteritis. Usually the stomach and intestine are involved, so the term *gastroenteritis* applies. The most common cause is a virus, which can be passed from person to person. This stomach flu usually lasts 24 to 36 hours. If the cause is a bacterial toxin, the condition is food poisoning. Occasionally, bacterial infection or, rarely, protozoal infection (dysentery) causes enteritis. Diarrhea and generalized cramping abdominal pain are symptoms of the condition. Food poisoning from toxic foods, poisonous mushrooms, and so on is implicated in many cases. The inflammation also may result from illness or dietary changes, especially when eating foods or drinking water while traveling to foreign countries, or may result from extended use of antibiotics. Primary treatment is rehydration and relaxing the hyperactive bowel. Fluids only for 24 hours relaxes the intestine because food stimulates gastrointestinal hormone release and peristalsis. Several compounds slow the bowel: bismuth subsalicylate (Pepto-Bismol), diphenoxylate with atropine (Lomotil), and anticholinergic antispasmodics such as dicyclomine (Bentyl). If a stool culture shows a bacterial or protozoal infection, an antibiotic or antiprotozoal is given.

Hemorrhoids

Hemorrhoids are dilated varicose veins of the anus. They often appear during pregnancy and delivery. External hemorrhoids lie distal to the anorectal margin; internal hemorrhoids lie proximal. Occasionally, a thrombus or clot forms, resulting in a painful, bluish mass. Hemorrhoids may cause pain, but the usual symptom is bleeding and itching caused by drying up of the protective mucus. Primary treatment is with sitz baths, suppositories, and stool softeners. The clot may be removed surgically under local anesthesia. Hemorrhoids also are treatable with a laser to seal the blood vessels, cryosurgery, injection, or surgical removal.

Hepatitis

Hepatitis is an infection of the liver and is discussed in the section on immunity in Chapter 11.

Hernia

A hernia is the protrusion of soft tissues through a tear or weak spot in a muscle wall. Herniae can occur anywhere but are most common in the abdomen. In a hiatal hernia the intestines bulge through an opening in the diaphragm. An inguinal hernia produces a bulging of the abdominal organs or the inguinal canal. A reducible hernia means that the bulge can be pressed back through the opening. An irreducible hernia cannot be repaired, and obstruction or strangulation may occur that creates a medical emergency.

Inflammatory Bowel Disease

Two inflammatory diseases of the gastrointestinal tract affect mainly young men and women, ages 20 to 40, causing ulcerative lesions and thickening of the intestinal wall. The cause for both is unknown, but an autoimmunity may be a factor. *Ulcerative colitis* primarily affects the sigmoid colon, with symptoms of lower abdominal pain and bloody diarrhea. Ulcers actually develop inside the large intestine. Regional enteritis is a chronic inflammation of the intestine, most commonly the ileum, is known as Crohn's disease, and presents symptoms of cramping, right lower quadrant pain, and intermittent diarrhea. One or two attacks may occur, or they may occur regularly. The body does not absorb nutrients and loses weight. Primary treatment for both is an adequate diet, antibiotic therapy, and steroids. Occasionally, surgical removal of the ileum is necessary.

Irritable Bowel Syndrome

Irritable bowel syndrome is also known as spastic, or irritable, colon. Symptoms include abdominal pain, alternating constipation and diarrhea, nausea, and gas. Poor diet, tension, and emotional problems can induce irritable bowel syndrome. Peristaltic action is not well coordinated and results in changes in the pattern of bowel movements. Primary treatment includes a diet high in fiber, restriction of alcohol and tobacco, a psyllium laxative such as Metamucil, and perhaps an anticholinergic tranquilizer such as Librax. A comprehensive stress management program is beneficial.

Malabsorption and Intolerance Syndromes

Malabsorption syndromes involve poor absorption of nutrients and can be caused by deficiency of digestive enzymes, inadequate transport of nutrients, or abnormalities in the structure of the intestine because of disease or surgery and hypersensitivity reaction to a particular food. Wheat, corn, and dairy products are the most common foods, and elimination diets may be beneficial. Malabsorption can result from cystic fibrosis, diabetes mellitus, or dietary intolerance such as celiac disease, a reaction to dietary gluten, or lactose intolerance as a result of lactase deficiency.

Obstructions

An obstruction is a partial or complete closure of the small or large intestine. As a result, chyme backs up, the intestinal walls expand, local arteries may be compressed, and ischemic bowel disease can result. Obstructions are caused by any of the following:

- Adhesion: Bands of fibrous tissue from previous inflammation or surgical scars that grow between and around the loops of intestine can cause strangulation.
- Hernia: A protrusion of the intestine through a weakness in the abdominal wall; if the loop of intestine becomes trapped or strangulated, a medical emergency exists.
- Tumors: Growths such as are seen in colon cancer can obstruct the intestine.
- Volvulus: A knotting or twisting can cause strangulation in the intestine.

Pancreatitis

Most cases of acute pancreatitis involve alcoholism and gallstones. Lipase, amylase, and trypsin (digestive enzymes) back up in the pancreas and are released into the surrounding tissue. This causes autodigestion of the pancreas and necrosis of tissues, including the peritoneum. Hemorrhage and shock may develop. Massive destruction of tissue accompanied by fluid and blood loss may lead to shock and death. Signs and symptoms include the following:

- Intense pain in the center of the upper abdomen radiating to the back
- Nausea and vomiting
- Distended, tender, and bruised abdomen; the person feels better sitting than lying.
- Elevated amylase and lipase levels in the bloodstream

Acute pancreatitis is a medical emergency. If one suspects the condition, immediate referral is necessary.

Chronic pancreatitis may occur after acute pancreatitis, gallstones, or alcohol abuse. Pancreatic function decreases and ultimately stops, no longer producing insulin and other pancreatic enzymes and hormones. Pain may be intense, and the person may require surgery to remove the pancreas or sever the nerves.

Peptic Ulcer Disease

A peptic ulcer is a gastric or duodenal ulcer that affects the lining of the esophagus, stomach, or duodenum. The sore can perforate the wall of the digestive tract. *Peptic ulcer disease* is the name given to the process. The term *peptic* means that pepsin is involved. Risk factors include being male, smoking, heredity, alcohol, and stress. An increased secretion of hydrochloric acid and pepsin, as well as decreased tissue resistance, contributes to the process. The normal protective mechanisms of the duodenal and gastric mucosa against hydrochloric acid and pepsin are blocked. Excessive vagal stimulation is present. The ulcer causes pain and may erode into a vessel and cause bleeding. The ulcer may perforate the intestinal or stomach wall, causing peritonitis and shock. Recent studies indicate a bacterial infection may cause many ulcers, and treatment involves the use of antibiotics.

Common signs and symptoms of peptic ulcer disease include the following:

- Heartburn or burning pain 1/2 hour to 2 hours after a meal, relieved by antacids
- Vomiting of brownish black material (the color of coffee grounds) or the passage of dark stools, indicating the presence of blood
- Tenderness on palpation of the epigastric region of the abdomen
- Nausea, weight loss, and decreased appetite

Antacids such as magnesium–aluminum hydroxide mixtures (Maalox, Mylanta) are useful. Cimetidine (Tagamet) or ranitidine (Zantac) inhibit gastric acid secretion. Stopping smoking, decreasing or stopping alcohol consumption, and using stress-management techniques also are indicated.

Reflux Esophagitis (Gastroesophageal Reflux)

Reflux esophagitis is the regurgitation of gastric acid up through an open esophageal sphincter, causing heartburn. This common and unpleasant problem usually is caused by problems with control of the esophageal sphincter that may be caused by hiatal hernia or other less common pathologic conditions. However, reflux esophagitis also may be caused by physical corrosion from components in the diet such as tobacco, alcohol, and acidic food. Lying flat or bending over often aggravates the discomfort, and sitting upright relieves it. Reflux esophagitis frequently occurs in obese persons. Inflammation or ulceration of the esophagus is present. Primary treatment is weight loss, to decrease the pressure on the abdominal structures and relieve the hiatal hernia, and use of an antacid.

Stomach Cancer

Stomach cancer is one of the more common causes of cancer death. Causal factors include exposure to environmental chemicals and chronic gastritis. Onset is slow and insidious with little advanced warning or detection mechanisms. Indigestion appears; other signs and symptoms are unexplained weight loss, epigastric pain, palpable upper abdominal mass, and iron-deficiency anemia from gastric bleeding.

INDICATIONS CONTRAINDICATIONS

For Therapeutic Massage

A client with shoulder pain (referred), abdominal pain, or referred back pain may have one of several gastrointestinal disorders. In such cases referral is necessary for proper diagnosis. Many gastrointestinal diseases are bacterial or viral and contagious. The practitioner should take appropriate precautions to maintain sanitary practice. Most chronic gastrointestinal diseases have a strong correlation to stress. The intestinal tract is highly responsive to changes in autonomic function and endocrine patterns. The influence of the vagus nerve is extensive, and research indicates therapeutic massage influences vagal function. Sympathetic arousal changes peristaltic action and can send the intestinal tract into all kinds of dysfunction. Comprehensive stress management programs, including therapeutic massage methods, are often effective in managing these conditions. Ginger is an herb that has been shown to soothe the digestive system.

A specific type of massage to the large intestine can assist in managing constipation. The practitioner can teach this method to the client for self-care. Such massage is contraindicated in inflammatory bowel disease, and the practitioner should obtain permission from the physician for any other conditions. The massage consists of short, scooping strokes firmly against the abdomen beginning on the left, always directed toward the rectum. Progress continues the length of the large intestine to the cecum in a fashion of two steps forward and one step back as the direction of the force is down and back toward the rectum. Beginning at the cecum on the right may push fecal material into a large mass, especially at the flexure (Figure 12-14, Activity 12-2). ■

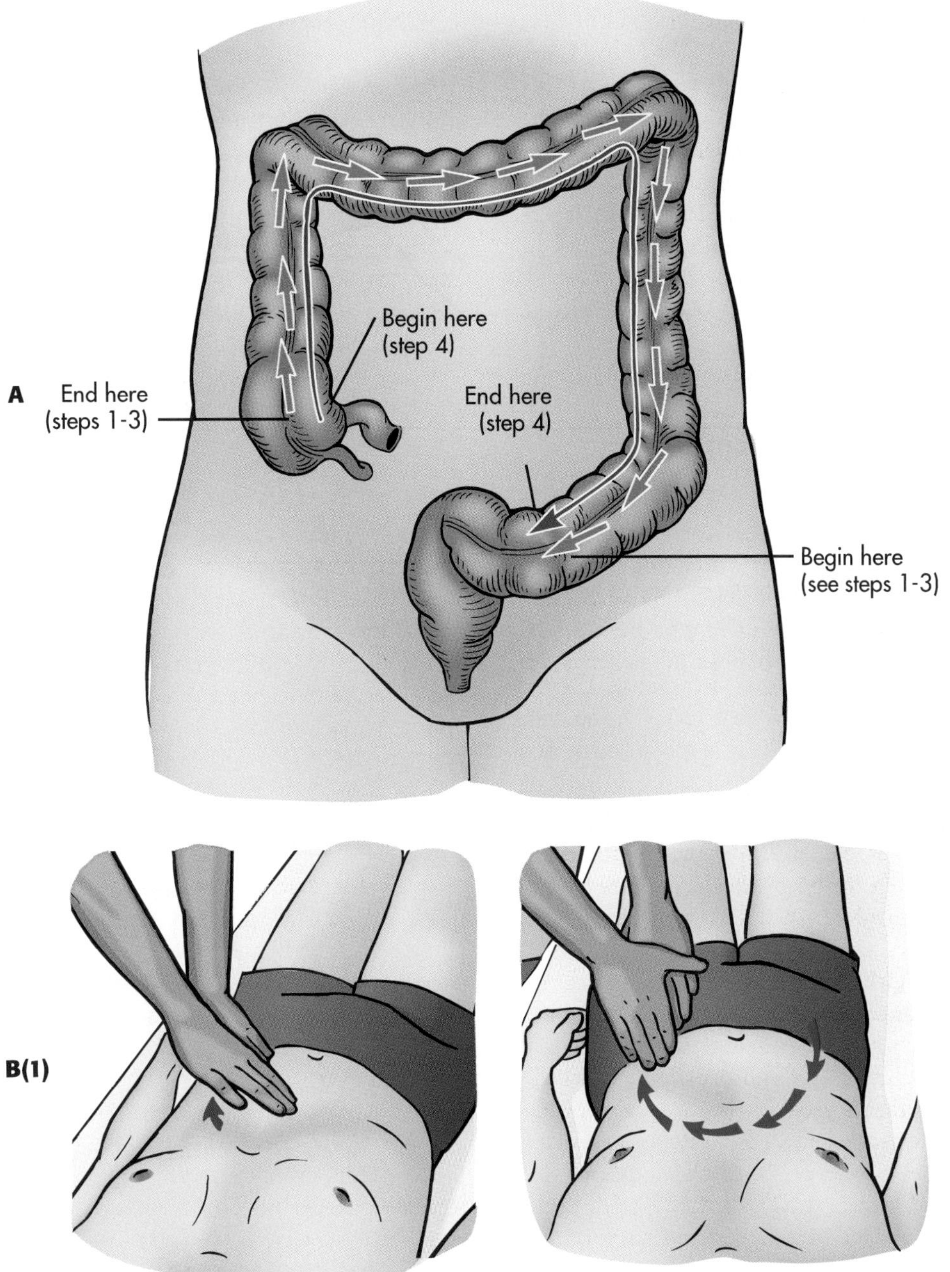

Figure 12-14

A, Colon with flow pattern arrows. All massage manipulations are directed in a clockwise fashion. The manipulations begin in the lower left-hand quadrant (on the left side as one views the illustration) at the sigmoid colon. The methods progressively contact all of the large intestine as they eventually end up encompassing the entire colon area. **B,** Abdominal sequence. The direction of flow for emptying of the large intestine and colon is as follows: *1,* Massage down the left side of the descending colon using short strokes directed to the sigmoid colon. *2,* Massage across the transverse colon to the left side using short strokes directed to the sigmoid colon. *3,* Massage up the ascending colon on the right side of the body using short strokes directed to the sigmoid colon. End at the right side ileocecal valve located in the lower right-hand quadrant of the abdomen. *4,* Massage entire flow pattern using long, light to moderate strokes from ileocecal valve to sigmoid colon. Repeat sequence. (Modified from Fritz S: *Mosby's fundamentals of therapeutic massage,* ed 3, St Louis, 2004, Mosby.)

Continued

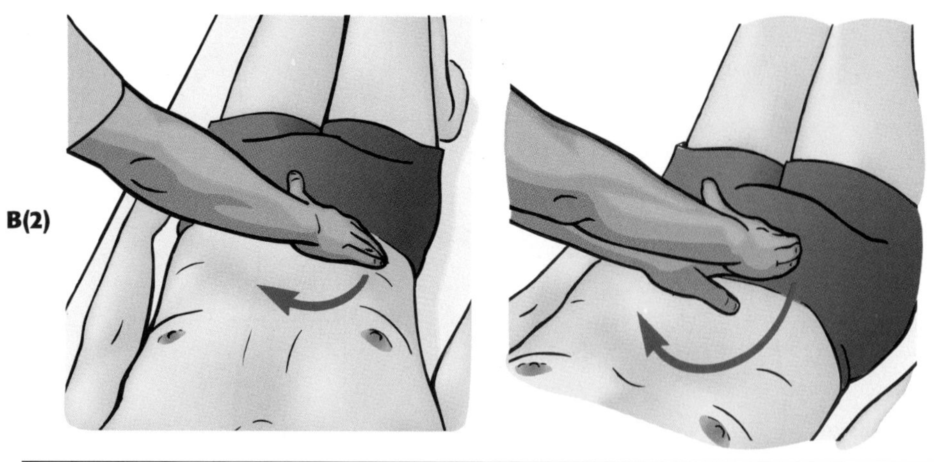

Figure 12-14—cont'd.

ACTIVITY 12-2

We must be able to explain and justify the therapeutic value of the work we do. The following activity will assist you in developing the skills to explain the effectiveness of therapeutic massage to clients and other health care professionals. Use the clinical reasoning model that follows to accomplish this task. The focus should be the primary modality or modalities applied to the digestive system.

Methods/Applications

1. What are the facts?

   a. Which system is involved, and which structures of that system can be reached directly or indirectly?

   b. Which of these structures are most affected by this modality?

   c. Which physiologic functions are affected by this approach?

   d. When the treatment is applied, what changes in function will occur in

      (1) this system?

      (2) the whole body?

   e. What is considered normal or balanced function?

   f. How are the functions of this system related to the homeostasis of the body?

ACTIVITY 12-2—cont'd

g. What has worked or has not worked?

h. Where could you find information that would support the use of this modality as a therapeutic intervention?

i. What research is available to support the use of the therapeutic intervention?

j. How does the intervention support a healthy state?

k. Under which pathologic or dysfunctional conditions is the therapeutic massage most likely to be beneficial?

2. What are the possibilities?

a. What do the data suggest?

b. What are the reasons for using the proposed methods?

c. What are the possible interventions?

d. List at least three applications of massage that would affect the structure and function of the system involved.

e. What are other ways to look at the situation?

f. What other methods could provide similar benefits?

3. What is the logical outcome of therapeutic intervention?

a. What would be the logical progression of the symptom pattern, contributing factors, and current behaviors?

Continued

ACTIVITY 12-2—cont'd

b. What are the benefits and drawbacks of each intervention suggested?

Benefits:

Drawbacks:

c. What are the costs in terms of time, resources, and finances?

d. What is likely to happen if the modality is not used?

e. What is likely to happen if the modality is used?

4. For the intervention proposed, what would be the effect on the persons involved, specifically the client, practitioner, and other professionals working with the client?

a. How does each person involved (including, besides the foregoing, the client's family and support system) feel about the possible interventions?

b. Does the practitioner feel qualified to work with the situation and apply the identified modality to the particular person?

c. Does a feeling of cooperation and agreement exist among all those involved, and how would the practitioner recognize this feeling?

Justification

Using the information developed in the clinical reasoning model, present a clear, concise statement of how the ways in which the particular soft tissue or movement modality would be beneficial in supporting the particular body system in a healthy condition or as part of a treatment plan for a pathologic or dysfunctional condition. Based on the foregoing information, give a brief summary of the effectiveness of the modality for this system.

Urinary System and Fluid Electrolyte Balances

The urinary system consists of two kidneys, two ureters, one bladder, and one urethra (Figure 12-15). The kidneys maintain homeostasis by filtering waste products from the blood and keeping the proper amount of water and nutrients in the blood. Urine passes out of the kidneys and down through the ureters to the bladder for storage. When the bladder reaches a certain volume, one has the urge to void. The bladder expels urine through the urethra.

Functions of the Urinary System

The important functions of the urinary system are as follows:

- Conservation of water
- Maintenance of the normal concentration of electrolytes
- Regulation of the acid-base balance
- Regulation of blood pressure
- Activation of vitamin D

The kidneys filter and eliminate most waste. In the average person the kidneys filter about 100 L of blood, reabsorbing 99 L of filtrate and leaving about 1 L of urine. Substances secreted from the capillaries into the tubular filtrate include hydrogen, potassium, and ammonia.

Micturition (voiding, urination) is a parasympathetic action, modified by voluntary control and is initiated when afferent impulses from stretch receptors in the bladder stimulate the sacral portion of the spinal cord. The detrusor muscle contracts and the sphincter relaxes.

Organs of the Urinary System

Kidneys

The kidneys are two reddish brown, bean-shaped organs located on the posterior wall of the abdomen against the back body wall musculature, just above the waist. The kidneys are imbedded in fat and located about the spinal level of T11 to L3 on each side of the vertebral column. The right kidney is lower than the left because of its displacement by the liver. On top of each kidney is an adrenal gland.

The inside of a kidney is divided into a cortex, medulla, and pelvis. The cortex and medulla contain approximately 1 million nephrons, specialized tube-shaped filters that reabsorb or excrete substances to form *urine.* A nephron consists of a Bowman's capsule; glomerulus, which is composed of a group of capillaries; and a renal tubule. Water and small solids from the blood pass across the membrane of the capillaries and enter the tubule. From there they travel through smaller loops and tubules to the collecting cups. Necessary substances such as water and electrolytes are returned to the blood while the urine drains through ducts and eventually reaches the ureters.

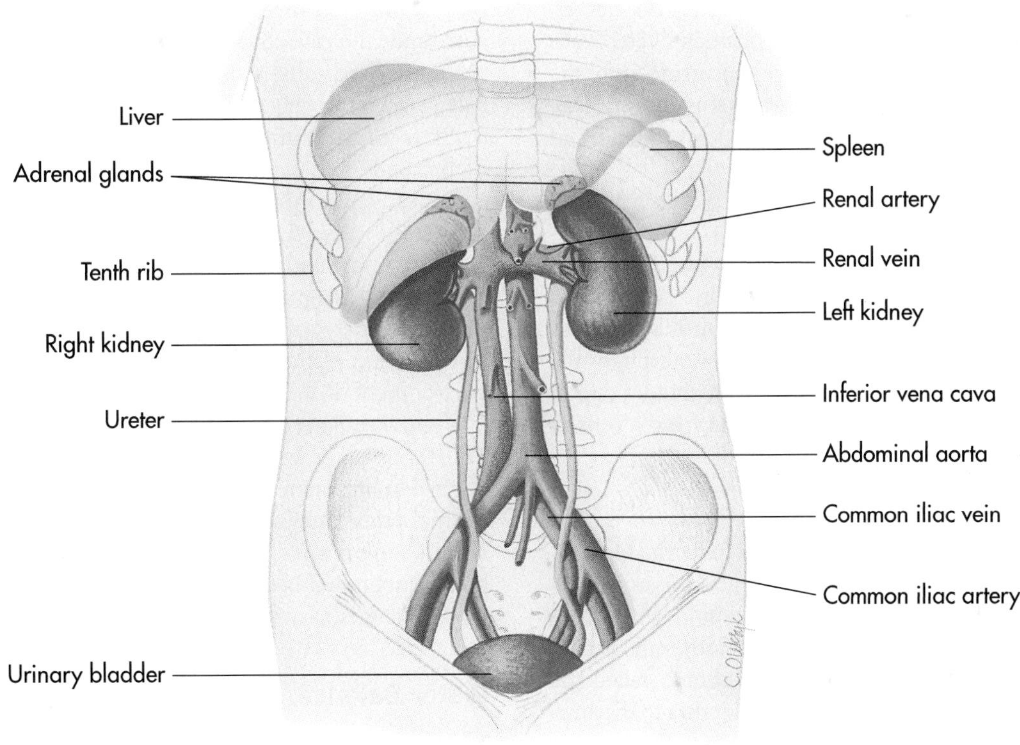

Figure 12-15
Urinary system. (From Thibodeau GA, Patton KT: *The human body in health and disease,* ed 3, St Louis, 2002, Mosby.)

The renal artery, renal vein, and ureters enter or exit the kidney at the renal hilus. Although sympathetic and parasympathetic nerve fibers are present in the kidney, the important component is sympathetic, causing vasoconstriction and the release of renin, a substance important in blood pressure control.

Kidneys and Homeostasis

Although we think of the kidney as an organ of excretion, it is more than that. The kidney does remove wastes, but it also removes normal components of the blood that are present in greater-than-normal concentrations. When excess water, sodium ions, calcium ions, and so on are present, the excess quickly passes out in the urine. Moreover, the kidneys step up their reclamation of these same substances when they are present in the blood in less-than-normal amounts. Thus the kidney continuously regulates the chemical composition of the blood within narrow limits. The kidney is one of the major homeostatic devices of the body.

Several hormones affect the kidneys. The kidneys also function as endocrine glands, producing *erythropoietin,* a hormone released in response to lowered levels of oxygen in the blood, and *calcitriol* (vitamin D_3), the active form of vitamin D that stimulates the bone marrow to produce more red blood cells. The kidneys also contribute to the acid-base balance.

Ureters

The ureters are two narrow tubes extending from the kidney and connecting to the bladder. The two ureters lie in the psoas muscles. Each is a tube about 12 inches long, $^1/_8$ to $^1/_4$ inch in diameter, and abundantly supplied with nerves. Peristalsis moves urine down into the bladder. Ureter walls contain muscle cells that help move the urine into the bladder. As the bladder fills, it presses against the ureters, compressing them, and thus preventing a reverse flow of urine.

Urinary Bladder

The bladder is a muscular, baglike organ that lies in the pelvis and acts as a reservoir for urine. Urine flows continuously into the bladder from the ureters until a sufficient quantity of urine is collected for disposal through the urethra. When the bladder is distended with about a cup of urine, the signal to empty the bladder occurs and a muscle called the detrusor muscle causes the bladder to contract.

Urethra

The urethra is the tube that carries urine from the bladder. The male urethra is about 8 inches long and serves to pass urine and semen. The female urethra is about $1^1/_2$ inches long, lies anterior to the vagina, and functions only to pass urine. The opening at the end of the urethra is called the meatus. The close proximity of the female urethra to the anus allows anal bacteria to migrate up the urethra to the bladder, ureters, and kidneys, predisposing females to ascending urinary tract infections.

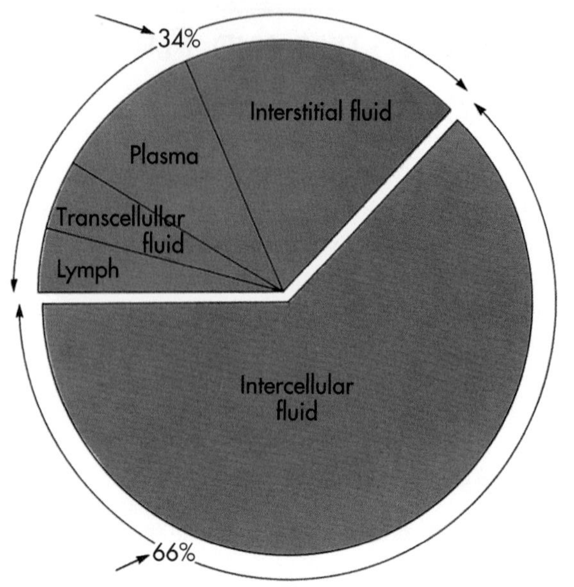

Figure 12-16
Distribution of total body water. (From Thibodeau GA, Patton KT: *Anatomy and physiology*, ed. 5, St. Louis, 2003, Mosby.)

Urinary Function

For the body to maintain homeostasis, input of water and electrolytes must be balanced by output.

The fluid or water content of the human body will range from 40% to 60% of its total weight. The total body water can be subdivided into two major fluid compartments called the extracellular and the intracellular fluid compartments (Figure 12-16). Extracellular fluid consists mainly of the plasma found in the blood vessels, the interstitial fluid that surrounds the cells, the lymph, the cerebrospinal fluid, and the specialized joint fluids. Intracellular fluid refers to the water inside the cells (Figure 12-17).

Extracellular fluid constitutes the internal environment of the body and serves the dual functions of providing a constant environment for cells and of transporting substances to and from them. Intracellular fluid functions to facilitate intracellular chemical reactions that maintain life. With the exception of plasma, fluid volumes are proportionately larger in infants and children than in adults. The function of the urinary system is to maintain the fluid environment of the body.

Fluid regulation is essential to homeostasis (Figure 12-18). If water or electrolyte levels rise or fall beyond normal limits, many bodily functions fail to proceed at their normal rates. Dehydration is the most common imbalance. Maintaining normal pH levels is also important for normal body functioning because small changes in pH can produce major changes in metabolism.

Water Balance

Water is a constituent of all living things and often is referred to as the *universal biologic solvent.* Only liquid ammonia is able to dissolve more substances than water.

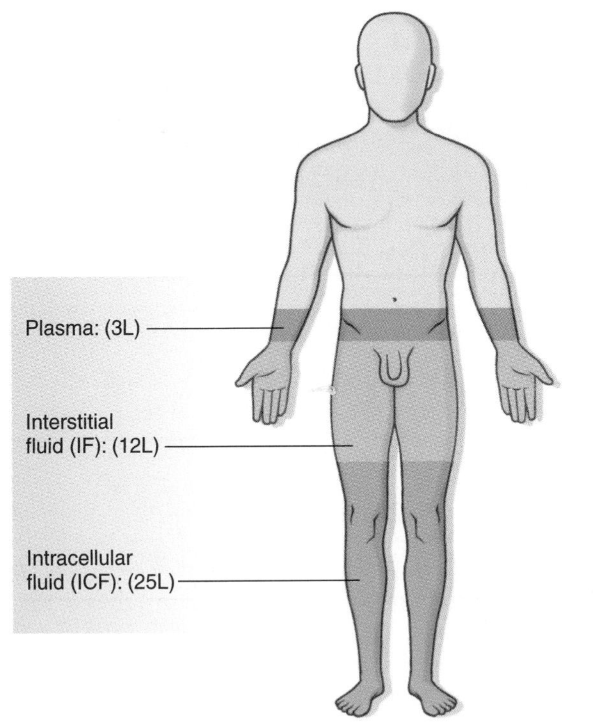

Figure 12-17
Relative volumes of three body fluids. Values represent fluid distribution in a young, adult male. (From Thibodeau GA, Patton KT: *Anatomy and physiology*, ed. 5, St. Louis, 2003, Mosby.)

Water acts to minimize temperature changes throughout the body because of its high specific heat.

A considerable amount of energy is needed to break the hydrogen bonds between water molecules to make the water molecules move faster (that is, increase the temperature of water). Therefore water can absorb much heat without rapidly changing its own temperature.

Box 12-3 lists the many important functions of water in the body.

The water content of the body tissues varies. Adipose tissue (fat) has the lowest percentage of water; the skeleton has the second lowest water content. Skeletal muscle, skin, and the blood are among the tissues that have the highest content of water in the body (Table 12-3).

The total water content of the body decreases most dramatically during the first 10 years and continues to decline through old age, at which time water content may be only 45% of the total body weight. Men tend to have higher percentages of water (about 65%) than women (about 55%), mainly because of their increased muscle mass and lower amount of subcutaneous fat.

Water in the body is in a constant state of motion, shifting between the two major fluid compartments of the body and being continuously lost from and taken into the body. In a normal, healthy human being water input equals water output. Maintaining this ratio is of prime importance in maintaining health. Approximately 90% of the water intake comes via the gastrointestinal tract (food and liquids). The remaining 10% is called metabolic water and is produced as the result of various chemical reactions in the cells of the tissues.

Table 12-4 shows the routes by which the normal healthy adult loses water.

The amount of water lost via the kidneys is under hormonal control. The average amount of water lost and consumed per day is around 2.5 L (approximately $4^{1}/_{4}$ pints) in a healthy adult.

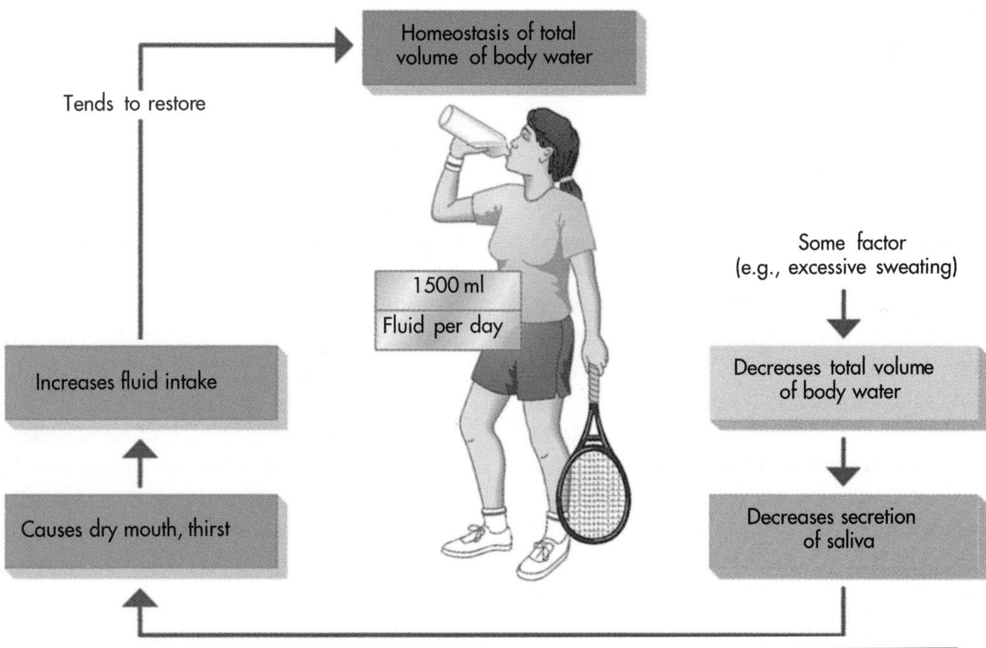

Figure 12-18
The role of coenzymes in transferring chemical energy. (From Thibodeau GA, Patton KT: *Anatomy and physiology*, ed. 5, St. Louis, 2003, Mosby.)

BOX 12-3

Functions of Water in Human Physiology

Provides medium for chemical reactions.
Is crucial for regulating chemical and bioelectric distributions within cells.
Transports substances such as hormones and nutrients.
Aids oxygen transport from lungs to body cells.
Aids carbon dioxide transport from body cells to lungs.
Dilutes toxic substances and waste products and transports them to the kidneys and the liver.
Distributes heat around the body.

TABLE 12-4
Where Water Is Lost from the Body (Healthy Adult)

ORGAN	MODE OF WATER LOSS	PERCENTAGE OF LOSS
Kidneys	Urine	62
Skin	Diffusion and sweat	19
Lungs	Water vapor	13
Gastrointestinal tract	Feces	6

TABLE 12-3
Percentage of Water in the Body Tissues

TISSUE	PERCENTAGE OF WATER
Blood	83.0
Kidneys	82.7
Heart	79.2
Lungs	79.0
Spleen	75.8
Muscle	75.6
Brain	74.8
Intestine	74.5
Skin	72.0
Liver	68.3
Skeleton	22.0
Adipose tissue	10.0

The walls of the blood vessels form a barrier to the free passage of fluid between interstitial fluid and blood plasma. At the capillaries, these walls are only one cell thick. These capillary walls are generally permeable to water and small solutes but impermeable to large organic molecules such as proteins. Thus the blood plasma tends to have a higher concentration of such molecules compared with the interstitial fluid. Much of this interstitial fluid is taken up by the lymphatic system and eventually finds its way back into the bloodstream. The section on the lymphatic system in Chapter 11 discusses this process.

Because water and small solutes such as sodium, potassium, and calcium can be exchanged freely between the blood plasma and the interstitial fluid, the action of the kidneys on the blood regulates these electrolytes. This exchange depends mainly on the hydrostatic and osmotic forces of these fluid compartments.

Hydrostatic Forces

Force exerted by water is caused by the weight of water pushing against a surface, such as a dam in a river or the wall of a blood vessel. The pressure of blood in the capillaries serves as a major hydrostatic force in the human body. The capillary hydrostatic pressure is a filtration force. This is due to the pressure of the fluid being higher at the arterial end of the capillary than at the venous end.

The pressure of the interstitial fluid is negative (–5 mm Hg) because of the lymphatic system continuously taking up the excess fluid forced out of the capillaries.

Osmotic Pressure

Osmotic pressure is the attraction of water to large molecules such as proteins. As already stated, proteins are more abundant in the blood vessels than outside them, and the concentration of proteins in the blood tends to attract water from the interstitial space.

Overall, near equilibrium exists between fluid forced out of the capillaries and the fluid reabsorbed, because the lymphatic system collects the excess fluid forced out at the artery end and eventually drains it back into the veins at the base of the neck.

A similar situation exists between the interstitial fluid and the intracellular fluid, although ion pumps and carriers complicate the process. Generally, water movement is substantial in both directions, but ion movement is restricted and depends on active transport via the pumps. Nutrients and oxygen, because they are dissolved in water, move passively into cells while waste products and carbon dioxide move out.

The mechanisms for regulating body fluids are centered in the *hypothalamus*. The hypothalamus also receives input from the digestive tract that helps to control thirst. Antidiuretic hormone (ADH) regulates body fluid volume and extracellular osmosis. ADH has many areas of influence in the body. One of the major functions of ADH is to increase the permeability of the collecting tubules in the kidneys, thus allowing more water to be reabsorbed in the kidneys. If the body is short of fluid intake (such as during sleep) the result is a concentrated, darker-colored urine of reduced volume. Absence of ADH occurs when the individual is overhydrated. The urine is dilute, pale, or colorless and of high volume.

Primary factors involved in the triggering of ADH production are osmoreceptors and baroreceptors (pressure receptors). Secondary factors include, stress, pain, hypoxia, and severe exercise.

Osmoreceptors

Dehydration produced by water loss or lack of fluid intake or relative dehydration in which the body loses no overall water content but rather gains sodium ions stimulates osmoreceptors.

The precise location of the osmoreceptors is as yet unclear, but they appear to be in the hypothalamus or the third ventricle of the brain.

The thirst response is connected to the response of the osmoreceptors. How in fact the response actually works is not yet understood completely. The moistening of the mucosal linings of the mouth and pharynx seems to initiate some sort of neurologic response, which sends a message to the thirst center of the hypothalamus. Perhaps more importantly, stretch receptors in the gastrointestinal tract also appear to transmit nerve messages to the thirst center of the hypothalamus that inhibit the thirst response.

Baroreceptors

Changes in the circulating volume of body fluid also stimulate ADH secretion that results in an increase or decrease of internal pressure monitored by baroreceptors.

A reduction of 8% to 10% from the normal body volume of water because of hemorrhage or excess perspiration results in ADH secretion. Pressure receptors located in the atria of the heart and the pulmonary artery and vein relay their messages to the hypothalamus via the vagus nerve.

Electrolyte Balance

An electrolyte is any chemical that dissociates into ions when dissolved in a solution. Ions can be positively charged (cations) or negatively charged (anions).

The major electrolytes found in the human body are these:

Sodium (Na^+)
Potassium (K^+)
Calcium (Ca^{2+})
Magnesium (Mg^{2+})
Chloride (Cl^-)
Phosphate (HPO_4^{2-})
Sulfate (SO_4^-)
Bicarbonate (HCO_3^-)

Interstitial fluid and blood plasma are similar in their electrolyte makeup, sodium and chloride being the major electrolytes. In the intracellular fluid, potassium and phosphate are the major electrolytes.

Sodium balance. Sodium balance plays an important role in the excitability of muscles and neurones and is also crucially important in regulating fluid balance in the body. The kidneys closely regulate sodium levels.

Potassium balance. Potassium is the major electrolyte of intracellular fluid. Concentration within the cells is 28 times that of the extracellular fluids. As with sodium, potassium is important in the correct functioning of excitable cells such as muscles, neurones, and sensory receptors. Potassium also is involved in the regulation of fluid levels within the cell and in maintaining the correct pH balance within the body.

The pH balance of the body also affects potassium levels. In acidosis, potassium excretion decreases, whereas the opposite occurs in alkalosis.

Calcium and phosphorus balance. Calcium is found mainly in the extracellular fluids, whereas phosphorus is found mostly in the intracellular fluids. Both are important in the maintenance of healthy bone and teeth.

Calcium is also important in the transmission of nerve impulses across synapses, the clotting of blood, and the contraction of muscles. If the levels of calcium fall below normal level, muscles and nerves become more excitable.

Phosphorus is required for the synthesis of nucleic acids and high-energy compounds such as adenosine triphosphate. Phophorus is also important in the maintenance of pH balance.

Decreased levels of calcium in the body stimulate the parathyroid gland to secrete parathyroid hormone, causing an increase in the calcium and phosphate levels of the interstitial fluids by releasing them from the reservoirs of these minerals lodged in the bones and the teeth. Parathyroid hormone also decreases calcium excretion by the kidneys.

If the levels of calcium in the body become too high, the thyroid gland releases a hormone called calcitonin that inhibits the release of calcium and potassium from the bones. Calcitonin also inhibits the absorption of calcium from the gastrointestinal tract and increases calcium excretion by the kidneys.

Magnesium balance. Most magnesium is found in the intracellular fluid and in bone. Within cells, magnesium functions in the sodium-potassium pump and as an aid to enzyme action. Magnesium plays a role in muscle contraction, action potential conduction, and bone and teeth production. Aldosterone controls magnesium concentrations in the extracellular fluid. Low magnesium levels result in an increased aldosterone secretion, and the aldosterone increases magnesium reabsorption by the kidneys.

Chloride balance. Chloride is the most plentiful extracellular electrolyte, with an extracellular concentration 26 times that of its intracellular concentration. Chloride ions are able to diffuse easily across plasma membranes, and their transport is linked closely to sodium movement, which also explains the indirect role of aldosterone in chloride regulation. When sodium is reabsorbed, chloride follows passively. Chloride helps to regulate osmotic pressure differences between fluid compartments and is essential in pH balance. The chloride shift within the blood helps to move bicarbonate ions out of the red blood cells and into the plasma for transport. In the gastric intestinal system, chlorine and hydrogen combine to form hydrochloric acid.

pH balance. pH is a measurement of the hydrogen concentration of a solution. Lower pH values indicate a higher hydrogen concentration, or a higher acidity. Higher pH values indicate a lower hydrogen concentration, or higher alkalinity.

Therefore hydrogen ion balance often is referred to as pH balance or acid-base balance. Hydrogen ion regulation in the fluid compartments of the body is critically important to health. Even a slight change in hydrogen ion concentration can result in a significant alteration in the rate of chemical reactions. Changes in hydrogen ion concentration also can affect the distribution of ions such as sodium, potassium, and calcium and can affect the structure and function of proteins.

The normal pH of the arterial blood is 7.4, whereas that of the venous blood is 7.35. The lower pH of the venous blood is caused by the higher concentration of carbon dioxide in the venous blood, which dissolves in water to make a weak acid called carbonic acid. When the pH changes in the arterial blood, two conditions may result: acidosis or alkalosis. *Acidosis* is a condition that occurs when the hydrogen ion concentration of the arterial blood increases and therefore the pH decreases. *Alkalosis* is the condition that occurs when the hydrogen ion concentration in the arterial blood decreases and the pH increases.

Sources of hydrogen ions in the body include carbonic acid formed as previously mentioned, sulfuric acid (a by-product in the breakdown of proteins), phosphoric acid (a by-product of protein and phospholipid metabolism), ketone bodies from fat metabolism, and lactic acid (a product formed in skeletal muscle during exercise).

About half of all the acid formed or introduced into the body is neutralized by the ingestion of alkaline foods. The remaining acid is neutralized by three major systems of the body; namely, chemical buffers, the respiratory system, and the kidneys.

Chemical buffers have an instantaneous effect on pH changes. They are effective in minimizing pH changes but do not entirely eliminate the change. Within cells, chemical buffers generally take about 2 to 4 hours to minimize changes in pH. The respiratory system also helps to minimize pH changes; the effects occur within minutes. Renal regulation of pH is able to return the pH to normal completely and requires from hours to several days.

Pathologic Conditions

Clinical Problems With Fluid Balance

The fluid balance of the body can be upset in many ways, resulting in severe problems and even death.

Dehydration. Dehydration obviously occurs in conditions in which water is unavailable (Figure 12-19). However, conditions such as diarrhea, severe vomiting, excessive sweating, bleeding, and surgical removal of body fluids also can result in dehydration. The foregoing may result in one of three types of dehydration. *Hypertonic dehydration* occurs when the fluid loss results in an increase in the electrolyte levels, causing the blood pressure to fall and the blood to become thicker, which can result in heart failure. *Isotonic dehydration* results in no perceptible difference from the normal electrolyte balance and may lead to hypotonic dehydration in which the fluid and electrolyte losses keep pace with each other. Any intake of pure water alters the fluid electrolyte balance (too much water, not enough electrolytes). Thus in cases of severe diarrhea, replacing the body fluid with a balanced preparation of electrolytes and water is important (Figure 12-20).

Problems with the production of urine also can lead to dehydration. Impaired ability to concentrate urine can be caused by the following:

Damage to the medulla of the kidneys: Inadequate water reabsorption occurs and the urine is too dilute, resulting in fluid loss.

Inadequate ADH production: Inadequate ADH production occurs in diabetes insipidus. Individuals suffering from this may eliminate as much as 5 to 20 L ($8^1/_2$ pints to 34 pints) of urine per day. A psychologic disorder known as polydipsia may occur in which the sufferer is obsessed with drinking (usually water), which results in dilution of the plasma, causing artificial lowering of the osmolarity and decreasing ADH secretion.

Solute diuresis in individuals suffering from diabetes mellitus: Elevated blood sugar levels can result in the inability of the kidney to reabsorb water, which then results in excess fluid loss.

In any of the aforementioned conditions, fluid balance must be maintained; otherwise, dehydration or even hypovolemic shock (because of insufficient volume of body fluid) may occur.

Edema. Edema is a condition in which an excess of fluid exists within the interstitial compartment. The condition often results in tissue swelling and is common whenever lymphatic blockage occurs. Other causes result from an impaired ability of the body to dilute the urine. Renal failure can lead to edema, especially the early stages of acute renal failure and the later stages of chronic renal failure.

Liver failure can result in inefficient metabolism of aldosterone, a hormone that controls sodium levels.

Heart failure means that the production of aldosterone is enhanced because of the lowering of the blood pressure. The result is the same as in liver failure.

Excessive ADH secretion is a rare condition that may occur because of tumors in the lung, brain, or pancreas, resulting in increased reabsorption of water.

To test for edema, one applies steady pressure of the thumb onto the lower leg for 10 to 20 seconds. If a depression

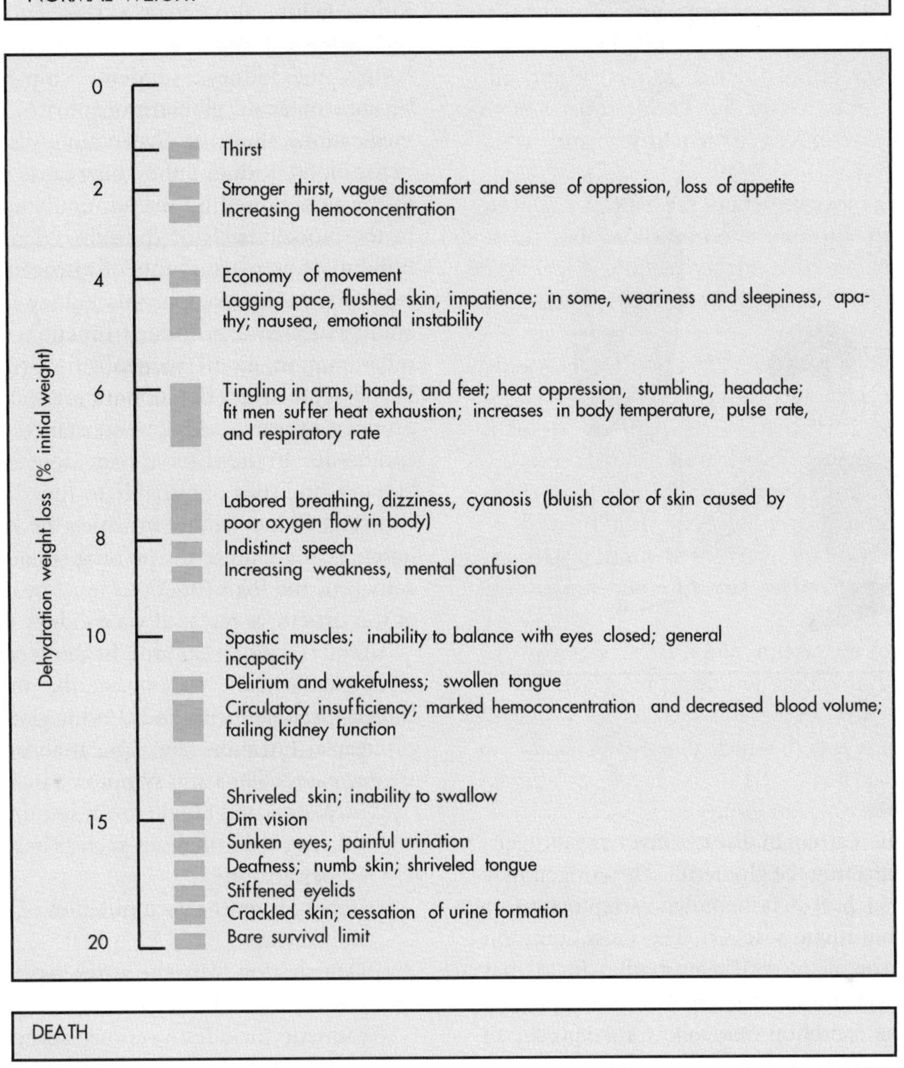

Figure 12-19
The effects of dehydration. (From Thibodeau GA, Patton KT: *Anatomy and physiology,* ed 5, St Louis, 2003, Mosby.)

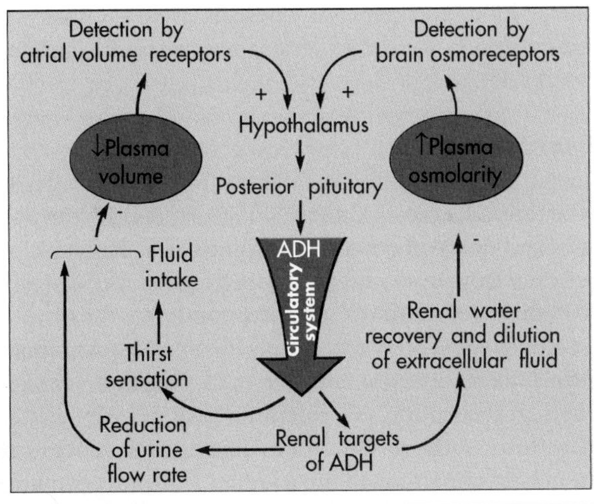

Figure 12-20
Mechanisms of fluid and electrolyte regulation. (From Thibodeau GA, Patton KT: *Anatomy and physiology,* ed 5, St Louis, 2003, Mosby.)

remains after removal of pressure, fluid retention is indicated (Figure 12-21).

Bladder Infections

A bladder infection (cystitis) is a common infection that occurs most often in females. In women the infection usually is caused by bacteria in the bladder that spread from the perineal region. Symptoms include pain in the lower abdomen, stinging or burning during urination, frequent urination (frequency) with only small amounts released, and a continuous, sometimes uncontrollable urge to urinate (urgency). Antibiotics such as nitrofurantoin (Macrodantin), sulfa-containing agents such as trimethoprim/sulfamethoxazole (Bactrim, Septra), and synthetic penicillins (ampicillin or amoxicillin) are effective. Cranberry juice also seems to be beneficial in managing bladder infection.

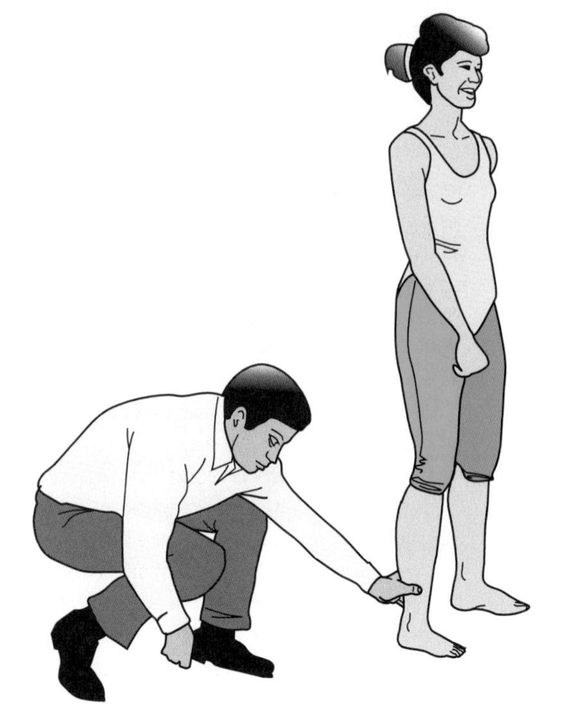

Figure 12-21
Test for edema.

Glomerulonephritis
Glomerulonephritis is a group of diseases involving antigen-antibody reactions affecting the glomeruli. The antigen may be an external one such as beta-hemolytic streptococci or may involve an autoimmune reaction. The most common type is post-streptococcal, in which antibodies form that react with streptococci. Immune complexes are deposited in the glomeruli. The condition may follow a streptococcal infection such as pharyngitis, tonsillitis, or impetigo. For mild cases without bacterial infections, treatment is bed rest and salt restriction. Streptococcal infections require antibiotic treatment, whereas autoimmune reactions require treatment with immunosuppressant medications or steroids.

Incontinence
Urinary incontinence is the inability to control urination and most often is caused by weak pelvic floor muscles or nerve damage. Causal factors include age, infection, obesity, brain or spinal cord lesion, damage to the nerves to the bladder, or injury to the sphincter usually occurring during childbirth. Stress incontinence is urine leakage during coughing, straining, sneezing, and so on when stress is placed on the muscles. This condition benefits from strengthening the pelvic floor muscles. Urge incontinence is a feeling of needing to void frequently and may be caused by irritation or infection. Urge incontinence also occurs in women during or after menopause because a decrease in the amount of estrogen in the body can weaken pelvic floor muscles and reduces the size of the mucous membranes, resulting in stress and urge incontinence.

Kidney Failure
Kidney failure, also known as renal failure, is the inability to excrete waste products and retain electrolytes. In acute kidney failure, the kidneys suddenly stop working, frequently because of acute glomerulonephritis, allergic reactions to medications, shock, or obstruction. Waste products back up in the blood. Kidney failure may cause hypertension, itching of the skin caused by the accumulation of waste products in the blood vessels of the skin, edema, and dehydration. Buildup of excess amounts of nitrogen wastes in the blood is known as uremia. Chronic kidney failure is caused by a gradual decrease in kidney function, often as a result of inflammation, glomerulonephritis, or diabetes mellitus. As in the acute stage, the kidneys are unable to excrete waste products or water, and these substances back up in the blood and tissues. In the chronic stage, scar tissue builds up in the kidneys, and they are unable to function. Scarring leads to end-stage kidney failure in which the kidneys are unable to function at all, a life-threatening situation. The kidneys are damaged, and their functions must be replaced with dialysis or the structures replaced via a kidney transplant.

Uremia (kidney failure) is the terminal stage of renal insufficiency from any cause, the most common being chronic pyelonephritis and chronic glomerulonephritis. The glomerular filtration rate, tubular absorption, and secretion are decreased. Signs and symptoms include the following:

- Weakness and fatigue from sodium, potassium, and calcium abnormalities such as anemia and acidosis
- Hypertension
- Itching from the accumulation of waste products in skin vessels
- Dehydration from the water loss
- Generalized edema

Treatment includes cautious administration of amino acids, adequate calories, sodium, and calcium, as well as antihypertensive medication. Blood transfusions may be necessary. Hemodialysis is the clearing of wastes from blood using an artificial kidney. Kidney transplants are among the most successful of organ transplants. Careful matching of similar blood and genetic types, as well as up-to-date immunosuppressive drug therapy, may result in long-term survival rates.

Kidney Stones
Kidney stones are small crystalline substances that develop in the kidney. Most kidney stones (calculi) consist of calcium, whereas others contain amino acids, uric acids, and other excretory products. The most frequent cause of stone formation is dehydration. Summer months are the time that most kidney stone problems occur. Other factors contributing to stone formation are urinary tract infection, impaired tubular reabsorption of calcium, gout, family history, medications such as diuretics, dietary imbalances, and immobilization. Although most kidney stones are composed of calcium, they usually result from the internal processing of calcium and not excessive intake. Kidney stones are usually undiscovered until one passes into a ureter, causing

sudden, excruciating flank pain. Nausea and vomiting also may occur. Treatment includes increasing fluid intake to help pass the stone if it is small enough to pass through the ureters. If the stone is too large, surgical removal may be necessary. As a substitute for surgery, the person may have the stones crushed with an ultrasonic beam or shock wave.

Obstruction

Obstruction of the urethra, causing retention of urine, is most common in older males who have prostate problems. (The reproductive section of this chapter dicusses the topic further.)

Pyelonephritis

Pyelonephritis is an infection of the kidney that affects the nephrons, or filtering units. Bacteria may reach the kidney from the bladder or by spreading through the bloodstream from another infected site such as the tonsils, middle ear, sinuses, or prostate. Common symptoms are flank and back pain, usually on one side, abdominal pain that moves into the groin, and fever, sometimes with chills and nausea. Treatment includes the use of an appropriate antibiotic. If not treated, pyelonephritis may become chronic and lead to kidney failure.

INDICATIONS CONTRAINDICATIONS

For Therapeutic Massage

Therapeutic massage tends to increase blood volume through the kidneys via mechanical and reflexive processes. In the healthy individual, massage therapy supports the filtration process. For those with kidney disease the increased volume can strain the kidney function. Therefore, general contraindications exist for anyone with kidney disease. Therapeutic massage modalities may be useful for pain and stress management, but only with the careful supervision of the treating physician.

Acute infectious processes contraindicate massage until the infection has run its course. Massage therapy may support chronic infection treatment as part of a supervised treatment plan. Stress is a contributing factor to incontinence. Any form of stress management helps somewhat with stress and urge incontinence. The practitioner needs to consider that incontinent clients require frequent and easy access to the restroom (Activity 12-3). ■

ACTIVITY 12-3

We must be able to explain and justify the therapeutic value of the work we do. The following activity will assist you in developing the skills to explain the effectiveness of therapeutic massage to clients and other health care professionals. Use the clinical reasoning model that follows to accomplish this task. The focus should be the primary modality or modalities applied to the urinary system.

Methods/Applications

1. What are the facts?

a. Which system is involved, and which structures of that system can be reached directly or indirectly?

b. Which of these structures are most affected by this massage?

c. Which physiologic functions are affected by this approach?

d. When the treatment is applied, what changes in function will occur in

(1) this system?

Continued

ACTIVITY 12-3—cont'd

(2) the whole body?

e. What is considered normal or balanced function?

f. How are the functions of this system related to the homeostasis of the body?

g. What has worked or has not worked?

h. Where could you find information that would support the use of this modality as a therapeutic intervention?

i. What research is available to support the use of the therapeutic intervention?

j. How does the intervention support a healthy state?

k. Under which pathologic or dysfunctional conditions is the therapeutic massage most likely to be beneficial?

2. What are the possibilities?

a. What do the data suggest?

b. What are the reasons for using the proposed methods?

c. What are the possible interventions?

d. List at least three applications of massage that would affect the structure and function of the system involved.

e. What are other ways to look at the situation?

ACTIVITY 12-3—cont'd

f. What other methods could provide similar benefits?

3. What is the logical outcome of therapeutic intervention?

a. What would be the logical progression of the symptom pattern, contributing factors, and current behaviors?

b. What are the benefits and drawbacks of each intervention suggested?

Benefits:

Drawbacks:

c. What are the costs in terms of time, resources, and finances?

d. What is likely to happen if the modality is not used?

e. What is likely to happen if the modality is used?

4. For the intervention proposed, what would be the effect on the persons involved, specifically the client, practitioner, and other professionals working with the client?

a. How does each person involved (including, besides the foregoing, the client's family and support system) feel about the possible interventions?

b. Does the practitioner feel qualified to work with the situation and apply the identified modality to the particular person?

c. Does a feeling of cooperation and agreement exist among all those involved, and how would the practitioner recognize this feeling?

Justification

Using the information developed in the clinical reasoning model, present a clear, concise statement of how the ways in which the particular soft tissue or movement modality would be beneficial in supporting the particular body system in a healthy condition or as part of a treatment plan for a pathologic or dysfunctional condition. Based on the foregoing information, give a brief summary of the effectiveness of the modality for this system.

REPRODUCTIVE SYSTEM

Continuation of the species is the biologic function of the reproductive system, yet our sexuality is more than reproduction and more than our genitals. This last section, the reproductive system, connects our study of the body to the beginning, to the cell. The essence of reproduction is the duality of yin/yang and male/female, when at the moment of conception two cells create one whole.

This section focuses on the anatomy of the reproductive organs and the functions of procreation. A study of human sexuality, in its more holistic body/mind/spirit form, is beyond the scope of this text, yet such study is important to raise the questions concerning the most intimate of physical acts in its expansive form as a communication of creative energy.

Along with the function of procreation, the sexual act is a pleasurable function, providing the same rewards as other pleasurable functions. The act of sex and orgasm stimulates the same feel-good neurochemicals as other forms of touch, food, and exercise. Sexual arousal is a physiologic response generated primarily through parasympathetic activation—the same pattern sought in most forms of stress management. Orgasm is a sympathetic autonomic nervous system tensing and relaxing of bodywide proportion.

Yet if the act of sex between human beings is viewed only as biologic, what is the motivation in society to elevate the bonds between persons who share sexual energy to a spiritual union? What makes sharing our bodies in a sexual union different than sharing a pizza? We do not have the answers, but we do know that the miracle and magic of the human experience is more than a sum of its parts. We acknowledge that compassion cannot be explained totally by neurotransmitters, healing only by the repair mechanism of connective tissue and cellular division, growth purely by digestion and growth hormone, pain only in terms of neuropathways, anger as autonomic nervous system survival responses, and connectedness as entrainment. The experience of living is more than the biology that supports life, just as the clinical study of reproduction and birth cannot explain love, new life, and the sharing of creative energy. With all this said, understanding the anatomy/form and physiology/function in the pure physical sense is necessary to be able to comprehend the beauty of the rest.

The human being is actually androgynous. Some generally recognized developmental behavioral differences exist between males and females in terms of brain development and function, social motivation, and communication styles, but these are insignificant in terms of general function. The gender differences do not limit what can be done. Differences are reflected more in the process than in the result. For example, the generic female is more interactive and tends to solve problems in a group with much discussion of the feelings and satisfaction of those involved. The generic male more likely solves problems independently, somewhat less concerned with the feelings of persons and more concerned with the outcome of the process. Neither process is right or wrong, and women certainly can make decisions independently and men can work effectively in social groups.

The strongest and most obvious differences between males and females are the function and construction of the reproductive systems. In this anatomy and physiology the gender differences are most evident. Even in the differentiation between male and female, a continuity of function exists. The same hormones from the hypothalamus stimulate ovaries and testes. Musculature is similar, as is nervous system distribution. The main difference lies in development of the sex cells (ovum and sperm), the anatomy required to deliver the sperm to the ovum, and the organs to house the developing infant. The difference is not so prevalent in young children before puberty or in those in their mature years after 60 or so, but during the reproductive years, the differences and in some ways the gender behaviors are more evident.

Male Reproductive System

The male reproductive system consists of the *testicles, epididymis, vas deferens, ejaculatory duct, urethra, penis,* and *scrotum* (Figure 12-22). The two testicles are enclosed in an external sac called the scrotum. Tiny seminiferous tubules in the testicles produce *sperm.*

Sperm travels from the testicles into the epididymis, where the sperm cells mature. Sperm then moves into the *vas deferens,* which extends upward into the body cavity, over the symphysis pubis and around the urinary bladder to connect with the two *seminal vesicles.*

The seminal vesicles produce and secrete a viscous fluid that makes up most of the semen and joins with the sperm to pass from the vas deferens into the ejaculatory duct. The *ejaculatory duct* passes through the *prostate gland* and joins with the urethra. The prostate gland is actually a group of small glands that surround the urethra as it exits the bladder and produces a milky alkaline fluid that becomes a component of semen.

The duct of the bulbourethral, or Cowper's, glands connects to the urethra below the prostate. These two small glands secrete a thick lubricating fluid, which is also a component of semen. On ejaculation, semen flows through the urethra to the outside of the body.

The penis is composed of a meshwork of erectile tissue (able to become firm by engorgement with blood) and consists of a shaft, the end of which is covered with a loose flap of skin called the prepuce, or foreskin. This foreskin often is removed in a surgical process called circumcision. The end of the penis is called the glans penis. In the reproductive system the penis functions to deposit sperm cells into the vagina.

Hormonal and Nervous System Control

Follicle-stimulating hormone (FSH) and luteinizing hormone (LH) from the pituitary gland control testicular

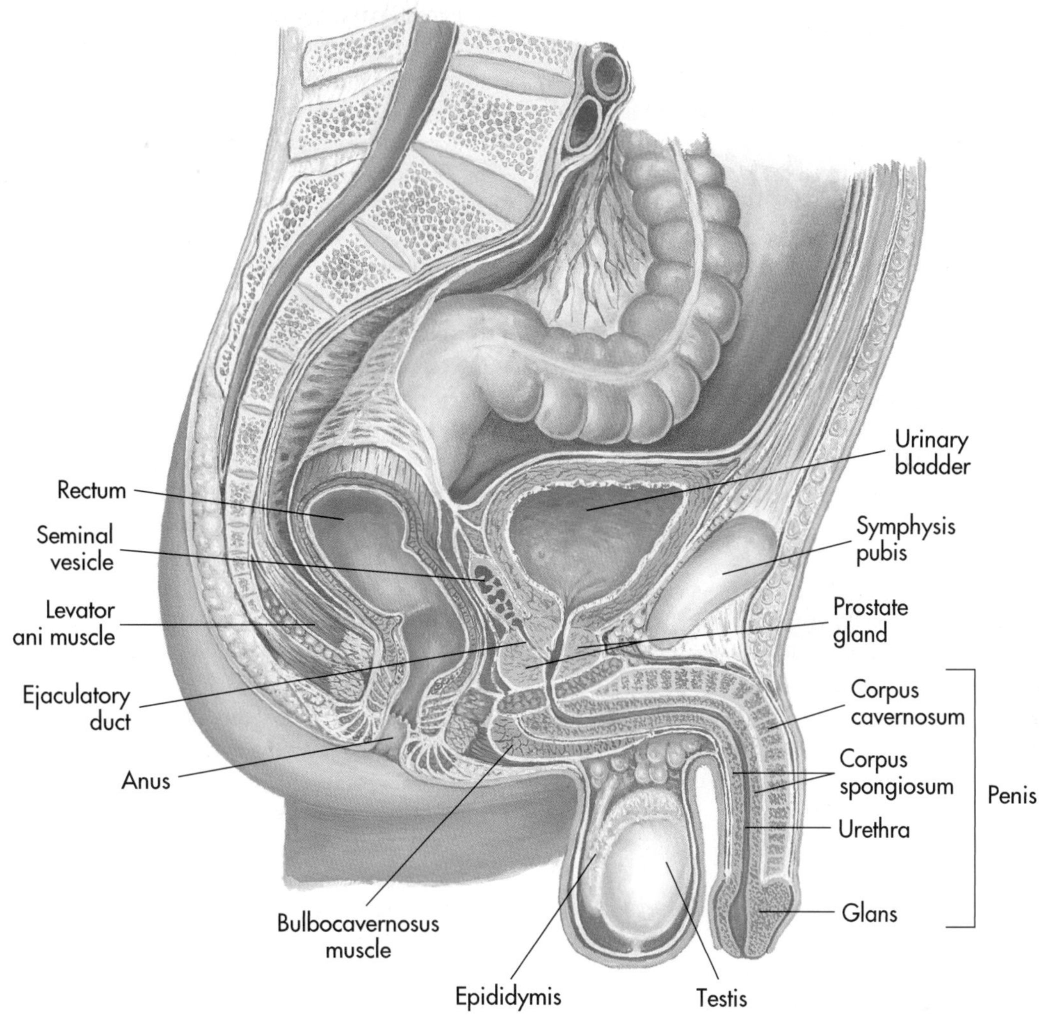

Figure 12-22
Male pelvic organs. (From Seidel HM et al: *Mosby's guide to physical examination,* ed 5, St Louis, 2003, Mosby.)

function. FSH stimulates sperm production, whereas LH stimulates the secretion of testosterone from interstitial cells. Gonadotropin-releasing hormone from the hypothalamus stimulates production of FSH and LH.

Before puberty, males produce little testosterone because no releasing hormone is secreted. During puberty or adolescence the hypothalamus matures and gonadotropin-releasing hormone stimulates the production of FSH and LH. LH increases the number of interstitial cells, and testosterone production accelerates. Testosterone increases the synthesis of protein in cells, creating an anabolic effect. Male secondary sex characteristics appear. Body growth accelerates, muscle and bone mass increase, the penis and scrotum enlarge, the larynx develops and the voice deepens, and hair appears on the face, chest, axillae, abdomen, and pubis.

Hormones stimulate the sebaceous glands of the skin, increasing the development of acne. Testosterone stimulates the male sexual drive or libido. Boys may begin to exhibit more aggressive social behavior. The production of sperm (spermatogenesis) accelerates. Testosterone and sperm are produced throughout life, gradually diminishing after age 40. Spermatogenesis takes place at a temperature lower than body temperature, so the testes are located in the scrotal sac, where the temperature is cooler. During cold weather, the cremaster muscle contracts and elevates the testes closer to the body.

Erection is a parasympathetic response in which arteries of the penis dilate and veins constrict; allowing blood flow into the erectile tissue but blocking venous outflow. A variety of stimuli cause erection. *Emission* involves the contraction of the epididymis, the vas deferens, the prostate, and the seminal vesicles. Semen moves into the urethra. *Ejaculation* consists of contraction of the muscles at the base of the penis (bulbocavernosus, ischiocavernosus). Ejaculation propels approximately 3 ml of semen at high pressure through the penile urethra.

Male Contraceptive Methods

For men, several contraceptive methods are available: abstinence, the condom, the condom with spermicidal jelly or foam, withdrawal, and vasectomy. The condom alone and the withdrawal method are not reliable. The condom with a spermicide is a fairly reliable method. In addition, the condom protects against venereal disease. *Vasectomy* is a procedure done in the physician's office with the area under local anesthesia and involves removal of a 2-cm piece of the vas deferens and tying of the remaining ends. The man should consider vasectomy a permanent method of sterilization, even though the cut ends can be rejoined. In most cases after rejoining, fertility is less than 50%.

Female Reproductive System

The female reproductive system is designed for childbearing. The system consists of two ovaries, two fallopian tubes, a uterus, and a vagina. Also included in the system are the external genitalia and mammary glands (Figure 12-23).

Internal Organs

The *ovaries* are solid glands that produce the hormones *estrogen* and *progesterone.* The cortex of the ovaries contains numerous small masses of cells called ovarian (graafian) follicles. Each follicle contains an *ovum.* The two ovaries are held in position, one on each side of the uterus, by several ligaments. The largest of these ligaments is called the broad ligament, which holds the ovaries in close proximity to the *fallopian tubes.*

Each funnel-shaped fallopian tube is about 4 inches long and serves as a duct to transport the ovum to the *uterus.* The uterus, or womb, is a hollow, muscular organ in the shape of an inverted pear. The uterus lies between the urinary bladder and rectum. The upper part of the uterus is called the fundus, and the middle part of the uterus is called the corpus. The lower, narrow portion of the uterus is the *cervix,* which opens into the *vagina.* The uterus receives the ovum and serves as the area in which the embryo grows and develops into a fetus. The inner lining is a soft, spongy layer, the *endometrium,* the surface of which is shed each month during *menstruation.* Uterine contractions at the end of the gestation period push the fetus into the vagina.

The vagina is a flexible, fibromuscular tube about $3^1/_2$ inches long that receives the sperm from the male and serves as the birth canal. The region between the vagina and anus is the *clinical perineum* and may tear during the birth process because of overstretching.

The vagina has a dual function: sexual intercourse and delivery of a baby. Mucus in the vagina during nonsexual times comes from *uterine glands.* During sexual arousal, *Bartholin's glands* secrete mucus into the vagina. During orgasm, the muscular layer of the vagina contracts, moving semen into the cervix. Changes in the vaginal mucosa reflect cyclic endocrine changes that may be used to determine times of increased fertility.

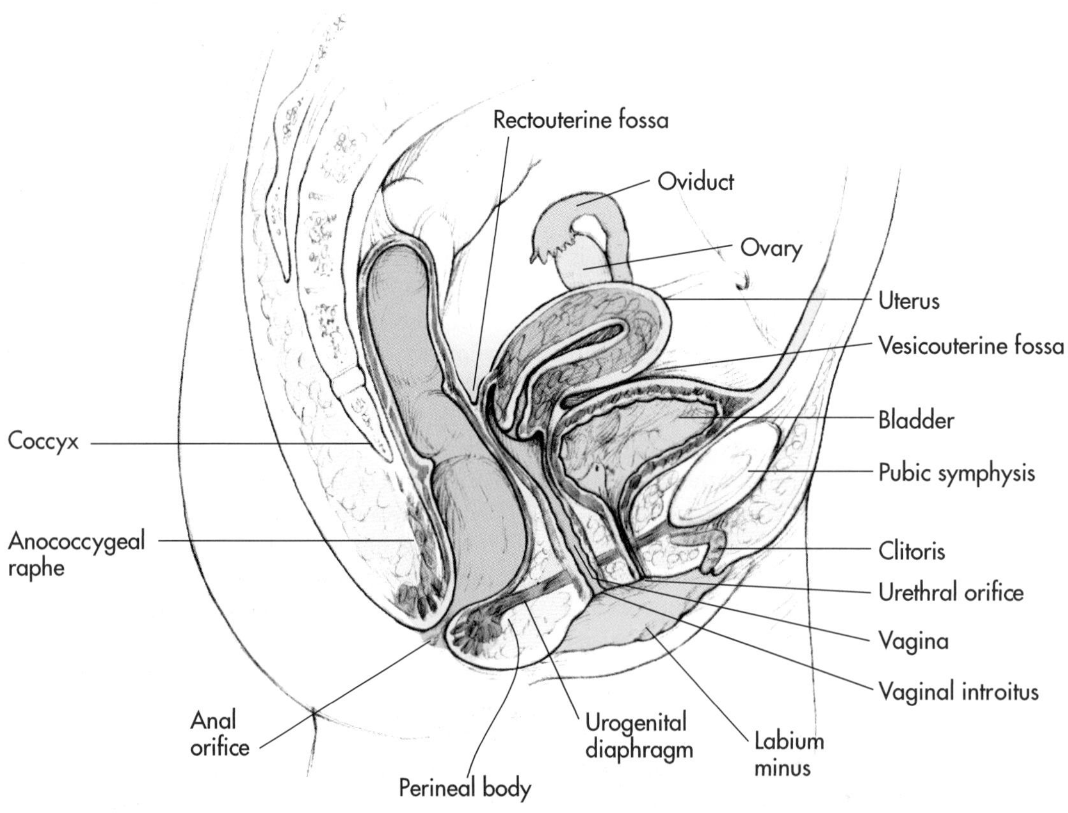

Figure 12-23
Female pelvic floor, midsagittal view. (From Mathers LH et al: *Clinical anatomy principles,* St Louis, 1995, Mosby.)

External Organs

The external organs of the female reproductive system include *the labia majora, labia minora, clitoris, mons pubis, vestibule, vaginal orifice,* and *Bartholin's (vestibular) glands.* The aforementioned external genitalia are known collectively as the vulva. The mons pubis, located over the symphysis pubis, becomes covered with hair after puberty.

Each Bartholin's gland opens into the mucosal surface near the superior portion of the labia minora. The gland discharges a clear secretion during sexual arousal. Cysts and abscesses are common in these glands.

The *mammary glands* (breasts) are accessory organs that produce and secrete milk after pregnancy. The mammary glands are included in the integument and are discussed in that section of this book.

Beginning with puberty and for the next 35 to 40 years, the ovaries undergo cyclic changes in which a certain number of ovarian follicles develop. When one ovum completes the developmental process, it is released into one of the fallopian tubes. If fertilization does not occur, the developed ovum disintegrates and a new cycle begins.

Hormonal and Nervous System Control

A series of hormonal events takes place approximately every 28 days. Known as the menstrual cycle, day number 1 begins with the first day of uterine bleeding, called menses or menstruation. Cyclic hormonal changes occur in the pituitary, uterus, ovaries, and vagina. As in the male, FSH and LH from the pituitary gland affect the gonads. FSH stimulates growth of the follicle containing the egg and the secretion of female hormones collectively called estrogen. The main estrogen is estradiol, responsible for female secondary sex characteristics, growth of the maturing follicle, growth of the uterine lining (endometrium), and negative feedback control of FSH. LH has two main functions: ovulation and formation of the corpus luteum (from the old follicle). The corpus luteum secretes estrogen and another group of hormones, the progestins. The main progestin, progesterone, is responsible for the secretory phase of the uterine cycle, glandular growth in the breast, and negative feedback control of LH.

In the female, as in the male, almost no gonadal hormones are formed before age 9 or 10. As the hypothalamus matures, gonadotropin-releasing hormone stimulates production of FSH and LH. In response the ovaries produce estradiol and then progesterone. Breast buds and pubic hair appear about age 11. The breasts grow, and axillary hair appears, with the adrenal cortex responsible for initial axillary and pubic hair growth in both sexes. The uterus and vagina enlarge. Uterine bleeding (the menarche) begins about 2 years after breast bud development and is often sporadic for several months. Ovulation takes place after the menarche.

As puberty progresses, the hips broaden, the forearms diverge more at the elbows, and scant body hair but much head hair are evident. The voice retains a high-pitched quality. Estradiol is not as anabolic as testosterone, and muscular development, bone size, and general body growth is not as great as in the male. Estrogens cause the skin to have a smooth texture. Prepubertal characteristics such as voice, head hairline, sparse body hair (compared with the male), and the distribution of body fat are retained and accentuated. Estradiol and testosterones are responsible for the female libido. In mammals, estrogens induce mating behavior, receptiveness of the female for the male, and nesting and maternal characteristics. As in the male, libido is influenced by cerebral control. Libido increases at ovulation and sometimes during menstruation.

After ages 40 to 50, a decrease in the responsiveness of the ovaries to FSH and LH, accompanied by irregular menstrual cycles, is the menopause. Although levels of estradiol and progesterone decrease, frequently little change in libido occurs.

The autonomic nervous system exerts influence over the female reproductive system; as in the male, sexual arousal is a parasympathetic function and orgasm is a sympathetic activation. Sympathetic deviances can interfere with ovulation and menstruation and thus are implicated in menstrual disorders and infertility.

Female Contraceptive Methods

In contrast to the male a multitude of contraceptive methods are available to the female. The woman should consider removal of the uterus (hysterectomy) and tying or cauterizing the fallopian tubes (tubal ligation) permanent procedures. As with the vasectomy, even though the ends of the cut and tied fallopian tubes may be rejoined later, fertility decreases. Tubal ligation by cauterization is almost impossible to reverse. Currently used methods of birth control are the birth control pill, injections of hormones, implanted hormone-releasing devices, the intrauterine device, the diaphragm, spermicidal agents, post-coital douche, abstinence, and the rhythm method. The most reliable methods are the pill, injections, implants, the condom plus a spermicidal agent, the intrauterine device, and the diaphragm with a spermicidal agent, in decreasing order of effectiveness. In some women the pill contributes to venous thromboembolism. In others the pill may cause weight gain. The condom with a spermicidal agent has the added benefit of protection from venereal disease.

Pregnancy

Fertilization is the penetration of the egg by a sperm, restoring the diploid number (46) of chromosomes. Fertilization usually occurs as the egg moves down the fallopian tube. The ovum contains one X chromosome. A sperm contains an X or a Y chromosome, so the male determines the sex of the baby. If a male sperm (Y) reaches the egg, a male baby results; if a female sperm (X) reaches the egg, a female baby is produced. After the head of the sperm enters the egg, the tail detaches, and the ovum prohibits the entrance of other sperm. The chromosomes of egg and sperm nuclei arrange themselves at the two poles of the fertilized egg, and it begins to divide.

Gestation takes approximately 10 lunar months (9 calendar months) and is divided into *trimesters.*

First trimester. Various physiologic changes occur during the first trimester along with radical hormonal changes. The changes influence mood, digestion, sleep, and energy levels.

Early pregnancy is a different experience for each woman. Actual menstruation stops, but slight bleeding may occur throughout the first trimester, which is why some women often do not realize they are pregnant until about 3 months into the pregnancy. About 7 days after conception, implantation bleeding may occur. This bleeding is rare but normal vaginal spotting caused by the formation of new blood vessels. The urge to urinate occurs more frequently. The uterus begins to enlarge and press down on the bladder. Hormonal changes such as megabursts of progesterone result in retention and release of more water.

Most women feel changes in their breasts. The breasts may swell, tingle, throb, or hurt from the breast developing milk glands and the increased blood supply to the breasts. The veins become more pronounced and visible. The nipples enlarge and become more erect, and the areolae darken and become broader. Some women notice early on that their nipples feel sensitive and sore.

Fatigue is another major symptom at this stage and begins after the first missed period and persists until the fourteenth to twentieth week of pregnancy. The need for sleep increases. About 10 hours of sleep a night is suggested during the first trimester.

Increased levels of progesterone also may cause the pregnant woman to feel faint and constipated. The progesterone dilates the smooth muscle of the blood vessels and causes blood to pool in the legs, and more blood begins to flow to the uterus, which can cause low blood pressure and may result in fainting. Standing or sitting for long periods of time tends to trigger faintness. Lying flat and doing exercises that get the blood circulating prevent this.

Progesterone relaxes the smooth muscles of the small and large intestines, slowing down the digestive process and leading to constipation. Lower back pain also occurs because the expanding uterus might put pressure on the sciatic nerve.

Between 60% and 80% of all women suffer nausea and vomiting in the first trimester. Discomfort that begins in the morning, often called morning sickness, often persists 24 hours a day for the first few weeks of pregnancy. Sometimes the nausea is not bad enough to cause vomiting and is an ever-present condition that can be controlled by dry crackers or juice.

Numerous other symptoms that accompany morning sickness include an aversion to certain tastes or smells. Changes in hormone levels somehow affect the stomach lining and stomach acids, causing the nausea. An empty stomach aggravates the nausea. A strong connection also exists between nausea and low blood sugar levels. Eating well is important during pregnancy. Some women require a vitamin supplement; some women must discontinue taking vitamin supplements to relieve or prevent other symptoms.

Fitness and exercise are important, but in moderation.

Second trimester. In the second trimester, the woman settles into the pregnant state, develops maternal feelings, and often has a general sense of well-being. Appetite increases, blood volume increases, and the body places additional workload on all physiologic functions.

Increased blood in the vaginal area causes an increase in vaginal secretions or discharge. A foul odor or itching or a yellow or green discharge may indicate a vaginal infection. A curdy white discharge with itching is probably a yeast infection and is treatable. A foul-smelling discharge or one that is yellow or green could indicate a more serious infection that could lead to premature labor if untreated.

Genital warts may begin to increase in number and in size. Moles, like warts, also are nourished through the hormones that increase in pregnancy, and they can grow in size, number, and color.

Progesterone depresses the central nervous system and may cause moodiness or depression.

The hormones that slow down the intestinal tract also relax the sphincter between the stomach and esophagus, allowing stomach juices to flow up into the esophagus. Reflux of stomach juices into the esophagus causes a burning sensation in the middle of the chest called *heartburn.* As the uterus grows, it crowds the intestines and heartburn may get much worse.

By week 15 the baby weighs almost 2 oz. The bones are growing and the muscle movement is increasing. The pregnant woman probably does not feel the baby moving yet, and the first movements feel like flutters. A soft, fine hair called lanugo covers the baby. The neck of the baby becomes longer and the head can move. The arms move freely in front of the body, and the hands can grasp one another. Ultrasound has picked up babies actually sucking their thumbs by this time.

Table 12-5 gives an approximation of weight distribution during pregnancy. This distribution varies with each mother and increases with twins, triplets, and quadruplets. The student should keep in mind that with multiple babies, the weight of each baby is less.

The amount of blood circulating throughout the body and especially in the areas of the vagina and rectum continues to increase. New vessels form, but they are not as strong and often bulge or swell in the vaginal area, rectum, and legs, and varicose veins form around the labia, vagina, and legs. When the vessels in the rectum swell, hemorrhoids develop and may protrude out of the rectum with strenuous bowel movements.

By 21 weeks, the baby weighs almost 1 lb and is nearly 10 to 11 inches long. Every system is progressing in development. The primitive structures of the brain have been developed for some time. Now the fine details of the nerve pathways in the brain are forming. Nerve cells that allow the baby's brain to receive and transmit messages are forming layers in the brain. This process continues at a much slower rate for another 3 months.

T cells and B cells are essential for the immune system development. The baby is able to hear sounds from outside

TABLE 12-5
Weight Gain During Pregnancy

Area of Gain	Amount of Gain
Mother (at Term)	
Uterus	2-3 lb
Breasts	1-3 lb
Blood volume	3-5 lb
Body fluid	1-3 lb
Fat, protein, etc.	5-8 lb
Baby (at 9 Months)	
Baby	7-8 lb
Amniotic fluid	2-2 1/2 lb
Placenta	1-1 1/2 lb
Total	22-32 lb

of the body and is aware of the constant rhythm created by the mother's beating heart as well as the switching and gurgling of fluids inside her body. The baby's eyes remain fused shut. By the end of week 21, the layers of the retina are developed and the skin is developing a white coating called vernix caseosa, a fatty film that protects the baby's skin from breakdown in the amniotic fluid. Vernix also prevents the loss of water and electrolytes from the baby into the amniotic fluid. The permanent ridges that form the fingers, hands, and feet are now developed and the fingernails and toenails are getting harder.

The baby is swallowing more than 2 tsp of amniotic fluid per day and by the end of the pregnancy may be swallowing nearly 2 cups of amniotic fluid per day. The digestive system is developed, and the digestive processes are beginning. Stool called meconium forms in the bowel. The air sacs in the lungs called alveoli are beginning to emerge.

In the pregnant woman the progesterone that has slowed the digestive system affects the gallbladder in much the same way. The gallbladder takes a longer time to empty, allowing bile salts to accumulate in the system and absorb through the skin. This causes significant itching noticeable around the navel, entire belly, chest, neck, face, and sometimes hands.

The growing uterus and baby put a lot of pressure on the two main blood vessels that lead into and out of the heart called the vena cava and aorta. Pressure occurs when lying flat on the back. The side-lying position is best.

As the pregnancy progresses, the capillaries become more permeable and have a tendency to leak water. When the capillaries leak water, the result is an increase in water retention, or edema. Some edema is normal in pregnancy, but edema that increases all over the body, particularly the legs, arms, lower back, and face, could indicate a serious problem requiring immediate referral to a physician.

Following are suggestions and cautions to ease the discomforts of swelling:

- Drink plenty of fluids to stimulate the kidneys.
- Avoid tight-fitting clothing, especially socks, hose, pant legs, and waistbands.
- Avoid standing or sitting in one place for long periods of time.
- Rest with the legs elevated on a chair or pillow.
- Lie down on the left side to increase kidney function.
- Increase the protein intake to pull the fluid back into the vessels.
- Exercise such as walking and swimming increases circulation and lymphatic movement of water back into the vessels.
- Do not take diuretics for water retention in pregnancy.

The renal system of pregnant women changes. The kidneys produce more urine, and the bladder has decreased tone. The same progesterone that alters other systems influences the urinary system to be less efficient. As a result, many pregnant women have a tendency to develop urinary tract infections. Urinary tract infections can become serious and cause not only pain and discomfort but also preterm labor. If untreated, a mild urinary tract infection can lead to a serious bladder or kidney infection that could require hospitalization and treatment with antibiotics intravenously.

The following are warning signs of urinary tract infection:

- Increased urge and frequency of urination (usually small amounts of urine)
- Pain or burning sensation with urination
- Pain in the lower abdomen or back
- Blood visible in the urine
- Fever and chills
- Rapid heart rate
- Nausea and vomiting

The following are suggestions to decrease chances of urinary tract infections:

- Drink plenty of fluids.
- Lie on the left side to increase kidney efficiency and output.
- Wear cotton panties.
- Avoid tight-fitting clothes.
- Keep the vaginal area clean: Always wipe from front to back after urinating or having a bowel movement.
- Avoid perfumed soaps and panty liners.

At the end of the second trimester the baby is at a milestone in development. The eyes are no longer fused shut; the fine details of optic nerve development, peripheral vision, and focus are present. Hearing is developed completely. The brain is functioning at a higher level, as are all of the baby's senses: sight, hearing, taste, touch, and smell. The baby has developed a schedule of sorts, moving while awake and being still while asleep. An early sucking reflex is present, although the ability to suck and swallow will not be present until about 34 weeks. The baby is also practicing the breathing motion.

Third trimester. The last trimester finds the mother-to-be heavy with the baby, and postural changes are evident. Internal organs are crowded. Physiologic systems are strained with sustaining mother and baby. The mother's connective tissue structure softens to allow for the expansion needed for the birth. This is a time of rest and waiting (Figure 12-24).

The third trimester begins after about 26 weeks of pregnancy. During these last 3 months, the baby continues to grow and develop. Although a baby might survive if born during the early to middle part of the last trimester, these months are critical to the development of organs such as the lungs and the brain.

The baby is now about 15 inches long and weighs around 3 pounds. He or she may be active. The baby may suck the thumb, hiccup, and respond to stimuli such as light, pain, and sounds.

In the mother the lower abdomen may hurt from time to time and may have an occasional, brief contraction in which the uterus hardens and then returns to normal. Vaginal discharge may become heavier, and the mother may feel breathless for no apparent reason and have difficulty sleeping. Colostrum, the early form of milk, may leak from the breasts, and the mother may feel apprehensive or excited about the coming labor and delivery.

By the eighth month the baby has grown to about 18 inches and weighs 5 lb. He or she can see and hear. The lungs are still immature, but many other organs are well developed. Brain growth is especially rapid during this time. At some point during the eighth month, the baby shifts into a position he or she will maintain until birth.

By 36 weeks, the baby is about 20 inches long and weighs 6 to 7 lb and will gain about $^1/_2$ lb a week until delivery. The baby's lungs are mature. Movement often slows down because of the cramped space and head-down position in the pelvis.

For the pregnant woman, backache and heaviness increase, the abdomen may itch, and the pelvis may be

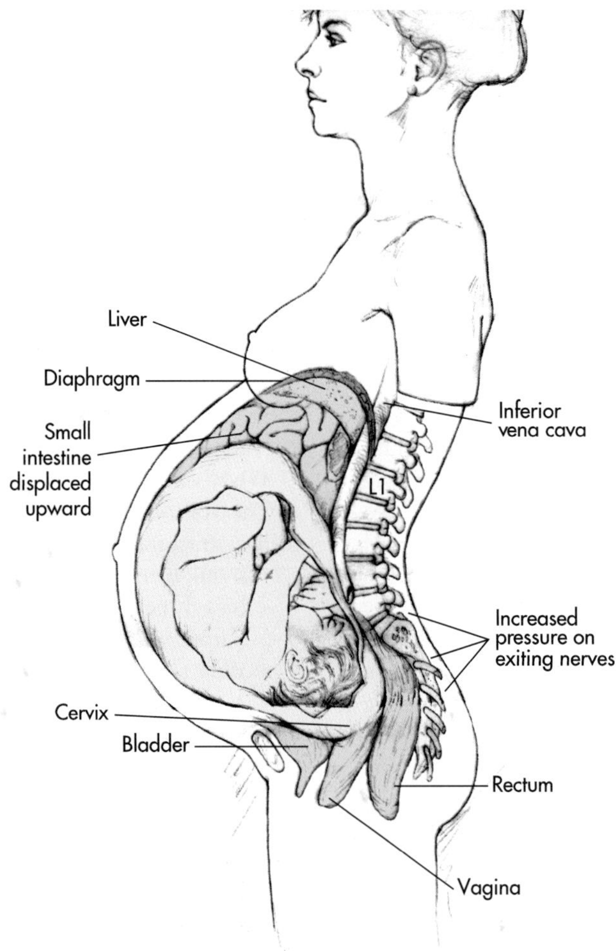

Figure 12-24
Fetus in utero. This illustration shows the impressive degree to which the pregnant uterus displaces other abdominopelvic structures and puts pressure on important regions such as the pelvic diaphragm and the respiratory diaphragm. Venous return from pelvic and lower limb structures is made more difficult by pressure on the inferior vena cava, and women commonly develop hemorrhoids and varicose veins in the lower limbs. Breathing may be difficult because of pressure on the diaphragm and the inability to depress it fully to permit filling of the lungs. Back and lower limb pain is common because of pressure on exiting nerves of the lumbar and sacral plexuses. (From Mathers LH et al: *Clinical anatomy principles,* St Louis, 1995, Mosby.)

uncomfortable. After the baby drops, breathing and eating become easier, but urinary urge increases. Uterine contractions may increase and feel more intense.

Birth

The exact stimulus for birth is unknown, but increased fetal activity seems to play a role. Oxytocin stimulates contraction of the uterus, causes delivery of the placenta after expulsion of the fetus, and promotes parental bonding with the baby.

Prelabor. Prelabor can begin anywhere in the last few weeks or last days of pregnancy. The mother also may get diarrhea and possibly a severe backache, both precursors to early labor. The diarrhea is nature's enema, a way of emptying the intestinal tract before actual labor begins, and Braxton Hicks contractions may begin to be more frequent (these are painless).

The cervix at this stage softens and may start to thin out a little, which allows it to dilate (open up) slightly. The woman also will experience some mucous, bloody discharge called bloody show, which means that the mucus plug sealing the cervical opening is now pink or blood-streaked and is leaking discharge.

As the baby's head presses down against the amniotic membranes containing fluid, the membranes may break in what is known as "breaking the water," the classic prelabor symptom. Women expect this event to be like a flood of water suddenly rushing out of their vaginas, and it frequently happens this way, but the fluid also may just trickle out. The fluid normally is clear and odorless. Some women think that they have wet their pants when this happens. If the water does not break at this point, it probably will during more active labor.

Early labor. Prelabor slowly unfolds into early labor. This phase lasts about 7 or 8 hours. Early labor and active labor also are known as the first stage of labor. Early labor is characterized by contractions that cause the cervix to dilate 3 to 4 cm. These contractions can feel wavelike. They build up and then recede. They are mildly intense and begin in the lower back. They also can feel like heavy menstrual cramps. The contractions are anywhere from 5 to 20 minutes apart, become more intense each time they occur, last anywhere from 30 to 45 seconds, get longer each time they occur, and get closer together.

Active labor. Active labor is similar to early labor but is far more pronounced. This phase lasts from 3 to 5 hours. Now the contractions occur every 2 to 4 minutes and last up to 60 seconds. They may be moderately or extremely painful, depending on the woman. The physician would administer an epidural, a painkiller that numbs from the breasts down, at this point. A natural childbirth does not use this type of procedure. Epidural or not, the mother will have an incredible urge to push, which mirrors the urge to push out a bowel movement. The mother may also start to feel warm or even get chills.

Transition phase. The transition phase proceeds to delivery and lasts anywhere from 30 to 90 minutes. Active labor has been in progress for approximately 3 hours. The mother may be tired, abusive, and frustrated; have no clue what time it is; may be shaking, hiccupping, vomiting, or having chills; have cold feet, dry mouth, and lips; and be hyperventilating, moaning, crying, or screaming. She has a tremendous urge to push and rectal pressure. Contractions are intense, occurring every 30 seconds and lasting 90 seconds. The cervix is almost fully dilated. Some women may want to use the bathroom, which will help them relax and encourage pushing.

Delivery: bearing down. Instead of holding back the urge to push, the woman actually gets to push. This is tough work. At this phase the hardest part is pushing out the head. As the head emerges, the woman may feel intense burning and stinging sensations. The vagina is like a huge elastic band that stretches for this.

Episiotomy. An episiotomy is a minor surgical procedure in which the physician makes an incision in the perineum, the area between the rectum and vagina. The episiotomy enlarges the opening for vaginal births, making it easier for the baby's head to come out. This procedure is usually not necessary.

Some women find this an uncomfortable procedure and a hindrance to the overall childbirth experience.

A routine episiotomy cuts through skin, vagina mucosa, and three layers of muscle in an otherwise sensitive area. The side effects include pain, bleeding, a breakdown of stitches, and delayed healing. Many doctors believe that a little natural tearing, which often takes place without the episiotomy, not only heals much quicker than a surgical procedure but is less painful.

When is an episiotomy necessary? Any medical emergency during delivery can be a reason for an episiotomy, for example, when the baby's heartbeat becomes abnormal during pushing; to facilitate the delivery of a premature or breech baby; and whenever forceps are necessary (for instance, if the head is in an awkward position). The procedure is also necessary when the delivery of the baby's head is progressing at a rate or manner that will badly tear the perineum, or when the vagina is not stretching. But for the majority of normal, vaginal deliveries, episiotomy is not necessary.

Cesarean birth. A cesarean section, or C-section, is a surgical procedure that is essentially abdominal delivery. Cesarean section is considered major pelvic surgery that usually involves a spinal or epidural anesthetic (only in some cases is a general anesthetic necessary). The surgeon makes a vertical or horizontal incision just above the pubic hair and then (usually) cuts horizontally through the uterine muscle and eases the baby out. Sometimes, this second cut is vertical, known as the "classic incision." The second cut, into the uterine muscle, affects the viability of a vaginal birth after cesarean. With a horizontal cut, women have gone on to have normal second vaginal births.

In some instances, the pregnant woman knows in advance whether she will have a cesarean section. The pelvis may be too small, or the cervix may have irreparable scarring from previous pelvic surgery that prevents dilation, or an emergency situation may be detected in utero (in the womb) that requires the fetus to be taken out immediately.

Usually the problem does not come up until labor, which entails a dizzying array of complications too numerous to list that necessitates a cesarean.

Placenta. The placenta is known as the *afterbirth, birth of placenta,* or just the *third stage of labor.* In a vaginal delivery, episiotomy or not, after the birth of the baby the uterus contracts enough to loosen the placenta from the uterine wall. These contractions may be painful, but they are mild in comparison to previous contractions. The placenta then slips out with one or two pushes. The uterus then continues to contract against exposed blood vessels from where the placenta used to be as a natural way to control bleeding.

Hormones secreted by the placenta, including chorionic gonadotropin and other substances having estrogenic, progestational, or adrenocorticoid activity, play an important function during pregnancy.

Parental bonding with the infant immediately after birth seems to be important. The touch, sound, and smell of parents and infant in the first hours of birth establish biologic and emotional bonds. The hormone oxytocin seems to play a role in this bonding process for mothers and fathers.

Lactation

The main physiologic function of the mammary glands is to provide proper nutrition for the baby, as well as to protect the infant from infections during the first few months of life by transferring antibodies from mother to baby. The breasts enlarge substantially after the second month of pregnancy because of increased amounts of estrogens and progesterone. Prolactin causes the production and secretion of milk. The actual ejection (letdown) of milk from the nipple requires suckling and the release of oxytocin from the posterior pituitary gland. The cry of the infant, and in some cases emotional responses, may cause oxytocin release and lactation. Because milk production is based on a demand, if suckling continues, lactation persists for months, even years. The breasts secrete a yellow fluid, colostrum, during the last part of pregnancy and for the first day or two after delivery. Colostrum has a high protein content and contains antibodies. The breasts secrete milk 1 to 3 days after delivery.

Pathologic Conditions

Abnormal Pregnancy

Bleeding. The student should remember that not all bleeding means that a miscarriage is imminent. Nevertheless, although some bleeding during early pregnancy is fairly common, it is still not normal.

A woman with heavy bleeding that requires heavy-duty pads that need to be changed frequently should report the condition immediately. Other signs and symptoms including cramps, pain in the abdomen, fever, weakness, and possibly vomiting are serious. The blood may have clumps of tissue in it and have an unusual odor. Another kind of bleeding is brown, intermittent, or continuous vaginal spotting or light bleeding accompanied by severe abdominal or shoulder pain. Finally, light bleeding that continues for more than 3 days is not a good sign.

Miscarriage. Heavy bleeding and cramping anywhere between the end of the second month to the end of the third month are classic signs. Cramps without any bleeding are also a danger sign of miscarrying. The bleeding can be heavy enough to soak several pads in an hour, or may be manageable and more like a heavy period. Cramping may occur with passing clots, which are dark red clumps that look like small pieces of raw beef liver. Sometimes grayish or pinkish tissue is passed. A miscarriage also can take place with persistent, light bleeding and milder cramping at this stage.

Several kinds of spontaneous abortions occur:

Threatened abortion: The cervix still is closed, but the woman has cramps, bleeding, or staining. The doctor will perform a physical examination and check the fetal heartbeat and may prescribe bed rest. In some cases the bleeding stops and the pregnancy continues normally.

Inevitable abortion: In this case, nature has taken its course already and the process of miscarriage has started. Bleeding is heavy, cramps increase, and the cervix begins to dilate, expelling everything still intact: the fetus, amniotic sac, and placenta, accompanied by much blood.

Incomplete abortion: In this condition the uterus has spontaneously expelled some, but not all, pregnancy tissue. Usually, what remains are fragments of the placenta. Only half of the fetus is expelled; the other half remains. The condition is correctable with a dilation and curettage procedure to clean out the uterus and help it to heal.

Complete abortion: Complete abortion occurs when all pregnancy tissue passes spontaneously. Although dilation and curettage may be indicated, this usually is not necessary.

Missed abortion: The fetus dies in the uterus but is not expelled. Symptoms that something is wrong may not occur. In this situation, all of the pregnancy symptoms gradually disappear. The physician diagnoses missed abortion frequently during a routine examination, when the fetal heartbeat is no longer audible. Treatment depends on the duration of the pregnancy.

Usually the reason for miscarriage has to do with a fetus self-terminating because of improper development or genetic problems.

Ectopic pregnancy. An ectopic pregnancy occurs when the fetus fails to implant itself in the uterus and starts to develop in the fallopian tube. Ectopic pregnancies are dangerous.

Rupture of the tube could be a life-threatening situation. The classic symptoms of ectopic pregnancy are sharp abdominal cramps or pains on one side. The pains may start out as a dull ache that gets more severe. Neck pains and shoulder pains are also common. The woman also may experience a menstrual type of bleeding along with the pain, but the pain is the most obvious sign.

The problem with ectopic pregnancies is that often women do not realize they are pregnant until they have one.

Women in high-risk groups for ectopic pregnancies generally have the following characteristics:

- Users of intrauterine devices
- A history of pelvic inflammatory disease
- A history of pelvic surgery (scarring may block the tube and prevent the egg from leaving)
- A history of ectopic pregnancy
- Pregnancy results from assisted contraception techniques in which gametes or embryos have been injected into the fallopian tubes

Preeclampsia, toxemia, and pregnancy-induced hypertension. Preeclampsia is a disease that only occurs during pregnancy. *Preeclampsia, pregnancy-induced hypertension,* and *toxemia* are essentially interchangeable terms used by care providers for this disease. This disease is characterized by swelling, high blood pressure, and the presence of protein in the urine. Obvious complications of preeclampsia are swelling, high blood pressure, poor kidney function, poor liver function, pulmonary edema (fluid in the lungs), and possible seizure. A poor blood supply to the baby decreases the baby's nutrients, interfering with development. Preeclampsia occurs in 5% to 10% of all pregnancies and can appear without warning any time throughout the pregnancy, labor, or in the early post-partum period. This disease also can be chronic, gradually becoming worse over time. Preeclampsia may be mild or severe, but the only cure is delivery of the baby.

Bartholin's Cyst

Bartholin's glands are located on each side of the vaginal opening. Obstruction of a duct sometimes occurs from a bacterial infection. The area is painful and swollen. Treatment may require drainage.

Breast Lumps

Most breast lumps are not cancerous, although the incidence increases with age. See Chapter 11 on the integumentary system.

Cervical Cancer

Cervical cancer is the third most common malignancy in women, after breast and colon cancer. Cervical dysplasia is a change in the cells of the cervix. Some of these abnormal cells can develop into cancerous cells. Early detection and treatment, by removing or destroying the cells, may prevent cancer. Factors contributing to the development of cervical cancer are becoming sexually active at an early age, multiple sexual partners, genital herpes, and a possible viral infection. Cervical cancer not treated in the early stages can spread into other tissues, especially lymph nodes and the uterus.

Cervicitis

Cervicitis is inflammation of the cervix. Acute cervicitis usually is caused by the same organisms that cause vaginitis (fungus, bacteria, or protozoa). Symptoms vary and can include redness, bleeding, pelvic pain, and discharge.

Chronic cervicitis is a recurrent inflammation of the cervix, frequently causing pelvic pain and often with a heavy discharge. Treatment of cervicitis includes medications if caused by organisms or cauterization if the condition becomes chronic.

Endometriosis

Endometriosis is a disease in which endometrial tissue is present in nonuterine locations, such as on the intestines, ovaries, or even in the fallopian tubes. Endometriosis most often occurs in young women between the ages of 25 and 50, especially if they have no children. Although symptoms may be mild, common symptoms are heavy menstrual periods, intense back or pelvic pain, painful menstruation (dysmenorrhea), and painful intercourse (dyspareunia). Pregnancy often eliminates the problem. Birth control pills may help because they cause a change in the endometrial tissue. Sometimes surgical intervention is necessary.

Infertility

Infertility is a decrease in the ability to conceive, whereas sterility is a total loss of the ability to conceive. Infertility may be temporary and can result from structural or functional problems with the male, the female, or both. In males, common causes are impotency (the inability to have an erection), a decrease in sperm number, or abnormalities of sperm anatomy and motility. In females, common causes include a lack of ovulation, disorders of the fallopian tubes (often from a previous infection), and abnormal mucus secretion from the cervix, creating an environment hostile to sperm. A low sperm count may be caused by excessive use of alcohol, tobacco, and caffeine; poor nutrition; and fatigue. Men should not wear tight underwear because they pull the testes close to the body, increasing the temperature and decreasing the sperm count. In females, clomiphene citrate is sometimes effective in inducing ovulation. Surgery may be beneficial to correct tubal scarring. The administration of estrogen may restore normal cervical mucus. Generalized stress can be one causal factor for infertility.

Hyperemesis Gravidarum

Hyperemesis gravidarum is severe nausea and vomiting in pregnancy resulting in dehydration and loss of at least 10 lb. Women often are unable to eat or drink anything for days. They often need intravenous hydration and have blood chemical level abnormalities. Hyperemesis gravidarum is exhausting and emotionally distressing but usually has no effect on the developing fetus.

Prostate Disorders

Prostatitis is an infection of the prostate, usually resulting from a urinary tract infection. Perineal pain, fever, chills, painful urination, and a tender prostate on rectal examination are common signs. If bacteria cause prostatitis, treatment with an antibiotic is indicated. Chronic prostatitis commonly occurs in older men with enlarged prostate glands.

Benign prostatic hypertrophy is the enlargement of the prostate, a disorder of males age 45 and older, possibly caused by a decrease in the ratio of testosterone to estrogen. As testosterone declines, estrogen produced by the adrenal cortex seems to stimulate the central portion of the prostate, causing an overgrowth of prostate tissue. The amount of the enlargement is not as important as its ability to compress the urethra, which causes problems with urination such as straining, dribbling, and sometimes urinary retention. Medical treatment, including catheterization and surgery, is indicated in the most severe cases. The herb saw palmetto has been shown to be beneficial in decreasing hypertrophy.

Prostatic cancer is the most common malignancy in males (other than skin cancer) and is slow growing and often asymptomatic and is found most frequently during a physical checkup. Early stage cancer is usually slow growing, whereas in later stages, metastasis to bone commonly occurs, particularly in the thoracic and lumbar vertebrae and the sacrum. Symptoms include urinary retention if obstruction has taken place and lower back pain if metastasis has occurred. Primary treatment depends on the age of the person and stage of the cancer and may focus on relieving symptoms or removing the cancer with methods such as prostatectomy, radiation therapy, and removal of the testes because testosterone stimulates cancer cells.

Sexually Transmitted Diseases

Sexually transmitted diseases include *vaginal infections, hepatitis B infection, nongonococcal urethritis* or *chlamydia, genital warts, herpes genitalis, acquired immunodeficiency syndrome, gonorrhea, syphilis,* and *body lice.* Most of these diseases have been discussed elsewhere in the text.

Gonorrhea is an infectious disease caused by a bacterium and is becoming more resistant to antibiotics because mutant strains have developed. Gonorrhea infects the urethra of both sexes, producing urethritis several days after exposure. The person may show no signs or mild symptoms, which the person ignores while the bacteria spread.

In men, gonorrhea primarily affects the urethra, where it can cause scarring. If untreated, the bacteria can infect and inflame the prostate or the epididymis. Symptoms include difficult urination and a cloudy discharge.

In the female, gonorrhea usually infects the cervix, causing cervicitis. Untreated gonorrhea may infect the uterus or fallopian tubes, causing scarring that may result in infertility. Involvement of the tubes and surrounding pelvic area is *pelvic inflammatory disease.* If gonorrhea travels to the abdominal cavity, it can cause peritonitis. Signs and symptoms of gonorrhea in women include fever, abnormal bleeding, cloudy vaginal discharge, bilateral pelvic pain (usually during the menses), and tenderness on movement of the cervix (stretching the broad ligament).

Untreated gonorrhea in both sexes can infect the bloodstream, causing blood poisoning, and can spread to the skin, bones, joints, and tendons.

Syphilis is a bacterial infection transmitted sexually or from mother to fetus. Frequency of infections declined with the discovery of penicillin, but as with gonorrhea, resistant strains are appearing. Syphilis appears in three stages:

Stage 1: Painless skin sores, treated primarily with antibiotics

Stage 2: Skin rash, which may be helped with antibiotics (stages 1 and 2 are highly contagious)

Stage 3: Referred to as late syphilis, stage 3 is not as contagious except for blood exchanged between two persons; if the person does not recognize the symptoms from stages 1 or 2, the third stage can flare at any time and affect the brain, nervous system, aorta, and other organs of the body; syphilis cannot be reversed in the third stage.

Herpes simplex is a DNA virus that causes painful blisters and small ulcers in and around the mouth and on the genital area. Type 1 usually infects the upper body, and type 2 affects the genital area. Type 2 is a common sexually transmitted disease. The primary infection lasts about 1 to 4 weeks. Recurrent lesions are less painful and debilitating, often emerge every month or two, and last 7 to 10 days. The blisters form, then break open, and remain open for 2 to 3 weeks. The open blisters are painful. Herpes is transmitted when it is active; that is, when the lesions are present and up to 7 days afterward. In some persons, lesions recur. In others, recurrence takes place once or twice, and never again. Fever, emotional stress, the menses, sunlight, infections, and trauma may activate herpes lesions. Genital lesions in women consist of painful vesicles and erosions on the labia, vagina, or cervix. In males the lesions often are located on the penis. The antiviral drug acyclovir (Zovirax) is effective.

Uterine Disorders

A *myoma,* or *fibroid,* is a benign tumor in the uterus that grows inside the uterine muscle wall or attaches to the wall. These tumors may be small, grow slowly, and be asymptomatic. Tumors that grow large or rapidly cause heavy bleeding. If blood loss is extensive, anemia may occur. Fibroids are the most common disorder of the uterus. Occurring in late reproductive years, the tumor is estrogen dependent. Prolonged or abnormal menstrual bleeding is usually the first sign. Treatment may be dietary for the anemia. In the rare case that the tumor grows large enough to cause severe bleeding, a hysterectomy is required.

Polyps are small growths of the endometrium extending into the body of the uterus. They are common in all age groups, especially in women with no children. The main symptom is increased menstrual bleeding between periods or post-menopausal bleeding. Removal of the polyps with a uterine curet (curettage) is indicated if symptoms are problematic. Cervical polyps occur when the lining of the cervix develops growths that hang outside the cervix.

Dysfunctional uterine bleeding is abnormal bleeding throughout much of the 28-day cycle. The main form of diagnosis and treatment is dilation and curettage.

Vaginitis

Vaginitis is inflammation of the vagina. Signs and symptoms are vaginal discharge, itching (pruritus), and irritation.

Yeast vaginitis (candidiasis, moniliasis) is a common fungal infection caused by the fungus *Candida albicans.* The infection responds to an antifungal ointment such as miconazole (Monistat) or nystatin.

Trichomonas vaginitis (trichomoniasis) is caused by a protozoal parasite that may infect the urinary tract of both sexes and is a sexually transmitted organism. Metronidazole (Flagyl) is effective. The sexual partner also may require treatment.

Gardnerella (Haemophilus) vaginitis is a bacterial infection of the vagina and responds to metronidazole.

INDICATIONS CONTRAINDICATIONS

For Therapeutic Massage

As with all acute infections, massage is contraindicated until any infectious diseases of the reproductive system run their course. Massage in clients with malignancies is contraindicated unless the appropriate health care professional provides approval and supervision. Therapeutic massage during a normal pregnancy is structured as part of a wellness program with accommodation for the changes in the pregnant woman. The practitioner should obtain permission from the supervising health care professional. Certainly anyone working with pregnant women regularly should learn more about pregnancy and fetal development than is provided in this text. Most reproductive system conditions present regional contraindications. As with most chronic illness and pain, therapeutic massage offers generalized support for homeostasis and can offer palliative or comfort care for the maintenance of these conditions (Activity 12-4). ■

ACTIVITY 12-4

We must be able to explain and justify the therapeutic value of the work we do. The following activity will assist you in developing the skills to explain the effectiveness of therapeutic massage to clients and other health care professionals. Use the clinical reasoning model that follows to accomplish this task. The focus should be the primary modality or modalities applied to the reproductive system.

Methods/Applications

1. What are the facts?

   a. Which system is involved, and which structures of that system can be reached directly or indirectly?

   b. Which of these structures are most affected by this massage?

   c. Which physiologic functions are affected by this approach?

   d. When the treatment is applied, what changes in function will occur in

      (1) this system?

      (2) the whole body?

Continued

ACTIVITY 12-4—cont'd

e. What is considered normal or balanced function?

f. How are the functions of this system related to the homeostasis of the body?

g. What has worked or has not worked?

h. Where could you find information that would support the use of this modality as a therapeutic intervention?

i. What research is available to support the use of the therapeutic intervention?

j. How does the intervention support a healthy state?

k. Under which pathologic or dysfunctional conditions is the therapeutic massage most likely to be beneficial?

2. What are the possibilities?

a. What do the data suggest?

b. What are the reasons for using the proposed method?

c. What are the possible interventions?

d. List at least three applications of massage that would affect the structure and function of the system involved.

e. What are other ways to look at the situation?

ACTIVITY 12-4—cont'd

f. What other methods could provide similar benefits?

3. What is the logical outcome of therapeutic intervention?

a. What would be the logical progression of the symptom pattern, contributing factors, and current behaviors?

b. What are the benefits and drawbacks of each intervention suggested?

Benefits:

Drawbacks:

c. What are the costs in terms of time, resources, and finances?

d. What is likely to happen if the modality is not used?

e. What is likely to happen if the modality is used?

4. For the intervention proposed, what would be the effect on the persons involved, specifically the client, practitioner, and other professionals working with the client?

a. How does each person involved (including, besides the foregoing, the client's family and support system) feel about the possible interventions?

b. Does the practitioner feel qualified to work with the situation and apply the identified modality to the particular person?

c. Does a feeling of cooperation and agreement exist among all those involved, and how would the practitioner recognize this feeling?

Justification

Using the information developed in the clinical reasoning model, present a clear, concise statement of how the ways in which the particular soft tissue or movement modality would be beneficial in supporting the particular body system in a healthy condition or as part of a treatment plan for a pathologic or dysfunctional condition. Based on the foregoing information, give a brief summary of the effectiveness of the modality for this system.

SUMMARY

On completion of the last set of justification exercises, the student should be familiar with a logical model of reasoning that honors intuition and the emotions and perceptions of the persons involved. As with all knowledge, you must question it, individualize the process, make it your own, and improve it. This model is only a framework; however, the model helps us be more objective and address questions and issues we may not think of on our own. This is good—to consider various perspectives and then make our own best decisions.

The respiratory, digestive, urinary, and reproductive systems contribute to the complete function of the body as a whole. These systems concern the movement of energy, water, and air and creation of new life in and out of the body. Again we see the interconnectedness of being alive and, with these systems, the need for interaction outside ourselves as we breathe in air, take in food and water, and connect with another to produce life.

evolve

Log on to your student account on the Fritz EVOLVE site and read the therapeutic massage case study under Course Materials Chapter 12. Then, list the reasons that justify the effectiveness of therapeutic massage in supporting health maintenance for the reproductive system.

Workbook Section

Section • Workbook Section • Workbook Section • Workbook Section • Workbook Section

Short Answer

1. What are the parts of the upper and lower respiratory tract?

2. How does the nose affect the breathing pattern when we sleep?

3. What happens in our bodies to prevent food from going into our lungs while we are swallowing?

4. How does the diaphragm work to help us breathe?

5. Describe the mechanics of relaxed breathing.

6. What is a normal respiratory rate and how can it be affected?

7. Where does digestion begin and end?

8. List the organs of digestion.

9. What are the steps in digestion and what does each involve?

WORKBOOK SECTION

10. What are the main food groups and why is each important? Give two examples of each.

11. What are the organs of the urinary system and where are they located?

12. How much urine does the average person produce per day?

13. What are the parts of the male reproductive system?

14. What are the parts of the female reproductive system?

15. What are the divisions of the gestational period in the human being, and what are the primary features of each period?

FILL IN THE BLANK

(1) Respiration is the movement of air in and out of the lungs, the exchange of oxygen and carbon dioxide between the lungs and blood, and the exchange between blood and body tissues.

(2) External respiration is the exchange of oxygen and carbon dioxide between the lungs and the bloodstream.

The lower two thirds of the (3) external nose is composed mostly of cartilage. The upper third, or bridge of the nose, is formed from two small hard nasal bones. The tip of the nose is the apex, and the nostrils are the (4) nares.

The (5) nasal cavity is the actual space inside the external and internal nose structures. It is separated into left and right sides by the septum, a partition composed of cartilage and bone. At the upper portion of the nasal cavity, three thin, curled bones, the (6) turbinates, or conchae, project inward from the two outer walls.

Venous areas called (7) swell bodies are located on the turbinates.

The (8) sinuses are four groups of air-filled spaces that open into the frontal, ethmoid, sphenoid, and maxillary bones of the skull. The (9) nasopharynx is the continuation of the nasal cavity into the throat, or pharynx. The (10) __larynx__, or voice box, connects the pharynx to the trachea. Its structure consists of cartilage, ligaments, connective tissue, muscles, and the vocal cords. The vocal cords and the spaces between the cords are located inside the (11) __glottis__.

The (12) __trachea__, or windpipe, is the main airway to the lungs. It is a 4- to 5-inch tube that begins at the glottis and ends at the junction of the two main bronchi near the level of the sternal angle.

The two (13) __lungs__ are the primary organs of respiration. These soft, spongy, highly vascular structures are separated into the left and right lungs by the mediastinum. The (14) __digphragm__ is a dome-shaped sheet of muscle attached to the thoracic wall that separates the lungs and thoracic cavity from the abdominal cavity.

The (15) __thorax__, or chest cavity, is the upper region of the torso enclosed by the sternum, ribs, and thoracic vertebrae. It contains the lungs, heart, and great vessels.

The (16) __~~adbom~~ abdomen__, or (17) __abdomonal cavity__, contains the major organs of digestion. The cavity is lined with a mucous membrane, the (18) __peritoneum__, the function of which is to prevent friction.

Products of digestion are propelled along the tract from the esophagus to the anus by the rhythmic contraction of smooth muscle called (19) __peristalsis__. Digestive secretion generally refers to the release of various substances from the (20) __exocrineglands__ that serve the digestive system. Digestive secretion includes the release of saliva, gastric juice, pancreatic juice, bile, and intestinal juice.

The citric acid cycle is the main pathway by which food energy is released by cells to manufacture their own energy-rich (21) __adenosine__ __triphosphate__ (ATP).

(22) __water__ is a constituent of all living things. The water content of the tissues of the body varies. Adipose tissue (fat) has the lowest percent of water; the (23) __skeleton__ has the second lowest water content.

The testicles contain tiny seminiferous tubules that produce (24) __sperm__. The (25) __prostate__ gland surrounds the urethra and produces a milky alkaline fluid.

The (26) __ovaries__ are solid glands that produce the hormones estrogen and progesterone. The external female genitalia are known collectively as the (27) __vulva__.

Gestation takes approximately 10 lunar months (9 calendar months) and is divided into (28) __trimesters__. The hormone (29) __oxytocin__ stimulates contraction of the uterus. Prelabor can begin anywhere in the last few weeks or last days of pregnancy. The (30) __cervix__ at this stage softens and may start to thin out a little, which allows it to dilate (open up) slightly. As the baby's head presses down against the amniotic membranes containing fluid, the membranes may break, producing what is known as "__breaking the water__." This is the classic prelabor symptom.

WORKBOOK SECTION

EXERCISE

In the illustration of the digestive system below, write the name of each part of the system next to its corresponding letter. Then color the illustration.

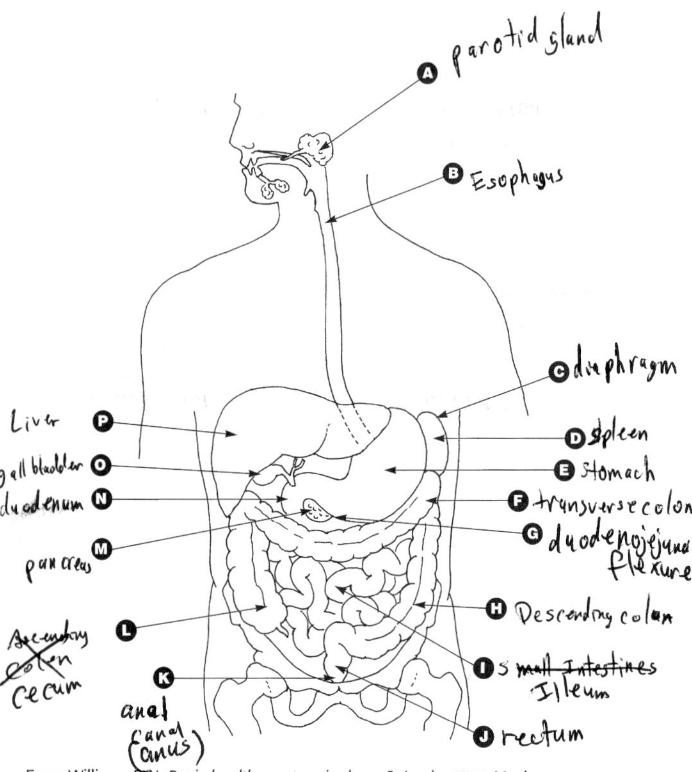

From Williams RW: *Basic healthcare terminology,* St Louis, 1995, Mosby.

PROFESSIONAL APPLICATION

What education and information does a massage practitioner need to work with pregnant women?

____

____

____

____

____

____

____

____

Answer Key

1. The upper respiratory tract consists of the nasal cavity and all its structures and the pharynx; the lower respiratory tract consists of the larynx and trachea and the bronchi and alveoli in the lungs.
2. When a person lies with his or her head to one side, the swell bodies of the lower nostril become congested. The chamber narrows and the lumen closes. When sleeping, we only breathe through one nostril at a time. The closure of the nostril then initiates movement of the head from one side to the other, which in turn causes a major movement and turning of the body. This head-body moving cycle initiated by the nose ensures maximal rest during sleep. A poorly functioning nose may allow the body and head to remain in one position and can cause symptoms such as backaches, numbness, cramps, and circulatory dysfunction.
3. The pharynx functions as a passageway for food between the mouth and the esophagus and as a passageway for air between the nose, mouth, and trachea. At the entrance to the larynx is a small cartilaginous flap, the epiglottis. As we swallow food, the epiglottis closes over the glottis, preventing food or fluids from entering the lungs.
4. The diaphragm is a dome-shaped sheet of muscle attached to the thoracic wall that separates the lungs and thoracic cavity from the abdominal cavity. As the chest cavity enlarges, the diaphragm moves downward and creates a vacuum that allows air to flow into the lungs. As the chest contracts and the diaphragm relaxes, the diaphragm arches upward, helping air to flow out of the lungs.
5. During the moments before we take a breath, the pressure inside the lungs and outside the body are equal, whereas the pressure inside the pleural space is slightly lower. When we begin to inhale, the external intercostal muscles between the ribs contract, lifting the lower ribs up and out. This creates a vacuum that expands the lungs, causing the pressure inside the lungs to decrease. The diaphragm moves down, increasing the volume of the pleural cavities and decreasing the pressure even more. Elastic fibers in the alveolar walls stretch, permitting expansion of the air sacs. The lungs draw in air until the pressure is equal again.

   As we exhale, the pressure inside the pleural cavity increases; the external intercostals, diaphragm, and alveolar walls relax; the volume inside the lungs decreases; and the pressure in the lungs increases until it again equals the air pressure.
6. The respiratory rate in adults is about 12 to 16 breaths per minute. In the newborn the respiratory rate is about 35 and gradually decreases to adult values at about age 20. Emotions are a powerful stimulus for respiratory changes. Fear, grief, and shock slow the respiratory rate; anger and sexual arousal increase the respiratory rate.
7. Digestion begins in the mouth and ends in the small intestine and is accompanied by digestive enzymes (protein catalysts) that split large substances into small ones. The gastrointestinal tract contains glands that secrete mucus and digestive enzymes.
8. The digestive tract consists of the mouth, pharynx, esophagus, stomach, small intestine, large intestine, rectum,

and anus. Accessory structures include the salivary glands, pancreas, liver, and gallbladder.

9. The four essential steps in the process of digestion are these:
   Ingestion: Food entering the mouth
   Digestion: The mechanical and chemical breakdown of food from its complex form into simple molecules
   Absorption: The movement of these simple molecules from the digestive tract to the circulatory or lymphatic systems; vitamins and minerals are absorbed in the small intestine; amino acids, simple sugars, and small fatty acids pass through the intestinal villi into the bloodstream; the larger fatty acids are reconstituted to fats in the intestinal wall and pass into the lymphatic system; capillaries of the intestinal villi become venules and then veins, and finally the large portal vein carries absorbed foodstuffs to the liver; the liver converts these substances into compounds required for bodily functions.
   Elimination (egestion): Removal and release of solid waste products from food that cannot be digested or absorbed
10. Proteins: Proteins are large, high-molecular-weight substances containing carbon, hydrogen, oxygen, and nitrogen and smaller amounts of other elements. Proteins break down into amino acids. The body uses 24 amino acids for its metabolic requirements. Dietary proteins include animal products and bean and grain combinations. Proteins are the chief structural components of the body.
    Carbohydrates: Complex carbohydrates are long chains of glucose molecules found in rice and vegetables. Glucose is the main fuel for the manufacture of adenosine triphosphate in the cell. Sugars are converted to glucose in the liver.
    Fats: In addition to serving as a reservoir of stored energy, fats are essential components of the cell membrane and myelin sheath of the nerve fiber. Dietary fats are found in nuts, seeds, oils, and animal products.
11. Kidneys: The kidneys are reddish brown, bean-shaped organs located on the posterior wall of the abdomen against the back body wall musculature, just above the waist. The kidneys are imbedded in fat and located about the spinal level of T11 to L3 on each side of the vertebral column. The right kidney is lower than the left because of its displacement by the liver. An adrenal gland sits on top of each kidney.
    Ureters: Ureters are two narrow tubes extending from the kidney and connecting to the bladder. The two ureters lie in the psoas muscles.
    Bladder (urinary bladder): The urinary bladder, a reservoir for urine, is a muscular, baglike organ that lies in the pelvis.
    Urethra: The urethra is the tube that carries urine from the bladder. The opening at the end of the urethra is called the meatus.
12. In the average person the kidneys filter about 100 L of blood per day, reabsorbing 99 L of filtrate and leaving about 1 L of urine.
13. The male reproductive system consists of the testicles, epididymis, vas deferens, ejaculatory duct, urethra, penis, and scrotum.
14. The female reproductive system is designed for child-bearing. The system consists of two ovaries, two fallopian tubes, a uterus, and a vagina. Also included in the system are the external genitalia and mammary glands.
15. Gestation takes approximately 10 lunar months (9 calendar months) and is divided into trimesters. In the beginning of the second trimester, the baby weighs almost 2 oz. The bones are growing and the muscle movement is increasing. The last trimester is mostly a weight-gaining and maturing process preparing the baby for life outside the womb. Various physiologic changes occur for the mother during these markers as well. The first trimester is a time of radical hormonal changes. Changes for the mother occur and could consist of moodiness, fatigue, possible back pain, constipation, and energy level changes. In the second trimester, appetite increases, blood volume increases, and the body places additional workload on all physiologic functions. The last trimester finds the mother heavy with the baby, and posture changes are evident. Internal organs are crowded. Physiologic systems are strained with sustaining mother and baby. The connective tissue structure of the body alters by softening to allow for the expansion needed for the birth. This is a time of rest and waiting.

Fill in the Blank

1. Respiration
2. External respiration
3. external nose
4. nares
5. nasal cavity
6. turbinates
7. swell bodies
8. sinuses
9. nasopharynx
10. larynx
11. glottis
12. trachea
13. lungs
14. diaphragm
15. thorax
16. abdomen
17. abdominal cavity
18. peritoneum
19. peristalsis
20. exocrine glands
21. adenosine triphosphate
22. Water
23. skeleton
24. sperm
25. prostate
26. ovaries
27. vulva
28. trimesters
29. oxytocin
30. cervix
31. breaking the water

Exercise

A. Parotid gland
B. Esophagus
C. Diaphragm
D. Spleen
E. Stomach
F. Transverse colon
G. Duodenojejunal flexure
H. Descending colon
I. Ileum
J. Rectum
K. Anus
L. Cecum
M. Pancreas
N. Duodenum
O. Gallbladder
P. Liver

FINAL WORD

The learning journey continues. The student would be well served to obtain a comprehensive anatomy and physiology text to pursue further self-study and take additional courses on these topics.

This text has provided a map for an introductory journey through the body. The information has been presented with the therapeutic massage student and future professional in mind and represents current scientific validation of the practice of therapeutic massage. The themes of dynamic balance, homeostasis, and clinical reasoning have been supported throughout the learning process. One goal has been to teach students to be their own teachers.

East/West philosophy and theory and ancient healing wisdom have been presented with a focus on science, but with a balance provided by acknowledging the body, mind, and spirit of being human. In the end, we can see that the concepts are similar, although the languages are different. The common ground is the body, and the anatomy and physiology are universal.

A competent integrated practice of therapeutic massage is what this text is based on. The knowledge coupled with practical application supports the ability to plan and organize an effective massage session to achieve long-term outcome goals for massage clients. Massage, if provided in an intelligent manner, can be effective for stress reduction, relaxation, comfort for the touch deprived, managing chronic conditions, providing therapeutic change for the movement from disease to wellness, or to ease suffering through compassionate palliative care. A successful professional practice is based on being effective for the client. This is what they pay for.

This text has also led you on a journey of yourself. Self-reflection and self-care are indications of a skilled professional practice. This leads to successful therapeutic relationships with clients and satisfying interactions with other professionals from many disciplines. To become an effective team member, you must be able to communicate with clients, and the language in this text provides the means for understanding. Maybe most important is the ongoing pursuit of professional development. This text is designed to teach you to be your own teacher. The ability to think, integrate, and apply knowledge in an intuitive compassionate way is the final determinant of a competent massage professional.

Another theme of this text can be recognized in retrospect: that the form and function of the human body can be wonderful examples and teachers for the form and function of life itself. The way in which the many systems of the body cooperate, and in so doing, support life, is similar to the way we as human beings can cooperate, respecting and supporting each other and other living creatures as we live and work together on this planet.

With just that vision, this text has been written.

Appendix A

Internet Resources

Foundations and Associations

American Massage Therapy Association (AMTA)
This site includes general information on AMTA, which represents more than 47,000 massage therapists in nearly 30 countries.
http://www.amtamassage.org

Associated Bodywork & Massage Professionals (ABMP)
Here you'll find general information on ABMP, which serves massage, bodywork, somatic, and esthetic professionals.
http://www.abmp.com

Centers for Disease Control and Prevention (CDC)
Visit this site to find general information on CDC, including publications, announcements, links, and health topics.
http://www.cdc.gov/

Commission on Massage Therapy Accreditation (COMTA)
COMTA is the independent accrediting body for the massage therapy profession.
http://www.comta.org/

Human Anatomy & Physiology Society (HAPS)
HAPS promotes communication among anatomy and physiology teachers and presents workshops and conferences to explain the latest developments in the field.
http://www.hapsweb.org/

The Massage & Bodywork Resource Center
This site contains information on massage and massage schools and also provides additional links of interest.
http://www.massageresource.com/

MedPortal
Click below for the medical research search engine with access to Medline.
http://www.medportal.com/

National Center for Complementary and Alternative Medicine (NCCAM)
Here you'll find general information on the NCCAM, including links to other resources.
http://altmed.od.nih.gov/

National Certification Board for Therapeutic Massage and Bodywork (NCBTMB)
NCBTMB's site includes general information on obtaining national certification in massage and bodywork and finding a nationally certified practitioner.
http://www.ncbtmb.com

Touch Research Institutes
Look up general information on the Touch Research Institutes, which study the effects of touch therapy on individuals in every stage of life.
http://www.miami.edu/touch-research/

United States Association for Small Business and Entrepreneurship (USASBE)
On this site you'll find general information on the USASBE, which is devoted to continued education for entrepreneurs and small business owners.
http://www.usasbe.org/index.asp

Anatomy and Physiology

Anatomy Teaching Models
Click on the link below for radiology exhibits from the University of Washington Department of Radiology.
http://www.rad.washington.edu/anatomy/index.html

Digital Anatomist Project
This is an online information system in anatomy from the Department of Biological Structure at the University of Washington.
http://sig.biostr.washington.edu/projects/da/

Functional Anatomy of the Knee
Knee anatomy, function, and related problems are described on this site.
http://ourworld.compuserve.com/homepages/Dr_John/kneeanat.htm#content

Gross Anatomy from Loyola University
Visit this site to find tutorials and curriculum from the Medical Education Network.
http://www.meddean.luc.edu/lumen/MedEd/GrossAnatomy/GA.html

Hosford Muscle Tables
Find detailed information on the skeletal muscles of the human body: origin, insertion, action, blood supply, and innervation.
http://www.ptcentral.com/muscles/

Human Anatomy Online
Great animations and graphics show any part of the human anatomy in color and 3-D on this website.
http://www.innerbody.com/htm/body.html

Illustrated Encyclopedia of Human Anatomic Variation
This site includes illustrations from the Virtual Hospital (University of Iowa).
http://www.vh.org/

Knee Anatomy
Southern California Orthopedic Institute provides a great knee anatomy lesson.
http://www.scoi.com/kneeanat.htm

Master Muscle List
If you need to know the origin, insertion, action, and nerve innervation for any and every muscle in the body, this is the place.
http://www.meddean.luc.edu/lumen/MedEd/GrossAnatomy/dissector/mml/index.htm

Muscle List
Here you'll find a nice outline of all the muscles and pain referral zones they encompass.
http://danke.com/Orthodoc/outline.html

Muscles in Action
Movies, images, and text descriptions of muscles and their action can be found on this site.
http://www.med.umich.edu/lrc/Hypermuscle/Hyper.html

Primal Pictures 3-D Anatomy Online
This site features 3-D images of anatomical and physiological subject matter.
http://www.anatomy.tv/Default.asp?bhcp=1

Shoulder Anatomy
The excellent graphics on this site help explain shoulder structure and function.
http://www.scoi.com/sholanat.htm

The Visible Human Project
Learn about anatomy in 3-D web technology.
http://www.nlm.nih.gov/research/visible/visible_human.html

Virtual Anatomy Explorer
The Visible Human Project was established by the National Library of Medicine to create anatomically detailed, 3-D representations of the human body.
http://www.med.uni-giessen.de/ipl/vae.html

APPENDIX B

MUSCLE QUICK REFERENCE GUIDE

This chart is an abbreviated, simplified description of the main muscles and referred pain patterns encountered during massage application. Detailed information is provided in Chapters 9 and 10.

MUSCLE NAME	FUNCTION	TRIGGER POINT REFERRED PAIN PATTERN*
MUSCLES OF THE FACE AND HEAD		
Muscles of Facial Expression	Move scalp forward and backward; assist in raising the eyebrows and wrinkling the forehead; draw the eyebrows downward and medially; and create transverse wrinkles over the bridge of the nose.	Galea aponeurotica, muscles over the eyebrows, eyes, ears, nose, and scalp above the ears
Auricular (ear) muscles	Move the ear.	None identified.
Eye muscles	Open and close the eyelids; provide intrinsic movement of the eye ball.	Superior orbital area above the eyelid
Muscles That Move the Mouth	Move lips; aid in mastication; force air out between the lips; and compress the cheek against the teeth.	
Muscles of Mastication (Chewing)	Move the mouth; close the jaw; provide side-to-side movement and biting; and elevate the mandible.	Near and in the zygomatic arch; anterior, medial, and posterior along the inferior aspect of the muscles near the tendinous junction at the coronoid process of the mandible; temporal region, eyebrow, upper teeth, cheek, and temporomandibular joint; back of the throat, into the ear; upper and lower jaw, the ear, and the eyebrow
MUSCLES OF THE NECK		
Anterior Triangle of the Neck		
Suprahyoid muscles	Affect movement of the tongue; elevate the hyoid bone; help produce sound and speech; draw the larynx and thyroid cartilage downward; depress the larynx; and elevate thyroid cartilage.	Neck and throat
Infrahyoid muscles	Depress the hyoid bone; influence swallowing; and help produce sound.	Neck and throat
Posterior Triangle of the Neck		
Longus colli and capitus	Bend the neck forward (flexion); oblique portion bends neck laterally; inferior portion rotates neck to the opposite side; control acceleration of cervical extension, lateral extension, and contralateral rotation; and provide dynamic stabilization of cervical spine.	These muscles are difficult to palpate and so no specific trigger point locations have been identified.

* The most common location of trigger points is in the belly of the muscles or at the attachments.

Continued

Muscle Name	Function	Trigger Point Referred Pain Pattern*
SCALENE GROUP		
Scalenus anterior	Bends the cervical portion of the vertebral column forward (flexion) and laterally; also rotates to the opposite side and assists in elevation of the first rib, thus functioning as an accessory muscle of respiration; checks (decelerates) cervical lateral flexion and rotation; and stabilizes cervical spine.	Pectoral region, rhomboid region, and the entire length of the arm into the hand
Scalenus medius	Acting from above, helps to raise the first rib, thus functioning as an accessory muscle of respiration; acting from below, bends the cervical part of the vertebral column to the same side; assists flexion of the neck; checks (decelerates) cervical lateral flexion and rotation; and stabilizes cervical spine.	Pectoral region, rhomboid region, and the entire length of the arm into the hand
Scalenus posterior	When the second rib is fixed, bends the lower end of the cervical portion of the vertebral column to the same side (lateral flexion); when the upper attachment is fixed, helps to elevate the second rib, thus functioning as an accessory muscle of respiration; checks (decelerates) cervical lateral flexion and rotation; and stabilizes cervical spine.	Pectoral region, rhomboid region, and the entire length of the arm into the hand
Sternocleidomastoideus	Assists in flexing the cervical portion of the vertebral column forward, elevating thorax, and extending the head at the atlantooccipital joint; stabilizes the head; and resists forceful backward movement of the head, tilts head, rotates the head, and simultaneously acts to control rotation.	Several trigger points are located in the entire length of both divisions of the muscle. Head and face, particularly the occipital region, ear, and forehead. Autonomic nervous system phenomena and proprioceptive disturbances are common.
Deep Posterior Cervical Muscles		
Splenius capitis and cervicis	Extend head and neck, draw head dorsally and laterally and rotate head to the same side; check and control cervical flexion and contralateral rotation; and stabilize cervical spine.	Belly of the muscles closer to the head; to the top of the skull (the pain often feels as if it is inside the head), to the eye, and into the shoulder
Erector Spinae Group		
Spinalis thoracis, cervicis, and capitis Longissimus thoracis, cervicis, and capitis Iliocostalis lumborum, thoracis, and cervicis	Extend, rotate, and laterally flex the vertebral column and head; assist with anterior tilt elevation and rotation of the pelvis and spinal stabilization; control and decelerate vertebral flexor rotation and lateral flexion; and stabilize lumbar spine primarily.	Scapular, lumbar, abdominal, and gluteal areas, bandlike headache into the eyes, stiff neck
Oblique muscles, transversospinalis group: Semispinalis thoracis, cervicis, and capitis Multifidus Rotatores Intertransversarii lumborum, thoracis, and cervicis Interspinales	This group of muscles extends the motion segments of the back; rotates the thoracic, cervical, and lumbar vertebral joints; and stabilizes the vertebral column.	Scapular, lumbar, abdominal, and gluteal areas, bandlike headache into the eyes, stiff neck

Muscle Name	Function	Trigger Point Referred Pain Pattern*
Suboccipital muscles Rectus capitis posterior major and minor Oblique capitis superior and inferior	As a group these muscles extend and rotate the head in small, precise movements. More often these muscles isometrically function as stabilizers of the head and provide proprioceptive input about head position. These muscles are also important postural muscles and are neuro-reporting stations on balance and proprioceptive monitors of cervical spine and neck position.	Belly of the muscle, located with deep palpation at the base of the skull, around the ear on the same side, sensation of compressed junction of skull and neck, bandlike headache
MUSCLES OF THE TORSO		
Muscles of the Thorax and Posterior Abdominal Wall		
Diaphragm	Participates in respiration; during inspiration (breathing in), diaphragmatic contractions increase the capacity of the thoracic cavity; controls expiration as the diaphragm relaxes; and during breath holding, assists in stabilizing the lumbar and pelvic floor.	None identified.
Serratus posterior superior	Assists in lifting the ribs during inspiration.	Under the scapula near the insertion of the muscle on the ribs and under the upper portion of the scapula
Serratus posterior inferior	Depresses last four ribs (9-12). Some studies disagree that this is the function, finding no electromyographic activity of this muscle during respiration. Seems to act as a stabilizer during forced expirations such as coughing.	Nagging ache in the area of the muscle
External intercostals	Elevate ribs and draw adjacent ribs together; lift ribs, increasing the volume of the thoracic cavity—contralateral torso rotation; and stabilize the thorax.	The intercostals can develop trigger points, which are located by palpating the muscles between the ribs. Pain spans the intercostal segment, especially noticed with deep breathing or rotational movement.
Internal intercostals	Depress ribs and draw adjacent ribs together, decreasing volume of thoracic cavity—ipsilateral torso rotation; stabilize the thorax.	The intercostals can develop trigger points, which are located by palpating the muscles between the ribs. Pain spans the intercostal segment, especially noticed with deep breathing or rotational movement.
Innermost intercostals	The muscles of this small group attach to the internal aspects of two adjoining ribs. They are believed to act with the internal intercostals.	The intercostals can develop trigger points, which are located by palpating the muscles between the ribs. Pain spans the intercostal segment, especially noticed with deep breathing or rotational movement.
Transversus thoracis	Draws anterior portion of the ribs caudally (reduces thoracic cavity); stabilizes rib cage.	None identified.
Quadratus lumborum	Draws last rib downward; flexes lumbar vertebral column laterally to the same side; acts to elevate and anteriorly tilt pelvis; acting bilaterally, extends the lumbar spine and assists forced exhalation, as when coughing; restrains and checks lateral flexion; and assists normal inhalation by stabilizing the diaphragm and the twelfth rib and stabilizing the lumbar area.	Gluteal and groin area, sacroiliac joint and greater trochanter: these points are implicated in most low back pain. The dual function of lumbar stabilization (isometric function) and respiration (concentric function) can cause severe pain in the low back with a cough or sneeze if these trigger points are active. Low back pain often is related more to maintenance of posture than trigger point activity; therefore one commonly finds corresponding pain patterns in the muscles that laterally flex the head and neck, such as the scalenes.

Continued

Muscle Name	Function	Trigger Point Referred Pain Pattern*
Psoas major and minor	With origin fixed, flex the hip joint by flexing the femur on the pelvis; may assist in lateral rotation of the hip joint; acting bilaterally, flex the hip joint by flexing the trunk on the pelvis; can assist extension of the lumbar spine, increasing lumbar lordosis; acting unilaterally, may assist in lateral flexion of the trunk toward the same side; restrain and check trunk and hip extension and contralateral flexion of the trunk; control tendency of lordosis; and stabilize lumbar spine and help to maintain upright posture.	Entire lumbar area into the superior gluteal region; front of the thigh; menstrual aching; and can mimic appendicitis. Shortening is a major cause of low back pain. If tension or trigger point activity is located at insertion, pain can mimic a groin pull. Because of postural reflexes, muscles that flex the head and neck are facilitated with psoas activation. A common correlation exists between neck pain and stiffness and psoas pain and low back stiffness. Massage often must address both areas in sequence to be effective.
Iliacus	Flexes the hip joint; may assist in lateral rotation and abduction of the hip joint; with insertion fixed and acting bilaterally, flexes the hip joint by flexing the trunk on the femur; tilts pelvis forward (anterior) when legs are fixed; decelerates hip extension; and stabilizes the pelvis.	Inner border of the ilium behind the anterior superior iliac spine
Muscles of the Anterior Abdominal Wall		
Transversus abdominis	Constricts and compresses the abdomen, increasing intraabdominal pressure, and supports the abdominal viscera; assists in forced expiration.	Pain located throughout the area but concentrated more in the external circle of the abdominal wall rather than toward the middle near the umbilicus
Obliquus internus abdominis	Compresses the abdominal cavity (some isometric activity); assists with posterior tilt of the pelvis; flexes the vertebral column, bringing the costal cartilage toward the pubis; laterally bends and ipsilaterally rotates the vertebral column (brings the shoulder of the opposite side forward); and restrains trunk extension.	Pain located throughout the area but concentrated more in the external circle of the abdominal wall rather than toward the middle near the umbilicus
Obliquus externus abdominis	Compresses the abdominal cavity (some isometric activity); assists in forced expiration; with both sides acting, flexes the vertebral column, bringing the pubis toward the xiphoid process of sternum; supports posterior pelvic rotation; laterally bends and brings the shoulder of the same side forward; and restrains trunk extension.	Pain located throughout the area but concentrated more in the external circle of the abdominal wall rather than toward the middle near the umbilicus
Rectus abdominis	Flexes the vertebral column, bringing the sternum toward the pelvis; compresses the abdominal cavity; assists with posterior tilt of the pelvis (some isometric activity); assists in forced expiration; and restrains trunk extension.	Trigger points often found in the rectus abdominis just below the umbilicus on either side of the linea alba and near the attachment on the ribs. Pain is referred in local area or to groin.
MUSCLES OF SCAPULAR STABILIZATION		
Trapezius	Upper trapezius elevates the shoulder and, with the shoulder fixed, can assist in drawing the head backward and laterally to tilt chin; the middle portion adducts (retracts) the scapula, draws back the acromion process, and rotates the scapula; lower fibers depress the scapula; the entire muscle, acting bilaterally, assists extension of the cervical and thoracic spine; upper trapezius restrains and controls flexion, lateral flexion, and rotation of the neck and head. Middle trapezius controls and restrains scapular abduction (protraction). Lower trapezius restrains scapular elevation. Trapezius stabilizes scapula and cervical spine.	Neck behind the ear and to the temple; subscapular area; acromial pain

Muscle Name	Function	Trigger Point Referred Pain Pattern*
Rhomboideus major and minor	Adduct (retract) and elevate the scapula and also rotate it downward so that the glenoid cavity faces down toward feet; restrain protraction and upward rotation of scapula; stabilize the scapula.	At the attachment point near the scapular border; scapular region
Levator scapulae	Raises the scapula and draws it medially; with the scapula fixed, extends the neck laterally and rotates it to the same side; bilaterally extends the neck; restrains and controls head and neck flexion, scapular depression, and lateral flexion of cervical spine; and stabilizes cervical/scapular function.	Belly of the muscle just as it begins the rotation and at the attachment near the scapula; angle of the neck and along the vertebral border of the scapula; stiff neck in rotation
Pectoralis minor	Assists in drawing the scapula forward (protraction) around the chest wall; rotates the scapula to depress the point of the shoulder; assists in forced inspiration; restrains scapular retraction; and stabilizes scapula during movement.	Near the attachment at the coracoid process and at the belly of the muscle. May mimic angina with pain in front of the chest from the shoulder and down the ulnar side of the arm into the fingers.
Serratus anterior	Abducts (protracts) the scapula; rotates the scapula so that the glenoid cavity faces cranially (toward the head); raises the ribs with the scapula fixed and therefore is an accessory muscle of respiration; controls scapular retraction; and holds the medial border of the scapula firmly against the thorax and prevents winging of the scapula.	Along the midaxillary line near the ribs; side and back of the chest and down the ulnar aspect of the arm into the hand. May result in shortness of breath and pain during inhalation.
MUSCLES OF THE MUSCULOTENDINOUS (ROTATOR) CUFF		
Supraspinatus	Abducts the arm; restrains adduction of the arm; and acts to stabilize the humeral head in the glenoid cavity during movements of the shoulder joint.	Shoulder, deltoid, and down the arm to the elbow, often experienced as a dull ache
Infraspinatus	Provides lateral or external rotation of the arm at the shoulder; restrains and controls internal (medial) rotation of the arm at the shoulder; and acts to stabilize the humeral head in the glenoid cavity during movements of the shoulder joint.	Deep into the shoulder and deltoid area, down the arm, suboccipital area, medial border of the scapula, with limits reaching behind back
Teres minor	Provides adduction and lateral (external) rotation of the arm; restrains internal (medial) rotation of the arm; and acts to stabilize the humeral head in the glenoid cavity during movements of the shoulder joint.	Posterior deltoid region; client often experiences limited range of motion when reaching behind the back, such as putting hands in back pocket of pants.
Subscapularis	Rotates humerus medially (internal rotation) and draws it forward and down when the arm is raised; restrains lateral (external) rotation of the arm; and stabilizes humeral head in the glenoid cavity during movement of the shoulder.	Access is through the axilla near the attachment at the humerus and in the belly of the muscle. Pain in posterior deltoid, scapular region, triceps area and into the wrist often is mistaken for bursitis because pain often refers to insertion at shoulder.
MUSCLES OF THE SHOULDER JOINT		
Deltoideus	Provides flexion and medial and lateral rotation of the arm and abduction of the arm. Anterior deltoid restrains and controls extension and external rotation of the arm. Middle deltoid restrains arm adduction. Posterior deltoid restrains flexion and internal rotators and horizontal adduction of the arm. Deltoid stabilizes glenohumeral joint during arm movement.	Deltoid region and down the lateral side of the arm

Continued

Muscle Name	Function	Trigger Point Referred Pain Pattern*
Pectoralis major	With proximal attachment (origin) fixed, adducts and draws the humerus forward (flexion) and horizontally and medially (internally) rotates it; with insertion fixed and arm abducted, assists in elevating the thorax (as in forced inspiration); controls arm extension, horizontal abduction, and external rotation; and stabilizes the shoulder during overhead activity.	Chest and breast and down the ulnar aspect of the arm to the fourth and fifth fingers
Subclavius	Draws the clavicle forward and down; stabilizes the clavicle.	Chest and breast and down the ulnar aspect of the arm to the fourth and fifth fingers
Latissimus dorsi	With proximal attachment (origin) fixed, medially or internally rotates, adducts, and extends the humerus; depresses the shoulder girdle and assists in lateral flexion of the trunk; with insertion fixed, assists in tilting the pelvis anteriorly and laterally; acting bilaterally, assists in hyperextending the spine and tilting the pelvis anteriorly; controls abduction, flexion, and external (lateral) rotation of humerus; and stabilizes the lumbar and pelvic area by maintaining tension on the thoracolumbar fascia.	Posterior axillary area just as the muscle begins to twist around the teres major; belly of the muscle near the rib attachments; just below the scapula and into the ulnar side of the arm; anterior deltoid region and abdominal oblique area.
Teres major	Medial or internal rotation, adduction, and extension of the arm; upward rotation of scapula; controls and restrains flexion, abduction, and external rotation of the arm; and stabilizes glenohumeral joint.	Near the musculotendinous junction at both attachments; posterior deltoid region and down the dorsal portion of the arm
Coracobrachialis	Flexion and adduction of the humerus; controls extension and abduction of the humerus; stabilizes the shoulder and scapula.	Front of shoulder, posterior aspect of the arm down the triceps and dorsal forearm into the dorsal hand
MUSCLES OF THE ELBOW AND RADIOULNAR JOINTS		
Biceps brachii	Provides flexion of the humerus. The long head may assist with abduction if the humerus is laterally rotated. The short head assists arm adduction. With proximal attachment (origin) fixed, flexes the forearm toward the humerus and supinates the forearm; with insertion fixed, flexes the elbow joint, moving the humerus toward the forearm, as in a pull-up or chin-up; restrains and controls elbow extension and extension of the humerus; stabilizes the humerus at the shoulder and the elbow joint during full extension; and stabilizes the elbow when flexed and holding a weight.	Front of the shoulder at the anterior deltoid region and into the scapular region; also into the antecubital space or the front of the elbow
Brachialis	Flexes the elbow joint; restrains and controls elbow extension; stabilizes elbow in full extension and fixed flexion.	Primarily to the thumb, with some pain in the anterior deltoid area and at the elbow
Brachioradialis	Flexes the elbow joint after brachialis and biceps initiate movement; assists in pronation and supination of the forearm to midposition; restrains and controls elbow extension; and stabilizes the elbow in full extension and fixed flexion.	Wrist and base of the thumb in the web space between the thumb and index finger and to the lateral epicondyle at the elbow

Muscle Name	Function	Trigger Point Referred Pain Pattern*
Pronator teres	Pronates the forearm; assists in flexing the elbow joint; controls supination of the forearm; and stabilizes the elbow joint and radioulnar joint.	Radial side of the forearm into the wrist and thumb. Pain may mimic carpal tunnel syndrome.
Supinator	Supinates the forearm; assists with flexion of the forearm at the elbow when the hand is held half way between supination and pronation; restrains and controls pronation of the forearm; and stabilizes the elbow and radioulnar joint.	Lateral epicondyle and dorsal aspect of the arm (pain mimics tennis elbow); near the radius in the antecubital space
Pronator quadratus	Provides pronation of the forearm; restrains and controls supination of the forearm.	Belly of muscle; active supination
Triceps brachii	Extension of the forearm; in addition, the long head adducts and assists in extension of the humerus; restrains elbow flexion and arm abduction and flexion; stabilizes the elbow in extension and fixed flexion to allow carrying weight in the hands; and assists in stabilizing the glenohumeral joint.	Length of posterior arm
Anconeus (elbow)	Assists the triceps in extension of the elbow joint; balances elbow flexion; and stabilizes the joint capsule of the elbow.	Elbow at lateral epicondyle
MUSCLES OF THE WRIST AND HAND JOINTS		
Anterior Flexor Group: Superficial Layer		
Flexor carpi radialis	Flexes and abducts the wrist (radial deviation); may assist in pronation of the forearm and flexion of the elbow; restrains and controls extension and adduction of the wrist; and stabilizes the wrist.	Into the wrist and fingers; occasionally into the elbow
Palmaris longus	Flexes the wrist; may assist in flexion of the elbow and pronation of the forearm; restrains wrist extension; and tenses the palmar fascia.	Into the wrist and fingers; occasionally into the elbow
Flexor carpi ulnaris	Flexes and adducts (ulnar deviation) the wrist; may assist in elbow flexion; controls and restrains wrist extension and abduction; and stabilizes wrist.	Into the wrist and fingers; occasionally into the elbow
Flexor digitorum superficialis	Flexes the proximal interphalangeal joints of the second through fifth digits; assists in flexion of the wrist; restrains and controls finger extension; and stabilizes wrist and hand joints.	Into the wrist and fingers; occasionally into the elbow
Flexor digitorum profundus	Flexes the distal interphalangeal joints of the second through fifth digits; assists in flexion of the proximal interphalangeal and metacarpophalangeal joints; assists in adduction of the index, ring, and little fingers and in flexion of the wrist; restrains and controls extension of the fingers; and stabilizes the fingers.	Into the wrist and fingers; occasionally into the elbow
Flexor pollicis longus	Flexes interphalangeal joint of the thumb; assists in flexion of the metacarpophalangeal and carpometacarpal joints; restrains thumb; and stabilizes the thumb.	Thumb
Posterior Extensor Group: Superficial Layer		
Extensor carpi radialis longus	Extends and adducts (ulnar deviation) the wrist; may assist in flexion of the elbow and pronation of the forearm; restrains and controls wrist flexion and abduction; and stabilizes wrist and elbow joints.	From the lateral epicondyle at the elbow down the dorsum of the forearm to various parts of the hand, especially to the web of the thumb

Continued

Muscle Name	Function	Trigger Point Referred Pain Pattern*
Extensor carpi radialis brevis	Extends the wrist and assists in abduction (radial deviation) of wrist and weak flexion of the forearm; restrains and controls wrist flexion and adduction; and stabilizes wrist.	From the lateral epicondyle at the elbow down the dorsum of the forearm to various parts of the hand, especially to the web of the thumb
Extensor digitorum	Extends the metacarpophalangeal joints; extends the interphalangeal joint of the second through fifth digits (with the lumbricales and interossei); assists in extension of the wrist; restrains and controls wrist and finger flexion; and stabilizes the wrist.	From the lateral epicondyle at the elbow down the dorsum of the forearm to various parts of the hand, especially to the web of the thumb
Extensor digiti minimi	Extends the metacarpophalangeal and (with the interosseous and lumbrical muscles) the interphalangeal joints of the little finger; assists in abduction of the little finger; controls and restrains flexion and adduction of the little finger; and stabilizes the joints of the little finger.	From the lateral epicondyle at the elbow down the dorsum of the forearm to various parts of the hand, especially to the web of the thumb
Extensor carpi ulnaris	Extends and abducts (ulnar deviation) the wrist; controls wrist flexion and adduction; and stabilizes wrist.	From the lateral epicondyle at the elbow down the dorsum of the forearm to various parts of the hand, especially to the web of the thumb
Extensor pollicis brevis	Extends and abducts the carpometacarpal joint of the thumb; extends the metacarpophalangeal joint; assists in abduction (radial deviation) of the wrist; assists supination of the forearm; restrains flexion of the thumb and adduction of the wrist; and stabilizes the thumb.	From the lateral epicondyle at the elbow down the dorsum of the forearm to various parts of the hand, especially to the web of the thumb
Posterior Extensor Group: Deep Layer		
Abductor pollicis longus	Abducts and extends the carpometacarpal joint of the thumb; abducts (radial deviation) and assists in wrist flexion and supination of the forearm; controls thumb adduction; and stabilizes thumb and wrist.	To the web of the thumb
Extensor pollicis longus	Extends the interphalangeal joint and assists in extension of the metacarpophalangeal and carpometacarpal joints of the thumb; assists in abduction (radial deviation) and extension of the wrist; restrains thumb and wrist flexion; and stabilizes thumb and wrist.	To the web of the thumb
Extensor indicis	Extends the metacarpophalangeal joint and, with the lumbrical and interosseous muscles, extends the interphalangeal joints of the index finger; may assist in adduction of the index finger and supination of the forearm; and restrains, stabilizes, and controls flexion of the index finger.	Dorsum of the forearm to various parts of the hand
INTRINSIC MUSCLES OF THE HAND		
Thenar Eminence Muscles		
Opponens pollicis	Adducts the carpometacarpal joint of the thumb; adducts and assists in flexion of the metacarpophalangeal joint; aids in opposition of the thumb to each of the other digits; controls and restrains abduction of the thumb; and stabilizes the thumb.	Into the thumb and the wrist

Muscle Name	Function	Trigger Point Referred Pain Pattern*
Abductor pollicis brevis	Abducts and aids in opposition of the thumb; controls and restrains adduction of the thumb; and stabilizes thumb.	Into the thumb and the wrist
Flexor pollicis brevis	Flexes the proximal phalanx of the thumb; assists in opposition of the thumb; restrains and controls extension of the thumb; and stabilizes the thumb.	Into the thumb and the wrist
Hypothenar Muscles		
Opponens digiti minimi	Provides flexion and slight rotation of the carpometacarpal joint of the little finger; helps to cup the palm of the hand; and stabilizes the little finger.	The little finger and wrist
Abductor digiti minimi	Abducts and assists in extension of the metacarpophalangeal joint of the little finger; controls and restrains adduction and flexion of the little finger; and stabilizes the little finger.	The little finger and wrist
Flexor digiti minimi (brevis)	Flexes the metacarpophalangeal joint of the little finger; assists in opposition of the little finger to the thumb; controls extension of the little finger; and stabilizes the little finger.	The little finger and wrist
Deep Muscles of the Hand		
Adductor pollicis	Adducts the thumb and aids in opposition; restrains thumb abduction; and stabilizes the thumb.	The thumb
Interossei palmares	Adducts the index, ring, and little fingers toward the middle digit; assists in restraining abduction of the fingers; and stabilizes the hand.	Into the associated finger
Interossei dorsales	Abducts the index, middle, and ring fingers from the midline of the hand.	Into the associated finger
Lumbricales	Extends the interphalangeal joints and simultaneously flexes the metacarpophalangeal joint of the second through fifth digits.	Into the associated finger
MUSCLES OF THE GLUTEAL REGION		
Gluteus maximus	Extends and laterally rotates the hip joint; upper fibers assist abduction of the hip; lower fibers assist in adduction of the hip joint; with femur fixed, assists in extension of the trunk and posterior tilt of the pelvis; the gluteus maximus is active primarily during strenuous activity, such as running, jumping, and climbing stairs; restrains and controls hip and trunk flexion and medial rotation and abduction/adduction of the hip.These muscles are important postural muscles that help maintain the upright posture, stabilize the pelvis, and provide tension to the iliotibial tract to keep the fascial band taut.	Regionally into the gluteal area, especially to the ischial tuberosity, the tip of the greater trochanter, and the sacrum
Gluteus medius	Abducts the hip joint; anterior fibers medially rotate and assist in flexion of the hip joint and anterior tilt of the pelvis; posterior fibers laterally rotate and assist in extension of the hip joint and posterior tilt of the pelvis; restrains adduction, medial/lateral rotation and flexion/extension of the hip; and stabilizes the pelvis when a person is standing on one foot.	Along the musculotendinous junction at the iliac crest; low back, posterior crest of the ilium to the sacrum, and to the posterior and lateral areas of the buttock into the upper thigh

Continued

MUSCLE NAME	FUNCTION	TRIGGER POINT REFERRED PAIN PATTERN*
Gluteus minimus	Abducts the hip joint and medially rotates the thigh when the limb is extended; restrains and controls hip adduction and lateral rotation; and keeps the pelvis level when a person is standing on one foot.	Lower lateral buttock and down the lateral to posterior aspect of the thigh, knee, and leg to the ankle
Tensor fasciae latae	Flexes, medially rotates, and may assist in abduction of the hip joint; assists in anterior pelvic tilt; extends the knee; restrains hip extension and lateral rotation; tenses the iliotibial tract, counterbalancing the backward pull of the gluteus maximus on the iliotibial tract; and stabilizes the pelvis and knee.	Localized in the hip and down the lateral side of the leg to the knee
Deep Lateral Rotators Piriformis Obturator internus and externus Gemellus superior and inferior	Provide lateral rotation and abduction of the hip joint when the thigh is flexed and posterior pelvic tilt; restrain medial rotation and adduction of the hip; and stabilize the hip joint.	The belly of each muscle can house trigger points. Sacroiliac region, entire buttock and down the posterior thigh to just above the knee
Quadratus femoris	Laterally rotates the hip joint and adducts the thigh; restrains internal rotation and abduction of the hip joint; and stabilizes the hip joint.	The main trigger points are near the attachments and the insertion. Tension in this muscle may cause deep hip and groin pain.
MUSCLES OF THE POSTERIOR THIGH		
Semimembranosus	Flexes the knee and medially rotates the knee joint when the knee is semiflexed; moves the medial meniscus posteriorly during knee flexion; extends and assists in medial rotation and adduction of the hip joint; posteriorly tilts the pelvis; restrains and controls knee extension and lateral rotation; assists in controlling flexion and lateral rotation of the hip; and stabilizes the knee and hip complex.	Several areas in the belly of each muscle and at the musculotendinous junction closer to the knee; ischial tuberosity, back of the knee, and the entire posterior leg to midcalf
Semitendinosus	Flexes the knee and medially rotates the knee joint when the knee is semiflexed; extends and assists in medial rotation and adduction of the hip joint; restrains and controls knee extension and lateral rotation; assists in controlling flexion and lateral rotation of the hip; and stabilizes the knee and hip complex.	Several areas in the belly of each muscle and at the musculotendinous junction closer to the knee; ischial tuberosity, back of the knee, and the entire posterior leg to midcalf
Biceps femoris	Flexes and laterally rotates the knee joint when the knee is semiflexed; long head also extends and assists in lateral rotation of the hip joint and posteriorly tilts the pelvis; restrains and controls knee extension and medial rotation; also restrains hip flexion and medial rotation; and stabilizes the hip and knee complex.	Several areas in the belly of each muscle and at the musculotendinous junction closer to the knee; ischial tuberosity, back of the knee, and the entire posterior leg to midcalf
MUSCLES OF THE MEDIAL THIGH		
Pectineus	Adducts, flexes, and assists in medial rotation of the hip joint and anterior tilt of the pelvis; restrains abduction, extension, and lateral rotation of hip; and stabilizes the hip.	Deep in the groin into the medial thigh and downward to the knee and shin. Pain may mimic hamstring tension.

Muscle Name	Function	Trigger Point Referred Pain Pattern*
Adductor brevis	Adducts and assists in flexing the hip joint anteriorly and tilts the pelvis; restrains and controls abduction and extension of the hip; and stabilizes the hip and trunk in the standing position.	Deep in the groin into the medial thigh and downward to the knee and shin. Pain may mimic hamstring tension.
Adductor longus	Adducts and assists in flexing the hip joint and anteriorly tilts the pelvis; restrains and controls abduction and extension of the hip; and stabilizes the hip and trunk in the standing position.	Deep in the groin into the medial thigh and downward to the knee and shin. Pain may mimic hamstring tension.
Adductor magnus	Adducts the hip joint and posteriorly tilts the pelvis; upper portion medially rotates and flexes, whereas the lower portion laterally rotates and extends the hip joint; restrains and controls hip abduction; and stabilizes the trunk, pelvis, and hip.	Deep in the groin into the medial thigh and downward to the knee and shin. Pain may mimic hamstring tension.
Gracilis	Adducts and flexes the hip joint; assists with anterior tilt of the pelvis; flexes the knee and medially rotates the knee joint when the knee is semiflexed; controls and restrains hip abduction and extension and knee extension and lateral rotation; and assists in controlling and stabilizing the valgus angulation of the knee and stabilizing the pelvic and knee complex.	Deep in the groin into the medial thigh and downward to the knee and shin. Pain may mimic hamstring tension.
MUSCLES OF THE ANTERIOR THIGH		
Sartorius	Flexes, laterally rotates, and abducts the hip joint; also weakly flexes the torso toward the pelvis when the leg is fixed and anteriorly and laterally tilts the pelvis; flexes and assists in medial rotation of the knee joint; controls and restrains extension, medial rotation, and adduction of the hip and assists in restraining trunk extension; at the knee, restrains and controls extension and lateral rotation of the knee; and stabilizes the knee and hip complex.	Into hip and medial knee
Quadriceps Femoris Group		
Rectus femoris	Extends the knee joint; flexes the hip joint; anteriorly tilts the pelvis; restrains and controls knee flexion and hip extension; and stabilizes the knee and hip complex.	Into hip and knee
Vastus lateralis	Extends the knee joint and exerts a lateral pull on the patella; controls and restrains knee flexion and medial pull of patella; and stabilizes iliotibial tract and knee.	Into hip and lateral knee
Vastus medialis	Extends the leg and draws the patella medially, particularly the lower oblique aspect of the muscle (vastus medialis oblique) with attachment into the adductor magnus; controls and restrains knee flexion and lateral movement of patella; and stabilizes the knee and patella.	Entire anterior thigh, with concentration at the knee
Vastus intermedius	Extends the knee joint; restrains and controls knee flexion; and stabilizes the knee and patella.	Into the knee
MUSCLES OF THE ANTERIOR AND LATERAL LEG		
Anterior Muscles		
Tibialis anterior	Provides dorsiflexion of the ankle joint; assists in inversion and adduction of the foot.	Down the leg to the ankle and into the toes

Continued

Muscle Name	Function	Trigger Point Referred Pain Pattern*
	Note: Combined action of inversion and adduction results in supination. Restrains and controls plantar flexion and eversion of the foot. Stabilizes the ankle.	
Extensor digitorum longus	Extends the phalanges of the second through fifth digits; assists in dorsiflexion of the ankle joint and eversion and abduction of the foot; restrains and controls flexion of the toes, plantar flexion, and inversion of the ankle and foot; and stabilizes the ankle and foot.	Down the leg to the ankle and into the toes
Extensor hallucis longus	Extends the metatarsophalangeal joint of the great toe; also assists in inverting and adducting (supination) the foot and dorsiflexing the ankle joint; restrains and controls flexion of the great toes, eversion of the foot, and plantar flexion of the ankle; and stabilizes the great toe and assists in stabilizing the ankle.	Down the leg to the ankle and into the toes
Fibularis (peroneus) tertius	Dorsiflexes the ankle joint; everts and abducts (pronates) the foot; assists in controlling and restraining plantar flexion of the ankle and inversion of the foot; and assists in stabilizing the ankle.	Down the leg to the ankle
Lateral Muscles		
Fibularis (peroneus) longus and brevis	Everts *and abducts (pronates)* the foot; assists in plantar flexion of the ankle joint; restrains and controls dorsiflexion of the ankle and inversion of the foot; and stabilizes the ankle.	To the malleolus lateralis and the heel
POSTERIOR LEG MUSCLES		
Popliteus	Assists in restraining knee extension; stabilizes the knee.	To the back of the knee
Tibialis posterior	Inverts the foot; assists in plantar flexion of the ankle joint; restrains and controls eversion of the foot and dorsiflexion of the ankle; and stabilizes the ankle.	Down the posterior leg to the heel and the sole of the foot into the plantar surface of the toes. Can be a factor in knee pain and restricted mobility of the knee and ankle.
Flexor digitorum longus	Flexes the joints of the second through fifth digits; assists in plantar flexion of the ankle joint and inversion and adduction (supination) of the foot; restrains and controls extension of the toes; assists in controlling dorsiflexion of the ankle and eversion of the foot; and stabilizes the ankle and toes.	Down the posterior leg to the heel and the sole of the foot into the plantar surface of the toes. Can be a factor in knee pain and restricted mobility of the knee and ankle.
Flexor hallucis longus	Flexes the joints of the great toe; provides plantar flexion of the ankle joint and inverts the foot; restrains extension of the great toe and assists in controlling dorsiflexion of the ankle and eversion of the foot; and stabilizes the great toe, ankle, and foot.	Down the posterior leg to the heel and the sole of the foot into the plantar surface of the great toe
Plantaris	Provides plantar flexion of the ankle joint; assists in flexion of the knee joint; restrains dorsiflexion of the ankle and assists in controlling extension of the knee; and assists in stabilizing the ankle/knee complex.	Can be a factor in knee pain and restricted mobility of the knee and ankle.

Muscle Name	Function	Trigger Point Referred Pain Pattern*
Soleus	Provides plantar flexion of the ankle joint and assists inversion of the foot at the ankle; restrains and controls dorsiflexion and eversion of the ankle; and stabilizes the leg over the foot and ankle.	Down the posterior leg to the heel and the sole of the foot into the plantar surface of the toes. Can restrict mobility of the ankle.
Gastrocnemius	Provides plantar flexion of the ankle joint; assists in flexion of the knee joint and inversion of the foot; restrains and controls dorsiflexion of the ankle and extension of the knee; stabilizes the knee and ankle complex and is involved in maintaining balance in static standing.	Down the posterior leg to the heel and the sole of the foot into the plantar surface of the toes. Can be a factor in knee pain and restricted mobility of the knee and ankle.
MUSCLES OF THE FOOT		
Dorsal Aspect		
Extensor digitorum brevis	Extends metatarsophalangeal joint of the first toe and extends the interphalangeal and metatarsophalangeal joints of the second through fourth toes.	The entire foot with areas concentrated at the toes, the ball of the foot, and the heel
Plantar Aspect: Superficial Layer		
Abductor hallucis	Abducts and assists in flexion of the metatarsophalangeal joint of the great toe.	The entire foot with areas concentrated at the large toe, the ball of the foot, and the heel
Flexor digitorum brevis	Flexes the proximal interphalangeal joints and assists in flexion of the metatarsophalangeal joints of the second through fifth toes.	The entire foot with areas concentrated at the toes, the ball of the foot, and the heel
Abductor digiti minimi	Abducts and assists in flexing the metatarsophalangeal joint of the fifth toe.	The entire foot with areas concentrated at the small toe
Plantar Aspect: Second Layer		
Quadratus plantae	Modifies the line of pull of the flexor digitorum longus and assists in flexion of the second through the fifth digits.	The entire foot
Lumbricales	These muscles flex the metatarsophalangeal joints and extend the interphalangeal joints of the second through the fifth digits.	Several areas concentrated in the belly of each muscle; the entire foot with areas concentrated at the large toe, the ball of the foot, and the heel
Plantar Aspect: Third Layer		
Flexor hallucis brevis	Flexes metatarsophalangeal joint of the great toe.	The entire foot with areas concentrated at the large toe
Adductor hallucis	Adducts and assists in flexion of the metatarsophalangeal joint of the great toe.	The entire foot with areas concentrated at the large toe
Flexor digiti minimi brevis	Flexes the metatarsophalangeal joint of the fifth toe.	The entire foot with areas concentrated at the little toe
Plantar Aspect: Fourth Layer		
Interossei plantares	These muscles adduct the third, fourth, and fifth toes toward an axis through the second toe; assist in flexion of the metatarsophalangeal joints of the third through fifth toes.	The entire foot
Interossei dorsales	These muscles abduct the second, third, and fourth toes from a longitudinal axis through the second toe; also assist in flexion of the metatarsophalangeal joints of the second through the fourth digits and extension of interphalangeal joints of the second through fourth digits.	The entire foot

* The most common location of trigger points is in the belly of the muscles or at the attachments.

Appendix C

Diseases and Indications/Contraindications to Massage Therapy

This appendix is arranged in alphabetical order

Disease	Indications/Contraindications of Massage Therapy	Chapter Reference
Alzheimer's disease	The degeneration of Alzheimer's disease may be slowed with therapeutic intervention and medication. Studies indicate that sensory stimulation modalities such as rhythmic massage and movement may provide calming and orienting influences.	4
Amyotrophic lateral sclerosis Also known as Lou Gehrig disease, ALS is a progressive disease beginning in the central nervous system that involves the degeneration of motor neurons and eventually results in the atrophy of voluntary muscle.	Massage is indicated for ALS, with caution and under a doctor's supervision. The degrees of pressure and intensity need to be adjusted as the disease progresses. General constitutional methods are indicated. The practitioner should avoid stressing the system and should work toward general restorative processes that reduce pain, support sleep, and create an overall sense of well-being.	4
Aneurysm An aneurysm is a weakening and bulging of any artery, including those in the brain.	Contraindicated. Refer client immediately to a physician.	4
Ankylosing spondylitis Also called rheumatoid inflammatory disorder, this disease destroys the articular hyaline cartilage, causing the bones to fuse and spinal ligaments to ossify, and tends to begin in the sacroiliac joints and progress up the spine.	Massage therapy modalities are effective in managing backache. The benefits derived are from reduction in protective muscle spasm compensation (guarding) and generalized pain-modulating effects. Be aware that protective spasm provides stabilization. The goal is not to eliminate protective spasm but to support the body in managing dysfunctional patterns. Complex backache involving the joint structures requires the practitioner to incorporate therapeutic massage into a total treatment program supervised by the appropriate health care professional.	8
Anterior compartment syndrome This syndrome covers any condition that increases pressure in the anterior compartment of the leg, interfering with blood flow and compressing the nerves.	Treatment is contraindicated regionally unless supervised by the diagnosing or treating health care provider. Massage methods may soften the connective tissue sheath, relieving some of the pressure, but could aggravate the flow to the area, thus increasing the pressure. Elevation and ice may help.	9
Anxiety Endogenous anxiety is a biochemical phenomenon usually unrelated to environmental stimuli. Reactive, or exogenous, anxiety is prompted by an anxiety-provoking stimulus such as specific events, situations, relationships, or conflicts.	Massage and exercise often are effective as part of a comprehensive management strategy dealing with anxiety symptoms.	5
Bartholin's cyst The cyst occurs in the Bartholin's glands located on each side of the vaginal opening.	Most reproductive system conditions present regional contraindications. As with most chronic illness and pain, therapeutic massage offers generalized support for homeostasis and can offer palliative or comfort care for the maintenance of these conditions.	12

Continued

Disease	Indications/Contraindications of Massage Therapy	Chapter Reference
Bell's palsy This palsy causes partial or total paralysis of the facial muscles on one side as the result of inflammation or injury to the seventh cranial nerve.	Massage approaches for infectious disease can be supportive and can reduce stress. The practitioner must gauge the intensity and duration of any therapeutic intervention so that the demand to adapt does not overtax an already stressed system, aggravating the condition. The less-is-more philosophy of intervention, which calls for shorter, more frequent interventions, often is indicated.	5
Bladder infection (cystitis) The bacteria in the bladder spread from the perineal region.	Therapeutic massage modalities may be useful for pain and stress management, but only with the careful supervision of the treating physician. Acute infectious processes contraindicate massage until the infection has run its course. Therapeutic massage may support chronic infection treatment as part of a supervised treatment plan. Stress is a contributing factor to incontinence. Any form of stress management helps somewhat with stress and urge incontinence. The practitioner needs to consider that incontinent clients require frequent and easy access to the restroom.	12
Breathing pattern disorder This is a complex, altered breathing function.	Therapeutic massage approaches and moderate application of movement therapies such as tai chi, yoga, or aerobic exercise assist with breathing. Almost every meditation or relaxation system uses breathing patterns because they are a direct link to altering autonomic nervous system patterns, which in turn alter mood, feelings, and behavior.	12
Bursitis The inflammation of the bursae, especially those located between the bony prominences and a muscle or tendon such as in the shoulder, elbow, hip, or knee, usually results from trauma and repetitive use.	Therapeutic massage can be a beneficial adjunct treatment, especially with the symptomatic management of pain in supporting increase in range of motion. Massage directly over the bursae is contraindicated.	8
Carpal tunnel syndrome This syndrome results from irritation of the meridian nerve as it passes under the transverse carpal ligament into the wrist.	Various forms of massage application reduce muscle spasm, lengthen shortened muscles, and soften and stretch connective tissue, restoring a more normal space around the nerve and alleviating impingement. When massage is combined with other appropriate methods, surgery is seldom necessary. If surgery is performed, the practitioner must manage adhesions appropriately to prevent reentrapment of the nerve by maintaining soft tissue suppleness around the healing surgical area and, as healing progresses, extending the soft tissue methods to deal with the forming scar more directly. Before doing any work near the site of a recent incision, one must obtain physician's approval. In general, work close to the surgical area can begin after the stitches have been removed and all inflammation is gone. Direct work on a new scar usually is safe 8 to 12 weeks into the healing period.	5
Cervical cancer Cervical dysplasia is a change in the cells of the cervix. Some of these abnormal cells can develop into cancerous cells.	Massage for clients with malignancies is contraindicated unless the appropriate health care professional gives approval and supervision. As with most chronic illness and pain, therapeutic massage offers generalized support for homeostasis and can offer palliative or comfort care for the maintenance of these conditions.	12
Cervicitis Cervicitis is inflammation of the cervix.	Most reproductive system conditions present regional contraindications. As with most chronic illness and pain, therapeutic massage offers generalized support for homeostasis and can offer palliative or comfort care for the maintenance of these conditions.	12

Disease	Indications/Contraindications of Massage Therapy	Chapter Reference
Chorea Chorea results from the degeneration of neurons in the basal ganglia.	Therapeutic massage is supportive in a multidisciplinary treatment. The practitioner can manage secondary muscle tension effectively with massage therapy and other forms of soft tissue manipulation.	4
Cirrhosis Cirrhosis is infiltration of connective tissue into the functioning cells of the liver, causing slow deterioration of the liver.	Caution is indicated depending on degree of liver function. Nonstressful general massage may be beneficial in stress management.	12
Club foot This deformity is evident in most cases when a child is born with one or both feet bent downward and adducted; in other cases the feet are pointed upward and abducted.	If skeletal problems create or are part of a permanent condition, supportive care is required. Massage methods are helpful in managing compensatory muscle spasms and connective tissue changes. Light, superficial methods, such as the gentle laying on of hands, are helpful.	8
Colon cancer This cancer usually affects the lowest part of the rectum.	Comprehensive stress management programs with medical supervision, including therapeutic massage methods, are often effective in managing these conditions.	12
Concussion A concussion is a brain trauma that may be mild, moderate, or severe.	Massage and bodywork is an effective part of a supervised comprehensive care program. Massage and other forms of bodywork can help manage secondary muscle tension.	4
Conn's syndrome If caused by an adrenal tumor, the disease is primary hyperaldosteronism. In rare cases, if caused by a nonspecific enlargement of the adrenal glands, the disease is called aldosteronism.	After these conditions are diagnosed, stress management can be an important part of ongoing therapeutic management.	6
Constipation Constipation is difficulty passing stools or an incomplete or infrequent passage of hard stools.	After these conditions are diagnosed, stress management can be an important part of ongoing therapeutic management. A specific type of massage to the large intestine can assist in managing constipation. The practitioner can teach this method to the client for self-care. The method is contraindicated in inflammatory bowel disease, and one should obtain permission from the physician for any other conditions.	12
Contracture Contracture is the chronic shortening of a muscle, especially the connective tissue component.	Gentle, slow intervention using connective tissue methods and stretching may improve contractures. Applying massage may prevent or slow the development of a contracture. The practitioner must consider the reason for the contracture when developing a treatment plan.	9
Contusion A muscle bruise results from trauma to the muscles and involves local internal bleeding and inflammation.	Direct work over the area of injury is contraindicated regionally until all signs of inflammation have dissipated.	9
Cramps Cramps are painful muscle contractions, may result from mild myositis or fibromyositis, and can be a symptom of any irritation or of an electrolyte imbalance.	The practitioner can manage simple cramps or spasms by firmly pushing the belly of the muscle together or by initiating reciprocal inhibition, which involves placing the attachment and insertion of the cramping muscle close together and then contracting the antagonist. The muscle lengthens gently after the cramp or spasm subsides.	9

Continued

Disease	Indications/Contraindications of Massage Therapy	Chapter Reference
Cushing's syndrome This syndrome is caused by excessive production of adrenocorticotropic hormone in the body.	After diagnosis of these conditions, stress management can be an important part of ongoing therapeutic management.	6
Cystic fibrosis This genetic disease involves exocrine gland dysfunction.	Percussion helps loosen the phlegm but should not be attempted without medical supervision and training.	12
Depression Depression is associated with a decrease in the neurotransmitters norepinephrine, serotonin, and dopamine.	Therapeutic massage is supportive in a multidisciplinary treatment of depression because such methods influence serotonin, among other neurotransmitters. In addition, the practitioner can manage secondary muscle tension effectively with massage therapy and other forms of soft tissue manipulation.	4
Diabetes mellitus This disease results from the pancreas not producing enough insulin or not producing any insulin.	A general stress management program is supportive in managing diabetes. Therapeutic massage can be an integral part of such a program. An important part of working with the diabetic client is that massage be a part of an overall treatment program with medical supervision. Careful observation of the feet during massage supports a hygiene program. The practitioner should refer the client for immediate medical care for any noted tissue changes. In pain management of diabetic neuropathy, massage approaches used as part of a supervised program can prove beneficial for short-term reduction of pain symptoms.	6
Disk degeneration Disk degeneration occurs when the fibrocartilage surrounding the intervertebral disk ruptures, releasing the nucleus pulposus, which cushions the vertebrae above and below.	Various forms of massage are important in managing the muscle spasm and pain. The muscle spasms serve a stabilizing and protective function called guarding. Without some protective spasm, the nerve could be damaged further, but too much muscle spasm increases the discomfort. Therapeutic intervention seeks to reduce pain and excessive tension and restore moderate mobility while allowing for the resourceful compensation produced by the muscle tension pattern.	5
Dislocation Dislocation is displacement of the bones of a joint; a subluxation is a partial dislocation.	Massage and bodywork are contraindicated locally over a trauma area until healing is complete. Light, subtle methods of touch therapies (e.g., a gentle laying on of hands) may be beneficial in diminishing pain. The process usually is calming and soothing, which encourages healing through stress management. Massage methods are beneficial in supporting the rest of the body during the healing process, especially in managing compensation patterns caused by immobilization of an area. Massage and other forms of bodywork can help manage secondary muscle tension.	8
Diverticula These small, saclike outpouchings of the intestinal wall occur in weak areas of the colon near where vessels are located.	Abdominal pain or referred back pain may indicate one of several gastrointestinal disorders. In such cases, referral is necessary for proper diagnosis.	12
Dupuytren's contracture This disorder is a thickened plaque overlying the tendon of the ring finger and occasionally the little finger at the level of the distal palmar crease.	Treatment is contraindicated regionally if methods increase symptoms.	9

Disease	Indications/Contraindications of Massage Therapy	Chapter Reference
Ectopic pregnancy Ectopic pregnancy occurs when the zygote fails to implant itself in the uterus and starts to develop in the fallopian tube.	Refer client immediately to a physician.	12
Edema Edema is a condition in which excess fluid accumulates within the interstitial spaces.	Therapeutic massage tends to increase blood volume through the kidneys via mechanical and reflexive processes. In the healthy individual, therapy supports the filtration process. For those with kidney disease the increased volume can strain the kidney function. General contraindications exist for anyone with kidney disease.	12
Emphysema This chronic pulmonary disease is marked by an abnormal increase in the size of air spaces distal to the terminal bronchiole, with destruction of the alveolar walls.	Simple palliative measures to provide comfort and encourage sleep are appropriate. In chronic conditions such as emphysema, general stress management and maintenance of normal function of the muscles of respiration are beneficial, again after one gauges the appropriate added stress levels caused by the massage stimulation.	12
Encephalitis Encephalitis is a bacterial or viral infection of the brain.	Infectious processes are contraindicated for massage intervention unless closely supervised by appropriate medical personnel. Refer a client with unusual or unexplained stiff neck immediately for diagnosis.	4
Endometriosis In this disease, endometrial tissue is present in nonuterine locations, such as on the intestines, ovaries, or even in the fallopian tubes.	Most reproductive system conditions present regional contraindications. As with most chronic illness and pain, therapeutic massage offers generalized support for homeostasis and can offer palliative or comfort care for the maintenance of these conditions.	12
Epicondylitis Epicondylitis is inflammation of the epicondyle of the humerus and surrounding tissues.	Therapeutic massage can be a beneficial adjunct treatment, especially with the symptomatic management of pain supporting increase in range of motion.	8
Fibromyalgia This syndrome has symptoms of widespread pain or aching, persistent fatigue, generalized morning stiffness, nonrestorative sleep, and multiple tender points.	General constitutional approaches seem to work best to aid in symptomatic pain reduction and restoration of the sleep pattern. The client should avoid any form of therapy that causes therapeutic inflammation, including intense exercise and stretching programs, until healing mechanisms in the body are functioning. If tender points have been injected with antiinflammatory medications, anesthetics, or other substances, the practitioner should not massage over these areas.	9
Flaccid muscles Muscles have decreased tone.	Flaccid or spastic muscles often are associated with motor neuron disorders. The reason for the change in tone determines the appropriateness of therapeutic massage. These conditions differ from general muscle tension or weakness in that the dysfunction has a physical cause rather than a functional one.	9
Fracture Fractures are breaks or ruptures in a bone.	Massage and bodywork is contraindicated locally over a trauma area until healing is complete. Light, subtle methods of touch therapies (e.g., a gentle laying on of hands) may be beneficial in diminishing pain. Stress fractures may not be readily detectable. Referral is indicated if the history points toward a mechanical stress condition such as participation in a recent athletic event.	8

Continued

Disease	Indications/Contraindications of Massage Therapy	Chapter Reference
Gallbladder disease (cholelithiasis) The disease almost always results from a gallstone composed of bile salts and/or cholesterol lodged in the cystic duct.	Abdominal pain or referred back pain may indicate one of several gastrointestinal disorders. In such cases, referral is necessary for proper diagnosis. Many gastrointestinal diseases are bacterial or viral and are contagious. The practitioner should take appropriate precautions to maintain sanitary practice. Most chronic gastrointestinal diseases have a strong correlation to stress. The intestinal tract is highly responsive to changes in autonomic function and endocrine patterns. Sympathetic arousal changes peristaltic action and can send the intestinal tract into all kinds of dysfunction. Comprehensive stress management programs, including therapeutic massage methods, are often effective in managing these conditions.	12
Gibbus Gibbus is an angular deformity of a collapsed vertebra.	Most backaches are preventable. Massage therapy modalities are effective in managing backache. The benefits derived are from reduced protective muscle spasm compensation (guarding) and the generalized pain modulating effects. Be aware that protective spasm provides stabilization. The goal is not to eliminate protective spasm but to support the body in managing dysfunctional patterns. The joint structures require that therapeutic massage be incorporated into a total treatment program with supervision by the appropriate health care professional.	8
Glomerulonephritis This group of diseases involves antigen-antibody reactions affecting the glomeruli.	Therapeutic massage tends to increase blood volume through the kidneys via mechanical and reflexive processes. In the healthy individual, therapy supports the filtration process. For those with kidney disease the increased volume can strain the kidney function. General contraindications exist for anyone with kidney disease. Therapeutic massage modalities may be useful for pain and stress management.	12
Gout Gout is a form of arthritis caused by a disturbance of metabolism.	Massage therapy is contraindicated regionally.	8
Growing pains These pains occur during growth spurts in children and adolescents when the bone grows faster than the attached muscles.	Treatment of local areas may be contraindicated if inflammation is present. Methods that do not introduce any sort of therapeutic inflammation often soothe general growing pains. The practitioner should avoid intense stretching and frictioning methods. Methods that relax and lengthen the muscle and soften the connective tissue are appropriate.	7
Headache Pain occurs in the forehead, eyes, jaw, temples, scalp, skull, occiput, or neck.	Massage therapy is effective in treating muscle tension headache but much less so with migraine or cluster headaches and can relieve secondary muscle tension headache caused by the pain of the primary headache. Headache is often stress induced. Stress management in all forms usually is indicated in chronic headache conditions.	4
Hepatitis Hepatitis is an infection of the liver.	Abdominal pain or referred back pain may indicate one of several gastrointestinal disorders. In such cases, referral is necessary for proper diagnosis. Many gastrointestinal diseases are bacterial or viral and are contagious. The practitioner should take appropriate precautions to maintain sanitary practice.	12
Hernia Hernia usually is caused by the weakness of abdominal muscles or protrusion of an abdominal organ (commonly the small intestine) through an opening in the abdominal wall.	Treatment of a client with a hernia is contraindicated regionally, and referral is indicated for initial diagnosis or for any change in a hernia.	9

Disease	Indications/Contraindications of Massage Therapy	Chapter Reference
Hyperparathyroidism Primary hyperparathyroidism usually results from a benign tumor, and secondary hyperparathyroidism results mostly from kidney disease.	The symptoms of hyperparathyroidism include mild to severe skeletal pain. Osteoporosis may result as well. The client may seek therapeutic massage for these conditions, and massage practitioners must take care to provide the appropriate referral to determine the underlying cause of the problem.	6
Hyperthyroidism or thyrotoxicosis These diseases result from overfunction of the thyroid.	Because thyroid conditions can go undiagnosed as a result of the symptoms being common to many stress-related conditions, referring clients for medical assessment to rule out thyroid dysfunction is important when they have any symptom of hyperthyroidism or hypothyroidism.	6
Hypothyroidism This condition results from underfunction of the thyroid.	Some studies suggest that mild cases of hypothyroidism respond to cold water therapy and moderate aerobic exercise. Exposure to cold triggers release of thyroid-stimulating hormone. Therapeutic massage may be beneficial in managing symptoms of hyperthyroidism and hypothyroidism. Because thyroid conditions can go undiagnosed as a result of the symptoms being common to many stress-related conditions, referring clients for medical assessment to rule out thyroid dysfunction is important when they have any symptom of hyperthyroidism or hypothyroidism.	6
Immobilization External restraint mechanisms such as casts may cause reactions such as pain and inflammation or paralysis.	Dynamic movable splinting devices such as air casts and continuous passive motion devices that are capable of moving joints passively and repeatedly through a specified position of the physiologic range of motion have been beneficial in reducing immobilization in joints. Therapeutic massage can maintain pliability in accessible connective tissue structures. Therapeutic massage methods and movement approaches are beneficial in assisting a return to normal function after removal of the splinting.	8
Immune system	Therapeutic massage approaches support immune function by supporting balanced homeostatic functions. No specific methods are used for the immune system, yet any behavior that supports wellness, including regular massage, supports immunity. Any modality that normalizes autonomic nervous system functions supports immunity.	11
Infectious arthritis Infections such as rheumatic fever, gonorrhea, and tuberculosis can cause infectious arthritis.	Infectious disease is a contraindication of massage unless the appropriate health care professionals directly supervise the massage therapy.	8
Infertility Infertility is a decrease in the ability to conceive.	Most reproductive system conditions present regional contraindications. Therapeutic massage offers generalized support for homeostasis.	12
Irritable bowel syndrome Also called spastic, or irritable, colon.	Referral is necessary for proper diagnosis. Most chronic gastrointestinal diseases have a strong correlation to stress. The intestinal tract is highly responsive to changes in autonomic function and endocrine patterns. Sympathetic arousal changes peristaltic action and can send the intestinal tract into all kinds of dysfunction. Comprehensive stress management programs, including therapeutic massage methods, are often effective in managing these conditions.	12

Continued

Disease	Indications/Contraindications of Massage Therapy	Chapter Reference
Joint injuries	Pain and swelling of joint injury can be overcome with the judicious and short-term use of pain medication, antiinflammatory medications, and appropriate rehabilitation exercise. Massage, myofascial release, and trigger point work are often effective after the acute phase (2-3 days). The application of ice along with rehabilitation exercise is beneficial. Management and rehabilitation of joint problems is a long-term process often requiring a multidisciplinary approach. Ice is contraindicated in some conditions and thus should be used with caution. Although direct work over an area that is actively healing is contraindicated, unless supervised, massage and other forms of soft tissue work, coupled with movement therapies, can manage compensatory patterns that develop because of casting and other forms of immobilization.	8
Kidney failure Also known as renal failure, the disease is the inability of the kidneys to excrete waste products and retain electrolytes.	Therapeutic massage tends to increase blood volume through the kidneys via mechanical and reflexive processes. In the healthy individual, therapy supports the filtration process. For those with kidney disease the increased volume can strain the kidney function. General contraindications exist for anyone with kidney disease.	12
Kidney stones These are small crystalline substances that develop in the kidney.	Therapeutic massage tends to increase blood volume through the kidneys via mechanical and reflexive processes. For those with kidney disease the increased volume can strain the kidney function. General contraindications exist for anyone with kidney disease. Therapeutic massage modalities may be useful for pain and stress management, but only with the careful supervision of the treating physician.	12
Kyphosis Kyphosis is a rounded thoracic convexity.	Massage therapy modalities are effective in managing backache. The benefits derived are from reduction in protective muscle spasm compensation (guarding) and generalized pain-modulating effects. Be aware that protective spasm provides stabilization. The goal is not to eliminate protective spasm but to support the body in managing dysfunctional patterns. Complex backache involving the joint structures requires the practitioner to incorporate therapeutic massage into a total treatment program supervised by the appropriate health care professional.	8
Legg-Calvé-Perthes disease This disease is the degeneration and necrosis of the head of the femur, followed by recalcification.	Necrosis usually is a localized condition that requires regional avoidance of the involved bone area. Because massage provides the generalized effect of enhanced circulation, indirect benefits might be realized with careful use of these methods. However, because these disorders are pathologic conditions, the primary health care provider must give permission for and supervise any massage.	7
List List is a lateral tilt of the spine.	Massage therapy modalities are effective in managing backache. The benefits derived are from reduction in protective muscle spasm compensation (guarding), and generalized pain-modulating effects. Be aware that protective spasm provides stabilization. The goal is not to eliminate protective spasm but to support the body in managing dysfunctional patterns. Complex backache involving the joint structures requires that therapeutic massage be incorporated into a total treatment program with supervision by the appropriate health care professional.	8

Disease	Indications/Contraindications of Massage Therapy	Chapter Reference
Lordosis Lordosis is an accentuation of the normal lumbar curve that develops to compensate for the protuberant abdomen of pregnancy or great obesity.	Massage therapy modalities are effective in managing backache. The benefits derived are from reduction in protective muscle spasm compensation (guarding) and generalized pain-modulating effects. Be aware that protective spasm provides stabilization. The goal is not to eliminate protective spasm but to support the body in managing dysfunctional patterns. Complex backache involving the joint structures requires that therapeutic massage be incorporated into a total treatment program with supervision by the appropriate health care professional.	8
Lymphatic system disorders	Massage is contraindicated for malignant and infectious conditions until the client's health care professional gives approval. Modification of massage application is necessary depending on the type of treatment the client is receiving and the stress and fatigue levels. Massage that relaxes the client supports well-being and is helpful. The practitioner can manage simple edema with massage application focused to support the lymphatic system. More complicated lymphedema requires support of the appropriate health professional concerning massage application.	11
Malabsorption syndromes These diseases involve poor absorption of nutrients.	The intestinal tract is highly responsive to changes in autonomic function and endocrine patterns. Sympathetic arousal changes peristaltic action and can send the intestinal tract into all kinds of dysfunction. Comprehensive stress management programs, including therapeutic massage methods, are often effective in managing these conditions.	12
Meningitis Meningitis is a bacterial or viral infection in the meninges, mainly in the subarachnoid fluid.	Infectious processes contraindicate massage intervention unless closely supervised by appropriate medical personnel. Immediately refer the client with unusual or unexplained stiff neck for diagnosis.	4
Miscarriage Miscarriage is termination of pregnancy.	Refer the client immediately to the appropriate physician or emergency room.	12
Multiple sclerosis MS is a disease of autoimmune or viral cause (or both) in which myelin degenerates in random areas of the central nervous system.	Massage can be an effective part of a comprehensive, long-term care program. Stress management also is an important component of an overall care program for any chronic disease. Massage and other forms of bodywork can help manage secondary muscle tension caused by the alteration of posture and the use of equipment such as wheelchairs, braces, and crutches. Because therapeutic massage produces some stress, the practitioner must gauge the intensity and duration of any therapeutic intervention so as not to aggravate the condition.	5
Muscle infection Infection of muscle is caused by several bacteria, viruses, and parasites, often producing local or widespread myositis (muscle inflammation).	Massage therapy is contraindicated until infection is no longer present.	9
Muscle strain Strain is an injury to skeletal muscles from overexertion or trauma and can range from mild to moderate to severe.	Direct work over the area of injury is contraindicated regionally until all signs of inflammation have dissipated. The use of ice and gentle range of motion can support healing. Methods to manage distortion in posture resulting from compensation in the rest of the body are helpful.	9

Continued

Disease	Indications/Contraindications of Massage Therapy	Chapter Reference
Muscle tension headache The contracted muscles exert pressure on the nerves and blood vessels in the area, causing the pain, which is a dull, persistent ache with feelings of tightness around the head, temples, forehead, and occipital areas.	Various strategies are available to treat stress-induced muscle tension headaches, including massage. Chronic patterns often indicate connective tissue shortening. Headaches respond best to whole-body therapy, which not only addresses the immediate areas but also relaxes the entire body.	9
Muscular dystrophy This group of disorders is characterized by atrophy of skeletal muscles with no malfunction of the nervous system.	Careful intervention may slow the atrophy process. Passive and active range of motion methods not only directly affect the muscles and joints but also aid in the circulation and elimination processes. Abdominal massage may help with constipation. The practitioner should avoid methods that cause any inflammation.	9
Myasthenia gravis In this autoimmune disease the immune system attacks muscle cells at the neuromuscular junction and interferes with the action of acetylcholine.	General constitutional massage methods are indicated. The practitioner should avoid stressing the system and should work toward general restorative processes that reduce pain, support sleep, and create an overall sense of well-being.	5
Myelitis Myelitis is an infection of the spinal cord and/or brainstem.	Infectious processes are contraindicated for massage intervention unless closely supervised by the appropriate medical personnel. Immediately refer clients with unusual or unexplained stiff neck for diagnosis.	4
Myofascial system disorders	Intervention focuses on reversing nonproductive processes and supporting resourceful compensation patterns that develop in response to chronic problems. The goal is to support circulation, connective tissue strength and pliability, and nervous system interaction. The compression and stroking of massage support circulation. Connective tissue responds to methods that affect the viscoelastic, plastic, and colloid properties. Muscle tension patterns respond to compression and drag that stimulate proprioceptors. Muscle energy methods systematically use contraction and relaxing of muscles combined with lengthening to restore normal length of the muscles. Trigger points respond to methods that reduce hyperactivity, such as muscle energy methods and compression. Calming the sympathetic arousal is also necessary.	9
Myoma Also called a fibroid, myoma is a benign tumor in the uterus that grows inside the uterine muscle wall or attaches to the wall.	Massage is contraindicated. Most reproductive system conditions present regional contraindications. As with most chronic illness and pain, therapeutic massage offers generalized support for homeostasis and can offer palliative or comfort care for the maintenance of these conditions.	12
Myopathies: metabolic and toxic	Treatment for these types of myopathy usually is not contraindicated, as long as the therapeutic approaches are general and focus on supporting body restoration and the healing processes. Massage can support detoxification efforts, because these methods enhance circulation. The practitioner must take care in toxic conditions not to tax an already overloaded system.	9
Myositis ossificans This disease involves an inflammatory process that stimulates the formation of osseous tissue in the fascial components of muscles.	Treatment is contraindicated regionally.	9

Disease	Indications/Contraindications of Massage Therapy	Chapter Reference
Neuropathy Neuropathy is the inflammation or degeneration of the peripheral nerves.	Nerve pain is difficult to manage, does not respond well to analgesics, and often is intractable. Massage, because of the interface with the nervous system, may provide short-term, symptomatic pain relief through shifts in neurotransmitters and stimulation of alternate nerve pathways, resulting in hyperstimulation analgesia and counterirritation. Any therapy that increases mood-elevating and pain-modulating mechanisms makes coping with nerve pain somewhat easier for short periods.	5
Obstruction of the urethra causing retention of urine	Refer the client to a physician for diagnosis.	12
Osgood-Schlatter disease This disease occurs when the tubercle becomes inflamed or separates from the tibia because of irritation caused by the patellar tendon pulling on the tubercle during periods of rapid growth or overuse of the quadriceps.	Treatment of local areas may be contraindicated if inflammation or necrosis is present. Methods that relax and lengthen the muscle and soften the connective tissue are appropriate.	7
Osteitis fibrosa cystica In this disease, fibrous tissue and cysts replace bone tissue, making the bones weak and prone to fracture.	The practitioner must exercise caution before using any massage and bodywork requiring any amount of compressive force on a client with a condition that causes demineralization of bone or that results in brittle, fragile bones. A fragile skeletal structure, regardless of the cause, is a contraindication for any type of compressive force or joint movement methods unless the appropriate medical professionals carefully supervise these methods. Light, superficial methods, such as the gentle laying on of hands used in some forms of touch systems, might be indicated with supervision. One may use massage methods on the unaffected areas and avoid the involved area.	7
Osteoarthritis A degenerative joint disease, osteoarthritis is the breakdown of joints caused by normal wear and tear.	Because the progression and flare-ups of the disease are often stress related, the generalized gentle stress reduction methods provided by massage therapy may be beneficial in long-term management of the condition, if supervised as part of a total care program. The practitioner should avoid frictioning techniques or any other forms of bodywork that cause inflammation. General systemic changes in the neurotransmitters and hormones that accompany exercise and many forms of bodywork can elevate mood and thus reduce pain perception.	8
Osteochondritis dissecans This condition affects a joint in which a fragment of cartilage and its underlying bone become detached from the articular surface.	Massage therapy is contraindicated regionally.	7
Osteogenesis imperfecta This group of hereditary disorders appears in newborns or young children. The bones are deformed and fragile as a result of demineralization and defective formation of connective tissue.	If skeletal problems create or are part of a permanent condition, supportive care is required. Massage methods are helpful in managing compensatory muscle spasms and connective tissue changes. Any type of compressive force or joint movement methods are contraindicated for a fragile skeletal structure, regardless of the cause, unless carefully supervised by the appropriate medical professionals. Light, superficial methods, such as the gentle laying on of hands used in some forms of touch systems, might be indicated, again with supervision.	7

Continued

Disease	Indications/Contraindications of Massage Therapy	Chapter Reference
Osteomyelitis Osteomyelitis is an inflammation in the bone, bone marrow, or periosteum, usually caused by pyogenic (pus-producing) bacteria.	Massage is contraindicated in infectious disease unless carefully supervised by medical personnel. The therapist always must refer clients with vague pain symptoms for proper diagnosis.	7
Osteonecrosis (ischemic necrosis) Osteonecrosis is the death of a segment of bone, usually caused by insufficient blood flow to a region of the skeleton.	Necrosis usually is a localized condition that requires regional avoidance of the involved bone area. Because massage provides the generalized effect of enhanced circulation, the practitioner might realize indirect benefits with careful use of these methods. However, because these disorders are pathologic conditions, one must give massage with the permission and supervision of the primary health care provider.	7
Osteoporosis In this disorder the bone lacks calcium and other minerals and bone protein.	The practitioner must exercise caution before using any massage and bodywork requiring any amount of compressive force on a client with a condition that causes demineralization of bone or that results in brittle, fragile bones. A fragile skeletal structure, regardless of the cause, is a contraindication for any type of compressive force or joint movement methods unless the appropriate medical professionals carefully supervise these methods. Light, superficial methods, such as the gentle laying on of hands used in some forms of touch systems, might be indicated with supervision. Bone involvement may be localized, such as with radiation treatment. In these cases, one can use bodywork methods on the unaffected areas and avoid the involved area.	7
Paget's disease (osteitis deformans) This disease occurs when the bones undergo normal periods of calcium loss followed by periods of excessive new cell growth.	The practitioner must exercise caution before using any massage and bodywork requiring any amount of compressive force on a client with a condition that causes demineralization of bone or that results in brittle, fragile bones. A fragile skeletal structure, regardless of the cause, is a contraindication for any type of compressive force or joint movement methods unless the appropriate medical professionals carefully supervise these methods. Light, superficial methods, such as the gentle laying on of hands used in some forms of touch systems, might be indicated with supervision.	7
Pancreatitis Pancreatitis is the inflammation of the pancreas.	Abdominal pain or referred back pain may indicate one of several gastrointestinal disorders. In such cases, referral is necessary for proper diagnosis.	12
Parkinson's disease In this disease, neurons that release the neurotransmitter dopamine in the brain degenerate, thus slowing or stopping its release.	Because massage has been shown to increase dopamine activity, its use is indicated for managing Parkinson's disease and tremor. In addition, the practitioner can manage secondary muscle tension effectively with massage therapy and other forms of soft tissue manipulation.	4
Peptic ulcer A gastric or duodenal ulcer affects the lining of the esophagus, stomach, or duodenum.	Abdominal pain or referred back pain may indicate one of several gastrointestinal disorders. In such cases, referral is necessary for proper diagnosis. Most chronic gastrointestinal diseases have a strong correlation to stress. The intestinal tract is highly responsive to changes in autonomic function and endocrine patterns. Sympathetic arousal changes peristaltic action and can send the intestinal tract into all kinds of dysfunction. Comprehensive stress management programs, including therapeutic massage methods, are often effective in managing these conditions.	12
Plantar fasciitis The condition is an inflammation of the plantar fascia and surrounding myofascial structures.	Acute-phase plantar fasciitis responds to rest and ice. After the inflammation has diminished, soft tissue methods that address the connective tissue and judicial use of stretching are beneficial.	9

Disease	Indications/Contraindications of Massage Therapy	Chapter Reference
Poliomyelitis—postpolio syndrome Poliomyelitis is a viral infection of the nerves that control skeletal muscle movement. Years later, postpolio syndrome can cause fatigue and muscle aching and weakness.	For postpolio syndrome, general constitutional approaches seem to work best to aid in overall pain reduction and restoration of the sleep pattern. The practitioner should avoid any form of therapy that causes therapeutic inflammation, including intense exercise and stretching programs.	9
Preeclampsia Also termed pregnancy-induced hypertension or toxemia, the condition is a complication of pregnancy characterized by increasing hypertension, proteinuria, and edema.	Refer the client immediately for medical treatment.	12
Pregnancy abnormality and bleeding during pregnancy	Refer the client immediately to the appropriate physician or emergency room.	12
Prostatitis Infection of the prostate usually results from a urinary tract infection.	Massage therapy is contraindicated until infection is no longer present.	12
Pyelonephritis Infection of the kidney affects the nephrons, or filtering units.	Therapeutic massage tends to increase blood volume through the kidneys via mechanical and reflexive processes. Acute infectious processes contraindicate massage until the infection has run its course. The appropriate health care professional may support chronic infection treatment as part of a supervised treatment plan.	12
Radiation therapy disorders	The practitioner must exercise caution before using any massage and bodywork requiring any amount of compressive force on a client with a condition that causes demineralization of bone or that results in brittle, fragile bones. A fragile skeletal structure, regardless of the cause, is a contraindication for any type of compressive force or joint movement methods unless the appropriate medical professionals carefully supervise these methods. Light, superficial methods, such as the gentle laying on of hands used in some forms of touch systems, might be indicated with supervision. One can use massage methods on the unaffected areas and avoid the involved area.	7
Reflux esophagitis Regurgitation of gastric acid up through an open esophageal sphincter causes heartburn.	Abdominal pain or referred back pain may indicate one of several gastrointestinal disorders. In such cases, referral is necessary for proper diagnosis. Most chronic gastrointestinal diseases have a strong correlation to stress. The intestinal tract is highly responsive to changes in autonomic function and endocrine patterns. Sympathetic arousal changes peristaltic action and can send the intestinal tract into all kinds of dysfunction. Comprehensive stress management programs, including therapeutic massage methods, are often effective in managing these conditions.	12
Regional enteritis Also called Crohn's disease, enteritis is a chronic inflammation of the intestine, most commonly the ileum.	Abdominal pain or referred back pain may indicate one of several gastrointestinal disorders. In such cases, referral is necessary for proper diagnosis. Many gastrointestinal diseases are bacterial or viral and are contagious. The intestinal tract is highly responsive to changes in autonomic function and endocrine patterns. Sympathetic arousal changes peristaltic action and can send the intestinal tract into all kinds of dysfunction. Comprehensive stress management programs, including therapeutic massage methods, are often effective in managing these conditions.	12

Continued

Disease	Indications/Contraindications of Massage Therapy	Chapter Reference
Rheumatoid arthritis This crippling condition is characterized by swelling of the joints in the hands, feet, and other parts of the body as a result of inflammation and overgrowth of the synovial membranes and other joint tissues.	Because the progression and flare-ups of the disease are often stress related, the generalized gentle stress reduction methods provided by massage therapy may be beneficial in long-term management of the condition, if supervised as part of a total care program. The practitioner should avoid frictioning techniques or any other forms of bodywork that cause inflammation.	8
Rickets This disease of bone formation in children most commonly results from vitamin D deficiency and is marked by inadequate mineralization of developing cartilage and newly formed bone, causing abnormalities in the shape, structure, and strength of the skeleton.	Regardless of the cause, a fragile skeletal structure is a contraindication for any type of compressive force or joint movement methods unless the appropriate medical professionals carefully supervise these methods. Light, superficial methods, such as the gentle laying on of hands used in some forms of touch systems, might be indicated with supervision.	7
Rotator cuff tear Tears often are caused by repeated impingement, overuse, or other conditions that weaken the rotator cuff and eventually cause partial or complete tears.	Work on acute myofascial tears is contraindicated. However, massage therapy may be indicated in the rehabilitative process and as part of a supervised treatment protocol. The practitioner can manage and improve compensatory patterns with massage.	9
Scheuermann's disease This disease most commonly is caused by necrosis or inflammation in bone or in a disk of the thoracic vertebrae.	Necrosis usually is a localized condition that requires regional avoidance of the involved bone area. Because massage provides the generalized effect of enhanced circulation, the practitioner might realize indirect benefits with careful use of these methods. However, because these disorders are pathologic conditions, one must give massage with the permission and supervision of the primary health care provider.	7
Schizophrenia Schizophrenia is the most common mental disorder and includes a large group of psychotic disorders characterized by gross distortion of reality; disturbances of language and communication; withdrawal from social interaction; and disorganization and fragmentation of thought, perception, and emotional reaction.	Therapeutic massage is supportive in a multidisciplinary treatment, approach for such methods influence neurotransmitters. Supervision is necessary.	4
Sciatica	Various forms of massage application reduce muscle spasm, lengthen shortened muscles, and soften and stretch connective tissue, restoring a more normal space around the nerve and alleviating impingement. When massage is combined with other appropriate methods, surgery is seldom necessary. If surgery is performed, the practitioner must manage adhesions appropriately to prevent reentrapment of the nerve by maintaining soft tissue suppleness around the healing surgical area and, as healing progresses, extending the soft tissue methods to deal with the forming scar more directly. Before doing any work near the site of a recent incision, one must obtain the physician's approval. In general, work close to the surgical area can begin after the stitches have been removed and all inflammation is gone. Direct work on a new scar usually is safe 8 to 12 weeks into the healing period.	5

Disease	Indications/Contraindications of Massage Therapy	Chapter Reference
Scoliosis Scoliosis is a lateral S-type curvature of the spine	Most backaches are preventable. One should not use the back muscles for lifting but should bring the weight close to the body, above the hips if possible, and allow the legs to do the actual lifting. An adequate exercise program is also important.	8
Scurvy Scurvy is the reduction of bone density caused by a vitamin C deficiency.	Regardless of the cause, a fragile skeletal structure is a contraindication for any type of compressive force or joint movement methods unless the appropriate medical professionals carefully supervise these methods. Light, superficial methods, such as the gentle laying on of hands used in some forms of touch systems, might be indicated with supervision.	7
Seizures	The application of massage techniques may decrease the side effects of medications. Massage therapists must remember to refer any clients with any exaggerated or increased symptoms to the prescribing physician.	4
Sexually transmitted diseases	As with all acute infections, massage is contraindicated until any disease of the reproductive system runs its course. Most reproductive system conditions present regional contraindications. As with most chronic illness and pain, therapeutic massage offers generalized support for homeostasis and can offer palliative or comfort care for the maintenance of these conditions	12
Shin splints Shin splints are an inflammation of the proximal portion of any of the musculotendinous structures originating from the lower part of the tibia.	Massage approaches may be beneficial as long as they do not increase inflammation and a stress fracture has been ruled out.	9
Skin conditions	Therapeutic massage usually is not contraindicated in localized skin conditions, but local (regional) avoidance of the affected area is necessary. Localized touch can irritate most skin disorders. Massage is contraindicated if the skin is inflamed or if the condition is contagious or transmissible through touch. Malignancy is a contraindication unless the appropriate medical personnel supervise the therapy.	11
Spinal abnormalities: scoliosis, kyphosis, and lordosis Abnormal curvatures of the spine may be congenital, may result from paralysis or weakness or tension in spinal muscles, or may result from rapid growth of the body, especially after puberty.	If skeletal problems create or are part of a permanent condition, supportive care is required. Massage methods are helpful in managing compensatory muscle spasms and connective tissue changes. Any type of compressive force or joint movement methods are contraindicated for fragile skeletal structure, regardless of the causes, unless carefully supervised by the appropriate medical professionals. Light, superficial methods, such as the gentle laying on of hands used in some forms of touch systems, might be indicated, again with supervision.	7
Spinal cord injury	Massage is an effective part of a comprehensive, supervised rehabilitation and long-term care program. Massage and other forms of bodywork can help manage secondary muscle tension resulting from the alteration of posture and the use of equipment such as wheelchairs, braces, and crutches. Specifically focused massage can help manage difficulties with bowel paralysis. The circulation enhancement of massage can assist in managing a decubitus ulcer.	4

Continued

Disease	Indications/Contraindications of Massage Therapy	Chapter Reference
Spondylitis Spondylitis is inflammation of more than one vertebra.	Massage therapy modalities are effective in managing backache. The benefits derived are from reduction in protective muscle spasm compensation (guarding) and generalized pain-modulating effects. Be aware that protective spasm provides stabilization. The goal is not to eliminate protective spasm but to support the body in managing dysfunctional patterns. Complex backache involving the joint structures requires the practitioner to incorporate therapeutic massage into a total treatment program supervised by the appropriate health care professional.	8
Spondylolisthesis In this condition a part of one vertebra moves forward on another.	Massage therapy modalities are effective in managing backache. The benefits derived are from reduction in protective muscle spasm compensation (guarding) and generalized pain-modulating effects. Be aware that protective spasm provides stabilization. The goal is not to eliminate protective spasm but to support the body in managing dysfunctional patterns. Complex backache involving the joint structures requires the practitioner to incorporate therapeutic massage into a total treatment program supervised by the appropriate health care professional.	8
Spondylosis Spondylosis is the formation of bony spurs at the disk margin of the vertebral bodies and causes degenerative changes in the intervertebral disks.	Massage therapy modalities are effective in managing backache. The benefits derived are from reduction in protective muscle spasm compensation (guarding) and generalized pain-modulating effects. Be aware that protective spasm provides stabilization. The goal is not to eliminate protective spasm but to support the body in managing dysfunctional patterns. Complex backache involving the joint structures requires the practitioner to incorporate therapeutic massage into a total treatment program supervised by the appropriate health care professional.	8
Stomach cancer	Abdominal pain or referred back pain may indicate one of several gastrointestinal disorders. In such cases, referral is necessary for proper diagnosis.	12
Stroke Stroke is sudden loss of neurologic function caused by a vascular injury to the brain.	Stroke is a medical emergency requiring immediate referral. Massage and bodywork is an effective part of a supervised comprehensive care program. Massage and other forms of bodywork can help manage secondary muscle tension resulting from the alteration of posture and the use of equipment such as wheelchairs, braces, and crutches.	4
Tendonitis/tenosynovitis Tendonitis is inflammation of a tendon; tenosynovitis is inflammation of a tendon sheath.	Any methods that could increase the inflammatory response are contraindicated for areas of inflammation. In the acute phase the use of ice and gentle movement are indicated. Chronic conditions may benefit from methods that elongate the connective tissue structures, relieving friction in the area.	9
Thoracic outlet syndrome This syndrome occurs because the brachial plexus and blood supply of the arm become impinged, resulting in shooting pains, weakness, and numbness.	Massage methods help relieve muscle impingement of nerves by relaxing and lengthening the muscles.	9

Disease	Indications/Contraindications of Massage Therapy	Chapter Reference
Thrombosis A thrombus (blood clot) forms within the lumen (open cavity) of the blood vessels or heart.	Thrombosis contraindicates massage. Because obstruction could be a medical emergency, immediate referral is indicated.	11
Thrombus A thrombus is a clot that forms inside a blood vessel. A clot is the conversion of blood from a liquid to a solid through the process of coagulation. A clot that moves inside the vessel is referred to as an embolus (embolism). The presence of atherosclerotic plaque lining blood vessel walls is a significant stimulus for clot formation. Blood clots form from platelets and other elements and may obstruct a blood vessel at its point of formation or travel to other areas of the body. A thrombus that forms in the more surface vessels may create the signs and symptoms of pain, heat, redness and swelling.	Massage therapy is contraindicated regionally and generally because of the potential to move the clot or increased bruising from the medication. Thrombosis can be a medical emergency, and immediate referral is indicated. Treatment may include elevation, the application of heat packs to the affected area and blood thinning medications (such as heparin or warfarin).	11
Torticollis Also called wry neck, the condition involves a spasm or shortening of one of the sternocleidomastoid muscles.	Management of torticollis with massage therapy involves relaxing the neck, releasing trigger points, stretching the contracted muscles, and improving range of motion. Avoiding pressure on the vessels under the sternocleidomastoid muscle is important.	9
Tremors Tremors are involuntary muscle twitches.	Because massage has been shown to increase dopamine activity, it is indicated in managing tremor. In addition, the practitioner can manage secondary muscle tension effectively with massage therapy and other forms of soft tissue manipulation.	4
Tuberculosis This systemic disease is caused by the tubercular bacillus.	Massage is contraindicated in infectious disease unless carefully supervised by medical personnel. The therapist always must refer clients with vague pain symptoms for proper diagnosis.	7
Ulcerative colitis This disease primarily affects the sigmoid colon, with symptoms of lower abdominal pain and bloody diarrhea.	Abdominal pain or referred back pain may indicate one of several gastrointestinal disorders. In such cases, referral is necessary for proper diagnosis. The intestinal tract is highly responsive to changes in autonomic function and endocrine patterns. Sympathetic arousal changes peristaltic action and can send the intestinal tract into all kinds of dysfunction. Comprehensive stress management programs, including therapeutic massage methods, are often effective in managing these conditions.	12
Urinary incontinence The inability to control urination most often is caused by weak pelvic floor muscles or nerve damage.	Stress is a contributing factor to incontinence. Any form of stress management helps somewhat with stress and urge incontinence. The practitioner needs to consider that incontinent clients require frequent and easy access to the restroom.	12

Continued

Disease	Indications/Contraindications of Massage Therapy	Chapter Reference
Vaginitis Vaginitis is inflammation of the vagina. Signs and symptoms are vaginal discharge, itching (pruritus), and irritation.	Most reproductive system conditions present regional contraindications. As with most chronic illness and pain, therapeutic massage offers generalized support for homeostasis and can offer palliative or comfort care for the maintenance of these conditions.	12
Vertebral subluxation; muscle spasms (entrapment) and shortening; disk degeneration; disk herniation	Various forms of massage are important in managing muscle spasm and pain associated with the aforementioned conditions. The student must remember that the muscle spasms serve a stabilizing and protective function called guarding. Without some protective spasm, the nerve could be damaged further, but too much muscle spasm increases the discomfort. Therapeutic intervention seeks to reduce pain and excessive tension and restore moderate mobility while allowing for the resourceful compensation produced by the muscle tension pattern. Because low back pain is a common disorder, the massage practitioner must be familiar with its causes and treatment protocols.	5
Vertigo Vertigo is the sensation that the body or environment is spinning or swaying.	Movement therapies can help or aggravate vertigo; therefore the practitioner must take care to design an individual therapeutic program based on the client's history. Massage methods can deal effectively with muscle tension and diminish anxiety and nausea, but the benefit is temporary because the symptoms return with a recurrence of vertigo.	5
Whiplash Whiplash is an injury to the soft tissues of the neck caused by sudden hyperextension or flexion (or both) of the neck.	Direct intervention during the acute phase is contraindicated unless closely supervised by a physician or other qualified health care professional. Massage methods are valuable as part of rehabilitation in the subacute phase and can help restore function if the condition is chronic. Extension injury is the more severe and requires careful intervention.	9

GLOSSARY

Abduction Lateral movement away from the midline of the trunk.

Absorption The movement of food molecules from the digestive tract to the circulatory or lymphatic systems.

Acetylcholine A neurotransmitter that stimulates the parasympathetic nervous system and the skeletal muscles and is involved in memory.

Acne A chronic inflammation of the sebaceous glands and hair follicles caused by interactions between bacteria, sebum, and sex hormones.

Active transport The transport of substances into or out of a cell using energy.

Acupuncture The practice of inserting needles at specific points on meridians, or channels, to stimulate or sedate energy flow to regulate or alter body function. A branch of Chinese medicine, acupuncture is the art and science of manipulating the flow of Qi, the basic life force, and xue, the blood, body fluids, and nourishing essences. Western medicine uses acupuncture primarily to reduce pain. Acupressure, which uses digital pressure, follows the same Asian principles.

Acute disease Disease that has a specific beginning, signs, and symptoms that develop quickly, last a short time, and then disappear.

Acute pain Pain that is usually temporary, of sudden onset, and easily localized. Acute pain can be a symptom of a disease process or a temporary aspect of medical treatment. Acting as a warning signal, acute pain activates the sympathetic nervous system.

Adduction A medial movement toward the midline of the body.

Adenosine triphosphate (ATP) A compound that stores energy in the muscles. When ATP is broken down during catabolic reactions, it releases energy.

Adrenergic Stimulation of the sympathetic nervous system causing a release of epinephrine and similar neurotransmitters and hormones.

Afferent Toward a center or point of reference.

Afferent nerves Sensory nerves that link sensory receptors with the central nervous system and transmit sensory information.

Agonist A muscle that causes or controls joint motion through a specified plane of motion; also known as the primary or prime mover.

Alimentary canal The tube-shaped portion of the digestive system known as the gastrointestinal tract; the alimentary canal is about 30 feet long and contains several special structures throughout its length.

All-or-none response The property of a muscle fiber (cell) contraction by which, when contraction is initiated, the fiber contracts to its full ability or does not contract at all.

Alopecia Hair loss or baldness on parts or all of the body

Amphiarthrosis A slightly movable joint that connects bone to bone with fibrocartilage or hyaline growth cartilage. The two types in the human body are symphyses and synchondroses.

Amyotrophic lateral sclerosis (ALS) A progressive disease that begins in the central nervous system and involves the degeneration of motor neurons and the subsequent atrophy of voluntary muscle. Also called Lou Gehrig's disease.

Anabolism Chemical processes in the body that join simple compounds to form more complex compounds of carbohydrates, lipids, proteins, and nucleic acids. The processes require energy supplied from adenosine triphosphate.

Anaplasia Meaning without shape, the term describes abnormal or undifferentiated cells that fail to mature into specialized cell types. Anaplasia is a characteristic of malignant cells.

Anatomic position A standard position in which the person stands upright with the feet slightly apart, arms hanging at the sides, and palms facing forward with thumbs outward.

Anatomic range of motion (ROM) The amount of motion available to a joint based on the structure of the joint and determined by the shape of the joint surfaces, joint capsule, ligaments, muscle bulk, and surrounding musculotendinous and bony structures.

Anatomy The study of the structures of the body and the relationship of its parts.

Androgens Male sex hormones.

Anemia A decrease in the normal number of red blood cells or in the amount of hemoglobin or iron in the blood.

Aneurysm A permanent dilation of part of a blood vessel caused by weakness or damage to its structure. The most common sites of aneurysms are the aorta and the arteries of the brain.

Antagonist A muscle usually located on the opposite side of a joint from the agonist and having the opposite action.

Anterior pelvic rotation Anterior movement of the upper pelvis; the iliac crest tilts forward in a sagittal plane.

Antibody A specific protein produced to destroy or suppress antigens.

Antigen Any substance that causes the body to produce antibodies.

Aorta The large artery that carries oxygen and nutrients out of the heart.

Apical surface The surface of epithelial cells that is exposed to the external surface such as the atmostphere or a passage in the body.

Apocrine A type of sweat gland that discharges a thicker and more odoriferous form of sweat.

Aponeurosis A broad, flat sheet of fibrous connective tissue.

Appendicular skeleton The part of the skeleton composed of the limbs and their attachments.

Arterioles The smallest arteries.

Arteriosclerosis A term meaning hardening of the arteries and referring to arteries that have become brittle and have lost their elasticity.

Artery A blood vessel that transports oxygenated blood from the heart to the body or deoxygenated blood from the heart to the lungs.

Arthritis The most common type of joint disorder, *arthritis* literally means inflammation of the joint.

Arthrokinematics Movement of bone surface in the joint capsule including roll, spin, and slide.

Articulation Another word for a joint, the structure created when bones connect to each other.

Ascending tracts Tracts that carry sensory information to the brain.

Atherosclerosis A condition in which fatty plaque is deposited in medium and large arteries.

Atom The smallest particle of an element that retains and exhibits the properties of that element. Atoms are made up of protons, neutrons, and electrons.

Atrium One of the two small, thin-walled, upper chambers of the heart; the right and left atria are separated by a thin interatrial septum.

Atrophy A decrease in the size of a body part or organ caused by a decrease in the size of the cells.

Attachments Connections of skeletal muscles to bones; often referred to as the origin and insertion.

Autonomic nervous system A division of the peripheral nervous system composed of nerves that connect the central nervous system to the glands, heart, and smooth muscles to maintain the internal body environment.

Avulsion Injury to a ligament or tendon involving tearing off of its attachment.

Axial skeleton The axis of the body; the axial skeleton consists of the head, vertebral column (the spine), and the ribs and sternum and provides the body with form and protection.

Axon A single elongated projection from the nerve cell body that transmits impulses away from the cell body.

Balance The ability to control equilibrium. Two types of balance are static or still balance and dynamic or moving balance.

Ball-and-socket joint Joint that allows movement in many directions around a central point. Ball-and-socket joints are ball-shaped convex surfaces fitted into concave sockets. This type of joint gives the greatest freedom of movement but also is the most easily dislocated.

Basal metabolic rate (BMR) The rate of energy expenditure of the body under normal, relaxed activities.

Basal surface The tissue surface that faces the inside of the body.

Basement membrane A permeable membrane that attaches epithelial tissues to the underlying connective tissues.

Benign A term usually describing a noncancerous tumor that is contained and does not spread.

Biologic rhythms The internal, periodic timing component of an organism, also known as a biorhythm. Circadian rhythms work on a 24-hour period to coordinate internal functions such as sleep. Ultradian rhythms repeat themselves from every 90 minutes to every few hours, whereas seasonal rhythms are annual functions.

Biomechanics The study of mechanical principles, movements, and actions applied to living bodies.

Blood A thick, red fluid that provides oxygen, nourishment, and protection to the cells and carries away waste products. Whole blood consists of two components: the formed cellular elements and the liquid plasma. Blood is a form of connective tissue.

Blood pressure The measurement of pressure exerted by the heart on the walls of the blood vessels. The highest pressure exerted is called systolic pressure, which results when the ventricles are contracted. Diastolic pressure, the lowest pressure, results when the ventricles are at rest. Blood forced into the aorta during systole sets up a pressure wave that travels down the arteries. The wave expands the arterial wall, and the expansion can be palpated by pressing the artery against tissue; the waves constitute the pulse rate.

Brain The largest and most complex unit of the nervous system, the brain is responsible for perception, sensation, emotion, intellect, and action.

Brainstem The primitive portion of the brain that contains centers for vital functions and reflex actions, such as vomiting, coughing, sneezing, posture, and basic movement patterns.

Breathing pattern disorder A complex set of behaviors that leads to overbreathing without a pathologic condition present.

Buffers Compounds that prevent the hydrogen ion concentration from fluctuating too much and too rapidly to alter the pH

Bursa A flat sac of synovial membrane in which the inner sides of the sac are separated by fluid film. Bursae are located where moving structures are apt to rub.

Bursitis Inflammation of a bursa.

Callus An area of thickened, hardened skin that develops in an area of friction or region of recurrent pressure.

Cancer Malignant, nonencapsulated cells that invade surrounding tissue. They often break away, or metastasize, from the primary tumor and form secondary cancer masses.

Capillary One of the small blood vessels found between arteries and veins that allows the exchange of gases, nutrients, and waste products. The walls of capillaries are thin, allowing molecules to diffuse easily.

Carbohydrates Sugars, starches, and cellulose composed of carbon, hydrogen, and oxygen.

Cardiac cycle A synchronized sequence of events that takes place during one full heartbeat.

Cardiac muscle fibers Smaller, striated, involuntary muscle fibers (cells) in the heart that contract to pump blood.

Cardiac output The amount of blood pumped by the left ventricle in 1 minute.

Carotene A yellow pigment found in the dermis that provides a natural yellow tint to the skin of some individuals.

Cartilage A form of flexible connective tissue. Types of cartilage include hyaline, fibrocartilage, and elastic cartilage.

Catabolism Chemical processes in the body that release energy as complex compounds are broken down into simpler ones.

Catecholamines A group of neurotransmitters involved in sleep, mood, pleasure, and motor function.

Cell The basic structural unit of a living organism. A cell contains a nucleus and cytoplasm and is surrounded by a membrane.

Center of gravity An imaginary midpoint or center of the weight of a body or object, where the body or object could balance on a point.

Central nervous system The brain and spinal cord and their coverings.

Cerebellum The second largest part of the brain, the cerebellum is involved with balance, posture, coordination, and movement.

Cerebrospinal fluid A clear, colorless fluid that flows throughout the brain and around the spinal cord, cushioning and protecting these structures and maintaining proper pH balance.

Cerebrum The largest of the brain divisions, the cerebrum consists of two hemispheres that occupy the uppermost region of the cranium. The cerebrum receives, interprets, and associates incoming information with past memories and then transmits the appropriate motor response.

Cerumen A sticky substance released by glands in the ear. Also known as earwax, cerumen protects the ear from the entry of foreign material and repels insects.

Ceruminous glands Modified apocrine glands found in the external ear canal that secrete cerumen.

Charting The process of keeping a written record of a client or patient. The most effective charting methods follow clinical reasoning, which emphasizes a problem-solving approach. Many systems of charting are used, but these models all have similar components: POMR (problem-oriented medical record) and SOAP (subjective, objective, analysis, and plan–the four parts of the written record).

Chemical properties Properties that demonstrate how a substance reacts with other substances or responds to a change in the environment.

Chronic disease Disease with a vague onset that develops slowly and lasts for a long time, sometimes for life.

Chronic pain Pain that continues or recurs over a prolonged time, usually for more than 6 months. The onset may be obscure, and the character and quality of the pain change over time. Chronic pain usually is poorly localized and not as intense as acute pain, although for some the pain is exhausting and depressing. Chronic pain usually does not activate the sympathetic nervous system.

Circumduction Circular movement of a limb, combining the movements of flexion, extension, abduction, and adduction, to create a cone shape.

Closed kinematic chain The positioning of joints in such a way that motion at one of the joints is accompanied by motion at an adjacent joint.

Close-packed position The only position of a synovial joint in which the surfaces fit precisely together and maximal contact between the opposing surfaces occurs. The compression of joint surfaces permits no movement, and the joint possesses its greatest stability.

Collagen A protein substance composed of small fibrils that combine to create the connective tissue of fasciae, tendons, and ligaments. When combined with water, it forms gelatin. Collagen constitutes approximately one fourth of the protein in the body.

Collagenous fibers Strong fibers with little capacity for stretch. They have a high degree of tensile strength, which allows them to withstand longitudinal stress.

Collaterals Branches from an axon that allow communication among neurons.

Combining vowel A vowel added between two roots or a root and a suffix to make pronunciation of the word easier.

Compact (dense) bone The hard portion of bone that protects spongy bone and provides the firm framework of the bone and the body. The osteocytes in this type of bone are located in concentric rings around a central haversian canal, through which nerves and blood vessels pass.

Concentric contraction The action of a prime mover or agonist by which a muscle develops tension as it shortens to provide enough force to overcome resistance, described as positive contraction.

Condyle A rounded projection at the end of a bone.

Condyloid (condylar) joint Joint that allows movement in two directions, but one motion predominates. The joint resembles a condyle, which is a rounded protuberance at the end of a bone forming an articulation.

Connective tissue The most abundant type of tissue in the body, connective tissue supports and holds together the body and its parts, protects the body from foreign matter, and is organized to transport substances throughout the body.

Contractility The ability of a muscle to shorten forcibly with adequate stimulation. This property sets muscle apart from all other types of tissue.

Contracture The chronic shortening of a muscle, especially the connective tissue component.

Contusion A bruise.

Corn A painful, conical thickening of skin over bony prominences of the feet caused by continued pressure and friction on normally thin skin. Soft corns are those located in moist areas, such as between the toes.

Coronary arteries The arteries that supply oxygenated blood to the heart muscle itself; they are located in grooves between the atria and ventricles and between the two ventricles.

Coronary veins Veins that return the deoxygenated blood from the heart to the right atrium.

Cortisol A glucocorticoid, also known as hydrocortisone. Levels of stress often are measured by cortisol levels.

Cramps Painful muscle spasms or involuntary twitches that involve the whole muscle.

Cranial nerves Twelve pairs of nerves that originate from the olfactory bulbs, thalamus, visual cortex, and brainstem. They transmit information to and from the sensory organs of the face and the muscles of the face, neck, and upper shoulders.

Creep The slow movement of viscoelastic materials back to their original state and tissue structure after release of a deforming force.

Cytoplasm Material enclosed by the cell membrane.

Cytoskeleton A framework of proteins inside the cell providing flexibility and strength.

Cytosol The fluid that surrounds the nucleus or organelles inside the cell membrane.

Deep fascia A coarse sheet of fibrous connective tissue that binds muscles into functional groups and forms partitions, called intermuscular septae, between muscle groups.

Degenerative joint disease Osteoarthritis.

Dendrites Branching projections from the nerve cell body that carry signals to the cell body.

Deoxyribonucleic acid (DNA) Genetic material of the cell that carries the chemical "blueprint" of the body

Depression Downward or inferior movement.

Dermatitis A general term for acute or chronic skin inflammation characterized by redness, eruptions, edema, scaling, and itching. The three main types are atopic dermatitis, seborrheic dermatitis, and contact dermatitis. Eczema is a form of dermatitis.

Dermatome A cutaneous (skin) section supplied by a single spinal nerve.

Dermis The inner layer of skin that contains collagen and elastin fibers, which provide much of the structure and strength of the skin, and is much thicker than the epidermis.

Descending tracts Tracts that carry motor information from the brain to the spinal cord.

Diagnosis A labeling of signs and symptoms by a licensed medical professional.

Diagonal abduction Movement of a limb through a diagonal plane directly across and away from the midline of the body.

Diagonal adduction Movement of a limb through a diagonal plane toward and across the midline of the body.

Diaphragm A dome-shaped sheet of muscle attached to the thoracic wall that separates the lungs and thoracic cavity from the abdominal cavity. As the chest cavity enlarges, the diaphragm moves downward and flattens to create a vacuum that allows air to flow into the lungs. As the chest contracts and the diaphragm relaxes, the diaphragm arches upward, helping air to flow out of the lungs.

Diarthrosis A freely movable synovial joint.

Diffusion Movement of ions and molecules from an area of higher concentration to that of a lower concentration.

Digestion The mechanical and chemical breakdown of food from its complex form into simple molecules.

Disease An abnormality in functions of the body, especially when the abnormality threatens well-being.

Disharmony Distortions in health that result when the functions or systems are neither balanced nor working at their optimum. In

Chinese medicine, disharmony can be created by the imbalance of the Six Pernicious Influences or the Seven Emotions.

Disk herniation A pathologic condition that occurs when the fibrocartilage that surrounds the intervertebral disk ruptures, releasing the nucleus pulposus that cushions the vertebrae above and below. The resultant pressure on spinal nerve roots may cause pain and damage the surrounding nerves.

Dopamine A catecholamine found in the brain and autonomic system. Generally a stimulant, dopamine is involved in emotions/moods and in regulating motor control and the executive functioning of the brain.

Dorsal root One of two roots that attaches a spinal nerve to the spinal cord.

Dorsiflexion (dorsal flexion) Movement of the ankle that results in the top of the foot moving toward the anterior tibia.

Dosha An Ayurvedic concept that describes chemical processes in the body. The three types are Vata, Pitta, and Kapha.

Dynamic force Force applied to an object that produces movement in or of the object.

Eccentric contraction The action of an antagonist by which a muscle lengthens while under tension and changes in tension to control the descent of the resistance. Eccentric contractions may be thought of as controlling movement against gravity or resistance and are described as negative contractions.

Eccrine A type of sweat gland that releases a watery fluid known as sweat, which cools the body and provides minor elimination of metabolic waste.

Edema The accumulation of abnormal amounts of fluid in tissue spaces.

Efferent Away from a center or point of reference.

Efferent nerves Motor nerves that link the central nervous system to the effectors outside it and transmit motor impulses.

Effort The force applied to overcome resistance.

Elastic fibers Connective tissue fibers that are extensible and elastic. They are made of a protein called elastin, which returns to its original length after being stretched.

Elasticity The ability of a muscle to recoil and resume its original resting length after being stretched.

Elastin A connective tissue fiber type that has elastic properties and allows flexibility of connective tissue structures.

Element Substance containing only a single kind of atom.

Elevation Upward or superior movement.

Elimination (egestion) Removal and release of solid waste products from food that cannot be digested or absorbed.

Endocrine gland A ductless gland that secretes hormones directly into the bloodstream.

Endocytosis The cellular process of engulfing particles located outside the cell membrane into a cell by forming vesicles.

Endoplasmic reticulum A network of intracellular membranes in the form of tubes that is connected to the nuclear membrane.

Endorphins Peptide hormones that mainly work like morphine to suppress pain. They influence mood, producing a mild euphoric feeling such as is seen in runner's high.

Endoskeleton The bony support structure found inside the human body that accommodates growth.

Endosteum A thin membrane of connective tissue that lines the marrow cavity of a bone.

Energy The capacity to work, and work is the movement of or a change in the physical structure of matter.

Entrainment A coordination or synchronization to an internal or external rhythm, especially when a person responds to certain patterns by moving in a coordinated manner to those patterns.

Epicondyle A bony projection above a condyle.

Epidermis The outer or top layer of skin composed of sublayers called strata. The epidermis contains no nerves or blood vessels.

Epilepticus A continuous seizure.

Epinephrine A catecholamine released by the nervous system and involved in fight-or-flight responses such as dilation of blood vessels to the skeletal muscles. Epinephrine is classified as a hormone when secreted by the adrenal gland.

Epithelial tissues A specialized group of tissues that cover and protect the surface of the body and its parts, line body cavities, and form glands. Epithelial tissue usually is found in areas that move substances into and out of the body during secretion, absorption, and excretion.

Erythrocytes Red blood cells that contain hemoglobin and function to transport oxygen to the cells and carbon dioxide away from the cells.

Essential tremor A chronic tremor that does not proceed from any other pathologic condition.

Etiology The study of the factors involved in the development of disease, including the nature of the disease and the susceptibility of the person.

Eversion Movement of the sole of the foot outward away from the midline.

Excitability The ability of a muscle to receive and respond to a stimulus.

Exocrine gland A gland that secretes hormones through ducts directly into specific areas. Exocrine glands are part of the endocrine system.

Exocytosis The movement of substances out of a cell.

Extensibility The ability of a muscle to be stretched or extended.

Extension A movement that increases the angle between two bones, usually moving the body part back toward the anatomic position.

External respiration The exchange of oxygen and carbon dioxide between the lungs and the bloodstream.

External rotation Rotary movement around the longitudinal axis of a bone away from the midline of the body. Also known as rotation laterally, outward rotation, and lateral rotation.

Facet A smooth, flat surface on a bone.

Facilitated diffusion The transport of substances by carriers to which the substance binds to move the substance into a cell along the concentration gradient without energy.

Fascia A fibrous membrane covering, supporting, and separating muscles; the subcutaneous tissue that connects the skin to the muscles.

Feedback loop A self-regulating control system in the body that receives information, integrates that information, and provides a response to maintain homeostasis. Negative feedback reverses the original stimulus, whereas positive feedback enhances and maintains the stimulus.

Fibrocartilage A connective tissue that permits little motion in joints and structures, is found in places such as the intervertebral disks, and forms our ears.

Fibromyalgia A syndrome with symptoms of widespread pain or aching, persistent fatigue, generalized morning stiffness, nonrestorative sleep, and multiple tender points. A disrupted sleep pattern, coupled with the dysfunction of myofascial repair mechanisms, seems to be a factor.

Fibrous joint An articulation in which fibrous tissue connects bone directly to bone.

Fistula A tract that is open at both ends through which abnormal connection occurs between two surfaces.

Fixator One of the stabilizing muscles surrounding a joint or body part that contracts to fixate, or stabilize, the area, enabling another limb or body segment to exert force and move.

Flaccid A term used to describe a muscle with decreased or absent tone.

Flexion A movement that decreases the angle between two bones as the body part moves out of the anatomic position.

Fontanels Areas of the skull of an infant in which the bone formation is incomplete. The fontanels allow for compression of the skull as the infant travels through the birth canal and expansion as the brain grows.

Foramen An opening in a bone, such as the foramen magnum of the skull.

Force Any push or pull on an object in an attempt to affect motion or shape.

Fossa A depression in the surface or at the end of a bone.

Free nerve endings Sensory receptors that detect itch and tickle sensations.

Frontal (coronal) plane A vertical plane that divides the body into anterior and posterior (front and back) parts.

Gait The rhythmic and alternating motions of the legs, trunk, and arms resulting in the propulsion of the body.

Gait cycle Subdivided into the stance phase and swing phase, this cycle begins when the heel of one foot strikes the floor and continues until the same heel strikes the floor again.

Gallbladder A small 3- to 4-inch sac that stores and concentrates bile.

Ganglion Cystic, round, usually nontender swellings located along tendon sheaths or joint capsules.

General adaptation syndrome The method the body uses to mobilize different defense mechanisms when threatened by actual or perceived harmful stimuli.

Gestation The period of fetal growth from conception until birth.

Gibbus An angular deformity of a collapsed vertebra, the causes of which include metastatic cancer and tuberculosis of the spine.

Gliding joints Known also as synovial planes, gliding joints allow only a gliding motion in various planes.

Gray matter Unmyelinated nervous tissue, particularly that found in the central nervous system.

Gross anatomy The study of body structures visible to the naked eye.

Ground substance The medium in which the cells and protein fibers are suspended. Ground substance is usually clear and colorless and has the consistency of thick syrup.

Half-life The amount of time required for half of a hormone to be eliminated from the bloodstream.

Health A condition of homeostasis resulting in a state of physical, emotional, social, and spiritual well-being.

Heart The pump of the cardiovascular system; the heart is hollow, cone-shaped, and about the size of a fist and is located in the mediastinum of the thoracic cavity. The myocardium is the heart muscle itself, the endocardium is the thin inner lining, and the epicardium is the outer membrane.

Heart rate The number of cardiac cycles in 1 minute. In the average, healthy person the rate works out to be 60 to 70 cycles or beats per minute.

Heart sounds The two main sounds resulting from the closure of the valves. Murmurs are extra sounds, such as those resulting from faulty valves.

Heart valves Four sets of valves that keep the blood flowing in the correct direction through the heart.

Hemoglobin The oxygen-carrying, red-colored molecule in the blood.

Hemorrhage The passage of blood outside of the cardiovascular system.

Hernia Weakness in a muscle or structure that allows for protrusion of a muscle, organ, or structure through the resulting opening.

Herpes simplex A DNA virus that causes painful blisters and small ulcers in and around the mouth and on the genital area.

High-energy bonds Covalent bonds created in specific organic substrates in the presence of enzymes.

Hinge joint Joint that allows flexion and extension in one direction, changing the angle of the bones at the joint, like a door hinge.

Histamine A neurotransmitter that is considered a stimulant. Histamine is released by the mast cells as part of the inflammatory process and can cause itching.

Homeostasis The relatively constant state of the internal environment of the body that is maintained by adaptive responses. Specific control and feedback mechanisms are responsible for adjusting body systems to maintain this state.

Horizontal abduction Movement of the humerus in the horizontal plane away from the midline of the body. Also known as the horizontal extension or transverse abduction.

Horizontal adduction Movement of the humerus in the horizontal plane toward the midline of the body. Also known as horizontal flexion or transverse adduction.

Hyaline cartilage The thin covering of articular connective tissue on the ends of the bones in freely movable joints in the adult skeleton. Hyaline cartilage forms a smooth, resilient, low-friction surface for the articulation of one bone with another, distributes forces, and helps absorb some of the pressure imposed on the joint surfaces.

Hyperalgesia An increased sensitivity to pain.

Hyperextension A movement that takes the body part further in the direction of the extension, further out of anatomic position.

Hypermobility A range of motion of a joint greater than would be permitted normally by the structure. Hypermobility results in instability.

Hyperplasia An uncontrolled increase in the number of cells of a body part.

Hypersecretion The excessive release of a hormone.

Hypertension An increase in systolic and diastolic pressures.

Hypertrophy An increase in the size of a cell, which results in an increase in the size of a body part or organ.

Hyperventilation Abnormally deep or rapid breathing in excess of physical demands.

Hypomobility A range of motion of a joint less than what would be permitted normally by the structure.

Hyposecretion The insufficient release of a hormone.

Hypotension A decrease in systolic and diastolic pressures. Hypotension is an important manifestation of shock, which causes inadequate blood supply to vital organs.

Immunity Resistance to disease provided by the body through specific or nonspecific immunity. The immune system is a functional system rather than an organ system in the anatomic sense. The most important immune cells are lymphocytes and macrophages. The key to immunity is the ability of the body to distinguish self from nonself.

Impermeable The quality of not permitting entry of a substance.

Incontinence The inability to control urination or defecation, most often because of weak pelvic floor muscles or nerve damage.

Inertia The reluctance of matter to change its state of motion.

Inflammation A protective response of the tissues to irritation or injury that may be chronic or acute. The four primary signs are redness, heat, swelling, and pain.

Inflammatory response A sequence of events that involves chemical and cellular activation that destroys pathogens and aids in repairing tissues.

Ingestion Taking food into the mouth.

Inorganic compounds Chemical structures that do not have carbon and hydrogen atoms as the primary structure.

Insertion The distal attachment of a muscle; the part of a muscle that attaches farthest from the midline, or center, of the body.

Integument The skin and its appendages: hair, sebaceous and sweat glands, nails, and breasts.

Internal respiration The exchange of gases between the tissues and blood.

Internal rotation Medial rotary movement of a bone. Also known as rotation medially, inward rotation, and medial rotation.

Interphase The period during which a cell grows and carries on its activities.

Intractable pain The continuation of chronic pain without active disease present or when chronic pain persists even with treatment.

Inversion Movement of the sole of the foot inward toward the midline.

Ion pumps Carriers that transport substances into or out of a cell using energy.

Ischemia A temporary deficiency or decreased supply of blood to a tissue.

Isometric contraction The action of the prime mover that occurs when tension develops within the muscle but no appreciable change occurs in the joint angle or the length of the muscle. Movement does not occur.

Isotonic contraction The action of the prime mover that occurs when tension develops in the muscle while it shortens or lengthens.

Joint capsule A connective tissue structure that indirectly connects the bony components of a joint.

Joint play The involuntary movement that occurs between articular surfaces are separate from the range of motion of a joint produced by muscles. Joint play is an essential component of joint motion and must occur for normal functioning of the joint.

Keratin The fibrous protein produced in the epidermis that protects our skin and makes it waterproof.

Kinematics A branch of mechanics that involves the time, space, and mass aspects of a moving system.

Kinesiology The study of movement that combines the fields of anatomy, physiology, physics, and geometry, and relates them to human movement.

Kinetic chain An integrated functional unit. The kinetic chain is made up of the myofascial system (muscle, ligament, tendon, and fascia), articular (joint) system, and nervous system. Each of these systems works interdependently to allow structural and functional efficiency in all three planes of motion: sagittal, frontal, and transverse.

Kinetics Those forces causing movement in a system.

Kyphosis A condition of exaggeration of the thoracic curve.

Lateral flexion (side bending) Movement of the head or trunk laterally away from the midline. Abduction of the spine.

Lateral recumbency (side lying) Lying horizontally on the right or left side.

Leukocytes White blood cells that protect the body from pathogens and remove dead cells and substances.

Lever A solid mass, such as a crowbar or a person's arm, that rotates around a fixed point called the fulcrum. The rotation is produced by a force applied to a lever at some distance from the fulcrum.

Ligaments Dense bundles of parallel connective tissue fibers, primarily collagen, that connect bones and strengthen and stabilize the joint.

Lipids Fats and oils; organic compounds that have carbon, hydrogen, and oxygen atoms but in a different proportion than that of carbohydrates.

List A lateral tilt of the spine.

Locomotion Moving from one place to another; walking.

Loose-packed position The position of a synovial joint in which the joint capsule is most lax. Joints tend to assume this position when inflammation occurs to accommodate the increased volume of synovial fluid.

Lordosis A condition of exaggeration of the normal lumbar curve.

Lower respiratory tract The larynx, trachea, bronchi, and alveoli.

Lungs The primary organs of respiration, the lungs are soft, spongy, highly vascular structures separated into the left and right lungs by the mediastinum. Each lung is separated into lobes. The right lung has three lobes: an upper, middle, and lower; the left, two lobes: an upper and lower.

Lymph A clear interstitial tissue fluid that bathes the cells. Lymph contains lymphocytes, which provide immune response; returns plasma proteins that have leaked out through capillary walls; and transports fats from the gastrointestinal system to the bloodstream.

Lymph nodes Small, round structures distributed along the network of lymph vessels that provide a filtering system for removing waste products and transferring them to the bloodstream for removal to the spleen, intestines, and kidneys for detoxification. Lymph nodes are centers for lymphocyte production. Their main function is to prevent bacteria and viruses from gaining access to the bloodstream. Generally clustered at the joints for assistance in pumping when the joint moves, they are especially numerous in the axillae, groin, and neck and along certain blood vessels of the pelvic, abdominal, and thoracic cavities.

Lysosome Cell organelle that is part of the intracellular digestive system.

Matrix The basic substance between the cells of a tissue. Matrix is composed of amorphous ground substance consisting of molecules that expand when water molecules and electrolytes bind to them. Up to 90% of connective tissue is ground substance. Fibers make up the other component of matrix.

Maximal stimulus The point at which all motor units of a muscle have been recruited and the muscle is unable to increase in strength.

Mechanical receptors Sensory receptors that detect changes in pressure, movement, temperature, or other mechanical forces.

Mechanics The branch of physics dealing with the study of forces and the motion produced by their actions.

Meiosis A type of cell division in which each daughter cell receives half the normal number of chromosomes, forming two reproductive cells.

Melanin The pigment that colors our skin and works as a natural sunscreen to protect us from ultraviolet rays by darkening our skin.

Membrane A thin, sheetlike layer of tissue that covers a cell, an organ, or some other structure; that lines a tube or a cavity; or that divides or separates one part from another.

Metabolism Chemical processes in the body that convert food and oxygen into energy to support growth, distribution of nutrients, and elimination of waste.

Metabolites Molecules synthesized or broken down inside the body by chemical reactions.

Microorganisms Small life forms that may be damaging to the body or interfere with its function.

Microvilli Small projections of the cell membrane that increase the surface area of the cell.

Micturition The clinical term for urination or voiding.

Mitochondria Cell organelles of rod or oval shape.

Mitosis Cell division in which the cell duplicates its DNA and divides into two identical daughter cells.

Mixed nerves Nerves that contain sensory and motor axons.

Mole Also known as a nevus, a mole is a benign pigmented skin growth formed of melanocytes.

Molecule A combination of two or more atoms. A molecule is the smallest portion of a substance that can exist separately without losing the physical and chemical properties of that substance.

Monoplegia Paralysis of a single limb or a single group of muscles.

Motor point The location where the motor neuron enters the muscle and where a visible contraction can be elicited with a minimal amount of stimulation. Motor points most often are located in the belly of the muscle.

Motor unit A motor neuron and all of the muscle fibers it controls.

Muscle tissue A specialized form of tissue that contracts and shortens to provide movement, maintain posture, and produce heat.

Myasthenia gravis A disorder that usually affects muscles in the face, lips, tongue, neck and throat, which are innervated by the cranial nerves, but that can affect any muscle group.

Myelin A white, fatty, insulating substance formed by the Schwann cells that surrounds some axons. Also produced in the central nervous system by oligodendrocytes.

Myotome A skeletal muscle or group of skeletal muscles that receives motor axons from a particular spinal nerve.

Negative feedback system A control mechanism that provides a stimulus to decrease a function, such as a fire alarm, which causes a series of reactions that work to reduce the fire.

Neoplasm The abnormal growth of new tissue. Also called a tumor, a neoplasm may be benign or malignant.

Nerve A bundle of axons or dendrites or both.

Nervous tissue A specialized tissue that coordinates and regulates body activity and can develop more excitability and conductivity than other types of tissue.

Neurilemma The outer cell membrane of a Schwann cell that is essential in the regeneration of injured axons. The thin membrane spirally wraps the myelin layers of certain fibers, especially of peripheral nerves, or the axons of certain unmyelinated nerve fibers. Also called Schwann's membrane, sheath of Schwann, and endoneural membrane.

Neuroglia Specialized connective tissue cells that support, protect, and hold neurons together.

Neurons Nerve cells that conduct impulses.

Neurotransmitters Chemical compounds that generate action potentials when released in the synapses from presynaptic cells.

Nociceptors Sensory receptors that detect painful or intense stimuli.

Norepinephrine A catecholamine primarily involved in emotional responses. Norepinephrine is found in the central nervous system and the sympathetic division of the autonomic nervous system and causes constriction of blood vessels in the skeletal muscles.

Nucleic acids The two types of nucleic acid are deoxyribonucleic acid (DNA) and ribonucleic acid (RNA).

Nutrients Essential elements and molecules obtained from the diet that are required by the body for normal body function.

Nutrition The use of food for growth and maintenance of the body.

Open kinematic chain A position in which the ends of the limbs or parts of the body are free to move without causing motion at another joint.

Opportunistic pathogens Organisms that cause disease only when the immunity is low in a host.

Opposition Movement of the thumb across the palmar aspect to make contact with the fingers.

Organelles The basic components of a cell that perform specific functions within the cell.

Organic compounds Substances that have carbon and hydrogen as part of their basic structure.

Origin The proximal attachment of a muscle; the part that attaches closest to the midline (center) of the body; the least movable part of a muscle.

Osmosis Diffusion of water from a region of lower concentration of solution to a region of higher concentration of solution across the semipermeable membrane of a cell.

Osteokinematics The movement of bones as opposed to the movement of articular surfaces; also known as range of motion.

Osteoporosis A disorder of the bones in which a lack of calcium and other minerals and a decrease in bone protein leaves the bones soft, fragile, and more likely to break.

Oxygen debt The extra amount of oxygen that must be taken in to convert lactic acid to glucose or glycogen.

Pain An unpleasant sensation. Pain is a complex, private experience with physiologic, psychologic, and social aspects. Because pain is subjective, it is often difficult to explain or describe.

Paraplegia Paralysis of the lower portion of the body and of both legs.

Parasympathetic nervous system The energy conservation and restorative system associated with what commonly is called the relaxation response.

Passive transport Transportation of a substance across the cell membrane without the use of energy

Pathogenesis The development of a disease.

Pathogenicity The ability of the infectious agent to cause disease.

Pathogens Microorganisms capable of producing disease.

Pathologic range of motion The amount of motion at a joint that fails to reach the normal physiologic range or exceeds normal anatomic limits of motion of that joint.

Pathology The study of disease as observed in the structure and function of the body.

Pericardium A double membranous, serous sac surrounding the heart. The pericardium secretes a lubricating fluid to prevent friction from the movement of the heart.

Periosteum The thin membrane of connective tissue that covers bones except at articulations.

Peripheral nervous system The system of somatic and autonomic neurons outside the central nervous system. The peripheral nervous system comprises the afferent (sensory) division and the efferent (motor) division.

Peristalsis Rhythmic contraction of smooth muscles that propel products of digestion along the tract from the esophagus to the anus.

Peritoneum The mucous membrane that lines the abdominal cavity to prevent friction from the organs.

Phagocytosis The process of endocytosis followed by digestion of the vesicle contents by enzymes present in the cytoplasm.

Phantom pain A form of pain or other sensation experienced in the missing extremity after a limb amputation.

Pharynx The throat.

Phospholipid bilayer Cell membrane made up of lipids, carbohydrates, and proteins.

Physiologic range of motion The amount of motion available to a joint determined by the nervous system from information provided by joint sensory receptors. This information usually prevents a joint from being positioned so that injury could occur.

Physiology The study of the processes and functions of the body involved in supporting life.

Piezoelectric The quality of bones that allows them to deform slightly and vibrate when electrical currents pass through them. Bone formation patterns follow lines of stress load directed by the piezoelectric currents.

Pivot joint A bony projection from one bone fits into a "ring" formed by another bone and ligament structure to allow rotation around its own axis.

Plantar flexion An extension movement of the ankle that results in the foot and toes moving away from the body.

Plasma A thick, straw-colored fluid that makes up about 55% of the blood.

Plastic range The range of movement of connective tissue that is taken beyond the elastic limits. In this range the tissue permanently deforms and cannot return to its original state.

Plexus A network of intertwining nerves that innervates a particular region of the body.

Polio (or poliomyelitis) A viral infection that affects the nerves that control skeletal muscle movement.

Posterior pelvic rotation Posterior movement of the upper pelvis; the iliac crest tilts backward in a sagittal plane.

Prefix A word element added to the beginning of a root to change the meaning of the word.

Pressure The amount of force on a specific area.

Process Any prominent bony growth that projects out from the bone.

Pronation Internal rotary movement of the radius on the ulna that results in the hand moving from the palm-up to the palm-down position.

Prone Lying horizontal with the face down.

Proprioceptors Sensory receptors that provide the body with information about position, movement, muscle tension, joint activity, and equilibrium.

Proteins Substances formed from amino acids.

Protraction Forward movement remaining in a horizontal plane.

Psoriasis A common, chronic skin disease characterized by reddened skin covered by dry, silvery scales. Psoriasis most often is found on the scalp, elbows, knees, back, or buttocks.

Pulmonary trunk The large artery that carries blood to the lungs to release carbon dioxide and take in oxygen.

Pulmonary veins The four veins from the lungs that bring oxygen-rich blood to the left atrium.

Qi Also known as Chi, Qi refers to the life force.

Quadriplegia Paralysis or loss of movement of all four limbs.

Reciprocal inhibition Stimulation of an antagonist muscle to inhibit action in the prime mover.

Reciprocal innervation The circuitry of neurons that allows reciprocal inhibition to take place. One can use reciprocal innervation therapeutically to assist in muscle relaxation.

Reduction Return of the spinal column to the anatomic position from lateral flexion. Adduction of the spine.

Referred pain Pain felt in a surface area far from the stimulated organ.

Reflex An automatic, involuntary reaction to a stimulus.

Reflex arc The pathway that a nerve impulse follows in a reflex action.

Regional anatomy The study of the structures of a particular area of the body.

Remission A reversal of signs and symptoms in chronic disease that can be temporary or permanent.

Respiration The movement of air in and out of the lungs, the exchange of oxygen and carbon dioxide between the lungs and blood, and the exchange between blood and body tissues.

Respiratory rate The number of breaths in 1 minute.

Reticular fibers Delicate, connective tissue fibers that occur in networks and support small structures, such as capillaries, nerve fibers, and the basement membrane. Reticular fibers are made of a specialized type of collagen called reticulin.

Retraction Backward movement in a horizontal plane.

Ribonucleic acid (RNA) Nucleic acids that transfer genetic information and control cellular chemical activities.

Root A word element that contains the basic meaning of the word.

Rotation Partial turning or pivoting in an arc around a central axis.

Rupture The tearing or disruption of connective tissue fibers that takes place when they exceed the limits of the plastic range.

Saddle joint Joint that is convex in one plane and concave in the other with the surfaces fitting together like a rider on a saddle.

Schwann cell A specialized cell that forms myelin.

Scoliosis A lateral curvature of the spine.

Sebaceous glands The oil glands found in the skin.

Sebum The oily substance secreted by sebaceous glands that prevents dehydration, softens skin and hair, and slows the growth of bacteria.

Serotonin A neurotransmitter that works primarily as an inhibitor in the central nervous system and is synthesized into melatonin and affects our sleep and moods.

Sesamoid bones Round bones that often are embedded in tendons and joint capsules.

Seven Emotions, The The Asian concept that joy, anger, fear, fright, sadness, worry, and grief are emotional responses that may trigger disharmony in the body, mind, or spirit under certain conditions.

Shock An inadequate blood supply to vital organs, causing reduced function in these organs.

Signs Objective changes that someone other than the client or patient can observe and measure.

Sinus Four groups of air-filled spaces that open into the internal nose. They are located in the frontal, ethmoid, sphenoid, and maxillary bones of the skull. Sinuses are lined with mucosa and function to lighten the weight of the skull, making it easier to hold the head up and help in the production of sound.

Six Pernicious Influences, The The Asian concept that heat, cold, wind, dampness, dryness, and summer heat, which are natural climate changes, may induce disease under certain conditions.

Skeletal muscle fibers Large, cross-striated cells that are connected to the skeleton and under voluntary control of the nervous system.

Smooth muscle fibers Muscle fibers that are neither striated nor voluntary. These muscle cells help regulate blood flow through the cardiovascular system, propel food through the gut, and squeeze secretions from glands.

SOAP notes The acronym refers to subjective, objective, analysis or assessment, and plan, the four parts of the written account of record keeping.

Somatic nervous system A system of nerves that keeps the body in balance with its external environment by transmitting impulses between the central nervous system, skeletal muscles, and skin.

Somatic pain Pain that arises from the body as opposed to the viscera. Superficial somatic pain comes from the stimulation of receptors in the skin, whereas deep somatic pain arises from stimulation of receptors in skeletal muscles, joints, tendons, and fasciae.

Spastic Term used to describe a muscle with excessive tone.

Spinal cord Portion of the central nervous system that exits the skull into the vertebral column. The two major functions of the spinal cord are to conduct nerve impulses and to be a center for spinal reflexes.

Spinal nerves Thirty-one pairs of mixed nerves, originating in the spinal cord and emerging from the vertebral column, that make sensation and movement possible.

Spongy (cancellous) bone The lighter-weight portion of bone made up of trabeculae.

Stabilizer A force or an object that helps maintain a position. Stabilization is essential to assess movement patterns accurately.

Standard Precautions Safety measures established by the Centers for Disease Control and Prevention. The precautions were instituted to prevent the spread of bacterial and viral infections by setting up specific methods of dealing with human fluids and waste products. Standard Precautions protect client and practitioner from pathogens.

Static force Force applied to an object in such a way that it does not produce movement.

Stress Any external or internal stimulus that requires a change or response to prevent an imbalance in the internal environment of the body, mind, or emotions. Stress may be any activity that makes demands on mental and emotional resources. Some responses to stress may stimulate neurons of the hypothalamus to release corticotropin-releasing hormone.

Subacute Diseases with characteristics between acute and chronic.

Suffix A word element added to the end of a root to change the meaning of the word.

Superficial fascia The subcutaneous tissue that composes the third layer of skin, consists of loose connective tissue, and contains fat or adipose tissue.

Supination External rotary movement of the radius on the ulna that results in the hand moving from the palm-down to the palm-up position.

Supine Lying horizontal with the face up.

Surface anatomy The study of internal organs and structures as they can be recognized and related to external features.

Suture A synarthrotic joint in which two bony components are united by a thin layer of dense fibrous tissue.

Sweat glands The sudoriferous glands in the skin; they are classified as apocrine or eccrine based on their location and structure.

Sympathetic nervous system The part of the autonomic nervous system that provides for most of the active function of the body; when the body is under stress, the sympathetic nervous system predominates with fight-or-flight responses.

Symphysis A cartilaginous joint in which the two bony components are joined directly by fibrocartilage in the form of a disk or plate.

Symptoms The subjective changes noticed or felt only by the client or patient.

Synapse Spaces between neurons or between a neuron and an effector organ.

Synarthrosis A limited-movement, nonsynovial joint.

Synchondrosis A joint in which the material used for connecting the two components is hyaline growth cartilage.

Syndesmosis A fibrous joint in which two bony components are joined directly by a ligament, cord, or aponeurotic membrane.

Syndrome A group of different signs and symptoms that identify a pathologic condition, especially when they have a common cause.

Synergist A muscle that aids or assists the action of the agonist but is not primarily responsible for the action; also known as a guiding muscle.

Synovial fluid A thick, colorless, lubricating fluid secreted by the joint cavity membrane.

Synovial joint A freely moving joint allowing motion in one or more planes of action.

Systemic anatomy The study of the structure of a particular body system.

Tao An ancient philosophic concept that represents the whole and its parts as one and the same.

Tendonitis Inflammation of a tendon.

Tenosynovitis Inflammation of a tendon sheath.

Thermal receptors Sensory receptors that detect changes in temperature.

Thorax Also known as the chest cavity, the thorax is the upper region of the torso enclosed by the sternum, ribs, and thoracic vertebrae and contains the lungs, heart, and great vessels.

Threshold stimulus The stimulus at which the first observable muscle contraction occurs.

Tissue A group of similar cells combined to perform a common function.

Tone The state of tension in resting muscles.

Trabeculae An irregular meshing of small, bony plates that makes up spongy bone; its spaces are filled with red marrow.

Tracts Collections of nerve fibers in the brain and spinal cord with a common function.

Trigger points A hyperirritable area within a taut band of skeletal muscle, located in the muscular tissue and/or its associated fascia. The spot is painful on compression and can cause characteristic referred pain and autonomic phenomena.

Trochanter One of two large bony processes found only on the femur.

Tropic (or trophic) hormones Hormones produced by the endocrine glands that affect other endocrine glands.

Tubercle A small rounded process on a bone.

Tuberosity A large rounded protuberance on a bone.

Tumor Also referred to as a neoplasm, a tumor is a growth of new tissues that may be benign (nonthreatening or noncancerous) or malignant (cancerous).

Ulcer A round, open sore of the skin or mucous membrane.

Upper respiratory tract The nasal cavity and all its structures and the pharynx.

Upward rotation Scapular motion that turns the glenoid fossa upward and moves the inferior angle superiorly and laterally away from the spinal column.

Vector The direction of force.

Veins Blood vessels that collect blood from the capillaries and transport it back to the heart. Seventy-five percent of the blood in the body is in the venous system. Larger veins often contain a set of valves that ensure that blood flows in the correct direction to the heart and also prevent backflow.

Vena cava One of two large arteries that returns poorly oxygenated blood to the right atrium of the heart.

Ventral root One of two roots that attaches a spinal nerve to the spinal cord.

Ventricles The two large, lower chambers of the heart; they are thick-walled and separated by a thick interventricular septum.

Venules The smallest veins.

Virulent A quality of organisms that readily cause disease.

Visceral pain Pain that results from the stimulation of receptors or an abnormal condition in the viscera (internal organs).

Viscoelasticity The combination of resistance offered by a fluid to a change of form and the ability of material to return to its original state after deformation. This term describes connective tissue.

Whiplash An injury to the soft tissues of the neck caused by sudden hyperextension and/or flexion of the neck.

Word elements The parts of a word; the prefix, root, and suffix.

Yellow elastic cartilage Cartilage that is more opaque, flexible, and elastic than hyaline cartilage and is distinguished further by its yellow color. The ground substance is penetrated in all directions by frequently branching fibers that give all of the reactions for elastin.

Yin/yang *Yin* and *yang* are terms used to describe polar relationships. Yin/yang refers to the dynamic balance between opposing forces and the continual process of creation and destruction. Yin/yang reflects the natural order and duality of the whole universe and everything in it, including the individual.

WORKS CONSULTED

1998 physician's GenRx, ed 8, St Louis, 1998, Mosby.

A practical dictionary of chinese medicine, Cohen, 1996; Ding, 1990

Advice for the patient: drug information in lay language, vol 2, Rockville, Maryland, 1990, United States Pharmaceutical Convention.

An outline of Chinese acupuncture: The Academy of Traditional Chinese Medicine, Foreign Languages Press, Peking, 1975.

Agur AMR: *Grant's atlas of anatomy*, ed 9, Baltimore, 1991, Williams & Wilkins.

Arnheim DD, Prentice WE: *Principles of athletic training*, ed 10, New York 2000, McGraw Hill.

Basmajian JV, DeLuca CJ: *Muscles alive: their functions revealed by electromyography*, ed 5, Baltimore, 1985, Williams & Wilkins.

Basmajian JV, Nyberg R: *Rational manual therapies*, Baltimore, 1993, Williams & Wilkins.

Bates B: *A guide to physical examination and history taking*, ed 6, Philadelphia, 1995, Lippincott-Raven.

Best ML et al, editors: *The physician's assistant compendium of drug therapy*, New Jersey, 1994, Compendium.

Birch SJ, Felt RL: *Understanding acupuncture*, New York, 1999, Churchill Livingston.

Born BA: *An introduction to practical pathology for the myomassologist*, ed 7, Southfield, Mich, 1993.

Brennan R: *The Alexander technique workbook*, Rockport, Massachusetts, 1992, Element.

Bullock BL, Rosendahl PP: *Pathophysiology: adaptations and alterations in function*, ed 3, Philadelphia, 1992, JB Lippincott.

Burkitt GH, Young B, Heath J: *Wheater's functional histology*, ed 3, New York, 1993, Churchill Livingstone.

Butler DS: *Mobilization of the nervous system*, Melbourne, 1991, Churchill Livingstone.

Cailliet R: *Foot and ankle pain*, ed 3, Philadelphia, 1997, FA Davis.

Cailliet R: *Hand pain and impairment*, ed 4, Philadelphia, 1994, FA Davis.

Cailliet R: *Knee pain and disability*, ed 3, Philadelphia, 1992, FA Davis.

Cailliet R: *Low back pain syndrome*, ed 5, Philadelphia, 1995, FA Davis.

Cailliet R: *Neck and arm pain*, ed 3, Philadelphia, 1991, FA Davis.

Cailliet R: *Shoulder pain*, ed 3, Philadelphia, 1991, FA Davis.

Cailliet R: *Soft tissue pain and disability*, Philadelphia, 1996, FA Davis.

Cassar M-P: *Handbook of massage therapy: a complete guide for the student and professional massage therapist,* Boston, 1999, Butterworth-Heinemann.

Castleman M: *Nature's cures*, Emmaus, Pa., 1996, Rodale Press.

Chaitow L: *Journal of bodywork and movement therapies*, New York, 1996, Churchill Livingstone.

Chaitow L: *Modern neuromuscular techniques*, New York, 1996, Churchill Livingstone.

Chaitow L: *Muscle energy techniques*, New York, 1996, Churchill Livingstone.

Chaitow L: *The acupuncture treatment of pain*, Rochester, Vermont, 1976, 1983, 1990, Healing Art Press.Chaitow L: *The book of natural pain relief*, New York, 1995, Harper Paperbacks.

Chaitow L: *The acupuncture treatment of pain*, Rochester, Vt, 1990, Healing Arts Press.

Chaitow L, Delany J: *Clinical application of neuromuscular techniques*, vol 1, *the upper body*, London, 2002, Churchill Livingstone.

Chaitow L, Delany J: *Clinical application of neuromuscular techniques*, vol 2, *the lower body*, London, 2002, Churchill Livingstone.

Chang MY, Wang SY, Chen CH: Effects of massage on pain and anxiety during labour: a randomized controlled trial in Taiwan, *J Adv Nurs* 38(1):68-73, 2000.

Chopra D: *Restful sleep*, New York, 1994, Crowne.

Clayton BD, Stock YN: *Basic pharmacology for nurses*, ed 11, St Louis, 1996, Mosby.

Colton H: *Touch therapy*, New York, 1983, Kensington.

Cooley C: *The book*, Scottsdale, Ariz, 1992, Big Guy Books!

Cowan P: *American Chronic Pain Association: staying well: advanced pain management for ACPA members*, 1994, California Dental Association.

Crawford AM: *The herbal menopause book*, Freedom, Calif, 1996, Crossing Press.

Damjanov I: *Pathology for the health-related professions*, ed 2, Philadelphia, 1996, Saunders.Daulby M, Mathison C: *Guide to spiritual healing*, London, 1996, Brockhampton Press.

Degenhardt B, Kuchera M: Update of osteopathic medical concepts and the lymphatic system, *J Am Osteopath Assoc* 96(2):97, 1996.

Di Lima SN, Painter SJ, Johns LT, editors: *Orthopaedic patient education resource manual*, Gaithersburg, Maryland, 1995, Aspen.

Doctor's little black bag of remedies and cures, vol 1, 1997, Boardroom.

Dossey L: *Space, time and medicine*, Boston, 1982, Random House.

Dvorak J, Vaclav D: *Medical checklists: manual medicine*, New York, 1991, Thieme Medical Publishers.

Editors of Consumers Guide: *Prescription drugs*, Lincolnwood, Ill, 1995, Publications International.

Falvo DR: *Medical and psychosocial aspects of chronic illness and disability*, Gaithersburg, Md, 1991, Aspen.

Freeman LW, Lawlis GF: *Mosby's complementary and alternative medicine: a research-based approach*, St Louis, 2001, Mosby.

Furlan AD, Brosseau L, Imamura M, Irvin E: Massage for low back pain, *Clin J Pain* 18(3):154-163, 2002.

Garofano JS: *Therapeutic massage and bodywork*, Stamford, Conn, 1997, Appleton & Lange.

Golan R: *Optimal wellness*, New York, 1995, Ballantine Books.

Gray's anatomy, the anatomical basis of medicine and surgery, ed 38, Edinburgh, 1996, Churchill Livingstone.Greenman PE: *Principles of manual medicine*, ed 2, Baltimore, 1996, Williams & Wilkins.

Gunn C: *Bones and joints*, ed 3, New York, 1996, Churchill Livingstone.

Gurevich D: *Russian medical massage*, Flint, Mich, 1992.

Hattan J, King L, Griffiths P: The impact of foot massage and guided relaxation following cardiac surgery: a randomized controlled trial, *Med Clin North Am* 86(1):163-171, 2002.

Heinerman J: *Healing powers of herbs*, Boca Raton, Fla, 1995, Globe Communications.

Hislop HJ, Montgomery J: *Daniel and Worthingham's muscle testing: techniques of manual examination*, ed 6, Philadelphia, 2002, WB Saunders.

Hoffman CJ: *HEV 370 nutrition*, ed 2, Mount Pleasant, Mich, 1996.

Hooper J, Teresi D: *The three pound universe*, New York, 1986, Dell.

Huan Z, Rose K: *Who can ride the dragon?*, Brookline, Mass, 1995, 1996, 1997, 1998, 1999, Paradigm Publications.

Isselbacher KJ et al: *Harrison's principles of internal medicine*, ed 13, New York, 1994, McGraw-Hill.

Jacobs PH, Anhalt TS: *Handbook of skin clues of systemic diseases*, ed 2, Philadelphia, 1992, Lea & Febiger.

Kapit W, Rober I, Macey EM: *The physiology coloring book*, ed 3, New York, 2001, HarperCollins.

Keen JH, Baird MS, Allen JH: *Mosby's critical care and emergency drug reference*, ed 2, St Louis, 1996, Mosby.

Keirsey D, Bates M: *Please understand me: character and temperament types*, ed 2, Del Mar, Calif, 1984, Prometheus Nemesis.

Keirsey D, Bates M: *Please understand me: temperament in leading*, Del Mar, Calif, 1996, Prometheus Nemesis.

Kendall F: *Florence Kendall's muscle testing video library*, vols 1-5, Baltimore, Williams & Wilkins (no date).

Kisner C, Colby LA: *Therapeutic exercise: foundations and techniques*, ed 3, Philadelphia, 1996, FA Davis.

Leadbeater CW: *The chakras*, Wheaton, Ill., 1927, Theosophical Publishing House.

Le Blanc-Louvry I, Costaglioli B, Boulon C, Leroi AM, Ducrotte PJ: Does mechanical massage of the abdominal wall after colectomy reduce postoperative pain and shorten the duration of ileus? Results of a randomized study, *J Adv Nurs* 38(1):68-73, 2002.

Lee D: *Manual therapy for the thorax: a biomechanical approach*, 1994, British Columbia.

Leflet DH: *HEMME approach to modalities*, Bonifay, Fla, 1996, Hemme Approach Publications.

Leflet DH: *HEMME approach to soft tissue therapy*, Bonifay, Fla, 1992, HEMME Approach Publications.

Lillis CA: *A concise introduction to medical terminology*, ed 4, Stamford, Conn, 1997, Appleton & Lange.

Lindsay DT: *Functional human anatomy*, St Louis, 1996, Mosby.

Lowe WW: *Functional assessment in massage therapy*, ed 2, Corvallis, Ore, 1995, Pacific Orthopedic Massage.

Maciocia G: *The foundations of Chinese medicine*, New York, 1994, Churchill Livingstone.

Macnab I, McCulloch J: *Neck ache and shoulder pain*, Baltimore, 1994, Williams & Wilkins

Marieb EN: *Human anatomy and physiology*, ed 4, Redwood City, Calif, 1997, Benjamin/Cummings.

Masunaga S, Ohashi W: *Zen Shiatsu: how to harmonize Yin and Yang for better health*, Tokyo, 1977, Japan Publications, Inc.

McCraty R, Tiller WA, Atkinson M: *Head-heart entrainment: a preliminary survey*, Institute of HeartMath, PO Box 1463, 14700 West Park Ave, Boulder Creek CA 95006 Hrtmath@netcom. com http://www.heartmath.org/researchpapers/Head/Hart/Headheart.html

McNaught AB, Callander R: *Illustrated physiology*, ed 4, New York, 1983, Churchill Livingstone.

Memmler RL, Cohen BH, Wood DL: *The human body in health and disease*, ed 7, Philadelphia, 1992, JB Lippincott.

Mennell JM: *The musculoskeletal system: differential diagnosis from symptoms and physical signs*, Gaithersburg, Md, 1992, Aspen.

Millenson JR: *Mind matters: psychological medicine in holistic practice*, Seattle, 1995, Eastland Press.

Muscolino JE: *The muscular system manual, the skeletal muscles of the human body*, St Louis, 2003, Mosby.

Myers TW: *Anatomy trains, myofascial meridians for manual and movement therapists*, New York, 2001, Churchill Livingstone.

Netter FH: *The CIBA collection of medical illustrations*, New Jersey, 1991, CIBA.

Netter FH: *The CIBA collection of medical illustrations*, ed 2, New Jersey, 1992, Hennegan.

Newton D: Pathology for massage therapists, ed 2, Portland, 1995, Simran Publications.

Nikola RJ: *Creatures of water: hydrotherapy textbook*, Salt Lake City, 1995, Europa Therapeutic.

Norkin CC, Levangie PK: *Joint structure and function*, ed 2, Philadelphia, 1992, FA Davis.

Northrup C: *Heal your symptoms naturally*, Potomac, Md, 1996, Phillips.

Northrup C: *Women's bodies, women's wisdom*, New York, 1994, Bantam Books.

Ornstein R, Sobel D: *The healing brain*, New York, 1987, Simon & Schuster.

Osborne-Sheets C: *Deep tissue sculpting: a technical and artistic manual for therapeutic bodywork practitioners*, Poway, Calif, 1990, Body Therapy Associates.

Oschman JL: *What is healing energy?* III. Silent pulses, *J Bodywork Movement Ther* 1(3):179, 1997.

Perry HM III, Morley JE, Coe RM: *Aging and musculoskeletal disorders*, New York, 1993, Springer.

Premkumar K: *Pathology A to Z: a handbook for massage therapists*, Calgary, Canada, 1996, VanPub Books.

Premkumar K: *The massage connection: anatomy, physiology & pathology*, Calgary, Alberta, 1997, VanPub Books.

Price SA, Wilson LM: *Pathophysiology, clinical concepts of disease processes*, ed 5, St. Louis, 1997, Mosby.

Rattray F, Ludwig L: *Clinical massage therapy: understanding, assessing, and treating over 70 Conditions*, Toronto, 2000, Talus, Inc.

Schlossberg L, Zuidema GD: *The Johns Hopkins atlas of human functional anatomy*, ed 2, Baltimore, 1981, Johns Hopkins University Press.

Schneider W, Tritschler T, Spring H: *Mobility: theory and practice*, New York, 1992, Thieme Medical Publishers.

Seeley RR, Stephens TD, Tate P: *Essentials of anatomy and physiology*, ed 2, St Louis, 1996, Mosby.

Selye H: *The stress of life*, New York, 1978, McGraw-Hill.

Sieg K, Adams S: *Illustrated essentials of musculoskeletal anatomy*, ed 3, 1996, Megabooks.

Simons D: Understanding effective treatments of myofascial trigger points, *J Bodywork Movement Ther* 6(2): 2002

Smith LK, Weiss E, Lehmkuhl L: *Brunnstrom's clinical kinesiology*, ed 5, Philadelphia, 1996, FA Davis.

Sorrentino SA: *Mosby's textbook for nursing assistants*, ed 4, St Louis, 1996, Mosby.

Stanway A: *The new natural family doctor*, Berkeley, Calif, 1987, North Atlantic Books.

Steefel L: Treating depression: helping the body heal the mind, *Alt Complem Ther* Jan/Feb 1996.

Stewart J: *Clinical anatomy and pathophysiology for the health professional*, Miami, 1994, MedMaster.

Sun C: *Chinese bodywork: a complete manual of Chinese therapeutic massage*, Berkeley, Calif, 1993, Pacific View Press.

Thibodeau GA, Patton KT: *Structure and function of the body*, ed 10, 1997, Mosby.

Thibodeau GA, Patton KT: *Anatomy and physiology*, ed 5, St Louis, 2003, Mosby.

Thibodeau GA, Patton KT: *The human body in health and disease*, ed 3, St Louis, 2001, Mosby.

Thomas CL: *Taber's cyclopedic medical dictionary*, ed 16, Philadelphia, 1985, FA Davis.
Thompson GW, Floyd RT: *Manual of structural kinesiology with dynamic movement*, ed 14, St Louis, 2000, Mosby.
Timmons BH, Ley R: *Behavioral and psychological approaches to breathing disorders*, New York, 1994, Plenum Press.
Tortora GJ, Anagnostakos NP: *Anatomy and physiological laboratory manual*, ed 4, New York, 1993, Macmillan.
Tortora GJ, Grabowski SR: *Principles of anatomy and physiology*, ed 7, New York, 1993, HarperCollins.
Trew M, Everett T: *Human movement: an introductory text*, ed 3, New York, 1997, Churchill Livingstone.
Vardaxis NJ: *Pathology for the health sciences*, New York, 1995, Churchill Livingstone.
Warfel JH: *The head, neck, and trunk*, ed 6, Philadelphia, 1993, Lea & Febiger.
Warfel JH: *The extremities: muscles and motor points*, ed 6, Philadelphia, 1992, Lea & Febiger.
Warfield CA: *Principles and practice of pain management*, New York, 1993, McGraw-Hill.
Warms CA, Turner JA, Marshall HM, Cardenas DD: Treatments for chronic pain associated with spinal cord injuries: many are tried, few are helpful, *J Gastro Surg* 6(1):43-49, 2002.
Wheater P, Burkitt G, Stevens A, et al.: *Basic histopathology*, ed 2, New York, 1993, Churchill Livingstone.
Whitney EN, Rolfes SR: *Understanding nutrition*, ed 7, Minneapolis, 1996, West Publishers.
Williams RW: *Basic healthcare terminology*, St Louis, 1995, Mosby.
Wilson KM, Klein JD: Adolescents' use of complementary and alternative medicine, *Anesth Analg* 94(4):872-875, 2002.
Witters W, Venturelli P, Hanson G: *Drugs and society*, ed 3, Boston, 1986, Jones & Bartlett.
Yates J: *A physician's guide to therapeutic massage: its physiological effects and their application to treatment*, Vancouver, British Columbia, 1990, Massage Therapist Association of British Columbia.
Zahourek J: *Myologik: an atlas of human musculature in clay*, vols 1-5, Zoologik Systems Kinesthetic Anatomy Maniken, Zahourek Stytems, Loveland, Colo, 1996.
Zi N: *The art of breathing*, Glendale, Calif, 1997, Vivi.
Zukav G: *The dancing wu li masters*, New York, 1980, Bantam Books.

Recommended Readings

1998 Physician's GenRx, ed 8, St Louis, 1998, Mosby.
Anderson KN, Anderson LE, Glanze WD, editors: *Mosby's medical, nursing, and allied health dictionary*, ed 5, St Louis, 1998, Mosby.
Calais-Germain B: *Anatomy of movement*, Seattle, 1993, Eastland Press.
Chaitow L: *Palpation skills: assessment and diagnosis through touch*, New York, 1997, Churchill Livingstone.
Cohen MR: *The Chinese way to healing: many paths to wholeness*, New York, 1996, Berkeley Publishing Group.
Edwards D: *Mosby's anatomy flash cards: musculature, bones, and joints*, St Louis, 1998, Mosby.
Fritz S: *Mosby's fundamentals of therapeutic massage*, St Louis, 1995, Mosby.
Hinkle CZ: *Fundamentals of anatomy and movement: a workbook and guide*, St Louis, 1997, Mosby.
Kapit W, Lawrence ME: *The anatomy coloring book*, ed 2, New York, 1993, Harper Collins.
Li D: *Acupuncture meridian theory and acupuncture points*, Beijing, San Francisco, 1990, China Books & Periodicals.
Lowe WW: *Functional assessment in massage therapy*, ed 2, Corvallis, Ore, 1995, Pacific Orthopedic Massage.
Maciocia G: *The foundations of Chinese medicine*, New York, 1994, Churchill Livingstone.
Olson TR: *ADAM student atlas of anatomy*, Baltimore, 1996, Williams & Wilkins.
Sieg K, Adams S: *Illustrated essentials of musculoskeletal anatomy*, ed 2, 1994, Megabooks.
Thompson DL: *Hands heal: documentation for massage therapy*, Seattle, 1993, Thompson.
Travell JG, Simons DG: *Myofascial pain and dysfunction: the trigger point manual (the lower extremities)*, Baltimore, 1992, Williams & Wilkins.
Travell JG, Simons DG: *Myofascial pain and dysfunction: the trigger point manual (upper half)*, vol 1, Baltimore, 1983, Williams & Wilkins.
Zahourek J: *Myologik: an atlas of human musculature in clay*, vols 1-5, Zoologik Systems Kinesthetic Anatomy Maniken, Zahourek Stytems, Loveland, Colo, 1996.

INDEX

Page numbers followed by b indicate boxes; f, figures; t, tables.

C

G

H

M

O

P

Q

R

U

V